HEALTH CARE STATE RANKINGS
1998

Health Care in the 50 United States

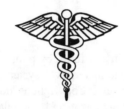

Kathleen O'Leary Morgan, Scott Morgan and Mark A. Uhlig, Editors

Associate Editor: Kim Tiffany

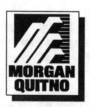

Morgan Quitno Press
© Copyright 1998, All Rights Reserved

512 East 9th Street, P.O. Box 1656
Lawrence, KS 66044-8656
USA
800-457-0742 or 785-841-3534
www.morganquitno.com

Sixth Edition

ISBN: 1-56692-330-1
ISSN: 1065-1403

Health Care State Rankings 1998 sells for $49.95 ($5.00 shipping) and is only available in paper binding. For those who prefer ranking information tailored to a particular state, we also offer *Health Care State Perspectives*, state-specific reports for each of the 50 states. These individual guides provide information on a state's data and rank for each of the categories featured in the national *Health Care State Rankings* volume. Perspectives sell for $19.00 or $9.50 if ordered with *Health Care State Rankings*. If crime statistics are your interest, please ask about our annual *Crime State Rankings* ($49.95 paper). If you are interested in city and metropolitan crime data, we offer *City Crime Rankings* ($37.95 paper). If you are interested in a general view of the states, please ask about our original annual *State Rankings* ($49.95 paper). All of our data sets are also available in machine readable format. Shipping and handling is $5.00 per order.

Sixth Edition
Printed in the United States of America
June 1998

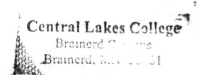

PREFACE

How healthy is your state? Discover the answer in *Health Care State Rankings 1998*. Now in its sixth edition, this popular reference volume compares states in births and reproductive health, deaths, disease, insurance and finance, health care providers, facilities and physical fitness. In all, more than 500 tables of state health comparisons give you all the information you need on virtually every aspect of health care in the 50 United States.

Important Notes About *Health Care State Rankings 1998*

Over the last year, we have collected data from a number of government and private sector health care sources. The end result of that research is *Health Care State Rankings 1998*. Each table has undergone a thorough review to ensure that our readers have access to the most up-to-date, reliable information available. Most tables were updated from last year, a few are new and a few others were deleted. In some cases updated information is not available and tables are repeated. Our regular readers will note that once again the finance chapter has a number of repeat tables. Unfortunately, the Health Care Financing Administration has not yet issued updates of its state estimates of health care expenditures (1993 are the latest). While we await the revised state numbers, we have included this year a table showing national health care expenditures for 1996 (see page 229).

Our annual review process may bring about a number of changes in our books, but there are many popular features that are retained. These include source information and other pertinent footnotes clearly shown at the bottom of each page and national totals, rates and percentages prominently displayed at the top of each table. In addition, every other line is shaded in gray for easier reading. We also provide numerous information finding tools: a thorough table of contents, table listings at the beginning of each chapter, a roster of sources with addresses and phone numbers, a detailed index and a chapter thumb index.

As in all of our reference books, the numbers shown in *Health Care State Rankings* are "complete," meaning that no additional calculations are required to convert them from millions, thousands, etc. All states are ranked on a high to low basis, with any ties among the states listed alphabetically for a given ranking. Negative numbers are shown in parentheses "( )." For tables with national totals (as opposed to rates, per capita's, etc.) a separate column is included showing what percent of the national total each individual state's total represents. This column is headed by "% of USA." This percentage figure is particularly interesting when compared with a state's share of the nation's population for a particular year (provided in an appendix).

If you are interested in looking for information for just one state, check out our *Health Care State Perspective* series of publications. These 21-page comb bound reports feature data and ranking information for an individual state, as reported in *Health Care State Rankings 1998*. (For example *California Health Care in Perspective* features information about the state of California only.) They serve as handy, quick reference guides for those who do not want to page through the entire *Health Care State Rankings* volume searching for information for their particular state. When purchased by themselves, *Health Care State Perspectives* sell for $19. When purchased with a copy of *Health Care State Rankings*, these handy quick reference guides are just $9.50.

Other Books From Morgan Quitno Press

In addition to *Health Care State Rankings*, our company offers three other rankings reference books. The first of these, *State Rankings*, provides a general view of the states. Statistics are featured in a wide variety of categories including agriculture, transportation, government finance, health, population, crime, education, social welfare, energy and environment. Our annual compilation of state crime data is featured in *Crime State Rankings*. In its fifth edition for 1998, this reference volume contains a huge collection of user friendly statistics on law enforcement personnel and expenditures, corrections, arrests and offenses. If city and metro area crime are your interest, *City Crime Rankings* compares crime in all metropolitan areas and cities of 75,000 or more population (approximately 300 cities). Numbers of crimes, crime rates, changes in crime rates over one and five years are presented for all major crime categories reported by the FBI. Final 1996 crime data are featured.

City Crime Rankings sells for $37.95. The *State Rankings* and *Crime State Rankings* books each are available for $49.95. (S/H $5 per order) All books are paperback. For true data aficionados, the information in our books also is available on diskette (PC format dBASE or Excel). This electronic format allows you to import our data into your computer program for tailor-made analysis.

Beginning in July of 1998, we will launch our new monthly journal, *State Statistical Trends*. This publication will highlight a different subject area each month and examine multi-year trends in taxation, education, crime, health and numerous other issues affecting American lives and government. If you would like a brochure or further information on *State Statistical Trends* or any of our other publications, please give us a call at 1-800-457-0742.

Finally, we want to thank the many librarians, government and health care industry officials who helped us each year with the development, design and production of this book. *Health Care State Rankings* is a truly usable reference volume because of your guidance. We always enjoy hearing from our readers, so please don't hesitate to keep sending us your comments and suggestions.

THE EDITORS

WHICH STATE IS HEALTHIEST?

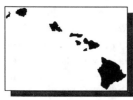

It's true — paradise is good for your health. Hawaii, home of beautiful beaches, volcanoes, hibiscus flowers and macadamia nuts, is the 1998 Healthiest State. This marks the second consecutive year that the Aloha State has earned this award. Also making a repeat appearance in our Healthiest State spotlight is Arkansas, placing last for the fifth straight year.

Each year we take a step back from our objective reporting of health statistics, throw some basic figures into our computer and determine which is the Healthiest State. Once again Hawaii hangs on as #1, with Minnesota, New Hampshire, Vermont and Utah rounding out the top five spots.

At the opposite end of the ranking scale (and with continued apologies to the Clintons) Arkansas ranks last for the fifth year in a row. It is preceded by Louisiana, Missouri, Tennessee and Alabama.

Admittedly the categories selected have a lot to do with the outcome of the award. While most factors remain consistent from year to year, we assess them annually to ensure that they remain relevant and continue

1998 HEALTHIEST STATE AWARD

RANK	STATE	AVG	'97	RANK	STATE	AVG	'97
1	Hawaii	35.30	1	26	Illinois	24.96	17
2	Minnesota	34.09	2	27	North Carolina	24.65	19
3	New Hampshire	33.55	4	28	New York	24.57	18
4	Vermont	33.17	6	29	North Dakota	24.48	24
5	Utah	32.91	5	30	Colorado	24.26	29
6	Kansas	31.48	26	31	Michigan	24.09	37
7	Iowa	30.74	8	32	Delaware	24.00	32
8	South Dakota	30.43	20	33	Ohio	23.83	31
9	Connecticut	30.09	3	34	New Mexico	23.48	27
10	Nebraska	29.87	9	35	Indiana	22.96	39
11	Montana	29.61	12	36	Texas	22.87	33
12	California	29.30	14	37	Pennsylvania	22.61	38
13	Washington	28.78	7	38	Oklahoma	22.00	34
14	Maine	28.74	27	39	Arizona	21.17	40
15	Idaho	28.65	11	39	Nevada	21.17	41
16	Massachusetts	28.52	10	41	West Virginia	20.52	49
16	Virginia	28.52	13	42	Florida	20.13	44
18	Maryland	28.48	15	43	South Carolina	19.57	36
18	Wyoming	28.48	25	44	Kentucky	18.35	45
20	Alaska	26.78	16	45	Mississippi	18.04	42
21	Georgia	26.70	35	46	Alabama	18.00	47
22	Rhode Island	26.26	30	47	Tennessee	17.87	46
23	Wisconsin	26.00	23	48	Missouri	17.52	43
24	Oregon	25.22	21	49	Louisiana	17.00	48
25	New Jersey	25.13	22	50	Arkansas	15.74	50

to reflect healthy living. Accordingly, for 1998 we have eliminated the combined notifiable disease rate and have added sexually transmitted disease rate. Overall, the factors chosen reflect affordability of health care, access to health care and a generally healthy population. All factors are given equal weight.

The methodology for determining the healthiest state has not changed. Once the factors were determined, we averaged each state's rankings for the 23 categories. Based on these averages, states were then ranked from "healthiest" (highest average ranking) to "least healthy" (lowest average ranking). The tables in *Health Care State Rankings 1998* list data from highest to lowest. However, for purposes of this award, we inverted rankings for those factors we determined to be "positive." Thus the state with the highest percent of its children immunized in the book (ranking 1st) would be given a "50" for purposes of this award.

The table above shows how each state fared in the 1998 Healthiest State Award as well as its placement in 1997. We are always pleased with the meaningful discussion generated by this award in many state capitals. Congratulations once again to the healthy citizens of Hawaii!

THE EDITORS

POSITIVE (+) AND NEGATIVE (-) FACTORS CONSIDERED:
1. Births of Low Birthweight as a Percent of All Births (Table 15) -
2. Births to Teenage Mothers as a Percent of Live Births (Table 27) -
3. Percent of Mothers Receiving Late or No Prenatal Care (Table 54) -
4. Death Rate (Table 77) -
5. Infant Mortality Rate (Table 84) -
6. Estimated Age Adjusted Death Rate by Cancer (Table 110) -
7. Death Rate by Suicide (Table 162) -
8. Percent of Population Not Covered by Health Insurance (Table 287) -
9. Change in Percent of Population Uninsured: 1991 to 1996 (Table 294) -
10. Health Care Expenditures as a Percent of Gross State Product (Table 231) -
11. Per Capita Personal Health Expenditures (Table 232) -
12. Estimated Rate of New Cancer Cases (Table 355) -

13. AIDS Rate (Table 377) -
14. Sexually Transmitted Disease Rate (Table 410) -
15. Percent of Population Lacking Access to Primary Care (Table 439) -
16. Percent of Adults Who Are Binge Drinkers (Table 501) -
17. Percent of Adults Who Smoke (Table 502) -
18. Percent of Adults Overweight (Table 505) -
19. Number of Days in Past Month When Physical Health was "Not Good" (Table 506) -
20. Community Hospitals per 1,000 Square Miles (Table 180) +
21. Beds in Community Hospitals per 100,000 Population (Table 185) +
22. Percent of Children Aged 19-35 Months Fully Immunized (Table 408) +
23. Safety Belt Usage Rate (Table 510) +

TABLE OF CONTENTS

I. Births and Reproductive Health

TABLE OF CONTENTS (continued)

Abortions

II. Deaths

TABLE OF CONTENTS (continued)

TABLE OF CONTENTS (continued)

III. Facilities

IV. Finance

TABLE OF CONTENTS (continued)

TABLE OF CONTENTS (continued)

TABLE OF CONTENTS (continued)

V. Incidence of Disease

TABLE OF CONTENTS (continued)

VI. Providers

TABLE OF CONTENTS (continued)

VII. Physical Fitness

VIII. Appendix

IX. Sources

X. Index

I. BIRTHS AND REPRODUCTIVE HEALTH

1   Births in 1996
2   Birth Rate in 1996
3   Births in 1995
4   Birth Rate in 1995
5   Births in 1990
6   Birth Rate in 1990
7   Births in 1980
8   Birth Rate in 1980
9   Fertility Rate in 1996
10 Births to White Women in 1996
11 White Births as a Percent of All Births in 1996
12 Births to Black Women in 1996
13 Black Births as a Percent of All Births in 1996
14 Births of Low Birthweight in 1996
15 Births of Low Birthweight as a Percent of All Births in 1996
16 Births of Low Birthweight to White Women in 1996
17 Births of Birthweight to White Women as a Percent of All Births to White Women in 1996
18 Births of Low Birthweight to Black Women in 1996
19 Births of Low Birthweight to Black Women as a Percent of All Births to Black Women in 1996
20 Births to Unmarried Women in 1996
21 Births to Unmarried Women as a Percent of All Births in 1996
22 Births to Unmarried White Women in 1996
23 Births to Unmarried White Women as a Percent of All Births to White Women in 1996
24 Births to Unmarried Black Women in 1996
25 Births to Unmarried Black Women as a Percent of All Births to Black Women in 1996
26 Births to Teenage Mothers in 1996
27 Percent of Births to Teenage Mothers in 1996
28 Births to Teenage Mothers in 1995
29 Teenage Birth Rate in 1995
30 Births to Teenage Mothers as a Percent of Live Births in 1995
31 Births to White Teenage Mothers in 1995
32 Births to White Teenage Mothers as a Percent of White Births in 1995
33 Births to Black Teenage Mothers in 1995
34 Births to Black Teenage Mothers as a Percent of Black Births in 1995
35 Pregnancy Rate for 15 to 19 Year Old Women in 1994
36 Percent Change in Pregnancy Rate for 15 to 19 Year Old Women: 1992 to 1994
37 Births to Teenage Mothers in 1990
38 Teenage Birth Rate in 1990
39 Percent Change in Teenage Birth Rate: 1990 to 1995
40 Births to Teenage Mothers in 1980
41 Teenage Birth Rate in 1980
42 Births to Women 35 to 49 Years Old in 1995
43 Births to Women 35 to 49 Years Old as a Percent of All Births in 1995
44 Births by Vaginal Delivery in 1995
45 Percent of Births by Vaginal Delivery in 1995
46 Births by Cesarean Delivery in 1995
47 Percent of Births by Cesarean Delivery in 1995
48 Percent Change in Rate of Cesarean Births: 1989 to 1995
49 Births by Vaginal Delivery After a Previous Cesarean Delivery (VBAC) in 1995
50 Percent of Vaginal Births After a Cesarean (VBAC) in 1995
51 Percent of Mothers Beginning Prenatal Care in First Trimester in 1996
52 Percent of White Mothers Beginning Prenatal Care in First Trimester in 1996
53 Percent of Black Mothers Beginning Prenatal Care in First Trimester in 1996
54 Percent of Mother Receiving Late or No Prenatal Care in 1995
55 Percent of White Mothers Receiving Late or No Prenatal Care in 1995
56 Percent of Black Mothers Receiving Late or No Prenatal Care in 1995
57 Percent of Births to Women Who Smoked During Pregnancy in 1995
58 Percent of Births Attended by Midwives in 1995

I. BIRTHS AND REPRODUCTIVE HEALTH
(CONTINUED)

Abortions

Births in 1996

National Total = 3,914,953 Live Births*

ALPHA ORDER				RANK ORDER			
RANK	STATE	BIRTHS	% of USA	RANK	STATE	BIRTHS	% of USA
23	Alabama	61,477	1.57%	1	California	539,789	13.79%
47	Alaska	10,161	0.26%	2	Texas	327,163	8.36%
16	Arizona	79,590	2.03%	3	New York	271,458	6.93%
34	Arkansas	36,418	0.93%	4	Florida	189,458	4.84%
1	California	539,789	13.79%	5	Illinois	184,369	4.71%
24	Colorado	55,840	1.43%	6	Ohio	152,664	3.90%
28	Connecticut	44,312	1.13%	7	Pennsylvania	149,962	3.83%
46	Delaware	10,243	0.26%	8	Michigan	137,471	3.51%
4	Florida	189,458	4.84%	9	Georgia	114,848	2.93%
9	Georgia	114,848	2.93%	10	New Jersey	113,902	2.91%
40	Hawaii	18,334	0.47%	11	North Carolina	105,741	2.70%
39	Idaho	19,059	0.49%	12	Virginia	92,400	2.36%
5	Illinois	184,369	4.71%	13	Indiana	83,303	2.13%
13	Indiana	83,303	2.13%	14	Massachusetts	80,457	2.06%
33	Iowa	37,120	0.95%	15	Washington	79,959	2.04%
32	Kansas	39,734	1.01%	16	Arizona	79,590	2.03%
25	Kentucky	52,632	1.34%	17	Missouri	73,782	1.88%
21	Louisiana	66,178	1.69%	18	Tennessee	73,779	1.88%
42	Maine	13,775	0.35%	19	Maryland	69,696	1.78%
19	Maryland	69,696	1.78%	20	Wisconsin	67,094	1.71%
14	Massachusetts	80,457	2.06%	21	Louisiana	66,178	1.69%
8	Michigan	137,471	3.51%	22	Minnesota	63,779	1.63%
22	Minnesota	63,779	1.63%	23	Alabama	61,477	1.57%
30	Mississippi	41,662	1.06%	24	Colorado	55,840	1.43%
17	Missouri	73,782	1.88%	25	Kentucky	52,632	1.34%
44	Montana	10,707	0.27%	26	South Carolina	50,807	1.30%
37	Nebraska	23,321	0.60%	27	Oklahoma	46,209	1.18%
36	Nevada	26,034	0.66%	28	Connecticut	44,312	1.13%
41	New Hampshire	14,548	0.37%	29	Oregon	43,677	1.12%
10	New Jersey	113,902	2.91%	30	Mississippi	41,662	1.06%
35	New Mexico	27,235	0.70%	31	Utah	41,388	1.06%
3	New York	271,458	6.93%	32	Kansas	39,734	1.01%
11	North Carolina	105,741	2.70%	33	Iowa	37,120	0.95%
48	North Dakota	8,358	0.21%	34	Arkansas	36,418	0.93%
6	Ohio	152,664	3.90%	35	New Mexico	27,235	0.70%
27	Oklahoma	46,209	1.18%	36	Nevada	26,034	0.66%
29	Oregon	43,677	1.12%	37	Nebraska	23,321	0.60%
7	Pennsylvania	149,962	3.83%	38	West Virginia	20,704	0.53%
43	Rhode Island	12,514	0.32%	39	Idaho	19,059	0.49%
26	South Carolina	50,807	1.30%	40	Hawaii	18,334	0.47%
45	South Dakota	10,475	0.27%	41	New Hampshire	14,548	0.37%
18	Tennessee	73,779	1.88%	42	Maine	13,775	0.35%
2	Texas	327,163	8.36%	43	Rhode Island	12,514	0.32%
31	Utah	41,388	1.06%	44	Montana	10,707	0.27%
49	Vermont	6,745	0.17%	45	South Dakota	10,475	0.27%
12	Virginia	92,400	2.36%	46	Delaware	10,243	0.26%
15	Washington	79,959	2.04%	47	Alaska	10,161	0.26%
38	West Virginia	20,704	0.53%	48	North Dakota	8,358	0.21%
20	Wisconsin	67,094	1.71%	49	Vermont	6,745	0.17%
50	Wyoming	6,285	0.16%	50	Wyoming	6,285	0.16%
					District of Columbia	8,336	0.21%

Source: U.S. Department of Health and Human Services, National Center for Health Statistics
"Monthly Vital Statistics Report" (Vol. 46, No. 1(S)2, September 11, 1997)
*Data are preliminary estimates by state of residence.

Birth Rate in 1996

National Rate = 14.8 Live Births per 1,000 Population*

ALPHA ORDER

RANK	STATE	RATE
19	Alabama	14.4
5	Alaska	16.7
2	Arizona	18.0
17	Arkansas	14.5
4	California	16.9
16	Colorado	14.6
37	Connecticut	13.5
25	Delaware	14.1
38	Florida	13.2
9	Georgia	15.6
11	Hawaii	15.5
7	Idaho	16.0
9	Illinois	15.6
21	Indiana	14.3
41	Iowa	13.0
12	Kansas	15.4
35	Kentucky	13.6
14	Louisiana	15.2
50	Maine	11.1
31	Maryland	13.7
38	Massachusetts	13.2
21	Michigan	14.3
31	Minnesota	13.7
13	Mississippi	15.3
29	Missouri	13.8
47	Montana	12.2
25	Nebraska	14.1
6	Nevada	16.2
45	New Hampshire	12.5
21	New Jersey	14.3
8	New Mexico	15.9
15	New York	14.9
19	North Carolina	14.4
41	North Dakota	13.0
31	Ohio	13.7
27	Oklahoma	14.0
35	Oregon	13.6
46	Pennsylvania	12.4
44	Rhode Island	12.6
31	South Carolina	13.7
21	South Dakota	14.3
28	Tennessee	13.9
3	Texas	17.1
1	Utah	20.7
48	Vermont	11.5
29	Virginia	13.8
17	Washington	14.5
49	West Virginia	11.3
41	Wisconsin	13.0
40	Wyoming	13.1

RANK ORDER

RANK	STATE	RATE
1	Utah	20.7
2	Arizona	18.0
3	Texas	17.1
4	California	16.9
5	Alaska	16.7
6	Nevada	16.2
7	Idaho	16.0
8	New Mexico	15.9
9	Georgia	15.6
9	Illinois	15.6
11	Hawaii	15.5
12	Kansas	15.4
13	Mississippi	15.3
14	Louisiana	15.2
15	New York	14.9
16	Colorado	14.6
17	Arkansas	14.5
17	Washington	14.5
19	Alabama	14.4
19	North Carolina	14.4
21	Indiana	14.3
21	Michigan	14.3
21	New Jersey	14.3
21	South Dakota	14.3
25	Delaware	14.1
25	Nebraska	14.1
27	Oklahoma	14.0
28	Tennessee	13.9
29	Missouri	13.8
29	Virginia	13.8
31	Maryland	13.7
31	Minnesota	13.7
31	Ohio	13.7
31	South Carolina	13.7
35	Kentucky	13.6
35	Oregon	13.6
37	Connecticut	13.5
38	Florida	13.2
38	Massachusetts	13.2
40	Wyoming	13.1
41	Iowa	13.0
41	North Dakota	13.0
41	Wisconsin	13.0
44	Rhode Island	12.6
45	New Hampshire	12.5
46	Pennsylvania	12.4
47	Montana	12.2
48	Vermont	11.5
49	West Virginia	11.3
50	Maine	11.1
	District of Columbia	15.3

Source: U.S. Department of Health and Human Services, National Center for Health Statistics
"Monthly Vital Statistics Report" (Vol. 46, No. 1(S)2, September 11, 1997)
*Data are preliminary estimates by state of residence.

Births in 1995

National Total = 3,899,589 Live Births*

ALPHA ORDER				RANK ORDER			
RANK	STATE	BIRTHS	% of USA	RANK	STATE	BIRTHS	% of USA
23	Alabama	60,329	1.55%	1	California	552,045	14.16%
47	Alaska	10,244	0.26%	2	Texas	322,753	8.28%
18	Arizona	72,463	1.86%	3	New York	271,369	6.96%
34	Arkansas	35,175	0.90%	4	Florida	188,723	4.84%
1	California	552,045	14.16%	5	Illinois	185,812	4.76%
24	Colorado	54,332	1.39%	6	Ohio	154,064	3.95%
28	Connecticut	44,334	1.14%	7	Pennsylvania	151,850	3.89%
46	Delaware	10,266	0.26%	8	Michigan	134,642	3.45%
4	Florida	188,723	4.84%	9	New Jersey	114,828	2.94%
10	Georgia	112,282	2.88%	10	Georgia	112,282	2.88%
39	Hawaii	18,595	0.48%	11	North Carolina	101,592	2.61%
40	Idaho	18,035	0.46%	12	Virginia	92,578	2.37%
5	Illinois	185,812	4.76%	13	Indiana	82,835	2.12%
13	Indiana	82,835	2.12%	14	Massachusetts	81,648	2.09%
33	Iowa	36,810	0.94%	15	Washington	77,228	1.98%
32	Kansas	37,201	0.95%	16	Tennessee	73,173	1.88%
25	Kentucky	52,377	1.34%	17	Missouri	73,028	1.87%
21	Louisiana	65,641	1.68%	18	Arizona	72,463	1.86%
42	Maine	13,896	0.36%	19	Maryland	72,396	1.86%
19	Maryland	72,396	1.86%	20	Wisconsin	67,479	1.73%
14	Massachusetts	81,648	2.09%	21	Louisiana	65,641	1.68%
8	Michigan	134,642	3.45%	22	Minnesota	63,263	1.62%
22	Minnesota	63,263	1.62%	23	Alabama	60,329	1.55%
30	Mississippi	41,344	1.06%	24	Colorado	54,332	1.39%
17	Missouri	73,028	1.87%	25	Kentucky	52,377	1.34%
44	Montana	11,142	0.29%	26	South Carolina	50,926	1.31%
37	Nebraska	23,243	0.60%	27	Oklahoma	45,672	1.17%
36	Nevada	25,056	0.64%	28	Connecticut	44,334	1.14%
41	New Hampshire	14,665	0.38%	29	Oregon	42,811	1.10%
9	New Jersey	114,828	2.94%	30	Mississippi	41,344	1.06%
35	New Mexico	26,920	0.69%	31	Utah	39,577	1.01%
3	New York	271,369	6.96%	32	Kansas	37,201	0.95%
11	North Carolina	101,592	2.61%	33	Iowa	36,810	0.94%
48	North Dakota	8,476	0.22%	34	Arkansas	35,175	0.90%
6	Ohio	154,064	3.95%	35	New Mexico	26,920	0.69%
27	Oklahoma	45,672	1.17%	36	Nevada	25,056	0.64%
29	Oregon	42,811	1.10%	37	Nebraska	23,243	0.60%
7	Pennsylvania	151,850	3.89%	38	West Virginia	21,162	0.54%
43	Rhode Island	12,776	0.33%	39	Hawaii	18,595	0.48%
26	South Carolina	50,926	1.31%	40	Idaho	18,035	0.46%
45	South Dakota	10,475	0.27%	41	New Hampshire	14,665	0.38%
16	Tennessee	73,173	1.88%	42	Maine	13,896	0.36%
2	Texas	322,753	8.28%	43	Rhode Island	12,776	0.33%
31	Utah	39,577	1.01%	44	Montana	11,142	0.29%
49	Vermont	6,783	0.17%	45	South Dakota	10,475	0.27%
12	Virginia	92,578	2.37%	46	Delaware	10,266	0.26%
15	Washington	77,228	1.98%	47	Alaska	10,244	0.26%
38	West Virginia	21,162	0.54%	48	North Dakota	8,476	0.22%
20	Wisconsin	67,479	1.73%	49	Vermont	6,783	0.17%
50	Wyoming	6,261	0.16%	50	Wyoming	6,261	0.16%
					District of Columbia	9,014	0.23%

Source: U.S. Department of Health and Human Services, National Center for Health Statistics
   "Monthly Vital Statistics Report" (Vol. 45, No. 11, Supplement, June 10, 1997)
*Final data by state of residence.

Birth Rate in 1995

National Rate = 14.8 Live Births per 1,000 Population*

RANK	STATE	RATE
22	Alabama	14.2
5	Alaska	17.0
3	Arizona	17.2
22	Arkansas	14.2
2	California	17.5
15	Colorado	14.5
37	Connecticut	13.5
20	Delaware	14.3
39	Florida	13.3
10	Georgia	15.6
8	Hawaii	15.7
11	Idaho	15.5
8	Illinois	15.7
20	Indiana	14.3
42	Iowa	13.0
15	Kansas	14.5
35	Kentucky	13.6
13	Louisiana	15.1
50	Maine	11.2
18	Maryland	14.4
38	Massachusetts	13.4
26	Michigan	14.1
33	Minnesota	13.7
12	Mississippi	15.3
33	Missouri	13.7
45	Montana	12.8
22	Nebraska	14.2
6	Nevada	16.4
45	New Hampshire	12.8
15	New Jersey	14.5
7	New Mexico	16.0
14	New York	15.0
26	North Carolina	14.1
40	North Dakota	13.2
32	Ohio	13.8
29	Oklahoma	13.9
35	Oregon	13.6
47	Pennsylvania	12.6
44	Rhode Island	12.9
29	South Carolina	13.9
18	South Dakota	14.4
29	Tennessee	13.9
3	Texas	17.2
1	Utah	20.3
48	Vermont	11.6
28	Virginia	14.0
22	Washington	14.2
48	West Virginia	11.6
40	Wisconsin	13.2
42	Wyoming	13.0

RANK	STATE	RATE
1	Utah	20.3
2	California	17.5
3	Arizona	17.2
3	Texas	17.2
5	Alaska	17.0
6	Nevada	16.4
7	New Mexico	16.0
8	Hawaii	15.7
8	Illinois	15.7
10	Georgia	15.6
11	Idaho	15.5
12	Mississippi	15.3
13	Louisiana	15.1
14	New York	15.0
15	Colorado	14.5
15	Kansas	14.5
15	New Jersey	14.5
18	Maryland	14.4
18	South Dakota	14.4
20	Delaware	14.3
20	Indiana	14.3
22	Alabama	14.2
22	Arkansas	14.2
22	Nebraska	14.2
22	Washington	14.2
26	Michigan	14.1
26	North Carolina	14.1
28	Virginia	14.0
29	Oklahoma	13.9
29	South Carolina	13.9
29	Tennessee	13.9
32	Ohio	13.8
33	Minnesota	13.7
33	Missouri	13.7
35	Kentucky	13.6
35	Oregon	13.6
37	Connecticut	13.5
38	Massachusetts	13.4
39	Florida	13.3
40	North Dakota	13.2
40	Wisconsin	13.2
42	Iowa	13.0
42	Wyoming	13.0
44	Rhode Island	12.9
45	Montana	12.8
45	New Hampshire	12.8
47	Pennsylvania	12.6
48	Vermont	11.6
48	West Virginia	11.6
50	Maine	11.2
	District of Columbia	16.3

Source: U.S. Department of Health and Human Services, National Center for Health Statistics
"Monthly Vital Statistics Report" (Vol. 45, No. 11, Supplement, June 10, 1997)
*Final data by state of residence.

Births in 1990

National Total = 4,158,212 Live Births*

ALPHA ORDER

RANK	STATE	BIRTHS	% of USA
23	Alabama	63,487	1.53%
44	Alaska	11,902	0.29%
21	Arizona	68,995	1.66%
33	Arkansas	36,457	0.88%
1	California	612,628	14.73%
26	Colorado	53,525	1.29%
27	Connecticut	50,123	1.21%
46	Delaware	11,113	0.27%
4	Florida	199,339	4.79%
10	Georgia	112,666	2.71%
39	Hawaii	20,489	0.49%
42	Idaho	16,433	0.40%
5	Illinois	195,790	4.71%
14	Indiana	86,214	2.07%
31	Iowa	39,409	0.95%
32	Kansas	39,020	0.94%
25	Kentucky	54,362	1.31%
20	Louisiana	72,192	1.74%
41	Maine	17,359	0.42%
15	Maryland	80,245	1.93%
13	Massachusetts	92,654	2.23%
8	Michigan	153,700	3.70%
22	Minnesota	68,013	1.64%
29	Mississippi	43,563	1.05%
16	Missouri	79,260	1.91%
45	Montana	11,613	0.28%
36	Nebraska	24,380	0.59%
38	Nevada	21,599	0.52%
40	New Hampshire	17,569	0.42%
9	New Jersey	122,289	2.94%
35	New Mexico	27,402	0.66%
3	New York	297,576	7.16%
11	North Carolina	104,525	2.51%
48	North Dakota	9,250	0.22%
7	Ohio	166,913	4.01%
28	Oklahoma	47,649	1.15%
30	Oregon	42,891	1.03%
6	Pennsylvania	171,961	4.14%
43	Rhode Island	15,195	0.37%
24	South Carolina	58,610	1.41%
47	South Dakota	10,999	0.26%
18	Tennessee	74,962	1.80%
2	Texas	316,423	7.61%
34	Utah	36,277	0.87%
49	Vermont	8,273	0.20%
12	Virginia	99,352	2.39%
17	Washington	79,251	1.91%
37	West Virginia	22,585	0.54%
19	Wisconsin	72,895	1.75%
50	Wyoming	6,985	0.17%

RANK ORDER

RANK	STATE	BIRTHS	% of USA
1	California	612,628	14.73%
2	Texas	316,423	7.61%
3	New York	297,576	7.16%
4	Florida	199,339	4.79%
5	Illinois	195,790	4.71%
6	Pennsylvania	171,961	4.14%
7	Ohio	166,913	4.01%
8	Michigan	153,700	3.70%
9	New Jersey	122,289	2.94%
10	Georgia	112,666	2.71%
11	North Carolina	104,525	2.51%
12	Virginia	99,352	2.39%
13	Massachusetts	92,654	2.23%
14	Indiana	86,214	2.07%
15	Maryland	80,245	1.93%
16	Missouri	79,260	1.91%
17	Washington	79,251	1.91%
18	Tennessee	74,962	1.80%
19	Wisconsin	72,895	1.75%
20	Louisiana	72,192	1.74%
21	Arizona	68,995	1.66%
22	Minnesota	68,013	1.64%
23	Alabama	63,487	1.53%
24	South Carolina	58,610	1.41%
25	Kentucky	54,362	1.31%
26	Colorado	53,525	1.29%
27	Connecticut	50,123	1.21%
28	Oklahoma	47,649	1.15%
29	Mississippi	43,563	1.05%
30	Oregon	42,891	1.03%
31	Iowa	39,409	0.95%
32	Kansas	39,020	0.94%
33	Arkansas	36,457	0.88%
34	Utah	36,277	0.87%
35	New Mexico	27,402	0.66%
36	Nebraska	24,380	0.59%
37	West Virginia	22,585	0.54%
38	Nevada	21,599	0.52%
39	Hawaii	20,489	0.49%
40	New Hampshire	17,569	0.42%
41	Maine	17,359	0.42%
42	Idaho	16,433	0.40%
43	Rhode Island	15,195	0.37%
44	Alaska	11,902	0.29%
45	Montana	11,613	0.28%
46	Delaware	11,113	0.27%
47	South Dakota	10,999	0.26%
48	North Dakota	9,250	0.22%
49	Vermont	8,273	0.20%
50	Wyoming	6,985	0.17%
	District of Columbia	11,850	0.28%

Source: U.S. Department of Health and Human Services, National Center for Health Statistics
"Monthly Vital Statistics Report" (Vol. 41, No. 9, Supplement, February 25, 1993)
*Final data by state of residence.

Birth Rate in 1990

National Rate = 16.7 Births per 1,000 Population*

<table>
<tr><td colspan="3">ALPHA ORDER</td><td colspan="3">RANK ORDER</td></tr>
<tr><th>RANK</th><th>STATE</th><th>RATE</th><th>RANK</th><th>STATE</th><th>RATE</th></tr>
<tr><td>26</td><td>Alabama</td><td>15.7</td><td>1</td><td>Alaska</td><td>21.6</td></tr>
<tr><td>1</td><td>Alaska</td><td>21.6</td><td>2</td><td>Utah</td><td>21.1</td></tr>
<tr><td>4</td><td>Arizona</td><td>18.8</td><td>3</td><td>California</td><td>20.6</td></tr>
<tr><td>29</td><td>Arkansas</td><td>15.5</td><td>4</td><td>Arizona</td><td>18.8</td></tr>
<tr><td>3</td><td>California</td><td>20.6</td><td>5</td><td>Texas</td><td>18.6</td></tr>
<tr><td>20</td><td>Colorado</td><td>16.2</td><td>6</td><td>Hawaii</td><td>18.5</td></tr>
<tr><td>38</td><td>Connecticut</td><td>15.2</td><td>7</td><td>New Mexico</td><td>18.1</td></tr>
<tr><td>15</td><td>Delaware</td><td>16.7</td><td>8</td><td>Nevada</td><td>18.0</td></tr>
<tr><td>32</td><td>Florida</td><td>15.4</td><td>9</td><td>Georgia</td><td>17.4</td></tr>
<tr><td>9</td><td>Georgia</td><td>17.4</td><td>10</td><td>Illinois</td><td>17.1</td></tr>
<tr><td>6</td><td>Hawaii</td><td>18.5</td><td>10</td><td>Louisiana</td><td>17.1</td></tr>
<tr><td>18</td><td>Idaho</td><td>16.3</td><td>12</td><td>Mississippi</td><td>16.9</td></tr>
<tr><td>10</td><td>Illinois</td><td>17.1</td><td>13</td><td>Maryland</td><td>16.8</td></tr>
<tr><td>28</td><td>Indiana</td><td>15.6</td><td>13</td><td>South Carolina</td><td>16.8</td></tr>
<tr><td>48</td><td>Iowa</td><td>14.2</td><td>15</td><td>Delaware</td><td>16.7</td></tr>
<tr><td>26</td><td>Kansas</td><td>15.7</td><td>16</td><td>Michigan</td><td>16.5</td></tr>
<tr><td>43</td><td>Kentucky</td><td>14.8</td><td>16</td><td>New York</td><td>16.5</td></tr>
<tr><td>10</td><td>Louisiana</td><td>17.1</td><td>18</td><td>Idaho</td><td>16.3</td></tr>
<tr><td>49</td><td>Maine</td><td>14.1</td><td>18</td><td>Washington</td><td>16.3</td></tr>
<tr><td>13</td><td>Maryland</td><td>16.8</td><td>20</td><td>Colorado</td><td>16.2</td></tr>
<tr><td>32</td><td>Massachusetts</td><td>15.4</td><td>21</td><td>Virginia</td><td>16.1</td></tr>
<tr><td>16</td><td>Michigan</td><td>16.5</td><td>22</td><td>New Hampshire</td><td>15.8</td></tr>
<tr><td>29</td><td>Minnesota</td><td>15.5</td><td>22</td><td>New Jersey</td><td>15.8</td></tr>
<tr><td>12</td><td>Mississippi</td><td>16.9</td><td>22</td><td>North Carolina</td><td>15.8</td></tr>
<tr><td>29</td><td>Missouri</td><td>15.5</td><td>22</td><td>South Dakota</td><td>15.8</td></tr>
<tr><td>45</td><td>Montana</td><td>14.5</td><td>26</td><td>Alabama</td><td>15.7</td></tr>
<tr><td>32</td><td>Nebraska</td><td>15.4</td><td>26</td><td>Kansas</td><td>15.7</td></tr>
<tr><td>8</td><td>Nevada</td><td>18.0</td><td>28</td><td>Indiana</td><td>15.6</td></tr>
<tr><td>22</td><td>New Hampshire</td><td>15.8</td><td>29</td><td>Arkansas</td><td>15.5</td></tr>
<tr><td>22</td><td>New Jersey</td><td>15.8</td><td>29</td><td>Minnesota</td><td>15.5</td></tr>
<tr><td>7</td><td>New Mexico</td><td>18.1</td><td>29</td><td>Missouri</td><td>15.5</td></tr>
<tr><td>16</td><td>New York</td><td>16.5</td><td>32</td><td>Florida</td><td>15.4</td></tr>
<tr><td>22</td><td>North Carolina</td><td>15.8</td><td>32</td><td>Massachusetts</td><td>15.4</td></tr>
<tr><td>45</td><td>North Dakota</td><td>14.5</td><td>32</td><td>Nebraska</td><td>15.4</td></tr>
<tr><td>32</td><td>Ohio</td><td>15.4</td><td>32</td><td>Ohio</td><td>15.4</td></tr>
<tr><td>39</td><td>Oklahoma</td><td>15.1</td><td>32</td><td>Tennessee</td><td>15.4</td></tr>
<tr><td>39</td><td>Oregon</td><td>15.1</td><td>32</td><td>Wyoming</td><td>15.4</td></tr>
<tr><td>45</td><td>Pennsylvania</td><td>14.5</td><td>38</td><td>Connecticut</td><td>15.2</td></tr>
<tr><td>39</td><td>Rhode Island</td><td>15.1</td><td>39</td><td>Oklahoma</td><td>15.1</td></tr>
<tr><td>13</td><td>South Carolina</td><td>16.8</td><td>39</td><td>Oregon</td><td>15.1</td></tr>
<tr><td>22</td><td>South Dakota</td><td>15.8</td><td>39</td><td>Rhode Island</td><td>15.1</td></tr>
<tr><td>32</td><td>Tennessee</td><td>15.4</td><td>42</td><td>Wisconsin</td><td>14.9</td></tr>
<tr><td>5</td><td>Texas</td><td>18.6</td><td>43</td><td>Kentucky</td><td>14.8</td></tr>
<tr><td>2</td><td>Utah</td><td>21.1</td><td>44</td><td>Vermont</td><td>14.7</td></tr>
<tr><td>44</td><td>Vermont</td><td>14.7</td><td>45</td><td>Montana</td><td>14.5</td></tr>
<tr><td>21</td><td>Virginia</td><td>16.1</td><td>45</td><td>North Dakota</td><td>14.5</td></tr>
<tr><td>18</td><td>Washington</td><td>16.3</td><td>45</td><td>Pennsylvania</td><td>14.5</td></tr>
<tr><td>50</td><td>West Virginia</td><td>12.6</td><td>48</td><td>Iowa</td><td>14.2</td></tr>
<tr><td>42</td><td>Wisconsin</td><td>14.9</td><td>49</td><td>Maine</td><td>14.1</td></tr>
<tr><td>32</td><td>Wyoming</td><td>15.4</td><td>50</td><td>West Virginia</td><td>12.6</td></tr>
<tr><td></td><td></td><td></td><td></td><td>District of Columbia</td><td>19.5</td></tr>
</table>

Source: U.S. Department of Health and Human Services, National Center for Health Statistics
  "Monthly Vital Statistics Report" (Vol. 41, No. 9, Supplement, February 25, 1993)
Final data by state of residence.

Births in 1980

National Total = 3,612,000 Births*

ALPHA ORDER						RANK ORDER			

RANK	STATE	BIRTHS	% of USA
21	Alabama	64,000	1.77%
48	Alaska	10,000	0.28%
26	Arizona	50,000	1.38%
34	Arkansas	37,000	1.02%
1	California	403,000	11.16%
26	Colorado	50,000	1.38%
33	Connecticut	39,000	1.08%
49	Delaware	9,000	0.25%
8	Florida	132,000	3.65%
10	Georgia	92,000	2.55%
39	Hawaii	18,000	0.50%
38	Idaho	20,000	0.55%
4	Illinois	190,000	5.26%
11	Indiana	88,000	2.44%
28	Iowa	48,000	1.33%
32	Kansas	41,000	1.14%
22	Kentucky	60,000	1.66%
13	Louisiana	82,000	2.27%
40	Maine	16,000	0.44%
22	Maryland	60,000	1.66%
17	Massachusetts	73,000	2.02%
7	Michigan	146,000	4.04%
19	Minnesota	68,000	1.88%
28	Mississippi	48,000	1.33%
14	Missouri	79,000	2.19%
41	Montana	14,000	0.39%
36	Nebraska	27,000	0.75%
43	Nevada	13,000	0.36%
41	New Hampshire	14,000	0.39%
9	New Jersey	97,000	2.69%
37	New Mexico	26,000	0.72%
3	New York	239,000	6.62%
12	North Carolina	84,000	2.33%
45	North Dakota	12,000	0.33%
5	Ohio	169,000	4.68%
24	Oklahoma	52,000	1.44%
30	Oregon	43,000	1.19%
6	Pennsylvania	159,000	4.40%
45	Rhode Island	12,000	0.33%
24	South Carolina	52,000	1.44%
43	South Dakota	13,000	0.36%
18	Tennessee	69,000	1.91%
2	Texas	274,000	7.59%
31	Utah	42,000	1.16%
50	Vermont	8,000	0.22%
15	Virginia	78,000	2.16%
19	Washington	68,000	1.88%
35	West Virginia	29,000	0.80%
16	Wisconsin	75,000	2.08%
47	Wyoming	11,000	0.30%

RANK	STATE	BIRTHS	% of USA
1	California	403,000	11.16%
2	Texas	274,000	7.59%
3	New York	239,000	6.62%
4	Illinois	190,000	5.26%
5	Ohio	169,000	4.68%
6	Pennsylvania	159,000	4.40%
7	Michigan	146,000	4.04%
8	Florida	132,000	3.65%
9	New Jersey	97,000	2.69%
10	Georgia	92,000	2.55%
11	Indiana	88,000	2.44%
12	North Carolina	84,000	2.33%
13	Louisiana	82,000	2.27%
14	Missouri	79,000	2.19%
15	Virginia	78,000	2.16%
16	Wisconsin	75,000	2.08%
17	Massachusetts	73,000	2.02%
18	Tennessee	69,000	1.91%
19	Minnesota	68,000	1.88%
19	Washington	68,000	1.88%
21	Alabama	64,000	1.77%
22	Kentucky	60,000	1.66%
22	Maryland	60,000	1.66%
24	Oklahoma	52,000	1.44%
24	South Carolina	52,000	1.44%
26	Arizona	50,000	1.38%
26	Colorado	50,000	1.38%
28	Iowa	48,000	1.33%
28	Mississippi	48,000	1.33%
30	Oregon	43,000	1.19%
31	Utah	42,000	1.16%
32	Kansas	41,000	1.14%
33	Connecticut	39,000	1.08%
34	Arkansas	37,000	1.02%
35	West Virginia	29,000	0.80%
36	Nebraska	27,000	0.75%
37	New Mexico	26,000	0.72%
38	Idaho	20,000	0.55%
39	Hawaii	18,000	0.50%
40	Maine	16,000	0.44%
41	Montana	14,000	0.39%
41	New Hampshire	14,000	0.39%
43	Nevada	13,000	0.36%
43	South Dakota	13,000	0.36%
45	North Dakota	12,000	0.33%
45	Rhode Island	12,000	0.33%
47	Wyoming	11,000	0.30%
48	Alaska	10,000	0.28%
49	Delaware	9,000	0.25%
50	Vermont	8,000	0.22%
	District of Columbia	9,000	0.25%

Source: U.S. Department of Health and Human Services, National Center for Health Statistics
"Vital Statistics of the United States, 1980" and "Monthly Vital Statistics Report"
*Live births by state of residence.

Birth Rate in 1980

National Rate = 15.9 Births per 1,000 Population*

<table>
<tr><td colspan="3">ALPHA ORDER</td><td colspan="3">RANK ORDER</td></tr>
<tr><td>RANK</td><td>STATE</td><td>RATE</td><td>RANK</td><td>STATE</td><td>RATE</td></tr>
<tr><td>27</td><td>Alabama</td><td>16.3</td><td>1</td><td>Utah</td><td>28.6</td></tr>
<tr><td>2</td><td>Alaska</td><td>23.7</td><td>2</td><td>Alaska</td><td>23.7</td></tr>
<tr><td>11</td><td>Arizona</td><td>18.4</td><td>3</td><td>Wyoming</td><td>22.5</td></tr>
<tr><td>27</td><td>Arkansas</td><td>16.3</td><td>4</td><td>Idaho</td><td>21.4</td></tr>
<tr><td>18</td><td>California</td><td>17.0</td><td>5</td><td>New Mexico</td><td>20.0</td></tr>
<tr><td>15</td><td>Colorado</td><td>17.2</td><td>6</td><td>Louisiana</td><td>19.5</td></tr>
<tr><td>50</td><td>Connecticut</td><td>12.5</td><td>7</td><td>South Dakota</td><td>19.2</td></tr>
<tr><td>33</td><td>Delaware</td><td>15.8</td><td>7</td><td>Texas</td><td>19.2</td></tr>
<tr><td>45</td><td>Florida</td><td>13.5</td><td>9</td><td>Mississippi</td><td>19.0</td></tr>
<tr><td>19</td><td>Georgia</td><td>16.9</td><td>10</td><td>Hawaii</td><td>18.8</td></tr>
<tr><td>10</td><td>Hawaii</td><td>18.8</td><td>11</td><td>Arizona</td><td>18.4</td></tr>
<tr><td>4</td><td>Idaho</td><td>21.4</td><td>11</td><td>North Dakota</td><td>18.4</td></tr>
<tr><td>20</td><td>Illinois</td><td>16.6</td><td>13</td><td>Montana</td><td>18.1</td></tr>
<tr><td>30</td><td>Indiana</td><td>16.1</td><td>14</td><td>Nebraska</td><td>17.4</td></tr>
<tr><td>24</td><td>Iowa</td><td>16.4</td><td>15</td><td>Colorado</td><td>17.2</td></tr>
<tr><td>15</td><td>Kansas</td><td>17.2</td><td>15</td><td>Kansas</td><td>17.2</td></tr>
<tr><td>27</td><td>Kentucky</td><td>16.3</td><td>15</td><td>Oklahoma</td><td>17.2</td></tr>
<tr><td>6</td><td>Louisiana</td><td>19.5</td><td>18</td><td>California</td><td>17.0</td></tr>
<tr><td>41</td><td>Maine</td><td>14.6</td><td>19</td><td>Georgia</td><td>16.9</td></tr>
<tr><td>43</td><td>Maryland</td><td>14.2</td><td>20</td><td>Illinois</td><td>16.6</td></tr>
<tr><td>49</td><td>Massachusetts</td><td>12.7</td><td>20</td><td>Minnesota</td><td>16.6</td></tr>
<tr><td>34</td><td>Michigan</td><td>15.7</td><td>20</td><td>Nevada</td><td>16.6</td></tr>
<tr><td>20</td><td>Minnesota</td><td>16.6</td><td>20</td><td>South Carolina</td><td>16.6</td></tr>
<tr><td>9</td><td>Mississippi</td><td>19.0</td><td>24</td><td>Iowa</td><td>16.4</td></tr>
<tr><td>30</td><td>Missouri</td><td>16.1</td><td>24</td><td>Oregon</td><td>16.4</td></tr>
<tr><td>13</td><td>Montana</td><td>18.1</td><td>24</td><td>Washington</td><td>16.4</td></tr>
<tr><td>14</td><td>Nebraska</td><td>17.4</td><td>27</td><td>Alabama</td><td>16.3</td></tr>
<tr><td>20</td><td>Nevada</td><td>16.6</td><td>27</td><td>Arkansas</td><td>16.3</td></tr>
<tr><td>39</td><td>New Hampshire</td><td>14.9</td><td>27</td><td>Kentucky</td><td>16.3</td></tr>
<tr><td>47</td><td>New Jersey</td><td>13.2</td><td>30</td><td>Indiana</td><td>16.1</td></tr>
<tr><td>5</td><td>New Mexico</td><td>20.0</td><td>30</td><td>Missouri</td><td>16.1</td></tr>
<tr><td>44</td><td>New York</td><td>13.6</td><td>32</td><td>Wisconsin</td><td>15.9</td></tr>
<tr><td>42</td><td>North Carolina</td><td>14.4</td><td>33</td><td>Delaware</td><td>15.8</td></tr>
<tr><td>11</td><td>North Dakota</td><td>18.4</td><td>34</td><td>Michigan</td><td>15.7</td></tr>
<tr><td>34</td><td>Ohio</td><td>15.7</td><td>34</td><td>Ohio</td><td>15.7</td></tr>
<tr><td>15</td><td>Oklahoma</td><td>17.2</td><td>36</td><td>Vermont</td><td>15.4</td></tr>
<tr><td>24</td><td>Oregon</td><td>16.4</td><td>37</td><td>Tennessee</td><td>15.1</td></tr>
<tr><td>46</td><td>Pennsylvania</td><td>13.4</td><td>37</td><td>West Virginia</td><td>15.1</td></tr>
<tr><td>48</td><td>Rhode Island</td><td>12.9</td><td>39</td><td>New Hampshire</td><td>14.9</td></tr>
<tr><td>20</td><td>South Carolina</td><td>16.6</td><td>40</td><td>Virginia</td><td>14.7</td></tr>
<tr><td>7</td><td>South Dakota</td><td>19.2</td><td>41</td><td>Maine</td><td>14.6</td></tr>
<tr><td>37</td><td>Tennessee</td><td>15.1</td><td>42</td><td>North Carolina</td><td>14.4</td></tr>
<tr><td>7</td><td>Texas</td><td>19.2</td><td>43</td><td>Maryland</td><td>14.2</td></tr>
<tr><td>1</td><td>Utah</td><td>28.6</td><td>44</td><td>New York</td><td>13.6</td></tr>
<tr><td>36</td><td>Vermont</td><td>15.4</td><td>45</td><td>Florida</td><td>13.5</td></tr>
<tr><td>40</td><td>Virginia</td><td>14.7</td><td>46</td><td>Pennsylvania</td><td>13.4</td></tr>
<tr><td>24</td><td>Washington</td><td>16.4</td><td>47</td><td>New Jersey</td><td>13.2</td></tr>
<tr><td>37</td><td>West Virginia</td><td>15.1</td><td>48</td><td>Rhode Island</td><td>12.9</td></tr>
<tr><td>32</td><td>Wisconsin</td><td>15.9</td><td>49</td><td>Massachusetts</td><td>12.7</td></tr>
<tr><td>3</td><td>Wyoming</td><td>22.5</td><td>50</td><td>Connecticut</td><td>12.5</td></tr>
<tr><td></td><td></td><td></td><td></td><td>District of Columbia</td><td>14.7</td></tr>
</table>

Source: U.S. Department of Health and Human Services, National Center for Health Statistics
  "Vital Statistics of the United States, 1980" and "Monthly Vital Statistics Report"
*Live births by state of residence.

Fertility Rate in 1996

National Rate = 65.7 Live Births per 1,000 Women 15 to 44 Years Old*

ALPHA ORDER

RANK	STATE	RATE
25	Alabama	63.1
7	Alaska	72.6
2	Arizona	81.4
12	Arkansas	67.2
4	California	74.8
23	Colorado	63.6
30	Connecticut	61.5
36	Delaware	60.3
19	Florida	64.6
18	Georgia	64.9
8	Hawaii	72.2
6	Idaho	72.9
11	Illinois	69.5
28	Indiana	62.6
35	Iowa	60.5
10	Kansas	70.5
38	Kentucky	59.3
16	Louisiana	66.1
50	Maine	49.5
40	Maryland	58.6
45	Massachusetts	57.2
26	Michigan	63.0
33	Minnesota	60.6
13	Mississippi	66.7
29	Missouri	62.1
43	Montana	57.7
21	Nebraska	64.3
3	Nevada	75.2
47	New Hampshire	53.4
19	New Jersey	64.6
9	New Mexico	71.7
15	New York	66.5
22	North Carolina	63.7
33	North Dakota	60.6
32	Ohio	60.7
17	Oklahoma	65.0
27	Oregon	62.7
44	Pennsylvania	57.6
46	Rhode Island	56.3
39	South Carolina	59.2
14	South Dakota	66.6
31	Tennessee	60.9
5	Texas	74.3
1	Utah	87.6
49	Vermont	50.1
41	Virginia	58.5
23	Washington	63.6
48	West Virginia	52.4
42	Wisconsin	58.2
37	Wyoming	59.8

RANK ORDER

RANK	STATE	RATE
1	Utah	87.6
2	Arizona	81.4
3	Nevada	75.2
4	California	74.8
5	Texas	74.3
6	Idaho	72.9
7	Alaska	72.6
8	Hawaii	72.2
9	New Mexico	71.7
10	Kansas	70.5
11	Illinois	69.5
12	Arkansas	67.2
13	Mississippi	66.7
14	South Dakota	66.6
15	New York	66.5
16	Louisiana	66.1
17	Oklahoma	65.0
18	Georgia	64.9
19	Florida	64.6
19	New Jersey	64.6
21	Nebraska	64.3
22	North Carolina	63.7
23	Colorado	63.6
23	Washington	63.6
25	Alabama	63.1
26	Michigan	63.0
27	Oregon	62.7
28	Indiana	62.6
29	Missouri	62.1
30	Connecticut	61.5
31	Tennessee	60.9
32	Ohio	60.7
33	Minnesota	60.6
33	North Dakota	60.6
35	Iowa	60.5
36	Delaware	60.3
37	Wyoming	59.8
38	Kentucky	59.3
39	South Carolina	59.2
40	Maryland	58.6
41	Virginia	58.5
42	Wisconsin	58.2
43	Montana	57.7
44	Pennsylvania	57.6
45	Massachusetts	57.2
46	Rhode Island	56.3
47	New Hampshire	53.4
48	West Virginia	52.4
49	Vermont	50.1
50	Maine	49.5
	District of Columbia	61.9

Source: U.S. Department of Health and Human Services, National Center for Health Statistics
     "Monthly Vital Statistics Report" (Vol. 46, No. 1(S)2, September 11, 1997)
*Data are preliminary estimates by state of residence.

Births to White Women in 1996

National Total = 3,113,014 Live Births to White Women*

<u>ALPHA ORDER</u>

RANK	STATE	BIRTHS	% of USA
24	Alabama	40,943	1.32%
47	Alaska	6,930	0.22%
13	Arizona	69,869	2.24%
33	Arkansas	27,915	0.90%
1	California	440,213	14.14%
21	Colorado	51,100	1.64%
28	Connecticut	37,755	1.21%
45	Delaware	7,620	0.24%
4	Florida	142,670	4.58%
11	Georgia	73,762	2.37%
50	Hawaii	4,790	0.15%
39	Idaho	18,446	0.59%
5	Illinois	141,603	4.55%
12	Indiana	73,237	2.35%
31	Iowa	35,125	1.13%
30	Kansas	35,518	1.14%
22	Kentucky	47,243	1.52%
27	Louisiana	37,983	1.22%
41	Maine	13,461	0.43%
23	Maryland	44,763	1.44%
14	Massachusetts	69,418	2.23%
8	Michigan	109,200	3.51%
19	Minnesota	57,003	1.83%
36	Mississippi	21,801	0.70%
17	Missouri	61,277	1.97%
43	Montana	9,390	0.30%
37	Nebraska	21,373	0.69%
35	Nevada	22,262	0.72%
40	New Hampshire	14,252	0.46%
9	New Jersey	86,407	2.78%
34	New Mexico	23,193	0.75%
3	New York	197,275	6.34%
10	North Carolina	74,710	2.40%
46	North Dakota	7,416	0.24%
6	Ohio	128,739	4.14%
29	Oklahoma	36,642	1.18%
25	Oregon	40,456	1.30%
7	Pennsylvania	125,639	4.04%
42	Rhode Island	11,049	0.35%
32	South Carolina	32,197	1.03%
44	South Dakota	8,662	0.28%
20	Tennessee	56,539	1.82%
2	Texas	278,760	8.95%
26	Utah	39,291	1.26%
48	Vermont	6,666	0.21%
16	Virginia	67,359	2.16%
15	Washington	69,329	2.23%
38	West Virginia	19,808	0.64%
18	Wisconsin	57,936	1.86%
49	Wyoming	5,956	0.19%

<u>RANK ORDER</u>

RANK	STATE	BIRTHS	% of USA
1	California	440,213	14.14%
2	Texas	278,760	8.95%
3	New York	197,275	6.34%
4	Florida	142,670	4.58%
5	Illinois	141,603	4.55%
6	Ohio	128,739	4.14%
7	Pennsylvania	125,639	4.04%
8	Michigan	109,200	3.51%
9	New Jersey	86,407	2.78%
10	North Carolina	74,710	2.40%
11	Georgia	73,762	2.37%
12	Indiana	73,237	2.35%
13	Arizona	69,869	2.24%
14	Massachusetts	69,418	2.23%
15	Washington	69,329	2.23%
16	Virginia	67,359	2.16%
17	Missouri	61,277	1.97%
18	Wisconsin	57,936	1.86%
19	Minnesota	57,003	1.83%
20	Tennessee	56,539	1.82%
21	Colorado	51,100	1.64%
22	Kentucky	47,243	1.52%
23	Maryland	44,763	1.44%
24	Alabama	40,943	1.32%
25	Oregon	40,456	1.30%
26	Utah	39,291	1.26%
27	Louisiana	37,983	1.22%
28	Connecticut	37,755	1.21%
29	Oklahoma	36,642	1.18%
30	Kansas	35,518	1.14%
31	Iowa	35,125	1.13%
32	South Carolina	32,197	1.03%
33	Arkansas	27,915	0.90%
34	New Mexico	23,193	0.75%
35	Nevada	22,262	0.72%
36	Mississippi	21,801	0.70%
37	Nebraska	21,373	0.69%
38	West Virginia	19,808	0.64%
39	Idaho	18,446	0.59%
40	New Hampshire	14,252	0.46%
41	Maine	13,461	0.43%
42	Rhode Island	11,049	0.35%
43	Montana	9,390	0.30%
44	South Dakota	8,662	0.28%
45	Delaware	7,620	0.24%
46	North Dakota	7,416	0.24%
47	Alaska	6,930	0.22%
48	Vermont	6,666	0.21%
49	Wyoming	5,956	0.19%
50	Hawaii	4,790	0.15%
	District of Columbia	2,062	0.07%

Source: U.S. Department of Health and Human Services, National Center for Health Statistics
"Monthly Vital Statistics Report" (Vol. 46, No. 1(S)2, September 11, 1997)
*Preliminary data by state of residence. By race of mother.

White Births as a Percent of All Births in 1996

National Percent = 79.5% of Live Births*

RANK	STATE	PERCENT
44	Alabama	66.6
43	Alaska	68.2
18	Arizona	87.8
35	Arkansas	76.7
31	California	81.6
11	Colorado	91.5
24	Connecticut	85.2
39	Delaware	74.4
38	Florida	75.3
45	Georgia	64.2
50	Hawaii	26.1
4	Idaho	96.8
34	Illinois	76.8
17	Indiana	87.9
8	Iowa	94.6
13	Kansas	89.4
12	Kentucky	89.8
48	Louisiana	57.4
3	Maine	97.7
45	Maryland	64.2
22	Massachusetts	86.3
32	Michigan	79.4
13	Minnesota	89.4
49	Mississippi	52.3
29	Missouri	83.1
19	Montana	87.7
10	Nebraska	91.6
23	Nevada	85.5
2	New Hampshire	98.0
37	New Jersey	75.9
24	New Mexico	85.2
41	New York	72.7
42	North Carolina	70.7
15	North Dakota	88.7
27	Ohio	84.3
33	Oklahoma	79.3
9	Oregon	92.6
28	Pennsylvania	83.8
16	Rhode Island	88.3
47	South Carolina	63.4
30	South Dakota	82.7
36	Tennessee	76.6
24	Texas	85.2
6	Utah	94.9
1	Vermont	98.8
40	Virginia	72.9
20	Washington	86.7
5	West Virginia	95.7
21	Wisconsin	86.4
7	Wyoming	94.8

RANK	STATE	PERCENT
1	Vermont	98.8
2	New Hampshire	98.0
3	Maine	97.7
4	Idaho	96.8
5	West Virginia	95.7
6	Utah	94.9
7	Wyoming	94.8
8	Iowa	94.6
9	Oregon	92.6
10	Nebraska	91.6
11	Colorado	91.5
12	Kentucky	89.8
13	Kansas	89.4
13	Minnesota	89.4
15	North Dakota	88.7
16	Rhode Island	88.3
17	Indiana	87.9
18	Arizona	87.8
19	Montana	87.7
20	Washington	86.7
21	Wisconsin	86.4
22	Massachusetts	86.3
23	Nevada	85.5
24	Connecticut	85.2
24	New Mexico	85.2
24	Texas	85.2
27	Ohio	84.3
28	Pennsylvania	83.8
29	Missouri	83.1
30	South Dakota	82.7
31	California	81.6
32	Michigan	79.4
33	Oklahoma	79.3
34	Illinois	76.8
35	Arkansas	76.7
36	Tennessee	76.6
37	New Jersey	75.9
38	Florida	75.3
39	Delaware	74.4
40	Virginia	72.9
41	New York	72.7
42	North Carolina	70.7
43	Alaska	68.2
44	Alabama	66.6
45	Georgia	64.2
45	Maryland	64.2
47	South Carolina	63.4
48	Louisiana	57.4
49	Mississippi	52.3
50	Hawaii	26.1
	District of Columbia	24.7

Source: Morgan Quitno Press using data from U.S. Dept. of Health and Human Services, Nat'l Center for Health Statistics "Monthly Vital Statistics Report" (Vol. 46, No. 1(S)2, September 11, 1997)
*Preliminary data by state of residence. By race of mother.

Births to Black Women in 1996

National Total = 596,039 Live Births to Black Women*

RANK	STATE (ALPHA ORDER)	BIRTHS	% of USA		RANK	STATE (RANK ORDER)	BIRTHS	% of USA
15	Alabama	19,833	3.33%		1	New York	55,805	9.36%
41	Alaska	425	0.07%		2	Florida	42,288	7.09%
31	Arizona	2,447	0.41%		3	Georgia	38,777	6.51%
21	Arkansas	7,921	1.33%		4	Texas	38,708	6.49%
5	California	37,695	6.32%		5	California	37,695	6.32%
30	Colorado	2,579	0.43%		6	Illinois	36,499	6.12%
24	Connecticut	5,224	0.88%		7	North Carolina	27,462	4.61%
32	Delaware	2,391	0.40%		8	Louisiana	26,860	4.51%
2	Florida	42,288	7.09%		9	Michigan	24,873	4.17%
3	Georgia	38,777	6.51%		10	Maryland	22,349	3.75%
39	Hawaii	508	0.09%		11	Ohio	21,705	3.64%
47	Idaho	76	0.01%		12	Virginia	20,920	3.51%
6	Illinois	36,499	6.12%		13	Pennsylvania	20,791	3.49%
20	Indiana	9,024	1.51%		14	New Jersey	20,101	3.37%
35	Iowa	1,047	0.18%		15	Alabama	19,833	3.33%
29	Kansas	3,006	0.50%		16	Mississippi	19,288	3.24%
25	Kentucky	4,862	0.82%		17	South Carolina	17,861	3.00%
8	Louisiana	26,860	4.51%		18	Tennessee	16,029	2.69%
45	Maine	85	0.01%		19	Missouri	11,091	1.86%
10	Maryland	22,349	3.75%		20	Indiana	9,024	1.51%
22	Massachusetts	7,329	1.23%		21	Arkansas	7,921	1.33%
9	Michigan	24,873	4.17%		22	Massachusetts	7,329	1.23%
28	Minnesota	3,034	0.51%		23	Wisconsin	6,425	1.08%
16	Mississippi	19,288	3.24%		24	Connecticut	5,224	0.88%
19	Missouri	11,091	1.86%		25	Kentucky	4,862	0.82%
49	Montana	37	0.01%		26	Oklahoma	4,486	0.75%
34	Nebraska	1,203	0.20%		27	Washington	3,187	0.53%
33	Nevada	1,972	0.33%		28	Minnesota	3,034	0.51%
43	New Hampshire	112	0.02%		29	Kansas	3,006	0.50%
14	New Jersey	20,101	3.37%		30	Colorado	2,579	0.43%
40	New Mexico	467	0.08%		31	Arizona	2,447	0.41%
1	New York	55,805	9.36%		32	Delaware	2,391	0.40%
7	North Carolina	27,462	4.61%		33	Nevada	1,972	0.33%
44	North Dakota	87	0.01%		34	Nebraska	1,203	0.20%
11	Ohio	21,705	3.64%		35	Iowa	1,047	0.18%
26	Oklahoma	4,486	0.75%		36	Rhode Island	931	0.16%
37	Oregon	893	0.15%		37	Oregon	893	0.15%
13	Pennsylvania	20,791	3.49%		38	West Virginia	744	0.12%
36	Rhode Island	931	0.16%		39	Hawaii	508	0.09%
17	South Carolina	17,861	3.00%		40	New Mexico	467	0.08%
46	South Dakota	83	0.01%		41	Alaska	425	0.07%
18	Tennessee	16,029	2.69%		42	Utah	331	0.06%
4	Texas	38,708	6.49%		43	New Hampshire	112	0.02%
42	Utah	331	0.06%		44	North Dakota	87	0.01%
50	Vermont	17	0.00%		45	Maine	85	0.01%
12	Virginia	20,920	3.51%		46	South Dakota	83	0.01%
27	Washington	3,187	0.53%		47	Idaho	76	0.01%
38	West Virginia	744	0.12%		48	Wyoming	49	0.01%
23	Wisconsin	6,425	1.08%		49	Montana	37	0.01%
48	Wyoming	49	0.01%		50	Vermont	17	0.00%
						District of Columbia	6,123	1.03%

Source: U.S. Department of Health and Human Services, National Center for Health Statistics
"Monthly Vital Statistics Report" (Vol. 46, No. 1(S)2, September 11, 1997)
*Preliminary data by state of residence. By race of mother.

Black Births as a Percent of All Births in 1996

National Percent = 15.2% of Live Births*

ALPHA ORDER			RANK ORDER		
RANK	STATE	PERCENT	RANK	STATE	PERCENT
5	Alabama	32.3	1	Mississippi	46.3
34	Alaska	4.2	2	Louisiana	40.6
37	Arizona	3.1	3	South Carolina	35.2
11	Arkansas	21.8	4	Georgia	33.8
30	California	7.0	5	Alabama	32.3
33	Colorado	4.6	6	Maryland	32.1
20	Connecticut	11.8	7	North Carolina	26.0
8	Delaware	23.3	8	Delaware	23.3
10	Florida	22.3	9	Virginia	22.6
4	Georgia	33.8	10	Florida	22.3
38	Hawaii	2.8	11	Arkansas	21.8
48	Idaho	0.4	12	Tennessee	21.7
14	Illinois	19.8	13	New York	20.6
22	Indiana	10.8	14	Illinois	19.8
38	Iowa	2.8	15	Michigan	18.1
27	Kansas	7.6	16	New Jersey	17.6
25	Kentucky	9.2	17	Missouri	15.0
2	Louisiana	40.6	18	Ohio	14.2
47	Maine	0.6	19	Pennsylvania	13.9
6	Maryland	32.1	20	Connecticut	11.8
26	Massachusetts	9.1	20	Texas	11.8
15	Michigan	18.1	22	Indiana	10.8
32	Minnesota	4.8	23	Oklahoma	9.7
1	Mississippi	46.3	24	Wisconsin	9.6
17	Missouri	15.0	25	Kentucky	9.2
49	Montana	0.3	26	Massachusetts	9.1
31	Nebraska	5.2	27	Kansas	7.6
27	Nevada	7.6	27	Nevada	7.6
43	New Hampshire	0.8	29	Rhode Island	7.4
16	New Jersey	17.6	30	California	7.0
41	New Mexico	1.7	31	Nebraska	5.2
13	New York	20.6	32	Minnesota	4.8
7	North Carolina	26.0	33	Colorado	4.6
42	North Dakota	1.0	34	Alaska	4.2
18	Ohio	14.2	35	Washington	4.0
23	Oklahoma	9.7	36	West Virginia	3.6
40	Oregon	2.0	37	Arizona	3.1
19	Pennsylvania	13.9	38	Hawaii	2.8
29	Rhode Island	7.4	38	Iowa	2.8
3	South Carolina	35.2	40	Oregon	2.0
43	South Dakota	0.8	41	New Mexico	1.7
12	Tennessee	21.7	42	North Dakota	1.0
20	Texas	11.8	43	New Hampshire	0.8
43	Utah	0.8	43	South Dakota	0.8
49	Vermont	0.3	43	Utah	0.8
9	Virginia	22.6	43	Wyoming	0.8
35	Washington	4.0	47	Maine	0.6
36	West Virginia	3.6	48	Idaho	0.4
24	Wisconsin	9.6	49	Montana	0.3
43	Wyoming	0.8	49	Vermont	0.3
				District of Columbia	73.5

Source: Morgan Quitno Press using data from U.S. Dept. of Health and Human Services, Nat'l Center for Health Statistics
"Monthly Vital Statistics Report" (Vol. 46, No. 1(S)2, September 11, 1997)
*Preliminary data by state of residence. By race of mother.

Births of Low Birthweight in 1996

National Total = 289,707 Live Births*

ALPHA ORDER

RANK	STATE	BIRTHS	% of USA
17	Alabama	5,717	1.97%
47	Alaska	559	0.19%
19	Arizona	5,253	1.81%
30	Arkansas	3,096	1.07%
1	California	32,387	11.18%
21	Colorado	4,914	1.70%
29	Connecticut	3,190	1.10%
41	Delaware	871	0.30%
4	Florida	14,967	5.17%
9	Georgia	9,762	3.37%
39	Hawaii	1,338	0.46%
40	Idaho	1,086	0.37%
5	Illinois	14,750	5.09%
15	Indiana	6,414	2.21%
33	Iowa	2,376	0.82%
31	Kansas	2,742	0.95%
26	Kentucky	4,105	1.42%
14	Louisiana	6,485	2.24%
43	Maine	813	0.28%
16	Maryland	5,924	2.04%
20	Massachusetts	5,069	1.75%
8	Michigan	10,448	3.61%
27	Minnesota	3,699	1.28%
25	Mississippi	4,125	1.42%
18	Missouri	5,534	1.91%
45	Montana	685	0.24%
38	Nebraska	1,469	0.51%
36	Nevada	1,953	0.67%
44	New Hampshire	698	0.24%
11	New Jersey	8,657	2.99%
35	New Mexico	2,043	0.71%
3	New York	20,631	7.12%
10	North Carolina	9,199	3.18%
49	North Dakota	476	0.16%
7	Ohio	11,144	3.85%
28	Oklahoma	3,419	1.18%
34	Oregon	2,315	0.80%
6	Pennsylvania	11,247	3.88%
42	Rhode Island	863	0.30%
22	South Carolina	4,674	1.61%
46	South Dakota	608	0.21%
13	Tennessee	6,493	2.24%
2	Texas	23,556	8.13%
32	Utah	2,690	0.93%
50	Vermont	418	0.14%
12	Virginia	7,115	2.46%
23	Washington	4,478	1.55%
37	West Virginia	1,636	0.56%
24	Wisconsin	4,160	1.44%
48	Wyoming	528	0.18%

RANK ORDER

RANK	STATE	BIRTHS	% of USA
1	California	32,387	11.18%
2	Texas	23,556	8.13%
3	New York	20,631	7.12%
4	Florida	14,967	5.17%
5	Illinois	14,750	5.09%
6	Pennsylvania	11,247	3.88%
7	Ohio	11,144	3.85%
8	Michigan	10,448	3.61%
9	Georgia	9,762	3.37%
10	North Carolina	9,199	3.18%
11	New Jersey	8,657	2.99%
12	Virginia	7,115	2.46%
13	Tennessee	6,493	2.24%
14	Louisiana	6,485	2.24%
15	Indiana	6,414	2.21%
16	Maryland	5,924	2.04%
17	Alabama	5,717	1.97%
18	Missouri	5,534	1.91%
19	Arizona	5,253	1.81%
20	Massachusetts	5,069	1.75%
21	Colorado	4,914	1.70%
22	South Carolina	4,674	1.61%
23	Washington	4,478	1.55%
24	Wisconsin	4,160	1.44%
25	Mississippi	4,125	1.42%
26	Kentucky	4,105	1.42%
27	Minnesota	3,699	1.28%
28	Oklahoma	3,419	1.18%
29	Connecticut	3,190	1.10%
30	Arkansas	3,096	1.07%
31	Kansas	2,742	0.95%
32	Utah	2,690	0.93%
33	Iowa	2,376	0.82%
34	Oregon	2,315	0.80%
35	New Mexico	2,043	0.71%
36	Nevada	1,953	0.67%
37	West Virginia	1,636	0.56%
38	Nebraska	1,469	0.51%
39	Hawaii	1,338	0.46%
40	Idaho	1,086	0.37%
41	Delaware	871	0.30%
42	Rhode Island	863	0.30%
43	Maine	813	0.28%
44	New Hampshire	698	0.24%
45	Montana	685	0.24%
46	South Dakota	608	0.21%
47	Alaska	559	0.19%
48	Wyoming	528	0.18%
49	North Dakota	476	0.16%
50	Vermont	418	0.14%
	District of Columbia	1,184	0.41%

Source: Morgan Quitno Press using data from U.S. Dept. of Health & Human Services, Nat'l Center for Health Statistics "Monthly Vital Statistics Report" (Vol. 46, No. 1(S)2, September 11, 1997)
Estimates based on preliminary data by state of residence. Births of less than 2,500 grams (5 pounds 8 ounces).

Births of Low Birthweight as a Percent of All Births in 1996

National Percent = 7.4% of Live Births*

RANK	STATE (ALPHA ORDER)	PERCENT		RANK	STATE (RANK ORDER)	PERCENT
3	Alabama	9.3		1	Mississippi	9.9
48	Alaska	5.5		2	Louisiana	9.8
33	Arizona	6.6		3	Alabama	9.3
8	Arkansas	8.5		4	South Carolina	9.2
41	California	6.0		5	Colorado	8.8
5	Colorado	8.8		5	Tennessee	8.8
29	Connecticut	7.2		7	North Carolina	8.7
8	Delaware	8.5		8	Arkansas	8.5
14	Florida	7.9		8	Delaware	8.5
8	Georgia	8.5		8	Georgia	8.5
27	Hawaii	7.3		8	Maryland	8.5
45	Idaho	5.7		12	Wyoming	8.4
13	Illinois	8.0		13	Illinois	8.0
17	Indiana	7.7		14	Florida	7.9
35	Iowa	6.4		14	West Virginia	7.9
31	Kansas	6.9		16	Kentucky	7.8
16	Kentucky	7.8		17	Indiana	7.7
2	Louisiana	9.8		17	Virginia	7.7
42	Maine	5.9		19	Michigan	7.6
8	Maryland	8.5		19	New Jersey	7.6
37	Massachusetts	6.3		19	New York	7.6
19	Michigan	7.6		22	Missouri	7.5
43	Minnesota	5.8		22	Nevada	7.5
1	Mississippi	9.9		22	New Mexico	7.5
22	Missouri	7.5		22	Pennsylvania	7.5
35	Montana	6.4		26	Oklahoma	7.4
37	Nebraska	6.3		27	Hawaii	7.3
22	Nevada	7.5		27	Ohio	7.3
50	New Hampshire	4.8		29	Connecticut	7.2
19	New Jersey	7.6		29	Texas	7.2
22	New Mexico	7.5		31	Kansas	6.9
19	New York	7.6		31	Rhode Island	6.9
7	North Carolina	8.7		33	Arizona	6.6
45	North Dakota	5.7		34	Utah	6.5
27	Ohio	7.3		35	Iowa	6.4
26	Oklahoma	7.4		35	Montana	6.4
49	Oregon	5.3		37	Massachusetts	6.3
22	Pennsylvania	7.5		37	Nebraska	6.3
31	Rhode Island	6.9		39	Vermont	6.2
4	South Carolina	9.2		39	Wisconsin	6.2
43	South Dakota	5.8		41	California	6.0
5	Tennessee	8.8		42	Maine	5.9
29	Texas	7.2		43	Minnesota	5.8
34	Utah	6.5		43	South Dakota	5.8
39	Vermont	6.2		45	Idaho	5.7
17	Virginia	7.7		45	North Dakota	5.7
47	Washington	5.6		47	Washington	5.6
14	West Virginia	7.9		48	Alaska	5.5
39	Wisconsin	6.2		49	Oregon	5.3
12	Wyoming	8.4		50	New Hampshire	4.8
					District of Columbia	14.2

*Source: U.S. Department of Health and Human Services, National Center for Health Statistics
"Monthly Vital Statistics Report" (Vol. 46, No. 1(S)2, September 11, 1997)
Preliminary data by state of residence. Births of less than 2,500 grams (5 pounds 8 ounces).

Births of Low Birthweight to White Women in 1996

National Total = 196,120 Live Births*

ALPHA ORDER

RANK	STATE	BIRTHS	% of USA
23	Alabama	2,948	1.50%
49	Alaska	347	0.18%
13	Arizona	4,472	2.28%
33	Arkansas	1,982	1.01%
1	California	23,772	12.12%
14	Colorado	4,344	2.21%
28	Connecticut	2,416	1.23%
44	Delaware	511	0.26%
4	Florida	9,416	4.80%
12	Georgia	4,721	2.41%
50	Hawaii	235	0.12%
39	Idaho	1,051	0.54%
5	Illinois	8,921	4.55%
10	Indiana	5,127	2.61%
31	Iowa	2,108	1.07%
29	Kansas	2,273	1.16%
20	Kentucky	3,496	1.78%
25	Louisiana	2,583	1.32%
40	Maine	781	0.40%
24	Maryland	2,820	1.44%
17	Massachusetts	4,096	2.09%
8	Michigan	6,880	3.51%
22	Minnesota	3,135	1.60%
35	Mississippi	1,591	0.81%
18	Missouri	3,983	2.03%
43	Montana	592	0.30%
38	Nebraska	1,282	0.65%
37	Nevada	1,514	0.77%
42	New Hampshire	670	0.34%
9	New Jersey	5,530	2.82%
34	New Mexico	1,739	0.89%
3	New York	12,823	6.54%
11	North Carolina	5,080	2.59%
47	North Dakota	423	0.22%
6	Ohio	8,239	4.20%
27	Oklahoma	2,492	1.27%
32	Oregon	2,104	1.07%
7	Pennsylvania	8,167	4.16%
41	Rhode Island	718	0.37%
30	South Carolina	2,254	1.15%
44	South Dakota	511	0.26%
16	Tennessee	4,127	2.10%
2	Texas	18,119	9.24%
26	Utah	2,554	1.30%
48	Vermont	413	0.21%
15	Virginia	4,244	2.16%
19	Washington	3,674	1.87%
36	West Virginia	1,545	0.79%
21	Wisconsin	3,186	1.62%
46	Wyoming	494	0.25%

RANK ORDER

RANK	STATE	BIRTHS	% of USA
1	California	23,772	12.12%
2	Texas	18,119	9.24%
3	New York	12,823	6.54%
4	Florida	9,416	4.80%
5	Illinois	8,921	4.55%
6	Ohio	8,239	4.20%
7	Pennsylvania	8,167	4.16%
8	Michigan	6,880	3.51%
9	New Jersey	5,530	2.82%
10	Indiana	5,127	2.61%
11	North Carolina	5,080	2.59%
12	Georgia	4,721	2.41%
13	Arizona	4,472	2.28%
14	Colorado	4,344	2.21%
15	Virginia	4,244	2.16%
16	Tennessee	4,127	2.10%
17	Massachusetts	4,096	2.09%
18	Missouri	3,983	2.03%
19	Washington	3,674	1.87%
20	Kentucky	3,496	1.78%
21	Wisconsin	3,186	1.62%
22	Minnesota	3,135	1.60%
23	Alabama	2,948	1.50%
24	Maryland	2,820	1.44%
25	Louisiana	2,583	1.32%
26	Utah	2,554	1.30%
27	Oklahoma	2,492	1.27%
28	Connecticut	2,416	1.23%
29	Kansas	2,273	1.16%
30	South Carolina	2,254	1.15%
31	Iowa	2,108	1.07%
32	Oregon	2,104	1.07%
33	Arkansas	1,982	1.01%
34	New Mexico	1,739	0.89%
35	Mississippi	1,591	0.81%
36	West Virginia	1,545	0.79%
37	Nevada	1,514	0.77%
38	Nebraska	1,282	0.65%
39	Idaho	1,051	0.54%
40	Maine	781	0.40%
41	Rhode Island	718	0.37%
42	New Hampshire	670	0.34%
43	Montana	592	0.30%
44	Delaware	511	0.26%
44	South Dakota	511	0.26%
46	Wyoming	494	0.25%
47	North Dakota	423	0.22%
48	Vermont	413	0.21%
49	Alaska	347	0.18%
50	Hawaii	235	0.12%
	District of Columbia	144	0.07%

Source: Morgan Quitno Press using data from U.S. Dept. of Health and Human Services, Nat'l Center for Health Statistics "Monthly Vital Statistics Report" (Vol. 46, No. 1(S)2, September 11, 1997)

*Preliminary data by state of residence. Births of less than 2,500 grams (5 pounds 8 ounces). Calculated by the editors by multiplying total number of births to white women by percent of such births reported as being of low birthweight.

Births of Birthweight to White Women
As a Percent of All Births to White Women in 1996
National Percent = 6.3% of Live Births to White Women*

ALPHA ORDER				RANK ORDER		
RANK	STATE	PERCENT		RANK	STATE	PERCENT
8	Alabama	7.2		1	Colorado	8.5
48	Alaska	5.0		2	Wyoming	8.3
24	Arizona	6.4		3	West Virginia	7.8
9	Arkansas	7.1		4	New Mexico	7.5
45	California	5.4		5	Kentucky	7.4
1	Colorado	8.5		6	Mississippi	7.3
24	Connecticut	6.4		6	Tennessee	7.3
16	Delaware	6.7		8	Alabama	7.2
17	Florida	6.6		9	Arkansas	7.1
24	Georgia	6.4		10	Indiana	7.0
49	Hawaii	4.9		10	South Carolina	7.0
41	Idaho	5.7		12	Louisiana	6.8
30	Illinois	6.3		12	Nevada	6.8
10	Indiana	7.0		12	North Carolina	6.8
36	Iowa	6.0		12	Oklahoma	6.8
24	Kansas	6.4		16	Delaware	6.7
5	Kentucky	7.4		17	Florida	6.6
12	Louisiana	6.8		18	Missouri	6.5
40	Maine	5.8		18	New York	6.5
30	Maryland	6.3		18	Pennsylvania	6.5
38	Massachusetts	5.9		18	Rhode Island	6.5
30	Michigan	6.3		18	Texas	6.5
43	Minnesota	5.5		18	Utah	6.5
6	Mississippi	7.3		24	Arizona	6.4
18	Missouri	6.5		24	Connecticut	6.4
30	Montana	6.3		24	Georgia	6.4
36	Nebraska	6.0		24	Kansas	6.4
12	Nevada	6.8		24	New Jersey	6.4
50	New Hampshire	4.7		24	Ohio	6.4
24	New Jersey	6.4		30	Illinois	6.3
4	New Mexico	7.5		30	Maryland	6.3
18	New York	6.5		30	Michigan	6.3
12	North Carolina	6.8		30	Montana	6.3
41	North Dakota	5.7		30	Virginia	6.3
24	Ohio	6.4		35	Vermont	6.2
12	Oklahoma	6.8		36	Iowa	6.0
47	Oregon	5.2		36	Nebraska	6.0
18	Pennsylvania	6.5		38	Massachusetts	5.9
18	Rhode Island	6.5		38	South Dakota	5.9
10	South Carolina	7.0		40	Maine	5.8
38	South Dakota	5.9		41	Idaho	5.7
6	Tennessee	7.3		41	North Dakota	5.7
18	Texas	6.5		43	Minnesota	5.5
18	Utah	6.5		43	Wisconsin	5.5
35	Vermont	6.2		45	California	5.4
30	Virginia	6.3		46	Washington	5.3
46	Washington	5.3		47	Oregon	5.2
3	West Virginia	7.8		48	Alaska	5.0
43	Wisconsin	5.5		49	Hawaii	4.9
2	Wyoming	8.3		50	New Hampshire	4.7
					District of Columbia	7.0

Source: U.S. Department of Health and Human Services, National Center for Health Statistics
"Monthly Vital Statistics Report" (Vol. 46, No. 1(S)2, September 11, 1997)
*Preliminary data by state of residence. Births of less than 2,500 grams (5 pounds 8 ounces).

Births of Low Birthweight to Black Women in 1996

National Total = 77,485 Live Births*

ALPHA ORDER

RANK ORDER

RANK	STATE	BIRTHS	% of USA
13	Alabama	2,717	3.51%
40	Alaska	53	0.07%
32	Arizona	301	0.39%
21	Arkansas	1,077	1.39%
6	California	4,448	5.74%
28	Colorado	387	0.50%
24	Connecticut	674	0.87%
31	Delaware	340	0.44%
3	Florida	5,159	6.66%
4	Georgia	4,925	6.36%
41	Hawaii	44	0.06%
NA	Idaho**	NA	NA
2	Illinois	5,292	6.83%
20	Indiana	1,263	1.63%
34	Iowa	153	0.20%
27	Kansas	403	0.52%
25	Kentucky	617	0.80%
8	Louisiana	3,814	4.92%
NA	Maine**	NA	NA
10	Maryland	2,950	3.81%
23	Massachusetts	755	0.97%
9	Michigan	3,383	4.37%
29	Minnesota	364	0.47%
16	Mississippi	2,488	3.21%
19	Missouri	1,420	1.83%
NA	Montana**	NA	NA
35	Nebraska	129	0.17%
33	Nevada	274	0.35%
NA	New Hampshire**	NA	NA
14	New Jersey	2,613	3.37%
39	New Mexico	64	0.08%
1	New York	6,641	8.57%
7	North Carolina	3,817	4.93%
NA	North Dakota**	NA	NA
12	Ohio	2,822	3.64%
26	Oklahoma	592	0.76%
37	Oregon	100	0.13%
11	Pennsylvania	2,932	3.78%
36	Rhode Island	112	0.14%
17	South Carolina	2,358	3.04%
NA	South Dakota**	NA	NA
18	Tennessee	2,276	2.94%
5	Texas	4,800	6.19%
42	Utah	39	0.05%
NA	Vermont**	NA	NA
15	Virginia	2,552	3.29%
30	Washington	344	0.44%
38	West Virginia	92	0.12%
22	Wisconsin	816	1.05%
NA	Wyoming**	NA	NA

RANK	STATE	BIRTHS	% of USA
1	New York	6,641	8.57%
2	Illinois	5,292	6.83%
3	Florida	5,159	6.66%
4	Georgia	4,925	6.36%
5	Texas	4,800	6.19%
6	California	4,448	5.74%
7	North Carolina	3,817	4.93%
8	Louisiana	3,814	4.92%
9	Michigan	3,383	4.37%
10	Maryland	2,950	3.81%
11	Pennsylvania	2,932	3.78%
12	Ohio	2,822	3.64%
13	Alabama	2,717	3.51%
14	New Jersey	2,613	3.37%
15	Virginia	2,552	3.29%
16	Mississippi	2,488	3.21%
17	South Carolina	2,358	3.04%
18	Tennessee	2,276	2.94%
19	Missouri	1,420	1.83%
20	Indiana	1,263	1.63%
21	Arkansas	1,077	1.39%
22	Wisconsin	816	1.05%
23	Massachusetts	755	0.97%
24	Connecticut	674	0.87%
25	Kentucky	617	0.80%
26	Oklahoma	592	0.76%
27	Kansas	403	0.52%
28	Colorado	387	0.50%
29	Minnesota	364	0.47%
30	Washington	344	0.44%
31	Delaware	340	0.44%
32	Arizona	301	0.39%
33	Nevada	274	0.35%
34	Iowa	153	0.20%
35	Nebraska	129	0.17%
36	Rhode Island	112	0.14%
37	Oregon	100	0.13%
38	West Virginia	92	0.12%
39	New Mexico	64	0.08%
40	Alaska	53	0.07%
41	Hawaii	44	0.06%
42	Utah	39	0.05%
NA	Idaho**	NA	NA
NA	Maine**	NA	NA
NA	Montana**	NA	NA
NA	New Hampshire**	NA	NA
NA	North Dakota**	NA	NA
NA	South Dakota**	NA	NA
NA	Vermont**	NA	NA
NA	Wyoming**	NA	NA

District of Columbia 1,029 1.33%

Source: Morgan Quitno Press using data from U.S. Dept. of Health and Human Services, Nat'l Center for Health Statistics
"Monthly Vital Statistics Report" (Vol. 46, No. 1(S)2, September 11, 1997)
*Preliminary data by state of residence. Births of less than 2,500 grams (5 pounds 8 ounces). Calculated by the editors by multiplying total number of births to black women by percent of such births reported as being of low birthweight.
**Not available.

Births of Low Birthweight to Black Women
As a Percent of All Births to Black Women in 1996
National Percent = 13.0% of Live Births to Black Women*

ALPHA ORDER

RANK	STATE	PERCENT
11	Alabama	13.7
27	Alaska	12.4
30	Arizona	12.3
12	Arkansas	13.6
36	California	11.8
1	Colorado	15.0
21	Connecticut	12.9
4	Delaware	14.2
31	Florida	12.2
24	Georgia	12.7
42	Hawaii	8.6
NA	Idaho**	NA
3	Illinois	14.5
8	Indiana	14.0
2	Iowa	14.6
15	Kansas	13.4
24	Kentucky	12.7
4	Louisiana	14.2
NA	Maine**	NA
16	Maryland	13.2
41	Massachusetts	10.3
12	Michigan	13.6
33	Minnesota	12.0
21	Mississippi	12.9
23	Missouri	12.8
NA	Montana**	NA
40	Nebraska	10.7
9	Nevada	13.9
NA	New Hampshire**	NA
19	New Jersey	13.0
12	New Mexico	13.6
35	New York	11.9
9	North Carolina	13.9
NA	North Dakota**	NA
19	Ohio	13.0
16	Oklahoma	13.2
38	Oregon	11.2
7	Pennsylvania	14.1
33	Rhode Island	12.0
16	South Carolina	13.2
NA	South Dakota**	NA
4	Tennessee	14.2
27	Texas	12.4
37	Utah	11.7
NA	Vermont**	NA
31	Virginia	12.2
39	Washington	10.8
27	West Virginia	12.4
24	Wisconsin	12.7
NA	Wyoming**	NA

RANK ORDER

RANK	STATE	PERCENT
1	Colorado	15.0
2	Iowa	14.6
3	Illinois	14.5
4	Delaware	14.2
4	Louisiana	14.2
4	Tennessee	14.2
7	Pennsylvania	14.1
8	Indiana	14.0
9	Nevada	13.9
9	North Carolina	13.9
11	Alabama	13.7
12	Arkansas	13.6
12	Michigan	13.6
12	New Mexico	13.6
15	Kansas	13.4
16	Maryland	13.2
16	Oklahoma	13.2
16	South Carolina	13.2
19	New Jersey	13.0
19	Ohio	13.0
21	Connecticut	12.9
21	Mississippi	12.9
23	Missouri	12.8
24	Georgia	12.7
24	Kentucky	12.7
24	Wisconsin	12.7
27	Alaska	12.4
27	Texas	12.4
27	West Virginia	12.4
30	Arizona	12.3
31	Florida	12.2
31	Virginia	12.2
33	Minnesota	12.0
33	Rhode Island	12.0
35	New York	11.9
36	California	11.8
37	Utah	11.7
38	Oregon	11.2
39	Washington	10.8
40	Nebraska	10.7
41	Massachusetts	10.3
42	Hawaii	8.6
NA	Idaho**	NA
NA	Maine**	NA
NA	Montana**	NA
NA	New Hampshire**	NA
NA	North Dakota**	NA
NA	South Dakota**	NA
NA	Vermont**	NA
NA	Wyoming**	NA
	District of Columbia	16.8

Source: U.S. Department of Health and Human Services, National Center for Health Statistics
"Monthly Vital Statistics Report" (Vol. 46, No. 1(S)2, September 11, 1997)
*Preliminary data by state of residence. Births of less than 2,500 grams (5 pounds 8 ounces).
**Insufficient data.

Births to Unmarried Women in 1996

National Total = 1,268,445 Live Births*

<u>ALPHA ORDER</u>

RANK	STATE	BIRTHS	% of USA
21	Alabama	20,595	1.62%
45	Alaska	3,180	0.25%
12	Arizona	31,040	2.45%
31	Arkansas	12,346	0.97%
1	California	170,573	13.45%
29	Colorado	13,848	1.09%
28	Connecticut	13,870	1.09%
43	Delaware	3,636	0.29%
4	Florida	68,205	5.38%
9	Georgia	40,197	3.17%
39	Hawaii	5,537	0.44%
41	Idaho	4,060	0.32%
5	Illinois	62,132	4.90%
14	Indiana	27,157	2.14%
35	Iowa	9,763	0.77%
34	Kansas	10,688	0.84%
25	Kentucky	15,684	1.24%
13	Louisiana	28,721	2.26%
42	Maine	3,953	0.31%
18	Maryland	23,278	1.84%
20	Massachusetts	20,597	1.62%
8	Michigan	46,465	3.66%
26	Minnesota	15,562	1.23%
23	Mississippi	18,790	1.48%
17	Missouri	24,422	1.93%
47	Montana	2,977	0.23%
38	Nebraska	5,760	0.45%
33	Nevada	11,117	0.88%
44	New Hampshire	3,404	0.27%
11	New Jersey	31,779	2.51%
32	New Mexico	11,466	0.90%
2	New York	105,326	8.30%
10	North Carolina	33,837	2.67%
48	North Dakota	2,106	0.17%
6	Ohio	50,226	3.96%
27	Oklahoma	14,279	1.13%
30	Oregon	12,972	1.02%
7	Pennsylvania	48,438	3.82%
40	Rhode Island	4,117	0.32%
22	South Carolina	18,900	1.49%
46	South Dakota	3,090	0.24%
16	Tennessee	24,642	1.94%
3	Texas	99,785	7.87%
36	Utah	6,622	0.52%
49	Vermont	1,781	0.14%
15	Virginia	26,611	2.10%
19	Washington	21,829	1.72%
37	West Virginia	6,501	0.51%
24	Wisconsin	18,384	1.45%
50	Wyoming	1,697	0.13%

<u>RANK ORDER</u>

RANK	STATE	BIRTHS	% of USA
1	California	170,573	13.45%
2	New York	105,326	8.30%
3	Texas	99,785	7.87%
4	Florida	68,205	5.38%
5	Illinois	62,132	4.90%
6	Ohio	50,226	3.96%
7	Pennsylvania	48,438	3.82%
8	Michigan	46,465	3.66%
9	Georgia	40,197	3.17%
10	North Carolina	33,837	2.67%
11	New Jersey	31,779	2.51%
12	Arizona	31,040	2.45%
13	Louisiana	28,721	2.26%
14	Indiana	27,157	2.14%
15	Virginia	26,611	2.10%
16	Tennessee	24,642	1.94%
17	Missouri	24,422	1.93%
18	Maryland	23,278	1.84%
19	Washington	21,829	1.72%
20	Massachusetts	20,597	1.62%
21	Alabama	20,595	1.62%
22	South Carolina	18,900	1.49%
23	Mississippi	18,790	1.48%
24	Wisconsin	18,384	1.45%
25	Kentucky	15,684	1.24%
26	Minnesota	15,562	1.23%
27	Oklahoma	14,279	1.13%
28	Connecticut	13,870	1.09%
29	Colorado	13,848	1.09%
30	Oregon	12,972	1.02%
31	Arkansas	12,346	0.97%
32	New Mexico	11,466	0.90%
33	Nevada	11,117	0.88%
34	Kansas	10,688	0.84%
35	Iowa	9,763	0.77%
36	Utah	6,622	0.52%
37	West Virginia	6,501	0.51%
38	Nebraska	5,760	0.45%
39	Hawaii	5,537	0.44%
40	Rhode Island	4,117	0.32%
41	Idaho	4,060	0.32%
42	Maine	3,953	0.31%
43	Delaware	3,636	0.29%
44	New Hampshire	3,404	0.27%
45	Alaska	3,180	0.25%
46	South Dakota	3,090	0.24%
47	Montana	2,977	0.23%
48	North Dakota	2,106	0.17%
49	Vermont	1,781	0.14%
50	Wyoming	1,697	0.13%
	District of Columbia	5,502	0.43%

Source: Morgan Quitno Press using data from U.S. Dept. of Health and Human Services, Nat'l Center for Health Statistics "Monthly Vital Statistics Report" (Vol. 46, No. 1(S)2, September 11, 1997)
Preliminary data by state of residence. Calculated by the editors by multiplying total number of births by reported percent of births to unmarried women.

Births to Unmarried Women as a Percent of All Births in 1996

National Percent = 32.4% of Live Births*

ALPHA ORDER

RANK	STATE	PERCENT
14	Alabama	33.5
25	Alaska	31.3
5	Arizona	39.0
11	Arkansas	33.9
23	California	31.6
45	Colorado	24.8
25	Connecticut	31.3
9	Delaware	35.5
8	Florida	36.0
10	Georgia	35.0
29	Hawaii	30.2
49	Idaho	21.3
13	Illinois	33.7
20	Indiana	32.6
42	Iowa	26.3
40	Kansas	26.9
30	Kentucky	29.8
2	Louisiana	43.4
34	Maine	28.7
15	Maryland	33.4
43	Massachusetts	25.6
12	Michigan	33.8
47	Minnesota	24.4
1	Mississippi	45.1
17	Missouri	33.1
36	Montana	27.8
46	Nebraska	24.7
3	Nevada	42.7
48	New Hampshire	23.4
35	New Jersey	27.9
4	New Mexico	42.1
6	New York	38.8
22	North Carolina	32.0
44	North Dakota	25.2
18	Ohio	32.9
27	Oklahoma	30.9
31	Oregon	29.7
21	Pennsylvania	32.3
18	Rhode Island	32.9
7	South Carolina	37.2
32	South Dakota	29.5
15	Tennessee	33.4
28	Texas	30.5
50	Utah	16.0
41	Vermont	26.4
33	Virginia	28.8
38	Washington	27.3
24	West Virginia	31.4
37	Wisconsin	27.4
39	Wyoming	27.0

RANK ORDER

RANK	STATE	PERCENT
1	Mississippi	45.1
2	Louisiana	43.4
3	Nevada	42.7
4	New Mexico	42.1
5	Arizona	39.0
6	New York	38.8
7	South Carolina	37.2
8	Florida	36.0
9	Delaware	35.5
10	Georgia	35.0
11	Arkansas	33.9
12	Michigan	33.8
13	Illinois	33.7
14	Alabama	33.5
15	Maryland	33.4
15	Tennessee	33.4
17	Missouri	33.1
18	Ohio	32.9
18	Rhode Island	32.9
20	Indiana	32.6
21	Pennsylvania	32.3
22	North Carolina	32.0
23	California	31.6
24	West Virginia	31.4
25	Alaska	31.3
25	Connecticut	31.3
27	Oklahoma	30.9
28	Texas	30.5
29	Hawaii	30.2
30	Kentucky	29.8
31	Oregon	29.7
32	South Dakota	29.5
33	Virginia	28.8
34	Maine	28.7
35	New Jersey	27.9
36	Montana	27.8
37	Wisconsin	27.4
38	Washington	27.3
39	Wyoming	27.0
40	Kansas	26.9
41	Vermont	26.4
42	Iowa	26.3
43	Massachusetts	25.6
44	North Dakota	25.2
45	Colorado	24.8
46	Nebraska	24.7
47	Minnesota	24.4
48	New Hampshire	23.4
49	Idaho	21.3
50	Utah	16.0
	District of Columbia	66.0

Source: U.S. Department of Health and Human Services, National Center for Health Statistics
"Monthly Vital Statistics Report" (Vol. 46, No. 1(S)2, September 11, 1997)
*Data are preliminary estimates by state of residence.

Births to Unmarried White Women in 1996

National Total = 800,045 Live Births*

ALPHA ORDER

RANK	STATE	BIRTHS	% of USA
32	Alabama	6,674	0.83%
47	Alaska	1,580	0.20%
9	Arizona	25,293	3.16%
34	Arkansas	6,337	0.79%
1	California	138,227	17.28%
22	Colorado	11,855	1.48%
24	Connecticut	9,665	1.21%
44	Delaware	1,859	0.23%
4	Florida	38,664	4.83%
16	Georgia	14,089	1.76%
50	Hawaii	814	0.10%
40	Idaho	3,837	0.48%
6	Illinois	33,277	4.16%
10	Indiana	20,067	2.51%
29	Iowa	8,711	1.09%
31	Kansas	8,347	1.04%
21	Kentucky	12,000	1.50%
30	Louisiana	8,660	1.08%
39	Maine	3,850	0.48%
26	Maryland	8,997	1.12%
13	Massachusetts	15,480	1.93%
8	Michigan	26,754	3.34%
20	Minnesota	12,085	1.51%
38	Mississippi	4,055	0.51%
14	Missouri	15,442	1.93%
43	Montana	2,160	0.27%
37	Nebraska	4,595	0.57%
28	Nevada	8,793	1.10%
41	New Hampshire	3,335	0.42%
12	New Jersey	17,713	2.21%
27	New Mexico	8,837	1.10%
3	New York	59,972	7.50%
15	North Carolina	14,270	1.78%
48	North Dakota	1,535	0.19%
5	Ohio	33,343	4.17%
25	Oklahoma	9,087	1.14%
23	Oregon	11,611	1.45%
7	Pennsylvania	31,410	3.93%
42	Rhode Island	3,248	0.41%
33	South Carolina	6,439	0.80%
45	South Dakota	1,845	0.23%
18	Tennessee	12,608	1.58%
2	Texas	73,871	9.23%
35	Utah	5,933	0.74%
46	Vermont	1,753	0.22%
17	Virginia	12,933	1.62%
11	Washington	17,887	2.24%
36	West Virginia	5,923	0.74%
19	Wisconsin	12,282	1.54%
49	Wyoming	1,525	0.19%

RANK ORDER

RANK	STATE	BIRTHS	% of USA
1	California	138,227	17.28%
2	Texas	73,871	9.23%
3	New York	59,972	7.50%
4	Florida	38,664	4.83%
5	Ohio	33,343	4.17%
6	Illinois	33,277	4.16%
7	Pennsylvania	31,410	3.93%
8	Michigan	26,754	3.34%
9	Arizona	25,293	3.16%
10	Indiana	20,067	2.51%
11	Washington	17,887	2.24%
12	New Jersey	17,713	2.21%
13	Massachusetts	15,480	1.93%
14	Missouri	15,442	1.93%
15	North Carolina	14,270	1.78%
16	Georgia	14,089	1.76%
17	Virginia	12,933	1.62%
18	Tennessee	12,608	1.58%
19	Wisconsin	12,282	1.54%
20	Minnesota	12,085	1.51%
21	Kentucky	12,000	1.50%
22	Colorado	11,855	1.48%
23	Oregon	11,611	1.45%
24	Connecticut	9,665	1.21%
25	Oklahoma	9,087	1.14%
26	Maryland	8,997	1.12%
27	New Mexico	8,837	1.10%
28	Nevada	8,793	1.10%
29	Iowa	8,711	1.09%
30	Louisiana	8,660	1.08%
31	Kansas	8,347	1.04%
32	Alabama	6,674	0.83%
33	South Carolina	6,439	0.80%
34	Arkansas	6,337	0.79%
35	Utah	5,933	0.74%
36	West Virginia	5,923	0.74%
37	Nebraska	4,595	0.57%
38	Mississippi	4,055	0.51%
39	Maine	3,850	0.48%
40	Idaho	3,837	0.48%
41	New Hampshire	3,335	0.42%
42	Rhode Island	3,248	0.41%
43	Montana	2,160	0.27%
44	Delaware	1,859	0.23%
45	South Dakota	1,845	0.23%
46	Vermont	1,753	0.22%
47	Alaska	1,580	0.20%
48	North Dakota	1,535	0.19%
49	Wyoming	1,525	0.19%
50	Hawaii	814	0.10%
	District of Columbia	573	0.07%

Source: Morgan Quitno Press using data from U.S. Dept. of Health and Human Services, Nat'l Center for Health Statistics "Monthly Vital Statistics Report" (Vol. 46, No. 1(S)2, September 11, 1997)
*Preliminary data by state of residence. Calculated by the editors by multiplying total number of births to white women by percent of such births reported as being to unmarried white women.

Births to Unmarried White Women
As a Percent of All Births to White Women in 1996
National Percent = 25.7% of Live Births*

<u>ALPHA ORDER</u>

RANK	STATE	PERCENT
49	Alabama	16.3
30	Alaska	22.8
3	Arizona	36.2
32	Arkansas	22.7
4	California	31.4
28	Colorado	23.2
16	Connecticut	25.6
24	Delaware	24.4
11	Florida	27.1
45	Georgia	19.1
48	Hawaii	17.0
39	Idaho	20.8
25	Illinois	23.5
10	Indiana	27.4
21	Iowa	24.8
25	Kansas	23.5
18	Kentucky	25.4
30	Louisiana	22.8
9	Maine	28.6
42	Maryland	20.1
33	Massachusetts	22.3
23	Michigan	24.5
37	Minnesota	21.2
47	Mississippi	18.6
19	Missouri	25.2
29	Montana	23.0
35	Nebraska	21.5
1	Nevada	39.5
27	New Hampshire	23.4
41	New Jersey	20.5
2	New Mexico	38.1
5	New York	30.4
45	North Carolina	19.1
40	North Dakota	20.7
14	Ohio	25.9
21	Oklahoma	24.8
8	Oregon	28.7
20	Pennsylvania	25.0
7	Rhode Island	29.4
43	South Carolina	20.0
36	South Dakota	21.3
33	Tennessee	22.3
12	Texas	26.5
50	Utah	15.1
13	Vermont	26.3
44	Virginia	19.2
15	Washington	25.8
6	West Virginia	29.9
37	Wisconsin	21.2
16	Wyoming	25.6

<u>RANK ORDER</u>

RANK	STATE	PERCENT
1	Nevada	39.5
2	New Mexico	38.1
3	Arizona	36.2
4	California	31.4
5	New York	30.4
6	West Virginia	29.9
7	Rhode Island	29.4
8	Oregon	28.7
9	Maine	28.6
10	Indiana	27.4
11	Florida	27.1
12	Texas	26.5
13	Vermont	26.3
14	Ohio	25.9
15	Washington	25.8
16	Connecticut	25.6
16	Wyoming	25.6
18	Kentucky	25.4
19	Missouri	25.2
20	Pennsylvania	25.0
21	Iowa	24.8
21	Oklahoma	24.8
23	Michigan	24.5
24	Delaware	24.4
25	Illinois	23.5
25	Kansas	23.5
27	New Hampshire	23.4
28	Colorado	23.2
29	Montana	23.0
30	Alaska	22.8
30	Louisiana	22.8
32	Arkansas	22.7
33	Massachusetts	22.3
33	Tennessee	22.3
35	Nebraska	21.5
36	South Dakota	21.3
37	Minnesota	21.2
37	Wisconsin	21.2
39	Idaho	20.8
40	North Dakota	20.7
41	New Jersey	20.5
42	Maryland	20.1
43	South Carolina	20.0
44	Virginia	19.2
45	Georgia	19.1
45	North Carolina	19.1
47	Mississippi	18.6
48	Hawaii	17.0
49	Alabama	16.3
50	Utah	15.1
	District of Columbia	27.8

Source: U.S. Department of Health and Human Services, National Center for Health Statistics
    "Monthly Vital Statistics Report" (Vol. 46, No. 1(S)2, September 11, 1997)
Data are preliminary estimates by state of residence. By race of mother.

Births to Unmarried Black Women in 1996

National Total = 416,035 Live Births*

ALPHA ORDER				RANK ORDER			
RANK	STATE	BIRTHS	% of USA	RANK	STATE	BIRTHS	% of USA
14	Alabama	13,804	3.32%	1	New York	39,566	9.51%
40	Alaska	171	0.04%	2	Florida	28,714	6.90%
31	Arizona	1,573	0.38%	3	Illinois	28,360	6.82%
21	Arkansas	5,869	1.41%	4	Georgia	25,825	6.21%
6	California	23,032	5.54%	5	Texas	24,502	5.89%
33	Colorado	1,496	0.36%	6	California	23,032	5.54%
24	Connecticut	3,688	0.89%	7	Louisiana	19,715	4.74%
30	Delaware	1,748	0.42%	8	Michigan	19,053	4.58%
2	Florida	28,714	6.90%	9	North Carolina	18,482	4.44%
4	Georgia	25,825	6.21%	10	Ohio	16,604	3.99%
42	Hawaii	110	0.03%	11	Pennsylvania	16,300	3.92%
46	Idaho	24	0.01%	12	Mississippi	14,505	3.49%
3	Illinois	28,360	6.82%	13	Maryland	14,035	3.37%
20	Indiana	6,948	1.67%	14	Alabama	13,804	3.32%
35	Iowa	753	0.18%	15	New Jersey	13,427	3.23%
27	Kansas	2,053	0.49%	16	Virginia	13,263	3.19%
25	Kentucky	3,583	0.86%	17	South Carolina	12,324	2.96%
7	Louisiana	19,715	4.74%	18	Tennessee	11,781	2.83%
44	Maine	37	0.01%	19	Missouri	8,651	2.08%
13	Maryland	14,035	3.37%	20	Indiana	6,948	1.67%
23	Massachusetts	4,324	1.04%	21	Arkansas	5,869	1.41%
8	Michigan	19,053	4.58%	22	Wisconsin	5,326	1.28%
28	Minnesota	2,042	0.49%	23	Massachusetts	4,324	1.04%
12	Mississippi	14,505	3.49%	24	Connecticut	3,688	0.89%
19	Missouri	8,651	2.08%	25	Kentucky	3,583	0.86%
NA	Montana**	NA	NA	26	Oklahoma	3,109	0.75%
34	Nebraska	860	0.21%	27	Kansas	2,053	0.49%
32	Nevada	1,511	0.36%	28	Minnesota	2,042	0.49%
43	New Hampshire	44	0.01%	29	Washington	1,794	0.43%
15	New Jersey	13,427	3.23%	30	Delaware	1,748	0.42%
39	New Mexico	286	0.07%	31	Arizona	1,573	0.38%
1	New York	39,566	9.51%	32	Nevada	1,511	0.36%
9	North Carolina	18,482	4.44%	33	Colorado	1,496	0.36%
48	North Dakota	20	0.00%	34	Nebraska	860	0.21%
10	Ohio	16,604	3.99%	35	Iowa	753	0.18%
26	Oklahoma	3,109	0.75%	36	Rhode Island	635	0.15%
37	Oregon	623	0.15%	37	Oregon	623	0.15%
11	Pennsylvania	16,300	3.92%	38	West Virginia	549	0.13%
36	Rhode Island	635	0.15%	39	New Mexico	286	0.07%
17	South Carolina	12,324	2.96%	40	Alaska	171	0.04%
45	South Dakota	25	0.01%	41	Utah	161	0.04%
18	Tennessee	11,781	2.83%	42	Hawaii	110	0.03%
5	Texas	24,502	5.89%	43	New Hampshire	44	0.01%
41	Utah	161	0.04%	44	Maine	37	0.01%
NA	Vermont**	NA	NA	45	South Dakota	25	0.01%
16	Virginia	13,263	3.19%	46	Idaho	24	0.01%
29	Washington	1,794	0.43%	47	Wyoming	22	0.01%
38	West Virginia	549	0.13%	48	North Dakota	20	0.00%
22	Wisconsin	5,326	1.28%	NA	Montana**	NA	NA
47	Wyoming	22	0.01%	NA	Vermont**	NA	NA
					District of Columbia	4,892	1.18%

Source: Morgan Quitno Press using data from U.S. Dept. of Health and Human Services, Nat'l Center for Health Statistics "Monthly Vital Statistics Report" (Vol. 46, No. 1(S)2, September 11, 1997)
Preliminary data by state of residence. Calculated by the editors by multiplying total number of births to black women by percent of such births reported as being to unmarried black women.

Births to Unmarried Black Women
As a Percent of All Births to Black Women in 1996
National Percent = 69.8% of Live Births*

ALPHA ORDER

RANK ORDER

RANK	STATE	PERCENT
21	Alabama	69.6
43	Alaska	40.3
31	Arizona	64.3
10	Arkansas	74.1
36	California	61.1
38	Colorado	58.0
19	Connecticut	70.6
15	Delaware	73.1
26	Florida	67.9
30	Georgia	66.6
48	Hawaii	21.7
45	Idaho	31.1
4	Illinois	77.7
5	Indiana	77.0
16	Iowa	71.9
24	Kansas	68.3
12	Kentucky	73.7
14	Louisiana	73.4
42	Maine	43.5
34	Maryland	62.8
37	Massachusetts	59.0
6	Michigan	76.6
27	Minnesota	67.3
9	Mississippi	75.2
3	Missouri	78.0
NA	Montana**	NA
17	Nebraska	71.5
6	Nevada	76.6
44	New Hampshire	39.2
29	New Jersey	66.8
35	New Mexico	61.3
18	New York	70.9
27	North Carolina	67.3
47	North Dakota	23.0
8	Ohio	76.5
22	Oklahoma	69.3
20	Oregon	69.8
2	Pennsylvania	78.4
25	Rhode Island	68.2
23	South Carolina	69.0
46	South Dakota	30.1
13	Tennessee	73.5
33	Texas	63.3
40	Utah	48.6
NA	Vermont**	NA
32	Virginia	63.4
39	Washington	56.3
11	West Virginia	73.8
1	Wisconsin	82.9
41	Wyoming	44.9

RANK	STATE	PERCENT
1	Wisconsin	82.9
2	Pennsylvania	78.4
3	Missouri	78.0
4	Illinois	77.7
5	Indiana	77.0
6	Michigan	76.6
6	Nevada	76.6
8	Ohio	76.5
9	Mississippi	75.2
10	Arkansas	74.1
11	West Virginia	73.8
12	Kentucky	73.7
13	Tennessee	73.5
14	Louisiana	73.4
15	Delaware	73.1
16	Iowa	71.9
17	Nebraska	71.5
18	New York	70.9
19	Connecticut	70.6
20	Oregon	69.8
21	Alabama	69.6
22	Oklahoma	69.3
23	South Carolina	69.0
24	Kansas	68.3
25	Rhode Island	68.2
26	Florida	67.9
27	Minnesota	67.3
27	North Carolina	67.3
29	New Jersey	66.8
30	Georgia	66.6
31	Arizona	64.3
32	Virginia	63.4
33	Texas	63.3
34	Maryland	62.8
35	New Mexico	61.3
36	California	61.1
37	Massachusetts	59.0
38	Colorado	58.0
39	Washington	56.3
40	Utah	48.6
41	Wyoming	44.9
42	Maine	43.5
43	Alaska	40.3
44	New Hampshire	39.2
45	Idaho	31.1
46	South Dakota	30.1
47	North Dakota	23.0
48	Hawaii	21.7
NA	Montana**	NA
NA	Vermont**	NA
	District of Columbia	79.9

Source: U.S. Department of Health and Human Services, National Center for Health Statistics
"Monthly Vital Statistics Report" (Vol. 46, No. 1(S)2, September 11, 1997)
*Data are preliminary estimates by state of residence. By race of mother.
**Too few births for a reliable figure.

Births to Teenage Mothers in 1996

National Total = 505,029 Live Births*

ALPHA ORDER

RANK	STATE	BIRTHS	% of USA
15	Alabama	11,250	2.23%
46	Alaska	1,138	0.23%
14	Arizona	11,939	2.36%
24	Arkansas	7,211	1.43%
1	California	64,775	12.83%
27	Colorado	6,645	1.32%
35	Connecticut	3,634	0.72%
41	Delaware	1,403	0.28%
3	Florida	25,387	5.03%
7	Georgia	18,261	3.62%
40	Hawaii	1,888	0.37%
38	Idaho	2,573	0.51%
5	Illinois	23,415	4.64%
13	Indiana	12,079	2.39%
34	Iowa	4,083	0.81%
31	Kansas	5,205	1.03%
19	Kentucky	8,947	1.77%
11	Louisiana	12,508	2.48%
43	Maine	1,336	0.26%
25	Maryland	7,179	1.42%
28	Massachusetts	5,873	1.16%
8	Michigan	16,771	3.32%
30	Minnesota	5,421	1.07%
20	Mississippi	8,874	1.76%
16	Missouri	10,403	2.06%
42	Montana	1,338	0.26%
39	Nebraska	2,472	0.49%
37	Nevada	3,463	0.69%
47	New Hampshire	1,077	0.21%
21	New Jersey	8,770	1.74%
32	New Mexico	4,875	0.97%
4	New York	24,974	4.95%
10	North Carolina	15,861	3.14%
49	North Dakota	802	0.16%
6	Ohio	20,304	4.02%
23	Oklahoma	7,948	1.57%
29	Oregon	5,765	1.14%
9	Pennsylvania	15,896	3.15%
44	Rhode Island	1,289	0.26%
22	South Carolina	8,536	1.69%
45	South Dakota	1,205	0.24%
12	Tennessee	12,395	2.45%
2	Texas	53,000	10.49%
33	Utah	4,387	0.87%
50	Vermont	600	0.12%
17	Virginia	10,164	2.01%
18	Washington	9,035	1.79%
36	West Virginia	3,478	0.69%
26	Wisconsin	7,112	1.41%
48	Wyoming	905	0.18%

RANK ORDER

RANK	STATE	BIRTHS	% of USA
1	California	64,775	12.83%
2	Texas	53,000	10.49%
3	Florida	25,387	5.03%
4	New York	24,974	4.95%
5	Illinois	23,415	4.64%
6	Ohio	20,304	4.02%
7	Georgia	18,261	3.62%
8	Michigan	16,771	3.32%
9	Pennsylvania	15,896	3.15%
10	North Carolina	15,861	3.14%
11	Louisiana	12,508	2.48%
12	Tennessee	12,395	2.45%
13	Indiana	12,079	2.39%
14	Arizona	11,939	2.36%
15	Alabama	11,250	2.23%
16	Missouri	10,403	2.06%
17	Virginia	10,164	2.01%
18	Washington	9,035	1.79%
19	Kentucky	8,947	1.77%
20	Mississippi	8,874	1.76%
21	New Jersey	8,770	1.74%
22	South Carolina	8,536	1.69%
23	Oklahoma	7,948	1.57%
24	Arkansas	7,211	1.43%
25	Maryland	7,179	1.42%
26	Wisconsin	7,112	1.41%
27	Colorado	6,645	1.32%
28	Massachusetts	5,873	1.16%
29	Oregon	5,765	1.14%
30	Minnesota	5,421	1.07%
31	Kansas	5,205	1.03%
32	New Mexico	4,875	0.97%
33	Utah	4,387	0.87%
34	Iowa	4,083	0.81%
35	Connecticut	3,634	0.72%
36	West Virginia	3,478	0.69%
37	Nevada	3,463	0.69%
38	Idaho	2,573	0.51%
39	Nebraska	2,472	0.49%
40	Hawaii	1,888	0.37%
41	Delaware	1,403	0.28%
42	Montana	1,338	0.26%
43	Maine	1,336	0.26%
44	Rhode Island	1,289	0.26%
45	South Dakota	1,205	0.24%
46	Alaska	1,138	0.23%
47	New Hampshire	1,077	0.21%
48	Wyoming	905	0.18%
49	North Dakota	802	0.16%
50	Vermont	600	0.12%
	District of Columbia	1,400	0.28%

Source: Morgan Quitno Press using data from U.S. Dept. of Health and Human Services, Nat'l Center for Health Statistics
"Monthly Vital Statistics Report" (Vol. 46, No. 1(S)2, September 11, 1997)
*Preliminary data. Live births to women under the age of 20 years old. These numbers were calculated by the editors by multiplying the percent of live births to teenage women times total births. These are rough estimates and differ from other teenage birth numbers in this book in that they include births to women under the age of 15.

Percent of Births to Teenage Mothers in 1996

National Percent = 12.9% of Live Births*

ALPHA ORDER		
RANK	STATE	PERCENT
4	Alabama	18.3
32	Alaska	11.2
13	Arizona	15.0
2	Arkansas	19.8
28	California	12.0
29	Colorado	11.9
47	Connecticut	8.2
18	Delaware	13.7
20	Florida	13.4
12	Georgia	15.9
39	Hawaii	10.3
19	Idaho	13.5
25	Illinois	12.7
15	Indiana	14.5
33	Iowa	11.0
24	Kansas	13.1
7	Kentucky	17.0
3	Louisiana	18.9
42	Maine	9.7
39	Maryland	10.3
50	Massachusetts	7.3
27	Michigan	12.2
46	Minnesota	8.5
1	Mississippi	21.3
17	Missouri	14.1
26	Montana	12.5
35	Nebraska	10.6
21	Nevada	13.3
49	New Hampshire	7.4
48	New Jersey	7.7
5	New Mexico	17.9
44	New York	9.2
13	North Carolina	15.0
43	North Dakota	9.6
21	Ohio	13.3
6	Oklahoma	17.2
23	Oregon	13.2
35	Pennsylvania	10.6
39	Rhode Island	10.3
8	South Carolina	16.8
30	South Dakota	11.5
8	Tennessee	16.8
11	Texas	16.2
35	Utah	10.6
45	Vermont	8.9
33	Virginia	11.0
31	Washington	11.3
8	West Virginia	16.8
35	Wisconsin	10.6
16	Wyoming	14.4

RANK ORDER		
RANK	STATE	PERCENT
1	Mississippi	21.3
2	Arkansas	19.8
3	Louisiana	18.9
4	Alabama	18.3
5	New Mexico	17.9
6	Oklahoma	17.2
7	Kentucky	17.0
8	South Carolina	16.8
8	Tennessee	16.8
8	West Virginia	16.8
11	Texas	16.2
12	Georgia	15.9
13	Arizona	15.0
13	North Carolina	15.0
15	Indiana	14.5
16	Wyoming	14.4
17	Missouri	14.1
18	Delaware	13.7
19	Idaho	13.5
20	Florida	13.4
21	Nevada	13.3
21	Ohio	13.3
23	Oregon	13.2
24	Kansas	13.1
25	Illinois	12.7
26	Montana	12.5
27	Michigan	12.2
28	California	12.0
29	Colorado	11.9
30	South Dakota	11.5
31	Washington	11.3
32	Alaska	11.2
33	Iowa	11.0
33	Virginia	11.0
35	Nebraska	10.6
35	Pennsylvania	10.6
35	Utah	10.6
35	Wisconsin	10.6
39	Hawaii	10.3
39	Maryland	10.3
39	Rhode Island	10.3
42	Maine	9.7
43	North Dakota	9.6
44	New York	9.2
45	Vermont	8.9
46	Minnesota	8.5
47	Connecticut	8.2
48	New Jersey	7.7
49	New Hampshire	7.4
50	Massachusetts	7.3
	District of Columbia	16.8

Source: U.S. Department of Health and Human Services, National Center for Health Statistics
   "Monthly Vital Statistics Report" (Vol. 46, No. 1(S)2, September 11, 1997)
*Births to women 19 years old and younger.

Births to Teenage Mothers in 1995

National Total = 499,873 Live Births*

ALPHA ORDER

RANK	STATE	BIRTHS	% of USA
14	Alabama	10,857	2.17%
46	Alaska	1,136	0.23%
15	Arizona	10,745	2.15%
26	Arkansas	6,710	1.34%
1	California	66,764	13.36%
27	Colorado	6,464	1.29%
35	Connecticut	3,716	0.74%
43	Delaware	1,301	0.26%
3	Florida	25,088	5.02%
7	Georgia	17,727	3.55%
40	Hawaii	1,841	0.37%
38	Idaho	2,489	0.50%
5	Illinois	23,467	4.69%
13	Indiana	11,933	2.39%
34	Iowa	4,024	0.81%
32	Kansas	4,801	0.96%
20	Kentucky	8,819	1.76%
11	Louisiana	12,208	2.44%
41	Maine	1,406	0.28%
24	Maryland	7,211	1.44%
28	Massachusetts	6,001	1.20%
8	Michigan	16,467	3.29%
30	Minnesota	5,241	1.05%
19	Mississippi	8,848	1.77%
16	Missouri	10,282	2.06%
42	Montana	1,395	0.28%
39	Nebraska	2,283	0.46%
37	Nevada	3,351	0.67%
47	New Hampshire	1,103	0.22%
18	New Jersey	9,151	1.83%
31	New Mexico	4,844	0.97%
4	New York	24,826	4.97%
10	North Carolina	15,049	3.01%
49	North Dakota	800	0.16%
6	Ohio	20,631	4.13%
23	Oklahoma	7,639	1.53%
29	Oregon	5,448	1.09%
9	Pennsylvania	15,979	3.20%
44	Rhode Island	1,267	0.25%
22	South Carolina	8,518	1.70%
45	South Dakota	1,179	0.24%
12	Tennessee	12,118	2.42%
2	Texas	52,135	10.43%
33	Utah	4,222	0.84%
50	Vermont	553	0.11%
17	Virginia	10,270	2.05%
21	Washington	8,709	1.74%
36	West Virginia	3,584	0.72%
25	Wisconsin	6,932	1.39%
48	Wyoming	937	0.19%

RANK ORDER

RANK	STATE	BIRTHS	% of USA
1	California	66,764	13.36%
2	Texas	52,135	10.43%
3	Florida	25,088	5.02%
4	New York	24,826	4.97%
5	Illinois	23,467	4.69%
6	Ohio	20,631	4.13%
7	Georgia	17,727	3.55%
8	Michigan	16,467	3.29%
9	Pennsylvania	15,979	3.20%
10	North Carolina	15,049	3.01%
11	Louisiana	12,208	2.44%
12	Tennessee	12,118	2.42%
13	Indiana	11,933	2.39%
14	Alabama	10,857	2.17%
15	Arizona	10,745	2.15%
16	Missouri	10,282	2.06%
17	Virginia	10,270	2.05%
18	New Jersey	9,151	1.83%
19	Mississippi	8,848	1.77%
20	Kentucky	8,819	1.76%
21	Washington	8,709	1.74%
22	South Carolina	8,518	1.70%
23	Oklahoma	7,639	1.53%
24	Maryland	7,211	1.44%
25	Wisconsin	6,932	1.39%
26	Arkansas	6,710	1.34%
27	Colorado	6,464	1.29%
28	Massachusetts	6,001	1.20%
29	Oregon	5,448	1.09%
30	Minnesota	5,241	1.05%
31	New Mexico	4,844	0.97%
32	Kansas	4,801	0.96%
33	Utah	4,222	0.84%
34	Iowa	4,024	0.81%
35	Connecticut	3,716	0.74%
36	West Virginia	3,584	0.72%
37	Nevada	3,351	0.67%
38	Idaho	2,489	0.50%
39	Nebraska	2,283	0.46%
40	Hawaii	1,841	0.37%
41	Maine	1,406	0.28%
42	Montana	1,395	0.28%
43	Delaware	1,301	0.26%
44	Rhode Island	1,267	0.25%
45	South Dakota	1,179	0.24%
46	Alaska	1,136	0.23%
47	New Hampshire	1,103	0.22%
48	Wyoming	937	0.19%
49	North Dakota	800	0.16%
50	Vermont	553	0.11%
	District of Columbia	1,404	0.28%

Source: U.S. Dept of Health & Human Services, National Center for Health Statistics
    (unpublished data)
Live births to women age 15 to 19 years old by state of residence.

Teenage Birth Rate in 1995

National Rate = 56.8 Births per 1,000 Teenage Women*

ALPHA ORDER

RANK ORDER

RANK	STATE	RATE		RANK	STATE	RATE
8	Alabama	70.3		1	Mississippi	80.6
26	Alaska	50.2		2	Texas	76.1
3	Arizona	75.7		3	Arizona	75.7
5	Arkansas	73.5		4	New Mexico	74.5
10	California	68.2		5	Arkansas	73.5
24	Colorado	51.3		6	Nevada	73.3
40	Connecticut	39.3		7	Georgia	71.1
19	Delaware	57.0		8	Alabama	70.3
16	Florida	61.7		9	Louisiana	69.9
7	Georgia	71.1		10	California	68.2
30	Hawaii	47.9		11	Tennessee	67.9
28	Idaho	49.0		12	South Carolina	65.1
17	Illinois	59.9		13	North Carolina	64.1
18	Indiana	57.5		14	Oklahoma	64.0
41	Iowa	38.6		15	Kentucky	62.5
23	Kansas	52.2		16	Florida	61.7
15	Kentucky	62.5		17	Illinois	59.9
9	Louisiana	69.9		18	Indiana	57.5
46	Maine	33.6		19	Delaware	57.0
31	Maryland	47.7		20	Missouri	55.5
45	Massachusetts	34.3		21	Ohio	53.4
27	Michigan	49.2		22	West Virginia	52.7
48	Minnesota	32.4		23	Kansas	52.2
1	Mississippi	80.6		24	Colorado	51.3
20	Missouri	55.5		25	Oregon	50.7
37	Montana	41.8		26	Alaska	50.2
44	Nebraska	37.6		27	Michigan	49.2
6	Nevada	73.3		28	Idaho	49.0
49	New Hampshire	30.5		29	Virginia	48.7
42	New Jersey	38.0		30	Hawaii	47.9
4	New Mexico	74.5		31	Maryland	47.7
34	New York	44.0		32	Washington	47.6
13	North Carolina	64.1		33	Wyoming	47.2
47	North Dakota	33.5		34	New York	44.0
21	Ohio	53.4		35	Rhode Island	43.1
14	Oklahoma	64.0		36	Utah	42.4
25	Oregon	50.7		37	Montana	41.8
38	Pennsylvania	41.7		38	Pennsylvania	41.7
35	Rhode Island	43.1		39	South Dakota	40.5
12	South Carolina	65.1		40	Connecticut	39.3
39	South Dakota	40.5		41	Iowa	38.6
11	Tennessee	67.9		42	New Jersey	38.0
2	Texas	76.1		43	Wisconsin	37.8
36	Utah	42.4		44	Nebraska	37.6
50	Vermont	28.6		45	Massachusetts	34.3
29	Virginia	48.7		46	Maine	33.6
32	Washington	47.6		47	North Dakota	33.5
22	West Virginia	52.7		48	Minnesota	32.4
43	Wisconsin	37.8		49	New Hampshire	30.5
33	Wyoming	47.2		50	Vermont	28.6
					District of Columbia	106.8

Source: U.S. Department of Health and Human Services, Centers for Disease Control and Prevention
"State-Specific Birth Rates for Teenagers" (Morbidity and Mortality Weekly Report, Vol. 46, No. 36, 9/12/97)
Women aged 15 to 19 years old.

Births to Teenage Mothers as a Percent of Live Births in 1995

National Percent = 12.8% of Live Births*

ALPHA ORDER

RANK	STATE	PERCENT
4	Alabama	18.0
32	Alaska	11.1
14	Arizona	14.8
2	Arkansas	19.1
28	California	12.1
29	Colorado	11.9
45	Connecticut	8.4
23	Delaware	12.7
21	Florida	13.3
12	Georgia	15.8
40	Hawaii	9.9
18	Idaho	13.8
25	Illinois	12.6
16	Indiana	14.4
34	Iowa	10.9
22	Kansas	12.9
7	Kentucky	16.8
3	Louisiana	18.6
38	Maine	10.1
39	Maryland	10.0
50	Massachusetts	7.3
27	Michigan	12.2
46	Minnesota	8.3
1	Mississippi	21.4
17	Missouri	14.1
26	Montana	12.5
42	Nebraska	9.8
19	Nevada	13.4
49	New Hampshire	7.5
48	New Jersey	8.0
4	New Mexico	18.0
44	New York	9.1
14	North Carolina	14.8
43	North Dakota	9.4
19	Ohio	13.4
8	Oklahoma	16.7
23	Oregon	12.7
36	Pennsylvania	10.5
40	Rhode Island	9.9
8	South Carolina	16.7
30	South Dakota	11.3
10	Tennessee	16.6
11	Texas	16.2
35	Utah	10.7
47	Vermont	8.2
32	Virginia	11.1
30	Washington	11.3
6	West Virginia	16.9
37	Wisconsin	10.3
13	Wyoming	15.0

RANK ORDER

RANK	STATE	PERCENT
1	Mississippi	21.4
2	Arkansas	19.1
3	Louisiana	18.6
4	Alabama	18.0
4	New Mexico	18.0
6	West Virginia	16.9
7	Kentucky	16.8
8	Oklahoma	16.7
8	South Carolina	16.7
10	Tennessee	16.6
11	Texas	16.2
12	Georgia	15.8
13	Wyoming	15.0
14	Arizona	14.8
14	North Carolina	14.8
16	Indiana	14.4
17	Missouri	14.1
18	Idaho	13.8
19	Nevada	13.4
19	Ohio	13.4
21	Florida	13.3
22	Kansas	12.9
23	Delaware	12.7
23	Oregon	12.7
25	Illinois	12.6
26	Montana	12.5
27	Michigan	12.2
28	California	12.1
29	Colorado	11.9
30	South Dakota	11.3
30	Washington	11.3
32	Alaska	11.1
32	Virginia	11.1
34	Iowa	10.9
35	Utah	10.7
36	Pennsylvania	10.5
37	Wisconsin	10.3
38	Maine	10.1
39	Maryland	10.0
40	Hawaii	9.9
40	Rhode Island	9.9
42	Nebraska	9.8
43	North Dakota	9.4
44	New York	9.1
45	Connecticut	8.4
46	Minnesota	8.3
47	Vermont	8.2
48	New Jersey	8.0
49	New Hampshire	7.5
50	Massachusetts	7.3
	District of Columbia	15.6

Source: U.S. Dept of Health & Human Services, National Center for Health Statistics
 (unpublished data)
*Live births to women age 15 to 19 years old by state of residence.

Births to White Teenage Mothers in 1995

National Total = 349,635 Live Births*

ALPHA ORDER					RANK ORDER			
RANK	STATE	BIRTHS	% of USA		RANK	STATE	BIRTHS	% of USA
19	Alabama	5,609	1.60%		1	California	55,461	15.86%
48	Alaska	599	0.17%		2	Texas	42,797	12.24%
10	Arizona	9,216	2.64%		3	New York	15,868	4.54%
26	Arkansas	4,325	1.24%		4	Florida	15,547	4.45%
1	California	55,461	15.86%		5	Ohio	14,979	4.28%
18	Colorado	5,746	1.64%		6	Illinois	13,842	3.96%
37	Connecticut	2,664	0.76%		7	Pennsylvania	10,896	3.12%
46	Delaware	721	0.21%		8	Michigan	10,396	2.97%
4	Florida	15,547	4.45%		9	Indiana	9,601	2.75%
11	Georgia	8,773	2.51%		10	Arizona	9,216	2.64%
50	Hawaii	263	0.08%		11	Georgia	8,773	2.51%
38	Idaho	2,407	0.69%		12	North Carolina	8,280	2.37%
6	Illinois	13,842	3.96%		13	Tennessee	7,946	2.27%
9	Indiana	9,601	2.75%		14	Kentucky	7,563	2.16%
32	Iowa	3,645	1.04%		15	Missouri	7,414	2.12%
31	Kansas	3,925	1.12%		16	Washington	7,360	2.11%
14	Kentucky	7,563	2.16%		17	Virginia	5,946	1.70%
23	Louisiana	4,962	1.42%		18	Colorado	5,746	1.64%
40	Maine	1,357	0.39%		19	Alabama	5,609	1.60%
35	Maryland	3,155	0.90%		20	Oklahoma	5,398	1.54%
25	Massachusetts	4,703	1.35%		21	New Jersey	5,215	1.49%
8	Michigan	10,396	2.97%		22	Oregon	4,995	1.43%
30	Minnesota	3,939	1.13%		23	Louisiana	4,962	1.42%
34	Mississippi	3,243	0.93%		24	Wisconsin	4,714	1.35%
15	Missouri	7,414	2.12%		25	Massachusetts	4,703	1.35%
42	Montana	1,074	0.31%		26	Arkansas	4,325	1.24%
39	Nebraska	1,898	0.54%		27	New Mexico	4,056	1.16%
36	Nevada	2,761	0.79%		28	South Carolina	4,037	1.15%
41	New Hampshire	1,080	0.31%		29	Utah	3,964	1.13%
21	New Jersey	5,215	1.49%		30	Minnesota	3,939	1.13%
27	New Mexico	4,056	1.16%		31	Kansas	3,925	1.12%
3	New York	15,868	4.54%		32	Iowa	3,645	1.04%
12	North Carolina	8,280	2.37%		33	West Virginia	3,371	0.96%
47	North Dakota	620	0.18%		34	Mississippi	3,243	0.93%
5	Ohio	14,979	4.28%		35	Maryland	3,155	0.90%
20	Oklahoma	5,398	1.54%		36	Nevada	2,761	0.79%
22	Oregon	4,995	1.43%		37	Connecticut	2,664	0.76%
7	Pennsylvania	10,896	3.12%		38	Idaho	2,407	0.69%
43	Rhode Island	990	0.28%		39	Nebraska	1,898	0.54%
28	South Carolina	4,037	1.15%		40	Maine	1,357	0.39%
45	South Dakota	790	0.23%		41	New Hampshire	1,080	0.31%
13	Tennessee	7,946	2.27%		42	Montana	1,074	0.31%
2	Texas	42,797	12.24%		43	Rhode Island	990	0.28%
29	Utah	3,964	1.13%		44	Wyoming	861	0.25%
49	Vermont	543	0.16%		45	South Dakota	790	0.23%
17	Virginia	5,946	1.70%		46	Delaware	721	0.21%
16	Washington	7,360	2.11%		47	North Dakota	620	0.18%
33	West Virginia	3,371	0.96%		48	Alaska	599	0.17%
24	Wisconsin	4,714	1.35%		49	Vermont	543	0.16%
44	Wyoming	861	0.25%		50	Hawaii	263	0.08%
						District of Columbia	120	0.03%

Source: U.S. Dept of Health & Human Services, National Center for Health Statistics
(unpublished data)
*Live births to women age 15 to 19 years old by state of residence.

Births to White Teenage Mothers as a Percent of White Births in 1995

National Percent = 11.3% of White Live Births*

ALPHA ORDER

RANK	STATE	PERCENT
11	Alabama	14.1
39	Alaska	8.5
9	Arizona	14.5
3	Arkansas	16.0
18	California	12.3
22	Colorado	11.6
45	Connecticut	7.1
33	Delaware	9.4
25	Florida	10.9
19	Georgia	12.2
50	Hawaii	5.3
12	Idaho	13.8
32	Illinois	9.7
14	Indiana	13.1
29	Iowa	10.4
21	Kansas	11.8
3	Kentucky	16.0
13	Louisiana	13.2
30	Maine	10.0
47	Maryland	6.7
47	Massachusetts	6.7
31	Michigan	9.8
46	Minnesota	6.9
6	Mississippi	15.0
19	Missouri	12.2
25	Montana	10.9
35	Nebraska	8.9
15	Nevada	12.8
44	New Hampshire	7.5
49	New Jersey	6.0
1	New Mexico	17.9
43	New York	8.0
22	North Carolina	11.6
41	North Dakota	8.1
22	Ohio	11.6
6	Oklahoma	15.0
17	Oregon	12.6
38	Pennsylvania	8.6
36	Rhode Island	8.8
16	South Carolina	12.7
34	South Dakota	9.1
10	Tennessee	14.2
5	Texas	15.6
28	Utah	10.5
40	Vermont	8.2
36	Virginia	8.8
25	Washington	10.9
2	West Virginia	16.7
41	Wisconsin	8.1
8	Wyoming	14.6

RANK ORDER

RANK	STATE	PERCENT
1	New Mexico	17.9
2	West Virginia	16.7
3	Arkansas	16.0
3	Kentucky	16.0
5	Texas	15.6
6	Mississippi	15.0
6	Oklahoma	15.0
8	Wyoming	14.6
9	Arizona	14.5
10	Tennessee	14.2
11	Alabama	14.1
12	Idaho	13.8
13	Louisiana	13.2
14	Indiana	13.1
15	Nevada	12.8
16	South Carolina	12.7
17	Oregon	12.6
18	California	12.3
19	Georgia	12.2
19	Missouri	12.2
21	Kansas	11.8
22	Colorado	11.6
22	North Carolina	11.6
22	Ohio	11.6
25	Florida	10.9
25	Montana	10.9
25	Washington	10.9
28	Utah	10.5
29	Iowa	10.4
30	Maine	10.0
31	Michigan	9.8
32	Illinois	9.7
33	Delaware	9.4
34	South Dakota	9.1
35	Nebraska	8.9
36	Rhode Island	8.8
36	Virginia	8.8
38	Pennsylvania	8.6
39	Alaska	8.5
40	Vermont	8.2
41	North Dakota	8.1
41	Wisconsin	8.1
43	New York	8.0
44	New Hampshire	7.5
45	Connecticut	7.1
46	Minnesota	6.9
47	Maryland	6.7
47	Massachusetts	6.7
49	New Jersey	6.0
50	Hawaii	5.3
	District of Columbia	5.9

Source: U.S. Dept of Health & Human Services, National Center for Health Statistics (unpublished data)
Live births to women age 15 to 19 years old by state of residence.

Births to Black Teenage Mothers in 1995

National Total = 133,694 Live Births*

ALPHA ORDER

RANK	STATE	BIRTHS	% of USA
12	Alabama	5,182	3.88%
40	Alaska	84	0.06%
32	Arizona	473	0.35%
20	Arkansas	2,315	1.73%
6	California	7,403	5.54%
31	Colorado	502	0.38%
26	Connecticut	992	0.74%
29	Delaware	571	0.43%
2	Florida	9,255	6.92%
4	Georgia	8,851	6.62%
41	Hawaii	60	0.04%
43	Idaho	16	0.01%
1	Illinois	9,457	7.07%
21	Indiana	2,262	1.69%
34	Iowa	289	0.22%
27	Kansas	745	0.56%
23	Kentucky	1,224	0.92%
7	Louisiana	7,127	5.33%
44	Maine	13	0.01%
17	Maryland	3,979	2.98%
25	Massachusetts	1,113	0.83%
9	Michigan	5,789	4.33%
28	Minnesota	667	0.50%
11	Mississippi	5,519	4.13%
19	Missouri	2,786	2.08%
48	Montana	8	0.01%
35	Nebraska	286	0.21%
33	Nevada	432	0.32%
46	New Hampshire	12	0.01%
18	New Jersey	3,827	2.86%
39	New Mexico	123	0.09%
5	New York	8,515	6.37%
8	North Carolina	6,309	4.72%
50	North Dakota	4	0.00%
10	Ohio	5,530	4.14%
24	Oklahoma	1,144	0.86%
36	Oregon	226	0.17%
13	Pennsylvania	4,905	3.67%
38	Rhode Island	197	0.15%
14	South Carolina	4,427	3.31%
47	South Dakota	10	0.01%
16	Tennessee	4,096	3.06%
3	Texas	8,882	6.64%
42	Utah	48	0.04%
49	Vermont	7	0.01%
15	Virginia	4,191	3.13%
30	Washington	565	0.42%
37	West Virginia	203	0.15%
22	Wisconsin	1,784	1.33%
44	Wyoming	13	0.01%

RANK ORDER

RANK	STATE	BIRTHS	% of USA
1	Illinois	9,457	7.07%
2	Florida	9,255	6.92%
3	Texas	8,882	6.64%
4	Georgia	8,851	6.62%
5	New York	8,515	6.37%
6	California	7,403	5.54%
7	Louisiana	7,127	5.33%
8	North Carolina	6,309	4.72%
9	Michigan	5,789	4.33%
10	Ohio	5,530	4.14%
11	Mississippi	5,519	4.13%
12	Alabama	5,182	3.88%
13	Pennsylvania	4,905	3.67%
14	South Carolina	4,427	3.31%
15	Virginia	4,191	3.13%
16	Tennessee	4,096	3.06%
17	Maryland	3,979	2.98%
18	New Jersey	3,827	2.86%
19	Missouri	2,786	2.08%
20	Arkansas	2,315	1.73%
21	Indiana	2,262	1.69%
22	Wisconsin	1,784	1.33%
23	Kentucky	1,224	0.92%
24	Oklahoma	1,144	0.86%
25	Massachusetts	1,113	0.83%
26	Connecticut	992	0.74%
27	Kansas	745	0.56%
28	Minnesota	667	0.50%
29	Delaware	571	0.43%
30	Washington	565	0.42%
31	Colorado	502	0.38%
32	Arizona	473	0.35%
33	Nevada	432	0.32%
34	Iowa	289	0.22%
35	Nebraska	286	0.21%
36	Oregon	226	0.17%
37	West Virginia	203	0.15%
38	Rhode Island	197	0.15%
39	New Mexico	123	0.09%
40	Alaska	84	0.06%
41	Hawaii	60	0.04%
42	Utah	48	0.04%
43	Idaho	16	0.01%
44	Maine	13	0.01%
44	Wyoming	13	0.01%
46	New Hampshire	12	0.01%
47	South Dakota	10	0.01%
48	Montana	8	0.01%
49	Vermont	7	0.01%
50	North Dakota	4	0.00%
	District of Columbia	1,276	0.95%

Source: U.S. Dept of Health & Human Services, National Center for Health Statistics
    (unpublished data)
Live births to women age 15 to 19 years old by state of residence.

Births to Black Teenage Mothers as a Percent of Black Births in 1995

National Percent = 22.2% of Black Live Births*

ALPHA ORDER				RANK ORDER		
RANK	STATE	PERCENT		RANK	STATE	PERCENT
6	Alabama	26.1		1	Arkansas	30.2
37	Alaska	18.9		2	Iowa	29.1
31	Arizona	21.1		3	Mississippi	28.7
1	Arkansas	30.2		4	Wisconsin	27.4
39	California	18.4		5	Louisiana	26.5
35	Colorado	19.2		6	Alabama	26.1
39	Connecticut	18.4		7	Indiana	25.9
17	Delaware	24.2		7	Oregon	25.9
28	Florida	22.0		9	Kansas	25.8
23	Georgia	23.0		10	Kentucky	25.6
48	Hawaii	10.6		11	Oklahoma	25.4
29	Idaho	21.6		11	Tennessee	25.4
14	Illinois	25.2		13	Missouri	25.3
7	Indiana	25.9		14	Illinois	25.2
2	Iowa	29.1		14	West Virginia	25.2
9	Kansas	25.8		16	Ohio	24.3
10	Kentucky	25.6		17	Delaware	24.2
5	Louisiana	26.5		17	New Mexico	24.2
44	Maine	16.5		19	South Carolina	24.0
43	Maryland	17.5		20	Nebraska	23.4
46	Massachusetts	14.3		20	North Carolina	23.4
22	Michigan	23.1		22	Michigan	23.1
23	Minnesota	23.0		23	Georgia	23.0
3	Mississippi	28.7		23	Minnesota	23.0
13	Missouri	25.3		25	Pennsylvania	22.9
32	Montana	20.0		25	Texas	22.9
20	Nebraska	23.4		27	Nevada	22.8
27	Nevada	22.8		28	Florida	22.0
47	New Hampshire	13.5		29	Idaho	21.6
41	New Jersey	18.2		30	Rhode Island	21.5
17	New Mexico	24.2		31	Arizona	21.1
45	New York	15.1		32	Montana	20.0
20	North Carolina	23.4		33	Utah	19.8
50	North Dakota	5.7		34	Virginia	19.7
16	Ohio	24.3		35	Colorado	19.2
11	Oklahoma	25.4		36	Washington	19.1
7	Oregon	25.9		37	Alaska	18.9
25	Pennsylvania	22.9		38	Wyoming	18.8
30	Rhode Island	21.5		39	California	18.4
19	South Carolina	24.0		39	Connecticut	18.4
49	South Dakota	10.0		41	New Jersey	18.2
11	Tennessee	25.4		42	Vermont	17.9
25	Texas	22.9		43	Maryland	17.5
33	Utah	19.8		44	Maine	16.5
42	Vermont	17.9		45	New York	15.1
34	Virginia	19.7		46	Massachusetts	14.3
36	Washington	19.1		47	New Hampshire	13.5
14	West Virginia	25.2		48	Hawaii	10.6
4	Wisconsin	27.4		49	South Dakota	10.0
38	Wyoming	18.8		50	North Dakota	5.7
					District of Columbia	18.8

Source: U.S. Dept of Health & Human Services, National Center for Health Statistics
        (unpublished data)
*Live births to women age 15 to 19 years old by state of residence.

Pregnancy Rate for 15 to 19 Year Old Women in 1994

National Rate = 80.2 Births and Abortions per 1,000 Women 15-19 Years Old*

ALPHA ORDER

RANK ORDER

RANK	STATE	RATE		RANK	STATE	RATE
7	Alabama	93.2		1	Texas	100.6
NA	Alaska**	NA		2	North Carolina	99.5
4	Arizona	98.6		3	Georgia	99.4
9	Arkansas	91.4		4	Arizona	98.6
NA	California**	NA		5	Nevada	98.3
25	Colorado	72.1		6	New York	94.5
24	Connecticut	72.5		7	Alabama	93.2
NA	Delaware**	NA		8	New Mexico	93.1
NA	Florida**	NA		9	Arkansas	91.4
3	Georgia	99.4		10	Tennessee	90.8
13	Hawaii	88.5		11	Mississippi	90.3
36	Idaho	51.6		12	Louisiana	89.3
NA	Illinois**	NA		13	Hawaii	88.5
27	Indiana	70.5		14	Rhode Island	85.7
NA	Iowa**	NA		15	South Carolina	84.1
16	Kansas	82.1		16	Kansas	82.1
17	Kentucky	79.0		17	Kentucky	79.0
12	Louisiana	89.3		18	Oregon	78.2
38	Maine	50.6		19	Washington	77.6
22	Maryland	72.8		20	Virginia	75.5
28	Massachusetts	67.3		21	Michigan	72.9
21	Michigan	72.9		22	Maryland	72.8
39	Minnesota	50.5		23	Ohio	72.7
11	Mississippi	90.3		24	Connecticut	72.5
26	Missouri	72.0		25	Colorado	72.1
31	Montana	62.4		26	Missouri	72.0
32	Nebraska	62.2		27	Indiana	70.5
5	Nevada	98.3		28	Massachusetts	67.3
NA	New Hampshire**	NA		29	Pennsylvania	64.6
30	New Jersey	64.2		30	New Jersey	64.2
8	New Mexico	93.1		31	Montana	62.4
6	New York	94.5		32	Nebraska	62.2
2	North Carolina	99.5		32	West Virginia	62.2
42	North Dakota	48.2		34	Vermont	60.4
23	Ohio	72.7		35	Wisconsin	52.7
NA	Oklahoma**	NA		36	Idaho	51.6
18	Oregon	78.2		36	South Dakota	51.6
29	Pennsylvania	64.6		38	Maine	50.6
14	Rhode Island	85.7		39	Minnesota	50.5
15	South Carolina	84.1		40	Utah	50.1
36	South Dakota	51.6		40	Wyoming	50.1
10	Tennessee	90.8		42	North Dakota	48.2
1	Texas	100.6		NA	Alaska**	NA
40	Utah	50.1		NA	California**	NA
34	Vermont	60.4		NA	Delaware**	NA
20	Virginia	75.5		NA	Florida**	NA
19	Washington	77.6		NA	Illinois**	NA
32	West Virginia	62.2		NA	Iowa**	NA
35	Wisconsin	52.7		NA	New Hampshire**	NA
40	Wyoming	50.1		NA	Oklahoma**	NA

District of Columbia   227.9

Source: Morgan Quitno Press using data from US Dept of Health & Human Serv's, Centers for Disease Control-Prevention "Abortion Surveillance-United States, 1994" (Morbidity and Mortality Weekly Report, Vol. 46, No. SS-4, 8/8/97)
The sum of live births and legal induced abortions per 1,000 women aged 15-19 years old. Births by state of residence, abortions by state of occurrence. National rate includes only states reporting abortions and births.
***Not available.*

Percent Change in Pregnancy Rate for 15 to 19 Year Old Women: 1992 to 1994

National Percent Change = 0.6% Increase*

ALPHA ORDER				RANK ORDER		
RANK	STATE	PERCENT CHANGE		RANK	STATE	PERCENT CHANGE
3	Alabama	0.0		1	Hawaii	2.4
NA	Alaska**	NA		2	Arkansas	0.8
17	Arizona	(4.7)		3	Alabama	0.0
2	Arkansas	0.8		4	Nebraska	(1.9)
NA	California**	NA		5	New York	(2.2)
32	Colorado	(9.6)		6	Indiana	(2.4)
NA	Connecticut**	NA		7	Ohio	(2.5)
NA	Delaware**	NA		8	Rhode Island	(2.7)
NA	Florida**	NA		9	Texas	(3.0)
23	Georgia	(7.0)		10	Massachusetts	(3.2)
1	Hawaii	2.4		11	Kentucky	(3.3)
41	Idaho	(13.6)		12	Tennessee	(3.4)
NA	Illinois**	NA		13	Oregon	(3.5)
6	Indiana	(2.4)		14	Louisiana	(3.6)
NA	Iowa**	NA		15	South Carolina	(4.4)
20	Kansas	(5.6)		15	Virginia	(4.4)
11	Kentucky	(3.3)		17	Arizona	(4.7)
14	Louisiana	(3.6)		18	North Carolina	(4.9)
27	Maine	(8.3)		19	Maryland	(5.3)
19	Maryland	(5.3)		20	Kansas	(5.6)
10	Massachusetts	(3.2)		21	West Virginia	(5.9)
28	Michigan	(8.5)		22	Wyoming	(6.7)
28	Minnesota	(8.5)		23	Georgia	(7.0)
35	Mississippi	(10.4)		24	Nevada	(7.3)
25	Missouri	(7.7)		25	Missouri	(7.7)
36	Montana	(11.1)		26	New Jersey	(7.9)
4	Nebraska	(1.9)		27	Maine	(8.3)
24	Nevada	(7.3)		28	Michigan	(8.5)
NA	New Hampshire**	NA		28	Minnesota	(8.5)
26	New Jersey	(7.9)		28	New Mexico	(8.5)
28	New Mexico	(8.5)		31	Washington	(8.8)
5	New York	(2.2)		32	Colorado	(9.6)
18	North Carolina	(4.9)		33	Pennsylvania	(9.9)
36	North Dakota	(11.1)		33	Utah	(9.9)
7	Ohio	(2.5)		35	Mississippi	(10.4)
NA	Oklahoma**	NA		36	Montana	(11.1)
13	Oregon	(3.5)		36	North Dakota	(11.1)
33	Pennsylvania	(9.9)		38	Vermont	(12.1)
8	Rhode Island	(2.7)		39	South Dakota	(13.1)
15	South Carolina	(4.4)		40	Wisconsin	(13.3)
39	South Dakota	(13.1)		41	Idaho	(13.6)
12	Tennessee	(3.4)		NA	Alaska**	NA
9	Texas	(3.0)		NA	California**	NA
33	Utah	(9.9)		NA	Connecticut**	NA
38	Vermont	(12.1)		NA	Delaware**	NA
15	Virginia	(4.4)		NA	Florida**	NA
31	Washington	(8.8)		NA	Illinois**	NA
21	West Virginia	(5.9)		NA	Iowa**	NA
40	Wisconsin	(13.3)		NA	New Hampshire**	NA
22	Wyoming	(6.7)		NA	Oklahoma**	NA
					District of Columbia	9.4

Source: Morgan Quitno Press using data from US Dept of Health & Human Serv's, Centers for Disease Control-Prevention "Abortion Surveillance-United States, 1994" (Morbidity and Mortality Weekly Report, Vol. 46, No. SS-4, 8/8/97)
*The sum of live births and legal induced abortions per 1,000 women aged 15-19 years old. Births by state of residence, abortions by state of occurrence. National rate includes only states reporting abortions and births.
**Not available.

Births to Teenage Mothers in 1990

National Total = 521,826 Live Births*

<table>
<tr><td colspan="4">ALPHA ORDER</td><td colspan="4">RANK ORDER</td></tr>
<tr><td>RANK</td><td>STATE</td><td>BIRTHS</td><td>% of USA</td><td>RANK</td><td>STATE</td><td>BIRTHS</td><td>% of USA</td></tr>
<tr><td>15</td><td>Alabama</td><td>11,252</td><td>2.16%</td><td>1</td><td>California</td><td>69,712</td><td>13.36%</td></tr>
<tr><td>47</td><td>Alaska</td><td>1,142</td><td>0.22%</td><td>2</td><td>Texas</td><td>48,302</td><td>9.26%</td></tr>
<tr><td>19</td><td>Arizona</td><td>9,612</td><td>1.84%</td><td>3</td><td>Florida</td><td>27,017</td><td>5.18%</td></tr>
<tr><td>27</td><td>Arkansas</td><td>7,011</td><td>1.34%</td><td>4</td><td>New York</td><td>26,608</td><td>5.10%</td></tr>
<tr><td>1</td><td>California</td><td>69,712</td><td>13.36%</td><td>5</td><td>Illinois</td><td>24,967</td><td>4.78%</td></tr>
<tr><td>28</td><td>Colorado</td><td>5,975</td><td>1.15%</td><td>6</td><td>Ohio</td><td>22,690</td><td>4.35%</td></tr>
<tr><td>33</td><td>Connecticut</td><td>4,038</td><td>0.77%</td><td>7</td><td>Michigan</td><td>20,312</td><td>3.89%</td></tr>
<tr><td>44</td><td>Delaware</td><td>1,277</td><td>0.24%</td><td>8</td><td>Georgia</td><td>18,369</td><td>3.52%</td></tr>
<tr><td>3</td><td>Florida</td><td>27,017</td><td>5.18%</td><td>9</td><td>Pennsylvania</td><td>18,216</td><td>3.49%</td></tr>
<tr><td>8</td><td>Georgia</td><td>18,369</td><td>3.52%</td><td>10</td><td>North Carolina</td><td>16,506</td><td>3.16%</td></tr>
<tr><td>39</td><td>Hawaii</td><td>2,122</td><td>0.41%</td><td>11</td><td>Tennessee</td><td>12,928</td><td>2.48%</td></tr>
<tr><td>40</td><td>Idaho</td><td>2,009</td><td>0.38%</td><td>12</td><td>Indiana</td><td>12,335</td><td>2.36%</td></tr>
<tr><td>5</td><td>Illinois</td><td>24,967</td><td>4.78%</td><td>13</td><td>Louisiana</td><td>12,270</td><td>2.35%</td></tr>
<tr><td>12</td><td>Indiana</td><td>12,335</td><td>2.36%</td><td>14</td><td>Virginia</td><td>11,353</td><td>2.18%</td></tr>
<tr><td>34</td><td>Iowa</td><td>3,989</td><td>0.76%</td><td>15</td><td>Alabama</td><td>11,252</td><td>2.16%</td></tr>
<tr><td>31</td><td>Kansas</td><td>4,722</td><td>0.90%</td><td>16</td><td>Missouri</td><td>11,227</td><td>2.15%</td></tr>
<tr><td>20</td><td>Kentucky</td><td>9,349</td><td>1.79%</td><td>17</td><td>New Jersey</td><td>10,068</td><td>1.93%</td></tr>
<tr><td>13</td><td>Louisiana</td><td>12,270</td><td>2.35%</td><td>18</td><td>South Carolina</td><td>9,721</td><td>1.86%</td></tr>
<tr><td>41</td><td>Maine</td><td>1,857</td><td>0.36%</td><td>19</td><td>Arizona</td><td>9,612</td><td>1.84%</td></tr>
<tr><td>23</td><td>Maryland</td><td>8,143</td><td>1.56%</td><td>20</td><td>Kentucky</td><td>9,349</td><td>1.79%</td></tr>
<tr><td>26</td><td>Massachusetts</td><td>7,266</td><td>1.39%</td><td>21</td><td>Mississippi</td><td>8,909</td><td>1.71%</td></tr>
<tr><td>7</td><td>Michigan</td><td>20,312</td><td>3.89%</td><td>22</td><td>Washington</td><td>8,397</td><td>1.61%</td></tr>
<tr><td>29</td><td>Minnesota</td><td>5,342</td><td>1.02%</td><td>23</td><td>Maryland</td><td>8,143</td><td>1.56%</td></tr>
<tr><td>21</td><td>Mississippi</td><td>8,909</td><td>1.71%</td><td>24</td><td>Oklahoma</td><td>7,590</td><td>1.45%</td></tr>
<tr><td>16</td><td>Missouri</td><td>11,227</td><td>2.15%</td><td>25</td><td>Wisconsin</td><td>7,281</td><td>1.40%</td></tr>
<tr><td>43</td><td>Montana</td><td>1,331</td><td>0.26%</td><td>26</td><td>Massachusetts</td><td>7,266</td><td>1.39%</td></tr>
<tr><td>38</td><td>Nebraska</td><td>2,352</td><td>0.45%</td><td>27</td><td>Arkansas</td><td>7,011</td><td>1.34%</td></tr>
<tr><td>37</td><td>Nevada</td><td>2,663</td><td>0.51%</td><td>28</td><td>Colorado</td><td>5,975</td><td>1.15%</td></tr>
<tr><td>45</td><td>New Hampshire</td><td>1,258</td><td>0.24%</td><td>29</td><td>Minnesota</td><td>5,342</td><td>1.02%</td></tr>
<tr><td>17</td><td>New Jersey</td><td>10,068</td><td>1.93%</td><td>30</td><td>Oregon</td><td>5,084</td><td>0.97%</td></tr>
<tr><td>32</td><td>New Mexico</td><td>4,367</td><td>0.84%</td><td>31</td><td>Kansas</td><td>4,722</td><td>0.90%</td></tr>
<tr><td>4</td><td>New York</td><td>26,608</td><td>5.10%</td><td>32</td><td>New Mexico</td><td>4,367</td><td>0.84%</td></tr>
<tr><td>10</td><td>North Carolina</td><td>16,506</td><td>3.16%</td><td>33</td><td>Connecticut</td><td>4,038</td><td>0.77%</td></tr>
<tr><td>49</td><td>North Dakota</td><td>793</td><td>0.15%</td><td>34</td><td>Iowa</td><td>3,989</td><td>0.76%</td></tr>
<tr><td>6</td><td>Ohio</td><td>22,690</td><td>4.35%</td><td>35</td><td>West Virginia</td><td>3,976</td><td>0.76%</td></tr>
<tr><td>24</td><td>Oklahoma</td><td>7,590</td><td>1.45%</td><td>36</td><td>Utah</td><td>3,707</td><td>0.71%</td></tr>
<tr><td>30</td><td>Oregon</td><td>5,084</td><td>0.97%</td><td>37</td><td>Nevada</td><td>2,663</td><td>0.51%</td></tr>
<tr><td>9</td><td>Pennsylvania</td><td>18,216</td><td>3.49%</td><td>38</td><td>Nebraska</td><td>2,352</td><td>0.45%</td></tr>
<tr><td>42</td><td>Rhode Island</td><td>1,564</td><td>0.30%</td><td>39</td><td>Hawaii</td><td>2,122</td><td>0.41%</td></tr>
<tr><td>18</td><td>South Carolina</td><td>9,721</td><td>1.86%</td><td>40</td><td>Idaho</td><td>2,009</td><td>0.38%</td></tr>
<tr><td>46</td><td>South Dakota</td><td>1,172</td><td>0.22%</td><td>41</td><td>Maine</td><td>1,857</td><td>0.36%</td></tr>
<tr><td>11</td><td>Tennessee</td><td>12,928</td><td>2.48%</td><td>42</td><td>Rhode Island</td><td>1,564</td><td>0.30%</td></tr>
<tr><td>2</td><td>Texas</td><td>48,302</td><td>9.26%</td><td>43</td><td>Montana</td><td>1,331</td><td>0.26%</td></tr>
<tr><td>36</td><td>Utah</td><td>3,707</td><td>0.71%</td><td>44</td><td>Delaware</td><td>1,277</td><td>0.24%</td></tr>
<tr><td>50</td><td>Vermont</td><td>702</td><td>0.13%</td><td>45</td><td>New Hampshire</td><td>1,258</td><td>0.24%</td></tr>
<tr><td>14</td><td>Virginia</td><td>11,353</td><td>2.18%</td><td>46</td><td>South Dakota</td><td>1,172</td><td>0.22%</td></tr>
<tr><td>22</td><td>Washington</td><td>8,397</td><td>1.61%</td><td>47</td><td>Alaska</td><td>1,142</td><td>0.22%</td></tr>
<tr><td>35</td><td>West Virginia</td><td>3,976</td><td>0.76%</td><td>48</td><td>Wyoming</td><td>943</td><td>0.18%</td></tr>
<tr><td>25</td><td>Wisconsin</td><td>7,281</td><td>1.40%</td><td>49</td><td>North Dakota</td><td>793</td><td>0.15%</td></tr>
<tr><td>48</td><td>Wyoming</td><td>943</td><td>0.18%</td><td>50</td><td>Vermont</td><td>702</td><td>0.13%</td></tr>
<tr><td></td><td></td><td></td><td></td><td></td><td>District of Columbia</td><td>2,030</td><td>0.39%</td></tr>
</table>

Source: U.S. Department of Health and Human Services, Centers for Disease Control and Prevention
   "Surveillance for Pregnancy and Birth Rates Among Teenagers" (MMWR, Vol. 42, No. SS-6, 12/17/93)
*Women aged 15 to 19 years old.

Teenage Birth Rate in 1990

National Rate = 59.9 Live Births per 1,000 Teenage Women*

ALPHA ORDER				RANK ORDER		
RANK	STATE	RATE		RANK	STATE	RATE
11	Alabama	71.0		1	Mississippi	81.0
17	Alaska	65.3		2	Arkansas	80.1
4	Arizona	75.5		3	New Mexico	78.2
2	Arkansas	80.1		4	Arizona	75.5
12	California	70.6		4	Georgia	75.5
28	Colorado	54.5		6	Texas	75.3
45	Connecticut	38.8		7	Louisiana	74.2
28	Delaware	54.5		8	Nevada	73.3
13	Florida	69.1		9	Tennessee	72.3
4	Georgia	75.5		10	South Carolina	71.3
20	Hawaii	61.2		11	Alabama	71.0
33	Idaho	50.6		12	California	70.6
18	Illinois	62.9		13	Florida	69.1
22	Indiana	58.6		14	Kentucky	67.6
43	Iowa	40.5		14	North Carolina	67.6
26	Kansas	56.1		16	Oklahoma	66.8
14	Kentucky	67.6		17	Alaska	65.3
7	Louisiana	74.2		18	Illinois	62.9
40	Maine	43.0		19	Missouri	62.8
30	Maryland	53.2		20	Hawaii	61.2
48	Massachusetts	35.1		21	Michigan	59.0
21	Michigan	59.0		22	Indiana	58.6
46	Minnesota	36.3		23	Ohio	57.9
1	Mississippi	81.0		24	West Virginia	57.3
19	Missouri	62.8		25	Wyoming	56.3
35	Montana	48.4		26	Kansas	56.1
42	Nebraska	42.3		27	Oregon	54.6
8	Nevada	73.3		28	Colorado	54.5
50	New Hampshire	33.0		28	Delaware	54.5
43	New Jersey	40.5		30	Maryland	53.2
3	New Mexico	78.2		31	Washington	53.1
39	New York	43.6		32	Virginia	52.9
14	North Carolina	67.6		33	Idaho	50.6
47	North Dakota	35.4		34	Utah	48.5
23	Ohio	57.9		35	Montana	48.4
16	Oklahoma	66.8		36	South Dakota	46.8
27	Oregon	54.6		37	Pennsylvania	44.9
37	Pennsylvania	44.9		38	Rhode Island	43.9
38	Rhode Island	43.9		39	New York	43.6
10	South Carolina	71.3		40	Maine	43.0
36	South Dakota	46.8		41	Wisconsin	42.6
9	Tennessee	72.3		42	Nebraska	42.3
6	Texas	75.3		43	Iowa	40.5
34	Utah	48.5		43	New Jersey	40.5
49	Vermont	34.0		45	Connecticut	38.8
32	Virginia	52.9		46	Minnesota	36.3
31	Washington	53.1		47	North Dakota	35.4
24	West Virginia	57.3		48	Massachusetts	35.1
41	Wisconsin	42.6		49	Vermont	34.0
25	Wyoming	56.3		50	New Hampshire	33.0
					District of Columbia	93.1

Source: U.S. Department of Health and Human Services, Centers for Disease Control and Prevention
"Surveillance for Pregnancy and Birth Rates Among Teenagers" (MMWR, Vol. 42, No. SS-6, 12/17/93)
*Women aged 15 to 19 years old.

Percent Change in Teenage Birth Rate: 1990 to 1995

National Percent Change = 5.2% Decrease*

ALPHA ORDER

RANK	STATE	PERCENT CHANGE
8	Alabama	(1.0)
50	Alaska	(23.1)
5	Arizona	0.3
33	Arkansas	(8.2)
13	California	(3.4)
22	Colorado	(5.9)
2	Connecticut	1.3
1	Delaware	4.6
37	Florida	(10.7)
20	Georgia	(5.8)
48	Hawaii	(21.7)
12	Idaho	(3.2)
17	Illinois	(4.8)
10	Indiana	(1.9)
15	Iowa	(4.7)
25	Kansas	(7.0)
28	Kentucky	(7.5)
20	Louisiana	(5.8)
49	Maine	(21.9)
35	Maryland	(10.3)
11	Massachusetts	(2.3)
47	Michigan	(16.6)
37	Minnesota	(10.7)
7	Mississippi	(0.5)
41	Missouri	(11.6)
44	Montana	(13.6)
39	Nebraska	(11.1)
6	Nevada	0.0
29	New Hampshire	(7.6)
24	New Jersey	(6.2)
15	New Mexico	(4.7)
4	New York	0.9
18	North Carolina	(5.2)
19	North Dakota	(5.4)
30	Ohio	(7.8)
14	Oklahoma	(4.2)
26	Oregon	(7.1)
26	Pennsylvania	(7.1)
9	Rhode Island	(1.8)
34	South Carolina	(8.7)
43	South Dakota	(13.5)
23	Tennessee	(6.1)
3	Texas	1.1
42	Utah	(12.6)
45	Vermont	(15.9)
31	Virginia	(7.9)
36	Washington	(10.4)
32	West Virginia	(8.0)
40	Wisconsin	(11.3)
46	Wyoming	(16.2)

RANK ORDER

RANK	STATE	PERCENT CHANGE
1	Delaware	4.6
2	Connecticut	1.3
3	Texas	1.1
4	New York	0.9
5	Arizona	0.3
6	Nevada	0.0
7	Mississippi	(0.5)
8	Alabama	(1.0)
9	Rhode Island	(1.8)
10	Indiana	(1.9)
11	Massachusetts	(2.3)
12	Idaho	(3.2)
13	California	(3.4)
14	Oklahoma	(4.2)
15	Iowa	(4.7)
15	New Mexico	(4.7)
17	Illinois	(4.8)
18	North Carolina	(5.2)
19	North Dakota	(5.4)
20	Georgia	(5.8)
20	Louisiana	(5.8)
22	Colorado	(5.9)
23	Tennessee	(6.1)
24	New Jersey	(6.2)
25	Kansas	(7.0)
26	Oregon	(7.1)
26	Pennsylvania	(7.1)
28	Kentucky	(7.5)
29	New Hampshire	(7.6)
30	Ohio	(7.8)
31	Virginia	(7.9)
32	West Virginia	(8.0)
33	Arkansas	(8.2)
34	South Carolina	(8.7)
35	Maryland	(10.3)
36	Washington	(10.4)
37	Florida	(10.7)
37	Minnesota	(10.7)
39	Nebraska	(11.1)
40	Wisconsin	(11.3)
41	Missouri	(11.6)
42	Utah	(12.6)
43	South Dakota	(13.5)
44	Montana	(13.6)
45	Vermont	(15.9)
46	Wyoming	(16.2)
47	Michigan	(16.6)
48	Hawaii	(21.7)
49	Maine	(21.9)
50	Alaska	(23.1)

District of Columbia   14.7

Source: Morgan Quitno Press using data from U.S. Department of Health and Human Services
 "State-Specific Birth Rates for Teenagers" (MMWR, Vol. 46, No. 36, 9/12/97)
 "Surveillance for Pregnancy and Birth Rates Among Teenagers" (MMWR, Vol. 42, No. SS-6, 12/17/93)
*Women aged 15 to 19 years old.

Births to Teenage Mothers in 1980

National Total = 562,330 Live Births*

ALPHA ORDER

RANK	STATE	BIRTHS	% of USA
15	Alabama	13,096	2.33%
49	Alaska	1,123	0.20%
25	Arizona	8,235	1.46%
26	Arkansas	8,060	1.43%
1	California	56,138	9.98%
29	Colorado	6,592	1.17%
36	Connecticut	4,408	0.78%
45	Delaware	1,572	0.28%
6	Florida	24,042	4.28%
9	Georgia	19,137	3.40%
40	Hawaii	2,085	0.37%
38	Idaho	2,645	0.47%
3	Illinois	29,798	5.30%
12	Indiana	15,331	2.73%
31	Iowa	5,962	1.06%
30	Kansas	6,090	1.08%
16	Kentucky	12,559	2.23%
10	Louisiana	16,504	2.93%
39	Maine	2,522	0.45%
23	Maryland	8,885	1.58%
27	Massachusetts	7,765	1.38%
8	Michigan	20,401	3.63%
28	Minnesota	7,048	1.25%
19	Mississippi	11,079	1.97%
14	Missouri	13,312	2.37%
43	Montana	1,761	0.31%
37	Nebraska	3,313	0.59%
41	Nevada	2,048	0.36%
47	New Hampshire	1,475	0.26%
18	New Jersey	11,904	2.12%
34	New Mexico	4,758	0.85%
4	New York	28,206	5.02%
11	North Carolina	16,192	2.88%
48	North Dakota	1,304	0.23%
5	Ohio	26,567	4.72%
21	Oklahoma	10,206	1.81%
33	Oregon	5,731	1.02%
7	Pennsylvania	22,029	3.92%
46	Rhode Island	1,502	0.27%
20	South Carolina	10,282	1.83%
42	South Dakota	1,797	0.32%
13	Tennessee	13,792	2.45%
2	Texas	50,125	8.91%
35	Utah	4,594	0.82%
50	Vermont	1,024	0.18%
17	Virginia	12,138	2.16%
24	Washington	8,495	1.51%
32	West Virginia	5,911	1.05%
22	Wisconsin	9,220	1.64%
44	Wyoming	1,634	0.29%

RANK ORDER

RANK	STATE	BIRTHS	% of USA
1	California	56,138	9.98%
2	Texas	50,125	8.91%
3	Illinois	29,798	5.30%
4	New York	28,206	5.02%
5	Ohio	26,567	4.72%
6	Florida	24,042	4.28%
7	Pennsylvania	22,029	3.92%
8	Michigan	20,401	3.63%
9	Georgia	19,137	3.40%
10	Louisiana	16,504	2.93%
11	North Carolina	16,192	2.88%
12	Indiana	15,331	2.73%
13	Tennessee	13,792	2.45%
14	Missouri	13,312	2.37%
15	Alabama	13,096	2.33%
16	Kentucky	12,559	2.23%
17	Virginia	12,138	2.16%
18	New Jersey	11,904	2.12%
19	Mississippi	11,079	1.97%
20	South Carolina	10,282	1.83%
21	Oklahoma	10,206	1.81%
22	Wisconsin	9,220	1.64%
23	Maryland	8,885	1.58%
24	Washington	8,495	1.51%
25	Arizona	8,235	1.46%
26	Arkansas	8,060	1.43%
27	Massachusetts	7,765	1.38%
28	Minnesota	7,048	1.25%
29	Colorado	6,592	1.17%
30	Kansas	6,090	1.08%
31	Iowa	5,962	1.06%
32	West Virginia	5,911	1.05%
33	Oregon	5,731	1.02%
34	New Mexico	4,758	0.85%
35	Utah	4,594	0.82%
36	Connecticut	4,408	0.78%
37	Nebraska	3,313	0.59%
38	Idaho	2,645	0.47%
39	Maine	2,522	0.45%
40	Hawaii	2,085	0.37%
41	Nevada	2,048	0.36%
42	South Dakota	1,797	0.32%
43	Montana	1,761	0.31%
44	Wyoming	1,634	0.29%
45	Delaware	1,572	0.28%
46	Rhode Island	1,502	0.27%
47	New Hampshire	1,475	0.26%
48	North Dakota	1,304	0.23%
49	Alaska	1,123	0.20%
50	Vermont	1,024	0.18%
	District of Columbia	1,933	0.34%

Source: U.S. Department of Health and Human Services, National Center for Health Statistics
    "Vital Statistics of the United States, 1980" (Vol. I-Natality, issued 1984)
*Births to women age 15 to 19 years old.

Teenage Birth Rate in 1980

National Rate = 53.0 Live Births per 1,000 Teenage Women*

ALPHA ORDER

RANK	STATE	RATE
10	Alabama	68.3
15	Alaska	64.4
12	Arizona	65.5
5	Arkansas	74.5
25	California	53.3
31	Colorado	49.9
49	Connecticut	30.5
28	Delaware	51.2
18	Florida	58.5
8	Georgia	71.9
30	Hawaii	50.7
17	Idaho	59.5
24	Illinois	55.8
21	Indiana	57.5
39	Iowa	43.0
23	Kansas	56.8
7	Kentucky	72.3
3	Louisiana	76.0
34	Maine	47.4
38	Maryland	43.4
50	Massachusetts	28.1
37	Michigan	45.0
44	Minnesota	35.4
1	Mississippi	83.7
20	Missouri	57.8
32	Montana	48.5
36	Nebraska	45.1
18	Nevada	58.5
47	New Hampshire	33.6
45	New Jersey	35.2
9	New Mexico	71.8
46	New York	34.8
21	North Carolina	57.5
40	North Dakota	41.7
27	Ohio	52.5
4	Oklahoma	74.6
29	Oregon	50.9
41	Pennsylvania	40.5
48	Rhode Island	33.0
14	South Carolina	64.8
26	South Dakota	52.6
16	Tennessee	64.1
6	Texas	74.3
13	Utah	65.2
42	Vermont	39.5
33	Virginia	48.3
35	Washington	46.7
11	West Virginia	67.8
42	Wisconsin	39.5
2	Wyoming	78.7

RANK ORDER

RANK	STATE	RATE
1	Mississippi	83.7
2	Wyoming	78.7
3	Louisiana	76.0
4	Oklahoma	74.6
5	Arkansas	74.5
6	Texas	74.3
7	Kentucky	72.3
8	Georgia	71.9
9	New Mexico	71.8
10	Alabama	68.3
11	West Virginia	67.8
12	Arizona	65.5
13	Utah	65.2
14	South Carolina	64.8
15	Alaska	64.4
16	Tennessee	64.1
17	Idaho	59.5
18	Florida	58.5
18	Nevada	58.5
20	Missouri	57.8
21	Indiana	57.5
21	North Carolina	57.5
23	Kansas	56.8
24	Illinois	55.8
25	California	53.3
26	South Dakota	52.6
27	Ohio	52.5
28	Delaware	51.2
29	Oregon	50.9
30	Hawaii	50.7
31	Colorado	49.9
32	Montana	48.5
33	Virginia	48.3
34	Maine	47.4
35	Washington	46.7
36	Nebraska	45.1
37	Michigan	45.0
38	Maryland	43.4
39	Iowa	43.0
40	North Dakota	41.7
41	Pennsylvania	40.5
42	Vermont	39.5
42	Wisconsin	39.5
44	Minnesota	35.4
45	New Jersey	35.2
46	New York	34.8
47	New Hampshire	33.6
48	Rhode Island	33.0
49	Connecticut	30.5
50	Massachusetts	28.1

District of Columbia   62.4

Source: U.S. Department of Health and Human Services, Centers for Disease Control and Prevention
"Surveillance for Pregnancy and Birth Rates Among Teenagers" (MMWR, Vol. 42, No. SS-6, 12/17/93)
*Women aged 15 to 19 years old.

Births to Women 35 to 49 Years Old in 1995

National Total = 453,722 Live Births*

ALPHA ORDER

RANK	STATE	BIRTHS	% of USA
26	Alabama	4,535	1.00%
44	Alaska	1,309	0.29%
18	Arizona	7,368	1.62%
38	Arkansas	2,360	0.52%
1	California	73,920	16.29%
20	Colorado	7,306	1.61%
19	Connecticut	7,319	1.61%
46	Delaware	1,071	0.24%
4	Florida	22,510	4.96%
12	Georgia	10,675	2.35%
36	Hawaii	2,572	0.57%
41	Idaho	1,702	0.38%
5	Illinois	22,314	4.92%
21	Indiana	7,177	1.58%
30	Iowa	3,585	0.79%
29	Kansas	3,806	0.84%
28	Kentucky	3,980	0.88%
24	Louisiana	5,439	1.20%
43	Maine	1,516	0.33%
13	Maryland	10,606	2.34%
10	Massachusetts	13,989	3.08%
9	Michigan	14,623	3.22%
16	Minnesota	8,275	1.82%
33	Mississippi	2,751	0.61%
22	Missouri	7,163	1.58%
45	Montana	1,294	0.29%
37	Nebraska	2,512	0.55%
35	Nevada	2,618	0.58%
39	New Hampshire	2,037	0.45%
7	New Jersey	19,156	4.22%
34	New Mexico	2,652	0.58%
2	New York	41,287	9.10%
15	North Carolina	9,439	2.08%
49	North Dakota	883	0.19%
8	Ohio	15,697	3.46%
32	Oklahoma	3,427	0.76%
25	Oregon	4,957	1.09%
6	Pennsylvania	19,458	4.29%
40	Rhode Island	1,738	0.38%
27	South Carolina	4,459	0.98%
47	South Dakota	1,010	0.22%
23	Tennessee	6,076	1.34%
3	Texas	29,817	6.57%
31	Utah	3,539	0.78%
48	Vermont	991	0.22%
11	Virginia	11,816	2.60%
14	Washington	9,853	2.17%
42	West Virginia	1,522	0.34%
17	Wisconsin	7,682	1.69%
50	Wyoming	605	0.13%

RANK ORDER

RANK	STATE	BIRTHS	% of USA
1	California	73,920	16.29%
2	New York	41,287	9.10%
3	Texas	29,817	6.57%
4	Florida	22,510	4.96%
5	Illinois	22,314	4.92%
6	Pennsylvania	19,458	4.29%
7	New Jersey	19,156	4.22%
8	Ohio	15,697	3.46%
9	Michigan	14,623	3.22%
10	Massachusetts	13,989	3.08%
11	Virginia	11,816	2.60%
12	Georgia	10,675	2.35%
13	Maryland	10,606	2.34%
14	Washington	9,853	2.17%
15	North Carolina	9,439	2.08%
16	Minnesota	8,275	1.82%
17	Wisconsin	7,682	1.69%
18	Arizona	7,368	1.62%
19	Connecticut	7,319	1.61%
20	Colorado	7,306	1.61%
21	Indiana	7,177	1.58%
22	Missouri	7,163	1.58%
23	Tennessee	6,076	1.34%
24	Louisiana	5,439	1.20%
25	Oregon	4,957	1.09%
26	Alabama	4,535	1.00%
27	South Carolina	4,459	0.98%
28	Kentucky	3,980	0.88%
29	Kansas	3,806	0.84%
30	Iowa	3,585	0.79%
31	Utah	3,539	0.78%
32	Oklahoma	3,427	0.76%
33	Mississippi	2,751	0.61%
34	New Mexico	2,652	0.58%
35	Nevada	2,618	0.58%
36	Hawaii	2,572	0.57%
37	Nebraska	2,512	0.55%
38	Arkansas	2,360	0.52%
39	New Hampshire	2,037	0.45%
40	Rhode Island	1,738	0.38%
41	Idaho	1,702	0.38%
42	West Virginia	1,522	0.34%
43	Maine	1,516	0.33%
44	Alaska	1,309	0.29%
45	Montana	1,294	0.29%
46	Delaware	1,071	0.24%
47	South Dakota	1,010	0.22%
48	Vermont	991	0.22%
49	North Dakota	883	0.19%
50	Wyoming	605	0.13%

| | District of Columbia | 1,326 | 0.29% |

Source: Morgan Quitno Press using data from U.S. Dept of Health & Human Services, National Center for Health Statistics (unpublished data)
*By state of residence.

Births to Women 35 to 49 Years Old as a Percent of All Births in 1995

National Percent = 11.6% of Live Births*

ALPHA ORDER

RANK ORDER

RANK	STATE	PERCENT		RANK	STATE	PERCENT
46	Alabama	7.5		1	Massachusetts	17.1
13	Alaska	12.8		2	New Jersey	16.7
28	Arizona	10.2		3	Connecticut	16.5
49	Arkansas	6.7		4	New York	15.2
11	California	13.4		5	Maryland	14.7
9	Colorado	13.5		6	Vermont	14.5
3	Connecticut	16.5		7	New Hampshire	13.9
25	Delaware	10.5		8	Hawaii	13.8
18	Florida	12.0		9	Colorado	13.5
36	Georgia	9.4		9	Rhode Island	13.5
8	Hawaii	13.8		11	California	13.4
36	Idaho	9.4		12	Minnesota	13.1
17	Illinois	12.1		13	Alaska	12.8
41	Indiana	8.7		13	Pennsylvania	12.8
32	Iowa	9.8		13	Washington	12.8
28	Kansas	10.2		16	Virginia	12.7
45	Kentucky	7.6		17	Illinois	12.1
43	Louisiana	8.3		18	Florida	12.0
22	Maine	10.9		19	Montana	11.7
5	Maryland	14.7		20	Oregon	11.6
1	Massachusetts	17.1		21	Wisconsin	11.4
22	Michigan	10.9		22	Maine	10.9
12	Minnesota	13.1		22	Michigan	10.9
49	Mississippi	6.7		24	Nebraska	10.8
32	Missouri	9.8		25	Delaware	10.5
19	Montana	11.7		25	Nevada	10.5
24	Nebraska	10.8		25	North Dakota	10.5
25	Nevada	10.5		28	Arizona	10.2
7	New Hampshire	13.9		28	Kansas	10.2
2	New Jersey	16.7		30	Ohio	10.1
31	New Mexico	9.9		31	New Mexico	9.9
4	New York	15.2		32	Iowa	9.8
38	North Carolina	9.2		32	Missouri	9.8
25	North Dakota	10.5		34	South Dakota	9.7
30	Ohio	10.1		35	Wyoming	9.6
46	Oklahoma	7.5		36	Georgia	9.4
20	Oregon	11.6		36	Idaho	9.4
13	Pennsylvania	12.8		38	North Carolina	9.2
9	Rhode Island	13.5		38	Texas	9.2
41	South Carolina	8.7		40	Utah	8.9
34	South Dakota	9.7		41	Indiana	8.7
43	Tennessee	8.3		41	South Carolina	8.7
38	Texas	9.2		43	Louisiana	8.3
40	Utah	8.9		43	Tennessee	8.3
6	Vermont	14.5		45	Kentucky	7.6
16	Virginia	12.7		46	Alabama	7.5
13	Washington	12.8		46	Oklahoma	7.5
48	West Virginia	7.2		48	West Virginia	7.2
21	Wisconsin	11.4		49	Arkansas	6.7
35	Wyoming	9.6		49	Mississippi	6.7

District of Columbia   14.7

Source: Morgan Quitno Press using data from U.S. Dept of Health & Human Services, National Center for Health Statistics
(unpublished data)
*By state of residence.

Births by Vaginal Delivery in 1995

National Total = 3,063,724 Live Births*

ALPHA ORDER

RANK	STATE	BIRTHS	% of USA
23	Alabama	46,163	1.51%
45	Alaska	8,743	0.29%
16	Arizona	60,141	1.96%
34	Arkansas	26,008	0.85%
1	California	438,222	14.30%
24	Colorado	46,078	1.50%
29	Connecticut	32,971	1.08%
47	Delaware	8,060	0.26%
5	Florida	147,294	4.81%
9	Georgia	88,356	2.88%
40	Hawaii	14,954	0.49%
39	Idaho	15,161	0.49%
4	Illinois	148,383	4.84%
13	Indiana	65,487	2.14%
31	Iowa	29,832	0.97%
32	Kansas	28,949	0.94%
25	Kentucky	39,420	1.29%
22	Louisiana	47,733	1.56%
42	Maine	10,921	0.36%
20	Maryland	56,348	1.84%
14	Massachusetts	64,537	2.11%
8	Michigan	106,656	3.48%
21	Minnesota	51,622	1.68%
30	Mississippi	30,584	1.00%
17	Missouri	57,825	1.89%
44	Montana	8,986	0.29%
37	Nebraska	18,756	0.61%
36	Nevada	20,099	0.66%
41	New Hampshire	11,706	0.38%
10	New Jersey	87,660	2.86%
35	New Mexico	21,938	0.72%
3	New York	207,920	6.79%
11	North Carolina	79,327	2.59%
48	North Dakota	6,823	0.22%
6	Ohio	123,366	4.03%
33	Oklahoma	28,617	0.93%
27	Oregon	35,281	1.15%
7	Pennsylvania	121,630	3.97%
43	Rhode Island	10,400	0.34%
26	South Carolina	39,352	1.28%
46	South Dakota	8,369	0.27%
18	Tennessee	57,374	1.87%
2	Texas	245,172	8.00%
28	Utah	33,092	1.08%
49	Vermont	5,647	0.18%
12	Virginia	72,564	2.37%
15	Washington	63,837	2.08%
38	West Virginia	16,156	0.53%
19	Wisconsin	57,039	1.86%
50	Wyoming	5,136	0.17%

RANK ORDER

RANK	STATE	BIRTHS	% of USA
1	California	438,222	14.30%
2	Texas	245,172	8.00%
3	New York	207,920	6.79%
4	Illinois	148,383	4.84%
5	Florida	147,294	4.81%
6	Ohio	123,366	4.03%
7	Pennsylvania	121,630	3.97%
8	Michigan	106,656	3.48%
9	Georgia	88,356	2.88%
10	New Jersey	87,660	2.86%
11	North Carolina	79,327	2.59%
12	Virginia	72,564	2.37%
13	Indiana	65,487	2.14%
14	Massachusetts	64,537	2.11%
15	Washington	63,837	2.08%
16	Arizona	60,141	1.96%
17	Missouri	57,825	1.89%
18	Tennessee	57,374	1.87%
19	Wisconsin	57,039	1.86%
20	Maryland	56,348	1.84%
21	Minnesota	51,622	1.68%
22	Louisiana	47,733	1.56%
23	Alabama	46,163	1.51%
24	Colorado	46,078	1.50%
25	Kentucky	39,420	1.29%
26	South Carolina	39,352	1.28%
27	Oregon	35,281	1.15%
28	Utah	33,092	1.08%
29	Connecticut	32,971	1.08%
30	Mississippi	30,584	1.00%
31	Iowa	29,832	0.97%
32	Kansas	28,949	0.94%
33	Oklahoma	28,617	0.93%
34	Arkansas	26,008	0.85%
35	New Mexico	21,938	0.72%
36	Nevada	20,099	0.66%
37	Nebraska	18,756	0.61%
38	West Virginia	16,156	0.53%
39	Idaho	15,161	0.49%
40	Hawaii	14,954	0.49%
41	New Hampshire	11,706	0.38%
42	Maine	10,921	0.36%
43	Rhode Island	10,400	0.34%
44	Montana	8,986	0.29%
45	Alaska	8,743	0.29%
46	South Dakota	8,369	0.27%
47	Delaware	8,060	0.26%
48	North Dakota	6,823	0.22%
49	Vermont	5,647	0.18%
50	Wyoming	5,136	0.17%
	District of Columbia	7,029	0.23%

Source: U.S. Department of Health and Human Services, National Center for Health Statistics unpublished data

Includes VBACs (vaginal births after cesarean).

Percent of Births by Vaginal Delivery in 1995

National Percent = 79.2% of Live Births*

ALPHA ORDER				RANK ORDER		
RANK	STATE	PERCENT		RANK	STATE	PERCENT
45	Alabama	76.6		1	Alaska	85.6
1	Alaska	85.6		2	Colorado	84.8
8	Arizona	83.2		3	Wisconsin	84.6
48	Arkansas	74.4		4	Idaho	84.3
29	California	79.4		5	Minnesota	83.7
2	Colorado	84.8		5	Utah	83.7
17	Connecticut	80.8		7	Vermont	83.3
36	Delaware	78.5		8	Arizona	83.2
37	Florida	78.3		9	Washington	82.9
33	Georgia	78.8		10	Oregon	82.6
14	Hawaii	81.5		11	Wyoming	82.1
4	Idaho	84.3		12	New Mexico	81.9
24	Illinois	80.1		13	Rhode Island	81.6
31	Indiana	79.3		14	Hawaii	81.5
15	Iowa	81.4		15	Iowa	81.4
22	Kansas	80.3		16	Montana	80.9
39	Kentucky	78.0		17	Connecticut	80.8
50	Louisiana	72.8		17	Nebraska	80.8
32	Maine	79.0		17	Nevada	80.8
39	Maryland	78.0		20	North Dakota	80.7
29	Massachusetts	79.4		21	Ohio	80.4
27	Michigan	79.7		22	Kansas	80.3
5	Minnesota	83.7		22	Pennsylvania	80.3
49	Mississippi	74.1		24	Illinois	80.1
28	Missouri	79.5		24	South Dakota	80.1
16	Montana	80.9		26	New Hampshire	80.0
17	Nebraska	80.8		27	Michigan	79.7
17	Nevada	80.8		28	Missouri	79.5
26	New Hampshire	80.0		29	California	79.4
44	New Jersey	76.7		29	Massachusetts	79.4
12	New Mexico	81.9		31	Indiana	79.3
42	New York	77.3		32	Maine	79.0
37	North Carolina	78.3		33	Georgia	78.8
20	North Dakota	80.7		33	Tennessee	78.8
21	Ohio	80.4		35	Virginia	78.7
43	Oklahoma	77.2		36	Delaware	78.5
10	Oregon	82.6		37	Florida	78.3
22	Pennsylvania	80.3		37	North Carolina	78.3
13	Rhode Island	81.6		39	Kentucky	78.0
41	South Carolina	77.6		39	Maryland	78.0
24	South Dakota	80.1		41	South Carolina	77.6
33	Tennessee	78.8		42	New York	77.3
47	Texas	76.4		43	Oklahoma	77.2
5	Utah	83.7		44	New Jersey	76.7
7	Vermont	83.3		45	Alabama	76.6
35	Virginia	78.7		46	West Virginia	76.5
9	Washington	82.9		47	Texas	76.4
46	West Virginia	76.5		48	Arkansas	74.4
3	Wisconsin	84.6		49	Mississippi	74.1
11	Wyoming	82.1		50	Louisiana	72.8
					District of Columbia	78.0

Source: U.S. Department of Health and Human Services, National Center for Health Statistics
unpublished data
*Of those births for which delivery data are available. Includes VBACs (vaginal births after cesarean).

Births by Cesarean Delivery in 1995

National Total = 806,722 Live Cesarean Births

ALPHA ORDER

RANK	STATE	BIRTHS	% of USA
19	Alabama	14,078	1.75%
48	Alaska	1,469	0.18%
21	Arizona	12,117	1.50%
27	Arkansas	8,927	1.11%
1	California	113,782	14.10%
29	Colorado	8,247	1.02%
30	Connecticut	7,850	0.97%
44	Delaware	2,205	0.27%
4	Florida	40,728	5.05%
10	Georgia	23,783	2.95%
39	Hawaii	3,389	0.42%
42	Idaho	2,814	0.35%
5	Illinois	36,839	4.57%
14	Indiana	17,066	2.12%
33	Iowa	6,824	0.85%
32	Kansas	7,108	0.88%
23	Kentucky	11,144	1.38%
13	Louisiana	17,826	2.21%
41	Maine	2,896	0.36%
16	Maryland	15,914	1.97%
15	Massachusetts	16,768	2.08%
8	Michigan	27,108	3.36%
26	Minnesota	10,053	1.25%
24	Mississippi	10,682	1.32%
18	Missouri	14,930	1.85%
45	Montana	2,119	0.26%
38	Nebraska	4,447	0.55%
37	Nevada	4,771	0.59%
40	New Hampshire	2,927	0.36%
9	New Jersey	26,644	3.30%
36	New Mexico	4,848	0.60%
3	New York	61,113	7.58%
11	North Carolina	21,963	2.72%
47	North Dakota	1,635	0.20%
6	Ohio	30,010	3.72%
28	Oklahoma	8,447	1.05%
31	Oregon	7,436	0.92%
7	Pennsylvania	29,840	3.70%
43	Rhode Island	2,342	0.29%
22	South Carolina	11,374	1.41%
46	South Dakota	2,084	0.26%
17	Tennessee	15,469	1.92%
2	Texas	75,875	9.41%
34	Utah	6,421	0.80%
49	Vermont	1,131	0.14%
12	Virginia	19,681	2.44%
20	Washington	13,127	1.63%
35	West Virginia	4,961	0.61%
25	Wisconsin	10,406	1.29%
50	Wyoming	1,120	0.14%

RANK ORDER

RANK	STATE	BIRTHS	% of USA
1	California	113,782	14.10%
2	Texas	75,875	9.41%
3	New York	61,113	7.58%
4	Florida	40,728	5.05%
5	Illinois	36,839	4.57%
6	Ohio	30,010	3.72%
7	Pennsylvania	29,840	3.70%
8	Michigan	27,108	3.36%
9	New Jersey	26,644	3.30%
10	Georgia	23,783	2.95%
11	North Carolina	21,963	2.72%
12	Virginia	19,681	2.44%
13	Louisiana	17,826	2.21%
14	Indiana	17,066	2.12%
15	Massachusetts	16,768	2.08%
16	Maryland	15,914	1.97%
17	Tennessee	15,469	1.92%
18	Missouri	14,930	1.85%
19	Alabama	14,078	1.75%
20	Washington	13,127	1.63%
21	Arizona	12,117	1.50%
22	South Carolina	11,374	1.41%
23	Kentucky	11,144	1.38%
24	Mississippi	10,682	1.32%
25	Wisconsin	10,406	1.29%
26	Minnesota	10,053	1.25%
27	Arkansas	8,927	1.11%
28	Oklahoma	8,447	1.05%
29	Colorado	8,247	1.02%
30	Connecticut	7,850	0.97%
31	Oregon	7,436	0.92%
32	Kansas	7,108	0.88%
33	Iowa	6,824	0.85%
34	Utah	6,421	0.80%
35	West Virginia	4,961	0.61%
36	New Mexico	4,848	0.60%
37	Nevada	4,771	0.59%
38	Nebraska	4,447	0.55%
39	Hawaii	3,389	0.42%
40	New Hampshire	2,927	0.36%
41	Maine	2,896	0.36%
42	Idaho	2,814	0.35%
43	Rhode Island	2,342	0.29%
44	Delaware	2,205	0.27%
45	Montana	2,119	0.26%
46	South Dakota	2,084	0.26%
47	North Dakota	1,635	0.20%
48	Alaska	1,469	0.18%
49	Vermont	1,131	0.14%
50	Wyoming	1,120	0.14%
	District of Columbia	1,984	0.25%

Source: U.S. Department of Health and Human Services, National Center for Health Statistics unpublished data

Percent of Births by Cesarean Delivery in 1995

National Percent = 20.8% of Live Births*

ALPHA ORDER

RANK	STATE	PERCENT
6	Alabama	23.4
50	Alaska	14.4
43	Arizona	16.8
3	Arkansas	25.6
21	California	20.6
49	Colorado	15.2
32	Connecticut	19.2
15	Delaware	21.5
13	Florida	21.7
17	Georgia	21.2
37	Hawaii	18.5
47	Idaho	15.7
26	Illinois	19.9
20	Indiana	20.7
36	Iowa	18.6
28	Kansas	19.7
11	Kentucky	22.0
1	Louisiana	27.2
19	Maine	21.0
11	Maryland	22.0
21	Massachusetts	20.6
24	Michigan	20.3
45	Minnesota	16.3
2	Mississippi	25.9
23	Missouri	20.5
35	Montana	19.1
32	Nebraska	19.2
32	Nevada	19.2
25	New Hampshire	20.0
7	New Jersey	23.3
39	New Mexico	18.1
9	New York	22.7
13	North Carolina	21.7
31	North Dakota	19.3
30	Ohio	19.6
8	Oklahoma	22.8
41	Oregon	17.4
28	Pennsylvania	19.7
38	Rhode Island	18.4
10	South Carolina	22.4
26	South Dakota	19.9
17	Tennessee	21.2
4	Texas	23.6
45	Utah	16.3
44	Vermont	16.7
16	Virginia	21.3
42	Washington	17.1
5	West Virginia	23.5
48	Wisconsin	15.4
40	Wyoming	17.9

RANK ORDER

RANK	STATE	PERCENT
1	Louisiana	27.2
2	Mississippi	25.9
3	Arkansas	25.6
4	Texas	23.6
5	West Virginia	23.5
6	Alabama	23.4
7	New Jersey	23.3
8	Oklahoma	22.8
9	New York	22.7
10	South Carolina	22.4
11	Kentucky	22.0
11	Maryland	22.0
13	Florida	21.7
13	North Carolina	21.7
15	Delaware	21.5
16	Virginia	21.3
17	Georgia	21.2
17	Tennessee	21.2
19	Maine	21.0
20	Indiana	20.7
21	California	20.6
21	Massachusetts	20.6
23	Missouri	20.5
24	Michigan	20.3
25	New Hampshire	20.0
26	Illinois	19.9
26	South Dakota	19.9
28	Kansas	19.7
28	Pennsylvania	19.7
30	Ohio	19.6
31	North Dakota	19.3
32	Connecticut	19.2
32	Nebraska	19.2
32	Nevada	19.2
35	Montana	19.1
36	Iowa	18.6
37	Hawaii	18.5
38	Rhode Island	18.4
39	New Mexico	18.1
40	Wyoming	17.9
41	Oregon	17.4
42	Washington	17.1
43	Arizona	16.8
44	Vermont	16.7
45	Minnesota	16.3
45	Utah	16.3
47	Idaho	15.7
48	Wisconsin	15.4
49	Colorado	15.2
50	Alaska	14.4

	District of Columbia	22.0

Source: U.S. Department of Health and Human Services, National Center for Health Statistics
unpublished data
*Of those births for which delivery data are available.

Percent Change in Rate of Cesarean Births: 1989 to 1995

National Percent Change = 8.8% Decrease*

ALPHA ORDER			RANK ORDER		
RANK	STATE	PERCENT CHANGE	RANK	STATE	PERCENT CHANGE
20	Alabama	(8.6)	1	Maine	7.1
10	Alaska	(5.3)	2	South Dakota	6.4
22	Arizona	(9.2)	3	Mississippi	0.0
9	Arkansas	(5.2)	4	Indiana	(1.0)
21	California	(8.8)	4	North Dakota	(1.0)
40	Colorado	(13.6)	6	South Carolina	(1.3)
24	Connecticut	(9.4)	7	New Mexico	(3.2)
27	Delaware	(10.4)	8	New York	(3.8)
42	Florida	(15.2)	9	Arkansas	(5.2)
17	Georgia	(7.8)	10	Alaska	(5.3)
33	Hawaii	(11.5)	10	Wyoming	(5.3)
45	Idaho	(19.9)	12	Montana	(5.4)
34	Illinois	(12.3)	13	Texas	(5.6)
4	Indiana	(1.0)	14	West Virginia	(6.7)
16	Iowa	(7.0)	15	North Carolina	(6.9)
43	Kansas	(17.9)	16	Iowa	(7.0)
30	Kentucky	(11.3)	17	Georgia	(7.8)
NA	Louisiana**	NA	18	Utah	(7.9)
1	Maine	7.1	19	Rhode Island	(8.5)
NA	Maryland**	NA	20	Alabama	(8.6)
26	Massachusetts	(10.0)	21	California	(8.8)
32	Michigan	(11.4)	22	Arizona	(9.2)
35	Minnesota	(12.4)	23	New Jersey	(9.3)
3	Mississippi	0.0	24	Connecticut	(9.4)
30	Missouri	(11.3)	25	New Hampshire	(9.9)
12	Montana	(5.4)	26	Massachusetts	(10.0)
NA	Nebraska**	NA	27	Delaware	(10.4)
NA	Nevada**	NA	28	Vermont	(10.7)
25	New Hampshire	(9.9)	29	Oregon	(11.2)
23	New Jersey	(9.3)	30	Kentucky	(11.3)
7	New Mexico	(3.2)	30	Missouri	(11.3)
8	New York	(3.8)	32	Michigan	(11.4)
15	North Carolina	(6.9)	33	Hawaii	(11.5)
4	North Dakota	(1.0)	34	Illinois	(12.3)
44	Ohio	(19.0)	35	Minnesota	(12.4)
NA	Oklahoma**	NA	35	Pennsylvania	(12.4)
29	Oregon	(11.2)	37	Tennessee	(12.8)
35	Pennsylvania	(12.4)	38	Wisconsin	(13.0)
19	Rhode Island	(8.5)	39	Virginia	(13.1)
6	South Carolina	(1.3)	40	Colorado	(13.6)
2	South Dakota	6.4	41	Washington	(14.9)
37	Tennessee	(12.8)	42	Florida	(15.2)
13	Texas	(5.6)	43	Kansas	(17.9)
18	Utah	(7.9)	44	Ohio	(19.0)
28	Vermont	(10.7)	45	Idaho	(19.9)
39	Virginia	(13.1)	NA	Louisiana**	NA
41	Washington	(14.9)	NA	Maryland**	NA
14	West Virginia	(6.7)	NA	Nebraska**	NA
38	Wisconsin	(13.0)	NA	Nevada**	NA
10	Wyoming	(5.3)	NA	Oklahoma**	NA
				District of Columbia	(18.8)

Source: Morgan Quitno Press using data from US Dept of Health & Human Services, National Center for Health Statistics unpublished data

*Of those births for which delivery data are available.

**Not available.

Births by Vaginal Delivery After a Previous Cesarean Delivery (VBAC) in 1995

National Total = 112,439 Live VBAC Births

ALPHA ORDER

RANK	STATE	BIRTHS	% of USA
27	Alabama	1,313	1.17%
46	Alaska	274	0.24%
21	Arizona	1,761	1.57%
33	Arkansas	832	0.74%
1	California	12,902	11.47%
22	Colorado	1,631	1.45%
24	Connecticut	1,433	1.27%
45	Delaware	361	0.32%
7	Florida	5,410	4.81%
13	Georgia	2,536	2.26%
38	Hawaii	598	0.53%
37	Idaho	599	0.53%
5	Illinois	5,708	5.08%
19	Indiana	2,170	1.93%
26	Iowa	1,344	1.20%
32	Kansas	955	0.85%
25	Kentucky	1,383	1.23%
30	Louisiana	1,040	0.92%
42	Maine	422	0.38%
15	Maryland	2,493	2.22%
12	Massachusetts	2,790	2.48%
9	Michigan	3,562	3.17%
20	Minnesota	2,131	1.90%
36	Mississippi	740	0.66%
14	Missouri	2,505	2.23%
44	Montana	388	0.35%
35	Nebraska	814	0.72%
40	Nevada	537	0.48%
39	New Hampshire	565	0.50%
8	New Jersey	3,675	3.27%
34	New Mexico	825	0.73%
2	New York	9,996	8.89%
11	North Carolina	2,842	2.53%
48	North Dakota	247	0.22%
6	Ohio	5,701	5.07%
31	Oklahoma	963	0.86%
23	Oregon	1,561	1.39%
4	Pennsylvania	5,843	5.20%
43	Rhode Island	394	0.35%
28	South Carolina	1,183	1.05%
47	South Dakota	272	0.24%
17	Tennessee	2,174	1.93%
3	Texas	7,891	7.02%
29	Utah	1,115	0.99%
49	Vermont	219	0.19%
10	Virginia	2,860	2.54%
16	Washington	2,319	2.06%
41	West Virginia	517	0.46%
18	Wisconsin	2,172	1.93%
50	Wyoming	203	0.18%

RANK ORDER

RANK	STATE	BIRTHS	% of USA
1	California	12,902	11.47%
2	New York	9,996	8.89%
3	Texas	7,891	7.02%
4	Pennsylvania	5,843	5.20%
5	Illinois	5,708	5.08%
6	Ohio	5,701	5.07%
7	Florida	5,410	4.81%
8	New Jersey	3,675	3.27%
9	Michigan	3,562	3.17%
10	Virginia	2,860	2.54%
11	North Carolina	2,842	2.53%
12	Massachusetts	2,790	2.48%
13	Georgia	2,536	2.26%
14	Missouri	2,505	2.23%
15	Maryland	2,493	2.22%
16	Washington	2,319	2.06%
17	Tennessee	2,174	1.93%
18	Wisconsin	2,172	1.93%
19	Indiana	2,170	1.93%
20	Minnesota	2,131	1.90%
21	Arizona	1,761	1.57%
22	Colorado	1,631	1.45%
23	Oregon	1,561	1.39%
24	Connecticut	1,433	1.27%
25	Kentucky	1,383	1.23%
26	Iowa	1,344	1.20%
27	Alabama	1,313	1.17%
28	South Carolina	1,183	1.05%
29	Utah	1,115	0.99%
30	Louisiana	1,040	0.92%
31	Oklahoma	963	0.86%
32	Kansas	955	0.85%
33	Arkansas	832	0.74%
34	New Mexico	825	0.73%
35	Nebraska	814	0.72%
36	Mississippi	740	0.66%
37	Idaho	599	0.53%
38	Hawaii	598	0.53%
39	New Hampshire	565	0.50%
40	Nevada	537	0.48%
41	West Virginia	517	0.46%
42	Maine	422	0.38%
43	Rhode Island	394	0.35%
44	Montana	388	0.35%
45	Delaware	361	0.32%
46	Alaska	274	0.24%
47	South Dakota	272	0.24%
48	North Dakota	247	0.22%
49	Vermont	219	0.19%
50	Wyoming	203	0.18%
	District of Columbia	270	0.24%

Source: U.S. Department of Health and Human Services, National Center for Health Statistics unpublished data

Percent of Vaginal Births After a Cesarean (VBAC) in 1995

National Percent = 27.5% of Live Births to Women Who Have Had a Cesarean*

ALPHA ORDER

RANK	STATE	PERCENT
47	Alabama	20.7
8	Alaska	35.3
31	Arizona	28.8
48	Arkansas	19.5
42	California	22.9
1	Colorado	40.4
11	Connecticut	33.8
25	Delaware	30.4
33	Florida	27.3
41	Georgia	23.2
12	Hawaii	33.7
4	Idaho	36.7
28	Illinois	29.1
37	Indiana	25.1
9	Iowa	34.4
39	Kansas	24.6
37	Kentucky	25.1
50	Louisiana	12.8
30	Maine	28.9
20	Maryland	32.0
20	Massachusetts	32.0
35	Michigan	26.0
3	Minnesota	37.0
49	Mississippi	15.1
22	Missouri	31.7
18	Montana	33.0
14	Nebraska	33.4
36	Nevada	25.2
7	New Hampshire	35.6
33	New Jersey	27.3
16	New Mexico	33.2
23	New York	31.0
29	North Carolina	29.0
32	North Dakota	28.7
14	Ohio	33.4
43	Oklahoma	22.7
2	Oregon	38.3
10	Pennsylvania	34.2
19	Rhode Island	32.6
44	South Carolina	22.6
40	South Dakota	24.1
27	Tennessee	29.5
46	Texas	21.0
26	Utah	30.1
6	Vermont	36.0
24	Virginia	30.5
12	Washington	33.7
45	West Virginia	21.9
5	Wisconsin	36.3
16	Wyoming	33.2

RANK ORDER

RANK	STATE	PERCENT
1	Colorado	40.4
2	Oregon	38.3
3	Minnesota	37.0
4	Idaho	36.7
5	Wisconsin	36.3
6	Vermont	36.0
7	New Hampshire	35.6
8	Alaska	35.3
9	Iowa	34.4
10	Pennsylvania	34.2
11	Connecticut	33.8
12	Hawaii	33.7
12	Washington	33.7
14	Nebraska	33.4
14	Ohio	33.4
16	New Mexico	33.2
16	Wyoming	33.2
18	Montana	33.0
19	Rhode Island	32.6
20	Maryland	32.0
20	Massachusetts	32.0
22	Missouri	31.7
23	New York	31.0
24	Virginia	30.5
25	Delaware	30.4
26	Utah	30.1
27	Tennessee	29.5
28	Illinois	29.1
29	North Carolina	29.0
30	Maine	28.9
31	Arizona	28.8
32	North Dakota	28.7
33	Florida	27.3
33	New Jersey	27.3
35	Michigan	26.0
36	Nevada	25.2
37	Indiana	25.1
37	Kentucky	25.1
39	Kansas	24.6
40	South Dakota	24.1
41	Georgia	23.2
42	California	22.9
43	Oklahoma	22.7
44	South Carolina	22.6
45	West Virginia	21.9
46	Texas	21.0
47	Alabama	20.7
48	Arkansas	19.5
49	Mississippi	15.1
50	Louisiana	12.8

	District of Columbia	27.5

Source: Morgan Quitno Press using data from US Dept of Health & Human Services, National Center for Health Statistics unpublished data

*Vaginal births after a cesarean delivery as a percent of all births to women with a previous cesarean delivery giving birth in 1995. Percent of births for which delivery data are available.

Percent of Mothers Beginning Prenatal Care in First Trimester in 1996

National Percent = 81.8% of Mothers*

ALPHA ORDER

RANK	STATE	PERCENT
32	Alabama	81.7
35	Alaska	81.2
49	Arizona	73.3
48	Arkansas	74.7
37	California	80.3
34	Colorado	81.4
5	Connecticut	88.2
23	Delaware	83.5
25	Florida	83.3
11	Georgia	85.2
16	Hawaii	84.2
43	Idaho	78.9
33	Illinois	81.5
42	Indiana	79.1
7	Iowa	87.2
8	Kansas	85.5
12	Kentucky	84.7
36	Louisiana	81.1
1	Maine	89.9
4	Maryland	88.3
21	Massachusetts	83.6
16	Michigan	84.2
21	Minnesota	83.6
45	Mississippi	78.4
8	Missouri	85.5
27	Montana	82.7
14	Nebraska	84.5
47	Nevada	77.6
3	New Hampshire	89.1
29	New Jersey	81.9
50	New Mexico	69.7
41	New York	79.2
23	North Carolina	83.5
12	North Dakota	84.7
8	Ohio	85.5
44	Oklahoma	78.7
39	Oregon	79.9
16	Pennsylvania	84.2
2	Rhode Island	89.6
40	South Carolina	79.4
31	South Dakota	81.8
25	Tennessee	83.3
46	Texas	78.2
19	Utah	84.1
6	Vermont	87.4
14	Virginia	84.5
38	Washington	80.2
28	West Virginia	82.0
19	Wisconsin	84.1
29	Wyoming	81.9

RANK ORDER

RANK	STATE	PERCENT
1	Maine	89.9
2	Rhode Island	89.6
3	New Hampshire	89.1
4	Maryland	88.3
5	Connecticut	88.2
6	Vermont	87.4
7	Iowa	87.2
8	Kansas	85.5
8	Missouri	85.5
8	Ohio	85.5
11	Georgia	85.2
12	Kentucky	84.7
12	North Dakota	84.7
14	Nebraska	84.5
14	Virginia	84.5
16	Hawaii	84.2
16	Michigan	84.2
16	Pennsylvania	84.2
19	Utah	84.1
19	Wisconsin	84.1
21	Massachusetts	83.6
21	Minnesota	83.6
23	Delaware	83.5
23	North Carolina	83.5
25	Florida	83.3
25	Tennessee	83.3
27	Montana	82.7
28	West Virginia	82.0
29	New Jersey	81.9
29	Wyoming	81.9
31	South Dakota	81.8
32	Alabama	81.7
33	Illinois	81.5
34	Colorado	81.4
35	Alaska	81.2
36	Louisiana	81.1
37	California	80.3
38	Washington	80.2
39	Oregon	79.9
40	South Carolina	79.4
41	New York	79.2
42	Indiana	79.1
43	Idaho	78.9
44	Oklahoma	78.7
45	Mississippi	78.4
46	Texas	78.2
47	Nevada	77.6
48	Arkansas	74.7
49	Arizona	73.3
50	New Mexico	69.7

District of Columbia   64.6

Source: U.S. Department of Health and Human Services, National Center for Health Statistics
    "Monthly Vital Statistics Report" (Vol. 46, No. 1(S)2, September 11, 1997)
*Preliminary data by state of residence.

Percent of White Mothers Beginning Prenatal Care in First Trimester in 1996

National Percent = 83.9% of White Mothers*

ALPHA ORDER				RANK ORDER		
RANK	STATE	PERCENT		RANK	STATE	PERCENT
11	Alabama	87.9		1	Maryland	92.4
35	Alaska	83.6		2	Rhode Island	90.8
49	Arizona	74.3		3	Maine	90.1
46	Arkansas	78.7		4	Connecticut	89.8
44	California	80.2		5	Hawaii	89.3
39	Colorado	81.9		5	New Hampshire	89.3
4	Connecticut	89.8		7	Georgia	89.0
18	Delaware	87.0		8	Louisiana	88.7
22	Florida	86.5		9	Virginia	88.4
7	Georgia	89.0		10	North Carolina	88.1
5	Hawaii	89.3		11	Alabama	87.9
45	Idaho	79.2		11	Mississippi	87.9
33	Illinois	84.7		11	Missouri	87.9
41	Indiana	81.1		14	Iowa	87.8
14	Iowa	87.8		15	Ohio	87.7
23	Kansas	86.4		16	Vermont	87.5
27	Kentucky	85.8		17	Pennsylvania	87.1
8	Louisiana	88.7		18	Delaware	87.0
3	Maine	90.1		18	Michigan	87.0
1	Maryland	92.4		18	Wisconsin	87.0
28	Massachusetts	85.5		21	Tennessee	86.7
18	Michigan	87.0		22	Florida	86.5
26	Minnesota	86.0		23	Kansas	86.4
11	Mississippi	87.9		24	North Dakota	86.3
11	Missouri	87.9		24	South Carolina	86.3
34	Montana	84.5		26	Minnesota	86.0
31	Nebraska	85.4		27	Kentucky	85.8
48	Nevada	78.5		28	Massachusetts	85.5
5	New Hampshire	89.3		28	New Jersey	85.5
28	New Jersey	85.5		28	South Dakota	85.5
50	New Mexico	71.9		31	Nebraska	85.4
36	New York	82.8		32	Utah	85.0
10	North Carolina	88.1		33	Illinois	84.7
24	North Dakota	86.3		34	Montana	84.5
15	Ohio	87.7		35	Alaska	83.6
41	Oklahoma	81.1		36	New York	82.8
43	Oregon	80.4		37	West Virginia	82.6
17	Pennsylvania	87.1		37	Wyoming	82.6
2	Rhode Island	90.8		39	Colorado	81.9
24	South Carolina	86.3		40	Washington	81.4
28	South Dakota	85.5		41	Indiana	81.1
21	Tennessee	86.7		41	Oklahoma	81.1
47	Texas	78.6		43	Oregon	80.4
32	Utah	85.0		44	California	80.2
16	Vermont	87.5		45	Idaho	79.2
9	Virginia	88.4		46	Arkansas	78.7
40	Washington	81.4		47	Texas	78.6
37	West Virginia	82.6		48	Nevada	78.5
18	Wisconsin	87.0		49	Arizona	74.3
37	Wyoming	82.6		50	New Mexico	71.9
					District of Columbia	77.1

Source: U.S. Department of Health and Human Services, National Center for Health Statistics
"Monthly Vital Statistics Report" (Vol. 46, No. 1(S)2, September 11, 1997)
*Preliminary data by state of residence.

Percent of Black Mothers Beginning Prenatal Care in First Trimester in 1996

National Percent = 71.3% of Black Mothers*

ALPHA ORDER

RANK	STATE	PERCENT
32	Alabama	68.9
3	Alaska	81.8
31	Arizona	69.7
48	Arkansas	61.0
6	California	78.5
15	Colorado	75.5
10	Connecticut	77.1
20	Delaware	72.8
22	Florida	72.3
9	Georgia	78.0
1	Hawaii	86.5
11	Idaho	76.8
33	Illinois	68.8
47	Indiana	62.6
16	Iowa	74.9
13	Kansas	76.4
17	Kentucky	74.4
29	Louisiana	70.3
2	Maine	85.5
6	Maryland	78.5
30	Massachusetts	70.2
26	Michigan	71.6
43	Minnesota	64.9
35	Mississippi	67.8
23	Missouri	72.2
4	Montana	80.6
19	Nebraska	73.4
36	Nevada	67.5
14	New Hampshire	75.7
42	New Jersey	65.6
49	New Mexico	60.9
34	New York	68.4
25	North Carolina	71.8
8	North Dakota	78.2
21	Ohio	72.4
38	Oklahoma	67.1
12	Oregon	76.6
38	Pennsylvania	67.1
5	Rhode Island	78.6
37	South Carolina	67.2
45	South Dakota	63.9
27	Tennessee	71.5
18	Texas	74.0
46	Utah	62.7
NA	Vermont**	NA
24	Virginia	72.1
28	Washington	71.0
41	West Virginia	66.0
40	Wisconsin	66.2
44	Wyoming	64.6

RANK ORDER

RANK	STATE	PERCENT
1	Hawaii	86.5
2	Maine	85.5
3	Alaska	81.8
4	Montana	80.6
5	Rhode Island	78.6
6	California	78.5
6	Maryland	78.5
8	North Dakota	78.2
9	Georgia	78.0
10	Connecticut	77.1
11	Idaho	76.8
12	Oregon	76.6
13	Kansas	76.4
14	New Hampshire	75.7
15	Colorado	75.5
16	Iowa	74.9
17	Kentucky	74.4
18	Texas	74.0
19	Nebraska	73.4
20	Delaware	72.8
21	Ohio	72.4
22	Florida	72.3
23	Missouri	72.2
24	Virginia	72.1
25	North Carolina	71.8
26	Michigan	71.6
27	Tennessee	71.5
28	Washington	71.0
29	Louisiana	70.3
30	Massachusetts	70.2
31	Arizona	69.7
32	Alabama	68.9
33	Illinois	68.8
34	New York	68.4
35	Mississippi	67.8
36	Nevada	67.5
37	South Carolina	67.2
38	Oklahoma	67.1
38	Pennsylvania	67.1
40	Wisconsin	66.2
41	West Virginia	66.0
42	New Jersey	65.6
43	Minnesota	64.9
44	Wyoming	64.6
45	South Dakota	63.9
46	Utah	62.7
47	Indiana	62.6
48	Arkansas	61.0
49	New Mexico	60.9
NA	Vermont**	NA
	District of Columbia	60.1

Source: U.S. Department of Health and Human Services, National Center for Health Statistics
   "Monthly Vital Statistics Report" (Vol. 46, No. 1(S)2, September 11, 1997)
Preliminary data by state of residence.
**Insufficient data.*

Percent of Mother Receiving Late or No Prenatal Care in 1995

National Percent = 4.2% of Mothers*

ALPHA ORDER				RANK ORDER		
RANK	STATE	PERCENT		RANK	STATE	PERCENT
18	Alabama	3.8		1	Arizona	8.2
29	Alaska	3.3		2	New Mexico	8.1
1	Arizona	8.2		3	Nevada	7.9
4	Arkansas	6.3		4	Arkansas	6.3
6	California	5.2		5	Texas	5.7
8	Colorado	5.1		6	California	5.2
43	Connecticut	2.5		6	New York	5.2
41	Delaware	2.8		8	Colorado	5.1
27	Florida	3.4		9	Oklahoma	4.9
32	Georgia	3.2		10	Mississippi	4.8
20	Hawaii	3.6		10	South Carolina	4.8
15	Idaho	4.1		12	Illinois	4.4
12	Illinois	4.4		13	Oregon	4.3
20	Indiana	3.6		14	New Jersey	4.2
44	Iowa	2.4		15	Idaho	4.1
42	Kansas	2.7		16	Louisiana	4.0
39	Kentucky	2.9		17	Pennsylvania	3.9
16	Louisiana	4.0		18	Alabama	3.8
49	Maine	1.7		18	Wyoming	3.8
34	Maryland	3.0		20	Hawaii	3.6
46	Massachusetts	1.9		20	Indiana	3.6
29	Michigan	3.3		20	South Dakota	3.6
34	Minnesota	3.0		20	Tennessee	3.6
10	Mississippi	4.8		24	Montana	3.5
34	Missouri	3.0		24	Ohio	3.5
24	Montana	3.5		24	Washington	3.5
39	Nebraska	2.9		27	Florida	3.4
3	Nevada	7.9		27	Wisconsin	3.4
48	New Hampshire	1.8		29	Alaska	3.3
14	New Jersey	4.2		29	Michigan	3.3
2	New Mexico	8.1		29	North Carolina	3.3
6	New York	5.2		32	Georgia	3.2
29	North Carolina	3.3		32	Virginia	3.2
45	North Dakota	2.3		34	Maryland	3.0
24	Ohio	3.5		34	Minnesota	3.0
9	Oklahoma	4.9		34	Missouri	3.0
13	Oregon	4.3		34	Utah	3.0
17	Pennsylvania	3.9		34	West Virginia	3.0
50	Rhode Island	1.3		39	Kentucky	2.9
10	South Carolina	4.8		39	Nebraska	2.9
20	South Dakota	3.6		41	Delaware	2.8
20	Tennessee	3.6		42	Kansas	2.7
5	Texas	5.7		43	Connecticut	2.5
34	Utah	3.0		44	Iowa	2.4
46	Vermont	1.9		45	North Dakota	2.3
32	Virginia	3.2		46	Massachusetts	1.9
24	Washington	3.5		46	Vermont	1.9
34	West Virginia	3.0		48	New Hampshire	1.8
27	Wisconsin	3.4		49	Maine	1.7
18	Wyoming	3.8		50	Rhode Island	1.3

District of Columbia 14.9

Source: U.S. Department of Health and Human Services, National Center for Health Statistics
"Monthly Vital Statistics Report" (Vol. 45, No. 11, June 10, 1997)
*Final data by state of residence. "Late" means care begun in third trimester.

Percent of White Mothers Receiving Late or No Prenatal Care in 1995

National Rate = 3.5% of White Mothers*

ALPHA ORDER

RANK	STATE	PERCENT
32	Alabama	2.2
20	Alaska	2.7
1	Arizona	7.8
7	Arkansas	4.7
5	California	5.2
6	Colorado	4.9
36	Connecticut	2.1
42	Delaware	1.9
23	Florida	2.6
36	Georgia	2.1
32	Hawaii	2.2
10	Idaho	4.0
14	Illinois	3.1
14	Indiana	3.1
30	Iowa	2.3
28	Kansas	2.4
23	Kentucky	2.6
42	Louisiana	1.9
47	Maine	1.7
48	Maryland	1.6
49	Massachusetts	1.5
30	Michigan	2.3
32	Minnesota	2.2
36	Mississippi	2.1
32	Missouri	2.2
16	Montana	2.8
23	Nebraska	2.6
2	Nevada	7.6
46	New Hampshire	1.8
16	New Jersey	2.8
3	New Mexico	7.2
9	New York	4.1
36	North Carolina	2.1
42	North Dakota	1.9
27	Ohio	2.5
11	Oklahoma	3.9
8	Oregon	4.2
20	Pennsylvania	2.7
50	Rhode Island	1.1
16	South Carolina	2.8
41	South Dakota	2.0
28	Tennessee	2.4
4	Texas	5.6
20	Utah	2.7
42	Vermont	1.9
36	Virginia	2.1
13	Washington	3.2
16	West Virginia	2.8
23	Wisconsin	2.6
12	Wyoming	3.5

RANK ORDER

RANK	STATE	PERCENT
1	Arizona	7.8
2	Nevada	7.6
3	New Mexico	7.2
4	Texas	5.6
5	California	5.2
6	Colorado	4.9
7	Arkansas	4.7
8	Oregon	4.2
9	New York	4.1
10	Idaho	4.0
11	Oklahoma	3.9
12	Wyoming	3.5
13	Washington	3.2
14	Illinois	3.1
14	Indiana	3.1
16	Montana	2.8
16	New Jersey	2.8
16	South Carolina	2.8
16	West Virginia	2.8
20	Alaska	2.7
20	Pennsylvania	2.7
20	Utah	2.7
23	Florida	2.6
23	Kentucky	2.6
23	Nebraska	2.6
23	Wisconsin	2.6
27	Ohio	2.5
28	Kansas	2.4
28	Tennessee	2.4
30	Iowa	2.3
30	Michigan	2.3
32	Alabama	2.2
32	Hawaii	2.2
32	Minnesota	2.2
32	Missouri	2.2
36	Connecticut	2.1
36	Georgia	2.1
36	Mississippi	2.1
36	North Carolina	2.1
36	Virginia	2.1
41	South Dakota	2.0
42	Delaware	1.9
42	Louisiana	1.9
42	North Dakota	1.9
42	Vermont	1.9
46	New Hampshire	1.8
47	Maine	1.7
48	Maryland	1.6
49	Massachusetts	1.5
50	Rhode Island	1.1

| | District of Columbia | 8.2 |

Source: U.S. Department of Health and Human Services, National Center for Health Statistics
"Monthly Vital Statistics Report" (Vol. 45, No. 11, Supplement, June 10, 1997)
*Final data by state of residence. "Late" means care begun in third trimester.

Percent of Black Mothers Receiving Late or No Prenatal Care in 1995

National Percent = 7.6% of Black Mothers*

ALPHA ORDER

RANK ORDER

RANK	STATE	PERCENT	RANK	STATE	PERCENT
23	Alabama	7.0	1	New Mexico	12.9
NA	Alaska**	NA	2	Arkansas	12.1
14	Arizona	8.2	3	Nevada	12.0
2	Arkansas	12.1	4	Pennsylvania	11.1
32	California	6.0	5	New Jersey	10.4
19	Colorado	7.5	6	Ohio	9.3
36	Connecticut	5.5	7	Illinois	9.2
34	Delaware	5.8	7	Minnesota	9.2
33	Florida	5.9	9	Wisconsin	9.1
37	Georgia	5.4	10	New York	9.0
NA	Hawaii**	NA	11	Oklahoma	8.7
NA	Idaho**	NA	12	South Carolina	8.4
7	Illinois	9.2	13	West Virginia	8.3
20	Indiana	7.2	14	Arizona	8.2
31	Iowa	6.2	15	Michigan	7.7
35	Kansas	5.6	15	Mississippi	7.7
26	Kentucky	6.5	15	Missouri	7.7
22	Louisiana	7.1	18	Tennessee	7.6
NA	Maine**	NA	19	Colorado	7.5
27	Maryland	6.4	20	Indiana	7.2
38	Massachusetts	4.7	20	Oregon	7.2
15	Michigan	7.7	22	Louisiana	7.1
7	Minnesota	9.2	23	Alabama	7.0
15	Mississippi	7.7	24	Virginia	6.7
15	Missouri	7.7	25	Texas	6.6
NA	Montana**	NA	26	Kentucky	6.5
29	Nebraska	6.3	27	Maryland	6.4
3	Nevada	12.0	27	North Carolina	6.4
NA	New Hampshire**	NA	29	Nebraska	6.3
5	New Jersey	10.4	29	Washington	6.3
1	New Mexico	12.9	31	Iowa	6.2
10	New York	9.0	32	California	6.0
27	North Carolina	6.4	33	Florida	5.9
NA	North Dakota**	NA	34	Delaware	5.8
6	Ohio	9.3	35	Kansas	5.6
11	Oklahoma	8.7	36	Connecticut	5.5
20	Oregon	7.2	37	Georgia	5.4
4	Pennsylvania	11.1	38	Massachusetts	4.7
39	Rhode Island	4.5	39	Rhode Island	4.5
12	South Carolina	8.4	NA	Alaska**	NA
NA	South Dakota**	NA	NA	Hawaii**	NA
18	Tennessee	7.6	NA	Idaho**	NA
25	Texas	6.6	NA	Maine**	NA
NA	Utah**	NA	NA	Montana**	NA
NA	Vermont**	NA	NA	New Hampshire**	NA
24	Virginia	6.7	NA	North Dakota**	NA
29	Washington	6.3	NA	South Dakota**	NA
13	West Virginia	8.3	NA	Utah**	NA
9	Wisconsin	9.1	NA	Vermont**	NA
NA	Wyoming**	NA	NA	Wyoming**	NA
				District of Columbia	17.0

Source: U.S. Department of Health and Human Services, National Center for Health Statistics
"Monthly Vital Statistics Report" (Vol. 45, No. 11, Supplement, June 10, 1997)
Final data by state of residence. "Late" means care begun in third trimester.
**Insufficient data.*

Percent of Births to Women Who Smoked During Pregnancy in 1995

National Percent = 13.9% of Live Births*

ALPHA ORDER			RANK ORDER		
RANK	**STATE**	**PERCENT**	**RANK**	**STATE**	**PERCENT**
28	Alabama	13.4	1	Kentucky	24.7
7	Alaska	19.2	2	West Virginia	24.6
38	Arizona	11.5	3	Ohio	20.2
6	Arkansas	19.3	4	Missouri	20.1
NA	California**	NA	5	Wyoming	19.8
35	Colorado	12.7	6	Arkansas	19.3
41	Connecticut	10.4	7	Alaska	19.2
30	Delaware	13.2	8	Wisconsin	18.9
33	Florida	12.9	9	Iowa	18.6
39	Georgia	11.2	9	Montana	18.6
45	Hawaii	8.4	9	Pennsylvania	18.6
26	Idaho	13.7	12	Michigan	18.3
33	Illinois	12.9	13	Maine	18.2
NA	Indiana**	NA	14	Tennessee	18.1
9	Iowa	18.6	15	North Dakota	17.9
36	Kansas	12.6	15	Oregon	17.9
1	Kentucky	24.7	17	Nebraska	17.5
40	Louisiana	11.1	17	New Hampshire	17.5
13	Maine	18.2	17	Oklahoma	17.5
37	Maryland	11.8	20	Vermont	17.0
27	Massachusetts	13.6	21	Rhode Island	16.6
12	Michigan	18.3	22	Washington	16.2
28	Minnesota	13.4	23	Nevada	16.1
31	Mississippi	13.0	24	North Carolina	15.9
4	Missouri	20.1	25	South Carolina	14.8
9	Montana	18.6	26	Idaho	13.7
17	Nebraska	17.5	27	Massachusetts	13.6
23	Nevada	16.1	28	Alabama	13.4
17	New Hampshire	17.5	28	Minnesota	13.4
44	New Jersey	8.9	30	Delaware	13.2
42	New Mexico	10.2	31	Mississippi	13.0
47	New York	5.6	31	Virginia	13.0
24	North Carolina	15.9	33	Florida	12.9
15	North Dakota	17.9	33	Illinois	12.9
3	Ohio	20.2	35	Colorado	12.7
17	Oklahoma	17.5	36	Kansas	12.6
15	Oregon	17.9	37	Maryland	11.8
9	Pennsylvania	18.6	38	Arizona	11.5
21	Rhode Island	16.6	39	Georgia	11.2
25	South Carolina	14.8	40	Louisiana	11.1
NA	South Dakota**	NA	41	Connecticut	10.4
14	Tennessee	18.1	42	New Mexico	10.2
46	Texas	7.9	43	Utah	9.2
43	Utah	9.2	44	New Jersey	8.9
20	Vermont	17.0	45	Hawaii	8.4
31	Virginia	13.0	46	Texas	7.9
22	Washington	16.2	47	New York	5.6
2	West Virginia	24.6	NA	California**	NA
8	Wisconsin	18.9	NA	Indiana**	NA
5	Wyoming	19.8	NA	South Dakota**	NA
				District of Columbia	8.3

Source: U.S. Department of Health and Human Services, National Center for Health Statistics
(unpublished data)
*HHS defines "Smoker" as averaging at least one cigarette a day.
**Not available.

Percent of Births Attended by Midwives in 1995

National Percent = 6.0% of Live Births*

ALPHA ORDER				RANK ORDER		
RANK	STATE	PERCENT		RANK	STATE	PERCENT
38	Alabama	3.4		1	New Mexico	17.9
2	Alaska	17.0		2	Alaska	17.0
14	Arizona	8.6		3	Oregon	12.9
43	Arkansas	1.9		4	Vermont	12.5
16	California	7.6		5	New Hampshire	12.2
17	Colorado	7.2		6	Georgia	12.0
23	Connecticut	6.3		7	Massachusetts	11.1
8	Delaware	10.8		8	Delaware	10.8
11	Florida	9.5		9	Maine	10.4
6	Georgia	12.0		10	Rhode Island	10.1
30	Hawaii	4.1		11	Florida	9.5
30	Idaho	4.1		12	New York	9.3
42	Illinois	2.5		13	Montana	8.7
43	Indiana	1.9		14	Arizona	8.6
45	Iowa	1.4		15	Washington	8.2
48	Kansas	0.7		16	California	7.6
39	Kentucky	3.3		17	Colorado	7.2
50	Louisiana	0.5		17	Utah	7.2
9	Maine	10.4		19	Maryland	6.6
19	Maryland	6.6		19	Minnesota	6.6
7	Massachusetts	11.1		21	Nevada	6.4
27	Michigan	5.1		21	South Carolina	6.4
19	Minnesota	6.6		23	Connecticut	6.3
46	Mississippi	1.1		24	Pennsylvania	6.0
49	Missouri	0.6		25	West Virginia	5.8
13	Montana	8.7		26	North Carolina	5.3
46	Nebraska	1.1		27	Michigan	5.1
21	Nevada	6.4		27	Wyoming	5.1
5	New Hampshire	12.2		29	North Dakota	4.8
32	New Jersey	3.7		30	Hawaii	4.1
1	New Mexico	17.9		30	Idaho	4.1
12	New York	9.3		32	New Jersey	3.7
26	North Carolina	5.3		32	Oklahoma	3.7
29	North Dakota	4.8		32	Tennessee	3.7
39	Ohio	3.3		32	Texas	3.7
32	Oklahoma	3.7		36	South Dakota	3.6
3	Oregon	12.9		37	Wisconsin	3.5
24	Pennsylvania	6.0		38	Alabama	3.4
10	Rhode Island	10.1		39	Kentucky	3.3
21	South Carolina	6.4		39	Ohio	3.3
36	South Dakota	3.6		41	Virginia	3.2
32	Tennessee	3.7		42	Illinois	2.5
32	Texas	3.7		43	Arkansas	1.9
17	Utah	7.2		43	Indiana	1.9
4	Vermont	12.5		45	Iowa	1.4
41	Virginia	3.2		46	Mississippi	1.1
15	Washington	8.2		46	Nebraska	1.1
25	West Virginia	5.8		48	Kansas	0.7
37	Wisconsin	3.5		49	Missouri	0.6
27	Wyoming	5.1		50	Louisiana	0.5
					District of Columbia	5.3

Source: Morgan Quitno Press using data from U.S. Dept of Health & Human Services, National Center for Health Statistics (unpublished data)

*Includes certified nurse midwives and other midwives.

Reported Legal Abortions in 1994

National Total = 1,267,415 Abortions*

ALPHA ORDER

RANK	STATE	ABORTIONS	% of USA
17	Alabama	14,825	1.17%
46	Alaska	1,585	0.13%
20	Arizona	13,930	1.10%
34	Arkansas	5,885	0.46%
1	California	308,564	24.35%
28	Colorado	9,584	0.76%
18	Connecticut	14,757	1.16%
36	Delaware	5,637	0.44%
4	Florida	73,394	5.79%
8	Georgia	36,374	2.87%
35	Hawaii	5,783	0.46%
48	Idaho	1,047	0.08%
5	Illinois	55,050	4.34%
23	Indiana	12,499	0.99%
33	Iowa	5,914	0.47%
27	Kansas	10,468	0.83%
29	Kentucky	8,145	0.64%
24	Louisiana	12,154	0.96%
41	Maine	3,089	0.24%
15	Maryland	17,627	1.39%
12	Massachusetts	32,195	2.54%
11	Michigan	33,061	2.61%
19	Minnesota	14,027	1.11%
39	Mississippi	3,979	0.31%
25	Missouri	11,879	0.94%
43	Montana	2,761	0.22%
37	Nebraska	5,324	0.42%
31	Nevada	6,736	0.53%
42	New Hampshire	3,008	0.24%
10	New Jersey	33,286	2.63%
38	New Mexico	4,929	0.39%
2	New York	149,598	11.80%
9	North Carolina	35,088	2.77%
47	North Dakota	1,301	0.10%
7	Ohio	37,742	2.98%
30	Oklahoma	6,774	0.53%
22	Oregon	13,392	1.06%
6	Pennsylvania	41,645	3.29%
32	Rhode Island	6,092	0.48%
26	South Carolina	10,922	0.86%
49	South Dakota	987	0.08%
16	Tennessee	16,837	1.33%
3	Texas	89,185	7.04%
40	Utah	3,609	0.28%
44	Vermont	2,321	0.18%
13	Virginia	26,369	2.08%
14	Washington	25,965	2.05%
45	West Virginia	2,085	0.16%
21	Wisconsin	13,396	1.06%
50	Wyoming	174	0.01%

RANK ORDER

RANK	STATE	ABORTIONS	% of USA
1	California	308,564	24.35%
2	New York	149,598	11.80%
3	Texas	89,185	7.04%
4	Florida	73,394	5.79%
5	Illinois	55,050	4.34%
6	Pennsylvania	41,645	3.29%
7	Ohio	37,742	2.98%
8	Georgia	36,374	2.87%
9	North Carolina	35,088	2.77%
10	New Jersey	33,286	2.63%
11	Michigan	33,061	2.61%
12	Massachusetts	32,195	2.54%
13	Virginia	26,369	2.08%
14	Washington	25,965	2.05%
15	Maryland	17,627	1.39%
16	Tennessee	16,837	1.33%
17	Alabama	14,825	1.17%
18	Connecticut	14,757	1.16%
19	Minnesota	14,027	1.11%
20	Arizona	13,930	1.10%
21	Wisconsin	13,396	1.06%
22	Oregon	13,392	1.06%
23	Indiana	12,499	0.99%
24	Louisiana	12,154	0.96%
25	Missouri	11,879	0.94%
26	South Carolina	10,922	0.86%
27	Kansas	10,468	0.83%
28	Colorado	9,584	0.76%
29	Kentucky	8,145	0.64%
30	Oklahoma	6,774	0.53%
31	Nevada	6,736	0.53%
32	Rhode Island	6,092	0.48%
33	Iowa	5,914	0.47%
34	Arkansas	5,885	0.46%
35	Hawaii	5,783	0.46%
36	Delaware	5,637	0.44%
37	Nebraska	5,324	0.42%
38	New Mexico	4,929	0.39%
39	Mississippi	3,979	0.31%
40	Utah	3,609	0.28%
41	Maine	3,089	0.24%
42	New Hampshire	3,008	0.24%
43	Montana	2,761	0.22%
44	Vermont	2,321	0.18%
45	West Virginia	2,085	0.16%
46	Alaska	1,585	0.13%
47	North Dakota	1,301	0.10%
48	Idaho	1,047	0.08%
49	South Dakota	987	0.08%
50	Wyoming	174	0.01%
	District of Columbia	16,437	1.30%

Source: U.S. Department of Health and Human Services, Centers for Disease Control and Prevention
"Abortion Surveillance-United States, 1993 & 1994" (Morbidity Mortality Weekly Report, Vol. 46, No. SS-4, 8/8/97)
*By state of occurrence.

Reported Legal Abortions per 1,000 Live Births in 1994

National Rate = 321 Abortions per 1,000 Live Births*

ALPHA ORDER

RANK	STATE	RATE
22	Alabama	244
44	Alaska	148
32	Arizona	196
37	Arkansas	169
2	California	544
36	Colorado	177
10	Connecticut	323
3	Delaware	543
5	Florida	385
9	Georgia	328
13	Hawaii	298
49	Idaho	60
14	Illinois	291
42	Indiana	151
39	Iowa	160
17	Kansas	281
40	Kentucky	154
34	Louisiana	179
29	Maine	215
25	Maryland	238
6	Massachusetts	384
24	Michigan	240
28	Minnesota	218
46	Mississippi	95
38	Missouri	162
21	Montana	250
26	Nebraska	230
16	Nevada	282
31	New Hampshire	199
15	New Jersey	283
34	New Mexico	179
1	New York	549
7	North Carolina	346
41	North Dakota	152
23	Ohio	242
43	Oklahoma	149
11	Oregon	320
20	Pennsylvania	266
4	Rhode Island	452
30	South Carolina	210
47	South Dakota	94
26	Tennessee	230
19	Texas	278
47	Utah	94
12	Vermont	314
18	Virginia	279
8	Washington	336
45	West Virginia	98
32	Wisconsin	196
50	Wyoming	27

RANK ORDER

RANK	STATE	RATE
1	New York	549
2	California	544
3	Delaware	543
4	Rhode Island	452
5	Florida	385
6	Massachusetts	384
7	North Carolina	346
8	Washington	336
9	Georgia	328
10	Connecticut	323
11	Oregon	320
12	Vermont	314
13	Hawaii	298
14	Illinois	291
15	New Jersey	283
16	Nevada	282
17	Kansas	281
18	Virginia	279
19	Texas	278
20	Pennsylvania	266
21	Montana	250
22	Alabama	244
23	Ohio	242
24	Michigan	240
25	Maryland	238
26	Nebraska	230
26	Tennessee	230
28	Minnesota	218
29	Maine	215
30	South Carolina	210
31	New Hampshire	199
32	Arizona	196
32	Wisconsin	196
34	Louisiana	179
34	New Mexico	179
36	Colorado	177
37	Arkansas	169
38	Missouri	162
39	Iowa	160
40	Kentucky	154
41	North Dakota	152
42	Indiana	151
43	Oklahoma	149
44	Alaska	148
45	West Virginia	98
46	Mississippi	95
47	South Dakota	94
47	Utah	94
49	Idaho	60
50	Wyoming	27
	District of Columbia**	NA

Source: U.S. Department of Health and Human Services, Centers for Disease Control and Prevention
    "Abortion Surveillance-United States, 1993 & 1994" (Morbidity Mortality Weekly Report, Vol. 46, No. SS-4, 8/8/97)
*By state of occurrence.
**The District of Columbia's ratio was not listed but was noted as being greater than 1,000 abortions per 1,000 live births.

Reported Legal Abortions per 1,000 Women Ages 15 to 44 in 1994

National Rate = 21 Reported Legal Abortions per 1,000 Women Ages 15 to 44*

ALPHA ORDER

RANK	STATE	RATE
22	Alabama	15
34	Alaska	11
20	Arizona	16
34	Arkansas	11
1	California	43
34	Colorado	11
14	Connecticut	20
3	Delaware	34
5	Florida	25
8	Georgia	21
7	Hawaii	22
49	Idaho	4
8	Illinois	21
42	Indiana	9
39	Iowa	10
16	Kansas	19
42	Kentucky	9
32	Louisiana	12
34	Maine	11
22	Maryland	15
6	Massachusetts	23
22	Michigan	15
29	Minnesota	13
46	Mississippi	6
39	Missouri	10
22	Montana	15
22	Nebraska	15
8	Nevada	21
34	New Hampshire	11
16	New Jersey	19
29	New Mexico	13
2	New York	36
8	North Carolina	21
42	North Dakota	9
22	Ohio	15
39	Oklahoma	10
14	Oregon	20
20	Pennsylvania	16
4	Rhode Island	27
29	South Carolina	13
46	South Dakota	6
28	Tennessee	14
8	Texas	21
45	Utah	8
18	Vermont	17
18	Virginia	17
8	Washington	21
48	West Virginia	5
32	Wisconsin	12
50	Wyoming	2

RANK ORDER

RANK	STATE	RATE
1	California	43
2	New York	36
3	Delaware	34
4	Rhode Island	27
5	Florida	25
6	Massachusetts	23
7	Hawaii	22
8	Georgia	21
8	Illinois	21
8	Nevada	21
8	North Carolina	21
8	Texas	21
8	Washington	21
14	Connecticut	20
14	Oregon	20
16	Kansas	19
16	New Jersey	19
18	Vermont	17
18	Virginia	17
20	Arizona	16
20	Pennsylvania	16
22	Alabama	15
22	Maryland	15
22	Michigan	15
22	Montana	15
22	Nebraska	15
22	Ohio	15
28	Tennessee	14
29	Minnesota	13
29	New Mexico	13
29	South Carolina	13
32	Louisiana	12
32	Wisconsin	12
34	Alaska	11
34	Arkansas	11
34	Colorado	11
34	Maine	11
34	New Hampshire	11
39	Iowa	10
39	Missouri	10
39	Oklahoma	10
42	Indiana	9
42	Kentucky	9
42	North Dakota	9
45	Utah	8
46	Mississippi	6
46	South Dakota	6
48	West Virginia	5
49	Idaho	4
50	Wyoming	2
	District of Columbia**	NA

Source: U.S. Department of Health and Human Services, Centers for Disease Control and Prevention
"Abortion Surveillance-United States, 1994" (Morbidity and Mortality Weekly Report, Vol. 46, No. SS-4, 8/8/97)
*By state of occurrence.
**The District of Columbia's rate was not listed but was noted as being greater than 100 abortions per 1,000 women ages 15 to 44 years.

Percent of Reported Legal Abortions Obtained by Out-Of-State Residents: 1994

National Percent = 8.5% of Reported Legal Abortions*

ALPHA ORDER				RANK ORDER		
RANK	STATE	PERCENT		RANK	STATE	PERCENT
16	Alabama	10.4		1	Kansas	40.6
NA	Alaska**	NA		2	Utah	29.9
38	Arizona	3.5		3	North Dakota	28.1
23	Arkansas	6.6		4	Vermont	25.3
NA	California**	NA		5	Kentucky	23.1
20	Colorado	7.7		6	Rhode Island	20.5
36	Connecticut	3.9		7	South Dakota	20.3
NA	Delaware**	NA		8	Nebraska	20.2
NA	Florida**	NA		9	Tennessee	17.5
17	Georgia	9.5		10	Montana	17.1
40	Hawaii	0.5		11	West Virginia	12.9
22	Idaho	7.2		12	Oregon	11.6
NA	Illinois**	NA		13	Nevada	11.3
33	Indiana	4.4		14	North Carolina	10.8
NA	Iowa**	NA		15	Missouri	10.6
1	Kansas	40.6		16	Alabama	10.4
5	Kentucky	23.1		17	Georgia	9.5
NA	Louisiana**	NA		18	Minnesota	9.2
27	Maine	5.0		19	Ohio	7.9
23	Maryland	6.6		20	Colorado	7.7
34	Massachusetts	4.3		21	South Carolina	7.6
37	Michigan	3.8		22	Idaho	7.2
18	Minnesota	9.2		23	Arkansas	6.6
35	Mississippi	4.1		23	Maryland	6.6
15	Missouri	10.6		25	Virginia	6.3
10	Montana	17.1		25	Wyoming	6.3
8	Nebraska	20.2		27	Maine	5.0
13	Nevada	11.3		27	Texas	5.0
NA	New Hampshire**	NA		27	Washington	5.0
39	New Jersey	2.1		30	New Mexico	4.9
30	New Mexico	4.9		31	Pennsylvania	4.8
NA	New York**	NA		32	Wisconsin	4.5
14	North Carolina	10.8		33	Indiana	4.4
3	North Dakota	28.1		34	Massachusetts	4.3
19	Ohio	7.9		35	Mississippi	4.1
NA	Oklahoma**	NA		36	Connecticut	3.9
12	Oregon	11.6		37	Michigan	3.8
31	Pennsylvania	4.8		38	Arizona	3.5
6	Rhode Island	20.5		39	New Jersey	2.1
21	South Carolina	7.6		40	Hawaii	0.5
7	South Dakota	20.3		NA	Alaska**	NA
9	Tennessee	17.5		NA	California**	NA
27	Texas	5.0		NA	Delaware**	NA
2	Utah	29.9		NA	Florida**	NA
4	Vermont	25.3		NA	Illinois**	NA
25	Virginia	6.3		NA	Iowa**	NA
27	Washington	5.0		NA	Louisiana**	NA
11	West Virginia	12.9		NA	New Hampshire**	NA
32	Wisconsin	4.5		NA	New York**	NA
25	Wyoming	6.3		NA	Oklahoma**	NA
				District of Columbia		51.9

Source: U.S. Department of Health and Human Services, Centers for Disease Control and Prevention
   "Abortion Surveillance-United States, 1994" (Morbidity and Mortality Weekly Report, Vol. 46, No. SS-4, 8/8/97)
*By state of occurrence.
**Not reported.

Percent of Reported Legal Abortions Obtained by White Women in 1994

Reporting States' Percent = 58.4% of Reported Legal Abortions*

ALPHA ORDER

RANK ORDER

RANK	STATE	PERCENT	RANK	STATE	PERCENT
28	Alabama	52.8	1	Vermont	96.4
NA	Alaska**	NA	2	Idaho	95.9
14	Arizona	79.1	3	Maine	94.3
20	Arkansas	63.9	4	North Dakota	90.3
NA	California**	NA	5	South Dakota	88.9
NA	Colorado**	NA	6	New Mexico	86.7
NA	Connecticut**	NA	7	Oregon	85.6
NA	Delaware**	NA	8	Utah	85.4
NA	Florida**	NA	9	Montana	84.4
30	Georgia	46.0	10	West Virginia	82.4
35	Hawaii	29.9	11	Minnesota	82.0
2	Idaho	95.9	12	Nevada	81.7
NA	Illinois**	NA	13	Rhode Island	79.8
19	Indiana	65.9	14	Arizona	79.1
NA	Iowa**	NA	15	Kansas	78.5
15	Kansas	78.5	16	Kentucky	77.0
16	Kentucky	77.0	17	Wisconsin	74.5
31	Louisiana	45.3	18	Texas	71.5
3	Maine	94.3	19	Indiana	65.9
32	Maryland	42.4	20	Arkansas	63.9
NA	Massachusetts**	NA	21	Missouri	63.3
NA	Michigan**	NA	22	Tennessee	63.1
11	Minnesota	82.0	23	Ohio	60.6
34	Mississippi	35.5	24	Pennsylvania	59.7
21	Missouri	63.3	25	Virginia	58.6
9	Montana	84.4	26	South Carolina	54.3
NA	Nebraska**	NA	27	North Carolina	53.9
12	Nevada	81.7	28	Alabama	52.8
NA	New Hampshire**	NA	29	New York	50.5
33	New Jersey	35.6	30	Georgia	46.0
6	New Mexico	86.7	31	Louisiana	45.3
29	New York	50.5	32	Maryland	42.4
27	North Carolina	53.9	33	New Jersey	35.6
4	North Dakota	90.3	34	Mississippi	35.5
23	Ohio	60.6	35	Hawaii	29.9
NA	Oklahoma**	NA	NA	Alaska**	NA
7	Oregon	85.6	NA	California**	NA
24	Pennsylvania	59.7	NA	Colorado**	NA
13	Rhode Island	79.8	NA	Connecticut**	NA
26	South Carolina	54.3	NA	Delaware**	NA
5	South Dakota	88.9	NA	Florida**	NA
22	Tennessee	63.1	NA	Illinois**	NA
18	Texas	71.5	NA	Iowa**	NA
8	Utah	85.4	NA	Massachusetts**	NA
1	Vermont	96.4	NA	Michigan**	NA
25	Virginia	58.6	NA	Nebraska**	NA
NA	Washington**	NA	NA	New Hampshire**	NA
10	West Virginia	82.4	NA	Oklahoma**	NA
17	Wisconsin	74.5	NA	Washington**	NA
NA	Wyoming**	NA	NA	Wyoming**	NA
				District of Columbia	19.1

Source: U.S. Department of Health and Human Services, Centers for Disease Control and Prevention
   "Abortion Surveillance-United States, 1994" (Morbidity and Mortality Weekly Report, Vol. 46, No. SS-4, 8/8/97)
*By state of occurrence. Includes those of Hispanic ethnicity. National percent is for reporting states only.
**Not reported.

Percent of Reported Legal Abortions Obtained by Black Women in 1994

Reporting States' Percent = 33.4% of Reported Legal Abortions*

ALPHA ORDER				RANK ORDER		
RANK	STATE	PERCENT		RANK	STATE	PERCENT
6	Alabama	44.0		1	Mississippi	63.3
NA	Alaska**	NA		2	Georgia	50.3
25	Arizona	5.2		2	Maryland	50.3
14	Arkansas	32.7		4	New York	46.2
NA	California**	NA		5	New Jersey	45.3
NA	Colorado**	NA		6	Alabama	44.0
NA	Connecticut**	NA		7	South Carolina	43.6
NA	Delaware**	NA		8	North Carolina	40.4
NA	Florida**	NA		9	Louisiana	40.3
2	Georgia	50.3		10	Pennsylvania	37.2
27	Hawaii	3.3		11	Virginia	36.7
34	Idaho	0.7		12	Tennessee	34.8
NA	Illinois**	NA		13	Missouri	33.5
16	Indiana	20.6		14	Arkansas	32.7
NA	Iowa**	NA		15	Ohio	29.9
20	Kansas	16.2		16	Indiana	20.6
19	Kentucky	19.1		17	Texas	20.3
9	Louisiana	40.3		17	Wisconsin	20.3
32	Maine	1.1		19	Kentucky	19.1
2	Maryland	50.3		20	Kansas	16.2
NA	Massachusetts**	NA		20	West Virginia	16.2
NA	Michigan**	NA		22	Rhode Island	13.7
23	Minnesota	9.4		23	Minnesota	9.4
1	Mississippi	63.3		24	Nevada	9.0
13	Missouri	33.5		25	Arizona	5.2
35	Montana	0.4		26	Oregon	4.8
NA	Nebraska**	NA		27	Hawaii	3.3
24	Nevada	9.0		28	New Mexico	2.9
NA	New Hampshire**	NA		29	Utah	1.8
5	New Jersey	45.3		30	South Dakota	1.4
28	New Mexico	2.9		31	North Dakota	1.2
4	New York	46.2		32	Maine	1.1
8	North Carolina	40.4		33	Vermont	1.0
31	North Dakota	1.2		34	Idaho	0.7
15	Ohio	29.9		35	Montana	0.4
NA	Oklahoma**	NA		NA	Alaska**	NA
26	Oregon	4.8		NA	California**	NA
10	Pennsylvania	37.2		NA	Colorado**	NA
22	Rhode Island	13.7		NA	Connecticut**	NA
7	South Carolina	43.6		NA	Delaware**	NA
30	South Dakota	1.4		NA	Florida**	NA
12	Tennessee	34.8		NA	Illinois**	NA
17	Texas	20.3		NA	Iowa**	NA
29	Utah	1.8		NA	Massachusetts**	NA
33	Vermont	1.0		NA	Michigan**	NA
11	Virginia	36.7		NA	Nebraska**	NA
NA	Washington**	NA		NA	New Hampshire**	NA
20	West Virginia	16.2		NA	Oklahoma**	NA
17	Wisconsin	20.3		NA	Washington**	NA
NA	Wyoming**	NA		NA	Wyoming**	NA
					District of Columbia	77.8

Source: U.S. Department of Health and Human Services, Centers for Disease Control and Prevention
   "Abortion Surveillance-United States, 1994" (Morbidity and Mortality Weekly Report, Vol. 46, No. SS-4, 8/8/97)
*By state of occurrence. National percent is for reporting states only.
**Not reported.

Percent of Reported Legal Abortions Obtained by Married Women in 1994

Reporting States' Percent = 19.3% of Reported Legal Abortions*

ALPHA ORDER			RANK ORDER		
RANK	**STATE**	**PERCENT**	**RANK**	**STATE**	**PERCENT**
31	Alabama	16.0	1	Utah	41.2
NA	Alaska**	NA	2	Idaho	24.7
NA	Arizona**	NA	3	Nevada	23.0
19	Arkansas	18.9	4	Vermont	22.6
NA	California**	NA	5	New York**	22.0
12	Colorado	20.0	6	Texas	21.5
NA	Connecticut**	NA	7	Hawaii	21.3
NA	Delaware**	NA	7	Rhode Island	21.3
NA	Florida**	NA	9	Oregon	21.0
26	Georgia	17.9	10	Missouri	20.6
7	Hawaii	21.3	11	Kansas	20.2
2	Idaho	24.7	12	Colorado	20.0
NA	Illinois**	NA	13	Tennessee	19.5
33	Indiana	15.5	13	West Virginia	19.5
NA	Iowa**	NA	13	Wyoming	19.5
11	Kansas	20.2	16	Maine	19.4
30	Kentucky	16.3	16	Maryland	19.4
NA	Louisiana**	NA	18	South Carolina	19.2
16	Maine	19.4	19	Arkansas	18.9
16	Maryland	19.4	20	North Dakota	18.8
NA	Massachusetts**	NA	21	North Carolina	18.7
36	Michigan	14.7	22	New Jersey	18.5
34	Minnesota	15.2	23	Montana	18.1
32	Mississippi	15.8	23	New Mexico	18.1
10	Missouri	20.6	23	Pennsylvania	18.1
23	Montana	18.1	26	Georgia	17.9
NA	Nebraska**	NA	27	South Dakota	17.6
3	Nevada	23.0	28	Ohio	17.5
NA	New Hampshire**	NA	29	Virginia	16.7
22	New Jersey	18.5	30	Kentucky	16.3
23	New Mexico	18.1	31	Alabama	16.0
5	New York**	22.0	32	Mississippi	15.8
21	North Carolina	18.7	33	Indiana	15.5
20	North Dakota	18.8	34	Minnesota	15.2
28	Ohio	17.5	35	Wisconsin	15.1
NA	Oklahoma**	NA	36	Michigan	14.7
9	Oregon	21.0	NA	Alaska**	NA
23	Pennsylvania	18.1	NA	Arizona**	NA
7	Rhode Island	21.3	NA	California**	NA
18	South Carolina	19.2	NA	Connecticut**	NA
27	South Dakota	17.6	NA	Delaware**	NA
13	Tennessee	19.5	NA	Florida**	NA
6	Texas	21.5	NA	Illinois**	NA
1	Utah	41.2	NA	Iowa**	NA
4	Vermont	22.6	NA	Louisiana**	NA
29	Virginia	16.7	NA	Massachusetts**	NA
NA	Washington**	NA	NA	Nebraska**	NA
13	West Virginia	19.5	NA	New Hampshire**	NA
35	Wisconsin	15.1	NA	Oklahoma**	NA
13	Wyoming	19.5	NA	Washington**	NA
				District of Columbia**	NA

Source: U.S. Department of Health and Human Services, Centers for Disease Control and Prevention
   "Abortion Surveillance-United States, 1994" (Morbidity and Mortality Weekly Report, Vol. 46, No. SS-4, 8/8/97)
*By state of occurrence. National percent is for reporting states only.
**Not reported. New York's percentage is for New York City only.

Percent of Reported Legal Abortions Obtained by Unmarried Women in 1994

Reporting States' Percent = 77.6% of Reported Legal Abortions*

ALPHA ORDER

RANK	STATE	PERCENT
5	Alabama	82.8
NA	Alaska**	NA
NA	Arizona**	NA
22	Arkansas	79.2
NA	California**	NA
18	Colorado	79.7
NA	Connecticut**	NA
NA	Delaware**	NA
NA	Florida**	NA
9	Georgia	81.2
23	Hawaii	78.2
29	Idaho	75.0
NA	Illinois**	NA
30	Indiana	74.6
NA	Iowa**	NA
20	Kansas	79.5
6	Kentucky	81.9
NA	Louisiana**	NA
31	Maine	74.5
24	Maryland	78.1
NA	Massachusetts**	NA
1	Michigan	84.5
4	Minnesota	83.4
3	Mississippi	84.0
25	Missouri	78.0
17	Montana	79.8
NA	Nebraska**	NA
28	Nevada	75.6
NA	New Hampshire**	NA
12	New Jersey	80.6
12	New Mexico	80.6
27	New York**	76.6
35	North Carolina	66.8
9	North Dakota	81.2
20	Ohio	79.5
NA	Oklahoma**	NA
34	Oregon	69.9
7	Pennsylvania	81.8
26	Rhode Island	77.1
11	South Carolina	80.8
8	South Dakota	81.7
16	Tennessee	80.2
32	Texas	72.2
36	Utah	58.8
33	Vermont	71.3
18	Virginia	79.7
NA	Washington**	NA
15	West Virginia	80.4
2	Wisconsin	84.1
14	Wyoming	80.5

RANK ORDER

RANK	STATE	PERCENT
1	Michigan	84.5
2	Wisconsin	84.1
3	Mississippi	84.0
4	Minnesota	83.4
5	Alabama	82.8
6	Kentucky	81.9
7	Pennsylvania	81.8
8	South Dakota	81.7
9	Georgia	81.2
9	North Dakota	81.2
11	South Carolina	80.8
12	New Jersey	80.6
12	New Mexico	80.6
14	Wyoming	80.5
15	West Virginia	80.4
16	Tennessee	80.2
17	Montana	79.8
18	Colorado	79.7
18	Virginia	79.7
20	Kansas	79.5
20	Ohio	79.5
22	Arkansas	79.2
23	Hawaii	78.2
24	Maryland	78.1
25	Missouri	78.0
26	Rhode Island	77.1
27	New York**	76.6
28	Nevada	75.6
29	Idaho	75.0
30	Indiana	74.6
31	Maine	74.5
32	Texas	72.2
33	Vermont	71.3
34	Oregon	69.9
35	North Carolina	66.8
36	Utah	58.8
NA	Alaska**	NA
NA	Arizona**	NA
NA	California**	NA
NA	Connecticut**	NA
NA	Delaware**	NA
NA	Florida**	NA
NA	Illinois**	NA
NA	Iowa**	NA
NA	Louisiana**	NA
NA	Massachusetts**	NA
NA	Nebraska**	NA
NA	New Hampshire**	NA
NA	Oklahoma**	NA
NA	Washington**	NA
	District of Columbia**	NA

Source: U.S. Department of Health and Human Services, Centers for Disease Control and Prevention
   "Abortion Surveillance-United States, 1994" (Morbidity and Mortality Weekly Report, Vol. 46, No. SS-4, 8/8/97)
By state of occurrence. National percent is for reporting states only.
**Not reported. New York's percentage is for New York City only.*

Reported Legal Abortions Obtained by Teenagers in 1994

National Total = 160,102 Legal Abortions Obtained by Teenagers*

ALPHA ORDER

RANK	STATE	ABORTIONS	% of USA
14	Alabama	3,423	2.14%
NA	Alaska**	NA	NA
17	Arizona	2,762	1.73%
27	Arkansas	1,448	0.90%
NA	California**	NA	NA
25	Colorado	2,222	1.39%
15	Connecticut	3,096	1.93%
NA	Delaware**	NA	NA
NA	Florida**	NA	NA
5	Georgia	7,207	4.50%
28	Hawaii	1,344	0.84%
40	Idaho	260	0.16%
NA	Illinois**	NA	NA
18	Indiana	2,714	1.70%
NA	Iowa**	NA	NA
20	Kansas	2,644	1.65%
26	Kentucky	2,139	1.34%
19	Louisiana	2,669	1.67%
36	Maine	644	0.40%
13	Maryland	3,589	2.24%
10	Massachusetts	5,358	3.35%
6	Michigan	7,110	4.44%
21	Minnesota	2,613	1.63%
33	Mississippi	867	0.54%
23	Missouri	2,483	1.55%
35	Montana	705	0.44%
29	Nebraska	1,178	0.74%
31	Nevada	1,123	0.70%
NA	New Hampshire**	NA	NA
8	New Jersey	6,207	3.88%
32	New Mexico	1,026	0.64%
1	New York	28,532	17.82%
4	North Carolina	8,053	5.03%
39	North Dakota	323	0.20%
7	Ohio	6,967	4.35%
NA	Oklahoma**	NA	NA
16	Oregon	2,936	1.83%
3	Pennsylvania	8,338	5.21%
30	Rhode Island	1,148	0.72%
24	South Carolina	2,357	1.47%
40	South Dakota	260	0.16%
12	Tennessee	3,669	2.29%
2	Texas	15,905	9.93%
34	Utah	719	0.45%
38	Vermont	528	0.33%
11	Virginia	5,356	3.35%
9	Washington	5,364	3.35%
37	West Virginia	574	0.36%
22	Wisconsin	2,588	1.62%
42	Wyoming	42	0.03%

RANK ORDER

RANK	STATE	ABORTIONS	% of USA
1	New York	28,532	17.82%
2	Texas	15,905	9.93%
3	Pennsylvania	8,338	5.21%
4	North Carolina	8,053	5.03%
5	Georgia	7,207	4.50%
6	Michigan	7,110	4.44%
7	Ohio	6,967	4.35%
8	New Jersey	6,207	3.88%
9	Washington	5,364	3.35%
10	Massachusetts	5,358	3.35%
11	Virginia	5,356	3.35%
12	Tennessee	3,669	2.29%
13	Maryland	3,589	2.24%
14	Alabama	3,423	2.14%
15	Connecticut	3,096	1.93%
16	Oregon	2,936	1.83%
17	Arizona	2,762	1.73%
18	Indiana	2,714	1.70%
19	Louisiana	2,669	1.67%
20	Kansas	2,644	1.65%
21	Minnesota	2,613	1.63%
22	Wisconsin	2,588	1.62%
23	Missouri	2,483	1.55%
24	South Carolina	2,357	1.47%
25	Colorado	2,222	1.39%
26	Kentucky	2,139	1.34%
27	Arkansas	1,448	0.90%
28	Hawaii	1,344	0.84%
29	Nebraska	1,178	0.74%
30	Rhode Island	1,148	0.72%
31	Nevada	1,123	0.70%
32	New Mexico	1,026	0.64%
33	Mississippi	867	0.54%
34	Utah	719	0.45%
35	Montana	705	0.44%
36	Maine	644	0.40%
37	West Virginia	574	0.36%
38	Vermont	528	0.33%
39	North Dakota	323	0.20%
40	Idaho	260	0.16%
40	South Dakota	260	0.16%
42	Wyoming	42	0.03%
NA	Alaska**	NA	NA
NA	California**	NA	NA
NA	Delaware**	NA	NA
NA	Florida**	NA	NA
NA	Illinois**	NA	NA
NA	Iowa**	NA	NA
NA	New Hampshire**	NA	NA
NA	Oklahoma**	NA	NA
	District of Columbia	1,612	1.01%

Source: U.S. Department of Health and Human Services, Centers for Disease Control and Prevention
    "Abortion Surveillance-United States, 1994" (Morbidity and Mortality Weekly Report, Vol. 46, No. SS-4, 8/8/97)
*Nineteen years old and younger by state of occurrence. National total is for reporting states only.
**Not reported.

Percent of Reported Legal Abortions Obtained by Teenagers in 1994

Reporting States' Percent = 19.8% of Legal Abortions*

ALPHA ORDER

RANK	STATE	PERCENT
12	Alabama	23.1
NA	Alaska**	NA
32	Arizona	19.8
8	Arkansas	24.6
NA	California**	NA
10	Colorado	23.2
23	Connecticut	21.0
NA	Delaware**	NA
NA	Florida**	NA
32	Georgia	19.8
10	Hawaii	23.2
6	Idaho	24.8
NA	Illinois**	NA
20	Indiana	21.7
NA	Iowa**	NA
5	Kansas	25.3
2	Kentucky	26.3
16	Louisiana	22.0
25	Maine	20.8
28	Maryland	20.4
42	Massachusetts	16.6
22	Michigan	21.5
37	Minnesota	18.6
18	Mississippi	21.8
24	Missouri	20.9
4	Montana	25.5
15	Nebraska	22.1
41	Nevada	16.7
NA	New Hampshire**	NA
37	New Jersey	18.6
25	New Mexico	20.8
35	New York	19.1
13	North Carolina	23.0
6	North Dakota	24.8
39	Ohio	18.5
NA	Oklahoma**	NA
17	Oregon	21.9
30	Pennsylvania	20.0
36	Rhode Island	18.8
21	South Carolina	21.6
2	South Dakota	26.3
18	Tennessee	21.8
40	Texas	17.8
31	Utah	19.9
14	Vermont	22.7
29	Virginia	20.3
27	Washington	20.7
1	West Virginia	27.5
34	Wisconsin	19.3
9	Wyoming	24.1

RANK ORDER

RANK	STATE	PERCENT
1	West Virginia	27.5
2	Kentucky	26.3
2	South Dakota	26.3
4	Montana	25.5
5	Kansas	25.3
6	Idaho	24.8
6	North Dakota	24.8
8	Arkansas	24.6
9	Wyoming	24.1
10	Colorado	23.2
10	Hawaii	23.2
12	Alabama	23.1
13	North Carolina	23.0
14	Vermont	22.7
15	Nebraska	22.1
16	Louisiana	22.0
17	Oregon	21.9
18	Mississippi	21.8
18	Tennessee	21.8
20	Indiana	21.7
21	South Carolina	21.6
22	Michigan	21.5
23	Connecticut	21.0
24	Missouri	20.9
25	Maine	20.8
25	New Mexico	20.8
27	Washington	20.7
28	Maryland	20.4
29	Virginia	20.3
30	Pennsylvania	20.0
31	Utah	19.9
32	Arizona	19.8
32	Georgia	19.8
34	Wisconsin	19.3
35	New York	19.1
36	Rhode Island	18.8
37	Minnesota	18.6
37	New Jersey	18.6
39	Ohio	18.5
40	Texas	17.8
41	Nevada	16.7
42	Massachusetts	16.6
NA	Alaska**	NA
NA	California**	NA
NA	Delaware**	NA
NA	Florida**	NA
NA	Illinois**	NA
NA	Iowa**	NA
NA	New Hampshire**	NA
NA	Oklahoma**	NA

District of Columbia 9.8

Source: Morgan Quitno Press using data from US Dept of Health & Human Serv's, Centers for Disease Control-Prevention
"Abortion Surveillance-United States, 1994" (Morbidity and Mortality Weekly Report, Vol. 46, No. SS-4, 8/8/97)
*Nineteen and younger by state of occurrence. National percent is for reporting states only.
**Not reported.

Reported Legal Abortions Obtained by Teenagers 17 Years and Younger in 1994

Reporting States' Total = 67,517 Reported Legal Abortions*

ALPHA ORDER

RANK ORDER

RANK	STATE	ABORTIONS	% of USA
15	Alabama	1,400	2.07%
NA	Alaska**	NA	NA
18	Arizona	1,135	1.68%
28	Arkansas	580	0.86%
NA	California**	NA	NA
21	Colorado	1,067	1.58%
14	Connecticut	1,453	2.15%
NA	Delaware**	NA	NA
NA	Florida**	NA	NA
5	Georgia	3,297	4.88%
27	Hawaii	618	0.92%
41	Idaho	101	0.15%
NA	Illinois**	NA	NA
23	Indiana	1,021	1.51%
NA	Iowa**	NA	NA
17	Kansas	1,247	1.85%
24	Kentucky	1,008	1.49%
19	Louisiana	1,096	1.62%
37	Maine	265	0.39%
12	Maryland	1,655	2.45%
11	Massachusetts	1,881	2.79%
6	Michigan	2,920	4.32%
26	Minnesota	994	1.47%
33	Mississippi	349	0.52%
25	Missouri	1,003	1.49%
34	Montana	310	0.46%
31	Nebraska	442	0.65%
29	Nevada	519	0.77%
NA	New Hampshire**	NA	NA
8	New Jersey	2,632	3.90%
30	New Mexico	463	0.69%
1	New York	12,786	18.94%
3	North Carolina	3,692	5.47%
40	North Dakota	117	0.17%
7	Ohio	2,808	4.16%
NA	Oklahoma**	NA	NA
16	Oregon	1,325	1.96%
4	Pennsylvania	3,480	5.15%
32	Rhode Island	391	0.58%
20	South Carolina	1,076	1.59%
39	South Dakota	121	0.18%
13	Tennessee	1,533	2.27%
2	Texas	6,151	9.11%
35	Utah	296	0.44%
38	Vermont	220	0.33%
10	Virginia	2,212	3.28%
9	Washington	2,506	3.71%
36	West Virginia	285	0.42%
22	Wisconsin	1,041	1.54%
42	Wyoming	21	0.03%

RANK	STATE	ABORTIONS	% of USA
1	New York	12,786	18.94%
2	Texas	6,151	9.11%
3	North Carolina	3,692	5.47%
4	Pennsylvania	3,480	5.15%
5	Georgia	3,297	4.88%
6	Michigan	2,920	4.32%
7	Ohio	2,808	4.16%
8	New Jersey	2,632	3.90%
9	Washington	2,506	3.71%
10	Virginia	2,212	3.28%
11	Massachusetts	1,881	2.79%
12	Maryland	1,655	2.45%
13	Tennessee	1,533	2.27%
14	Connecticut	1,453	2.15%
15	Alabama	1,400	2.07%
16	Oregon	1,325	1.96%
17	Kansas	1,247	1.85%
18	Arizona	1,135	1.68%
19	Louisiana	1,096	1.62%
20	South Carolina	1,076	1.59%
21	Colorado	1,067	1.58%
22	Wisconsin	1,041	1.54%
23	Indiana	1,021	1.51%
24	Kentucky	1,008	1.49%
25	Missouri	1,003	1.49%
26	Minnesota	994	1.47%
27	Hawaii	618	0.92%
28	Arkansas	580	0.86%
29	Nevada	519	0.77%
30	New Mexico	463	0.69%
31	Nebraska	442	0.65%
32	Rhode Island	391	0.58%
33	Mississippi	349	0.52%
34	Montana	310	0.46%
35	Utah	296	0.44%
36	West Virginia	285	0.42%
37	Maine	265	0.39%
38	Vermont	220	0.33%
39	South Dakota	121	0.18%
40	North Dakota	117	0.17%
41	Idaho	101	0.15%
42	Wyoming	21	0.03%
NA	Alaska**	NA	NA
NA	California**	NA	NA
NA	Delaware**	NA	NA
NA	Florida**	NA	NA
NA	Illinois**	NA	NA
NA	Iowa**	NA	NA
NA	New Hampshire**	NA	NA
NA	Oklahoma**	NA	NA
	District of Columbia**	NA	NA

Source: Morgan Quitno Press using data from US Dept of Health & Human Serv's, Centers for Disease Control-Prevention "Abortion Surveillance-United States, 1994" (Morbidity and Mortality Weekly Report, Vol. 46, No. SS-4, 8/8/97)
By state of occurrence. National total is for reporting states only.
**Not reported.*

Percent of Reported Legal Abortions Obtained
By Teenagers 17 Years and Younger in 1994
Reporting States' Total = 8.5% of Reported Legal Abortions*

ALPHA ORDER

RANK ORDER

RANK	STATE	PERCENT
17	Alabama	9.4
NA	Alaska**	NA
34	Arizona	8.1
10	Arkansas	9.9
NA	California**	NA
7	Colorado	11.1
13	Connecticut	9.8
NA	Delaware**	NA
NA	Florida**	NA
20	Georgia	9.1
8	Hawaii	10.7
15	Idaho	9.6
NA	Illinois**	NA
32	Indiana	8.2
NA	Iowa**	NA
5	Kansas	11.9
2	Kentucky	12.4
22	Louisiana	9.0
26	Maine	8.6
17	Maryland	9.4
42	Massachusetts	5.8
24	Michigan	8.8
39	Minnesota	7.1
24	Mississippi	8.8
28	Missouri	8.4
6	Montana	11.2
31	Nebraska	8.3
37	Nevada	7.7
NA	New Hampshire**	NA
35	New Jersey	7.9
17	New Mexico	9.4
27	New York	8.5
9	North Carolina	10.5
22	North Dakota	9.0
38	Ohio	7.4
NA	Oklahoma**	NA
10	Oregon	9.9
28	Pennsylvania	8.4
41	Rhode Island	6.4
10	South Carolina	9.9
3	South Dakota	12.3
20	Tennessee	9.1
40	Texas	6.9
32	Utah	8.2
16	Vermont	9.5
28	Virginia	8.4
14	Washington	9.7
1	West Virginia	13.7
36	Wisconsin	7.8
4	Wyoming	12.1

RANK	STATE	PERCENT
1	West Virginia	13.7
2	Kentucky	12.4
3	South Dakota	12.3
4	Wyoming	12.1
5	Kansas	11.9
6	Montana	11.2
7	Colorado	11.1
8	Hawaii	10.7
9	North Carolina	10.5
10	Arkansas	9.9
10	Oregon	9.9
10	South Carolina	9.9
13	Connecticut	9.8
14	Washington	9.7
15	Idaho	9.6
16	Vermont	9.5
17	Alabama	9.4
17	Maryland	9.4
17	New Mexico	9.4
20	Georgia	9.1
20	Tennessee	9.1
22	Louisiana	9.0
22	North Dakota	9.0
24	Michigan	8.8
24	Mississippi	8.8
26	Maine	8.6
27	New York	8.5
28	Missouri	8.4
28	Pennsylvania	8.4
28	Virginia	8.4
31	Nebraska	8.3
32	Indiana	8.2
32	Utah	8.2
34	Arizona	8.1
35	New Jersey	7.9
36	Wisconsin	7.8
37	Nevada	7.7
38	Ohio	7.4
39	Minnesota	7.1
40	Texas	6.9
41	Rhode Island	6.4
42	Massachusetts	5.8
NA	Alaska**	NA
NA	California**	NA
NA	Delaware**	NA
NA	Florida**	NA
NA	Illinois**	NA
NA	Iowa**	NA
NA	New Hampshire**	NA
NA	Oklahoma**	NA
	District of Columbia**	NA

Source: Morgan Quitno Press using data from US Dept of Health & Human Serv's, Centers for Disease Control-Prevention
"Abortion Surveillance-United States, 1994" (Morbidity and Mortality Weekly Report, Vol. 46, No. SS-4, 8/8/97)
*By state of occurrence. National percent is for reporting states only.
**Not reported.

Percent of Teenage Abortions Obtained
By Teenagers 17 Years and Younger in 1994
Reporting States' Percent = 42.6% of Teenage Abortions*

ALPHA ORDER

RANK ORDER

RANK	STATE	PERCENT		RANK	STATE	PERCENT
29	Alabama	40.9		1	Wyoming	50.0
NA	Alaska**	NA		2	West Virginia	49.7
25	Arizona	41.1		3	Colorado	48.0
34	Arkansas	40.1		4	Kansas	47.2
NA	California**	NA		5	Kentucky	47.1
3	Colorado	48.0		6	Connecticut	46.9
6	Connecticut	46.9		7	Washington	46.7
NA	Delaware**	NA		8	South Dakota	46.5
NA	Florida**	NA		9	Nevada	46.2
13	Georgia	45.7		10	Maryland	46.1
11	Hawaii	46.0		11	Hawaii	46.0
35	Idaho	38.8		12	North Carolina	45.8
NA	Illinois**	NA		13	Georgia	45.7
38	Indiana	37.6		13	South Carolina	45.7
NA	Iowa**	NA		15	New Mexico	45.1
4	Kansas	47.2		15	Oregon	45.1
5	Kentucky	47.1		17	New York	44.8
25	Louisiana	41.1		18	Montana	44.0
25	Maine	41.1		19	New Jersey	42.4
10	Maryland	46.1		20	Tennessee	41.8
41	Massachusetts	35.1		21	Pennsylvania	41.7
25	Michigan	41.1		21	Vermont	41.7
37	Minnesota	38.0		23	Virginia	41.3
31	Mississippi	40.3		24	Utah	41.2
30	Missouri	40.4		25	Arizona	41.1
18	Montana	44.0		25	Louisiana	41.1
39	Nebraska	37.5		25	Maine	41.1
9	Nevada	46.2		25	Michigan	41.1
NA	New Hampshire**	NA		29	Alabama	40.9
19	New Jersey	42.4		30	Missouri	40.4
15	New Mexico	45.1		31	Mississippi	40.3
17	New York	44.8		31	Ohio	40.3
12	North Carolina	45.8		33	Wisconsin	40.2
40	North Dakota	36.2		34	Arkansas	40.1
31	Ohio	40.3		35	Idaho	38.8
NA	Oklahoma**	NA		36	Texas	38.7
15	Oregon	45.1		37	Minnesota	38.0
21	Pennsylvania	41.7		38	Indiana	37.6
42	Rhode Island	34.1		39	Nebraska	37.5
13	South Carolina	45.7		40	North Dakota	36.2
8	South Dakota	46.5		41	Massachusetts	35.1
20	Tennessee	41.8		42	Rhode Island	34.1
36	Texas	38.7		NA	Alaska**	NA
24	Utah	41.2		NA	California**	NA
21	Vermont	41.7		NA	Delaware**	NA
23	Virginia	41.3		NA	Florida**	NA
7	Washington	46.7		NA	Illinois**	NA
2	West Virginia	49.7		NA	Iowa**	NA
33	Wisconsin	40.2		NA	New Hampshire**	NA
1	Wyoming	50.0		NA	Oklahoma**	NA

District of Columbia**   NA

*Source: Morgan Quitno Press using data from US Dept of Health & Human Serv's, Centers for Disease Control-Prevention
"Abortion Surveillance-United States, 1994" (Morbidity and Mortality Weekly Report, Vol. 46, No. SS-4, 8/8/97)*
By state of occurrence. National percent is for reporting states only.
*Not reported.

Reported Legal Abortions Performed at 12 Weeks or Less of Gestation in 1994

Reporting States' Total = 617,663 Abortions*

ALPHA ORDER

RANK	STATE	ABORTIONS	% of USA
13	Alabama	12,927	2.09%
NA	Alaska**	NA	NA
15	Arizona	12,038	1.95%
27	Arkansas	5,047	0.82%
NA	California**	NA	NA
22	Colorado	8,166	1.32%
12	Connecticut	13,071	2.12%
NA	Delaware**	NA	NA
NA	Florida**	NA	NA
4	Georgia	30,521	4.94%
28	Hawaii	4,957	0.80%
37	Idaho	987	0.16%
NA	Illinois**	NA	NA
16	Indiana	11,949	1.93%
NA	Iowa**	NA	NA
23	Kansas	8,155	1.32%
24	Kentucky	6,519	1.06%
21	Louisiana	10,094	1.63%
32	Maine	2,956	0.48%
10	Maryland	16,099	2.61%
NA	Massachusetts**	NA	NA
6	Michigan	28,900	4.68%
14	Minnesota	12,296	1.99%
30	Mississippi	3,458	0.56%
20	Missouri	10,542	1.71%
33	Montana	2,474	0.40%
NA	Nebraska**	NA	NA
25	Nevada	6,060	0.98%
NA	New Hampshire**	NA	NA
7	New Jersey	25,831	4.18%
29	New Mexico	3,858	0.62%
1	New York	124,981	20.23%
5	North Carolina	29,444	4.77%
36	North Dakota	1,176	0.19%
NA	Ohio**	NA	NA
NA	Oklahoma**	NA	NA
18	Oregon	10,839	1.75%
3	Pennsylvania	36,583	5.92%
26	Rhode Island	5,551	0.90%
19	South Carolina	10,710	1.73%
38	South Dakota	980	0.16%
11	Tennessee	16,005	2.59%
2	Texas	77,891	12.61%
31	Utah	3,338	0.54%
34	Vermont	2,210	0.36%
8	Virginia	25,194	4.08%
9	Washington	22,569	3.65%
35	West Virginia	1,832	0.30%
17	Wisconsin	11,282	1.83%
39	Wyoming	173	0.03%

RANK ORDER

RANK	STATE	ABORTIONS	% of USA
1	New York	124,981	20.23%
2	Texas	77,891	12.61%
3	Pennsylvania	36,583	5.92%
4	Georgia	30,521	4.94%
5	North Carolina	29,444	4.77%
6	Michigan	28,900	4.68%
7	New Jersey	25,831	4.18%
8	Virginia	25,194	4.08%
9	Washington	22,569	3.65%
10	Maryland	16,099	2.61%
11	Tennessee	16,005	2.59%
12	Connecticut	13,071	2.12%
13	Alabama	12,927	2.09%
14	Minnesota	12,296	1.99%
15	Arizona	12,038	1.95%
16	Indiana	11,949	1.93%
17	Wisconsin	11,282	1.83%
18	Oregon	10,839	1.75%
19	South Carolina	10,710	1.73%
20	Missouri	10,542	1.71%
21	Louisiana	10,094	1.63%
22	Colorado	8,166	1.32%
23	Kansas	8,155	1.32%
24	Kentucky	6,519	1.06%
25	Nevada	6,060	0.98%
26	Rhode Island	5,551	0.90%
27	Arkansas	5,047	0.82%
28	Hawaii	4,957	0.80%
29	New Mexico	3,858	0.62%
30	Mississippi	3,458	0.56%
31	Utah	3,338	0.54%
32	Maine	2,956	0.48%
33	Montana	2,474	0.40%
34	Vermont	2,210	0.36%
35	West Virginia	1,832	0.30%
36	North Dakota	1,176	0.19%
37	Idaho	987	0.16%
38	South Dakota	980	0.16%
39	Wyoming	173	0.03%
NA	Alaska**	NA	NA
NA	California**	NA	NA
NA	Delaware**	NA	NA
NA	Florida**	NA	NA
NA	Illinois**	NA	NA
NA	Iowa**	NA	NA
NA	Massachusetts**	NA	NA
NA	Nebraska**	NA	NA
NA	New Hampshire**	NA	NA
NA	Ohio**	NA	NA
NA	Oklahoma**	NA	NA
	District of Columbia**	NA	NA

Source: Morgan Quitno Press using data from US Dept of Health & Human Serv's, Centers for Disease Control-Prevention "Abortion Surveillance-United States, 1994" (Morbidity and Mortality Weekly Report, Vol. 46, No. SS-4, 8/8/97)
By state of occurrence. National total is for reporting states only.
**Not reported.*

Percent of Reported Legal Abortions Performed at 12 Weeks Or Less of Gestation in 1994
Reporting States' Percent = 86.3% of Reported Legal Abortions*

ALPHA ORDER

RANK	STATE	PERCENT
23	Alabama	87.2
NA	Alaska**	NA
26	Arizona	86.4
27	Arkansas	85.8
NA	California**	NA
29	Colorado	85.2
17	Connecticut	88.6
NA	Delaware**	NA
NA	Florida**	NA
31	Georgia	83.9
28	Hawaii	85.7
9	Idaho	94.3
NA	Illinois**	NA
5	Indiana	95.6
NA	Iowa**	NA
38	Kansas	77.9
36	Kentucky	80.0
34	Louisiana	83.1
4	Maine	95.7
11	Maryland	91.3
NA	Massachusetts**	NA
21	Michigan	87.4
20	Minnesota	87.7
24	Mississippi	86.9
16	Missouri	88.7
15	Montana	89.6
NA	Nebraska**	NA
14	Nevada	90.0
NA	New Hampshire**	NA
39	New Jersey	77.6
37	New Mexico	78.3
33	New York	83.5
31	North Carolina	83.9
13	North Dakota	90.4
NA	Ohio**	NA
NA	Oklahoma**	NA
35	Oregon	80.9
19	Pennsylvania	87.8
12	Rhode Island	91.1
3	South Carolina	98.1
2	South Dakota	99.3
8	Tennessee	95.1
22	Texas	87.3
10	Utah	92.5
7	Vermont	95.2
6	Virginia	95.5
24	Washington	86.9
18	West Virginia	87.9
30	Wisconsin	84.2
1	Wyoming	99.4

RANK ORDER

RANK	STATE	PERCENT
1	Wyoming	99.4
2	South Dakota	99.3
3	South Carolina	98.1
4	Maine	95.7
5	Indiana	95.6
6	Virginia	95.5
7	Vermont	95.2
8	Tennessee	95.1
9	Idaho	94.3
10	Utah	92.5
11	Maryland	91.3
12	Rhode Island	91.1
13	North Dakota	90.4
14	Nevada	90.0
15	Montana	89.6
16	Missouri	88.7
17	Connecticut	88.6
18	West Virginia	87.9
19	Pennsylvania	87.8
20	Minnesota	87.7
21	Michigan	87.4
22	Texas	87.3
23	Alabama	87.2
24	Mississippi	86.9
24	Washington	86.9
26	Arizona	86.4
27	Arkansas	85.8
28	Hawaii	85.7
29	Colorado	85.2
30	Wisconsin	84.2
31	Georgia	83.9
31	North Carolina	83.9
33	New York	83.5
34	Louisiana	83.1
35	Oregon	80.9
36	Kentucky	80.0
37	New Mexico	78.3
38	Kansas	77.9
39	New Jersey	77.6
NA	Alaska**	NA
NA	California**	NA
NA	Delaware**	NA
NA	Florida**	NA
NA	Illinois**	NA
NA	Iowa**	NA
NA	Massachusetts**	NA
NA	Nebraska**	NA
NA	New Hampshire**	NA
NA	Ohio**	NA
NA	Oklahoma**	NA
	District of Columbia**	NA

Source: Morgan Quitno Press using data from US Dept of Health & Human Serv's, Centers for Disease Control-Prevention "Abortion Surveillance-United States, 1994" (Morbidity and Mortality Weekly Report, Vol. 46, No. SS-4, 8/8/97)
*By state of occurrence. National percent is for reporting states only.
**Not reported.

Reported Legal Abortions Performed At or After 21 Weeks of Gestation in 1994

Reporting States' Total = 9,260 Abortions*

ALPHA ORDER

RANK	STATE	ABORTIONS	% of USA
12	Alabama	124	1.34%
NA	Alaska**	NA	NA
25	Arizona	21	0.23%
26	Arkansas	18	0.19%
NA	California**	NA	NA
12	Colorado	124	1.34%
28	Connecticut	6	0.06%
NA	Delaware**	NA	NA
NA	Florida**	NA	NA
3	Georgia	1,217	13.14%
18	Hawaii	58	0.63%
28	Idaho	6	0.06%
NA	Illinois**	NA	NA
36	Indiana	0	0.00%
NA	Iowa**	NA	NA
4	Kansas	854	9.22%
11	Kentucky	179	1.93%
8	Louisiana	233	2.52%
30	Maine	3	0.03%
32	Maryland	1	0.01%
NA	Massachusetts**	NA	NA
9	Michigan	225	2.43%
14	Minnesota	111	1.20%
23	Mississippi	27	0.29%
19	Missouri	56	0.60%
21	Montana	29	0.31%
NA	Nebraska**	NA	NA
36	Nevada	0	0.00%
NA	New Hampshire**	NA	NA
5	New Jersey	467	5.04%
20	New Mexico	39	0.42%
1	New York	2,830	30.56%
17	North Carolina	88	0.95%
32	North Dakota	1	0.01%
NA	Ohio**	NA	NA
NA	Oklahoma**	NA	NA
10	Oregon	186	2.01%
7	Pennsylvania	328	3.54%
27	Rhode Island	10	0.11%
24	South Carolina	24	0.26%
36	South Dakota	0	0.00%
21	Tennessee	29	0.31%
2	Texas	1,297	14.01%
32	Utah	1	0.01%
31	Vermont	2	0.02%
15	Virginia	108	1.17%
6	Washington	449	4.85%
32	West Virginia	1	0.01%
15	Wisconsin	108	1.17%
36	Wyoming	0	0.00%

RANK ORDER

RANK	STATE	ABORTIONS	% of USA
1	New York	2,830	30.56%
2	Texas	1,297	14.01%
3	Georgia	1,217	13.14%
4	Kansas	854	9.22%
5	New Jersey	467	5.04%
6	Washington	449	4.85%
7	Pennsylvania	328	3.54%
8	Louisiana	233	2.52%
9	Michigan	225	2.43%
10	Oregon	186	2.01%
11	Kentucky	179	1.93%
12	Alabama	124	1.34%
12	Colorado	124	1.34%
14	Minnesota	111	1.20%
15	Virginia	108	1.17%
15	Wisconsin	108	1.17%
17	North Carolina	88	0.95%
18	Hawaii	58	0.63%
19	Missouri	56	0.60%
20	New Mexico	39	0.42%
21	Montana	29	0.31%
21	Tennessee	29	0.31%
23	Mississippi	27	0.29%
24	South Carolina	24	0.26%
25	Arizona	21	0.23%
26	Arkansas	18	0.19%
27	Rhode Island	10	0.11%
28	Connecticut	6	0.06%
28	Idaho	6	0.06%
30	Maine	3	0.03%
31	Vermont	2	0.02%
32	Maryland	1	0.01%
32	North Dakota	1	0.01%
32	Utah	1	0.01%
32	West Virginia	1	0.01%
36	Indiana	0	0.00%
36	Nevada	0	0.00%
36	South Dakota	0	0.00%
36	Wyoming	0	0.00%
NA	Alaska**	NA	NA
NA	California**	NA	NA
NA	Delaware**	NA	NA
NA	Florida**	NA	NA
NA	Illinois**	NA	NA
NA	Iowa**	NA	NA
NA	Massachusetts**	NA	NA
NA	Nebraska**	NA	NA
NA	New Hampshire**	NA	NA
NA	Ohio**	NA	NA
NA	Oklahoma**	NA	NA
	District of Columbia**	NA	NA

Source: U.S. Department of Health and Human Services, Centers for Disease Control and Prevention
"Abortion Surveillance-United States, 1994" (Morbidity and Mortality Weekly Report, Vol. 46, No. SS-4, 8/8/97)
*By state of occurrence. National total is for reporting states only.
**Not reported.

Percent of Reported Legal Abortions Performed At or After 21 Weeks of Gestation in 1994
Reporting States' Percent = 1.3% of Reported Legal Abortions*

ALPHA ORDER

RANK ORDER

RANK	STATE	PERCENT		RANK	STATE	PERCENT
13	Alabama	0.8		1	Kansas	8.2
NA	Alaska**	NA		2	Georgia	3.3
25	Arizona	0.2		3	Kentucky	2.2
23	Arkansas	0.3		4	Louisiana	1.9
NA	California**	NA		4	New York	1.9
10	Colorado	1.3		6	Washington	1.7
32	Connecticut	0.0		7	Texas	1.5
NA	Delaware**	NA		8	New Jersey	1.4
NA	Florida**	NA		8	Oregon	1.4
2	Georgia	3.3		10	Colorado	1.3
12	Hawaii	1.0		11	Montana	1.1
20	Idaho	0.6		12	Hawaii	1.0
NA	Illinois**	NA		13	Alabama	0.8
32	Indiana	0.0		13	Minnesota	0.8
NA	Iowa**	NA		13	New Mexico	0.8
1	Kansas	8.2		13	Pennsylvania	0.8
3	Kentucky	2.2		13	Wisconsin	0.8
4	Louisiana	1.9		18	Michigan	0.7
29	Maine	0.1		18	Mississippi	0.7
32	Maryland	0.0		20	Idaho	0.6
NA	Massachusetts**	NA		21	Missouri	0.5
18	Michigan	0.7		22	Virginia	0.4
13	Minnesota	0.8		23	Arkansas	0.3
18	Mississippi	0.7		23	North Carolina	0.3
21	Missouri	0.5		25	Arizona	0.2
11	Montana	1.1		25	Rhode Island	0.2
NA	Nebraska**	NA		25	South Carolina	0.2
32	Nevada	0.0		25	Tennessee	0.2
NA	New Hampshire**	NA		29	Maine	0.1
8	New Jersey	1.4		29	North Dakota	0.1
13	New Mexico	0.8		29	Vermont	0.1
4	New York	1.9		32	Connecticut	0.0
23	North Carolina	0.3		32	Indiana	0.0
29	North Dakota	0.1		32	Maryland	0.0
NA	Ohio**	NA		32	Nevada	0.0
NA	Oklahoma**	NA		32	South Dakota	0.0
8	Oregon	1.4		32	Utah	0.0
13	Pennsylvania	0.8		32	West Virginia	0.0
25	Rhode Island	0.2		32	Wyoming	0.0
25	South Carolina	0.2		NA	Alaska**	NA
32	South Dakota	0.0		NA	California**	NA
25	Tennessee	0.2		NA	Delaware**	NA
7	Texas	1.5		NA	Florida**	NA
32	Utah	0.0		NA	Illinois**	NA
29	Vermont	0.1		NA	Iowa**	NA
22	Virginia	0.4		NA	Massachusetts**	NA
6	Washington	1.7		NA	Nebraska**	NA
32	West Virginia	0.0		NA	New Hampshire**	NA
13	Wisconsin	0.8		NA	Ohio**	NA
32	Wyoming	0.0		NA	Oklahoma**	NA
					District of Columbia**	NA

Source: Morgan Quitno Press using data from US Dept of Health & Human Serv's, Centers for Disease Control-Prevention "Abortion Surveillance-United States, 1994" (Morbidity and Mortality Weekly Report, Vol. 46, No. SS-4, 8/8/97)
*By state of occurrence. National percent is for reporting states only.
**Not reported.

II. DEATHS

II. DEATHS (Continued)

Deaths in 1996

National Total = 2,322,265 Deaths*

ALPHA ORDER

RANK	STATE	DEATHS	% of USA
18	Alabama	42,840	1.84%
50	Alaska	2,581	0.11%
22	Arizona	38,950	1.68%
31	Arkansas	26,525	1.14%
1	California	230,601	9.93%
32	Colorado	25,951	1.12%
27	Connecticut	29,594	1.27%
46	Delaware	6,507	0.28%
3	Florida	153,564	6.61%
11	Georgia	58,849	2.53%
43	Hawaii	7,929	0.34%
42	Idaho	8,716	0.38%
6	Illinois	106,358	4.58%
13	Indiana	54,568	2.35%
29	Iowa	27,787	1.20%
33	Kansas	23,967	1.03%
23	Kentucky	37,343	1.61%
21	Louisiana	40,482	1.74%
39	Maine	11,070	0.48%
20	Maryland	41,631	1.79%
12	Massachusetts	55,341	2.38%
8	Michigan	83,893	3.61%
24	Minnesota	37,102	1.60%
30	Mississippi	26,739	1.15%
14	Missouri	53,903	2.32%
44	Montana	7,667	0.33%
35	Nebraska	15,548	0.67%
36	Nevada	13,192	0.57%
41	New Hampshire	9,411	0.41%
9	New Jersey	71,812	3.09%
37	New Mexico	12,556	0.54%
2	New York	162,714	7.01%
10	North Carolina	66,322	2.86%
47	North Dakota	5,994	0.26%
7	Ohio	105,335	4.54%
26	Oklahoma	33,135	1.43%
28	Oregon	28,930	1.25%
5	Pennsylvania	129,588	5.58%
40	Rhode Island	9,546	0.41%
25	South Carolina	34,484	1.48%
45	South Dakota	6,785	0.29%
16	Tennessee	51,483	2.22%
4	Texas	138,451	5.96%
38	Utah	11,075	0.48%
48	Vermont	4,863	0.21%
15	Virginia	52,746	2.27%
19	Washington	42,164	1.82%
34	West Virginia	20,401	0.88%
17	Wisconsin	45,100	1.94%
49	Wyoming	3,619	0.16%

RANK ORDER

RANK	STATE	DEATHS	% of USA
1	California	230,601	9.93%
2	New York	162,714	7.01%
3	Florida	153,564	6.61%
4	Texas	138,451	5.96%
5	Pennsylvania	129,588	5.58%
6	Illinois	106,358	4.58%
7	Ohio	105,335	4.54%
8	Michigan	83,893	3.61%
9	New Jersey	71,812	3.09%
10	North Carolina	66,322	2.86%
11	Georgia	58,849	2.53%
12	Massachusetts	55,341	2.38%
13	Indiana	54,568	2.35%
14	Missouri	53,903	2.32%
15	Virginia	52,746	2.27%
16	Tennessee	51,483	2.22%
17	Wisconsin	45,100	1.94%
18	Alabama	42,840	1.84%
19	Washington	42,164	1.82%
20	Maryland	41,631	1.79%
21	Louisiana	40,482	1.74%
22	Arizona	38,950	1.68%
23	Kentucky	37,343	1.61%
24	Minnesota	37,102	1.60%
25	South Carolina	34,484	1.48%
26	Oklahoma	33,135	1.43%
27	Connecticut	29,594	1.27%
28	Oregon	28,930	1.25%
29	Iowa	27,787	1.20%
30	Mississippi	26,739	1.15%
31	Arkansas	26,525	1.14%
32	Colorado	25,951	1.12%
33	Kansas	23,967	1.03%
34	West Virginia	20,401	0.88%
35	Nebraska	15,548	0.67%
36	Nevada	13,192	0.57%
37	New Mexico	12,556	0.54%
38	Utah	11,075	0.48%
39	Maine	11,070	0.48%
40	Rhode Island	9,546	0.41%
41	New Hampshire	9,411	0.41%
42	Idaho	8,716	0.38%
43	Hawaii	7,929	0.34%
44	Montana	7,667	0.33%
45	South Dakota	6,785	0.29%
46	Delaware	6,507	0.28%
47	North Dakota	5,994	0.26%
48	Vermont	4,863	0.21%
49	Wyoming	3,619	0.16%
50	Alaska	2,581	0.11%
	District of Columbia	6,551	0.28%

Source: U.S. Department of Health and Human Services, National Center for Health Statistics
"Monthly Vital Statistics Report" (Vol. 46, No. 1(S)2, September 11, 1997)
*Preliminary data by state of residence.

Death Rate in 1996

National Rate = 875.4 Deaths per 100,000 Population*

ALPHA ORDER

RANK ORDER

RANK	STATE	RATE	RANK	STATE	RATE
7	Alabama	1,002.6	1	West Virginia	1,117.4
50	Alaska	425.2	2	Pennsylvania	1,074.9
30	Arizona	879.6	3	Florida	1,066.4
4	Arkansas	1,056.9	4	Arkansas	1,056.9
46	California	723.4	5	Missouri	1,005.9
47	Colorado	678.9	6	Oklahoma	1,003.8
23	Connecticut	903.8	7	Alabama	1,002.6
27	Delaware	897.7	8	Mississippi	984.5
3	Florida	1,066.4	9	Iowa	974.4
38	Georgia	800.3	10	Tennessee	967.8
48	Hawaii	669.8	11	Rhode Island	964.0
43	Idaho	732.9	12	Kentucky	961.5
26	Illinois	897.8	13	Ohio	942.8
15	Indiana	934.3	14	Nebraska	941.1
9	Iowa	974.4	15	Indiana	934.3
17	Kansas	931.8	16	South Carolina	932.3
12	Kentucky	961.5	17	Kansas	931.8
19	Louisiana	930.5	18	North Dakota	931.4
29	Maine	890.4	19	Louisiana	930.5
36	Maryland	820.9	20	South Dakota	926.4
21	Massachusetts	908.4	21	Massachusetts	908.4
31	Michigan	874.4	22	North Carolina	905.7
39	Minnesota	796.6	23	Connecticut	903.8
8	Mississippi	984.5	24	Oregon	903.0
5	Missouri	1,005.9	25	New Jersey	899.0
33	Montana	871.9	26	Illinois	897.8
14	Nebraska	941.1	27	Delaware	897.7
35	Nevada	822.9	28	New York	894.8
37	New Hampshire	809.6	29	Maine	890.4
25	New Jersey	899.0	30	Arizona	879.6
44	New Mexico	732.8	31	Michigan	874.4
28	New York	894.8	32	Wisconsin	874.1
22	North Carolina	905.7	33	Montana	871.9
18	North Dakota	931.4	34	Vermont	826.1
13	Ohio	942.8	35	Nevada	822.9
6	Oklahoma	1,003.8	36	Maryland	820.9
24	Oregon	903.0	37	New Hampshire	809.6
2	Pennsylvania	1,074.9	38	Georgia	800.3
11	Rhode Island	964.0	39	Minnesota	796.6
16	South Carolina	932.3	40	Virginia	790.1
20	South Dakota	926.4	41	Washington	762.1
10	Tennessee	967.8	42	Wyoming	751.8
45	Texas	723.8	43	Idaho	732.9
49	Utah	553.6	44	New Mexico	732.8
34	Vermont	826.1	45	Texas	723.8
40	Virginia	790.1	46	California	723.4
41	Washington	762.1	47	Colorado	678.9
1	West Virginia	1,117.4	48	Hawaii	669.8
32	Wisconsin	874.1	49	Utah	553.6
42	Wyoming	751.8	50	Alaska	425.2
				District of Columbia	1,206.0

Source: U.S. Department of Health and Human Services, National Center for Health Statistics
    "Monthly Vital Statistics Report" (Vol. 46, No. 1(S)2, September 11, 1997)
*Preliminary data by state of residence. Not age adjusted.

Births to Deaths Ratio in 1996

National Ratio = 1.69 Births for Every Death in 1996

ALPHA ORDER

RANK	STATE	RATIO
36	Alabama	1.44
1	Alaska	3.94
9	Arizona	2.04
43	Arkansas	1.37
4	California	2.34
8	Colorado	2.15
30	Connecticut	1.50
24	Delaware	1.57
48	Florida	1.23
11	Georgia	1.95
5	Hawaii	2.31
6	Idaho	2.19
15	Illinois	1.73
28	Indiana	1.53
45	Iowa	1.34
19	Kansas	1.66
38	Kentucky	1.41
21	Louisiana	1.63
47	Maine	1.24
17	Maryland	1.67
34	Massachusetts	1.45
20	Michigan	1.64
16	Minnesota	1.72
25	Mississippi	1.56
43	Missouri	1.37
39	Montana	1.40
30	Nebraska	1.50
10	Nevada	1.97
26	New Hampshire	1.55
22	New Jersey	1.59
7	New Mexico	2.17
17	New York	1.67
22	North Carolina	1.59
40	North Dakota	1.39
34	Ohio	1.45
40	Oklahoma	1.39
29	Oregon	1.51
49	Pennsylvania	1.16
46	Rhode Island	1.31
33	South Carolina	1.47
27	South Dakota	1.54
37	Tennessee	1.43
3	Texas	2.36
2	Utah	3.74
40	Vermont	1.39
13	Virginia	1.75
12	Washington	1.90
50	West Virginia	1.01
32	Wisconsin	1.49
14	Wyoming	1.74

RANK ORDER

RANK	STATE	RATIO
1	Alaska	3.94
2	Utah	3.74
3	Texas	2.36
4	California	2.34
5	Hawaii	2.31
6	Idaho	2.19
7	New Mexico	2.17
8	Colorado	2.15
9	Arizona	2.04
10	Nevada	1.97
11	Georgia	1.95
12	Washington	1.90
13	Virginia	1.75
14	Wyoming	1.74
15	Illinois	1.73
16	Minnesota	1.72
17	Maryland	1.67
17	New York	1.67
19	Kansas	1.66
20	Michigan	1.64
21	Louisiana	1.63
22	New Jersey	1.59
22	North Carolina	1.59
24	Delaware	1.57
25	Mississippi	1.56
26	New Hampshire	1.55
27	South Dakota	1.54
28	Indiana	1.53
29	Oregon	1.51
30	Connecticut	1.50
30	Nebraska	1.50
32	Wisconsin	1.49
33	South Carolina	1.47
34	Massachusetts	1.45
34	Ohio	1.45
36	Alabama	1.44
37	Tennessee	1.43
38	Kentucky	1.41
39	Montana	1.40
40	North Dakota	1.39
40	Oklahoma	1.39
40	Vermont	1.39
43	Arkansas	1.37
43	Missouri	1.37
45	Iowa	1.34
46	Rhode Island	1.31
47	Maine	1.24
48	Florida	1.23
49	Pennsylvania	1.16
50	West Virginia	1.01

| | District of Columbia | 1.27 |

Source: Morgan Quitno Press using data from U.S. Dept. of Health & Human Services, National Center for Health Statistics
"Monthly Vital Statistics Report" (Vol. 46, No. 1(S)2, September 11, 1997)
*Preliminary data by state of residence.

Deaths in 1990

National Total = 2,148,463 Deaths*

RANK	STATE	DEATHS	% of USA
18	Alabama	39,381	1.83%
50	Alaska	2,188	0.10%
26	Arizona	28,789	1.34%
31	Arkansas	24,652	1.15%
1	California	214,369	9.98%
33	Colorado	21,583	1.00%
27	Connecticut	27,607	1.28%
46	Delaware	5,764	0.27%
3	Florida	134,385	6.25%
12	Georgia	51,810	2.41%
44	Hawaii	6,782	0.32%
42	Idaho	7,452	0.35%
6	Illinois	103,006	4.79%
14	Indiana	49,569	2.31%
28	Iowa	26,884	1.25%
32	Kansas	22,279	1.04%
22	Kentucky	35,078	1.63%
20	Louisiana	37,571	1.75%
36	Maine	11,106	0.52%
19	Maryland	38,413	1.79%
11	Massachusetts	53,179	2.48%
8	Michigan	78,744	3.67%
23	Minnesota	34,776	1.62%
30	Mississippi	25,127	1.17%
13	Missouri	50,377	2.34%
43	Montana	6,861	0.32%
35	Nebraska	14,769	0.69%
39	Nevada	9,318	0.43%
41	New Hampshire	8,488	0.40%
9	New Jersey	70,383	3.28%
37	New Mexico	10,625	0.49%
2	New York	168,936	7.86%
10	North Carolina	57,315	2.67%
47	North Dakota	5,678	0.26%
7	Ohio	98,822	4.60%
24	Oklahoma	30,378	1.41%
29	Oregon	25,136	1.17%
5	Pennsylvania	121,951	5.68%
38	Rhode Island	9,576	0.45%
25	South Carolina	29,715	1.38%
45	South Dakota	6,326	0.29%
16	Tennessee	46,315	2.16%
4	Texas	125,479	5.84%
40	Utah	9,192	0.43%
48	Vermont	4,595	0.21%
15	Virginia	48,013	2.23%
21	Washington	37,087	1.73%
34	West Virginia	19,385	0.90%
17	Wisconsin	42,733	1.99%
49	Wyoming	3,203	0.15%

RANK	STATE	DEATHS	% of USA
1	California	214,369	9.98%
2	New York	168,936	7.86%
3	Florida	134,385	6.25%
4	Texas	125,479	5.84%
5	Pennsylvania	121,951	5.68%
6	Illinois	103,006	4.79%
7	Ohio	98,822	4.60%
8	Michigan	78,744	3.67%
9	New Jersey	70,383	3.28%
10	North Carolina	57,315	2.67%
11	Massachusetts	53,179	2.48%
12	Georgia	51,810	2.41%
13	Missouri	50,377	2.34%
14	Indiana	49,569	2.31%
15	Virginia	48,013	2.23%
16	Tennessee	46,315	2.16%
17	Wisconsin	42,733	1.99%
18	Alabama	39,381	1.83%
19	Maryland	38,413	1.79%
20	Louisiana	37,571	1.75%
21	Washington	37,087	1.73%
22	Kentucky	35,078	1.63%
23	Minnesota	34,776	1.62%
24	Oklahoma	30,378	1.41%
25	South Carolina	29,715	1.38%
26	Arizona	28,789	1.34%
27	Connecticut	27,607	1.28%
28	Iowa	26,884	1.25%
29	Oregon	25,136	1.17%
30	Mississippi	25,127	1.17%
31	Arkansas	24,652	1.15%
32	Kansas	22,279	1.04%
33	Colorado	21,583	1.00%
34	West Virginia	19,385	0.90%
35	Nebraska	14,769	0.69%
36	Maine	11,106	0.52%
37	New Mexico	10,625	0.49%
38	Rhode Island	9,576	0.45%
39	Nevada	9,318	0.43%
40	Utah	9,192	0.43%
41	New Hampshire	8,488	0.40%
42	Idaho	7,452	0.35%
43	Montana	6,861	0.32%
44	Hawaii	6,782	0.32%
45	South Dakota	6,326	0.29%
46	Delaware	5,764	0.27%
47	North Dakota	5,678	0.26%
48	Vermont	4,595	0.21%
49	Wyoming	3,203	0.15%
50	Alaska	2,188	0.10%
	District of Columbia	7,313	0.34%

Source: U.S. Department of Health and Human Services, National Center for Health Statistics
"Monthly Vital Statistics Report" (Vol. 41, No. 7(S), January 7, 1993)
*Final data by state of residence.

Death Rate in 1990

National Rate = 8.63 Deaths per 1,000 Population*

ALPHA ORDER

RANK	STATE	RATE
7	Alabama	9.74
50	Alaska	3.98
37	Arizona	7.84
2	Arkansas	10.48
44	California	7.19
47	Colorado	6.55
32	Connecticut	8.40
27	Delaware	8.64
3	Florida	10.38
35	Georgia	7.99
48	Hawaii	6.11
42	Idaho	7.40
19	Illinois	9.00
21	Indiana	8.94
8	Iowa	9.68
20	Kansas	8.99
11	Kentucky	9.51
22	Louisiana	8.90
18	Maine	9.05
34	Maryland	8.03
24	Massachusetts	8.84
31	Michigan	8.47
36	Minnesota	7.95
6	Mississippi	9.76
5	Missouri	9.84
29	Montana	8.59
14	Nebraska	9.36
38	Nevada	7.75
40	New Hampshire	7.65
16	New Jersey	9.10
46	New Mexico	7.01
13	New York	9.38
27	North Carolina	8.64
22	North Dakota	8.90
15	Ohio	9.11
9	Oklahoma	9.66
24	Oregon	8.84
4	Pennsylvania	10.26
10	Rhode Island	9.54
30	South Carolina	8.52
17	South Dakota	9.09
12	Tennessee	9.49
43	Texas	7.38
49	Utah	5.33
33	Vermont	8.17
38	Virginia	7.75
41	Washington	7.62
1	West Virginia	10.80
26	Wisconsin	8.74
45	Wyoming	7.06

RANK ORDER

RANK	STATE	RATE
1	West Virginia	10.80
2	Arkansas	10.48
3	Florida	10.38
4	Pennsylvania	10.26
5	Missouri	9.84
6	Mississippi	9.76
7	Alabama	9.74
8	Iowa	9.68
9	Oklahoma	9.66
10	Rhode Island	9.54
11	Kentucky	9.51
12	Tennessee	9.49
13	New York	9.38
14	Nebraska	9.36
15	Ohio	9.11
16	New Jersey	9.10
17	South Dakota	9.09
18	Maine	9.05
19	Illinois	9.00
20	Kansas	8.99
21	Indiana	8.94
22	Louisiana	8.90
22	North Dakota	8.90
24	Massachusetts	8.84
24	Oregon	8.84
26	Wisconsin	8.74
27	Delaware	8.64
27	North Carolina	8.64
29	Montana	8.59
30	South Carolina	8.52
31	Michigan	8.47
32	Connecticut	8.40
33	Vermont	8.17
34	Maryland	8.03
35	Georgia	7.99
36	Minnesota	7.95
37	Arizona	7.84
38	Nevada	7.75
38	Virginia	7.75
40	New Hampshire	7.65
41	Washington	7.62
42	Idaho	7.40
43	Texas	7.38
44	California	7.19
45	Wyoming	7.06
46	New Mexico	7.01
47	Colorado	6.55
48	Hawaii	6.11
49	Utah	5.33
50	Alaska	3.98
	District of Columbia	12.00

Source: U.S. Department of Health and Human Services, National Center for Health Statistics
"Monthly Vital Statistics Report" (Vol. 41, No. 7(S), January 7, 1993)
*Final data by state of residence. Not age adjusted.

Deaths in 1980

National Total = 1,989,841 Deaths*

<u>ALPHA ORDER</u>

RANK	STATE	DEATHS	% of USA
19	Alabama	35,542	1.79%
50	Alaska	1,714	0.09%
32	Arizona	21,367	1.07%
29	Arkansas	22,744	1.14%
1	California	186,624	9.38%
34	Colorado	18,956	0.95%
25	Connecticut	27,275	1.37%
46	Delaware	5,044	0.25%
5	Florida	104,670	5.26%
14	Georgia	44,262	2.22%
47	Hawaii	4,981	0.25%
41	Idaho	6,763	0.34%
6	Illinois	102,935	5.17%
13	Indiana	47,345	2.38%
26	Iowa	27,120	1.36%
30	Kansas	22,034	1.11%
21	Kentucky	33,796	1.70%
18	Louisiana	35,651	1.79%
36	Maine	10,800	0.54%
20	Maryland	34,016	1.71%
10	Massachusetts	55,070	2.77%
8	Michigan	75,187	3.78%
22	Minnesota	33,366	1.68%
28	Mississippi	23,656	1.19%
11	Missouri	49,660	2.50%
42	Montana	6,666	0.34%
35	Nebraska	14,474	0.73%
44	Nevada	5,896	0.30%
40	New Hampshire	7,647	0.38%
9	New Jersey	68,943	3.46%
38	New Mexico	9,093	0.46%
2	New York	172,853	8.69%
12	North Carolina	48,440	2.43%
45	North Dakota	5,596	0.28%
7	Ohio	98,421	4.95%
24	Oklahoma	28,234	1.42%
31	Oregon	21,798	1.10%
3	Pennsylvania	123,594	6.21%
37	Rhode Island	9,325	0.47%
27	South Carolina	25,154	1.26%
43	South Dakota	6,556	0.33%
17	Tennessee	40,774	2.05%
4	Texas	108,180	5.44%
39	Utah	8,120	0.41%
48	Vermont	4,582	0.23%
15	Virginia	42,506	2.14%
23	Washington	32,007	1.61%
33	West Virginia	19,237	0.97%
16	Wisconsin	40,838	2.05%
49	Wyoming	3,221	0.16%

<u>RANK ORDER</u>

RANK	STATE	DEATHS	% of USA
1	California	186,624	9.38%
2	New York	172,853	8.69%
3	Pennsylvania	123,594	6.21%
4	Texas	108,180	5.44%
5	Florida	104,670	5.26%
6	Illinois	102,935	5.17%
7	Ohio	98,421	4.95%
8	Michigan	75,187	3.78%
9	New Jersey	68,943	3.46%
10	Massachusetts	55,070	2.77%
11	Missouri	49,660	2.50%
12	North Carolina	48,440	2.43%
13	Indiana	47,345	2.38%
14	Georgia	44,262	2.22%
15	Virginia	42,506	2.14%
16	Wisconsin	40,838	2.05%
17	Tennessee	40,774	2.05%
18	Louisiana	35,651	1.79%
19	Alabama	35,542	1.79%
20	Maryland	34,016	1.71%
21	Kentucky	33,796	1.70%
22	Minnesota	33,366	1.68%
23	Washington	32,007	1.61%
24	Oklahoma	28,234	1.42%
25	Connecticut	27,275	1.37%
26	Iowa	27,120	1.36%
27	South Carolina	25,154	1.26%
28	Mississippi	23,656	1.19%
29	Arkansas	22,744	1.14%
30	Kansas	22,034	1.11%
31	Oregon	21,798	1.10%
32	Arizona	21,367	1.07%
33	West Virginia	19,237	0.97%
34	Colorado	18,956	0.95%
35	Nebraska	14,474	0.73%
36	Maine	10,800	0.54%
37	Rhode Island	9,325	0.47%
38	New Mexico	9,093	0.46%
39	Utah	8,120	0.41%
40	New Hampshire	7,647	0.38%
41	Idaho	6,763	0.34%
42	Montana	6,666	0.34%
43	South Dakota	6,556	0.33%
44	Nevada	5,896	0.30%
45	North Dakota	5,596	0.28%
46	Delaware	5,044	0.25%
47	Hawaii	4,981	0.25%
48	Vermont	4,582	0.23%
49	Wyoming	3,221	0.16%
50	Alaska	1,714	0.09%
	District of Columbia	7,108	0.36%

*Source: U.S. Department of Health and Human Services, National Center for Health Statistics
"Vital Statistics of the United States 1980" and "Monthly Vital Statistics Report"
Final data by state of residence.

Death Rate in 1980

National Rate = 8.77 Deaths per 1,000 Population*

RANK	STATE	RATE
18	Alabama	9.12
50	Alaska	4.25
40	Arizona	7.84
4	Arkansas	9.94
39	California	7.86
47	Colorado	6.54
23	Connecticut	8.77
27	Delaware	8.47
1	Florida	10.72
35	Georgia	8.09
49	Hawaii	5.15
44	Idaho	7.15
20	Illinois	8.99
25	Indiana	8.62
14	Iowa	9.30
14	Kansas	9.30
16	Kentucky	9.22
28	Louisiana	8.46
8	Maine	9.60
36	Maryland	8.06
9	Massachusetts	9.59
34	Michigan	8.11
33	Minnesota	8.17
11	Mississippi	9.37
3	Missouri	10.08
28	Montana	8.46
17	Nebraska	9.20
43	Nevada	7.35
30	New Hampshire	8.30
12	New Jersey	9.36
45	New Mexico	6.96
6	New York	9.84
32	North Carolina	8.23
26	North Dakota	8.56
19	Ohio	9.11
13	Oklahoma	9.32
31	Oregon	8.27
2	Pennsylvania	10.41
6	Rhode Island	9.84
37	South Carolina	8.05
10	South Dakota	9.47
22	Tennessee	8.87
42	Texas	7.58
48	Utah	5.54
21	Vermont	8.95
38	Virginia	7.94
41	Washington	7.73
5	West Virginia	9.87
24	Wisconsin	8.67
46	Wyoming	6.84

RANK	STATE	RATE
1	Florida	10.72
2	Pennsylvania	10.41
3	Missouri	10.08
4	Arkansas	9.94
5	West Virginia	9.87
6	New York	9.84
6	Rhode Island	9.84
8	Maine	9.60
9	Massachusetts	9.59
10	South Dakota	9.47
11	Mississippi	9.37
12	New Jersey	9.36
13	Oklahoma	9.32
14	Iowa	9.30
14	Kansas	9.30
16	Kentucky	9.22
17	Nebraska	9.20
18	Alabama	9.12
19	Ohio	9.11
20	Illinois	8.99
21	Vermont	8.95
22	Tennessee	8.87
23	Connecticut	8.77
24	Wisconsin	8.67
25	Indiana	8.62
26	North Dakota	8.56
27	Delaware	8.47
28	Louisiana	8.46
28	Montana	8.46
30	New Hampshire	8.30
31	Oregon	8.27
32	North Carolina	8.23
33	Minnesota	8.17
34	Michigan	8.11
35	Georgia	8.09
36	Maryland	8.06
37	South Carolina	8.05
38	Virginia	7.94
39	California	7.86
40	Arizona	7.84
41	Washington	7.73
42	Texas	7.58
43	Nevada	7.35
44	Idaho	7.15
45	New Mexico	6.96
46	Wyoming	6.84
47	Colorado	6.54
48	Utah	5.54
49	Hawaii	5.15
50	Alaska	4.25
	District of Columbia	11.09

Source: U.S. Department of Health and Human Services, National Center for Health Statistics
"Vital Statistics of the United States 1980" and "Monthly Vital Statistics Report"
*Final data by state of residence. Not age adjusted.

Infant Deaths in 1997

National Total = 27,000 Infant Deaths*

RANK	STATE	DEATHS	% of USA
18	Alabama	564	2.09%
45	Alaska	62	0.23%
12	Arizona	767	2.84%
30	Arkansas	303	1.12%
1	California	3,059	11.33%
27	Colorado	394	1.46%
29	Connecticut	307	1.14%
42	Delaware	75	0.28%
5	Florida	1,339	4.96%
10	Georgia	968	3.59%
40	Hawaii	96	0.36%
38	Idaho	134	0.50%
4	Illinois	1,429	5.29%
19	Indiana	558	2.07%
35	Iowa	189	0.70%
31	Kansas	292	1.08%
22	Kentucky	442	1.64%
17	Louisiana	584	2.16%
48	Maine	52	0.19%
16	Maryland	594	2.20%
26	Massachusetts	399	1.48%
6	Michigan	1,077	3.99%
25	Minnesota	401	1.49%
21	Mississippi	444	1.64%
15	Missouri	596	2.21%
41	Montana	78	0.29%
34	Nebraska	197	0.73%
38	Nevada	134	0.50%
44	New Hampshire	69	0.26%
11	New Jersey	786	2.91%
36	New Mexico	176	0.65%
3	New York	1,654	6.13%
9	North Carolina	1,019	3.77%
47	North Dakota	55	0.20%
7	Ohio	1,060	3.93%
28	Oklahoma	386	1.43%
32	Oregon	265	0.98%
8	Pennsylvania	1,048	3.88%
42	Rhode Island	75	0.28%
23	South Carolina	430	1.59%
46	South Dakota	57	0.21%
13	Tennessee	642	2.38%
2	Texas	1,898	7.03%
33	Utah	220	0.81%
49	Vermont	42	0.16%
14	Virginia	630	2.33%
24	Washington	418	1.55%
37	West Virginia	159	0.59%
20	Wisconsin	468	1.73%
50	Wyoming	32	0.12%

RANK	STATE	DEATHS	% of USA
1	California	3,059	11.33%
2	Texas	1,898	7.03%
3	New York	1,654	6.13%
4	Illinois	1,429	5.29%
5	Florida	1,339	4.96%
6	Michigan	1,077	3.99%
7	Ohio	1,060	3.93%
8	Pennsylvania	1,048	3.88%
9	North Carolina	1,019	3.77%
10	Georgia	968	3.59%
11	New Jersey	786	2.91%
12	Arizona	767	2.84%
13	Tennessee	642	2.38%
14	Virginia	630	2.33%
15	Missouri	596	2.21%
16	Maryland	594	2.20%
17	Louisiana	584	2.16%
18	Alabama	564	2.09%
19	Indiana	558	2.07%
20	Wisconsin	468	1.73%
21	Mississippi	444	1.64%
22	Kentucky	442	1.64%
23	South Carolina	430	1.59%
24	Washington	418	1.55%
25	Minnesota	401	1.49%
26	Massachusetts	399	1.48%
27	Colorado	394	1.46%
28	Oklahoma	386	1.43%
29	Connecticut	307	1.14%
30	Arkansas	303	1.12%
31	Kansas	292	1.08%
32	Oregon	265	0.98%
33	Utah	220	0.81%
34	Nebraska	197	0.73%
35	Iowa	189	0.70%
36	New Mexico	176	0.65%
37	West Virginia	159	0.59%
38	Idaho	134	0.50%
38	Nevada	134	0.50%
40	Hawaii	96	0.36%
41	Montana	78	0.29%
42	Delaware	75	0.28%
42	Rhode Island	75	0.28%
44	New Hampshire	69	0.26%
45	Alaska	62	0.23%
46	South Dakota	57	0.21%
47	North Dakota	55	0.20%
48	Maine	52	0.19%
49	Vermont	42	0.16%
50	Wyoming	32	0.12%
	District of Columbia	104	0.39%

Source: U.S. Department of Health and Human Services, National Center for Health Statistics
   "Monthly Vital Statistics Report" (Vol. 46, No. 7, March 17, 1998)
*For 12 months ending July 1997. Provisional data. Deaths under 1 year old by state of residence.

Infant Mortality Rate in 1997

National Rate = 7.0 Infant Deaths per 1,000 Live Births*

ALPHA ORDER

RANK	STATE	RATE
3	Alabama	9.3
36	Alaska	6.1
5	Arizona	9.0
8	Arkansas	8.4
40	California	5.9
17	Colorado	7.5
32	Connecticut	6.4
17	Delaware	7.5
24	Florida	7.0
11	Georgia	8.3
41	Hawaii	5.5
17	Idaho	7.5
16	Illinois	7.8
28	Indiana	6.9
46	Iowa	5.1
23	Kansas	7.1
8	Kentucky	8.4
4	Louisiana	9.1
50	Maine	3.8
7	Maryland	8.6
48	Massachusetts	4.9
15	Michigan	8.1
34	Minnesota	6.2
1	Mississippi	10.9
13	Missouri	8.2
21	Montana	7.4
8	Nebraska	8.4
44	Nevada	5.3
48	New Hampshire	4.9
29	New Jersey	6.8
30	New Mexico	6.6
34	New York	6.2
2	North Carolina	9.4
31	North Dakota	6.5
24	Ohio	7.0
13	Oklahoma	8.2
36	Oregon	6.1
22	Pennsylvania	7.3
38	Rhode Island	6.0
11	South Carolina	8.3
41	South Dakota	5.5
6	Tennessee	8.7
38	Texas	6.0
43	Utah	5.4
33	Vermont	6.3
24	Virginia	7.0
44	Washington	5.3
17	West Virginia	7.5
24	Wisconsin	7.0
46	Wyoming	5.1

RANK ORDER

RANK	STATE	RATE
1	Mississippi	10.9
2	North Carolina	9.4
3	Alabama	9.3
4	Louisiana	9.1
5	Arizona	9.0
6	Tennessee	8.7
7	Maryland	8.6
8	Arkansas	8.4
8	Kentucky	8.4
8	Nebraska	8.4
11	Georgia	8.3
11	South Carolina	8.3
13	Missouri	8.2
13	Oklahoma	8.2
15	Michigan	8.1
16	Illinois	7.8
17	Colorado	7.5
17	Delaware	7.5
17	Idaho	7.5
17	West Virginia	7.5
21	Montana	7.4
22	Pennsylvania	7.3
23	Kansas	7.1
24	Florida	7.0
24	Ohio	7.0
24	Virginia	7.0
24	Wisconsin	7.0
28	Indiana	6.9
29	New Jersey	6.8
30	New Mexico	6.6
31	North Dakota	6.5
32	Connecticut	6.4
33	Vermont	6.3
34	Minnesota	6.2
34	New York	6.2
36	Alaska	6.1
36	Oregon	6.1
38	Rhode Island	6.0
38	Texas	6.0
40	California	5.9
41	Hawaii	5.5
41	South Dakota	5.5
43	Utah	5.4
44	Nevada	5.3
44	Washington	5.3
46	Iowa	5.1
46	Wyoming	5.1
48	Massachusetts	4.9
48	New Hampshire	4.9
50	Maine	3.8
	District of Columbia	12.5

Source: U.S. Department of Health and Human Services, National Center for Health Statistics
   "Monthly Vital Statistics Report" (Vol. 46, No. 7, March 17, 1998)
*For 12 months ending July 1997. Provisional data. Deaths under 1 year old by state of residence.

Infant Deaths in 1996

National Total = 28,100 Infant Deaths*

ALPHA ORDER					RANK ORDER			
RANK	STATE		DEATHS	% of USA	RANK	STATE	DEATHS	% of USA
13	Alabama		631	2.25%	1	California	3,287	11.70%
42	Alaska		80	0.28%	2	Texas	1,913	6.81%
17	Arizona		605	2.15%	3	New York	1,828	6.51%
30	Arkansas		288	1.02%	4	Illinois	1,502	5.35%
1	California		3,287	11.70%	5	Florida	1,415	5.04%
28	Colorado		362	1.29%	6	Ohio	1,178	4.19%
31	Connecticut		273	0.97%	7	Pennsylvania	1,114	3.96%
44	Delaware		78	0.28%	8	Michigan	1,082	3.85%
5	Florida		1,415	5.04%	9	Georgia	1,035	3.68%
9	Georgia		1,035	3.68%	10	North Carolina	975	3.47%
40	Hawaii		106	0.38%	11	New Jersey	826	2.94%
39	Idaho		134	0.48%	12	Virginia	660	2.35%
4	Illinois		1,502	5.35%	13	Alabama	631	2.25%
14	Indiana		626	2.23%	14	Indiana	626	2.23%
34	Iowa		227	0.81%	15	Tennessee	622	2.21%
29	Kansas		358	1.27%	16	Louisiana	612	2.18%
26	Kentucky		397	1.41%	17	Arizona	605	2.15%
16	Louisiana		612	2.18%	18	Missouri	595	2.12%
46	Maine		60	0.21%	19	Maryland	594	2.11%
19	Maryland		594	2.11%	20	Wisconsin	500	1.78%
27	Massachusetts		390	1.39%	21	Washington	425	1.51%
8	Michigan		1,082	3.85%	22	Minnesota	407	1.45%
22	Minnesota		407	1.45%	23	Oklahoma	403	1.43%
25	Mississippi		401	1.43%	24	South Carolina	402	1.43%
18	Missouri		595	2.12%	25	Mississippi	401	1.43%
43	Montana		79	0.28%	26	Kentucky	397	1.41%
35	Nebraska		203	0.72%	27	Massachusetts	390	1.39%
38	Nevada		146	0.52%	28	Colorado	362	1.29%
41	New Hampshire		81	0.29%	29	Kansas	358	1.27%
11	New Jersey		826	2.94%	30	Arkansas	288	1.02%
37	New Mexico		160	0.57%	31	Connecticut	273	0.97%
3	New York		1,828	6.51%	32	Oregon	244	0.87%
10	North Carolina		975	3.47%	33	Utah	242	0.86%
50	North Dakota		36	0.13%	34	Iowa	227	0.81%
6	Ohio		1,178	4.19%	35	Nebraska	203	0.72%
23	Oklahoma		403	1.43%	36	West Virginia	161	0.57%
32	Oregon		244	0.87%	37	New Mexico	160	0.57%
7	Pennsylvania		1,114	3.96%	38	Nevada	146	0.52%
45	Rhode Island		66	0.23%	39	Idaho	134	0.48%
24	South Carolina		402	1.43%	40	Hawaii	106	0.38%
48	South Dakota		54	0.19%	41	New Hampshire	81	0.29%
15	Tennessee		622	2.21%	42	Alaska	80	0.28%
2	Texas		1,913	6.81%	43	Montana	79	0.28%
33	Utah		242	0.86%	44	Delaware	78	0.28%
46	Vermont		60	0.21%	45	Rhode Island	66	0.23%
12	Virginia		660	2.35%	46	Maine	60	0.21%
21	Washington		425	1.51%	46	Vermont	60	0.21%
36	West Virginia		161	0.57%	48	South Dakota	54	0.19%
20	Wisconsin		500	1.78%	49	Wyoming	37	0.13%
49	Wyoming		37	0.13%	50	North Dakota	36	0.13%
						District of Columbia	123	0.44%

Source: U.S. Department of Health and Human Services, National Center for Health Statistics
"Monthly Vital Statistics Report" (Vol. 45, No. 12, July 17, 1997)
*Provisional data. Deaths under 1 year old by state of residence.

Infant Mortality Rate in 1996

National Rate = 7.2 Infant Deaths per 1,000 Live Births*

ALPHA ORDER

RANK	STATE	RATE
1	Alabama	10.3
16	Alaska	7.9
21	Arizona	7.6
15	Arkansas	8.0
38	California	6.0
21	Colorado	7.6
35	Connecticut	6.2
19	Delaware	7.7
24	Florida	7.5
5	Georgia	9.0
42	Hawaii	5.8
31	Idaho	7.1
13	Illinois	8.1
24	Indiana	7.5
33	Iowa	6.5
6	Kansas	8.9
21	Kentucky	7.6
3	Louisiana	9.2
49	Maine	4.4
10	Maryland	8.4
48	Massachusetts	4.9
16	Michigan	7.9
34	Minnesota	6.4
2	Mississippi	9.7
13	Missouri	8.1
29	Montana	7.3
9	Nebraska	8.7
35	Nevada	6.2
43	New Hampshire	5.7
29	New Jersey	7.3
40	New Mexico	5.9
32	New York	6.7
3	North Carolina	9.2
50	North Dakota	4.3
19	Ohio	7.7
6	Oklahoma	8.9
44	Oregon	5.6
27	Pennsylvania	7.4
47	Rhode Island	5.2
16	South Carolina	7.9
45	South Dakota	5.4
10	Tennessee	8.4
37	Texas	6.1
40	Utah	5.9
6	Vermont	8.9
27	Virginia	7.4
46	Washington	5.3
12	West Virginia	8.2
24	Wisconsin	7.5
38	Wyoming	6.0

RANK ORDER

RANK	STATE	RATE
1	Alabama	10.3
2	Mississippi	9.7
3	Louisiana	9.2
3	North Carolina	9.2
5	Georgia	9.0
6	Kansas	8.9
6	Oklahoma	8.9
6	Vermont	8.9
9	Nebraska	8.7
10	Maryland	8.4
10	Tennessee	8.4
12	West Virginia	8.2
13	Illinois	8.1
13	Missouri	8.1
15	Arkansas	8.0
16	Alaska	7.9
16	Michigan	7.9
16	South Carolina	7.9
19	Delaware	7.7
19	Ohio	7.7
21	Arizona	7.6
21	Colorado	7.6
21	Kentucky	7.6
24	Florida	7.5
24	Indiana	7.5
24	Wisconsin	7.5
27	Pennsylvania	7.4
27	Virginia	7.4
29	Montana	7.3
29	New Jersey	7.3
31	Idaho	7.1
32	New York	6.7
33	Iowa	6.5
34	Minnesota	6.4
35	Connecticut	6.2
35	Nevada	6.2
37	Texas	6.1
38	California	6.0
38	Wyoming	6.0
40	New Mexico	5.9
40	Utah	5.9
42	Hawaii	5.8
43	New Hampshire	5.7
44	Oregon	5.6
45	South Dakota	5.4
46	Washington	5.3
47	Rhode Island	5.2
48	Massachusetts	4.9
49	Maine	4.4
50	North Dakota	4.3
	District of Columbia	14.9

Source: U.S. Department of Health and Human Services, National Center for Health Statistics
"Monthly Vital Statistics Report" (Vol. 45, No. 12, July 17, 1997)
*Provisional data. Deaths under 1 year old by state of residence.

Infant Deaths in 1990

National Total = 38,351 Infant Deaths*

ALPHA ORDER

RANK	STATE	DEATHS	% of USA
18	Alabama	688	1.79%
41	Alaska	125	0.33%
22	Arizona	610	1.59%
31	Arkansas	336	0.88%
1	California	4,844	12.63%
26	Colorado	472	1.23%
29	Connecticut	398	1.04%
44	Delaware	112	0.29%
5	Florida	1,918	5.00%
9	Georgia	1,392	3.63%
40	Hawaii	138	0.36%
39	Idaho	143	0.37%
4	Illinois	2,104	5.49%
13	Indiana	831	2.17%
33	Iowa	319	0.83%
32	Kansas	329	0.86%
27	Kentucky	461	1.20%
14	Louisiana	799	2.08%
46	Maine	108	0.28%
16	Maryland	766	2.00%
20	Massachusetts	650	1.69%
7	Michigan	1,641	4.28%
25	Minnesota	496	1.29%
24	Mississippi	529	1.38%
17	Missouri	748	1.95%
47	Montana	105	0.27%
37	Nebraska	202	0.53%
38	Nevada	181	0.47%
41	New Hampshire	125	0.33%
11	New Jersey	1,102	2.87%
35	New Mexico	246	0.64%
2	New York	2,851	7.43%
10	North Carolina	1,109	2.89%
48	North Dakota	74	0.19%
8	Ohio	1,640	4.28%
28	Oklahoma	438	1.14%
30	Oregon	354	0.92%
6	Pennsylvania	1,643	4.28%
43	Rhode Island	123	0.32%
19	South Carolina	683	1.78%
45	South Dakota	111	0.29%
15	Tennessee	771	2.01%
3	Texas	2,552	6.65%
34	Utah	271	0.71%
50	Vermont	53	0.14%
12	Virginia	1,013	2.64%
21	Washington	621	1.62%
36	West Virginia	223	0.58%
23	Wisconsin	598	1.56%
49	Wyoming	60	0.16%

RANK ORDER

RANK	STATE	DEATHS	% of USA
1	California	4,844	12.63%
2	New York	2,851	7.43%
3	Texas	2,552	6.65%
4	Illinois	2,104	5.49%
5	Florida	1,918	5.00%
6	Pennsylvania	1,643	4.28%
7	Michigan	1,641	4.28%
8	Ohio	1,640	4.28%
9	Georgia	1,392	3.63%
10	North Carolina	1,109	2.89%
11	New Jersey	1,102	2.87%
12	Virginia	1,013	2.64%
13	Indiana	831	2.17%
14	Louisiana	799	2.08%
15	Tennessee	771	2.01%
16	Maryland	766	2.00%
17	Missouri	748	1.95%
18	Alabama	688	1.79%
19	South Carolina	683	1.78%
20	Massachusetts	650	1.69%
21	Washington	621	1.62%
22	Arizona	610	1.59%
23	Wisconsin	598	1.56%
24	Mississippi	529	1.38%
25	Minnesota	496	1.29%
26	Colorado	472	1.23%
27	Kentucky	461	1.20%
28	Oklahoma	438	1.14%
29	Connecticut	398	1.04%
30	Oregon	354	0.92%
31	Arkansas	336	0.88%
32	Kansas	329	0.86%
33	Iowa	319	0.83%
34	Utah	271	0.71%
35	New Mexico	246	0.64%
36	West Virginia	223	0.58%
37	Nebraska	202	0.53%
38	Nevada	181	0.47%
39	Idaho	143	0.37%
40	Hawaii	138	0.36%
41	Alaska	125	0.33%
41	New Hampshire	125	0.33%
43	Rhode Island	123	0.32%
44	Delaware	112	0.29%
45	South Dakota	111	0.29%
46	Maine	108	0.28%
47	Montana	105	0.27%
48	North Dakota	74	0.19%
49	Wyoming	60	0.16%
50	Vermont	53	0.14%
	District of Columbia	245	0.64%

Source: U.S. Department of Health and Human Services, National Center for Health Statistics
    "Monthly Vital Statistics Report" (Vol. 41, No. 7(S), January 7, 1993)
Final data by state of residence. Infant deaths are those under 1 year old.

Infant Mortality Rate in 1990

National Rate = 9.22 Infant Deaths per 1,000 Live Births*

ALPHA ORDER

RANK	STATE	RATE
5	Alabama	10.84
9	Alaska	10.50
27	Arizona	8.84
22	Arkansas	9.22
42	California	7.91
28	Colorado	8.82
41	Connecticut	7.94
13	Delaware	10.08
17	Florida	9.62
1	Georgia	12.36
48	Hawaii	6.74
29	Idaho	8.70
6	Illinois	10.75
16	Indiana	9.64
37	Iowa	8.09
32	Kansas	8.43
31	Kentucky	8.48
4	Louisiana	11.07
50	Maine	6.22
19	Maryland	9.55
47	Massachusetts	7.02
7	Michigan	10.68
45	Minnesota	7.29
2	Mississippi	12.14
21	Missouri	9.44
24	Montana	9.04
34	Nebraska	8.29
33	Nevada	8.38
46	New Hampshire	7.11
25	New Jersey	9.01
26	New Mexico	8.98
18	New York	9.58
8	North Carolina	10.61
40	North Dakota	8.00
15	Ohio	9.83
23	Oklahoma	9.19
35	Oregon	8.25
19	Pennsylvania	9.55
37	Rhode Island	8.09
3	South Carolina	11.65
12	South Dakota	10.09
10	Tennessee	10.29
39	Texas	8.07
44	Utah	7.47
49	Vermont	6.41
11	Virginia	10.20
43	Washington	7.84
14	West Virginia	9.87
36	Wisconsin	8.20
30	Wyoming	8.59

RANK ORDER

RANK	STATE	RATE
1	Georgia	12.36
2	Mississippi	12.14
3	South Carolina	11.65
4	Louisiana	11.07
5	Alabama	10.84
6	Illinois	10.75
7	Michigan	10.68
8	North Carolina	10.61
9	Alaska	10.50
10	Tennessee	10.29
11	Virginia	10.20
12	South Dakota	10.09
13	Delaware	10.08
14	West Virginia	9.87
15	Ohio	9.83
16	Indiana	9.64
17	Florida	9.62
18	New York	9.58
19	Maryland	9.55
19	Pennsylvania	9.55
21	Missouri	9.44
22	Arkansas	9.22
23	Oklahoma	9.19
24	Montana	9.04
25	New Jersey	9.01
26	New Mexico	8.98
27	Arizona	8.84
28	Colorado	8.82
29	Idaho	8.70
30	Wyoming	8.59
31	Kentucky	8.48
32	Kansas	8.43
33	Nevada	8.38
34	Nebraska	8.29
35	Oregon	8.25
36	Wisconsin	8.20
37	Iowa	8.09
37	Rhode Island	8.09
39	Texas	8.07
40	North Dakota	8.00
41	Connecticut	7.94
42	California	7.91
43	Washington	7.84
44	Utah	7.47
45	Minnesota	7.29
46	New Hampshire	7.11
47	Massachusetts	7.02
48	Hawaii	6.74
49	Vermont	6.41
50	Maine	6.22

	District of Columbia	20.68

Source: U.S. Department of Health and Human Services, National Center for Health Statistics
   "Monthly Vital Statistics Report" (Vol. 41, No. 7(S), January 7, 1993)
*Final data by state of residence. Infant deaths are those under 1 year old.

Infant Deaths in 1980

National Total = 45,526 Infant Deaths*

ALPHA ORDER

RANK	STATE	DEATHS	% of USA
16	Alabama	962	2.11%
48	Alaska	117	0.26%
27	Arizona	620	1.36%
31	Arkansas	472	1.04%
1	California	4,454	9.78%
30	Colorado	501	1.10%
33	Connecticut	433	0.95%
47	Delaware	131	0.29%
7	Florida	1,921	4.22%
9	Georgia	1,337	2.94%
39	Hawaii	187	0.41%
38	Idaho	216	0.47%
4	Illinois	2,812	6.18%
14	Indiana	1,050	2.31%
28	Iowa	565	1.24%
34	Kansas	424	0.93%
23	Kentucky	766	1.68%
12	Louisiana	1,178	2.59%
41	Maine	152	0.33%
18	Maryland	842	1.85%
24	Massachusetts	763	1.68%
8	Michigan	1,862	4.09%
25	Minnesota	678	1.49%
19	Mississippi	814	1.79%
15	Missouri	980	2.15%
40	Montana	176	0.39%
36	Nebraska	314	0.69%
44	Nevada	143	0.31%
45	New Hampshire	136	0.30%
11	New Jersey	1,215	2.67%
37	New Mexico	301	0.66%
3	New York	2,994	6.58%
10	North Carolina	1,224	2.69%
42	North Dakota	145	0.32%
5	Ohio	2,160	4.74%
26	Oklahoma	663	1.46%
29	Oregon	525	1.15%
6	Pennsylvania	2,101	4.61%
46	Rhode Island	134	0.29%
20	South Carolina	812	1.78%
42	South Dakota	145	0.32%
17	Tennessee	935	2.05%
2	Texas	3,326	7.31%
32	Utah	436	0.96%
50	Vermont	84	0.18%
13	Virginia	1,067	2.34%
21	Washington	798	1.75%
35	West Virginia	348	0.76%
22	Wisconsin	770	1.69%
49	Wyoming	103	0.23%

RANK ORDER

RANK	STATE	DEATHS	% of USA
1	California	4,454	9.78%
2	Texas	3,326	7.31%
3	New York	2,994	6.58%
4	Illinois	2,812	6.18%
5	Ohio	2,160	4.74%
6	Pennsylvania	2,101	4.61%
7	Florida	1,921	4.22%
8	Michigan	1,862	4.09%
9	Georgia	1,337	2.94%
10	North Carolina	1,224	2.69%
11	New Jersey	1,215	2.67%
12	Louisiana	1,178	2.59%
13	Virginia	1,067	2.34%
14	Indiana	1,050	2.31%
15	Missouri	980	2.15%
16	Alabama	962	2.11%
17	Tennessee	935	2.05%
18	Maryland	842	1.85%
19	Mississippi	814	1.79%
20	South Carolina	812	1.78%
21	Washington	798	1.75%
22	Wisconsin	770	1.69%
23	Kentucky	766	1.68%
24	Massachusetts	763	1.68%
25	Minnesota	678	1.49%
26	Oklahoma	663	1.46%
27	Arizona	620	1.36%
28	Iowa	565	1.24%
29	Oregon	525	1.15%
30	Colorado	501	1.10%
31	Arkansas	472	1.04%
32	Utah	436	0.96%
33	Connecticut	433	0.95%
34	Kansas	424	0.93%
35	West Virginia	348	0.76%
36	Nebraska	314	0.69%
37	New Mexico	301	0.66%
38	Idaho	216	0.47%
39	Hawaii	187	0.41%
40	Montana	176	0.39%
41	Maine	152	0.33%
42	North Dakota	145	0.32%
42	South Dakota	145	0.32%
44	Nevada	143	0.31%
45	New Hampshire	136	0.30%
46	Rhode Island	134	0.29%
47	Delaware	131	0.29%
48	Alaska	117	0.26%
49	Wyoming	103	0.23%
50	Vermont	84	0.18%
	District of Columbia	234	0.51%

Source: U.S. Department of Health and Human Services, National Center for Health Statistics "Monthly Vital Statistics Report"
Final data by state of residence. Deaths under 1 year old, exclusive of fetal deaths.

Infant Mortality Rate in 1980

National Rate = 12.60 Infant Deaths per 1,000 Live Births*

ALPHA ORDER				RANK ORDER		
RANK	STATE	RATE		RANK	STATE	RATE
3	Alabama	15.15		1	Mississippi	17.01
24	Alaska	12.28		2	South Carolina	15.62
22	Arizona	12.39		3	Alabama	15.15
18	Arkansas	12.66		4	Illinois	14.80
35	California	11.05		5	Florida	14.58
46	Colorado	10.07		6	North Carolina	14.49
34	Connecticut	11.17		7	Georgia	14.48
10	Delaware	13.92		8	Louisiana	14.34
5	Florida	14.58		9	Maryland	14.05
7	Georgia	14.48		10	Delaware	13.92
44	Hawaii	10.30		11	Virginia	13.60
39	Idaho	10.71		12	Tennessee	13.51
4	Illinois	14.80		13	Pennsylvania	13.23
28	Indiana	11.87		14	Kentucky	12.86
29	Iowa	11.82		15	Michigan	12.80
43	Kansas	10.41		16	Ohio	12.77
14	Kentucky	12.86		17	Oklahoma	12.72
8	Louisiana	14.34		18	Arkansas	12.66
50	Maine	9.23		19	New Jersey	12.54
9	Maryland	14.05		20	New York	12.53
41	Massachusetts	10.51		21	Missouri	12.42
15	Michigan	12.80		22	Arizona	12.39
47	Minnesota	10.00		22	Montana	12.39
1	Mississippi	17.01		24	Alaska	12.28
21	Missouri	12.42		25	Oregon	12.17
22	Montana	12.39		26	Texas	12.16
33	Nebraska	11.48		27	North Dakota	12.10
38	Nevada	10.74		28	Indiana	11.87
48	New Hampshire	9.89		29	Iowa	11.82
19	New Jersey	12.54		30	West Virginia	11.81
32	New Mexico	11.53		31	Washington	11.76
20	New York	12.53		32	New Mexico	11.53
6	North Carolina	14.49		33	Nebraska	11.48
27	North Dakota	12.10		34	Connecticut	11.17
16	Ohio	12.77		35	California	11.05
17	Oklahoma	12.72		36	Rhode Island	10.99
25	Oregon	12.17		37	South Dakota	10.92
13	Pennsylvania	13.23		38	Nevada	10.74
36	Rhode Island	10.99		39	Idaho	10.71
2	South Carolina	15.62		40	Vermont	10.65
37	South Dakota	10.92		41	Massachusetts	10.51
12	Tennessee	13.51		42	Utah	10.43
26	Texas	12.16		43	Kansas	10.41
42	Utah	10.43		44	Hawaii	10.30
40	Vermont	10.65		45	Wisconsin	10.29
11	Virginia	13.60		46	Colorado	10.07
31	Washington	11.76		47	Minnesota	10.00
30	West Virginia	11.81		48	New Hampshire	9.89
45	Wisconsin	10.29		49	Wyoming	9.75
49	Wyoming	9.75		50	Maine	9.23
					District of Columbia	25.00

Source: U.S. Department of Health and Human Services, National Center for Health Statistics
   "Monthly Vital Statistics Report"
*Final data by state of residence. Deaths under 1 year old, exclusive of fetal deaths.

Percent Change in Infant Mortality Rate: 1990 to 1996

National Percent Change = 21.7% Decrease*

ALPHA ORDER

RANK ORDER

RANK	STATE	PERCENT CHANGE	RANK	STATE	PERCENT CHANGE
5	Alabama	(4.6)	1	Vermont	39.1
34	Alaska	(24.8)	2	Kansas	6.0
13	Arizona	(13.6)	3	Nebraska	4.8
10	Arkansas	(13.0)	4	Oklahoma	(3.3)
32	California	(24.1)	5	Alabama	(4.6)
13	Colorado	(13.6)	6	Wisconsin	(8.5)
27	Connecticut	(21.5)	7	Kentucky	(10.6)
31	Delaware	(23.8)	8	Minnesota	(12.3)
28	Florida	(21.9)	9	Maryland	(12.5)
38	Georgia	(27.4)	10	Arkansas	(13.0)
12	Hawaii	(13.4)	11	North Carolina	(13.2)
18	Idaho	(18.4)	12	Hawaii	(13.4)
35	Illinois	(25.0)	13	Arizona	(13.6)
28	Indiana	(21.9)	13	Colorado	(13.6)
23	Iowa	(19.8)	15	Missouri	(13.8)
2	Kansas	6.0	16	Louisiana	(17.1)
7	Kentucky	(10.6)	17	West Virginia	(17.2)
16	Louisiana	(17.1)	18	Idaho	(18.4)
40	Maine	(29.0)	18	Tennessee	(18.4)
9	Maryland	(12.5)	20	Montana	(18.9)
41	Massachusetts	(30.0)	20	New Jersey	(18.9)
36	Michigan	(26.2)	22	New Hampshire	(19.7)
8	Minnesota	(12.3)	23	Iowa	(19.8)
23	Mississippi	(19.8)	23	Mississippi	(19.8)
15	Missouri	(13.8)	25	Utah	(21.3)
20	Montana	(18.9)	26	Ohio	(21.4)
3	Nebraska	4.8	27	Connecticut	(21.5)
36	Nevada	(26.2)	28	Florida	(21.9)
22	New Hampshire	(19.7)	28	Indiana	(21.9)
20	New Jersey	(18.9)	30	Pennsylvania	(22.9)
47	New Mexico	(34.4)	31	Delaware	(23.8)
42	New York	(30.2)	32	California	(24.1)
11	North Carolina	(13.2)	33	Texas	(24.7)
49	North Dakota	(46.3)	34	Alaska	(24.8)
26	Ohio	(21.4)	35	Illinois	(25.0)
4	Oklahoma	(3.3)	36	Michigan	(26.2)
45	Oregon	(32.5)	36	Nevada	(26.2)
30	Pennsylvania	(22.9)	38	Georgia	(27.4)
48	Rhode Island	(35.8)	39	Virginia	(27.5)
45	South Carolina	(32.5)	40	Maine	(29.0)
50	South Dakota	(46.5)	41	Massachusetts	(30.0)
18	Tennessee	(18.4)	42	New York	(30.2)
33	Texas	(24.7)	42	Wyoming	(30.2)
25	Utah	(21.3)	44	Washington	(32.1)
1	Vermont	39.1	45	Oregon	(32.5)
39	Virginia	(27.5)	45	South Carolina	(32.5)
44	Washington	(32.1)	47	New Mexico	(34.4)
17	West Virginia	(17.2)	48	Rhode Island	(35.8)
6	Wisconsin	(8.5)	49	North Dakota	(46.3)
42	Wyoming	(30.2)	50	South Dakota	(46.5)

District of Columbia   (28.0)

Source: Morgan Quitno Press using data from US Dept of Health & Human Services, National Center for Health Statistics "Monthly Vital Statistics Report" (Vol. 41, No. 7(S), January 7, 1993; Vol. 45, No. 12, July 17, 1997)
By state of residence. Infant deaths are those under 1 year old.

Percent Change in Infant Mortality Rate: 1980 to 1990

National Percent Change = 26.83% Decrease in Infant Mortality Rate*

ALPHA ORDER

RANK ORDER

RANK	STATE	RATE		RANK	STATE	RATE
35	Alabama	(28.45)		1	South Dakota	(7.60)
4	Alaska	(14.50)		2	Wyoming	(11.90)
37	Arizona	(28.65)		3	Colorado	(12.41)
25	Arkansas	(27.17)		4	Alaska	(14.50)
34	California	(28.42)		5	Georgia	(14.64)
3	Colorado	(12.41)		6	West Virginia	(16.43)
38	Connecticut	(28.92)		7	Michigan	(16.56)
27	Delaware	(27.59)		8	Idaho	(18.77)
47	Florida	(34.02)		9	Indiana	(18.79)
5	Georgia	(14.64)		10	Kansas	(19.02)
49	Hawaii	(34.56)		11	Wisconsin	(20.31)
8	Idaho	(18.77)		12	Nevada	(21.97)
26	Illinois	(27.36)		13	New Mexico	(22.12)
9	Indiana	(18.79)		14	Louisiana	(22.80)
39	Iowa	(31.56)		15	Ohio	(23.02)
10	Kansas	(19.02)		16	New York	(23.54)
48	Kentucky	(34.06)		17	Tennessee	(23.83)
14	Louisiana	(22.80)		18	Missouri	(23.99)
42	Maine	(32.61)		19	Virginia	(25.00)
40	Maryland	(32.03)		20	South Carolina	(25.42)
43	Massachusetts	(33.21)		21	Rhode Island	(26.39)
7	Michigan	(16.56)		22	North Carolina	(26.78)
24	Minnesota	(27.10)		23	Montana	(27.04)
36	Mississippi	(28.63)		24	Minnesota	(27.10)
18	Missouri	(23.99)		25	Arkansas	(27.17)
23	Montana	(27.04)		26	Illinois	(27.36)
29	Nebraska	(27.79)		27	Delaware	(27.59)
12	Nevada	(21.97)		28	Oklahoma	(27.75)
31	New Hampshire	(28.11)		29	Nebraska	(27.79)
32	New Jersey	(28.15)		30	Pennsylvania	(27.82)
13	New Mexico	(22.12)		31	New Hampshire	(28.11)
16	New York	(23.54)		32	New Jersey	(28.15)
22	North Carolina	(26.78)		33	Utah	(28.38)
46	North Dakota	(33.88)		34	California	(28.42)
15	Ohio	(23.02)		35	Alabama	(28.45)
28	Oklahoma	(27.75)		36	Mississippi	(28.63)
41	Oregon	(32.21)		37	Arizona	(28.65)
30	Pennsylvania	(27.82)		38	Connecticut	(28.92)
21	Rhode Island	(26.39)		39	Iowa	(31.56)
20	South Carolina	(25.42)		40	Maryland	(32.03)
1	South Dakota	(7.60)		41	Oregon	(32.21)
17	Tennessee	(23.83)		42	Maine	(32.61)
45	Texas	(33.63)		43	Massachusetts	(33.21)
33	Utah	(28.38)		44	Washington	(33.33)
50	Vermont	(39.81)		45	Texas	(33.63)
19	Virginia	(25.00)		46	North Dakota	(33.88)
44	Washington	(33.33)		47	Florida	(34.02)
6	West Virginia	(16.43)		48	Kentucky	(34.06)
11	Wisconsin	(20.31)		49	Hawaii	(34.56)
2	Wyoming	(11.90)		50	Vermont	(39.81)

District of Columbia   (17.28)

Source: Morgan Quitno Press using data from US Dept of Health & Human Services, National Center for Health Statistics
"Monthly Vital Statistics Report" (Vol. 41, No. 7(S), January 7, 1993)
"Vital Statistics of the United States, 1980" (Vol. I-Natality, issued 1984) and unpublished data
*Final data by state of residence. Infant deaths are those occurring under 1 year, exclusive of fetal deaths.

White Infant Deaths in 1995

National Total = 19,490 Deaths*

ALPHA ORDER

RANK	STATE	DEATHS	% of USA
24	Alabama	284	1.46%
47	Alaska	43	0.22%
13	Arizona	457	2.34%
33	Arkansas	195	1.00%
1	California	2,625	13.47%
22	Colorado	300	1.54%
27	Connecticut	245	1.26%
46	Delaware	46	0.24%
6	Florida	857	4.40%
11	Georgia	468	2.40%
50	Hawaii	17	0.09%
39	Idaho	102	0.52%
4	Illinois	1,019	5.23%
9	Indiana	534	2.74%
26	Iowa	273	1.40%
31	Kansas	207	1.06%
19	Kentucky	347	1.78%
29	Louisiana	231	1.19%
40	Maine	86	0.44%
25	Maryland	282	1.45%
21	Massachusetts	330	1.69%
8	Michigan	661	3.39%
20	Minnesota	338	1.73%
36	Mississippi	151	0.77%
14	Missouri	386	1.98%
43	Montana	69	0.35%
34	Nebraska	155	0.80%
38	Nevada	119	0.61%
41	New Hampshire	79	0.41%
12	New Jersey	465	2.39%
37	New Mexico	138	0.71%
3	New York	1,241	6.37%
10	North Carolina	480	2.46%
45	North Dakota	51	0.26%
5	Ohio	940	4.82%
23	Oklahoma	287	1.47%
28	Oregon	235	1.21%
7	Pennsylvania	793	4.07%
41	Rhode Island	79	0.41%
30	South Carolina	215	1.10%
43	South Dakota	69	0.35%
16	Tennessee	383	1.97%
2	Texas	1,633	8.38%
32	Utah	200	1.03%
48	Vermont	41	0.21%
15	Virginia	385	1.98%
17	Washington	375	1.92%
35	West Virginia	154	0.79%
18	Wisconsin	367	1.88%
49	Wyoming	40	0.21%

RANK ORDER

RANK	STATE	DEATHS	% of USA
1	California	2,625	13.47%
2	Texas	1,633	8.38%
3	New York	1,241	6.37%
4	Illinois	1,019	5.23%
5	Ohio	940	4.82%
6	Florida	857	4.40%
7	Pennsylvania	793	4.07%
8	Michigan	661	3.39%
9	Indiana	534	2.74%
10	North Carolina	480	2.46%
11	Georgia	468	2.40%
12	New Jersey	465	2.39%
13	Arizona	457	2.34%
14	Missouri	386	1.98%
15	Virginia	385	1.98%
16	Tennessee	383	1.97%
17	Washington	375	1.92%
18	Wisconsin	367	1.88%
19	Kentucky	347	1.78%
20	Minnesota	338	1.73%
21	Massachusetts	330	1.69%
22	Colorado	300	1.54%
23	Oklahoma	287	1.47%
24	Alabama	284	1.46%
25	Maryland	282	1.45%
26	Iowa	273	1.40%
27	Connecticut	245	1.26%
28	Oregon	235	1.21%
29	Louisiana	231	1.19%
30	South Carolina	215	1.10%
31	Kansas	207	1.06%
32	Utah	200	1.03%
33	Arkansas	195	1.00%
34	Nebraska	155	0.80%
35	West Virginia	154	0.79%
36	Mississippi	151	0.77%
37	New Mexico	138	0.71%
38	Nevada	119	0.61%
39	Idaho	102	0.52%
40	Maine	86	0.44%
41	New Hampshire	79	0.41%
41	Rhode Island	79	0.41%
43	Montana	69	0.35%
43	South Dakota	69	0.35%
45	North Dakota	51	0.26%
46	Delaware	46	0.24%
47	Alaska	43	0.22%
48	Vermont	41	0.21%
49	Wyoming	40	0.21%
50	Hawaii	17	0.09%
	District of Columbia	13	0.07%

Source: U.S. Department of Health and Human Services, National Center for Health Statistics
"Monthly Vital Statistics Report" (Vol. 45, No. 11(S)2, June 12, 1997)
Final data. Deaths of infants under 1 year old, exclusive of fetal deaths. Based on race of the mother.

White Infant Mortality Rate in 1995

National Rate = 6.3 White Infant Deaths per 1,000 White Live Births*

ALPHA ORDER				RANK ORDER		
RANK	STATE	RATE		RANK	STATE	RATE
12	Alabama	7.1		1	Oklahoma	8.0
32	Alaska	6.1		2	South Dakota	7.9
9	Arizona	7.2		3	Iowa	7.8
9	Arkansas	7.2		4	West Virginia	7.6
41	California	5.8		5	Kentucky	7.4
34	Colorado	6.0		6	Indiana	7.3
21	Connecticut	6.5		6	Nebraska	7.3
34	Delaware	6.0		6	Ohio	7.3
34	Florida	6.0		9	Arizona	7.2
21	Georgia	6.5		9	Arkansas	7.2
NA	Hawaii**	NA		9	Illinois	7.2
41	Idaho	5.8		12	Alabama	7.1
9	Illinois	7.2		13	Mississippi	7.0
6	Indiana	7.3		13	Montana	7.0
3	Iowa	7.8		13	Rhode Island	7.0
26	Kansas	6.2		16	Tennessee	6.8
5	Kentucky	7.4		16	Wyoming	6.8
26	Louisiana	6.2		18	North Carolina	6.7
24	Maine	6.3		18	North Dakota	6.7
34	Maryland	6.0		18	South Carolina	6.7
49	Massachusetts	4.7		21	Connecticut	6.5
26	Michigan	6.2		21	Georgia	6.5
34	Minnesota	6.0		23	Missouri	6.4
13	Mississippi	7.0		24	Maine	6.3
23	Missouri	6.4		24	Wisconsin	6.3
13	Montana	7.0		26	Kansas	6.2
6	Nebraska	7.3		26	Louisiana	6.2
45	Nevada	5.5		26	Michigan	6.2
45	New Hampshire	5.5		26	New York	6.2
47	New Jersey	5.3		26	Pennsylvania	6.2
32	New Mexico	6.1		26	Vermont	6.2
26	New York	6.2		32	Alaska	6.1
18	North Carolina	6.7		32	New Mexico	6.1
18	North Dakota	6.7		34	Colorado	6.0
6	Ohio	7.3		34	Delaware	6.0
1	Oklahoma	8.0		34	Florida	6.0
39	Oregon	5.9		34	Maryland	6.0
26	Pennsylvania	6.2		34	Minnesota	6.0
13	Rhode Island	7.0		39	Oregon	5.9
18	South Carolina	6.7		39	Texas	5.9
2	South Dakota	7.9		41	California	5.8
16	Tennessee	6.8		41	Idaho	5.8
39	Texas	5.9		43	Virginia	5.7
47	Utah	5.3		44	Washington	5.6
26	Vermont	6.2		45	Nevada	5.5
43	Virginia	5.7		45	New Hampshire	5.5
44	Washington	5.6		47	New Jersey	5.3
4	West Virginia	7.6		47	Utah	5.3
24	Wisconsin	6.3		49	Massachusetts	4.7
16	Wyoming	6.8		NA	Hawaii**	NA
					District of Columbia**	NA

Source: U.S. Department of Health and Human Services, National Center for Health Statistics
    "Monthly Vital Statistics Report" (Vol. 45, No. 11(S)2, June 12, 1997)
*Final data. Deaths of infants under 1 year old, exclusive of fetal deaths. Based on race of the mother.
**Not available, fewer than 20 white infant deaths.

Black Infant Deaths in 1995

National Total = 9,118 Deaths*

ALPHA ORDER					RANK ORDER			
RANK	STATE	DEATHS	% of USA		RANK	STATE	DEATHS	% of USA
14	Alabama	302	3.31%		1	New York	783	8.59%
39	Alaska	11	0.12%		2	Illinois	702	7.70%
31	Arizona	38	0.42%		3	California	580	6.36%
22	Arkansas	110	1.21%		3	Georgia	580	6.36%
3	California	580	6.36%		5	Florida	549	6.02%
30	Colorado	44	0.48%		6	Texas	454	4.98%
24	Connecticut	68	0.75%		7	Michigan	434	4.76%
32	Delaware	31	0.34%		8	North Carolina	428	4.69%
5	Florida	549	6.02%		9	Louisiana	410	4.50%
3	Georgia	580	6.36%		10	Ohio	399	4.38%
37	Hawaii	13	0.14%		11	Pennsylvania	378	4.15%
41	Idaho	6	0.07%		12	Maryland	348	3.82%
2	Illinois	702	7.70%		13	Virginia	326	3.58%
19	Indiana	153	1.68%		14	Alabama	302	3.31%
33	Iowa	21	0.23%		15	Tennessee	290	3.18%
26	Kansas	51	0.56%		16	Mississippi	282	3.09%
26	Kentucky	51	0.56%		17	New Jersey	278	3.05%
9	Louisiana	410	4.50%		18	South Carolina	268	2.94%
44	Maine	2	0.02%		19	Indiana	153	1.68%
12	Maryland	348	3.82%		20	Missouri	152	1.67%
23	Massachusetts	70	0.77%		21	Wisconsin	121	1.33%
7	Michigan	434	4.76%		22	Arkansas	110	1.21%
26	Minnesota	51	0.56%		23	Massachusetts	70	0.77%
16	Mississippi	282	3.09%		24	Connecticut	68	0.75%
20	Missouri	152	1.67%		24	Oklahoma	68	0.75%
45	Montana	1	0.01%		26	Kansas	51	0.56%
37	Nebraska	13	0.14%		26	Kentucky	51	0.56%
34	Nevada	19	0.21%		26	Minnesota	51	0.56%
45	New Hampshire	1	0.01%		29	Washington	48	0.53%
17	New Jersey	278	3.05%		30	Colorado	44	0.48%
43	New Mexico	3	0.03%		31	Arizona	38	0.42%
1	New York	783	8.59%		32	Delaware	31	0.34%
8	North Carolina	428	4.69%		33	Iowa	21	0.23%
48	North Dakota	0	0.00%		34	Nevada	19	0.21%
10	Ohio	399	4.38%		35	Oregon	18	0.20%
24	Oklahoma	68	0.75%		36	West Virginia	14	0.15%
35	Oregon	18	0.20%		37	Hawaii	13	0.14%
11	Pennsylvania	378	4.15%		37	Nebraska	13	0.14%
39	Rhode Island	11	0.12%		39	Alaska	11	0.12%
18	South Carolina	268	2.94%		39	Rhode Island	11	0.12%
48	South Dakota	0	0.00%		41	Idaho	6	0.07%
15	Tennessee	290	3.18%		42	Utah	4	0.04%
6	Texas	454	4.98%		43	New Mexico	3	0.03%
42	Utah	4	0.04%		44	Maine	2	0.02%
48	Vermont	0	0.00%		45	Montana	1	0.01%
13	Virginia	326	3.58%		45	New Hampshire	1	0.01%
29	Washington	48	0.53%		45	Wyoming	1	0.01%
36	West Virginia	14	0.15%		48	North Dakota	0	0.00%
21	Wisconsin	121	1.33%		48	South Dakota	0	0.00%
45	Wyoming	1	0.01%		48	Vermont	0	0.00%
						District of Columbia	133	1.46%

Source: U.S. Department of Health and Human Services, National Center for Health Statistics
   "Monthly Vital Statistics Report" (Vol. 45, No. 11(S)2, June 12, 1997)
*Final data. Deaths of infants under 1 year old, exclusive of fetal deaths. Based on race of the mother.

Black Infant Mortality Rate in 1995

National Rate = 15.1 Black Infant Deaths per 1,000 Black Live Births*

ALPHA ORDER

RANK	STATE	RATE
18	Alabama	15.2
NA	Alaska**	NA
11	Arizona	17.0
24	Arkansas	14.3
23	California	14.4
12	Colorado	16.8
30	Connecticut	12.6
28	Delaware	13.1
29	Florida	13.0
19	Georgia	15.1
NA	Hawaii**	NA
NA	Idaho**	NA
2	Illinois	18.7
8	Indiana	17.5
1	Iowa	21.2
5	Kansas	17.6
32	Kentucky	10.7
15	Louisiana	15.3
NA	Maine**	NA
15	Maryland	15.3
33	Massachusetts	9.0
10	Michigan	17.3
5	Minnesota	17.6
21	Mississippi	14.7
26	Missouri	13.8
NA	Montana**	NA
NA	Nebraska**	NA
NA	Nevada**	NA
NA	New Hampshire**	NA
27	New Jersey	13.3
NA	New Mexico**	NA
25	New York	13.9
14	North Carolina	15.9
NA	North Dakota**	NA
8	Ohio	17.5
19	Oklahoma	15.1
NA	Oregon**	NA
5	Pennsylvania	17.6
NA	Rhode Island**	NA
22	South Carolina	14.6
NA	South Dakota**	NA
4	Tennessee	17.9
31	Texas	11.7
NA	Utah**	NA
NA	Vermont**	NA
15	Virginia	15.3
13	Washington	16.2
NA	West Virginia**	NA
3	Wisconsin	18.6
NA	Wyoming**	NA

RANK ORDER

RANK	STATE	RATE
1	Iowa	21.2
2	Illinois	18.7
3	Wisconsin	18.6
4	Tennessee	17.9
5	Kansas	17.6
5	Minnesota	17.6
5	Pennsylvania	17.6
8	Indiana	17.5
8	Ohio	17.5
10	Michigan	17.3
11	Arizona	17.0
12	Colorado	16.8
13	Washington	16.2
14	North Carolina	15.9
15	Louisiana	15.3
15	Maryland	15.3
15	Virginia	15.3
18	Alabama	15.2
19	Georgia	15.1
19	Oklahoma	15.1
21	Mississippi	14.7
22	South Carolina	14.6
23	California	14.4
24	Arkansas	14.3
25	New York	13.9
26	Missouri	13.8
27	New Jersey	13.3
28	Delaware	13.1
29	Florida	13.0
30	Connecticut	12.6
31	Texas	11.7
32	Kentucky	10.7
33	Massachusetts	9.0
NA	Alaska**	NA
NA	Hawaii**	NA
NA	Idaho**	NA
NA	Maine**	NA
NA	Montana**	NA
NA	Nebraska**	NA
NA	Nevada**	NA
NA	New Hampshire**	NA
NA	New Mexico**	NA
NA	North Dakota**	NA
NA	Oregon**	NA
NA	Rhode Island**	NA
NA	South Dakota**	NA
NA	Utah**	NA
NA	Vermont**	NA
NA	West Virginia**	NA
NA	Wyoming**	NA

District of Columbia	19.6

Source: U.S. Department of Health and Human Services, National Center for Health Statistics
   "Monthly Vital Statistics Report" (Vol. 45, No. 11(S)2, June 12, 1997)
*Final data. Deaths of infants under 1 year old, exclusive of fetal deaths. Based on race of the mother.
**Not available, fewer than 20 black infant deaths.

White Infant Mortality Rate in 1990

National Rate = 7.7 White Infant Deaths per 1,000 Live Births*

ALPHA ORDER

RANK	STATE	RATE
13	Alabama	8.3
10	Alaska	8.5
17	Arizona	8.2
21	Arkansas	8.0
32	California	7.6
12	Colorado	8.4
46	Connecticut	6.6
37	Delaware	7.3
32	Florida	7.6
4	Georgia	9.1
50	Hawaii	5.1
7	Idaho	8.7
29	Illinois	7.7
5	Indiana	8.9
26	Iowa	7.8
29	Kansas	7.7
21	Kentucky	8.0
37	Louisiana	7.3
49	Maine	6.2
47	Maryland	6.5
44	Massachusetts	6.7
24	Michigan	7.9
44	Minnesota	6.7
10	Mississippi	8.5
26	Missouri	7.8
8	Montana	8.6
39	Nebraska	7.2
19	Nevada	8.1
39	New Hampshire	7.2
43	New Jersey	6.8
3	New Mexico	9.3
29	New York	7.7
13	North Carolina	8.3
24	North Dakota	7.9
17	Ohio	8.2
2	Oklahoma	9.4
19	Oregon	8.1
26	Pennsylvania	7.8
13	Rhode Island	8.3
13	South Carolina	8.3
8	South Dakota	8.6
21	Tennessee	8.0
42	Texas	7.1
36	Utah	7.4
47	Vermont	6.5
35	Virginia	7.5
32	Washington	7.6
1	West Virginia	9.6
39	Wisconsin	7.2
6	Wyoming	8.8

RANK ORDER

RANK	STATE	RATE
1	West Virginia	9.6
2	Oklahoma	9.4
3	New Mexico	9.3
4	Georgia	9.1
5	Indiana	8.9
6	Wyoming	8.8
7	Idaho	8.7
8	Montana	8.6
8	South Dakota	8.6
10	Alaska	8.5
10	Mississippi	8.5
12	Colorado	8.4
13	Alabama	8.3
13	North Carolina	8.3
13	Rhode Island	8.3
13	South Carolina	8.3
17	Arizona	8.2
17	Ohio	8.2
19	Nevada	8.1
19	Oregon	8.1
21	Arkansas	8.0
21	Kentucky	8.0
21	Tennessee	8.0
24	Michigan	7.9
24	North Dakota	7.9
26	Iowa	7.8
26	Missouri	7.8
26	Pennsylvania	7.8
29	Illinois	7.7
29	Kansas	7.7
29	New York	7.7
32	California	7.6
32	Florida	7.6
32	Washington	7.6
35	Virginia	7.5
36	Utah	7.4
37	Delaware	7.3
37	Louisiana	7.3
39	Nebraska	7.2
39	New Hampshire	7.2
39	Wisconsin	7.2
42	Texas	7.1
43	New Jersey	6.8
44	Massachusetts	6.7
44	Minnesota	6.7
46	Connecticut	6.6
47	Maryland	6.5
47	Vermont	6.5
49	Maine	6.2
50	Hawaii	5.1

District of Columbia		12.1

Source: U.S. Department of Health and Human Services, National Center for Health Statistics,
   "Vital Statistics of the United States"
*Deaths of infants under 1 year old, exclusive of fetal deaths. Final data by state of residence.

Black Infant Mortality Rate in 1990

National Rate = 17.0 Black Infant Deaths per 1,000 Live Births*

ALPHA ORDER				RANK ORDER		
RANK	STATE	RATE		RANK	STATE	RATE
27	Alabama	15.9		1	Illinois	21.5
41	Alaska	11.2		2	Michigan	21.0
17	Arizona	16.7		3	Minnesota	19.7
33	Arkansas	13.6		4	Delaware	19.4
31	California	14.2		5	Pennsylvania	18.8
19	Colorado	16.5		5	Virginia	18.8
24	Connecticut	16.0		7	Ohio	18.3
4	Delaware	19.4		8	Wisconsin	18.1
22	Florida	16.2		9	Georgia	18.0
9	Georgia	18.0		9	Iowa	18.0
40	Hawaii	11.5		11	Missouri	17.5
42	Idaho	10.9		11	Tennessee	17.5
1	Illinois	21.5		13	New Jersey	17.3
24	Indiana	16.0		13	New York	17.3
9	Iowa	18.0		15	South Carolina	17.1
28	Kansas	15.4		16	Nebraska	16.8
33	Kentucky	13.6		17	Arizona	16.7
19	Louisiana	16.5		18	West Virginia	16.6
46	Maine	6.1		19	Colorado	16.5
21	Maryland	16.3		19	Louisiana	16.5
43	Massachusetts	10.4		21	Maryland	16.3
2	Michigan	21.0		22	Florida	16.2
3	Minnesota	19.7		23	Mississippi	16.1
23	Mississippi	16.1		24	Connecticut	16.0
11	Missouri	17.5		24	Indiana	16.0
35	Montana	13.3		24	North Carolina	16.0
16	Nebraska	16.8		27	Alabama	15.9
39	Nevada	12.5		28	Kansas	15.4
47	New Hampshire	5.4		29	Oregon	15.1
13	New Jersey	17.3		30	Washington	14.5
38	New Mexico	12.8		31	California	14.2
13	New York	17.3		32	Texas	13.9
24	North Carolina	16.0		33	Arkansas	13.6
NA	North Dakota**	NA		33	Kentucky	13.6
7	Ohio	18.3		35	Montana	13.3
36	Oklahoma	13.2		36	Oklahoma	13.2
29	Oregon	15.1		37	Utah	13.0
5	Pennsylvania	18.8		38	New Mexico	12.8
44	Rhode Island	9.7		39	Nevada	12.5
15	South Carolina	17.1		40	Hawaii	11.5
45	South Dakota	7.4		41	Alaska	11.2
11	Tennessee	17.5		42	Idaho	10.9
32	Texas	13.9		43	Massachusetts	10.4
37	Utah	13.0		44	Rhode Island	9.7
NA	Vermont**	NA		45	South Dakota	7.4
5	Virginia	18.8		46	Maine	6.1
30	Washington	14.5		47	New Hampshire	5.4
18	West Virginia	16.6		NA	North Dakota**	NA
8	Wisconsin	18.1		NA	Vermont**	NA
NA	Wyoming**	NA		NA	Wyoming**	NA
					District of Columbia	24.4

Source: U.S. Department of Health and Human Services, National Center for Health Statistics,
    "Vital Statistics of the United States"
*Deaths of infants under 1 year old, exclusive of fetal deaths. Final data by state of residence.
**Not available.

Neonatal Deaths in 1995

National Total = 19,155 Deaths*

ALPHA ORDER

RANK	STATE	DEATHS	% of USA
17	Alabama	389	2.03%
45	Alaska	48	0.25%
18	Arizona	351	1.83%
31	Arkansas	185	0.97%
1	California	2,169	11.32%
29	Colorado	219	1.14%
27	Connecticut	232	1.21%
46	Delaware	47	0.25%
6	Florida	884	4.61%
9	Georgia	697	3.64%
38	Hawaii	74	0.39%
41	Idaho	64	0.33%
4	Illinois	1,175	6.13%
13	Indiana	473	2.47%
30	Iowa	193	1.01%
32	Kansas	172	0.90%
26	Kentucky	240	1.25%
15	Louisiana	425	2.22%
42	Maine	60	0.31%
14	Maryland	444	2.32%
22	Massachusetts	299	1.56%
8	Michigan	727	3.80%
25	Minnesota	254	1.33%
24	Mississippi	255	1.33%
19	Missouri	336	1.75%
47	Montana	41	0.21%
35	Nebraska	121	0.63%
40	Nevada	71	0.37%
43	New Hampshire	54	0.28%
11	New Jersey	531	2.77%
36	New Mexico	112	0.58%
2	New York	1,471	7.68%
10	North Carolina	653	3.41%
48	North Dakota	35	0.18%
5	Ohio	918	4.79%
28	Oklahoma	223	1.16%
33	Oregon	137	0.72%
7	Pennsylvania	811	4.23%
39	Rhode Island	72	0.38%
19	South Carolina	336	1.75%
43	South Dakota	54	0.28%
16	Tennessee	398	2.08%
3	Texas	1,224	6.39%
34	Utah	126	0.66%
49	Vermont	29	0.15%
12	Virginia	505	2.64%
23	Washington	263	1.37%
36	West Virginia	112	0.58%
21	Wisconsin	312	1.63%
50	Wyoming	23	0.12%

RANK ORDER

RANK	STATE	DEATHS	% of USA
1	California	2,169	11.32%
2	New York	1,471	7.68%
3	Texas	1,224	6.39%
4	Illinois	1,175	6.13%
5	Ohio	918	4.79%
6	Florida	884	4.61%
7	Pennsylvania	811	4.23%
8	Michigan	727	3.80%
9	Georgia	697	3.64%
10	North Carolina	653	3.41%
11	New Jersey	531	2.77%
12	Virginia	505	2.64%
13	Indiana	473	2.47%
14	Maryland	444	2.32%
15	Louisiana	425	2.22%
16	Tennessee	398	2.08%
17	Alabama	389	2.03%
18	Arizona	351	1.83%
19	Missouri	336	1.75%
19	South Carolina	336	1.75%
21	Wisconsin	312	1.63%
22	Massachusetts	299	1.56%
23	Washington	263	1.37%
24	Mississippi	255	1.33%
25	Minnesota	254	1.33%
26	Kentucky	240	1.25%
27	Connecticut	232	1.21%
28	Oklahoma	223	1.16%
29	Colorado	219	1.14%
30	Iowa	193	1.01%
31	Arkansas	185	0.97%
32	Kansas	172	0.90%
33	Oregon	137	0.72%
34	Utah	126	0.66%
35	Nebraska	121	0.63%
36	New Mexico	112	0.58%
36	West Virginia	112	0.58%
38	Hawaii	74	0.39%
39	Rhode Island	72	0.38%
40	Nevada	71	0.37%
41	Idaho	64	0.33%
42	Maine	60	0.31%
43	New Hampshire	54	0.28%
43	South Dakota	54	0.28%
45	Alaska	48	0.25%
46	Delaware	47	0.25%
47	Montana	41	0.21%
48	North Dakota	35	0.18%
49	Vermont	29	0.15%
50	Wyoming	23	0.12%
	District of Columbia	111	0.58%

Source: U.S. Department of Health and Human Services, National Center for Health Statistics
    "Monthly Vital Statistics Report" (Vol. 45, No. 11(S)2, June 12, 1997)
*Final data. Deaths of infants under 28 days, exclusive of fetal deaths.

Neonatal Death Rate in 1995

National Rate = 4.9 Neonatal Deaths per 1,000 Live Births*

ALPHA ORDER

RANK	STATE	RATE
3	Alabama	6.4
25	Alaska	4.7
24	Arizona	4.8
16	Arkansas	5.3
40	California	3.9
37	Colorado	4.0
19	Connecticut	5.2
27	Delaware	4.6
25	Florida	4.7
6	Georgia	6.2
37	Hawaii	4.0
46	Idaho	3.5
5	Illinois	6.3
10	Indiana	5.7
19	Iowa	5.2
27	Kansas	4.6
27	Kentucky	4.6
2	Louisiana	6.5
33	Maine	4.3
8	Maryland	6.1
42	Massachusetts	3.7
13	Michigan	5.4
37	Minnesota	4.0
6	Mississippi	6.2
27	Missouri	4.6
42	Montana	3.7
19	Nebraska	5.2
50	Nevada	2.8
42	New Hampshire	3.7
27	New Jersey	4.6
35	New Mexico	4.2
13	New York	5.4
3	North Carolina	6.4
36	North Dakota	4.1
9	Ohio	6.0
23	Oklahoma	4.9
48	Oregon	3.2
16	Pennsylvania	5.3
11	Rhode Island	5.6
1	South Carolina	6.6
19	South Dakota	5.2
13	Tennessee	5.4
41	Texas	3.8
48	Utah	3.2
33	Vermont	4.3
12	Virginia	5.5
47	Washington	3.4
16	West Virginia	5.3
27	Wisconsin	4.6
42	Wyoming	3.7

RANK ORDER

RANK	STATE	RATE
1	South Carolina	6.6
2	Louisiana	6.5
3	Alabama	6.4
3	North Carolina	6.4
5	Illinois	6.3
6	Georgia	6.2
6	Mississippi	6.2
8	Maryland	6.1
9	Ohio	6.0
10	Indiana	5.7
11	Rhode Island	5.6
12	Virginia	5.5
13	Michigan	5.4
13	New York	5.4
13	Tennessee	5.4
16	Arkansas	5.3
16	Pennsylvania	5.3
16	West Virginia	5.3
19	Connecticut	5.2
19	Iowa	5.2
19	Nebraska	5.2
19	South Dakota	5.2
23	Oklahoma	4.9
24	Arizona	4.8
25	Alaska	4.7
25	Florida	4.7
27	Delaware	4.6
27	Kansas	4.6
27	Kentucky	4.6
27	Missouri	4.6
27	New Jersey	4.6
27	Wisconsin	4.6
33	Maine	4.3
33	Vermont	4.3
35	New Mexico	4.2
36	North Dakota	4.1
37	Colorado	4.0
37	Hawaii	4.0
37	Minnesota	4.0
40	California	3.9
41	Texas	3.8
42	Massachusetts	3.7
42	Montana	3.7
42	New Hampshire	3.7
42	Wyoming	3.7
46	Idaho	3.5
47	Washington	3.4
48	Oregon	3.2
48	Utah	3.2
50	Nevada	2.8
	District of Columbia	12.3

Source: U.S. Department of Health and Human Services, National Center for Health Statistics
"Monthly Vital Statistics Report" (Vol. 45, No. 11(S)2, June 12, 1997)
Final data. Deaths of infants under 28 days, exclusive of fetal deaths.

White Neonatal Deaths in 1995

National Total = 12,644 Deaths*

ALPHA ORDER

RANK ORDER

RANK	STATE	DEATHS	% of USA
24	Alabama	182	1.44%
47	Alaska	27	0.21%
12	Arizona	310	2.45%
33	Arkansas	119	0.94%
1	California	1,650	13.05%
23	Colorado	185	1.46%
25	Connecticut	180	1.42%
48	Delaware	26	0.21%
7	Florida	533	4.22%
13	Georgia	299	2.36%
50	Hawaii	11	0.09%
38	Idaho	62	0.49%
4	Illinois	705	5.58%
9	Indiana	358	2.83%
26	Iowa	174	1.38%
30	Kansas	139	1.10%
21	Kentucky	207	1.64%
28	Louisiana	154	1.22%
41	Maine	58	0.46%
22	Maryland	187	1.48%
17	Massachusetts	233	1.84%
8	Michigan	429	3.39%
20	Minnesota	211	1.67%
37	Mississippi	90	0.71%
16	Missouri	239	1.89%
44	Montana	36	0.28%
34	Nebraska	109	0.86%
38	Nevada	62	0.49%
42	New Hampshire	53	0.42%
10	New Jersey	340	2.69%
36	New Mexico	99	0.78%
3	New York	906	7.17%
11	North Carolina	331	2.62%
45	North Dakota	31	0.25%
5	Ohio	643	5.09%
27	Oklahoma	171	1.35%
31	Oregon	126	1.00%
6	Pennsylvania	555	4.39%
40	Rhode Island	61	0.48%
29	South Carolina	142	1.12%
43	South Dakota	40	0.32%
19	Tennessee	213	1.68%
2	Texas	958	7.58%
32	Utah	122	0.96%
46	Vermont	29	0.23%
14	Virginia	257	2.03%
18	Washington	220	1.74%
35	West Virginia	100	0.79%
15	Wisconsin	240	1.90%
49	Wyoming	20	0.16%

RANK	STATE	DEATHS	% of USA
1	California	1,650	13.05%
2	Texas	958	7.58%
3	New York	906	7.17%
4	Illinois	705	5.58%
5	Ohio	643	5.09%
6	Pennsylvania	555	4.39%
7	Florida	533	4.22%
8	Michigan	429	3.39%
9	Indiana	358	2.83%
10	New Jersey	340	2.69%
11	North Carolina	331	2.62%
12	Arizona	310	2.45%
13	Georgia	299	2.36%
14	Virginia	257	2.03%
15	Wisconsin	240	1.90%
16	Missouri	239	1.89%
17	Massachusetts	233	1.84%
18	Washington	220	1.74%
19	Tennessee	213	1.68%
20	Minnesota	211	1.67%
21	Kentucky	207	1.64%
22	Maryland	187	1.48%
23	Colorado	185	1.46%
24	Alabama	182	1.44%
25	Connecticut	180	1.42%
26	Iowa	174	1.38%
27	Oklahoma	171	1.35%
28	Louisiana	154	1.22%
29	South Carolina	142	1.12%
30	Kansas	139	1.10%
31	Oregon	126	1.00%
32	Utah	122	0.96%
33	Arkansas	119	0.94%
34	Nebraska	109	0.86%
35	West Virginia	100	0.79%
36	New Mexico	99	0.78%
37	Mississippi	90	0.71%
38	Idaho	62	0.49%
38	Nevada	62	0.49%
40	Rhode Island	61	0.48%
41	Maine	58	0.46%
42	New Hampshire	53	0.42%
43	South Dakota	40	0.32%
44	Montana	36	0.28%
45	North Dakota	31	0.25%
46	Vermont	29	0.23%
47	Alaska	27	0.21%
48	Delaware	26	0.21%
49	Wyoming	20	0.16%
50	Hawaii	11	0.09%
	District of Columbia	12	0.09%

Source: U.S. Department of Health and Human Services, National Center for Health Statistics
"Monthly Vital Statistics Report" (Vol. 45, No. 11(S)2, June 12, 1997)
*Final data. Deaths of infants under 28 days, exclusive of fetal deaths. Based on race of the mother.

White Neonatal Death Rate in 1995

National Rate = 4.1 White Neonatal Deaths per 1,000 White Live Births*

ALPHA ORDER

RANK	STATE	RATE
11	Alabama	4.6
32	Alaska	3.8
6	Arizona	4.9
16	Arkansas	4.4
35	California	3.7
35	Colorado	3.7
9	Connecticut	4.8
43	Delaware	3.4
35	Florida	3.7
22	Georgia	4.2
NA	Hawaii**	NA
41	Idaho	3.5
3	Illinois	5.0
6	Indiana	4.9
3	Iowa	5.0
22	Kansas	4.2
16	Kentucky	4.4
25	Louisiana	4.1
21	Maine	4.3
28	Maryland	4.0
45	Massachusetts	3.3
28	Michigan	4.0
35	Minnesota	3.7
22	Mississippi	4.2
30	Missouri	3.9
35	Montana	3.7
2	Nebraska	5.1
49	Nevada	2.9
35	New Hampshire	3.7
30	New Jersey	3.9
16	New Mexico	4.4
11	New York	4.6
11	North Carolina	4.6
25	North Dakota	4.1
3	Ohio	5.0
10	Oklahoma	4.7
47	Oregon	3.2
16	Pennsylvania	4.4
1	Rhode Island	5.4
15	South Carolina	4.5
11	South Dakota	4.6
32	Tennessee	3.8
41	Texas	3.5
47	Utah	3.2
16	Vermont	4.4
32	Virginia	3.8
45	Washington	3.3
6	West Virginia	4.9
25	Wisconsin	4.1
43	Wyoming	3.4

RANK ORDER

RANK	STATE	RATE
1	Rhode Island	5.4
2	Nebraska	5.1
3	Illinois	5.0
3	Iowa	5.0
3	Ohio	5.0
6	Arizona	4.9
6	Indiana	4.9
6	West Virginia	4.9
9	Connecticut	4.8
10	Oklahoma	4.7
11	Alabama	4.6
11	New York	4.6
11	North Carolina	4.6
11	South Dakota	4.6
15	South Carolina	4.5
16	Arkansas	4.4
16	Kentucky	4.4
16	New Mexico	4.4
16	Pennsylvania	4.4
16	Vermont	4.4
21	Maine	4.3
22	Georgia	4.2
22	Kansas	4.2
22	Mississippi	4.2
25	Louisiana	4.1
25	North Dakota	4.1
25	Wisconsin	4.1
28	Maryland	4.0
28	Michigan	4.0
30	Missouri	3.9
30	New Jersey	3.9
32	Alaska	3.8
32	Tennessee	3.8
32	Virginia	3.8
35	California	3.7
35	Colorado	3.7
35	Florida	3.7
35	Minnesota	3.7
35	Montana	3.7
35	New Hampshire	3.7
41	Idaho	3.5
41	Texas	3.5
43	Delaware	3.4
43	Wyoming	3.4
45	Massachusetts	3.3
45	Washington	3.3
47	Oregon	3.2
47	Utah	3.2
49	Nevada	2.9
NA	Hawaii**	NA
	District of Columbia**	NA

Source: U.S. Department of Health and Human Services, National Center for Health Statistics
"Monthly Vital Statistics Report" (Vol. 45, No. 11(S)2, June 12, 1997)
*Final data. Deaths of infants under 28 days, exclusive of fetal deaths. Based on race of the mother.
**Not available. Fewer than 20 white neonatal deaths.

Black Neonatal Deaths in 1995

National Total = 5,940 Deaths*

<table>
<tr><td colspan="4">ALPHA ORDER</td><td colspan="4">RANK ORDER</td></tr>
<tr><td>RANK</td><td>STATE</td><td>DEATHS</td><td>% of USA</td><td>RANK</td><td>STATE</td><td>DEATHS</td><td>% of USA</td></tr>
</table>

RANK	STATE	DEATHS	% of USA	RANK	STATE	DEATHS	% of USA
14	Alabama	203	3.42%	1	New York	520	8.75%
40	Alaska	4	0.07%	2	Illinois	457	7.69%
32	Arizona	20	0.34%	3	Georgia	391	6.58%
22	Arkansas	63	1.06%	4	California	346	5.82%
4	California	346	5.82%	5	Florida	344	5.79%
28	Colorado	29	0.49%	6	North Carolina	304	5.12%
24	Connecticut	49	0.82%	7	Michigan	288	4.85%
31	Delaware	21	0.35%	8	Louisiana	270	4.55%
5	Florida	344	5.79%	9	Ohio	269	4.53%
3	Georgia	391	6.58%	10	Texas	251	4.23%
35	Hawaii	11	0.19%	11	Pennsylvania	249	4.19%
41	Idaho	1	0.02%	12	Maryland	245	4.12%
2	Illinois	457	7.69%	13	Virginia	237	3.99%
19	Indiana	114	1.92%	14	Alabama	203	3.42%
33	Iowa	14	0.24%	15	South Carolina	191	3.22%
27	Kansas	31	0.52%	16	Tennessee	183	3.08%
26	Kentucky	32	0.54%	17	New Jersey	179	3.01%
8	Louisiana	270	4.55%	18	Mississippi	164	2.76%
41	Maine	1	0.02%	19	Indiana	114	1.92%
12	Maryland	245	4.12%	20	Missouri	96	1.62%
23	Massachusetts	54	0.91%	21	Wisconsin	69	1.16%
7	Michigan	288	4.85%	22	Arkansas	63	1.06%
30	Minnesota	24	0.40%	23	Massachusetts	54	0.91%
18	Mississippi	164	2.76%	24	Connecticut	49	0.82%
20	Missouri	96	1.62%	25	Oklahoma	38	0.64%
41	Montana	1	0.02%	26	Kentucky	32	0.54%
35	Nebraska	11	0.19%	27	Kansas	31	0.52%
39	Nevada	5	0.08%	28	Colorado	29	0.49%
41	New Hampshire	1	0.02%	28	Washington	29	0.49%
17	New Jersey	179	3.01%	30	Minnesota	24	0.40%
41	New Mexico	1	0.02%	31	Delaware	21	0.35%
1	New York	520	8.75%	32	Arizona	20	0.34%
6	North Carolina	304	5.12%	33	Iowa	14	0.24%
47	North Dakota	0	0.00%	34	West Virginia	12	0.20%
9	Ohio	269	4.53%	35	Hawaii	11	0.19%
25	Oklahoma	38	0.64%	35	Nebraska	11	0.19%
38	Oregon	8	0.13%	37	Rhode Island	10	0.17%
11	Pennsylvania	249	4.19%	38	Oregon	8	0.13%
37	Rhode Island	10	0.17%	39	Nevada	5	0.08%
15	South Carolina	191	3.22%	40	Alaska	4	0.07%
47	South Dakota	0	0.00%	41	Idaho	1	0.02%
16	Tennessee	183	3.08%	41	Maine	1	0.02%
10	Texas	251	4.23%	41	Montana	1	0.02%
41	Utah	1	0.02%	41	New Hampshire	1	0.02%
47	Vermont	0	0.00%	41	New Mexico	1	0.02%
13	Virginia	237	3.99%	41	Utah	1	0.02%
28	Washington	29	0.49%	47	North Dakota	0	0.00%
34	West Virginia	12	0.20%	47	South Dakota	0	0.00%
21	Wisconsin	69	1.16%	47	Vermont	0	0.00%
47	Wyoming	0	0.00%	47	Wyoming	0	0.00%
					District of Columbia	99	1.67%

Source: U.S. Department of Health and Human Services, National Center for Health Statistics
"Monthly Vital Statistics Report" (Vol. 45, No. 11(S)2, June 12, 1997)
*Final data. Deaths of infants under 28 days, exclusive of fetal deaths. Based on race of the mother.

Black Neonatal Death Rate in 1995

National Rate = 9.8 Black Neonatal Deaths per 1,000 Black Live Births*

<table>
<tr><td colspan="3">ALPHA ORDER</td><td colspan="3">RANK ORDER</td></tr>
<tr><td>RANK</td><td>STATE</td><td>RATE</td><td>RANK</td><td>STATE</td><td>RATE</td></tr>
<tr><td>14</td><td>Alabama</td><td>10.2</td><td>1</td><td>Indiana</td><td>13.0</td></tr>
<tr><td>NA</td><td>Alaska**</td><td>NA</td><td>2</td><td>Illinois</td><td>12.2</td></tr>
<tr><td>20</td><td>Arizona</td><td>8.9</td><td>3</td><td>Ohio</td><td>11.8</td></tr>
<tr><td>28</td><td>Arkansas</td><td>8.2</td><td>4</td><td>Pennsylvania</td><td>11.6</td></tr>
<tr><td>23</td><td>California</td><td>8.6</td><td>5</td><td>Michigan</td><td>11.5</td></tr>
<tr><td>8</td><td>Colorado</td><td>11.1</td><td>6</td><td>North Carolina</td><td>11.3</td></tr>
<tr><td>19</td><td>Connecticut</td><td>9.1</td><td>6</td><td>Tennessee</td><td>11.3</td></tr>
<tr><td>20</td><td>Delaware</td><td>8.9</td><td>8</td><td>Colorado</td><td>11.1</td></tr>
<tr><td>28</td><td>Florida</td><td>8.2</td><td>8</td><td>Virginia</td><td>11.1</td></tr>
<tr><td>14</td><td>Georgia</td><td>10.2</td><td>10</td><td>Maryland</td><td>10.8</td></tr>
<tr><td>NA</td><td>Hawaii**</td><td>NA</td><td>11</td><td>Kansas</td><td>10.7</td></tr>
<tr><td>NA</td><td>Idaho**</td><td>NA</td><td>12</td><td>Wisconsin</td><td>10.6</td></tr>
<tr><td>2</td><td>Illinois</td><td>12.2</td><td>13</td><td>South Carolina</td><td>10.4</td></tr>
<tr><td>1</td><td>Indiana</td><td>13.0</td><td>14</td><td>Alabama</td><td>10.2</td></tr>
<tr><td>NA</td><td>Iowa**</td><td>NA</td><td>14</td><td>Georgia</td><td>10.2</td></tr>
<tr><td>11</td><td>Kansas</td><td>10.7</td><td>16</td><td>Louisiana</td><td>10.1</td></tr>
<tr><td>31</td><td>Kentucky</td><td>6.7</td><td>17</td><td>Washington</td><td>9.8</td></tr>
<tr><td>16</td><td>Louisiana</td><td>10.1</td><td>18</td><td>New York</td><td>9.3</td></tr>
<tr><td>NA</td><td>Maine**</td><td>NA</td><td>19</td><td>Connecticut</td><td>9.1</td></tr>
<tr><td>10</td><td>Maryland</td><td>10.8</td><td>20</td><td>Arizona</td><td>8.9</td></tr>
<tr><td>30</td><td>Massachusetts</td><td>6.9</td><td>20</td><td>Delaware</td><td>8.9</td></tr>
<tr><td>5</td><td>Michigan</td><td>11.5</td><td>22</td><td>Missouri</td><td>8.7</td></tr>
<tr><td>27</td><td>Minnesota</td><td>8.3</td><td>23</td><td>California</td><td>8.6</td></tr>
<tr><td>24</td><td>Mississippi</td><td>8.5</td><td>24</td><td>Mississippi</td><td>8.5</td></tr>
<tr><td>22</td><td>Missouri</td><td>8.7</td><td>24</td><td>New Jersey</td><td>8.5</td></tr>
<tr><td>NA</td><td>Montana**</td><td>NA</td><td>24</td><td>Oklahoma</td><td>8.5</td></tr>
<tr><td>NA</td><td>Nebraska**</td><td>NA</td><td>27</td><td>Minnesota</td><td>8.3</td></tr>
<tr><td>NA</td><td>Nevada**</td><td>NA</td><td>28</td><td>Arkansas</td><td>8.2</td></tr>
<tr><td>NA</td><td>New Hampshire**</td><td>NA</td><td>28</td><td>Florida</td><td>8.2</td></tr>
<tr><td>24</td><td>New Jersey</td><td>8.5</td><td>30</td><td>Massachusetts</td><td>6.9</td></tr>
<tr><td>NA</td><td>New Mexico**</td><td>NA</td><td>31</td><td>Kentucky</td><td>6.7</td></tr>
<tr><td>18</td><td>New York</td><td>9.3</td><td>32</td><td>Texas</td><td>6.5</td></tr>
<tr><td>6</td><td>North Carolina</td><td>11.3</td><td>NA</td><td>Alaska**</td><td>NA</td></tr>
<tr><td>NA</td><td>North Dakota**</td><td>NA</td><td>NA</td><td>Hawaii**</td><td>NA</td></tr>
<tr><td>3</td><td>Ohio</td><td>11.8</td><td>NA</td><td>Idaho**</td><td>NA</td></tr>
<tr><td>24</td><td>Oklahoma</td><td>8.5</td><td>NA</td><td>Iowa**</td><td>NA</td></tr>
<tr><td>NA</td><td>Oregon**</td><td>NA</td><td>NA</td><td>Maine**</td><td>NA</td></tr>
<tr><td>4</td><td>Pennsylvania</td><td>11.6</td><td>NA</td><td>Montana**</td><td>NA</td></tr>
<tr><td>NA</td><td>Rhode Island**</td><td>NA</td><td>NA</td><td>Nebraska**</td><td>NA</td></tr>
<tr><td>13</td><td>South Carolina</td><td>10.4</td><td>NA</td><td>Nevada**</td><td>NA</td></tr>
<tr><td>NA</td><td>South Dakota**</td><td>NA</td><td>NA</td><td>New Hampshire**</td><td>NA</td></tr>
<tr><td>6</td><td>Tennessee</td><td>11.3</td><td>NA</td><td>New Mexico**</td><td>NA</td></tr>
<tr><td>32</td><td>Texas</td><td>6.5</td><td>NA</td><td>North Dakota**</td><td>NA</td></tr>
<tr><td>NA</td><td>Utah**</td><td>NA</td><td>NA</td><td>Oregon**</td><td>NA</td></tr>
<tr><td>NA</td><td>Vermont**</td><td>NA</td><td>NA</td><td>Rhode Island**</td><td>NA</td></tr>
<tr><td>8</td><td>Virginia</td><td>11.1</td><td>NA</td><td>South Dakota**</td><td>NA</td></tr>
<tr><td>17</td><td>Washington</td><td>9.8</td><td>NA</td><td>Utah**</td><td>NA</td></tr>
<tr><td>NA</td><td>West Virginia**</td><td>NA</td><td>NA</td><td>Vermont**</td><td>NA</td></tr>
<tr><td>12</td><td>Wisconsin</td><td>10.6</td><td>NA</td><td>West Virginia**</td><td>NA</td></tr>
<tr><td>NA</td><td>Wyoming**</td><td>NA</td><td>NA</td><td>Wyoming**</td><td>NA</td></tr>
</table>

District of Columbia   14.6

Source: U.S. Department of Health and Human Services, National Center for Health Statistics
"Monthly Vital Statistics Report" (Vol. 45, No. 11(S)2, June 12, 1997)
*Final data. Deaths of infants under 28 days, exclusive of fetal deaths. Based on race of the mother.
**Not available. Fewer than 20 black neonatal deaths.

Deaths by AIDS Through 1995

National Total = 262,957 Deaths*

ALPHA ORDER

RANK	STATE	DEATHS	% of USA
23	Alabama	2,023	0.77%
46	Alaska	144	0.05%
21	Arizona	2,642	1.00%
33	Arkansas	833	0.32%
2	California	46,310	17.61%
20	Colorado	2,733	1.04%
17	Connecticut	3,325	1.26%
37	Delaware	667	0.25%
3	Florida	24,695	9.39%
6	Georgia	8,691	3.31%
34	Hawaii	832	0.32%
44	Idaho	206	0.08%
7	Illinois	8,548	3.25%
24	Indiana	1,991	0.76%
39	Iowa	506	0.19%
32	Kansas	864	0.33%
31	Kentucky	1,032	0.39%
15	Louisiana	4,177	1.59%
40	Maine	409	0.16%
9	Maryland	6,254	2.38%
10	Massachusetts	5,414	2.06%
14	Michigan	4,388	1.67%
26	Minnesota	1,483	0.56%
28	Mississippi	1,368	0.52%
18	Missouri	2,930	1.11%
47	Montana	137	0.05%
42	Nebraska	387	0.15%
30	Nevada	1,140	0.43%
43	New Hampshire	272	0.10%
5	New Jersey	16,057	6.11%
35	New Mexico	795	0.30%
1	New York	52,269	19.88%
11	North Carolina	5,084	1.93%
50	North Dakota	52	0.02%
12	Ohio	4,707	1.79%
27	Oklahoma	1,430	0.54%
25	Oregon	1,754	0.67%
8	Pennsylvania	7,877	3.00%
36	Rhode Island	668	0.25%
19	South Carolina	2,904	1.10%
48	South Dakota	71	0.03%
22	Tennessee	2,382	0.91%
4	Texas	17,990	6.84%
38	Utah	520	0.20%
45	Vermont	164	0.06%
13	Virginia	4,433	1.69%
16	Washington	3,561	1.35%
41	West Virginia	392	0.15%
29	Wisconsin	1,361	0.52%
49	Wyoming	68	0.03%

RANK ORDER

RANK	STATE	DEATHS	% of USA
1	New York	52,269	19.88%
2	California	46,310	17.61%
3	Florida	24,695	9.39%
4	Texas	17,990	6.84%
5	New Jersey	16,057	6.11%
6	Georgia	8,691	3.31%
7	Illinois	8,548	3.25%
8	Pennsylvania	7,877	3.00%
9	Maryland	6,254	2.38%
10	Massachusetts	5,414	2.06%
11	North Carolina	5,084	1.93%
12	Ohio	4,707	1.79%
13	Virginia	4,433	1.69%
14	Michigan	4,388	1.67%
15	Louisiana	4,177	1.59%
16	Washington	3,561	1.35%
17	Connecticut	3,325	1.26%
18	Missouri	2,930	1.11%
19	South Carolina	2,904	1.10%
20	Colorado	2,733	1.04%
21	Arizona	2,642	1.00%
22	Tennessee	2,382	0.91%
23	Alabama	2,023	0.77%
24	Indiana	1,991	0.76%
25	Oregon	1,754	0.67%
26	Minnesota	1,483	0.56%
27	Oklahoma	1,430	0.54%
28	Mississippi	1,368	0.52%
29	Wisconsin	1,361	0.52%
30	Nevada	1,140	0.43%
31	Kentucky	1,032	0.39%
32	Kansas	864	0.33%
33	Arkansas	833	0.32%
34	Hawaii	832	0.32%
35	New Mexico	795	0.30%
36	Rhode Island	668	0.25%
37	Delaware	667	0.25%
38	Utah	520	0.20%
39	Iowa	506	0.19%
40	Maine	409	0.16%
41	West Virginia	392	0.15%
42	Nebraska	387	0.15%
43	New Hampshire	272	0.10%
44	Idaho	206	0.08%
45	Vermont	164	0.06%
46	Alaska	144	0.05%
47	Montana	137	0.05%
48	South Dakota	71	0.03%
49	Wyoming	68	0.03%
50	North Dakota	52	0.02%
	District of Columbia	4,017	1.53%

Source: U.S. Department of Health and Human Services, National Center for Health Statistics
(http://wonder.cdc.gov/WONDER/)
Cumulative deaths through 1995. However, due to reporting delays, these totals should increase. AIDS is Acquired Immunodeficiency Syndrome. The definition of what is AIDS was expanded in 1985, 1987 and 1993.

Deaths by AIDS in 1995

National Total = 43,115 Deaths*

ALPHA ORDER

RANK	STATE	DEATHS	% of USA
23	Alabama	393	0.91%
45	Alaska	30	0.07%
20	Arizona	483	1.12%
32	Arkansas	170	0.39%
2	California	6,455	14.97%
22	Colorado	407	0.94%
16	Connecticut	603	1.40%
33	Delaware	163	0.38%
3	Florida	4,368	10.13%
6	Georgia	1,586	3.68%
36	Hawaii	124	0.29%
44	Idaho	43	0.10%
7	Illinois	1,427	3.31%
24	Indiana	389	0.90%
39	Iowa	89	0.21%
35	Kansas	143	0.33%
30	Kentucky	218	0.51%
15	Louisiana	731	1.70%
41	Maine	76	0.18%
9	Maryland	1,290	2.99%
11	Massachusetts	944	2.19%
14	Michigan	801	1.86%
26	Minnesota	260	0.60%
27	Mississippi	255	0.59%
21	Missouri	469	1.09%
47	Montana	23	0.05%
42	Nebraska	60	0.14%
31	Nevada	202	0.47%
43	New Hampshire	47	0.11%
5	New Jersey	2,438	5.65%
34	New Mexico	153	0.35%
1	New York	7,997	18.55%
10	North Carolina	1,015	2.35%
50	North Dakota	6	0.01%
12	Ohio	884	2.05%
28	Oklahoma	234	0.54%
25	Oregon	288	0.67%
8	Pennsylvania	1,385	3.21%
37	Rhode Island	99	0.23%
18	South Carolina	557	1.29%
48	South Dakota	21	0.05%
19	Tennessee	508	1.18%
4	Texas	2,769	6.42%
38	Utah	94	0.22%
46	Vermont	27	0.06%
13	Virginia	834	1.93%
17	Washington	593	1.38%
40	West Virginia	79	0.18%
29	Wisconsin	220	0.51%
49	Wyoming	12	0.03%

RANK ORDER

RANK	STATE	DEATHS	% of USA
1	New York	7,997	18.55%
2	California	6,455	14.97%
3	Florida	4,368	10.13%
4	Texas	2,769	6.42%
5	New Jersey	2,438	5.65%
6	Georgia	1,586	3.68%
7	Illinois	1,427	3.31%
8	Pennsylvania	1,385	3.21%
9	Maryland	1,290	2.99%
10	North Carolina	1,015	2.35%
11	Massachusetts	944	2.19%
12	Ohio	884	2.05%
13	Virginia	834	1.93%
14	Michigan	801	1.86%
15	Louisiana	731	1.70%
16	Connecticut	603	1.40%
17	Washington	593	1.38%
18	South Carolina	557	1.29%
19	Tennessee	508	1.18%
20	Arizona	483	1.12%
21	Missouri	469	1.09%
22	Colorado	407	0.94%
23	Alabama	393	0.91%
24	Indiana	389	0.90%
25	Oregon	288	0.67%
26	Minnesota	260	0.60%
27	Mississippi	255	0.59%
28	Oklahoma	234	0.54%
29	Wisconsin	220	0.51%
30	Kentucky	218	0.51%
31	Nevada	202	0.47%
32	Arkansas	170	0.39%
33	Delaware	163	0.38%
34	New Mexico	153	0.35%
35	Kansas	143	0.33%
36	Hawaii	124	0.29%
37	Rhode Island	99	0.23%
38	Utah	94	0.22%
39	Iowa	89	0.21%
40	West Virginia	79	0.18%
41	Maine	76	0.18%
42	Nebraska	60	0.14%
43	New Hampshire	47	0.11%
44	Idaho	43	0.10%
45	Alaska	30	0.07%
46	Vermont	27	0.06%
47	Montana	23	0.05%
48	South Dakota	21	0.05%
49	Wyoming	12	0.03%
50	North Dakota	6	0.01%
	District of Columbia	653	1.51%

Source: U.S. Department of Health and Human Services, National Center for Health Statistics
   "Monthly Vital Statistics Report" (Vol. 45, No. 11(S)2, June 12, 1997)
*AIDS is Acquired Immunodeficiency Syndrome. It is a specific group of diseases or conditions which are indicative of severe immunosuppression related to infection with the Human Immunodeficiency Virus (HIV).

Death Rate by AIDS in 1995

National Rate = 16.4 Deaths per 100,000 Population*

ALPHA ORDER			RANK ORDER		
RANK	STATE	RATE	RANK	STATE	RATE
25	Alabama	9.2	1	New York	44.1
38	Alaska	5.0	2	Florida	30.8
17	Arizona	11.5	3	New Jersey	30.7
32	Arkansas	6.8	4	Maryland	25.6
7	California	20.4	5	Delaware	22.7
19	Colorado	10.9	6	Georgia	22.0
8	Connecticut	18.4	7	California	20.4
5	Delaware	22.7	8	Connecticut	18.4
2	Florida	30.8	9	Louisiana	16.8
6	Georgia	22.0	10	Massachusetts	15.5
21	Hawaii	10.4	11	South Carolina	15.2
44	Idaho	3.7	12	Texas	14.8
16	Illinois	12.1	13	North Carolina	14.1
33	Indiana	6.7	14	Nevada	13.2
46	Iowa	3.1	15	Virginia	12.6
35	Kansas	5.6	16	Illinois	12.1
35	Kentucky	5.6	17	Arizona	11.5
9	Louisiana	16.8	17	Pennsylvania	11.5
34	Maine	6.1	19	Colorado	10.9
4	Maryland	25.6	19	Washington	10.9
10	Massachusetts	15.5	21	Hawaii	10.4
29	Michigan	8.4	22	Rhode Island	10.0
35	Minnesota	5.6	23	Tennessee	9.7
24	Mississippi	9.5	24	Mississippi	9.5
28	Missouri	8.8	25	Alabama	9.2
48	Montana	2.6	25	Oregon	9.2
44	Nebraska	3.7	27	New Mexico	9.1
14	Nevada	13.2	28	Missouri	8.8
43	New Hampshire	4.1	29	Michigan	8.4
3	New Jersey	30.7	30	Ohio	7.9
27	New Mexico	9.1	31	Oklahoma	7.1
1	New York	44.1	32	Arkansas	6.8
13	North Carolina	14.1	33	Indiana	6.7
NA	North Dakota**	NA	34	Maine	6.1
30	Ohio	7.9	35	Kansas	5.6
31	Oklahoma	7.1	35	Kentucky	5.6
25	Oregon	9.2	35	Minnesota	5.6
17	Pennsylvania	11.5	38	Alaska	5.0
22	Rhode Island	10.0	39	Utah	4.8
11	South Carolina	15.2	40	Vermont	4.6
47	South Dakota	2.9	41	West Virginia	4.3
23	Tennessee	9.7	41	Wisconsin	4.3
12	Texas	14.8	43	New Hampshire	4.1
39	Utah	4.8	44	Idaho	3.7
40	Vermont	4.6	44	Nebraska	3.7
15	Virginia	12.6	46	Iowa	3.1
19	Washington	10.9	47	South Dakota	2.9
41	West Virginia	4.3	48	Montana	2.6
41	Wisconsin	4.3	NA	North Dakota**	NA
NA	Wyoming**	NA	NA	Wyoming**	NA
				District of Columbia	117.8

Source: U.S. Department of Health and Human Services, National Center for Health Statistics
   "Monthly Vital Statistics Report" (Vol. 45, No. 11(S)2, June 12, 1997)
*AIDS is Acquired Immunodeficiency Syndrome. It is a specific group of diseases or conditions which are indicative
of severe immunosuppression related to infection with the Human Immunodeficiency Virus (HIV).
**Not available as fewer than 20 deaths by AIDS, insufficient for a reliable rate.

Estimated Deaths by Cancer in 1998

National Estimated Total = 564,800 Deaths

ALPHA ORDER

RANK	STATE	DEATHS	% of USA
20	Alabama	9,500	1.68%
50	Alaska	600	0.11%
23	Arizona	9,000	1.59%
30	Arkansas	6,400	1.13%
1	California	52,100	9.22%
31	Colorado	6,100	1.08%
28	Connecticut	7,100	1.26%
45	Delaware	1,800	0.32%
2	Florida	40,500	7.17%
13	Georgia	13,000	2.30%
42	Hawaii	2,000	0.35%
42	Idaho	2,000	0.35%
6	Illinois	26,700	4.73%
14	Indiana	12,900	2.28%
29	Iowa	6,800	1.20%
33	Kansas	5,500	0.97%
20	Kentucky	9,500	1.68%
22	Louisiana	9,400	1.66%
37	Maine	3,300	0.58%
19	Maryland	10,500	1.86%
11	Massachusetts	14,500	2.57%
8	Michigan	20,700	3.67%
23	Minnesota	9,000	1.59%
31	Mississippi	6,100	1.08%
14	Missouri	12,900	2.28%
44	Montana	1,900	0.34%
36	Nebraska	3,400	0.60%
35	Nevada	3,500	0.62%
39	New Hampshire	2,600	0.46%
9	New Jersey	18,600	3.29%
38	New Mexico	2,900	0.51%
3	New York	38,400	6.80%
10	North Carolina	16,100	2.85%
47	North Dakota	1,500	0.27%
7	Ohio	26,000	4.60%
27	Oklahoma	7,200	1.27%
26	Oregon	7,300	1.29%
5	Pennsylvania	31,600	5.59%
40	Rhode Island	2,400	0.42%
25	South Carolina	8,100	1.43%
46	South Dakota	1,600	0.28%
16	Tennessee	11,900	2.11%
4	Texas	35,600	6.30%
40	Utah	2,400	0.42%
48	Vermont	1,200	0.21%
12	Virginia	13,300	2.35%
18	Washington	11,100	1.97%
34	West Virginia	4,900	0.87%
17	Wisconsin	11,300	2.00%
49	Wyoming	800	0.14%

RANK ORDER

RANK	STATE	DEATHS	% of USA
1	California	52,100	9.22%
2	Florida	40,500	7.17%
3	New York	38,400	6.80%
4	Texas	35,600	6.30%
5	Pennsylvania	31,600	5.59%
6	Illinois	26,700	4.73%
7	Ohio	26,000	4.60%
8	Michigan	20,700	3.67%
9	New Jersey	18,600	3.29%
10	North Carolina	16,100	2.85%
11	Massachusetts	14,500	2.57%
12	Virginia	13,300	2.35%
13	Georgia	13,000	2.30%
14	Indiana	12,900	2.28%
14	Missouri	12,900	2.28%
16	Tennessee	11,900	2.11%
17	Wisconsin	11,300	2.00%
18	Washington	11,100	1.97%
19	Maryland	10,500	1.86%
20	Alabama	9,500	1.68%
20	Kentucky	9,500	1.68%
22	Louisiana	9,400	1.66%
23	Arizona	9,000	1.59%
23	Minnesota	9,000	1.59%
25	South Carolina	8,100	1.43%
26	Oregon	7,300	1.29%
27	Oklahoma	7,200	1.27%
28	Connecticut	7,100	1.26%
29	Iowa	6,800	1.20%
30	Arkansas	6,400	1.13%
31	Colorado	6,100	1.08%
31	Mississippi	6,100	1.08%
33	Kansas	5,500	0.97%
34	West Virginia	4,900	0.87%
35	Nevada	3,500	0.62%
36	Nebraska	3,400	0.60%
37	Maine	3,300	0.58%
38	New Mexico	2,900	0.51%
39	New Hampshire	2,600	0.46%
40	Rhode Island	2,400	0.42%
40	Utah	2,400	0.42%
42	Hawaii	2,000	0.35%
42	Idaho	2,000	0.35%
44	Montana	1,900	0.34%
45	Delaware	1,800	0.32%
46	South Dakota	1,600	0.28%
47	North Dakota	1,500	0.27%
48	Vermont	1,200	0.21%
49	Wyoming	800	0.14%
50	Alaska	600	0.11%
	District of Columbia	1,400	0.25%

Source: American Cancer Society
"Cancer Facts & Figures-1998" (Copyright 1998, Reprinted with permission from the American Cancer Society)

Estimated Death Rate by Cancer in 1998

National Estimated Rate = 211.0 Deaths by Cancer per 100,000 Population*

ALPHA ORDER

RANK	STATE	RATE
20	Alabama	220.0
50	Alaska	98.5
38	Arizona	197.6
5	Arkansas	253.7
47	California	161.5
48	Colorado	156.7
23	Connecticut	217.1
6	Delaware	246.0
1	Florida	276.4
42	Georgia	173.7
43	Hawaii	168.5
46	Idaho	165.3
16	Illinois	224.4
20	Indiana	220.0
10	Iowa	238.4
30	Kansas	212.0
7	Kentucky	243.1
28	Louisiana	216.0
3	Maine	265.7
34	Maryland	206.1
11	Massachusetts	237.0
31	Michigan	211.8
40	Minnesota	192.1
17	Mississippi	223.4
9	Missouri	238.8
27	Montana	216.2
35	Nebraska	205.2
33	Nevada	208.7
18	New Hampshire	221.7
14	New Jersey	231.0
44	New Mexico	167.7
32	New York	211.7
25	North Carolina	216.8
12	North Dakota	234.1
13	Ohio	232.4
23	Oklahoma	217.1
15	Oregon	225.1
4	Pennsylvania	262.9
7	Rhode Island	243.1
29	South Carolina	215.4
25	South Dakota	216.8
18	Tennessee	221.7
41	Texas	183.1
49	Utah	116.6
36	Vermont	203.7
39	Virginia	197.5
37	Washington	197.8
2	West Virginia	269.9
22	Wisconsin	218.6
45	Wyoming	166.8

RANK ORDER

RANK	STATE	RATE
1	Florida	276.4
2	West Virginia	269.9
3	Maine	265.7
4	Pennsylvania	262.9
5	Arkansas	253.7
6	Delaware	246.0
7	Kentucky	243.1
7	Rhode Island	243.1
9	Missouri	238.8
10	Iowa	238.4
11	Massachusetts	237.0
12	North Dakota	234.1
13	Ohio	232.4
14	New Jersey	231.0
15	Oregon	225.1
16	Illinois	224.4
17	Mississippi	223.4
18	New Hampshire	221.7
18	Tennessee	221.7
20	Alabama	220.0
20	Indiana	220.0
22	Wisconsin	218.6
23	Connecticut	217.1
23	Oklahoma	217.1
25	North Carolina	216.8
25	South Dakota	216.8
27	Montana	216.2
28	Louisiana	216.0
29	South Carolina	215.4
30	Kansas	212.0
31	Michigan	211.8
32	New York	211.7
33	Nevada	208.7
34	Maryland	206.1
35	Nebraska	205.2
36	Vermont	203.7
37	Washington	197.8
38	Arizona	197.6
39	Virginia	197.5
40	Minnesota	192.1
41	Texas	183.1
42	Georgia	173.7
43	Hawaii	168.5
44	New Mexico	167.7
45	Wyoming	166.8
46	Idaho	165.3
47	California	161.5
48	Colorado	156.7
49	Utah	116.6
50	Alaska	98.5
	District of Columbia	264.7

Source: Morgan Quitno Press using data from American Cancer Society
"Cancer Facts & Figures-1998" (Copyright 1998, Reprinted with permission from the American Cancer Society)
Rates calculated using 1997 Census resident population estimates. Not age adjusted.

Estimated Age-Adjusted Death Rate by Cancer in 1998

National Rate = 173 Deaths per 100,000 Population*

ALPHA ORDER

RANK	STATE	RATE
16	Alabama	179
28	Alaska	171
38	Arizona	160
12	Arkansas	180
36	California	162
47	Colorado	147
33	Connecticut	165
1	Delaware	196
31	Florida	167
24	Georgia	176
49	Hawaii	136
46	Idaho	148
12	Illinois	180
21	Indiana	177
38	Iowa	160
40	Kansas	159
3	Kentucky	192
2	Louisiana	194
5	Maine	186
4	Maryland	189
12	Massachusetts	180
21	Michigan	177
41	Minnesota	156
9	Mississippi	181
21	Missouri	177
37	Montana	161
41	Nebraska	156
6	Nevada	185
9	New Hampshire	181
8	New Jersey	183
48	New Mexico	146
27	New York	172
25	North Carolina	175
41	North Dakota	156
9	Ohio	181
30	Oklahoma	170
31	Oregon	167
16	Pennsylvania	179
20	Rhode Island	178
16	South Carolina	179
44	South Dakota	154
12	Tennessee	180
28	Texas	171
50	Utah	125
26	Vermont	174
16	Virginia	179
33	Washington	165
7	West Virginia	184
33	Wisconsin	165
45	Wyoming	151

RANK ORDER

RANK	STATE	RATE
1	Delaware	196
2	Louisiana	194
3	Kentucky	192
4	Maryland	189
5	Maine	186
6	Nevada	185
7	West Virginia	184
8	New Jersey	183
9	Mississippi	181
9	New Hampshire	181
9	Ohio	181
12	Arkansas	180
12	Illinois	180
12	Massachusetts	180
12	Tennessee	180
16	Alabama	179
16	Pennsylvania	179
16	South Carolina	179
16	Virginia	179
20	Rhode Island	178
21	Indiana	177
21	Michigan	177
21	Missouri	177
24	Georgia	176
25	North Carolina	175
26	Vermont	174
27	New York	172
28	Alaska	171
28	Texas	171
30	Oklahoma	170
31	Florida	167
31	Oregon	167
33	Connecticut	165
33	Washington	165
33	Wisconsin	165
36	California	162
37	Montana	161
38	Arizona	160
38	Iowa	160
40	Kansas	159
41	Minnesota	156
41	Nebraska	156
41	North Dakota	156
44	South Dakota	154
45	Wyoming	151
46	Idaho	148
47	Colorado	147
48	New Mexico	146
49	Hawaii	136
50	Utah	125

	District of Columbia	218

Source: American Cancer Society
   "Cancer Facts & Figures-1998" (Copyright 1998, Reprinted with permission from the American Cancer Society)
*National rate is for 1997. Age-adjusted rates eliminate the distorting effects of the aging of the population.

Estimated Deaths by Female Breast Cancer in 1998

National Estimated Total = 43,500 Deaths*

ALPHA ORDER

RANK	STATE	DEATHS	% of USA
24	Alabama	600	1.38%
43	Alaska	100	0.23%
21	Arizona	700	1.61%
31	Arkansas	400	0.92%
1	California	4,300	9.89%
27	Colorado	500	1.15%
27	Connecticut	500	1.15%
43	Delaware	100	0.23%
3	Florida	2,900	6.67%
13	Georgia	1,000	2.30%
43	Hawaii	100	0.23%
37	Idaho	200	0.46%
6	Illinois	2,200	5.06%
13	Indiana	1,000	2.30%
24	Iowa	600	1.38%
31	Kansas	400	0.92%
21	Kentucky	700	1.61%
17	Louisiana	800	1.84%
37	Maine	200	0.46%
17	Maryland	800	1.84%
10	Massachusetts	1,100	2.53%
8	Michigan	1,500	3.45%
21	Minnesota	700	1.61%
31	Mississippi	400	0.92%
17	Missouri	800	1.84%
43	Montana	100	0.23%
34	Nebraska	300	0.69%
34	Nevada	300	0.69%
37	New Hampshire	200	0.46%
8	New Jersey	1,500	3.45%
37	New Mexico	200	0.46%
2	New York	3,300	7.59%
10	North Carolina	1,100	2.53%
43	North Dakota	100	0.23%
7	Ohio	2,100	4.83%
27	Oklahoma	500	1.15%
27	Oregon	500	1.15%
5	Pennsylvania	2,600	5.98%
37	Rhode Island	200	0.46%
24	South Carolina	600	1.38%
43	South Dakota	100	0.23%
15	Tennessee	900	2.07%
4	Texas	2,800	6.44%
37	Utah	200	0.46%
43	Vermont	100	0.23%
10	Virginia	1,100	2.53%
17	Washington	800	1.84%
34	West Virginia	300	0.69%
15	Wisconsin	900	2.07%
43	Wyoming	100	0.23%

RANK ORDER

RANK	STATE	DEATHS	% of USA
1	California	4,300	9.89%
2	New York	3,300	7.59%
3	Florida	2,900	6.67%
4	Texas	2,800	6.44%
5	Pennsylvania	2,600	5.98%
6	Illinois	2,200	5.06%
7	Ohio	2,100	4.83%
8	Michigan	1,500	3.45%
8	New Jersey	1,500	3.45%
10	Massachusetts	1,100	2.53%
10	North Carolina	1,100	2.53%
10	Virginia	1,100	2.53%
13	Georgia	1,000	2.30%
13	Indiana	1,000	2.30%
15	Tennessee	900	2.07%
15	Wisconsin	900	2.07%
17	Louisiana	800	1.84%
17	Maryland	800	1.84%
17	Missouri	800	1.84%
17	Washington	800	1.84%
21	Arizona	700	1.61%
21	Kentucky	700	1.61%
21	Minnesota	700	1.61%
24	Alabama	600	1.38%
24	Iowa	600	1.38%
24	South Carolina	600	1.38%
27	Colorado	500	1.15%
27	Connecticut	500	1.15%
27	Oklahoma	500	1.15%
27	Oregon	500	1.15%
31	Arkansas	400	0.92%
31	Kansas	400	0.92%
31	Mississippi	400	0.92%
34	Nebraska	300	0.69%
34	Nevada	300	0.69%
34	West Virginia	300	0.69%
37	Idaho	200	0.46%
37	Maine	200	0.46%
37	New Hampshire	200	0.46%
37	New Mexico	200	0.46%
37	Rhode Island	200	0.46%
37	Utah	200	0.46%
43	Alaska	100	0.23%
43	Delaware	100	0.23%
43	Hawaii	100	0.23%
43	Montana	100	0.23%
43	North Dakota	100	0.23%
43	South Dakota	100	0.23%
43	Vermont	100	0.23%
43	Wyoming	100	0.23%
	District of Columbia	100	0.23%

Source: American Cancer Society

"Cancer Facts & Figures-1998" (Copyright 1998, Reprinted with permission from the American Cancer Society)

*National total does not include an estimated 400 deaths of males by breast cancer.

Estimated Death Rate by Female Breast Cancer in 1998

National Estimated Rate = 32.1 Deaths per 100,000 Female Population*

ALPHA ORDER

RANK	STATE	RATE
41	Alabama	27.0
15	Alaska	34.8
26	Arizona	31.3
28	Arkansas	30.9
41	California	27.0
46	Colorado	26.0
33	Connecticut	29.7
43	Delaware	26.9
4	Florida	39.2
45	Georgia	26.5
50	Hawaii	17.1
18	Idaho	33.6
9	Illinois	36.3
20	Indiana	33.4
3	Iowa	41.0
31	Kansas	30.6
12	Kentucky	35.1
11	Louisiana	35.5
24	Maine	31.4
30	Maryland	30.7
14	Massachusetts	34.9
32	Michigan	30.5
33	Minnesota	29.7
40	Mississippi	28.3
37	Missouri	29.0
48	Montana	22.7
10	Nebraska	35.6
6	Nevada	38.2
17	New Hampshire	33.9
7	New Jersey	36.5
47	New Mexico	23.0
13	New York	35.0
36	North Carolina	29.2
27	North Dakota	31.0
8	Ohio	36.4
33	Oklahoma	29.7
28	Oregon	30.9
2	Pennsylvania	41.6
5	Rhode Island	38.9
24	South Carolina	31.4
43	South Dakota	26.9
21	Tennessee	32.8
38	Texas	28.9
49	Utah	19.9
19	Vermont	33.5
22	Virginia	32.3
39	Washington	28.8
23	West Virginia	31.8
16	Wisconsin	34.3
1	Wyoming	41.8

RANK ORDER

RANK	STATE	RATE
1	Wyoming	41.8
2	Pennsylvania	41.6
3	Iowa	41.0
4	Florida	39.2
5	Rhode Island	38.9
6	Nevada	38.2
7	New Jersey	36.5
8	Ohio	36.4
9	Illinois	36.3
10	Nebraska	35.6
11	Louisiana	35.5
12	Kentucky	35.1
13	New York	35.0
14	Massachusetts	34.9
15	Alaska	34.8
16	Wisconsin	34.3
17	New Hampshire	33.9
18	Idaho	33.6
19	Vermont	33.5
20	Indiana	33.4
21	Tennessee	32.8
22	Virginia	32.3
23	West Virginia	31.8
24	Maine	31.4
24	South Carolina	31.4
26	Arizona	31.3
27	North Dakota	31.0
28	Arkansas	30.9
28	Oregon	30.9
30	Maryland	30.7
31	Kansas	30.6
32	Michigan	30.5
33	Connecticut	29.7
33	Minnesota	29.7
33	Oklahoma	29.7
36	North Carolina	29.2
37	Missouri	29.0
38	Texas	28.9
39	Washington	28.8
40	Mississippi	28.3
41	Alabama	27.0
41	California	27.0
43	Delaware	26.9
43	South Dakota	26.9
45	Georgia	26.5
46	Colorado	26.0
47	New Mexico	23.0
48	Montana	22.7
49	Utah	19.9
50	Hawaii	17.1
	District of Columbia	34.6

Source: Morgan Quitno Press using data from American Cancer Society
  "Cancer Facts & Figures-1998" (Copyright 1998, Reprinted with permission from the American Cancer Society)
  *Rates calculated using 1996 Census resident female population estimates. Not age adjusted.

Estimated Deaths by Colon and Rectum Cancer in 1998

National Estimated Total = 56,500 Deaths

ALPHA ORDER

RANK ORDER

RANK	STATE	DEATHS	% of USA
26	Alabama	700	1.24%
47	Alaska	100	0.18%
20	Arizona	900	1.59%
29	Arkansas	600	1.06%
1	California	5,000	8.85%
29	Colorado	600	1.06%
26	Connecticut	700	1.24%
39	Delaware	200	0.35%
3	Florida	4,000	7.08%
16	Georgia	1,100	1.95%
39	Hawaii	200	0.35%
39	Idaho	200	0.35%
6	Illinois	2,800	4.96%
12	Indiana	1,300	2.30%
24	Iowa	800	1.42%
29	Kansas	600	1.06%
20	Kentucky	900	1.59%
20	Louisiana	900	1.59%
37	Maine	300	0.53%
16	Maryland	1,100	1.95%
10	Massachusetts	1,600	2.83%
8	Michigan	2,100	3.72%
24	Minnesota	800	1.42%
33	Mississippi	500	0.88%
12	Missouri	1,300	2.30%
39	Montana	200	0.35%
35	Nebraska	400	0.71%
35	Nevada	400	0.71%
39	New Hampshire	200	0.35%
9	New Jersey	2,000	3.54%
39	New Mexico	200	0.35%
2	New York	4,200	7.43%
10	North Carolina	1,600	2.83%
39	North Dakota	200	0.35%
7	Ohio	2,600	4.60%
26	Oklahoma	700	1.24%
29	Oregon	600	1.06%
5	Pennsylvania	3,400	6.02%
37	Rhode Island	300	0.53%
20	South Carolina	900	1.59%
47	South Dakota	100	0.18%
15	Tennessee	1,200	2.12%
4	Texas	3,600	6.37%
39	Utah	200	0.35%
47	Vermont	100	0.18%
12	Virginia	1,300	2.30%
19	Washington	1,000	1.77%
33	West Virginia	500	0.88%
16	Wisconsin	1,100	1.95%
47	Wyoming	100	0.18%

RANK	STATE	DEATHS	% of USA
1	California	5,000	8.85%
2	New York	4,200	7.43%
3	Florida	4,000	7.08%
4	Texas	3,600	6.37%
5	Pennsylvania	3,400	6.02%
6	Illinois	2,800	4.96%
7	Ohio	2,600	4.60%
8	Michigan	2,100	3.72%
9	New Jersey	2,000	3.54%
10	Massachusetts	1,600	2.83%
10	North Carolina	1,600	2.83%
12	Indiana	1,300	2.30%
12	Missouri	1,300	2.30%
12	Virginia	1,300	2.30%
15	Tennessee	1,200	2.12%
16	Georgia	1,100	1.95%
16	Maryland	1,100	1.95%
16	Wisconsin	1,100	1.95%
19	Washington	1,000	1.77%
20	Arizona	900	1.59%
20	Kentucky	900	1.59%
20	Louisiana	900	1.59%
20	South Carolina	900	1.59%
24	Iowa	800	1.42%
24	Minnesota	800	1.42%
26	Alabama	700	1.24%
26	Connecticut	700	1.24%
26	Oklahoma	700	1.24%
29	Arkansas	600	1.06%
29	Colorado	600	1.06%
29	Kansas	600	1.06%
29	Oregon	600	1.06%
33	Mississippi	500	0.88%
33	West Virginia	500	0.88%
35	Nebraska	400	0.71%
35	Nevada	400	0.71%
37	Maine	300	0.53%
37	Rhode Island	300	0.53%
39	Delaware	200	0.35%
39	Hawaii	200	0.35%
39	Idaho	200	0.35%
39	Montana	200	0.35%
39	New Hampshire	200	0.35%
39	New Mexico	200	0.35%
39	North Dakota	200	0.35%
39	Utah	200	0.35%
47	Alaska	100	0.18%
47	South Dakota	100	0.18%
47	Vermont	100	0.18%
47	Wyoming	100	0.18%
	District of Columbia	100	0.18%

Source: American Cancer Society
"Cancer Facts & Figures-1998" (Copyright 1998, Reprinted with permission from the American Cancer Society)

Estimated Death Rate by Colon and Rectum Cancer in 1998

National Estimated Rate = 21.1 Deaths per 100,000 Population*

ALPHA ORDER

RANK	STATE	RATE
44	Alabama	16.2
43	Alaska	16.4
32	Arizona	19.8
15	Arkansas	23.8
45	California	15.5
46	Colorado	15.4
27	Connecticut	21.4
6	Delaware	27.3
6	Florida	27.3
47	Georgia	14.7
41	Hawaii	16.9
42	Idaho	16.5
16	Illinois	23.5
23	Indiana	22.2
4	Iowa	28.0
19	Kansas	23.1
20	Kentucky	23.0
31	Louisiana	20.7
10	Maine	24.2
24	Maryland	21.6
8	Massachusetts	26.2
25	Michigan	21.5
38	Minnesota	17.1
36	Mississippi	18.3
11	Missouri	24.1
21	Montana	22.8
11	Nebraska	24.1
13	Nevada	23.9
38	New Hampshire	17.1
9	New Jersey	24.8
49	New Mexico	11.6
17	New York	23.2
25	North Carolina	21.5
1	North Dakota	31.2
17	Ohio	23.2
29	Oklahoma	21.1
34	Oregon	18.5
3	Pennsylvania	28.3
2	Rhode Island	30.4
13	South Carolina	23.9
48	South Dakota	13.6
22	Tennessee	22.4
34	Texas	18.5
50	Utah	9.7
40	Vermont	17.0
33	Virginia	19.3
37	Washington	17.8
5	West Virginia	27.5
28	Wisconsin	21.3
30	Wyoming	20.8

RANK ORDER

RANK	STATE	RATE
1	North Dakota	31.2
2	Rhode Island	30.4
3	Pennsylvania	28.3
4	Iowa	28.0
5	West Virginia	27.5
6	Delaware	27.3
6	Florida	27.3
8	Massachusetts	26.2
9	New Jersey	24.8
10	Maine	24.2
11	Missouri	24.1
11	Nebraska	24.1
13	Nevada	23.9
13	South Carolina	23.9
15	Arkansas	23.8
16	Illinois	23.5
17	New York	23.2
17	Ohio	23.2
19	Kansas	23.1
20	Kentucky	23.0
21	Montana	22.8
22	Tennessee	22.4
23	Indiana	22.2
24	Maryland	21.6
25	Michigan	21.5
25	North Carolina	21.5
27	Connecticut	21.4
28	Wisconsin	21.3
29	Oklahoma	21.1
30	Wyoming	20.8
31	Louisiana	20.7
32	Arizona	19.8
33	Virginia	19.3
34	Oregon	18.5
34	Texas	18.5
36	Mississippi	18.3
37	Washington	17.8
38	Minnesota	17.1
38	New Hampshire	17.1
40	Vermont	17.0
41	Hawaii	16.9
42	Idaho	16.5
43	Alaska	16.4
44	Alabama	16.2
45	California	15.5
46	Colorado	15.4
47	Georgia	14.7
48	South Dakota	13.6
49	New Mexico	11.6
50	Utah	9.7

| | District of Columbia | 18.9 |

Source: Morgan Quitno Press using data from American Cancer Society
   "Cancer Facts & Figures-1998" (Copyright 1998, Reprinted with permission from the American Cancer Society)
*Rates calculated using 1997 Census resident population estimates. Not age adjusted.

Estimated Deaths by Esophagus Cancer in 1998

National Estimated Total = 11,900 Deaths

ALPHA ORDER

RANK	STATE	DEATHS	% of USA
18	Alabama	200	1.68%
NA	Alaska*	NA	NA
18	Arizona	200	1.68%
26	Arkansas	100	0.84%
1	California	1,100	9.24%
26	Colorado	100	0.84%
18	Connecticut	200	1.68%
NA	Delaware*	NA	NA
3	Florida	800	6.72%
11	Georgia	300	2.52%
NA	Hawaii*	NA	NA
NA	Idaho*	NA	NA
6	Illinois	600	5.04%
11	Indiana	300	2.52%
26	Iowa	100	0.84%
26	Kansas	100	0.84%
18	Kentucky	200	1.68%
26	Louisiana	100	0.84%
26	Maine	100	0.84%
18	Maryland	200	1.68%
11	Massachusetts	300	2.52%
8	Michigan	500	4.20%
26	Minnesota	100	0.84%
26	Mississippi	100	0.84%
11	Missouri	300	2.52%
NA	Montana*	NA	NA
26	Nebraska	100	0.84%
26	Nevada	100	0.84%
26	New Hampshire	100	0.84%
9	New Jersey	400	3.36%
26	New Mexico	100	0.84%
2	New York	900	7.56%
9	North Carolina	400	3.36%
NA	North Dakota*	NA	NA
6	Ohio	600	5.04%
26	Oklahoma	100	0.84%
18	Oregon	200	1.68%
4	Pennsylvania	700	5.88%
NA	Rhode Island*	NA	NA
18	South Carolina	200	1.68%
NA	South Dakota*	NA	NA
18	Tennessee	200	1.68%
4	Texas	700	5.88%
NA	Utah*	NA	NA
NA	Vermont*	NA	NA
11	Virginia	300	2.52%
11	Washington	300	2.52%
26	West Virginia	100	0.84%
11	Wisconsin	300	2.52%
NA	Wyoming*	NA	NA

RANK ORDER

RANK	STATE	DEATHS	% of USA
1	California	1,100	9.24%
2	New York	900	7.56%
3	Florida	800	6.72%
4	Pennsylvania	700	5.88%
4	Texas	700	5.88%
6	Illinois	600	5.04%
6	Ohio	600	5.04%
8	Michigan	500	4.20%
9	New Jersey	400	3.36%
9	North Carolina	400	3.36%
11	Georgia	300	2.52%
11	Indiana	300	2.52%
11	Massachusetts	300	2.52%
11	Missouri	300	2.52%
11	Virginia	300	2.52%
11	Washington	300	2.52%
11	Wisconsin	300	2.52%
18	Alabama	200	1.68%
18	Arizona	200	1.68%
18	Connecticut	200	1.68%
18	Kentucky	200	1.68%
18	Maryland	200	1.68%
18	Oregon	200	1.68%
18	South Carolina	200	1.68%
18	Tennessee	200	1.68%
26	Arkansas	100	0.84%
26	Colorado	100	0.84%
26	Iowa	100	0.84%
26	Kansas	100	0.84%
26	Louisiana	100	0.84%
26	Maine	100	0.84%
26	Minnesota	100	0.84%
26	Mississippi	100	0.84%
26	Nebraska	100	0.84%
26	Nevada	100	0.84%
26	New Hampshire	100	0.84%
26	New Mexico	100	0.84%
26	Oklahoma	100	0.84%
26	West Virginia	100	0.84%
NA	Alaska*	NA	NA
NA	Delaware*	NA	NA
NA	Hawaii*	NA	NA
NA	Idaho*	NA	NA
NA	Montana*	NA	NA
NA	North Dakota*	NA	NA
NA	Rhode Island*	NA	NA
NA	South Dakota*	NA	NA
NA	Utah*	NA	NA
NA	Vermont*	NA	NA
NA	Wyoming*	NA	NA
	District of Columbia*	NA	NA

Source: American Cancer Society
   "Cancer Facts & Figures-1998" (Copyright 1998, Reprinted with permission from the American Cancer Society)
*Fewer than 50 deaths.

Estimated Death Rate by Esophagus Cancer in 1998

National Estimated Rate = 4.4 Deaths per 100,000 Population*

ALPHA ORDER

RANK ORDER

RANK	STATE	RATE		RANK	STATE	RATE
24	Alabama	4.6		1	New Hampshire	8.5
NA	Alaska**	NA		2	Maine	8.1
26	Arizona	4.4		3	Oregon	6.2
27	Arkansas	4.0		4	Connecticut	6.1
35	California	3.4		5	Nebraska	6.0
37	Colorado	2.6		5	Nevada	6.0
4	Connecticut	6.1		7	New Mexico	5.8
NA	Delaware**	NA		7	Pennsylvania	5.8
11	Florida	5.5		7	Wisconsin	5.8
27	Georgia	4.0		10	Missouri	5.6
NA	Hawaii**	NA		11	Florida	5.5
NA	Idaho**	NA		11	West Virginia	5.5
20	Illinois	5.0		13	North Carolina	5.4
17	Indiana	5.1		13	Ohio	5.4
34	Iowa	3.5		15	South Carolina	5.3
29	Kansas	3.9		15	Washington	5.3
17	Kentucky	5.1		17	Indiana	5.1
38	Louisiana	2.3		17	Kentucky	5.1
2	Maine	8.1		17	Michigan	5.1
29	Maryland	3.9		20	Illinois	5.0
23	Massachusetts	4.9		20	New Jersey	5.0
17	Michigan	5.1		20	New York	5.0
39	Minnesota	2.1		23	Massachusetts	4.9
31	Mississippi	3.7		24	Alabama	4.6
10	Missouri	5.6		25	Virginia	4.5
NA	Montana**	NA		26	Arizona	4.4
5	Nebraska	6.0		27	Arkansas	4.0
5	Nevada	6.0		27	Georgia	4.0
1	New Hampshire	8.5		29	Kansas	3.9
20	New Jersey	5.0		29	Maryland	3.9
7	New Mexico	5.8		31	Mississippi	3.7
20	New York	5.0		31	Tennessee	3.7
13	North Carolina	5.4		33	Texas	3.6
NA	North Dakota**	NA		34	Iowa	3.5
13	Ohio	5.4		35	California	3.4
36	Oklahoma	3.0		36	Oklahoma	3.0
3	Oregon	6.2		37	Colorado	2.6
7	Pennsylvania	5.8		38	Louisiana	2.3
NA	Rhode Island**	NA		39	Minnesota	2.1
15	South Carolina	5.3		NA	Alaska**	NA
NA	South Dakota**	NA		NA	Delaware**	NA
31	Tennessee	3.7		NA	Hawaii**	NA
33	Texas	3.6		NA	Idaho**	NA
NA	Utah**	NA		NA	Montana**	NA
NA	Vermont**	NA		NA	North Dakota**	NA
25	Virginia	4.5		NA	Rhode Island**	NA
15	Washington	5.3		NA	South Dakota**	NA
11	West Virginia	5.5		NA	Utah**	NA
7	Wisconsin	5.8		NA	Vermont**	NA
NA	Wyoming**	NA		NA	Wyoming**	NA
					District of Columbia**	NA

Source: Morgan Quitno Press using data from American Cancer Society
  "Cancer Facts & Figures-1998" (Copyright 1998, Reprinted with permission from the American Cancer Society)
*Rates calculated using 1997 Census resident population estimates. Not age adjusted.
**Fewer than 50 deaths.

Estimated Deaths by Leukemia in 1998

National Estimated Total = 21,600 Deaths

ALPHA ORDER

RANK	STATE	DEATHS	% of USA
19	Alabama	400	1.85%
NA	Alaska*	NA	NA
19	Arizona	400	1.85%
31	Arkansas	200	0.93%
1	California	2,100	9.72%
23	Colorado	300	1.39%
23	Connecticut	300	1.39%
35	Delaware	100	0.46%
2	Florida	1,400	6.48%
11	Georgia	500	2.31%
35	Hawaii	100	0.46%
35	Idaho	100	0.46%
6	Illinois	1,100	5.09%
11	Indiana	500	2.31%
23	Iowa	300	1.39%
31	Kansas	200	0.93%
23	Kentucky	300	1.39%
19	Louisiana	400	1.85%
35	Maine	100	0.46%
23	Maryland	300	1.39%
11	Massachusetts	500	2.31%
8	Michigan	800	3.70%
19	Minnesota	400	1.85%
31	Mississippi	200	0.93%
11	Missouri	500	2.31%
35	Montana	100	0.46%
35	Nebraska	100	0.46%
35	Nevada	100	0.46%
35	New Hampshire	100	0.46%
8	New Jersey	800	3.70%
35	New Mexico	100	0.46%
2	New York	1,400	6.48%
10	North Carolina	600	2.78%
35	North Dakota	100	0.46%
7	Ohio	900	4.17%
23	Oklahoma	300	1.39%
23	Oregon	300	1.39%
5	Pennsylvania	1,200	5.56%
35	Rhode Island	100	0.46%
23	South Carolina	300	1.39%
35	South Dakota	100	0.46%
11	Tennessee	500	2.31%
2	Texas	1,400	6.48%
35	Utah	100	0.46%
NA	Vermont*	NA	NA
11	Virginia	500	2.31%
11	Washington	500	2.31%
31	West Virginia	200	0.93%
11	Wisconsin	500	2.31%
NA	Wyoming*	NA	NA

RANK ORDER

RANK	STATE	DEATHS	% of USA
1	California	2,100	9.72%
2	Florida	1,400	6.48%
2	New York	1,400	6.48%
2	Texas	1,400	6.48%
5	Pennsylvania	1,200	5.56%
6	Illinois	1,100	5.09%
7	Ohio	900	4.17%
8	Michigan	800	3.70%
8	New Jersey	800	3.70%
10	North Carolina	600	2.78%
11	Georgia	500	2.31%
11	Indiana	500	2.31%
11	Massachusetts	500	2.31%
11	Missouri	500	2.31%
11	Tennessee	500	2.31%
11	Virginia	500	2.31%
11	Washington	500	2.31%
11	Wisconsin	500	2.31%
19	Alabama	400	1.85%
19	Arizona	400	1.85%
19	Louisiana	400	1.85%
19	Minnesota	400	1.85%
23	Colorado	300	1.39%
23	Connecticut	300	1.39%
23	Iowa	300	1.39%
23	Kentucky	300	1.39%
23	Maryland	300	1.39%
23	Oklahoma	300	1.39%
23	Oregon	300	1.39%
23	South Carolina	300	1.39%
31	Arkansas	200	0.93%
31	Kansas	200	0.93%
31	Mississippi	200	0.93%
31	West Virginia	200	0.93%
35	Delaware	100	0.46%
35	Hawaii	100	0.46%
35	Idaho	100	0.46%
35	Maine	100	0.46%
35	Montana	100	0.46%
35	Nebraska	100	0.46%
35	Nevada	100	0.46%
35	New Hampshire	100	0.46%
35	New Mexico	100	0.46%
35	North Dakota	100	0.46%
35	Rhode Island	100	0.46%
35	South Dakota	100	0.46%
35	Utah	100	0.46%
NA	Alaska*	NA	NA
NA	Vermont*	NA	NA
NA	Wyoming*	NA	NA
	District of Columbia*	NA	NA

Source: American Cancer Society
"Cancer Facts & Figures-1998" (Copyright 1998, Reprinted with permission from the American Cancer Society)
*Fewer than 50 deaths.

Estimated Death Rate by Leukemia in 1998

National Estimated Rate = 8.1 Deaths per 100,000 Population*

ALPHA ORDER

RANK	STATE	RATE
12	Alabama	9.3
NA	Alaska**	NA
21	Arizona	8.8
33	Arkansas	7.9
42	California	6.5
34	Colorado	7.7
15	Connecticut	9.2
2	Delaware	13.7
11	Florida	9.6
41	Georgia	6.7
25	Hawaii	8.4
26	Idaho	8.3
15	Illinois	9.2
22	Indiana	8.5
6	Iowa	10.5
34	Kansas	7.7
34	Kentucky	7.7
15	Louisiana	9.2
29	Maine	8.1
45	Maryland	5.9
27	Massachusetts	8.2
27	Michigan	8.2
22	Minnesota	8.5
39	Mississippi	7.3
12	Missouri	9.3
4	Montana	11.4
43	Nebraska	6.0
43	Nevada	6.0
22	New Hampshire	8.5
9	New Jersey	9.9
46	New Mexico	5.8
34	New York	7.7
29	North Carolina	8.1
1	North Dakota	15.6
31	Ohio	8.0
19	Oklahoma	9.0
15	Oregon	9.2
8	Pennsylvania	10.0
7	Rhode Island	10.1
31	South Carolina	8.0
3	South Dakota	13.6
12	Tennessee	9.3
40	Texas	7.2
47	Utah	4.9
NA	Vermont**	NA
38	Virginia	7.4
20	Washington	8.9
5	West Virginia	11.0
10	Wisconsin	9.7
NA	Wyoming**	NA

RANK ORDER

RANK	STATE	RATE
1	North Dakota	15.6
2	Delaware	13.7
3	South Dakota	13.6
4	Montana	11.4
5	West Virginia	11.0
6	Iowa	10.5
7	Rhode Island	10.1
8	Pennsylvania	10.0
9	New Jersey	9.9
10	Wisconsin	9.7
11	Florida	9.6
12	Alabama	9.3
12	Missouri	9.3
12	Tennessee	9.3
15	Connecticut	9.2
15	Illinois	9.2
15	Louisiana	9.2
15	Oregon	9.2
19	Oklahoma	9.0
20	Washington	8.9
21	Arizona	8.8
22	Indiana	8.5
22	Minnesota	8.5
22	New Hampshire	8.5
25	Hawaii	8.4
26	Idaho	8.3
27	Massachusetts	8.2
27	Michigan	8.2
29	Maine	8.1
29	North Carolina	8.1
31	Ohio	8.0
31	South Carolina	8.0
33	Arkansas	7.9
34	Colorado	7.7
34	Kansas	7.7
34	Kentucky	7.7
34	New York	7.7
38	Virginia	7.4
39	Mississippi	7.3
40	Texas	7.2
41	Georgia	6.7
42	California	6.5
43	Nebraska	6.0
43	Nevada	6.0
45	Maryland	5.9
46	New Mexico	5.8
47	Utah	4.9
NA	Alaska**	NA
NA	Vermont**	NA
NA	Wyoming**	NA
	District of Columbia**	NA

Source: Morgan Quitno Press using data from American Cancer Society
"Cancer Facts & Figures-1998" (Copyright 1998, Reprinted with permission from the American Cancer Society)
*Rates calculated using 1997 Census resident population estimates. Not age adjusted.
**Fewer than 50 deaths.

Estimated Deaths by Lung Cancer in 1998

National Estimated Total = 160,100 Deaths

ALPHA ORDER

RANK	STATE	DEATHS	% of USA
21	Alabama	2,800	1.75%
50	Alaska	200	0.12%
23	Arizona	2,600	1.62%
26	Arkansas	2,200	1.37%
1	California	13,700	8.56%
33	Colorado	1,500	0.94%
29	Connecticut	1,900	1.19%
41	Delaware	600	0.37%
2	Florida	12,000	7.50%
12	Georgia	3,900	2.44%
42	Hawaii	500	0.31%
42	Idaho	500	0.31%
7	Illinois	7,300	4.56%
12	Indiana	3,900	2.44%
29	Iowa	1,900	1.19%
33	Kansas	1,500	0.94%
17	Kentucky	3,300	2.06%
20	Louisiana	2,900	1.81%
36	Maine	1,000	0.62%
19	Maryland	3,000	1.87%
15	Massachusetts	3,800	2.37%
8	Michigan	5,900	3.69%
26	Minnesota	2,200	1.37%
31	Mississippi	1,700	1.06%
11	Missouri	4,000	2.50%
42	Montana	500	0.31%
37	Nebraska	900	0.56%
35	Nevada	1,100	0.69%
38	New Hampshire	700	0.44%
10	New Jersey	4,600	2.87%
38	New Mexico	700	0.44%
4	New York	10,100	6.31%
9	North Carolina	5,000	3.12%
48	North Dakota	300	0.19%
6	Ohio	7,700	4.81%
25	Oklahoma	2,300	1.44%
28	Oregon	2,100	1.31%
5	Pennsylvania	8,500	5.31%
38	Rhode Island	700	0.44%
24	South Carolina	2,400	1.50%
45	South Dakota	400	0.25%
12	Tennessee	3,900	2.44%
3	Texas	10,800	6.75%
45	Utah	400	0.25%
45	Vermont	400	0.25%
15	Virginia	3,800	2.37%
18	Washington	3,200	2.00%
32	West Virginia	1,600	1.00%
22	Wisconsin	2,700	1.69%
48	Wyoming	300	0.19%

RANK ORDER

RANK	STATE	DEATHS	% of USA
1	California	13,700	8.56%
2	Florida	12,000	7.50%
3	Texas	10,800	6.75%
4	New York	10,100	6.31%
5	Pennsylvania	8,500	5.31%
6	Ohio	7,700	4.81%
7	Illinois	7,300	4.56%
8	Michigan	5,900	3.69%
9	North Carolina	5,000	3.12%
10	New Jersey	4,600	2.87%
11	Missouri	4,000	2.50%
12	Georgia	3,900	2.44%
12	Indiana	3,900	2.44%
12	Tennessee	3,900	2.44%
15	Massachusetts	3,800	2.37%
15	Virginia	3,800	2.37%
17	Kentucky	3,300	2.06%
18	Washington	3,200	2.00%
19	Maryland	3,000	1.87%
20	Louisiana	2,900	1.81%
21	Alabama	2,800	1.75%
22	Wisconsin	2,700	1.69%
23	Arizona	2,600	1.62%
24	South Carolina	2,400	1.50%
25	Oklahoma	2,300	1.44%
26	Arkansas	2,200	1.37%
26	Minnesota	2,200	1.37%
28	Oregon	2,100	1.31%
29	Connecticut	1,900	1.19%
29	Iowa	1,900	1.19%
31	Mississippi	1,700	1.06%
32	West Virginia	1,600	1.00%
33	Colorado	1,500	0.94%
33	Kansas	1,500	0.94%
35	Nevada	1,100	0.69%
36	Maine	1,000	0.62%
37	Nebraska	900	0.56%
38	New Hampshire	700	0.44%
38	New Mexico	700	0.44%
38	Rhode Island	700	0.44%
41	Delaware	600	0.37%
42	Hawaii	500	0.31%
42	Idaho	500	0.31%
42	Montana	500	0.31%
45	South Dakota	400	0.25%
45	Utah	400	0.25%
45	Vermont	400	0.25%
48	North Dakota	300	0.19%
48	Wyoming	300	0.19%
50	Alaska	200	0.12%
	District of Columbia	400	0.25%

Source: American Cancer Society
"Cancer Facts & Figures-1998" (Copyright 1998, Reprinted with permission from the American Cancer Society)

Estimated Death Rate by Lung Cancer in 1998

National Estimated Rate = 59.8 Deaths per 100,000 Population*

ALPHA ORDER

RANK	STATE	RATE
19	Alabama	64.8
49	Alaska	32.8
31	Arizona	57.1
2	Arkansas	87.2
44	California	42.5
48	Colorado	38.5
29	Connecticut	58.1
4	Delaware	82.0
5	Florida	81.9
41	Georgia	52.1
45	Hawaii	42.1
46	Idaho	41.3
25	Illinois	61.4
17	Indiana	66.5
15	Iowa	66.6
30	Kansas	57.8
3	Kentucky	84.4
15	Louisiana	66.6
6	Maine	80.5
28	Maryland	58.9
24	Massachusetts	62.1
26	Michigan	60.4
42	Minnesota	47.0
23	Mississippi	62.3
7	Missouri	74.0
34	Montana	56.9
38	Nebraska	54.3
18	Nevada	65.6
27	New Hampshire	59.7
31	New Jersey	57.1
47	New Mexico	40.5
36	New York	55.7
14	North Carolina	67.3
43	North Dakota	46.8
12	Ohio	68.8
11	Oklahoma	69.3
20	Oregon	64.7
10	Pennsylvania	70.7
9	Rhode Island	70.9
21	South Carolina	63.8
39	South Dakota	54.2
8	Tennessee	72.7
37	Texas	55.6
50	Utah	19.4
13	Vermont	67.9
35	Virginia	56.4
33	Washington	57.0
1	West Virginia	88.1
40	Wisconsin	52.2
22	Wyoming	62.5

RANK ORDER

RANK	STATE	RATE
1	West Virginia	88.1
2	Arkansas	87.2
3	Kentucky	84.4
4	Delaware	82.0
5	Florida	81.9
6	Maine	80.5
7	Missouri	74.0
8	Tennessee	72.7
9	Rhode Island	70.9
10	Pennsylvania	70.7
11	Oklahoma	69.3
12	Ohio	68.8
13	Vermont	67.9
14	North Carolina	67.3
15	Iowa	66.6
15	Louisiana	66.6
17	Indiana	66.5
18	Nevada	65.6
19	Alabama	64.8
20	Oregon	64.7
21	South Carolina	63.8
22	Wyoming	62.5
23	Mississippi	62.3
24	Massachusetts	62.1
25	Illinois	61.4
26	Michigan	60.4
27	New Hampshire	59.7
28	Maryland	58.9
29	Connecticut	58.1
30	Kansas	57.8
31	Arizona	57.1
31	New Jersey	57.1
33	Washington	57.0
34	Montana	56.9
35	Virginia	56.4
36	New York	55.7
37	Texas	55.6
38	Nebraska	54.3
39	South Dakota	54.2
40	Wisconsin	52.2
41	Georgia	52.1
42	Minnesota	47.0
43	North Dakota	46.8
44	California	42.5
45	Hawaii	42.1
46	Idaho	41.3
47	New Mexico	40.5
48	Colorado	38.5
49	Alaska	32.8
50	Utah	19.4
	District of Columbia	75.6

Source: Morgan Quitno Press using data from American Cancer Society
"Cancer Facts & Figures-1998" (Copyright 1998, Reprinted with permission from the American Cancer Society)
Rates calculated using 1997 Census resident population estimates. Not age adjusted.

Estimated Deaths by Non-Hodgkin's Lymphoma in 1998

National Estimated Total = 24,900 Deaths

<u>ALPHA ORDER</u>

RANK	STATE	DEATHS	% of USA
19	Alabama	400	1.61%
NA	Alaska*	NA	NA
19	Arizona	400	1.61%
32	Arkansas	200	0.80%
1	California	2,200	8.84%
27	Colorado	300	1.20%
27	Connecticut	300	1.20%
38	Delaware	100	0.40%
2	Florida	1,800	7.23%
19	Georgia	400	1.61%
38	Hawaii	100	0.40%
38	Idaho	100	0.40%
6	Illinois	1,200	4.82%
14	Indiana	500	2.01%
19	Iowa	400	1.61%
27	Kansas	300	1.20%
27	Kentucky	300	1.20%
19	Louisiana	400	1.61%
32	Maine	200	0.80%
19	Maryland	400	1.61%
10	Massachusetts	700	2.81%
8	Michigan	900	3.61%
14	Minnesota	500	2.01%
32	Mississippi	200	0.80%
14	Missouri	500	2.01%
38	Montana	100	0.40%
32	Nebraska	200	0.80%
38	Nevada	100	0.40%
38	New Hampshire	100	0.40%
9	New Jersey	800	3.21%
38	New Mexico	100	0.40%
2	New York	1,800	7.23%
11	North Carolina	600	2.41%
38	North Dakota	100	0.40%
6	Ohio	1,200	4.82%
19	Oklahoma	400	1.61%
19	Oregon	400	1.61%
5	Pennsylvania	1,400	5.62%
38	Rhode Island	100	0.40%
27	South Carolina	300	1.20%
38	South Dakota	100	0.40%
14	Tennessee	500	2.01%
4	Texas	1,700	6.83%
32	Utah	200	0.80%
38	Vermont	100	0.40%
11	Virginia	600	2.41%
14	Washington	500	2.01%
32	West Virginia	200	0.80%
11	Wisconsin	600	2.41%
NA	Wyoming*	NA	NA

<u>RANK ORDER</u>

RANK	STATE	DEATHS	% of USA
1	California	2,200	8.84%
2	Florida	1,800	7.23%
2	New York	1,800	7.23%
4	Texas	1,700	6.83%
5	Pennsylvania	1,400	5.62%
6	Illinois	1,200	4.82%
6	Ohio	1,200	4.82%
8	Michigan	900	3.61%
9	New Jersey	800	3.21%
10	Massachusetts	700	2.81%
11	North Carolina	600	2.41%
11	Virginia	600	2.41%
11	Wisconsin	600	2.41%
14	Indiana	500	2.01%
14	Minnesota	500	2.01%
14	Missouri	500	2.01%
14	Tennessee	500	2.01%
14	Washington	500	2.01%
19	Alabama	400	1.61%
19	Arizona	400	1.61%
19	Georgia	400	1.61%
19	Iowa	400	1.61%
19	Louisiana	400	1.61%
19	Maryland	400	1.61%
19	Oklahoma	400	1.61%
19	Oregon	400	1.61%
27	Colorado	300	1.20%
27	Connecticut	300	1.20%
27	Kansas	300	1.20%
27	Kentucky	300	1.20%
27	South Carolina	300	1.20%
32	Arkansas	200	0.80%
32	Maine	200	0.80%
32	Mississippi	200	0.80%
32	Nebraska	200	0.80%
32	Utah	200	0.80%
32	West Virginia	200	0.80%
38	Delaware	100	0.40%
38	Hawaii	100	0.40%
38	Idaho	100	0.40%
38	Montana	100	0.40%
38	Nevada	100	0.40%
38	New Hampshire	100	0.40%
38	New Mexico	100	0.40%
38	North Dakota	100	0.40%
38	Rhode Island	100	0.40%
38	South Dakota	100	0.40%
38	Vermont	100	0.40%
NA	Alaska*	NA	NA
NA	Wyoming*	NA	NA
	District of Columbia*	NA	NA

Source: American Cancer Society
"Cancer Facts & Figures-1998" (Copyright 1998, Reprinted with permission from the American Cancer Society)
*Fewer than 50 deaths.

Estimated Death Rate by Non-Hodgkin's Lymphoma in 1998

National Estimated Rate = 9.3 Deaths per 100,000 Population*

ALPHA ORDER

RANK	STATE	RATE
24	Alabama	9.3
NA	Alaska**	NA
32	Arizona	8.8
40	Arkansas	7.9
45	California	6.8
42	Colorado	7.7
27	Connecticut	9.2
5	Delaware	13.7
7	Florida	12.3
48	Georgia	5.3
36	Hawaii	8.4
37	Idaho	8.3
19	Illinois	10.1
34	Indiana	8.5
4	Iowa	14.0
11	Kansas	11.6
42	Kentucky	7.7
27	Louisiana	9.2
2	Maine	16.1
40	Maryland	7.9
14	Massachusetts	11.4
27	Michigan	9.2
17	Minnesota	10.7
44	Mississippi	7.3
24	Missouri	9.3
14	Montana	11.4
9	Nebraska	12.1
46	Nevada	6.0
34	New Hampshire	8.5
21	New Jersey	9.9
47	New Mexico	5.8
21	New York	9.9
38	North Carolina	8.1
3	North Dakota	15.6
17	Ohio	10.7
9	Oklahoma	12.1
7	Oregon	12.3
11	Pennsylvania	11.6
19	Rhode Island	10.1
39	South Carolina	8.0
6	South Dakota	13.6
24	Tennessee	9.3
33	Texas	8.7
23	Utah	9.7
1	Vermont	17.0
30	Virginia	8.9
30	Washington	8.9
16	West Virginia	11.0
11	Wisconsin	11.6
NA	Wyoming**	NA

RANK ORDER

RANK	STATE	RATE
1	Vermont	17.0
2	Maine	16.1
3	North Dakota	15.6
4	Iowa	14.0
5	Delaware	13.7
6	South Dakota	13.6
7	Florida	12.3
7	Oregon	12.3
9	Nebraska	12.1
9	Oklahoma	12.1
11	Kansas	11.6
11	Pennsylvania	11.6
11	Wisconsin	11.6
14	Massachusetts	11.4
14	Montana	11.4
16	West Virginia	11.0
17	Minnesota	10.7
17	Ohio	10.7
19	Illinois	10.1
19	Rhode Island	10.1
21	New Jersey	9.9
21	New York	9.9
23	Utah	9.7
24	Alabama	9.3
24	Missouri	9.3
24	Tennessee	9.3
27	Connecticut	9.2
27	Louisiana	9.2
27	Michigan	9.2
30	Virginia	8.9
30	Washington	8.9
32	Arizona	8.8
33	Texas	8.7
34	Indiana	8.5
34	New Hampshire	8.5
36	Hawaii	8.4
37	Idaho	8.3
38	North Carolina	8.1
39	South Carolina	8.0
40	Arkansas	7.9
40	Maryland	7.9
42	Colorado	7.7
42	Kentucky	7.7
44	Mississippi	7.3
45	California	6.8
46	Nevada	6.0
47	New Mexico	5.8
48	Georgia	5.3
NA	Alaska**	NA
NA	Wyoming**	NA
	District of Columbia**	NA

Source: Morgan Quitno Press using data from American Cancer Society
   "Cancer Facts & Figures-1998" (Copyright 1998, Reprinted with permission from the American Cancer Society)
Rates calculated using 1997 Census resident population estimates. Not age adjusted.
**Fewer than 50 deaths.*

Estimated Deaths by Stomach Cancer in 1998

National Estimated Total = 13,700 Deaths

ALPHA ORDER

RANK	STATE	DEATHS	% of USA
16	Alabama	200	1.46%
NA	Alaska*	NA	NA
16	Arizona	200	1.46%
27	Arkansas	100	0.73%
1	California	1,600	11.68%
27	Colorado	100	0.73%
16	Connecticut	200	1.46%
NA	Delaware*	NA	NA
4	Florida	900	6.57%
11	Georgia	300	2.19%
27	Hawaii	100	0.73%
NA	Idaho*	NA	NA
6	Illinois	600	4.38%
16	Indiana	200	1.46%
27	Iowa	100	0.73%
27	Kansas	100	0.73%
16	Kentucky	200	1.46%
11	Louisiana	300	2.19%
27	Maine	100	0.73%
16	Maryland	200	1.46%
11	Massachusetts	300	2.19%
7	Michigan	500	3.65%
16	Minnesota	200	1.46%
16	Mississippi	200	1.46%
11	Missouri	300	2.19%
NA	Montana*	NA	NA
27	Nebraska	100	0.73%
27	Nevada	100	0.73%
NA	New Hampshire*	NA	NA
7	New Jersey	500	3.65%
27	New Mexico	100	0.73%
2	New York	1,300	9.49%
10	North Carolina	400	2.92%
NA	North Dakota*	NA	NA
7	Ohio	500	3.65%
27	Oklahoma	100	0.73%
27	Oregon	100	0.73%
5	Pennsylvania	800	5.84%
27	Rhode Island	100	0.73%
27	South Carolina	100	0.73%
NA	South Dakota*	NA	NA
16	Tennessee	200	1.46%
3	Texas	1,000	7.30%
NA	Utah*	NA	NA
NA	Vermont*	NA	NA
16	Virginia	200	1.46%
16	Washington	200	1.46%
27	West Virginia	100	0.73%
11	Wisconsin	300	2.19%
NA	Wyoming*	NA	NA

RANK ORDER

RANK	STATE	DEATHS	% of USA
1	California	1,600	11.68%
2	New York	1,300	9.49%
3	Texas	1,000	7.30%
4	Florida	900	6.57%
5	Pennsylvania	800	5.84%
6	Illinois	600	4.38%
7	Michigan	500	3.65%
7	New Jersey	500	3.65%
7	Ohio	500	3.65%
10	North Carolina	400	2.92%
11	Georgia	300	2.19%
11	Louisiana	300	2.19%
11	Massachusetts	300	2.19%
11	Missouri	300	2.19%
11	Wisconsin	300	2.19%
16	Alabama	200	1.46%
16	Arizona	200	1.46%
16	Connecticut	200	1.46%
16	Indiana	200	1.46%
16	Kentucky	200	1.46%
16	Maryland	200	1.46%
16	Minnesota	200	1.46%
16	Mississippi	200	1.46%
16	Tennessee	200	1.46%
16	Virginia	200	1.46%
16	Washington	200	1.46%
27	Arkansas	100	0.73%
27	Colorado	100	0.73%
27	Hawaii	100	0.73%
27	Iowa	100	0.73%
27	Kansas	100	0.73%
27	Maine	100	0.73%
27	Nebraska	100	0.73%
27	Nevada	100	0.73%
27	New Mexico	100	0.73%
27	Oklahoma	100	0.73%
27	Oregon	100	0.73%
27	Rhode Island	100	0.73%
27	South Carolina	100	0.73%
27	West Virginia	100	0.73%
NA	Alaska*	NA	NA
NA	Delaware*	NA	NA
NA	Idaho*	NA	NA
NA	Montana*	NA	NA
NA	New Hampshire*	NA	NA
NA	North Dakota*	NA	NA
NA	South Dakota*	NA	NA
NA	Utah*	NA	NA
NA	Vermont*	NA	NA
NA	Wyoming*	NA	NA
	District of Columbia	100	0.73%

Source: American Cancer Society
   "Cancer Facts & Figures-1998" (Copyright 1998, Reprinted with permission from the American Cancer Society)
*Fewer than 50 deaths.

Estimated Death Rate by Stomach Cancer in 1998

National Estimated Rate = 5.1 Deaths per 100,000 Population*

ALPHA ORDER

RANK	STATE	RATE
24	Alabama	4.6
NA	Alaska**	NA
26	Arizona	4.4
28	Arkansas	4.0
21	California	5.0
40	Colorado	2.6
9	Connecticut	6.1
NA	Delaware**	NA
9	Florida	6.1
28	Georgia	4.0
2	Hawaii	8.4
NA	Idaho**	NA
21	Illinois	5.0
35	Indiana	3.4
34	Iowa	3.5
30	Kansas	3.9
18	Kentucky	5.1
6	Louisiana	6.9
3	Maine	8.1
30	Maryland	3.9
23	Massachusetts	4.9
18	Michigan	5.1
27	Minnesota	4.3
4	Mississippi	7.3
15	Missouri	5.6
NA	Montana**	NA
11	Nebraska	6.0
11	Nevada	6.0
NA	New Hampshire**	NA
8	New Jersey	6.2
13	New Mexico	5.8
5	New York	7.2
17	North Carolina	5.4
NA	North Dakota**	NA
25	Ohio	4.5
37	Oklahoma	3.0
36	Oregon	3.1
7	Pennsylvania	6.7
1	Rhode Island	10.1
39	South Carolina	2.7
NA	South Dakota**	NA
32	Tennessee	3.7
18	Texas	5.1
NA	Utah**	NA
NA	Vermont**	NA
37	Virginia	3.0
33	Washington	3.6
16	West Virginia	5.5
13	Wisconsin	5.8
NA	Wyoming**	NA

RANK ORDER

RANK	STATE	RATE
1	Rhode Island	10.1
2	Hawaii	8.4
3	Maine	8.1
4	Mississippi	7.3
5	New York	7.2
6	Louisiana	6.9
7	Pennsylvania	6.7
8	New Jersey	6.2
9	Connecticut	6.1
9	Florida	6.1
11	Nebraska	6.0
11	Nevada	6.0
13	New Mexico	5.8
13	Wisconsin	5.8
15	Missouri	5.6
16	West Virginia	5.5
17	North Carolina	5.4
18	Kentucky	5.1
18	Michigan	5.1
18	Texas	5.1
21	California	5.0
21	Illinois	5.0
23	Massachusetts	4.9
24	Alabama	4.6
25	Ohio	4.5
26	Arizona	4.4
27	Minnesota	4.3
28	Arkansas	4.0
28	Georgia	4.0
30	Kansas	3.9
30	Maryland	3.9
32	Tennessee	3.7
33	Washington	3.6
34	Iowa	3.5
35	Indiana	3.4
36	Oregon	3.1
37	Oklahoma	3.0
37	Virginia	3.0
39	South Carolina	2.7
40	Colorado	2.6
NA	Alaska**	NA
NA	Delaware**	NA
NA	Idaho**	NA
NA	Montana**	NA
NA	New Hampshire**	NA
NA	North Dakota**	NA
NA	South Dakota**	NA
NA	Utah**	NA
NA	Vermont**	NA
NA	Wyoming**	NA

District of Columbia   18.9

Source: Morgan Quitno Press using data from American Cancer Society
    "Cancer Facts & Figures-1998" (Copyright 1998, Reprinted with permission from the American Cancer Society)
*Rates calculated using 1997 Census resident population estimates. Not age adjusted.
**Fewer than 50 deaths.

Estimated Deaths by Pancreatic Cancer in 1998

National Estimated Total = 28,900 Deaths

ALPHA ORDER

RANK	STATE	DEATHS	% of USA
18	Alabama	500	1.73%
NA	Alaska*	NA	NA
18	Arizona	500	1.73%
28	Arkansas	300	1.04%
1	California	2,800	9.69%
28	Colorado	300	1.04%
25	Connecticut	400	1.38%
39	Delaware	100	0.35%
2	Florida	2,200	7.61%
11	Georgia	700	2.42%
39	Hawaii	100	0.35%
39	Idaho	100	0.35%
6	Illinois	1,300	4.50%
11	Indiana	700	2.42%
28	Iowa	300	1.04%
28	Kansas	300	1.04%
18	Kentucky	500	1.73%
18	Louisiana	500	1.73%
34	Maine	200	0.69%
18	Maryland	500	1.73%
11	Massachusetts	700	2.42%
8	Michigan	1,100	3.81%
18	Minnesota	500	1.73%
28	Mississippi	300	1.04%
15	Missouri	600	2.08%
39	Montana	100	0.35%
34	Nebraska	200	0.69%
34	Nevada	200	0.69%
39	New Hampshire	100	0.35%
9	New Jersey	1,000	3.46%
34	New Mexico	200	0.69%
2	New York	2,200	7.61%
10	North Carolina	800	2.77%
39	North Dakota	100	0.35%
7	Ohio	1,200	4.15%
28	Oklahoma	300	1.04%
25	Oregon	400	1.38%
5	Pennsylvania	1,500	5.19%
39	Rhode Island	100	0.35%
25	South Carolina	400	1.38%
39	South Dakota	100	0.35%
15	Tennessee	600	2.08%
4	Texas	1,900	6.57%
39	Utah	100	0.35%
NA	Vermont*	NA	NA
11	Virginia	700	2.42%
18	Washington	500	1.73%
34	West Virginia	200	0.69%
15	Wisconsin	600	2.08%
NA	Wyoming*	NA	NA

RANK ORDER

RANK	STATE	DEATHS	% of USA
1	California	2,800	9.69%
2	Florida	2,200	7.61%
2	New York	2,200	7.61%
4	Texas	1,900	6.57%
5	Pennsylvania	1,500	5.19%
6	Illinois	1,300	4.50%
7	Ohio	1,200	4.15%
8	Michigan	1,100	3.81%
9	New Jersey	1,000	3.46%
10	North Carolina	800	2.77%
11	Georgia	700	2.42%
11	Indiana	700	2.42%
11	Massachusetts	700	2.42%
11	Virginia	700	2.42%
15	Missouri	600	2.08%
15	Tennessee	600	2.08%
15	Wisconsin	600	2.08%
18	Alabama	500	1.73%
18	Arizona	500	1.73%
18	Kentucky	500	1.73%
18	Louisiana	500	1.73%
18	Maryland	500	1.73%
18	Minnesota	500	1.73%
18	Washington	500	1.73%
25	Connecticut	400	1.38%
25	Oregon	400	1.38%
25	South Carolina	400	1.38%
28	Arkansas	300	1.04%
28	Colorado	300	1.04%
28	Iowa	300	1.04%
28	Kansas	300	1.04%
28	Mississippi	300	1.04%
28	Oklahoma	300	1.04%
34	Maine	200	0.69%
34	Nebraska	200	0.69%
34	Nevada	200	0.69%
34	New Mexico	200	0.69%
34	West Virginia	200	0.69%
39	Delaware	100	0.35%
39	Hawaii	100	0.35%
39	Idaho	100	0.35%
39	Montana	100	0.35%
39	New Hampshire	100	0.35%
39	North Dakota	100	0.35%
39	Rhode Island	100	0.35%
39	South Dakota	100	0.35%
39	Utah	100	0.35%
NA	Alaska*	NA	NA
NA	Vermont*	NA	NA
NA	Wyoming*	NA	NA
	District of Columbia	100	0.35%

Source: American Cancer Society
"Cancer Facts & Figures-1998" (Copyright 1998, Reprinted with permission from the American Cancer Society)
*Fewer than 50 deaths.

Estimated Death Rate by Pancreatic Cancer in 1998

National Estimated Rate = 10.8 Deaths per 100,000 Population*

ALPHA ORDER

RANK	STATE	RATE
16	Alabama	11.6
NA	Alaska**	NA
26	Arizona	11.0
13	Arkansas	11.9
42	California	8.7
46	Colorado	7.7
10	Connecticut	12.2
4	Delaware	13.7
3	Florida	15.0
39	Georgia	9.4
44	Hawaii	8.4
45	Idaho	8.3
29	Illinois	10.9
13	Indiana	11.9
34	Iowa	10.5
16	Kansas	11.6
6	Kentucky	12.8
20	Louisiana	11.5
1	Maine	16.1
37	Maryland	9.8
21	Massachusetts	11.4
23	Michigan	11.3
31	Minnesota	10.7
26	Mississippi	11.0
25	Missouri	11.1
21	Montana	11.4
11	Nebraska	12.1
13	Nevada	11.9
43	New Hampshire	8.5
8	New Jersey	12.4
16	New Mexico	11.6
11	New York	12.1
30	North Carolina	10.8
2	North Dakota	15.6
31	Ohio	10.7
40	Oklahoma	9.0
9	Oregon	12.3
7	Pennsylvania	12.5
36	Rhode Island	10.1
33	South Carolina	10.6
5	South Dakota	13.6
24	Tennessee	11.2
37	Texas	9.8
47	Utah	4.9
NA	Vermont**	NA
35	Virginia	10.4
41	Washington	8.9
26	West Virginia	11.0
16	Wisconsin	11.6
NA	Wyoming**	NA

RANK ORDER

RANK	STATE	RATE
1	Maine	16.1
2	North Dakota	15.6
3	Florida	15.0
4	Delaware	13.7
5	South Dakota	13.6
6	Kentucky	12.8
7	Pennsylvania	12.5
8	New Jersey	12.4
9	Oregon	12.3
10	Connecticut	12.2
11	Nebraska	12.1
11	New York	12.1
13	Arkansas	11.9
13	Indiana	11.9
13	Nevada	11.9
16	Alabama	11.6
16	Kansas	11.6
16	New Mexico	11.6
16	Wisconsin	11.6
20	Louisiana	11.5
21	Massachusetts	11.4
21	Montana	11.4
23	Michigan	11.3
24	Tennessee	11.2
25	Missouri	11.1
26	Arizona	11.0
26	Mississippi	11.0
26	West Virginia	11.0
29	Illinois	10.9
30	North Carolina	10.8
31	Minnesota	10.7
31	Ohio	10.7
33	South Carolina	10.6
34	Iowa	10.5
35	Virginia	10.4
36	Rhode Island	10.1
37	Maryland	9.8
37	Texas	9.8
39	Georgia	9.4
40	Oklahoma	9.0
41	Washington	8.9
42	California	8.7
43	New Hampshire	8.5
44	Hawaii	8.4
45	Idaho	8.3
46	Colorado	7.7
47	Utah	4.9
NA	Alaska**	NA
NA	Vermont**	NA
NA	Wyoming**	NA
	District of Columbia	18.9

Source: Morgan Quitno Press using data from American Cancer Society
"Cancer Facts & Figures-1998" (Copyright 1998, Reprinted with permission from the American Cancer Society)
*Rates calculated using 1997 Census resident population estimates. Not age adjusted.
**Fewer than 50 deaths.

Estimated Deaths by Prostate Cancer in 1998

National Estimated Total = 39,200 Deaths

ALPHA ORDER				RANK ORDER			
RANK	STATE	DEATHS	% of USA	RANK	STATE	DEATHS	% of USA
23	Alabama	600	1.53%	1	California	3,700	9.44%
NA	Alaska*	NA	NA	2	Florida	3,000	7.65%
17	Arizona	700	1.79%	3	New York	2,500	6.38%
25	Arkansas	500	1.28%	3	Texas	2,500	6.38%
1	California	3,700	9.44%	5	Pennsylvania	2,200	5.61%
25	Colorado	500	1.28%	6	Illinois	1,800	4.59%
25	Connecticut	500	1.28%	7	Ohio	1,700	4.34%
42	Delaware	100	0.26%	8	Michigan	1,400	3.57%
2	Florida	3,000	7.65%	9	New Jersey	1,200	3.06%
11	Georgia	1,000	2.55%	9	North Carolina	1,200	3.06%
42	Hawaii	100	0.26%	11	Georgia	1,000	2.55%
35	Idaho	200	0.51%	12	Massachusetts	900	2.30%
6	Illinois	1,800	4.59%	12	Virginia	900	2.30%
15	Indiana	800	2.04%	12	Wisconsin	900	2.30%
25	Iowa	500	1.28%	15	Indiana	800	2.04%
33	Kansas	400	1.02%	15	Missouri	800	2.04%
25	Kentucky	500	1.28%	17	Arizona	700	1.79%
17	Louisiana	700	1.79%	17	Louisiana	700	1.79%
35	Maine	200	0.51%	17	Maryland	700	1.79%
17	Maryland	700	1.79%	17	Minnesota	700	1.79%
12	Massachusetts	900	2.30%	17	Tennessee	700	1.79%
8	Michigan	1,400	3.57%	17	Washington	700	1.79%
17	Minnesota	700	1.79%	23	Alabama	600	1.53%
25	Mississippi	500	1.28%	23	South Carolina	600	1.53%
15	Missouri	800	2.04%	25	Arkansas	500	1.28%
35	Montana	200	0.51%	25	Colorado	500	1.28%
35	Nebraska	200	0.51%	25	Connecticut	500	1.28%
35	Nevada	200	0.51%	25	Iowa	500	1.28%
42	New Hampshire	100	0.26%	25	Kentucky	500	1.28%
9	New Jersey	1,200	3.06%	25	Mississippi	500	1.28%
35	New Mexico	200	0.51%	25	Oklahoma	500	1.28%
3	New York	2,500	6.38%	25	Oregon	500	1.28%
9	North Carolina	1,200	3.06%	33	Kansas	400	1.02%
42	North Dakota	100	0.26%	34	West Virginia	300	0.77%
7	Ohio	1,700	4.34%	35	Idaho	200	0.51%
25	Oklahoma	500	1.28%	35	Maine	200	0.51%
25	Oregon	500	1.28%	35	Montana	200	0.51%
5	Pennsylvania	2,200	5.61%	35	Nebraska	200	0.51%
42	Rhode Island	100	0.26%	35	Nevada	200	0.51%
23	South Carolina	600	1.53%	35	New Mexico	200	0.51%
42	South Dakota	100	0.26%	35	Utah	200	0.51%
17	Tennessee	700	1.79%	42	Delaware	100	0.26%
3	Texas	2,500	6.38%	42	Hawaii	100	0.26%
35	Utah	200	0.51%	42	New Hampshire	100	0.26%
42	Vermont	100	0.26%	42	North Dakota	100	0.26%
12	Virginia	900	2.30%	42	Rhode Island	100	0.26%
17	Washington	700	1.79%	42	South Dakota	100	0.26%
34	West Virginia	300	0.77%	42	Vermont	100	0.26%
12	Wisconsin	900	2.30%	42	Wyoming	100	0.26%
42	Wyoming	100	0.26%	NA	Alaska*	NA	NA
					District of Columbia	100	0.26%

Source: American Cancer Society
"Cancer Facts & Figures-1998" (Copyright 1998, Reprinted with permission from the American Cancer Society)
*Fewer than 50 deaths.

Estimated Death Rate by Prostate Cancer in 1998

National Estimated Rate = 30.2 Deaths per 100,000 Male Population*

ALPHA ORDER

RANK	STATE	RATE
29	Alabama	29.2
NA	Alaska**	NA
16	Arizona	31.9
4	Arkansas	41.2
45	California	23.2
40	Colorado	26.4
19	Connecticut	31.4
31	Delaware	28.3
2	Florida	42.9
34	Georgia	27.9
49	Hawaii	16.7
12	Idaho	33.6
21	Illinois	31.1
33	Indiana	28.1
7	Iowa	36.0
17	Kansas	31.6
38	Kentucky	26.5
14	Louisiana	33.4
15	Maine	32.9
31	Maryland	28.3
26	Massachusetts	30.6
28	Michigan	29.9
27	Minnesota	30.5
5	Mississippi	38.3
25	Missouri	30.8
1	Montana	45.7
42	Nebraska	24.7
43	Nevada	24.5
48	New Hampshire	17.5
23	New Jersey	31.0
44	New Mexico	23.7
30	New York	28.5
11	North Carolina	33.7
21	North Dakota	31.1
19	Ohio	31.4
23	Oklahoma	31.0
17	Oregon	31.6
6	Pennsylvania	37.9
46	Rhode Island	21.0
12	South Carolina	33.6
35	South Dakota	27.7
37	Tennessee	27.2
38	Texas	26.5
47	Utah	20.1
9	Vermont	34.5
36	Virginia	27.5
41	Washington	25.4
10	West Virginia	34.0
8	Wisconsin	35.5
3	Wyoming	41.3

RANK ORDER

RANK	STATE	RATE
1	Montana	45.7
2	Florida	42.9
3	Wyoming	41.3
4	Arkansas	41.2
5	Mississippi	38.3
6	Pennsylvania	37.9
7	Iowa	36.0
8	Wisconsin	35.5
9	Vermont	34.5
10	West Virginia	34.0
11	North Carolina	33.7
12	Idaho	33.6
12	South Carolina	33.6
14	Louisiana	33.4
15	Maine	32.9
16	Arizona	31.9
17	Kansas	31.6
17	Oregon	31.6
19	Connecticut	31.4
19	Ohio	31.4
21	Illinois	31.1
21	North Dakota	31.1
23	New Jersey	31.0
23	Oklahoma	31.0
25	Missouri	30.8
26	Massachusetts	30.6
27	Minnesota	30.5
28	Michigan	29.9
29	Alabama	29.2
30	New York	28.5
31	Delaware	28.3
31	Maryland	28.3
33	Indiana	28.1
34	Georgia	27.9
35	South Dakota	27.7
36	Virginia	27.5
37	Tennessee	27.2
38	Kentucky	26.5
38	Texas	26.5
40	Colorado	26.4
41	Washington	25.4
42	Nebraska	24.7
43	Nevada	24.5
44	New Mexico	23.7
45	California	23.2
46	Rhode Island	21.0
47	Utah	20.1
48	New Hampshire	17.5
49	Hawaii	16.7
NA	Alaska**	NA
	District of Columbia	39.3

Source: Morgan Quitno Press using data from American Cancer Society
    "Cancer Facts & Figures-1998" (Copyright 1998, Reprinted with permission from the American Cancer Society)
*Rates calculated using 1996 Census resident male population estimates. Not age adjusted.
**Fewer than 50 deaths.

Estimated Deaths by Ovarian Cancer in 1998

National Estimated Total = 14,500 Deaths

ALPHA ORDER

RANK	STATE	DEATHS	% of USA
20	Alabama	200	1.38%
NA	Alaska*	NA	NA
12	Arizona	300	2.07%
20	Arkansas	200	1.38%
1	California	1,500	10.34%
32	Colorado	100	0.69%
20	Connecticut	200	1.38%
NA	Delaware*	NA	NA
2	Florida	1,100	7.59%
12	Georgia	300	2.07%
32	Hawaii	100	0.69%
32	Idaho	100	0.69%
6	Illinois	700	4.83%
10	Indiana	400	2.76%
20	Iowa	200	1.38%
20	Kansas	200	1.38%
20	Kentucky	200	1.38%
20	Louisiana	200	1.38%
32	Maine	100	0.69%
20	Maryland	200	1.38%
12	Massachusetts	300	2.07%
9	Michigan	500	3.45%
20	Minnesota	200	1.38%
32	Mississippi	100	0.69%
12	Missouri	300	2.07%
NA	Montana*	NA	NA
32	Nebraska	100	0.69%
32	Nevada	100	0.69%
32	New Hampshire	100	0.69%
7	New Jersey	600	4.14%
32	New Mexico	100	0.69%
3	New York	1,000	6.90%
12	North Carolina	300	2.07%
NA	North Dakota*	NA	NA
7	Ohio	600	4.14%
20	Oklahoma	200	1.38%
20	Oregon	200	1.38%
5	Pennsylvania	800	5.52%
32	Rhode Island	100	0.69%
20	South Carolina	200	1.38%
NA	South Dakota*	NA	NA
12	Tennessee	300	2.07%
4	Texas	900	6.21%
32	Utah	100	0.69%
NA	Vermont*	NA	NA
12	Virginia	300	2.07%
12	Washington	300	2.07%
32	West Virginia	100	0.69%
10	Wisconsin	400	2.76%
NA	Wyoming*	NA	NA

RANK ORDER

RANK	STATE	DEATHS	% of USA
1	California	1,500	10.34%
2	Florida	1,100	7.59%
3	New York	1,000	6.90%
4	Texas	900	6.21%
5	Pennsylvania	800	5.52%
6	Illinois	700	4.83%
7	New Jersey	600	4.14%
7	Ohio	600	4.14%
9	Michigan	500	3.45%
10	Indiana	400	2.76%
10	Wisconsin	400	2.76%
12	Arizona	300	2.07%
12	Georgia	300	2.07%
12	Massachusetts	300	2.07%
12	Missouri	300	2.07%
12	North Carolina	300	2.07%
12	Tennessee	300	2.07%
12	Virginia	300	2.07%
12	Washington	300	2.07%
20	Alabama	200	1.38%
20	Arkansas	200	1.38%
20	Connecticut	200	1.38%
20	Iowa	200	1.38%
20	Kansas	200	1.38%
20	Kentucky	200	1.38%
20	Louisiana	200	1.38%
20	Maryland	200	1.38%
20	Minnesota	200	1.38%
20	Oklahoma	200	1.38%
20	Oregon	200	1.38%
20	South Carolina	200	1.38%
32	Colorado	100	0.69%
32	Hawaii	100	0.69%
32	Idaho	100	0.69%
32	Maine	100	0.69%
32	Mississippi	100	0.69%
32	Nebraska	100	0.69%
32	Nevada	100	0.69%
32	New Hampshire	100	0.69%
32	New Mexico	100	0.69%
32	Rhode Island	100	0.69%
32	Utah	100	0.69%
32	West Virginia	100	0.69%
NA	Alaska*	NA	NA
NA	Delaware*	NA	NA
NA	Montana*	NA	NA
NA	North Dakota*	NA	NA
NA	South Dakota*	NA	NA
NA	Vermont*	NA	NA
NA	Wyoming*	NA	NA
	District of Columbia*	NA	NA

Source: American Cancer Society
   "Cancer Facts & Figures-1998" (Copyright 1998, Reprinted with permission from the American Cancer Society)
*Fewer than 50 deaths.

Estimated Death Rate by Ovarian Cancer in 1998

National Estimated Rate = 10.7 Deaths per 100,000 Female Population*

ALPHA ORDER

RANK	STATE	RATE
35	Alabama	9.0
NA	Alaska**	NA
12	Arizona	13.4
6	Arkansas	15.4
33	California	9.4
43	Colorado	5.2
17	Connecticut	11.9
NA	Delaware**	NA
9	Florida	14.9
39	Georgia	8.0
2	Hawaii	17.1
4	Idaho	16.8
20	Illinois	11.5
12	Indiana	13.4
11	Iowa	13.7
7	Kansas	15.3
30	Kentucky	10.0
36	Louisiana	8.9
5	Maine	15.7
41	Maryland	7.7
32	Massachusetts	9.5
29	Michigan	10.2
38	Minnesota	8.5
42	Mississippi	7.1
22	Missouri	10.9
NA	Montana**	NA
17	Nebraska	11.9
15	Nevada	12.7
3	New Hampshire	16.9
10	New Jersey	14.6
20	New Mexico	11.5
25	New York	10.6
39	North Carolina	8.0
NA	North Dakota**	NA
28	Ohio	10.4
17	Oklahoma	11.9
16	Oregon	12.3
14	Pennsylvania	12.8
1	Rhode Island	19.5
27	South Carolina	10.5
NA	South Dakota**	NA
22	Tennessee	10.9
34	Texas	9.3
30	Utah	10.0
NA	Vermont**	NA
37	Virginia	8.8
24	Washington	10.8
25	West Virginia	10.6
7	Wisconsin	15.3
NA	Wyoming**	NA

RANK ORDER

RANK	STATE	RATE
1	Rhode Island	19.5
2	Hawaii	17.1
3	New Hampshire	16.9
4	Idaho	16.8
5	Maine	15.7
6	Arkansas	15.4
7	Kansas	15.3
7	Wisconsin	15.3
9	Florida	14.9
10	New Jersey	14.6
11	Iowa	13.7
12	Arizona	13.4
12	Indiana	13.4
14	Pennsylvania	12.8
15	Nevada	12.7
16	Oregon	12.3
17	Connecticut	11.9
17	Nebraska	11.9
17	Oklahoma	11.9
20	Illinois	11.5
20	New Mexico	11.5
22	Missouri	10.9
22	Tennessee	10.9
24	Washington	10.8
25	New York	10.6
25	West Virginia	10.6
27	South Carolina	10.5
28	Ohio	10.4
29	Michigan	10.2
30	Kentucky	10.0
30	Utah	10.0
32	Massachusetts	9.5
33	California	9.4
34	Texas	9.3
35	Alabama	9.0
36	Louisiana	8.9
37	Virginia	8.8
38	Minnesota	8.5
39	Georgia	8.0
39	North Carolina	8.0
41	Maryland	7.7
42	Mississippi	7.1
43	Colorado	5.2
NA	Alaska**	NA
NA	Delaware**	NA
NA	Montana**	NA
NA	North Dakota**	NA
NA	South Dakota**	NA
NA	Vermont**	NA
NA	Wyoming**	NA
	District of Columbia**	NA

Source: Morgan Quitno Press using data from American Cancer Society
   "Cancer Facts & Figures-1998" (Copyright 1998, Reprinted with permission from the American Cancer Society)
*Rates calculated using 1996 Census resident female population estimates. Not age adjusted.
**Fewer than 50 deaths.

Deaths by Alzheimer's Disease in 1995

National Total = 20,606 Deaths*

ALPHA ORDER

RANK	STATE	DEATHS	% of USA
20	Alabama	435	2.11%
50	Alaska	12	0.06%
23	Arizona	383	1.86%
33	Arkansas	187	0.91%
1	California	1,720	8.35%
27	Colorado	280	1.36%
30	Connecticut	240	1.16%
49	Delaware	41	0.20%
3	Florida	1,391	6.75%
15	Georgia	508	2.47%
46	Hawaii	47	0.23%
42	Idaho	89	0.43%
4	Illinois	1,043	5.06%
11	Indiana	544	2.64%
26	Iowa	335	1.63%
29	Kansas	241	1.17%
21	Kentucky	394	1.91%
24	Louisiana	366	1.78%
34	Maine	176	0.85%
25	Maryland	345	1.67%
7	Massachusetts	689	3.34%
10	Michigan	594	2.88%
17	Minnesota	486	2.36%
35	Mississippi	168	0.82%
18	Missouri	464	2.25%
38	Montana	126	0.61%
32	Nebraska	190	0.92%
43	Nevada	86	0.42%
40	New Hampshire	116	0.56%
12	New Jersey	528	2.56%
41	New Mexico	109	0.53%
9	New York	660	3.20%
8	North Carolina	662	3.21%
44	North Dakota	74	0.36%
5	Ohio	1,001	4.86%
31	Oklahoma	205	0.99%
21	Oregon	394	1.91%
6	Pennsylvania	906	4.40%
39	Rhode Island	121	0.59%
28	South Carolina	278	1.35%
45	South Dakota	72	0.35%
19	Tennessee	463	2.25%
2	Texas	1,477	7.17%
37	Utah	135	0.66%
48	Vermont	43	0.21%
14	Virginia	522	2.53%
16	Washington	489	2.37%
36	West Virginia	158	0.77%
13	Wisconsin	523	2.54%
47	Wyoming	45	0.22%

RANK ORDER

RANK	STATE	DEATHS	% of USA
1	California	1,720	8.35%
2	Texas	1,477	7.17%
3	Florida	1,391	6.75%
4	Illinois	1,043	5.06%
5	Ohio	1,001	4.86%
6	Pennsylvania	906	4.40%
7	Massachusetts	689	3.34%
8	North Carolina	662	3.21%
9	New York	660	3.20%
10	Michigan	594	2.88%
11	Indiana	544	2.64%
12	New Jersey	528	2.56%
13	Wisconsin	523	2.54%
14	Virginia	522	2.53%
15	Georgia	508	2.47%
16	Washington	489	2.37%
17	Minnesota	486	2.36%
18	Missouri	464	2.25%
19	Tennessee	463	2.25%
20	Alabama	435	2.11%
21	Kentucky	394	1.91%
21	Oregon	394	1.91%
23	Arizona	383	1.86%
24	Louisiana	366	1.78%
25	Maryland	345	1.67%
26	Iowa	335	1.63%
27	Colorado	280	1.36%
28	South Carolina	278	1.35%
29	Kansas	241	1.17%
30	Connecticut	240	1.16%
31	Oklahoma	205	0.99%
32	Nebraska	190	0.92%
33	Arkansas	187	0.91%
34	Maine	176	0.85%
35	Mississippi	168	0.82%
36	West Virginia	158	0.77%
37	Utah	135	0.66%
38	Montana	126	0.61%
39	Rhode Island	121	0.59%
40	New Hampshire	116	0.56%
41	New Mexico	109	0.53%
42	Idaho	89	0.43%
43	Nevada	86	0.42%
44	North Dakota	74	0.36%
45	South Dakota	72	0.35%
46	Hawaii	47	0.23%
47	Wyoming	45	0.22%
48	Vermont	43	0.21%
49	Delaware	41	0.20%
50	Alaska	12	0.06%
	District of Columbia	45	0.22%

Source: U.S. Department of Health and Human Services, National Center for Health Statistics
    "Monthly Vital Statistics Report" (Vol. 45, No. 11(S)2, June 12, 1997)
*Final data by state of residence. A degenerative disease of the brain cells producing loss of memory and general intellectual impairment. It usually affects people over age 65. As the disease progresses, a variety of symptoms may become apparent, including confusion, irritability, and restlessness, as well as disorientation and impaired judgment and concentration.

Death Rate by Alzheimer's Disease in 1995

National Rate = 7.8 Deaths per 100,000 Population*

ALPHA ORDER

RANK	STATE	RATE
10	Alabama	10.2
NA	Alaska**	NA
20	Arizona	9.1
32	Arkansas	7.5
47	California	5.4
32	Colorado	7.5
36	Connecticut	7.3
45	Delaware	5.7
15	Florida	9.8
37	Georgia	7.1
48	Hawaii	4.0
30	Idaho	7.7
23	Illinois	8.8
16	Indiana	9.4
5	Iowa	11.8
16	Kansas	9.4
10	Kentucky	10.2
27	Louisiana	8.4
2	Maine	14.2
39	Maryland	6.8
8	Massachusetts	11.3
43	Michigan	6.2
9	Minnesota	10.5
43	Mississippi	6.2
25	Missouri	8.7
1	Montana	14.5
6	Nebraska	11.6
46	Nevada	5.6
13	New Hampshire	10.1
40	New Jersey	6.6
41	New Mexico	6.5
49	New York	3.6
19	North Carolina	9.2
7	North Dakota	11.5
21	Ohio	9.0
42	Oklahoma	6.3
3	Oregon	12.5
32	Pennsylvania	7.5
4	Rhode Island	12.2
31	South Carolina	7.6
14	South Dakota	9.9
23	Tennessee	8.8
28	Texas	7.9
38	Utah	6.9
35	Vermont	7.4
28	Virginia	7.9
21	Washington	9.0
26	West Virginia	8.6
10	Wisconsin	10.2
16	Wyoming	9.4

RANK ORDER

RANK	STATE	RATE
1	Montana	14.5
2	Maine	14.2
3	Oregon	12.5
4	Rhode Island	12.2
5	Iowa	11.8
6	Nebraska	11.6
7	North Dakota	11.5
8	Massachusetts	11.3
9	Minnesota	10.5
10	Alabama	10.2
10	Kentucky	10.2
10	Wisconsin	10.2
13	New Hampshire	10.1
14	South Dakota	9.9
15	Florida	9.8
16	Indiana	9.4
16	Kansas	9.4
16	Wyoming	9.4
19	North Carolina	9.2
20	Arizona	9.1
21	Ohio	9.0
21	Washington	9.0
23	Illinois	8.8
23	Tennessee	8.8
25	Missouri	8.7
26	West Virginia	8.6
27	Louisiana	8.4
28	Texas	7.9
28	Virginia	7.9
30	Idaho	7.7
31	South Carolina	7.6
32	Arkansas	7.5
32	Colorado	7.5
32	Pennsylvania	7.5
35	Vermont	7.4
36	Connecticut	7.3
37	Georgia	7.1
38	Utah	6.9
39	Maryland	6.8
40	New Jersey	6.6
41	New Mexico	6.5
42	Oklahoma	6.3
43	Michigan	6.2
43	Mississippi	6.2
45	Delaware	5.7
46	Nevada	5.6
47	California	5.4
48	Hawaii	4.0
49	New York	3.6
NA	Alaska**	NA

District of Columbia   8.1

Source: U.S. Department of Health and Human Services, National Center for Health Statistics
    "Monthly Vital Statistics Report" (Vol. 45, No. 11(S)2, June 12, 1997)
*Final data by state of residence. A degenerative disease of the brain cells producing loss of memory and general intellectual impairment. It usually affects people over age 65. As the disease progresses, a variety of symptoms may become apparent, including confusion, irritability, and restlessness, as well as disorientation and impaired judgment and concentration. Not age adjusted. **Insufficient data for a reliable rate.*

Deaths by Atherosclerosis in 1995

National Total = 16,723 Deaths*

ALPHA ORDER

RANK	STATE	DEATHS	% of USA
27	Alabama	281	1.68%
49	Alaska	17	0.10%
23	Arizona	293	1.75%
32	Arkansas	174	1.04%
1	California	1,936	11.58%
17	Colorado	370	2.21%
31	Connecticut	175	1.05%
50	Delaware	13	0.08%
2	Florida	1,041	6.22%
9	Georgia	507	3.03%
48	Hawaii	22	0.13%
45	Idaho	48	0.29%
7	Illinois	673	4.02%
10	Indiana	484	2.89%
13	Iowa	421	2.52%
25	Kansas	289	1.73%
29	Kentucky	201	1.20%
21	Louisiana	321	1.92%
41	Maine	75	0.45%
30	Maryland	185	1.11%
15	Massachusetts	382	2.28%
6	Michigan	752	4.50%
22	Minnesota	297	1.78%
34	Mississippi	115	0.69%
20	Missouri	322	1.93%
40	Montana	77	0.46%
28	Nebraska	224	1.34%
38	Nevada	79	0.47%
37	New Hampshire	93	0.56%
11	New Jersey	452	2.70%
35	New Mexico	114	0.68%
5	New York	780	4.66%
12	North Carolina	428	2.56%
39	North Dakota	78	0.47%
8	Ohio	650	3.89%
16	Oklahoma	381	2.28%
26	Oregon	288	1.72%
4	Pennsylvania	790	4.72%
42	Rhode Island	70	0.42%
36	South Carolina	109	0.65%
44	South Dakota	52	0.31%
14	Tennessee	417	2.49%
3	Texas	980	5.86%
43	Utah	65	0.39%
46	Vermont	31	0.19%
19	Virginia	329	1.97%
18	Washington	345	2.06%
33	West Virginia	151	0.90%
24	Wisconsin	292	1.75%
47	Wyoming	24	0.14%

RANK ORDER

RANK	STATE	DEATHS	% of USA
1	California	1,936	11.58%
2	Florida	1,041	6.22%
3	Texas	980	5.86%
4	Pennsylvania	790	4.72%
5	New York	780	4.66%
6	Michigan	752	4.50%
7	Illinois	673	4.02%
8	Ohio	650	3.89%
9	Georgia	507	3.03%
10	Indiana	484	2.89%
11	New Jersey	452	2.70%
12	North Carolina	428	2.56%
13	Iowa	421	2.52%
14	Tennessee	417	2.49%
15	Massachusetts	382	2.28%
16	Oklahoma	381	2.28%
17	Colorado	370	2.21%
18	Washington	345	2.06%
19	Virginia	329	1.97%
20	Missouri	322	1.93%
21	Louisiana	321	1.92%
22	Minnesota	297	1.78%
23	Arizona	293	1.75%
24	Wisconsin	292	1.75%
25	Kansas	289	1.73%
26	Oregon	288	1.72%
27	Alabama	281	1.68%
28	Nebraska	224	1.34%
29	Kentucky	201	1.20%
30	Maryland	185	1.11%
31	Connecticut	175	1.05%
32	Arkansas	174	1.04%
33	West Virginia	151	0.90%
34	Mississippi	115	0.69%
35	New Mexico	114	0.68%
36	South Carolina	109	0.65%
37	New Hampshire	93	0.56%
38	Nevada	79	0.47%
39	North Dakota	78	0.47%
40	Montana	77	0.46%
41	Maine	75	0.45%
42	Rhode Island	70	0.42%
43	Utah	65	0.39%
44	South Dakota	52	0.31%
45	Idaho	48	0.29%
46	Vermont	31	0.19%
47	Wyoming	24	0.14%
48	Hawaii	22	0.13%
49	Alaska	17	0.10%
50	Delaware	13	0.08%
	District of Columbia	30	0.18%

Source: U.S. Department of Health and Human Services, National Center for Health Statistics
(http://wonder.cdc.gov/WONDER/)
*Final data by state of residence. Atherosclerosis is a form of hardening of the arteries.

Death Rate by Atherosclerosis in 1995

National Rate = 6.4 Deaths per 100,000 Population*

<u>ALPHA ORDER</u>

RANK	STATE	RATE
22	Alabama	6.6
48	Alaska	2.8
20	Arizona	6.8
18	Arkansas	7.0
27	California	6.1
6	Colorado	9.9
35	Connecticut	5.4
50	Delaware	1.8
15	Florida	7.3
18	Georgia	7.0
49	Hawaii	1.9
44	Idaho	4.1
32	Illinois	5.7
9	Indiana	8.3
1	Iowa	14.8
5	Kansas	11.3
37	Kentucky	5.2
14	Louisiana	7.4
27	Maine	6.1
45	Maryland	3.7
25	Massachusetts	6.3
12	Michigan	7.9
24	Minnesota	6.4
42	Mississippi	4.3
27	Missouri	6.1
8	Montana	8.8
2	Nebraska	13.7
37	Nevada	5.2
11	New Hampshire	8.1
32	New Jersey	5.7
21	New Mexico	6.7
42	New York	4.3
30	North Carolina	5.9
3	North Dakota	12.2
31	Ohio	5.8
4	Oklahoma	11.6
7	Oregon	9.1
23	Pennsylvania	6.5
16	Rhode Island	7.1
47	South Carolina	3.0
16	South Dakota	7.1
12	Tennessee	7.9
37	Texas	5.2
46	Utah	3.3
36	Vermont	5.3
40	Virginia	5.0
25	Washington	6.3
9	West Virginia	8.3
32	Wisconsin	5.7
40	Wyoming	5.0

<u>RANK ORDER</u>

RANK	STATE	RATE
1	Iowa	14.8
2	Nebraska	13.7
3	North Dakota	12.2
4	Oklahoma	11.6
5	Kansas	11.3
6	Colorado	9.9
7	Oregon	9.1
8	Montana	8.8
9	Indiana	8.3
9	West Virginia	8.3
11	New Hampshire	8.1
12	Michigan	7.9
12	Tennessee	7.9
14	Louisiana	7.4
15	Florida	7.3
16	Rhode Island	7.1
16	South Dakota	7.1
18	Arkansas	7.0
18	Georgia	7.0
20	Arizona	6.8
21	New Mexico	6.7
22	Alabama	6.6
23	Pennsylvania	6.5
24	Minnesota	6.4
25	Massachusetts	6.3
25	Washington	6.3
27	California	6.1
27	Maine	6.1
27	Missouri	6.1
30	North Carolina	5.9
31	Ohio	5.8
32	Illinois	5.7
32	New Jersey	5.7
32	Wisconsin	5.7
35	Connecticut	5.4
36	Vermont	5.3
37	Kentucky	5.2
37	Nevada	5.2
37	Texas	5.2
40	Virginia	5.0
40	Wyoming	5.0
42	Mississippi	4.3
42	New York	4.3
44	Idaho	4.1
45	Maryland	3.7
46	Utah	3.3
47	South Carolina	3.0
48	Alaska	2.8
49	Hawaii	1.9
50	Delaware	1.8
	District of Columbia	5.4

Source: U.S. Department of Health and Human Services, National Center for Health Statistics
(http://wonder.cdc.gov/WONDER/)
*Final data by state of residence. Atherosclerosis is a form of hardening of the arteries. Not age adjusted.

Deaths by Cerebrovascular Diseases in 1995

National Total = 157,991 Deaths*

ALPHA ORDER

RANK	STATE	DEATHS	% of USA
20	Alabama	2,774	1.76%
50	Alaska	145	0.09%
29	Arizona	2,185	1.38%
27	Arkansas	2,272	1.44%
1	California	16,239	10.28%
33	Colorado	1,600	1.01%
30	Connecticut	1,873	1.19%
47	Delaware	343	0.22%
2	Florida	9,895	6.26%
12	Georgia	4,044	2.56%
43	Hawaii	611	0.39%
41	Idaho	637	0.40%
6	Illinois	7,488	4.74%
13	Indiana	3,996	2.53%
28	Iowa	2,201	1.39%
32	Kansas	1,811	1.15%
24	Kentucky	2,467	1.56%
23	Louisiana	2,544	1.61%
37	Maine	744	0.47%
22	Maryland	2,645	1.67%
17	Massachusetts	3,459	2.19%
8	Michigan	5,865	3.71%
19	Minnesota	3,125	1.98%
31	Mississippi	1,870	1.18%
14	Missouri	3,883	2.46%
44	Montana	594	0.38%
35	Nebraska	1,165	0.74%
39	Nevada	710	0.45%
42	New Hampshire	634	0.40%
10	New Jersey	4,244	2.69%
38	New Mexico	719	0.46%
5	New York	8,119	5.14%
9	North Carolina	5,204	3.29%
46	North Dakota	496	0.31%
7	Ohio	6,688	4.23%
26	Oklahoma	2,377	1.50%
25	Oregon	2,440	1.54%
4	Pennsylvania	8,287	5.25%
40	Rhode Island	641	0.41%
21	South Carolina	2,761	1.75%
45	South Dakota	534	0.34%
11	Tennessee	4,193	2.65%
3	Texas	9,802	6.20%
36	Utah	778	0.49%
48	Vermont	334	0.21%
15	Virginia	3,803	2.41%
18	Washington	3,294	2.08%
34	West Virginia	1,242	0.79%
16	Wisconsin	3,578	2.26%
49	Wyoming	268	0.17%

RANK ORDER

RANK	STATE	DEATHS	% of USA
1	California	16,239	10.28%
2	Florida	9,895	6.26%
3	Texas	9,802	6.20%
4	Pennsylvania	8,287	5.25%
5	New York	8,119	5.14%
6	Illinois	7,488	4.74%
7	Ohio	6,688	4.23%
8	Michigan	5,865	3.71%
9	North Carolina	5,204	3.29%
10	New Jersey	4,244	2.69%
11	Tennessee	4,193	2.65%
12	Georgia	4,044	2.56%
13	Indiana	3,996	2.53%
14	Missouri	3,883	2.46%
15	Virginia	3,803	2.41%
16	Wisconsin	3,578	2.26%
17	Massachusetts	3,459	2.19%
18	Washington	3,294	2.08%
19	Minnesota	3,125	1.98%
20	Alabama	2,774	1.76%
21	South Carolina	2,761	1.75%
22	Maryland	2,645	1.67%
23	Louisiana	2,544	1.61%
24	Kentucky	2,467	1.56%
25	Oregon	2,440	1.54%
26	Oklahoma	2,377	1.50%
27	Arkansas	2,272	1.44%
28	Iowa	2,201	1.39%
29	Arizona	2,185	1.38%
30	Connecticut	1,873	1.19%
31	Mississippi	1,870	1.18%
32	Kansas	1,811	1.15%
33	Colorado	1,600	1.01%
34	West Virginia	1,242	0.79%
35	Nebraska	1,165	0.74%
36	Utah	778	0.49%
37	Maine	744	0.47%
38	New Mexico	719	0.46%
39	Nevada	710	0.45%
40	Rhode Island	641	0.41%
41	Idaho	637	0.40%
42	New Hampshire	634	0.40%
43	Hawaii	611	0.39%
44	Montana	594	0.38%
45	South Dakota	534	0.34%
46	North Dakota	496	0.31%
47	Delaware	343	0.22%
48	Vermont	334	0.21%
49	Wyoming	268	0.17%
50	Alaska	145	0.09%
	District of Columbia	370	0.23%

Source: U.S. Department of Health and Human Services, National Center for Health Statistics
    "Monthly Vital Statistics Report" (Vol. 45, No. 11(S)2, June 12, 1997)
*Final data by state of residence. Cerebrovascular diseases include stroke and other disorders of the blood
vessels of the brain.

Death Rate by Cerebrovascular Diseases in 1995

National Rate = 60.1 Deaths per 100,000 Population*

ALPHA ORDER

RANK	STATE	RATE
21	Alabama	65.2
50	Alaska	24.0
41	Arizona	51.8
1	Arkansas	91.5
43	California	51.4
47	Colorado	42.7
31	Connecticut	57.2
44	Delaware	47.8
13	Florida	69.9
34	Georgia	56.2
42	Hawaii	51.5
37	Idaho	54.8
24	Illinois	63.3
16	Indiana	68.9
4	Iowa	77.5
12	Kansas	70.6
23	Kentucky	63.9
29	Louisiana	58.6
28	Maine	59.9
39	Maryland	52.5
33	Massachusetts	57.0
25	Michigan	61.4
20	Minnesota	67.8
15	Mississippi	69.3
8	Missouri	72.9
18	Montana	68.3
11	Nebraska	71.2
45	Nevada	46.4
36	New Hampshire	55.2
38	New Jersey	53.4
47	New Mexico	42.7
46	New York	44.8
10	North Carolina	72.3
5	North Dakota	77.3
27	Ohio	60.0
9	Oklahoma	72.5
3	Oregon	77.7
17	Pennsylvania	68.6
22	Rhode Island	64.8
6	South Carolina	75.2
7	South Dakota	73.2
2	Tennessee	79.8
40	Texas	52.3
49	Utah	39.9
32	Vermont	57.1
30	Virginia	57.5
26	Washington	60.7
19	West Virginia	67.9
14	Wisconsin	69.8
35	Wyoming	55.8

RANK ORDER

RANK	STATE	RATE
1	Arkansas	91.5
2	Tennessee	79.8
3	Oregon	77.7
4	Iowa	77.5
5	North Dakota	77.3
6	South Carolina	75.2
7	South Dakota	73.2
8	Missouri	72.9
9	Oklahoma	72.5
10	North Carolina	72.3
11	Nebraska	71.2
12	Kansas	70.6
13	Florida	69.9
14	Wisconsin	69.8
15	Mississippi	69.3
16	Indiana	68.9
17	Pennsylvania	68.6
18	Montana	68.3
19	West Virginia	67.9
20	Minnesota	67.8
21	Alabama	65.2
22	Rhode Island	64.8
23	Kentucky	63.9
24	Illinois	63.3
25	Michigan	61.4
26	Washington	60.7
27	Ohio	60.0
28	Maine	59.9
29	Louisiana	58.6
30	Virginia	57.5
31	Connecticut	57.2
32	Vermont	57.1
33	Massachusetts	57.0
34	Georgia	56.2
35	Wyoming	55.8
36	New Hampshire	55.2
37	Idaho	54.8
38	New Jersey	53.4
39	Maryland	52.5
40	Texas	52.3
41	Arizona	51.8
42	Hawaii	51.5
43	California	51.4
44	Delaware	47.8
45	Nevada	46.4
46	New York	44.8
47	Colorado	42.7
47	New Mexico	42.7
49	Utah	39.9
50	Alaska	24.0
	District of Columbia	66.8

*Source: U.S. Department of Health and Human Services, National Center for Health Statistics
"Monthly Vital Statistics Report" (Vol. 45, No. 11(S)2, June 12, 1997)*
Final data by state of residence. Cerebrovascular diseases include stroke and other disorders of the blood vessels of the brain. Not age adjusted.

Deaths by Chronic Liver Disease and Cirrhosis in 1995

National Total = 25,222 Deaths*

ALPHA ORDER

RANK ORDER

RANK	STATE	DEATHS	% of USA
21	Alabama	372	1.47%
46	Alaska	61	0.24%
13	Arizona	553	2.19%
32	Arkansas	214	0.85%
1	California	3,564	14.13%
26	Colorado	322	1.28%
25	Connecticut	324	1.28%
47	Delaware	60	0.24%
3	Florida	1,845	7.32%
11	Georgia	583	2.31%
45	Hawaii	75	0.30%
42	Idaho	87	0.34%
5	Illinois	1,181	4.68%
19	Indiana	401	1.59%
36	Iowa	154	0.61%
35	Kansas	163	0.65%
24	Kentucky	347	1.38%
23	Louisiana	352	1.40%
38	Maine	117	0.46%
17	Maryland	422	1.67%
12	Massachusetts	568	2.25%
7	Michigan	995	3.94%
28	Minnesota	307	1.22%
31	Mississippi	233	0.92%
18	Missouri	420	1.67%
43	Montana	83	0.33%
40	Nebraska	97	0.38%
32	Nevada	214	0.85%
40	New Hampshire	97	0.38%
9	New Jersey	842	3.34%
30	New Mexico	259	1.03%
4	New York	1,799	7.13%
10	North Carolina	678	2.69%
49	North Dakota	41	0.16%
8	Ohio	952	3.77%
27	Oklahoma	317	1.26%
29	Oregon	289	1.15%
6	Pennsylvania	1,136	4.50%
37	Rhode Island	118	0.47%
20	South Carolina	373	1.48%
44	South Dakota	76	0.30%
14	Tennessee	491	1.95%
2	Texas	1,871	7.42%
39	Utah	103	0.41%
50	Vermont	35	0.14%
15	Virginia	477	1.89%
16	Washington	446	1.77%
34	West Virginia	202	0.80%
22	Wisconsin	353	1.40%
47	Wyoming	60	0.24%

RANK	STATE	DEATHS	% of USA
1	California	3,564	14.13%
2	Texas	1,871	7.42%
3	Florida	1,845	7.32%
4	New York	1,799	7.13%
5	Illinois	1,181	4.68%
6	Pennsylvania	1,136	4.50%
7	Michigan	995	3.94%
8	Ohio	952	3.77%
9	New Jersey	842	3.34%
10	North Carolina	678	2.69%
11	Georgia	583	2.31%
12	Massachusetts	568	2.25%
13	Arizona	553	2.19%
14	Tennessee	491	1.95%
15	Virginia	477	1.89%
16	Washington	446	1.77%
17	Maryland	422	1.67%
18	Missouri	420	1.67%
19	Indiana	401	1.59%
20	South Carolina	373	1.48%
21	Alabama	372	1.47%
22	Wisconsin	353	1.40%
23	Louisiana	352	1.40%
24	Kentucky	347	1.38%
25	Connecticut	324	1.28%
26	Colorado	322	1.28%
27	Oklahoma	317	1.26%
28	Minnesota	307	1.22%
29	Oregon	289	1.15%
30	New Mexico	259	1.03%
31	Mississippi	233	0.92%
32	Arkansas	214	0.85%
32	Nevada	214	0.85%
34	West Virginia	202	0.80%
35	Kansas	163	0.65%
36	Iowa	154	0.61%
37	Rhode Island	118	0.47%
38	Maine	117	0.46%
39	Utah	103	0.41%
40	Nebraska	97	0.38%
40	New Hampshire	97	0.38%
42	Idaho	87	0.34%
43	Montana	83	0.33%
44	South Dakota	76	0.30%
45	Hawaii	75	0.30%
46	Alaska	61	0.24%
47	Delaware	60	0.24%
47	Wyoming	60	0.24%
49	North Dakota	41	0.16%
50	Vermont	35	0.14%
	District of Columbia	93	0.37%

Source: U.S. Department of Health and Human Services, National Center for Health Statistics
    "Monthly Vital Statistics Report" (Vol. 45, No. 11(S)2, June 12, 1997)
*Final data by state of residence. Cirrhosis of the liver is characterized by the replacement of normal tissue with fibrous tissue and the loss of functional liver cells. It can result from alcohol abuse, nutritional deprivation, or infection especially by the hepatitis virus.

Death Rate by Chronic Liver Disease and Cirrhosis in 1995

National Rate = 9.6 Deaths per 100,000 Population*

ALPHA ORDER

RANK	STATE	RATE
27	Alabama	8.7
13	Alaska	10.1
3	Arizona	13.1
28	Arkansas	8.6
7	California	11.3
28	Colorado	8.6
16	Connecticut	9.9
32	Delaware	8.4
4	Florida	13.0
36	Georgia	8.1
46	Hawaii	6.3
39	Idaho	7.5
14	Illinois	10.0
41	Indiana	6.9
49	Iowa	5.4
44	Kansas	6.4
26	Kentucky	9.0
36	Louisiana	8.1
20	Maine	9.4
32	Maryland	8.4
20	Massachusetts	9.4
10	Michigan	10.4
43	Minnesota	6.7
28	Mississippi	8.6
38	Missouri	7.9
19	Montana	9.5
48	Nebraska	5.9
2	Nevada	14.0
32	New Hampshire	8.4
9	New Jersey	10.6
1	New Mexico	15.4
16	New York	9.9
20	North Carolina	9.4
44	North Dakota	6.4
31	Ohio	8.5
18	Oklahoma	9.7
25	Oregon	9.2
20	Pennsylvania	9.4
6	Rhode Island	11.9
12	South Carolina	10.2
10	South Dakota	10.4
24	Tennessee	9.3
14	Texas	10.0
50	Utah	5.3
47	Vermont	6.0
40	Virginia	7.2
35	Washington	8.2
8	West Virginia	11.0
41	Wisconsin	6.9
5	Wyoming	12.5

RANK ORDER

RANK	STATE	RATE
1	New Mexico	15.4
2	Nevada	14.0
3	Arizona	13.1
4	Florida	13.0
5	Wyoming	12.5
6	Rhode Island	11.9
7	California	11.3
8	West Virginia	11.0
9	New Jersey	10.6
10	Michigan	10.4
10	South Dakota	10.4
12	South Carolina	10.2
13	Alaska	10.1
14	Illinois	10.0
14	Texas	10.0
16	Connecticut	9.9
16	New York	9.9
18	Oklahoma	9.7
19	Montana	9.5
20	Maine	9.4
20	Massachusetts	9.4
20	North Carolina	9.4
20	Pennsylvania	9.4
24	Tennessee	9.3
25	Oregon	9.2
26	Kentucky	9.0
27	Alabama	8.7
28	Arkansas	8.6
28	Colorado	8.6
28	Mississippi	8.6
31	Ohio	8.5
32	Delaware	8.4
32	Maryland	8.4
32	New Hampshire	8.4
35	Washington	8.2
36	Georgia	8.1
36	Louisiana	8.1
38	Missouri	7.9
39	Idaho	7.5
40	Virginia	7.2
41	Indiana	6.9
41	Wisconsin	6.9
43	Minnesota	6.7
44	Kansas	6.4
44	North Dakota	6.4
46	Hawaii	6.3
47	Vermont	6.0
48	Nebraska	5.9
49	Iowa	5.4
50	Utah	5.3

| | District of Columbia | 16.8 |

Source: U.S. Department of Health and Human Services, National Center for Health Statistics
"Monthly Vital Statistics Report" (Vol. 45, No. 11(S)2, June 12, 1997)
*Final data by state of residence. Cirrhosis of the liver is characterized by the replacement of normal tissue with fibrous tissue and the loss of functional liver cells. It can result from alcohol abuse, nutritional deprivation, or infection especially by the hepatitis virus. Not age adjusted.

Deaths by Chronic Obstructive Pulmonary Diseases in 1995

National Total = 102,899 Deaths*

ALPHA ORDER

RANK	STATE	DEATHS	% of USA
21	Alabama	1,681	1.63%
50	Alaska	107	0.10%
18	Arizona	2,036	1.98%
32	Arkansas	1,118	1.09%
1	California	10,792	10.49%
24	Colorado	1,585	1.54%
30	Connecticut	1,164	1.13%
46	Delaware	258	0.25%
2	Florida	7,493	7.28%
11	Georgia	2,461	2.39%
48	Hawaii	242	0.24%
42	Idaho	444	0.43%
7	Illinois	4,492	4.37%
13	Indiana	2,395	2.33%
29	Iowa	1,372	1.33%
31	Kansas	1,151	1.12%
20	Kentucky	1,858	1.81%
27	Louisiana	1,421	1.38%
38	Maine	674	0.66%
23	Maryland	1,595	1.55%
14	Massachusetts	2,354	2.29%
8	Michigan	3,584	3.48%
22	Minnesota	1,675	1.63%
34	Mississippi	1,021	0.99%
12	Missouri	2,454	2.38%
39	Montana	480	0.47%
36	Nebraska	730	0.71%
35	Nevada	796	0.77%
40	New Hampshire	476	0.46%
10	New Jersey	2,745	2.67%
37	New Mexico	700	0.68%
4	New York	6,137	5.96%
9	North Carolina	2,853	2.77%
47	North Dakota	243	0.24%
6	Ohio	4,926	4.79%
25	Oklahoma	1,575	1.53%
26	Oregon	1,425	1.38%
5	Pennsylvania	5,294	5.14%
43	Rhode Island	416	0.40%
28	South Carolina	1,412	1.37%
44	South Dakota	324	0.31%
16	Tennessee	2,201	2.14%
3	Texas	6,237	6.06%
41	Utah	470	0.46%
49	Vermont	241	0.23%
15	Virginia	2,258	2.19%
17	Washington	2,155	2.09%
33	West Virginia	1,097	1.07%
19	Wisconsin	1,881	1.83%
45	Wyoming	266	0.26%

RANK ORDER

RANK	STATE	DEATHS	% of USA
1	California	10,792	10.49%
2	Florida	7,493	7.28%
3	Texas	6,237	6.06%
4	New York	6,137	5.96%
5	Pennsylvania	5,294	5.14%
6	Ohio	4,926	4.79%
7	Illinois	4,492	4.37%
8	Michigan	3,584	3.48%
9	North Carolina	2,853	2.77%
10	New Jersey	2,745	2.67%
11	Georgia	2,461	2.39%
12	Missouri	2,454	2.38%
13	Indiana	2,395	2.33%
14	Massachusetts	2,354	2.29%
15	Virginia	2,258	2.19%
16	Tennessee	2,201	2.14%
17	Washington	2,155	2.09%
18	Arizona	2,036	1.98%
19	Wisconsin	1,881	1.83%
20	Kentucky	1,858	1.81%
21	Alabama	1,681	1.63%
22	Minnesota	1,675	1.63%
23	Maryland	1,595	1.55%
24	Colorado	1,585	1.54%
25	Oklahoma	1,575	1.53%
26	Oregon	1,425	1.38%
27	Louisiana	1,421	1.38%
28	South Carolina	1,412	1.37%
29	Iowa	1,372	1.33%
30	Connecticut	1,164	1.13%
31	Kansas	1,151	1.12%
32	Arkansas	1,118	1.09%
33	West Virginia	1,097	1.07%
34	Mississippi	1,021	0.99%
35	Nevada	796	0.77%
36	Nebraska	730	0.71%
37	New Mexico	700	0.68%
38	Maine	674	0.66%
39	Montana	480	0.47%
40	New Hampshire	476	0.46%
41	Utah	470	0.46%
42	Idaho	444	0.43%
43	Rhode Island	416	0.40%
44	South Dakota	324	0.31%
45	Wyoming	266	0.26%
46	Delaware	258	0.25%
47	North Dakota	243	0.24%
48	Hawaii	242	0.24%
49	Vermont	241	0.23%
50	Alaska	107	0.10%
	District of Columbia	134	0.13%

Source: U.S. Department of Health and Human Services, National Center for Health Statistics
"Monthly Vital Statistics Report" (Vol. 45, No. 11(S)2, June 12, 1997)
*Final data by state of residence. Chronic obstructive pulmonary diseases are diseases of the lungs including bronchitis, emphysema and asthma. Includes allied conditions.

Death Rate by Chronic Obstructive Pulmonary Diseases in 1995

National Rate = 39.2 Deaths per 100,000 Population*

ALPHA ORDER

RANK	STATE	RATE
28	Alabama	39.5
50	Alaska	17.7
7	Arizona	48.3
13	Arkansas	45.0
41	California	34.2
19	Colorado	42.3
39	Connecticut	35.5
38	Delaware	36.0
5	Florida	52.9
41	Georgia	34.2
49	Hawaii	20.4
31	Idaho	38.2
32	Illinois	38.0
24	Indiana	41.3
7	Iowa	48.3
14	Kansas	44.9
9	Kentucky	48.1
46	Louisiana	32.7
4	Maine	54.3
47	Maryland	31.6
29	Massachusetts	38.8
35	Michigan	37.5
37	Minnesota	36.3
33	Mississippi	37.9
11	Missouri	46.1
3	Montana	55.2
15	Nebraska	44.6
6	Nevada	52.0
22	New Hampshire	41.5
40	New Jersey	34.5
22	New Mexico	41.5
44	New York	33.8
26	North Carolina	39.7
33	North Dakota	37.9
17	Ohio	44.2
9	Oklahoma	48.1
12	Oregon	45.4
18	Pennsylvania	43.9
20	Rhode Island	42.0
30	South Carolina	38.4
16	South Dakota	44.4
21	Tennessee	41.9
45	Texas	33.3
48	Utah	24.1
25	Vermont	41.2
43	Virginia	34.1
26	Washington	39.7
1	West Virginia	60.0
36	Wisconsin	36.7
2	Wyoming	55.4

RANK ORDER

RANK	STATE	RATE
1	West Virginia	60.0
2	Wyoming	55.4
3	Montana	55.2
4	Maine	54.3
5	Florida	52.9
6	Nevada	52.0
7	Arizona	48.3
7	Iowa	48.3
9	Kentucky	48.1
9	Oklahoma	48.1
11	Missouri	46.1
12	Oregon	45.4
13	Arkansas	45.0
14	Kansas	44.9
15	Nebraska	44.6
16	South Dakota	44.4
17	Ohio	44.2
18	Pennsylvania	43.9
19	Colorado	42.3
20	Rhode Island	42.0
21	Tennessee	41.9
22	New Hampshire	41.5
22	New Mexico	41.5
24	Indiana	41.3
25	Vermont	41.2
26	North Carolina	39.7
26	Washington	39.7
28	Alabama	39.5
29	Massachusetts	38.8
30	South Carolina	38.4
31	Idaho	38.2
32	Illinois	38.0
33	Mississippi	37.9
33	North Dakota	37.9
35	Michigan	37.5
36	Wisconsin	36.7
37	Minnesota	36.3
38	Delaware	36.0
39	Connecticut	35.5
40	New Jersey	34.5
41	California	34.2
41	Georgia	34.2
43	Virginia	34.1
44	New York	33.8
45	Texas	33.3
46	Louisiana	32.7
47	Maryland	31.6
48	Utah	24.1
49	Hawaii	20.4
50	Alaska	17.7
	District of Columbia	24.2

Source: U.S. Department of Health and Human Services, National Center for Health Statistics
"Monthly Vital Statistics Report" (Vol. 45, No. 11(S)2, June 12, 1997)
*Final data by state of residence. Chronic obstructive pulmonary diseases are diseases of the lungs including bronchitis, emphysema and asthma. Includes allied conditions. Not age adjusted.

Deaths by Diabetes Mellitus in 1995

National Total = 59,254 Deaths*

ALPHA ORDER

RANK	STATE	DEATHS	% of USA
19	Alabama	1,159	1.96%
50	Alaska	56	0.09%
25	Arizona	824	1.39%
32	Arkansas	556	0.94%
1	California	5,104	8.61%
33	Colorado	535	0.90%
30	Connecticut	594	1.00%
44	Delaware	193	0.33%
3	Florida	3,680	6.21%
17	Georgia	1,205	2.03%
45	Hawaii	168	0.28%
43	Idaho	206	0.35%
7	Illinois	2,663	4.49%
12	Indiana	1,437	2.43%
28	Iowa	637	1.08%
31	Kansas	577	0.97%
23	Kentucky	970	1.64%
11	Louisiana	1,495	2.52%
37	Maine	315	0.53%
13	Maryland	1,360	2.30%
14	Massachusetts	1,326	2.24%
9	Michigan	2,235	3.77%
24	Minnesota	862	1.45%
34	Mississippi	489	0.83%
15	Missouri	1,244	2.10%
42	Montana	210	0.35%
38	Nebraska	286	0.48%
41	Nevada	235	0.40%
39	New Hampshire	260	0.44%
8	New Jersey	2,393	4.04%
35	New Mexico	440	0.74%
4	New York	3,525	5.95%
10	North Carolina	1,747	2.95%
47	North Dakota	156	0.26%
6	Ohio	3,350	5.65%
27	Oklahoma	640	1.08%
26	Oregon	682	1.15%
5	Pennsylvania	3,408	5.75%
40	Rhode Island	244	0.41%
22	South Carolina	1,008	1.70%
45	South Dakota	168	0.28%
16	Tennessee	1,230	2.08%
2	Texas	4,576	7.72%
36	Utah	415	0.70%
48	Vermont	143	0.24%
18	Virginia	1,166	1.97%
21	Washington	1,052	1.78%
29	West Virginia	600	1.01%
20	Wisconsin	1,105	1.86%
49	Wyoming	106	0.18%

RANK ORDER

RANK	STATE	DEATHS	% of USA
1	California	5,104	8.61%
2	Texas	4,576	7.72%
3	Florida	3,680	6.21%
4	New York	3,525	5.95%
5	Pennsylvania	3,408	5.75%
6	Ohio	3,350	5.65%
7	Illinois	2,663	4.49%
8	New Jersey	2,393	4.04%
9	Michigan	2,235	3.77%
10	North Carolina	1,747	2.95%
11	Louisiana	1,495	2.52%
12	Indiana	1,437	2.43%
13	Maryland	1,360	2.30%
14	Massachusetts	1,326	2.24%
15	Missouri	1,244	2.10%
16	Tennessee	1,230	2.08%
17	Georgia	1,205	2.03%
18	Virginia	1,166	1.97%
19	Alabama	1,159	1.96%
20	Wisconsin	1,105	1.86%
21	Washington	1,052	1.78%
22	South Carolina	1,008	1.70%
23	Kentucky	970	1.64%
24	Minnesota	862	1.45%
25	Arizona	824	1.39%
26	Oregon	682	1.15%
27	Oklahoma	640	1.08%
28	Iowa	637	1.08%
29	West Virginia	600	1.01%
30	Connecticut	594	1.00%
31	Kansas	577	0.97%
32	Arkansas	556	0.94%
33	Colorado	535	0.90%
34	Mississippi	489	0.83%
35	New Mexico	440	0.74%
36	Utah	415	0.70%
37	Maine	315	0.53%
38	Nebraska	286	0.48%
39	New Hampshire	260	0.44%
40	Rhode Island	244	0.41%
41	Nevada	235	0.40%
42	Montana	210	0.35%
43	Idaho	206	0.35%
44	Delaware	193	0.33%
45	Hawaii	168	0.28%
45	South Dakota	168	0.28%
47	North Dakota	156	0.26%
48	Vermont	143	0.24%
49	Wyoming	106	0.18%
50	Alaska	56	0.09%
	District of Columbia	219	0.37%

Source: U.S. Department of Health and Human Services, National Center for Health Statistics
   "Monthly Vital Statistics Report" (Vol. 45, No. 11(S)2, June 12, 1997)
*Final data by state of residence. A severe, chronic form of diabetes caused by insufficient production of insulin and resulting in abnormal metabolism of carbohydrates, fats, and proteins. The disease, which typically appears in childhood or adolescence, is characterized by increased sugar levels in the blood and urine, excessive thirst and frequent urination.

Death Rate by Diabetes Mellitus in 1995

National Rate = 22.6 Deaths per 100,000 Population*

ALPHA ORDER

RANK ORDER

RANK	STATE	RATE		RANK	STATE	RATE
7	Alabama	27.3		1	Louisiana	34.4
50	Alaska	9.3		2	West Virginia	32.8
35	Arizona	19.5		3	New Jersey	30.1
28	Arkansas	22.4		4	Ohio	30.0
46	California	16.2		5	Pennsylvania	28.2
48	Colorado	14.3		6	South Carolina	27.4
40	Connecticut	18.1		7	Alabama	27.3
9	Delaware	26.9		8	Maryland	27.0
11	Florida	26.0		9	Delaware	26.9
45	Georgia	16.7		10	New Mexico	26.1
49	Hawaii	14.2		11	Florida	26.0
42	Idaho	17.7		12	Maine	25.4
26	Illinois	22.5		13	Kentucky	25.1
14	Indiana	24.8		14	Indiana	24.8
28	Iowa	22.4		15	Rhode Island	24.7
26	Kansas	22.5		16	Vermont	24.5
13	Kentucky	25.1		17	Texas	24.4
1	Louisiana	34.4		18	North Carolina	24.3
12	Maine	25.4		18	North Dakota	24.3
8	Maryland	27.0		20	Montana	24.1
31	Massachusetts	21.8		21	Michigan	23.4
21	Michigan	23.4		21	Missouri	23.4
39	Minnesota	18.7		21	Tennessee	23.4
40	Mississippi	18.1		24	South Dakota	23.0
21	Missouri	23.4		25	New Hampshire	22.6
20	Montana	24.1		26	Illinois	22.5
44	Nebraska	17.5		26	Kansas	22.5
47	Nevada	15.4		28	Arkansas	22.4
25	New Hampshire	22.6		28	Iowa	22.4
3	New Jersey	30.1		30	Wyoming	22.1
10	New Mexico	26.1		31	Massachusetts	21.8
37	New York	19.4		32	Oregon	21.7
18	North Carolina	24.3		33	Wisconsin	21.6
18	North Dakota	24.3		34	Utah	21.3
4	Ohio	30.0		35	Arizona	19.5
35	Oklahoma	19.5		35	Oklahoma	19.5
32	Oregon	21.7		37	New York	19.4
5	Pennsylvania	28.2		37	Washington	19.4
15	Rhode Island	24.7		39	Minnesota	18.7
6	South Carolina	27.4		40	Connecticut	18.1
24	South Dakota	23.0		40	Mississippi	18.1
21	Tennessee	23.4		42	Idaho	17.7
17	Texas	24.4		43	Virginia	17.6
34	Utah	21.3		44	Nebraska	17.5
16	Vermont	24.5		45	Georgia	16.7
43	Virginia	17.6		46	California	16.2
37	Washington	19.4		47	Nevada	15.4
2	West Virginia	32.8		48	Colorado	14.3
33	Wisconsin	21.6		49	Hawaii	14.2
30	Wyoming	22.1		50	Alaska	9.3
					District of Columbia	39.5

Source: U.S. Department of Health and Human Services, National Center for Health Statistics "Monthly Vital Statistics Report" (Vol. 45, No. 11(S)2, June 12, 1997)

Final data by state of residence. A severe, chronic form of diabetes caused by insufficient production of insulin and resulting in abnormal metabolism of carbohydrates, fats, and proteins. The disease, which typically appears in childhood or adolescence, is characterized by increased sugar levels in the blood and urine, excessive thirst and frequent urination. Not age adjusted.

Deaths by Diseases of the Heart in 1995

National Total = 737,563 Deaths*

ALPHA ORDER

RANK	STATE	DEATHS	% of USA
18	Alabama	13,361	1.81%
50	Alaska	547	0.07%
25	Arizona	10,234	1.39%
30	Arkansas	8,440	1.14%
1	California	68,329	9.26%
34	Colorado	6,448	0.87%
27	Connecticut	9,787	1.33%
46	Delaware	1,980	0.27%
3	Florida	49,804	6.75%
12	Georgia	17,452	2.37%
43	Hawaii	2,326	0.32%
42	Idaho	2,470	0.33%
6	Illinois	36,010	4.88%
13	Indiana	17,082	2.32%
29	Iowa	9,436	1.28%
31	Kansas	7,638	1.04%
19	Kentucky	12,190	1.65%
20	Louisiana	12,131	1.64%
37	Maine	3,648	0.49%
21	Maryland	11,922	1.62%
14	Massachusetts	16,750	2.27%
8	Michigan	28,153	3.82%
24	Minnesota	10,381	1.41%
28	Mississippi	9,603	1.30%
11	Missouri	18,380	2.49%
45	Montana	2,004	0.27%
35	Nebraska	5,108	0.69%
36	Nevada	3,778	0.51%
40	New Hampshire	2,950	0.40%
9	New Jersey	24,102	3.27%
39	New Mexico	3,305	0.45%
2	New York	63,518	8.61%
10	North Carolina	19,390	2.63%
47	North Dakota	1,952	0.26%
7	Ohio	35,391	4.80%
23	Oklahoma	11,157	1.51%
32	Oregon	7,539	1.02%
4	Pennsylvania	43,419	5.89%
38	Rhode Island	3,307	0.45%
26	South Carolina	10,197	1.38%
44	South Dakota	2,277	0.31%
15	Tennessee	16,197	2.20%
5	Texas	41,730	5.66%
41	Utah	2,891	0.39%
48	Vermont	1,627	0.22%
16	Virginia	15,896	2.16%
22	Washington	11,330	1.54%
33	West Virginia	6,927	0.94%
17	Wisconsin	14,417	1.95%
49	Wyoming	976	0.13%

RANK ORDER

RANK	STATE	DEATHS	% of USA
1	California	68,329	9.26%
2	New York	63,518	8.61%
3	Florida	49,804	6.75%
4	Pennsylvania	43,419	5.89%
5	Texas	41,730	5.66%
6	Illinois	36,010	4.88%
7	Ohio	35,391	4.80%
8	Michigan	28,153	3.82%
9	New Jersey	24,102	3.27%
10	North Carolina	19,390	2.63%
11	Missouri	18,380	2.49%
12	Georgia	17,452	2.37%
13	Indiana	17,082	2.32%
14	Massachusetts	16,750	2.27%
15	Tennessee	16,197	2.20%
16	Virginia	15,896	2.16%
17	Wisconsin	14,417	1.95%
18	Alabama	13,361	1.81%
19	Kentucky	12,190	1.65%
20	Louisiana	12,131	1.64%
21	Maryland	11,922	1.62%
22	Washington	11,330	1.54%
23	Oklahoma	11,157	1.51%
24	Minnesota	10,381	1.41%
25	Arizona	10,234	1.39%
26	South Carolina	10,197	1.38%
27	Connecticut	9,787	1.33%
28	Mississippi	9,603	1.30%
29	Iowa	9,436	1.28%
30	Arkansas	8,440	1.14%
31	Kansas	7,638	1.04%
32	Oregon	7,539	1.02%
33	West Virginia	6,927	0.94%
34	Colorado	6,448	0.87%
35	Nebraska	5,108	0.69%
36	Nevada	3,778	0.51%
37	Maine	3,648	0.49%
38	Rhode Island	3,307	0.45%
39	New Mexico	3,305	0.45%
40	New Hampshire	2,950	0.40%
41	Utah	2,891	0.39%
42	Idaho	2,470	0.33%
43	Hawaii	2,326	0.32%
44	South Dakota	2,277	0.31%
45	Montana	2,004	0.27%
46	Delaware	1,980	0.27%
47	North Dakota	1,952	0.26%
48	Vermont	1,627	0.22%
49	Wyoming	976	0.13%
50	Alaska	547	0.07%
	District of Columbia	1,676	0.23%

Source: U.S. Department of Health and Human Services, National Center for Health Statistics "Monthly Vital Statistics Report" (Vol. 45, No. 11(S)2, June 12, 1997)
Final data by state of residence.

Death Rate by Diseases of the Heart in 1995

National Rate = 280.7 Deaths per 100,000 Population*

ALPHA ORDER				RANK ORDER		
RANK	STATE	RATE		RANK	STATE	RATE
13	Alabama	314.2		1	West Virginia	378.9
50	Alaska	90.6		2	Pennsylvania	359.7
34	Arizona	242.6		3	Mississippi	356.0
8	Arkansas	339.8		4	Florida	351.6
42	California	216.3		5	New York	350.2
48	Colorado	172.1		6	Missouri	345.3
20	Connecticut	298.9		7	Oklahoma	340.4
29	Delaware	276.1		8	Arkansas	339.8
4	Florida	351.6		9	Rhode Island	334.1
35	Georgia	242.4		10	Iowa	332.0
47	Hawaii	196.0		11	Ohio	317.4
43	Idaho	212.3		12	Kentucky	315.8
17	Illinois	304.4		13	Alabama	314.2
23	Indiana	294.3		14	South Dakota	312.3
10	Iowa	332.0		15	Nebraska	312.0
21	Kansas	297.7		16	Tennessee	308.2
12	Kentucky	315.8		17	Illinois	304.4
26	Louisiana	279.4		18	North Dakota	304.3
24	Maine	293.9		19	New Jersey	303.3
38	Maryland	236.4		20	Connecticut	298.9
30	Massachusetts	275.8		21	Kansas	297.7
22	Michigan	294.8		22	Michigan	294.8
40	Minnesota	225.2		23	Indiana	294.3
3	Mississippi	356.0		24	Maine	293.9
6	Missouri	345.3		25	Wisconsin	281.4
39	Montana	230.3		26	Louisiana	279.4
15	Nebraska	312.0		27	Vermont	278.2
33	Nevada	246.9		28	South Carolina	277.6
32	New Hampshire	256.9		29	Delaware	276.1
19	New Jersey	303.3		30	Massachusetts	275.8
46	New Mexico	196.1		31	North Carolina	269.5
5	New York	350.2		32	New Hampshire	256.9
31	North Carolina	269.5		33	Nevada	246.9
18	North Dakota	304.3		34	Arizona	242.6
11	Ohio	317.4		35	Georgia	242.4
7	Oklahoma	340.4		36	Virginia	240.2
37	Oregon	240.1		37	Oregon	240.1
2	Pennsylvania	359.7		38	Maryland	236.4
9	Rhode Island	334.1		39	Montana	230.3
28	South Carolina	277.6		40	Minnesota	225.2
14	South Dakota	312.3		41	Texas	222.9
16	Tennessee	308.2		42	California	216.3
41	Texas	222.9		43	Idaho	212.3
49	Utah	148.1		44	Washington	208.6
27	Vermont	278.2		45	Wyoming	203.3
36	Virginia	240.2		46	New Mexico	196.1
44	Washington	208.6		47	Hawaii	196.0
1	West Virginia	378.9		48	Colorado	172.1
25	Wisconsin	281.4		49	Utah	148.1
45	Wyoming	203.3		50	Alaska	90.6
					District of Columbia	302.4

Source: U.S. Department of Health and Human Services, National Center for Health Statistics
"Monthly Vital Statistics Report" (Vol. 45, No. 11(S)2, June 12, 1997)
Final data by state of residence. Not age adjusted.

Deaths by Malignant Neoplasms in 1995

National Total = 538,455 Deaths*

ALPHA ORDER

RANK	STATE	DEATHS	% of USA
20	Alabama	9,414	1.75%
50	Alaska	574	0.11%
24	Arizona	8,020	1.49%
30	Arkansas	6,079	1.13%
1	California	51,423	9.55%
32	Colorado	5,467	1.02%
27	Connecticut	7,060	1.31%
45	Delaware	1,630	0.30%
3	Florida	37,321	6.93%
12	Georgia	12,765	2.37%
43	Hawaii	1,856	0.34%
42	Idaho	2,006	0.37%
7	Illinois	25,100	4.66%
14	Indiana	12,554	2.33%
29	Iowa	6,226	1.16%
33	Kansas	5,283	0.98%
22	Kentucky	8,847	1.64%
21	Louisiana	9,304	1.73%
36	Maine	3,015	0.56%
18	Maryland	10,181	1.89%
11	Massachusetts	14,083	2.62%
8	Michigan	19,430	3.61%
23	Minnesota	8,693	1.61%
31	Mississippi	5,748	1.07%
15	Missouri	12,282	2.28%
44	Montana	1,770	0.33%
35	Nebraska	3,375	0.63%
37	Nevada	2,976	0.55%
40	New Hampshire	2,356	0.44%
9	New Jersey	18,427	3.42%
38	New Mexico	2,689	0.50%
2	New York	38,684	7.18%
10	North Carolina	14,879	2.76%
47	North Dakota	1,375	0.26%
6	Ohio	25,208	4.68%
26	Oklahoma	7,142	1.33%
28	Oregon	6,744	1.25%
5	Pennsylvania	30,267	5.62%
39	Rhode Island	2,478	0.46%
25	South Carolina	7,416	1.38%
46	South Dakota	1,564	0.29%
16	Tennessee	11,611	2.16%
4	Texas	31,622	5.87%
41	Utah	2,119	0.39%
48	Vermont	1,163	0.22%
13	Virginia	12,600	2.34%
19	Washington	9,938	1.85%
34	West Virginia	4,743	0.88%
17	Wisconsin	10,571	1.96%
49	Wyoming	896	0.17%

RANK ORDER

RANK	STATE	DEATHS	% of USA
1	California	51,423	9.55%
2	New York	38,684	7.18%
3	Florida	37,321	6.93%
4	Texas	31,622	5.87%
5	Pennsylvania	30,267	5.62%
6	Ohio	25,208	4.68%
7	Illinois	25,100	4.66%
8	Michigan	19,430	3.61%
9	New Jersey	18,427	3.42%
10	North Carolina	14,879	2.76%
11	Massachusetts	14,083	2.62%
12	Georgia	12,765	2.37%
13	Virginia	12,600	2.34%
14	Indiana	12,554	2.33%
15	Missouri	12,282	2.28%
16	Tennessee	11,611	2.16%
17	Wisconsin	10,571	1.96%
18	Maryland	10,181	1.89%
19	Washington	9,938	1.85%
20	Alabama	9,414	1.75%
21	Louisiana	9,304	1.73%
22	Kentucky	8,847	1.64%
23	Minnesota	8,693	1.61%
24	Arizona	8,020	1.49%
25	South Carolina	7,416	1.38%
26	Oklahoma	7,142	1.33%
27	Connecticut	7,060	1.31%
28	Oregon	6,744	1.25%
29	Iowa	6,226	1.16%
30	Arkansas	6,079	1.13%
31	Mississippi	5,748	1.07%
32	Colorado	5,467	1.02%
33	Kansas	5,283	0.98%
34	West Virginia	4,743	0.88%
35	Nebraska	3,375	0.63%
36	Maine	3,015	0.56%
37	Nevada	2,976	0.55%
38	New Mexico	2,689	0.50%
39	Rhode Island	2,478	0.46%
40	New Hampshire	2,356	0.44%
41	Utah	2,119	0.39%
42	Idaho	2,006	0.37%
43	Hawaii	1,856	0.34%
44	Montana	1,770	0.33%
45	Delaware	1,630	0.30%
46	South Dakota	1,564	0.29%
47	North Dakota	1,375	0.26%
48	Vermont	1,163	0.22%
49	Wyoming	896	0.17%
50	Alaska	574	0.11%
	District of Columbia	1,481	0.28%

Source: U.S. Department of Health and Human Services, National Center for Health Statistics
"Monthly Vital Statistics Report" (Vol. 45, No. 11(S)2, June 12, 1997)
*Final data by state of residence. Neoplasms are abnormal tissue, tumors. Includes many cancers.

Death Rate by Malignant Neoplasms in 1995

National Rate = 204.9 Deaths per 100,000 Population*

ALPHA ORDER

RANK	STATE	RATE
13	Alabama	221.4
50	Alaska	95.1
38	Arizona	190.1
5	Arkansas	244.7
45	California	162.8
48	Colorado	145.9
18	Connecticut	215.6
11	Delaware	227.3
1	Florida	263.5
42	Georgia	177.3
47	Hawaii	156.4
43	Idaho	172.4
25	Illinois	212.2
17	Indiana	216.3
15	Iowa	219.1
29	Kansas	205.9
10	Kentucky	229.2
22	Louisiana	214.3
6	Maine	242.9
33	Maryland	201.9
7	Massachusetts	231.9
31	Michigan	203.5
39	Minnesota	188.6
24	Mississippi	213.1
9	Missouri	230.7
32	Montana	203.4
28	Nebraska	206.2
36	Nevada	194.5
30	New Hampshire	205.2
7	New Jersey	231.9
46	New Mexico	159.5
23	New York	213.3
26	North Carolina	206.8
21	North Dakota	214.4
12	Ohio	226.1
16	Oklahoma	217.9
19	Oregon	214.7
3	Pennsylvania	250.7
4	Rhode Island	250.4
33	South Carolina	201.9
20	South Dakota	214.5
14	Tennessee	220.9
44	Texas	168.9
49	Utah	108.6
35	Vermont	198.9
37	Virginia	190.4
41	Washington	183.0
2	West Virginia	259.4
27	Wisconsin	206.3
40	Wyoming	186.6

RANK ORDER

RANK	STATE	RATE
1	Florida	263.5
2	West Virginia	259.4
3	Pennsylvania	250.7
4	Rhode Island	250.4
5	Arkansas	244.7
6	Maine	242.9
7	Massachusetts	231.9
7	New Jersey	231.9
9	Missouri	230.7
10	Kentucky	229.2
11	Delaware	227.3
12	Ohio	226.1
13	Alabama	221.4
14	Tennessee	220.9
15	Iowa	219.1
16	Oklahoma	217.9
17	Indiana	216.3
18	Connecticut	215.6
19	Oregon	214.7
20	South Dakota	214.5
21	North Dakota	214.4
22	Louisiana	214.3
23	New York	213.3
24	Mississippi	213.1
25	Illinois	212.2
26	North Carolina	206.8
27	Wisconsin	206.3
28	Nebraska	206.2
29	Kansas	205.9
30	New Hampshire	205.2
31	Michigan	203.5
32	Montana	203.4
33	Maryland	201.9
33	South Carolina	201.9
35	Vermont	198.9
36	Nevada	194.5
37	Virginia	190.4
38	Arizona	190.1
39	Minnesota	188.6
40	Wyoming	186.6
41	Washington	183.0
42	Georgia	177.3
43	Idaho	172.4
44	Texas	168.9
45	California	162.8
46	New Mexico	159.5
47	Hawaii	156.4
48	Colorado	145.9
49	Utah	108.6
50	Alaska	95.1
	District of Columbia	267.2

Source: U.S. Department of Health and Human Services, National Center for Health Statistics
"Monthly Vital Statistics Report" (Vol. 45, No. 11(S)2, June 12, 1997)
Final data by state of residence. Neoplasms are abnormal tissue, tumors. Includes many cancers. Not age adjusted.

Deaths by Pneumonia and Influenza in 1995

National Total = 82,923 Deaths*

ALPHA ORDER

RANK	STATE	DEATHS	% of USA
21	Alabama	1,368	1.65%
50	Alaska	55	0.07%
25	Arizona	1,170	1.41%
31	Arkansas	942	1.14%
1	California	10,556	12.73%
30	Colorado	948	1.14%
26	Connecticut	1,110	1.34%
46	Delaware	209	0.25%
5	Florida	3,849	4.64%
13	Georgia	1,991	2.40%
42	Hawaii	317	0.38%
40	Idaho	320	0.39%
4	Illinois	3,860	4.65%
16	Indiana	1,836	2.21%
24	Iowa	1,217	1.47%
33	Kansas	878	1.06%
20	Kentucky	1,457	1.76%
27	Louisiana	1,027	1.24%
39	Maine	343	0.41%
23	Maryland	1,357	1.64%
9	Massachusetts	2,718	3.28%
8	Michigan	2,978	3.59%
19	Minnesota	1,513	1.82%
29	Mississippi	953	1.15%
12	Missouri	2,212	2.67%
40	Montana	320	0.39%
34	Nebraska	651	0.79%
38	Nevada	370	0.45%
45	New Hampshire	225	0.27%
10	New Jersey	2,516	3.03%
37	New Mexico	403	0.49%
2	New York	6,551	7.90%
11	North Carolina	2,437	2.94%
47	North Dakota	206	0.25%
7	Ohio	3,423	4.13%
22	Oklahoma	1,364	1.64%
32	Oregon	906	1.09%
3	Pennsylvania	4,286	5.17%
44	Rhode Island	308	0.37%
28	South Carolina	997	1.20%
43	South Dakota	312	0.38%
14	Tennessee	1,894	2.28%
6	Texas	3,830	4.62%
36	Utah	478	0.58%
48	Vermont	172	0.21%
15	Virginia	1,888	2.28%
18	Washington	1,526	1.84%
35	West Virginia	620	0.75%
17	Wisconsin	1,698	2.05%
49	Wyoming	137	0.17%

RANK ORDER

RANK	STATE	DEATHS	% of USA
1	California	10,556	12.73%
2	New York	6,551	7.90%
3	Pennsylvania	4,286	5.17%
4	Illinois	3,860	4.65%
5	Florida	3,849	4.64%
6	Texas	3,830	4.62%
7	Ohio	3,423	4.13%
8	Michigan	2,978	3.59%
9	Massachusetts	2,718	3.28%
10	New Jersey	2,516	3.03%
11	North Carolina	2,437	2.94%
12	Missouri	2,212	2.67%
13	Georgia	1,991	2.40%
14	Tennessee	1,894	2.28%
15	Virginia	1,888	2.28%
16	Indiana	1,836	2.21%
17	Wisconsin	1,698	2.05%
18	Washington	1,526	1.84%
19	Minnesota	1,513	1.82%
20	Kentucky	1,457	1.76%
21	Alabama	1,368	1.65%
22	Oklahoma	1,364	1.64%
23	Maryland	1,357	1.64%
24	Iowa	1,217	1.47%
25	Arizona	1,170	1.41%
26	Connecticut	1,110	1.34%
27	Louisiana	1,027	1.24%
28	South Carolina	997	1.20%
29	Mississippi	953	1.15%
30	Colorado	948	1.14%
31	Arkansas	942	1.14%
32	Oregon	906	1.09%
33	Kansas	878	1.06%
34	Nebraska	651	0.79%
35	West Virginia	620	0.75%
36	Utah	478	0.58%
37	New Mexico	403	0.49%
38	Nevada	370	0.45%
39	Maine	343	0.41%
40	Idaho	320	0.39%
40	Montana	320	0.39%
42	Hawaii	317	0.38%
43	South Dakota	312	0.38%
44	Rhode Island	308	0.37%
45	New Hampshire	225	0.27%
46	Delaware	209	0.25%
47	North Dakota	206	0.25%
48	Vermont	172	0.21%
49	Wyoming	137	0.17%
50	Alaska	55	0.07%
	District of Columbia	221	0.27%

Source: U.S. Department of Health and Human Services, National Center for Health Statistics
"Monthly Vital Statistics Report" (Vol. 45, No. 11(S)2, June 12, 1997)
*Final data by state of residence.

Death Rate by Pneumonia and Influenza in 1995

National Rate = 31.6 Deaths per 100,000 Population*

ALPHA ORDER

RANK	STATE	RATE
22	Alabama	32.2
50	Alaska	9.1
35	Arizona	27.7
7	Arkansas	37.9
18	California	33.4
43	Colorado	25.3
15	Connecticut	33.9
29	Delaware	29.1
39	Florida	27.2
36	Georgia	27.6
42	Hawaii	26.7
38	Idaho	27.5
21	Illinois	32.6
25	Indiana	31.6
2	Iowa	42.8
14	Kansas	34.2
8	Kentucky	37.7
47	Louisiana	23.7
36	Maine	27.6
41	Maryland	26.9
1	Massachusetts	44.8
26	Michigan	31.2
20	Minnesota	32.8
13	Mississippi	35.3
4	Missouri	41.6
9	Montana	36.8
6	Nebraska	39.8
45	Nevada	24.2
49	New Hampshire	19.0
24	New Jersey	31.7
46	New Mexico	23.9
10	New York	36.1
15	North Carolina	33.9
23	North Dakota	32.1
28	Ohio	30.7
4	Oklahoma	41.6
31	Oregon	28.8
12	Pennsylvania	35.5
27	Rhode Island	31.1
40	South Carolina	27.1
3	South Dakota	42.0
11	Tennessee	36.0
48	Texas	20.5
44	Utah	24.5
30	Vermont	29.0
32	Virginia	28.5
34	Washington	28.1
15	West Virginia	33.9
19	Wisconsin	33.1
32	Wyoming	28.5

RANK ORDER

RANK	STATE	RATE
1	Massachusetts	44.8
2	Iowa	42.8
3	South Dakota	42.0
4	Missouri	41.6
4	Oklahoma	41.6
6	Nebraska	39.8
7	Arkansas	37.9
8	Kentucky	37.7
9	Montana	36.8
10	New York	36.1
11	Tennessee	36.0
12	Pennsylvania	35.5
13	Mississippi	35.3
14	Kansas	34.2
15	Connecticut	33.9
15	North Carolina	33.9
15	West Virginia	33.9
18	California	33.4
19	Wisconsin	33.1
20	Minnesota	32.8
21	Illinois	32.6
22	Alabama	32.2
23	North Dakota	32.1
24	New Jersey	31.7
25	Indiana	31.6
26	Michigan	31.2
27	Rhode Island	31.1
28	Ohio	30.7
29	Delaware	29.1
30	Vermont	29.0
31	Oregon	28.8
32	Virginia	28.5
32	Wyoming	28.5
34	Washington	28.1
35	Arizona	27.7
36	Georgia	27.6
36	Maine	27.6
38	Idaho	27.5
39	Florida	27.2
40	South Carolina	27.1
41	Maryland	26.9
42	Hawaii	26.7
43	Colorado	25.3
44	Utah	24.5
45	Nevada	24.2
46	New Mexico	23.9
47	Louisiana	23.7
48	Texas	20.5
49	New Hampshire	19.0
50	Alaska	9.1
	District of Columbia	39.9

Source: U.S. Department of Health and Human Services, National Center for Health Statistics
"Monthly Vital Statistics Report" (Vol. 45, No. 11(S)2, June 12, 1997)
Final data by state of residence. Not age adjusted.

Deaths by Complications of Pregnancy and Childbirth in 1995

National Total = 277 Deaths*

ALPHA ORDER

RANK	STATE	DEATHS	% of USA
16	Alabama	4	1.44%
38	Alaska	0	0.00%
23	Arizona	3	1.08%
16	Arkansas	4	1.44%
1	California	44	15.88%
38	Colorado	0	0.00%
29	Connecticut	1	0.36%
38	Delaware	0	0.00%
4	Florida	18	6.50%
6	Georgia	11	3.97%
29	Hawaii	1	0.36%
24	Idaho	2	0.72%
6	Illinois	11	3.97%
12	Indiana	7	2.53%
29	Iowa	1	0.36%
24	Kansas	2	0.72%
16	Kentucky	4	1.44%
16	Louisiana	4	1.44%
29	Maine	1	0.36%
11	Maryland	8	2.89%
29	Massachusetts	1	0.36%
10	Michigan	9	3.25%
38	Minnesota	0	0.00%
14	Mississippi	5	1.81%
9	Missouri	10	3.61%
38	Montana	0	0.00%
29	Nebraska	1	0.36%
24	Nevada	2	0.72%
38	New Hampshire	0	0.00%
16	New Jersey	4	1.44%
29	New Mexico	1	0.36%
2	New York	32	11.55%
5	North Carolina	15	5.42%
29	North Dakota	1	0.36%
12	Ohio	7	2.53%
38	Oklahoma	0	0.00%
38	Oregon	0	0.00%
6	Pennsylvania	11	3.97%
29	Rhode Island	1	0.36%
16	South Carolina	4	1.44%
38	South Dakota	0	0.00%
24	Tennessee	2	0.72%
3	Texas	28	10.11%
24	Utah	2	0.72%
38	Vermont	0	0.00%
16	Virginia	4	1.44%
38	Washington	0	0.00%
38	West Virginia	0	0.00%
14	Wisconsin	5	1.81%
38	Wyoming	0	0.00%

RANK ORDER

RANK	STATE	DEATHS	% of USA
1	California	44	15.88%
2	New York	32	11.55%
3	Texas	28	10.11%
4	Florida	18	6.50%
5	North Carolina	15	5.42%
6	Georgia	11	3.97%
6	Illinois	11	3.97%
6	Pennsylvania	11	3.97%
9	Missouri	10	3.61%
10	Michigan	9	3.25%
11	Maryland	8	2.89%
12	Indiana	7	2.53%
12	Ohio	7	2.53%
14	Mississippi	5	1.81%
14	Wisconsin	5	1.81%
16	Alabama	4	1.44%
16	Arkansas	4	1.44%
16	Kentucky	4	1.44%
16	Louisiana	4	1.44%
16	New Jersey	4	1.44%
16	South Carolina	4	1.44%
16	Virginia	4	1.44%
23	Arizona	3	1.08%
24	Idaho	2	0.72%
24	Kansas	2	0.72%
24	Nevada	2	0.72%
24	Tennessee	2	0.72%
24	Utah	2	0.72%
29	Connecticut	1	0.36%
29	Hawaii	1	0.36%
29	Iowa	1	0.36%
29	Maine	1	0.36%
29	Massachusetts	1	0.36%
29	Nebraska	1	0.36%
29	New Mexico	1	0.36%
29	North Dakota	1	0.36%
29	Rhode Island	1	0.36%
38	Alaska	0	0.00%
38	Colorado	0	0.00%
38	Delaware	0	0.00%
38	Minnesota	0	0.00%
38	Montana	0	0.00%
38	New Hampshire	0	0.00%
38	Oklahoma	0	0.00%
38	Oregon	0	0.00%
38	South Dakota	0	0.00%
38	Vermont	0	0.00%
38	Washington	0	0.00%
38	West Virginia	0	0.00%
38	Wyoming	0	0.00%
	District of Columbia	6	2.17%

Source: U.S. Department of Health and Human Services, National Center for Health Statistics
   (http://wonder.cdc.gov/WONDER/)
*By state of residence.

Death Rate by Complications of Pregnancy and Childbirth in 1995

National Rate = 0.21 Deaths per 100,000 Female Population*

ALPHA ORDER

RANK	STATE	RATE
20	Alabama	0.18
38	Alaska	0.00
28	Arizona	0.14
6	Arkansas	0.31
11	California	0.28
38	Colorado	0.00
36	Connecticut	0.06
38	Delaware	0.00
13	Florida	0.25
9	Georgia	0.30
25	Hawaii	0.17
4	Idaho	0.34
20	Illinois	0.18
14	Indiana	0.23
34	Iowa	0.07
27	Kansas	0.15
16	Kentucky	0.20
20	Louisiana	0.18
26	Maine	0.16
6	Maryland	0.31
37	Massachusetts	0.03
20	Michigan	0.18
38	Minnesota	0.00
2	Mississippi	0.36
2	Missouri	0.36
38	Montana	0.00
29	Nebraska	0.12
12	Nevada	0.27
38	New Hampshire	0.00
33	New Jersey	0.10
29	New Mexico	0.12
4	New York	0.34
1	North Carolina	0.40
6	North Dakota	0.31
29	Ohio	0.12
38	Oklahoma	0.00
38	Oregon	0.00
20	Pennsylvania	0.18
18	Rhode Island	0.19
15	South Carolina	0.21
38	South Dakota	0.00
34	Tennessee	0.07
9	Texas	0.30
16	Utah	0.20
38	Vermont	0.00
29	Virginia	0.12
38	Washington	0.00
38	West Virginia	0.00
18	Wisconsin	0.19
38	Wyoming	0.00

RANK ORDER

RANK	STATE	RATE
1	North Carolina	0.40
2	Mississippi	0.36
2	Missouri	0.36
4	Idaho	0.34
4	New York	0.34
6	Arkansas	0.31
6	Maryland	0.31
6	North Dakota	0.31
9	Georgia	0.30
9	Texas	0.30
11	California	0.28
12	Nevada	0.27
13	Florida	0.25
14	Indiana	0.23
15	South Carolina	0.21
16	Kentucky	0.20
16	Utah	0.20
18	Rhode Island	0.19
18	Wisconsin	0.19
20	Alabama	0.18
20	Illinois	0.18
20	Louisiana	0.18
20	Michigan	0.18
20	Pennsylvania	0.18
25	Hawaii	0.17
26	Maine	0.16
27	Kansas	0.15
28	Arizona	0.14
29	Nebraska	0.12
29	New Mexico	0.12
29	Ohio	0.12
29	Virginia	0.12
33	New Jersey	0.10
34	Iowa	0.07
34	Tennessee	0.07
36	Connecticut	0.06
37	Massachusetts	0.03
38	Alaska	0.00
38	Colorado	0.00
38	Delaware	0.00
38	Minnesota	0.00
38	Montana	0.00
38	New Hampshire	0.00
38	Oklahoma	0.00
38	Oregon	0.00
38	South Dakota	0.00
38	Vermont	0.00
38	Washington	0.00
38	West Virginia	0.00
38	Wyoming	0.00

District of Columbia   2.04

Source: Morgan Quitno Press using data from U.S. Dept. of Health & Human Services, National Center for Health Statistics unpublished (http://wonder.cdc.gov/WONDER/)
By state of residence. Not age adjusted.

Deaths by Tuberculosis in 1995

National Total = 1,336 Deaths*

<table>
<tr><td colspan="4">ALPHA ORDER</td><td colspan="4">RANK ORDER</td></tr>
<tr><td>RANK</td><td>STATE</td><td>DEATHS</td><td>% of USA</td><td>RANK</td><td>STATE</td><td>DEATHS</td><td>% of USA</td></tr>
<tr><td>10</td><td>Alabama</td><td>41</td><td>3.07%</td><td>1</td><td>California</td><td>194</td><td>14.52%</td></tr>
<tr><td>34</td><td>Alaska</td><td>6</td><td>0.45%</td><td>2</td><td>New York</td><td>117</td><td>8.76%</td></tr>
<tr><td>16</td><td>Arizona</td><td>27</td><td>2.02%</td><td>3</td><td>Texas</td><td>113</td><td>8.46%</td></tr>
<tr><td>22</td><td>Arkansas</td><td>21</td><td>1.57%</td><td>4</td><td>Florida</td><td>83</td><td>6.21%</td></tr>
<tr><td>1</td><td>California</td><td>194</td><td>14.52%</td><td>5</td><td>Illinois</td><td>66</td><td>4.94%</td></tr>
<tr><td>31</td><td>Colorado</td><td>9</td><td>0.67%</td><td>6</td><td>Pennsylvania</td><td>54</td><td>4.04%</td></tr>
<tr><td>29</td><td>Connecticut</td><td>11</td><td>0.82%</td><td>7</td><td>Georgia</td><td>44</td><td>3.29%</td></tr>
<tr><td>44</td><td>Delaware</td><td>2</td><td>0.15%</td><td>8</td><td>Louisiana</td><td>43</td><td>3.22%</td></tr>
<tr><td>4</td><td>Florida</td><td>83</td><td>6.21%</td><td>9</td><td>Michigan</td><td>42</td><td>3.14%</td></tr>
<tr><td>7</td><td>Georgia</td><td>44</td><td>3.29%</td><td>10</td><td>Alabama</td><td>41</td><td>3.07%</td></tr>
<tr><td>36</td><td>Hawaii</td><td>5</td><td>0.37%</td><td>11</td><td>Tennessee</td><td>39</td><td>2.92%</td></tr>
<tr><td>47</td><td>Idaho</td><td>1</td><td>0.07%</td><td>12</td><td>New Jersey</td><td>38</td><td>2.84%</td></tr>
<tr><td>5</td><td>Illinois</td><td>66</td><td>4.94%</td><td>13</td><td>Ohio</td><td>33</td><td>2.47%</td></tr>
<tr><td>19</td><td>Indiana</td><td>24</td><td>1.80%</td><td>14</td><td>North Carolina</td><td>32</td><td>2.40%</td></tr>
<tr><td>36</td><td>Iowa</td><td>5</td><td>0.37%</td><td>15</td><td>South Carolina</td><td>29</td><td>2.17%</td></tr>
<tr><td>33</td><td>Kansas</td><td>7</td><td>0.52%</td><td>16</td><td>Arizona</td><td>27</td><td>2.02%</td></tr>
<tr><td>19</td><td>Kentucky</td><td>24</td><td>1.80%</td><td>17</td><td>Maryland</td><td>25</td><td>1.87%</td></tr>
<tr><td>8</td><td>Louisiana</td><td>43</td><td>3.22%</td><td>17</td><td>Virginia</td><td>25</td><td>1.87%</td></tr>
<tr><td>40</td><td>Maine</td><td>3</td><td>0.22%</td><td>19</td><td>Indiana</td><td>24</td><td>1.80%</td></tr>
<tr><td>17</td><td>Maryland</td><td>25</td><td>1.87%</td><td>19</td><td>Kentucky</td><td>24</td><td>1.80%</td></tr>
<tr><td>26</td><td>Massachusetts</td><td>15</td><td>1.12%</td><td>21</td><td>Oregon</td><td>22</td><td>1.65%</td></tr>
<tr><td>9</td><td>Michigan</td><td>42</td><td>3.14%</td><td>22</td><td>Arkansas</td><td>21</td><td>1.57%</td></tr>
<tr><td>27</td><td>Minnesota</td><td>13</td><td>0.97%</td><td>23</td><td>Missouri</td><td>18</td><td>1.35%</td></tr>
<tr><td>25</td><td>Mississippi</td><td>16</td><td>1.20%</td><td>23</td><td>Oklahoma</td><td>18</td><td>1.35%</td></tr>
<tr><td>23</td><td>Missouri</td><td>18</td><td>1.35%</td><td>25</td><td>Mississippi</td><td>16</td><td>1.20%</td></tr>
<tr><td>44</td><td>Montana</td><td>2</td><td>0.15%</td><td>26</td><td>Massachusetts</td><td>15</td><td>1.12%</td></tr>
<tr><td>40</td><td>Nebraska</td><td>3</td><td>0.22%</td><td>27</td><td>Minnesota</td><td>13</td><td>0.97%</td></tr>
<tr><td>34</td><td>Nevada</td><td>6</td><td>0.45%</td><td>27</td><td>Washington</td><td>13</td><td>0.97%</td></tr>
<tr><td>38</td><td>New Hampshire</td><td>4</td><td>0.30%</td><td>29</td><td>Connecticut</td><td>11</td><td>0.82%</td></tr>
<tr><td>12</td><td>New Jersey</td><td>38</td><td>2.84%</td><td>30</td><td>Wisconsin</td><td>10</td><td>0.75%</td></tr>
<tr><td>38</td><td>New Mexico</td><td>4</td><td>0.30%</td><td>31</td><td>Colorado</td><td>9</td><td>0.67%</td></tr>
<tr><td>2</td><td>New York</td><td>117</td><td>8.76%</td><td>32</td><td>West Virginia</td><td>8</td><td>0.60%</td></tr>
<tr><td>14</td><td>North Carolina</td><td>32</td><td>2.40%</td><td>33</td><td>Kansas</td><td>7</td><td>0.52%</td></tr>
<tr><td>44</td><td>North Dakota</td><td>2</td><td>0.15%</td><td>34</td><td>Alaska</td><td>6</td><td>0.45%</td></tr>
<tr><td>13</td><td>Ohio</td><td>33</td><td>2.47%</td><td>34</td><td>Nevada</td><td>6</td><td>0.45%</td></tr>
<tr><td>23</td><td>Oklahoma</td><td>18</td><td>1.35%</td><td>36</td><td>Hawaii</td><td>5</td><td>0.37%</td></tr>
<tr><td>21</td><td>Oregon</td><td>22</td><td>1.65%</td><td>36</td><td>Iowa</td><td>5</td><td>0.37%</td></tr>
<tr><td>6</td><td>Pennsylvania</td><td>54</td><td>4.04%</td><td>38</td><td>New Hampshire</td><td>4</td><td>0.30%</td></tr>
<tr><td>40</td><td>Rhode Island</td><td>3</td><td>0.22%</td><td>38</td><td>New Mexico</td><td>4</td><td>0.30%</td></tr>
<tr><td>15</td><td>South Carolina</td><td>29</td><td>2.17%</td><td>40</td><td>Maine</td><td>3</td><td>0.22%</td></tr>
<tr><td>50</td><td>South Dakota</td><td>0</td><td>0.00%</td><td>40</td><td>Nebraska</td><td>3</td><td>0.22%</td></tr>
<tr><td>11</td><td>Tennessee</td><td>39</td><td>2.92%</td><td>40</td><td>Rhode Island</td><td>3</td><td>0.22%</td></tr>
<tr><td>3</td><td>Texas</td><td>113</td><td>8.46%</td><td>40</td><td>Utah</td><td>3</td><td>0.22%</td></tr>
<tr><td>40</td><td>Utah</td><td>3</td><td>0.22%</td><td>44</td><td>Delaware</td><td>2</td><td>0.15%</td></tr>
<tr><td>47</td><td>Vermont</td><td>1</td><td>0.07%</td><td>44</td><td>Montana</td><td>2</td><td>0.15%</td></tr>
<tr><td>17</td><td>Virginia</td><td>25</td><td>1.87%</td><td>44</td><td>North Dakota</td><td>2</td><td>0.15%</td></tr>
<tr><td>27</td><td>Washington</td><td>13</td><td>0.97%</td><td>47</td><td>Idaho</td><td>1</td><td>0.07%</td></tr>
<tr><td>32</td><td>West Virginia</td><td>8</td><td>0.60%</td><td>47</td><td>Vermont</td><td>1</td><td>0.07%</td></tr>
<tr><td>30</td><td>Wisconsin</td><td>10</td><td>0.75%</td><td>47</td><td>Wyoming</td><td>1</td><td>0.07%</td></tr>
<tr><td>47</td><td>Wyoming</td><td>1</td><td>0.07%</td><td>50</td><td>South Dakota</td><td>0</td><td>0.00%</td></tr>
<tr><td></td><td></td><td></td><td></td><td></td><td>District of Columbia</td><td>11</td><td>0.82%</td></tr>
</table>

Source: U.S. Department of Health and Human Services, National Center for Health Statistics
    (http://wonder.cdc.gov/WONDER/)
*By state of residence.

Death Rate by Tuberculosis in 1995

National Rate = 0.50 Deaths per 100,000 Population*

ALPHA ORDER			RANK ORDER		
RANK	STATE	RATE	RANK	STATE	RATE
3	Alabama	0.96	1	Alaska	0.99
1	Alaska	0.99	1	Louisiana	0.99
9	Arizona	0.62	3	Alabama	0.96
4	Arkansas	0.84	4	Arkansas	0.84
11	California	0.61	5	South Carolina	0.79
37	Colorado	0.24	6	Tennessee	0.74
29	Connecticut	0.33	7	Oregon	0.69
35	Delaware	0.27	8	New York	0.64
15	Florida	0.58	9	Arizona	0.62
11	Georgia	0.61	9	Kentucky	0.62
24	Hawaii	0.42	11	California	0.61
49	Idaho	0.08	11	Georgia	0.61
16	Illinois	0.55	13	Texas	0.60
25	Indiana	0.41	14	Mississippi	0.59
46	Iowa	0.17	15	Florida	0.58
35	Kansas	0.27	16	Illinois	0.55
9	Kentucky	0.62	17	Oklahoma	0.54
1	Louisiana	0.99	18	Maryland	0.49
37	Maine	0.24	19	New Jersey	0.47
18	Maryland	0.49	20	Michigan	0.44
37	Massachusetts	0.24	20	North Carolina	0.44
20	Michigan	0.44	20	Pennsylvania	0.44
34	Minnesota	0.28	23	West Virginia	0.43
14	Mississippi	0.59	24	Hawaii	0.42
29	Missouri	0.33	25	Indiana	0.41
42	Montana	0.22	26	Nevada	0.39
45	Nebraska	0.18	27	Virginia	0.37
26	Nevada	0.39	28	New Hampshire	0.34
28	New Hampshire	0.34	29	Connecticut	0.33
19	New Jersey	0.47	29	Missouri	0.33
40	New Mexico	0.23	31	North Dakota	0.31
8	New York	0.64	32	Rhode Island	0.30
20	North Carolina	0.44	33	Ohio	0.29
31	North Dakota	0.31	34	Minnesota	0.28
33	Ohio	0.29	35	Delaware	0.27
17	Oklahoma	0.54	35	Kansas	0.27
7	Oregon	0.69	37	Colorado	0.24
20	Pennsylvania	0.44	37	Maine	0.24
32	Rhode Island	0.30	37	Massachusetts	0.24
5	South Carolina	0.79	40	New Mexico	0.23
50	South Dakota	0.00	40	Washington	0.23
6	Tennessee	0.74	42	Montana	0.22
13	Texas	0.60	43	Wyoming	0.20
48	Utah	0.15	44	Wisconsin	0.19
46	Vermont	0.17	45	Nebraska	0.18
27	Virginia	0.37	46	Iowa	0.17
40	Washington	0.23	46	Vermont	0.17
23	West Virginia	0.43	48	Utah	0.15
44	Wisconsin	0.19	49	Idaho	0.08
43	Wyoming	0.20	50	South Dakota	0.00
				District of Columbia	1.97

Source: U.S. Department of Health and Human Services, National Center for Health Statistics
unpublished (http://wonder.cdc.gov/WONDER/)
*By state of residence. Not age adjusted.

Deaths by Injury in 1995

National Total = 150,809 Deaths*

ALPHA ORDER

RANK	STATE	DEATHS	% of USA
16	Alabama	3,378	2.24%
43	Alaska	504	0.33%
17	Arizona	3,364	2.23%
30	Arkansas	1,921	1.27%
1	California	16,768	11.12%
23	Colorado	2,441	1.62%
32	Connecticut	1,558	1.03%
47	Delaware	389	0.26%
3	Florida	8,882	5.89%
9	Georgia	4,595	3.05%
42	Hawaii	556	0.37%
39	Idaho	771	0.51%
6	Illinois	6,546	4.34%
15	Indiana	3,414	2.26%
31	Iowa	1,581	1.05%
33	Kansas	1,454	0.96%
22	Kentucky	2,461	1.63%
18	Louisiana	3,219	2.13%
41	Maine	582	0.39%
20	Maryland	3,015	2.00%
28	Massachusetts	2,294	1.52%
7	Michigan	5,228	3.47%
26	Minnesota	2,404	1.59%
27	Mississippi	2,390	1.58%
13	Missouri	3,559	2.36%
40	Montana	640	0.42%
38	Nebraska	854	0.57%
35	Nevada	1,197	0.79%
44	New Hampshire	463	0.31%
14	New Jersey	3,441	2.28%
34	New Mexico	1,389	0.92%
4	New York	8,060	5.34%
10	North Carolina	4,573	3.03%
49	North Dakota	318	0.21%
8	Ohio	4,937	3.27%
24	Oklahoma	2,432	1.61%
29	Oregon	2,050	1.36%
5	Pennsylvania	6,698	4.44%
46	Rhode Island	398	0.26%
25	South Carolina	2,417	1.60%
45	South Dakota	433	0.29%
11	Tennessee	3,819	2.53%
2	Texas	10,627	7.05%
37	Utah	1,072	0.71%
50	Vermont	291	0.19%
12	Virginia	3,592	2.38%
19	Washington	3,070	2.04%
36	West Virginia	1,125	0.75%
21	Wisconsin	2,743	1.82%
48	Wyoming	342	0.23%

RANK ORDER

RANK	STATE	DEATHS	% of USA
1	California	16,768	11.12%
2	Texas	10,627	7.05%
3	Florida	8,882	5.89%
4	New York	8,060	5.34%
5	Pennsylvania	6,698	4.44%
6	Illinois	6,546	4.34%
7	Michigan	5,228	3.47%
8	Ohio	4,937	3.27%
9	Georgia	4,595	3.05%
10	North Carolina	4,573	3.03%
11	Tennessee	3,819	2.53%
12	Virginia	3,592	2.38%
13	Missouri	3,559	2.36%
14	New Jersey	3,441	2.28%
15	Indiana	3,414	2.26%
16	Alabama	3,378	2.24%
17	Arizona	3,364	2.23%
18	Louisiana	3,219	2.13%
19	Washington	3,070	2.04%
20	Maryland	3,015	2.00%
21	Wisconsin	2,743	1.82%
22	Kentucky	2,461	1.63%
23	Colorado	2,441	1.62%
24	Oklahoma	2,432	1.61%
25	South Carolina	2,417	1.60%
26	Minnesota	2,404	1.59%
27	Mississippi	2,390	1.58%
28	Massachusetts	2,294	1.52%
29	Oregon	2,050	1.36%
30	Arkansas	1,921	1.27%
31	Iowa	1,581	1.05%
32	Connecticut	1,558	1.03%
33	Kansas	1,454	0.96%
34	New Mexico	1,389	0.92%
35	Nevada	1,197	0.79%
36	West Virginia	1,125	0.75%
37	Utah	1,072	0.71%
38	Nebraska	854	0.57%
39	Idaho	771	0.51%
40	Montana	640	0.42%
41	Maine	582	0.39%
42	Hawaii	556	0.37%
43	Alaska	504	0.33%
44	New Hampshire	463	0.31%
45	South Dakota	433	0.29%
46	Rhode Island	398	0.26%
47	Delaware	389	0.26%
48	Wyoming	342	0.23%
49	North Dakota	318	0.21%
50	Vermont	291	0.19%
	District of Columbia	554	0.37%

Source: U.S. Department of Health and Human Services, National Center for Health Statistics
    unpublished (http://wonder.cdc.gov/WONDER/)
*By state of residence. Injury as used here includes Accidents (including motor vehicle), Suicides, Homicides and "Other" undetermined.

Death Rate by Injury in 1995

National Rate = 57.4 Deaths by Injury per 100,000 Population*

ALPHA ORDER

RANK	STATE	RATE		RANK	STATE	RATE
4	Alabama	79.5		1	Mississippi	88.6
2	Alaska	83.6		2	Alaska	83.6
5	Arizona	78.1		3	New Mexico	82.2
7	Arkansas	77.3		4	Alabama	79.5
37	California	53.1		5	Arizona	78.1
16	Colorado	65.1		6	Nevada	78.0
42	Connecticut	47.6		7	Arkansas	77.3
35	Delaware	54.2		8	Louisiana	74.2
21	Florida	62.6		8	Oklahoma	74.2
19	Georgia	63.7		10	Montana	73.5
43	Hawaii	47.1		11	Tennessee	72.8
14	Idaho	66.1		12	Wyoming	71.4
30	Illinois	55.5		13	Missouri	66.9
25	Indiana	58.9		14	Idaho	66.1
29	Iowa	55.6		15	South Carolina	65.9
26	Kansas	56.7		16	Colorado	65.1
18	Kentucky	63.8		16	Oregon	65.1
8	Louisiana	74.2		18	Kentucky	63.8
44	Maine	47.0		19	Georgia	63.7
23	Maryland	59.8		20	North Carolina	63.5
50	Massachusetts	37.7		21	Florida	62.6
32	Michigan	54.8		22	West Virginia	61.6
38	Minnesota	52.1		23	Maryland	59.8
1	Mississippi	88.6		24	South Dakota	59.3
13	Missouri	66.9		25	Indiana	58.9
10	Montana	73.5		26	Kansas	56.7
38	Nebraska	52.1		27	Texas	56.5
6	Nevada	78.0		28	Washington	56.3
48	New Hampshire	40.3		29	Iowa	55.6
47	New Jersey	43.3		30	Illinois	55.5
3	New Mexico	82.2		30	Pennsylvania	55.5
45	New York	44.3		32	Michigan	54.8
20	North Carolina	63.5		33	Utah	54.5
41	North Dakota	49.6		34	Virginia	54.3
45	Ohio	44.3		35	Delaware	54.2
8	Oklahoma	74.2		36	Wisconsin	53.5
16	Oregon	65.1		37	California	53.1
30	Pennsylvania	55.5		38	Minnesota	52.1
49	Rhode Island	40.1		38	Nebraska	52.1
15	South Carolina	65.9		40	Vermont	49.8
24	South Dakota	59.3		41	North Dakota	49.6
11	Tennessee	72.8		42	Connecticut	47.6
27	Texas	56.5		43	Hawaii	47.1
33	Utah	54.5		44	Maine	47.0
40	Vermont	49.8		45	New York	44.3
34	Virginia	54.3		45	Ohio	44.3
28	Washington	56.3		47	New Jersey	43.3
22	West Virginia	61.6		48	New Hampshire	40.3
36	Wisconsin	53.5		49	Rhode Island	40.1
12	Wyoming	71.4		50	Massachusetts	37.7
					District of Columbia	99.5

Source: U.S. Department of Health and Human Services, National Center for Health Statistics
   unpublished (http://wonder.cdc.gov/WONDER/)
*By state of residence. Injury as used here includes Accidents (including motor vehicle), Suicides, Homicides and "Other" undetermined. Not age adjusted.

Deaths by Accidents in 1995

National Total = 93,320 Deaths*

ALPHA ORDER

RANK	STATE	DEATHS	% of USA
14	Alabama	2,234	2.39%
42	Alaska	339	0.36%
17	Arizona	1,984	2.13%
30	Arkansas	1,213	1.30%
1	California	9,253	9.92%
25	Colorado	1,491	1.60%
32	Connecticut	1,077	1.15%
46	Delaware	266	0.29%
3	Florida	5,398	5.78%
9	Georgia	2,963	3.18%
43	Hawaii	327	0.35%
39	Idaho	526	0.56%
6	Illinois	4,013	4.30%
16	Indiana	2,206	2.36%
31	Iowa	1,168	1.25%
33	Kansas	993	1.06%
21	Kentucky	1,707	1.83%
19	Louisiana	1,841	1.97%
40	Maine	399	0.43%
27	Maryland	1,393	1.49%
29	Massachusetts	1,218	1.31%
8	Michigan	3,168	3.39%
22	Minnesota	1,666	1.79%
24	Mississippi	1,608	1.72%
13	Missouri	2,315	2.48%
41	Montana	380	0.41%
37	Nebraska	576	0.62%
38	Nevada	551	0.59%
45	New Hampshire	287	0.31%
12	New Jersey	2,316	2.48%
34	New Mexico	920	0.99%
4	New York	4,989	5.35%
10	North Carolina	2,951	3.16%
49	North Dakota	210	0.23%
7	Ohio	3,250	3.48%
26	Oklahoma	1,473	1.58%
28	Oregon	1,366	1.46%
5	Pennsylvania	4,266	4.57%
48	Rhode Island	217	0.23%
23	South Carolina	1,635	1.75%
44	South Dakota	324	0.35%
11	Tennessee	2,485	2.66%
2	Texas	6,431	6.89%
36	Utah	633	0.68%
50	Vermont	192	0.21%
15	Virginia	2,212	2.37%
18	Washington	1,894	2.03%
35	West Virginia	739	0.79%
20	Wisconsin	1,824	1.95%
47	Wyoming	240	0.26%

RANK ORDER

RANK	STATE	DEATHS	% of USA
1	California	9,253	9.92%
2	Texas	6,431	6.89%
3	Florida	5,398	5.78%
4	New York	4,989	5.35%
5	Pennsylvania	4,266	4.57%
6	Illinois	4,013	4.30%
7	Ohio	3,250	3.48%
8	Michigan	3,168	3.39%
9	Georgia	2,963	3.18%
10	North Carolina	2,951	3.16%
11	Tennessee	2,485	2.66%
12	New Jersey	2,316	2.48%
13	Missouri	2,315	2.48%
14	Alabama	2,234	2.39%
15	Virginia	2,212	2.37%
16	Indiana	2,206	2.36%
17	Arizona	1,984	2.13%
18	Washington	1,894	2.03%
19	Louisiana	1,841	1.97%
20	Wisconsin	1,824	1.95%
21	Kentucky	1,707	1.83%
22	Minnesota	1,666	1.79%
23	South Carolina	1,635	1.75%
24	Mississippi	1,608	1.72%
25	Colorado	1,491	1.60%
26	Oklahoma	1,473	1.58%
27	Maryland	1,393	1.49%
28	Oregon	1,366	1.46%
29	Massachusetts	1,218	1.31%
30	Arkansas	1,213	1.30%
31	Iowa	1,168	1.25%
32	Connecticut	1,077	1.15%
33	Kansas	993	1.06%
34	New Mexico	920	0.99%
35	West Virginia	739	0.79%
36	Utah	633	0.68%
37	Nebraska	576	0.62%
38	Nevada	551	0.59%
39	Idaho	526	0.56%
40	Maine	399	0.43%
41	Montana	380	0.41%
42	Alaska	339	0.36%
43	Hawaii	327	0.35%
44	South Dakota	324	0.35%
45	New Hampshire	287	0.31%
46	Delaware	266	0.29%
47	Wyoming	240	0.26%
48	Rhode Island	217	0.23%
49	North Dakota	210	0.23%
50	Vermont	192	0.21%
	District of Columbia	193	0.21%

Source: U.S. Department of Health and Human Services, National Center for Health Statistics
"Monthly Vital Statistics Report" (Vol. 45, No. 11(S)2, June 12, 1997)
Final data by state of residence. Includes motor vehicle deaths, poisoning, falls, drowning and other accidents.

Death Rate by Accidents in 1995

National Rate = 35.5 Deaths per 100,000 Population*

ALPHA ORDER

RANK	STATE	RATE
4	Alabama	52.5
2	Alaska	56.2
8	Arizona	47.0
6	Arkansas	48.8
42	California	29.3
22	Colorado	39.8
37	Connecticut	32.9
26	Delaware	37.1
24	Florida	38.1
18	Georgia	41.1
45	Hawaii	27.6
9	Idaho	45.2
34	Illinois	33.9
25	Indiana	38.0
18	Iowa	41.1
23	Kansas	38.7
13	Kentucky	44.2
17	Louisiana	42.4
41	Maine	32.1
45	Maryland	27.6
50	Massachusetts	20.1
36	Michigan	33.2
27	Minnesota	36.1
1	Mississippi	59.6
15	Missouri	43.5
14	Montana	43.7
31	Nebraska	35.2
28	Nevada	36.0
48	New Hampshire	25.0
43	New Jersey	29.1
3	New Mexico	54.6
47	New York	27.5
20	North Carolina	41.0
39	North Dakota	32.7
43	Ohio	29.1
10	Oklahoma	44.9
15	Oregon	43.5
30	Pennsylvania	35.3
49	Rhode Island	21.9
11	South Carolina	44.5
12	South Dakota	44.4
7	Tennessee	47.3
33	Texas	34.3
40	Utah	32.4
38	Vermont	32.8
35	Virginia	33.4
32	Washington	34.9
21	West Virginia	40.4
29	Wisconsin	35.6
5	Wyoming	50.0

RANK ORDER

RANK	STATE	RATE
1	Mississippi	59.6
2	Alaska	56.2
3	New Mexico	54.6
4	Alabama	52.5
5	Wyoming	50.0
6	Arkansas	48.8
7	Tennessee	47.3
8	Arizona	47.0
9	Idaho	45.2
10	Oklahoma	44.9
11	South Carolina	44.5
12	South Dakota	44.4
13	Kentucky	44.2
14	Montana	43.7
15	Missouri	43.5
15	Oregon	43.5
17	Louisiana	42.4
18	Georgia	41.1
18	Iowa	41.1
20	North Carolina	41.0
21	West Virginia	40.4
22	Colorado	39.8
23	Kansas	38.7
24	Florida	38.1
25	Indiana	38.0
26	Delaware	37.1
27	Minnesota	36.1
28	Nevada	36.0
29	Wisconsin	35.6
30	Pennsylvania	35.3
31	Nebraska	35.2
32	Washington	34.9
33	Texas	34.3
34	Illinois	33.9
35	Virginia	33.4
36	Michigan	33.2
37	Connecticut	32.9
38	Vermont	32.8
39	North Dakota	32.7
40	Utah	32.4
41	Maine	32.1
42	California	29.3
43	New Jersey	29.1
43	Ohio	29.1
45	Hawaii	27.6
45	Maryland	27.6
47	New York	27.5
48	New Hampshire	25.0
49	Rhode Island	21.9
50	Massachusetts	20.1
	District of Columbia	34.8

Source: U.S. Department of Health and Human Services, National Center for Health Statistics
   "Monthly Vital Statistics Report" (Vol. 45, No. 11(S)2, June 12, 1997)
*Final data by state of residence. Includes motor vehicle deaths, poisoning, falls, drowning and other accidents.
Not age adjusted.

Deaths by Motor Vehicle Accidents in 1995

National Total = 43,363 Deaths*

ALPHA ORDER

RANK ORDER

RANK	STATE	DEATHS	% of USA		RANK	STATE	DEATHS	% of USA
12	Alabama	1,139	2.63%		1	California	4,439	10.24%
47	Alaska	97	0.22%		2	Texas	3,328	7.67%
15	Arizona	990	2.28%		3	Florida	2,806	6.47%
28	Arkansas	652	1.50%		4	New York	1,798	4.15%
1	California	4,439	10.24%		5	Illinois	1,737	4.01%
25	Colorado	696	1.61%		6	Michigan	1,623	3.74%
35	Connecticut	349	0.80%		7	Pennsylvania	1,578	3.64%
46	Delaware	126	0.29%		8	Georgia	1,539	3.55%
3	Florida	2,806	6.47%		9	North Carolina	1,490	3.44%
8	Georgia	1,539	3.55%		10	Ohio	1,387	3.20%
43	Hawaii	142	0.33%		11	Tennessee	1,288	2.97%
38	Idaho	264	0.61%		12	Alabama	1,139	2.63%
5	Illinois	1,737	4.01%		13	Missouri	1,098	2.53%
14	Indiana	995	2.29%		14	Indiana	995	2.29%
30	Iowa	547	1.26%		15	Arizona	990	2.28%
32	Kansas	451	1.04%		16	Virginia	922	2.13%
19	Kentucky	851	1.96%		17	Louisiana	910	2.10%
17	Louisiana	910	2.10%		18	Mississippi	904	2.08%
41	Maine	182	0.42%		19	Kentucky	851	1.96%
26	Maryland	679	1.57%		20	South Carolina	849	1.96%
31	Massachusetts	487	1.12%		21	New Jersey	842	1.94%
6	Michigan	1,623	3.74%		22	Wisconsin	775	1.79%
27	Minnesota	664	1.53%		23	Washington	743	1.71%
18	Mississippi	904	2.08%		24	Oklahoma	725	1.67%
13	Missouri	1,098	2.53%		25	Colorado	696	1.61%
40	Montana	195	0.45%		26	Maryland	679	1.57%
39	Nebraska	254	0.59%		27	Minnesota	664	1.53%
37	Nevada	305	0.70%		28	Arkansas	652	1.50%
44	New Hampshire	135	0.31%		29	Oregon	593	1.37%
21	New Jersey	842	1.94%		30	Iowa	547	1.26%
33	New Mexico	450	1.04%		31	Massachusetts	487	1.12%
4	New York	1,798	4.15%		32	Kansas	451	1.04%
9	North Carolina	1,490	3.44%		33	New Mexico	450	1.04%
49	North Dakota	84	0.19%		34	West Virginia	387	0.89%
10	Ohio	1,387	3.20%		35	Connecticut	349	0.80%
24	Oklahoma	725	1.67%		36	Utah	335	0.77%
29	Oregon	593	1.37%		37	Nevada	305	0.70%
7	Pennsylvania	1,578	3.64%		38	Idaho	264	0.61%
50	Rhode Island	80	0.18%		39	Nebraska	254	0.59%
20	South Carolina	849	1.96%		40	Montana	195	0.45%
42	South Dakota	161	0.37%		41	Maine	182	0.42%
11	Tennessee	1,288	2.97%		42	South Dakota	161	0.37%
2	Texas	3,328	7.67%		43	Hawaii	142	0.33%
36	Utah	335	0.77%		44	New Hampshire	135	0.31%
48	Vermont	94	0.22%		45	Wyoming	130	0.30%
16	Virginia	922	2.13%		46	Delaware	126	0.29%
23	Washington	743	1.71%		47	Alaska	97	0.22%
34	West Virginia	387	0.89%		48	Vermont	94	0.22%
22	Wisconsin	775	1.79%		49	North Dakota	84	0.19%
45	Wyoming	130	0.30%		50	Rhode Island	80	0.18%
						District of Columbia	68	0.16%

Source: U.S. Department of Health and Human Services, National Center for Health Statistics
   "Monthly Vital Statistics Report" (Vol. 45, No. 11(S)2, June 12, 1997)
*Final data by state of residence. These numbers are compiled from death certificates by the Centers for Disease Control and Prevention. They may differ from motor vehicle deaths collected by the U.S. Department of Transportation from other sources.

Death Rate by Motor Vehicle Accidents in 1995

National Rate = 16.5 Deaths per 100,000 Population*

ALPHA ORDER

RANK	STATE	RATE
3	Alabama	26.8
30	Alaska	16.1
7	Arizona	23.5
5	Arkansas	26.3
37	California	14.1
23	Colorado	18.6
46	Connecticut	10.7
25	Delaware	17.6
20	Florida	19.8
14	Georgia	21.4
44	Hawaii	12.0
9	Idaho	22.7
34	Illinois	14.7
28	Indiana	17.1
21	Iowa	19.2
25	Kansas	17.6
13	Kentucky	22.0
16	Louisiana	21.0
34	Maine	14.7
40	Maryland	13.5
50	Massachusetts	8.0
29	Michigan	17.0
36	Minnesota	14.4
1	Mississippi	33.5
18	Missouri	20.6
10	Montana	22.4
32	Nebraska	15.5
19	Nevada	19.9
45	New Hampshire	11.8
47	New Jersey	10.6
4	New Mexico	26.7
48	New York	9.9
17	North Carolina	20.7
41	North Dakota	13.1
43	Ohio	12.4
11	Oklahoma	22.1
22	Oregon	18.9
41	Pennsylvania	13.1
49	Rhode Island	8.1
8	South Carolina	23.1
11	South Dakota	22.1
6	Tennessee	24.5
24	Texas	17.8
27	Utah	17.2
30	Vermont	16.1
38	Virginia	13.9
39	Washington	13.7
15	West Virginia	21.2
33	Wisconsin	15.1
2	Wyoming	27.1

RANK ORDER

RANK	STATE	RATE
1	Mississippi	33.5
2	Wyoming	27.1
3	Alabama	26.8
4	New Mexico	26.7
5	Arkansas	26.3
6	Tennessee	24.5
7	Arizona	23.5
8	South Carolina	23.1
9	Idaho	22.7
10	Montana	22.4
11	Oklahoma	22.1
11	South Dakota	22.1
13	Kentucky	22.0
14	Georgia	21.4
15	West Virginia	21.2
16	Louisiana	21.0
17	North Carolina	20.7
18	Missouri	20.6
19	Nevada	19.9
20	Florida	19.8
21	Iowa	19.2
22	Oregon	18.9
23	Colorado	18.6
24	Texas	17.8
25	Delaware	17.6
25	Kansas	17.6
27	Utah	17.2
28	Indiana	17.1
29	Michigan	17.0
30	Alaska	16.1
30	Vermont	16.1
32	Nebraska	15.5
33	Wisconsin	15.1
34	Illinois	14.7
34	Maine	14.7
36	Minnesota	14.4
37	California	14.1
38	Virginia	13.9
39	Washington	13.7
40	Maryland	13.5
41	North Dakota	13.1
41	Pennsylvania	13.1
43	Ohio	12.4
44	Hawaii	12.0
45	New Hampshire	11.8
46	Connecticut	10.7
47	New Jersey	10.6
48	New York	9.9
49	Rhode Island	8.1
50	Massachusetts	8.0
	District of Columbia	12.3

Source: U.S. Department of Health and Human Services, National Center for Health Statistics
"Monthly Vital Statistics Report" (Vol. 45, No. 11(S)2, June 12, 1997)
Final data by state of residence. These numbers are compiled from death certificates by the Centers for Disease Control and Prevention. They may differ from motor vehicle deaths collected by the U.S. Department of Transportation from other sources. Not age adjusted.

Deaths by Homicide in 1995

National Total = 22,895 Homicides*

RANK	STATE	HOMICIDES	% of USA
15	Alabama	530	2.31%
40	Alaska	54	0.24%
14	Arizona	537	2.35%
24	Arkansas	287	1.25%
1	California	3,649	15.94%
28	Colorado	213	0.93%
33	Connecticut	149	0.65%
43	Delaware	42	0.18%
5	Florida	1,244	5.43%
9	Georgia	741	3.24%
39	Hawaii	58	0.25%
41	Idaho	47	0.21%
4	Illinois	1,296	5.66%
18	Indiana	450	1.97%
38	Iowa	66	0.29%
32	Kansas	162	0.71%
25	Kentucky	250	1.09%
8	Louisiana	763	3.33%
45	Maine	21	0.09%
11	Maryland	640	2.80%
27	Massachusetts	226	0.99%
6	Michigan	946	4.13%
29	Minnesota	177	0.77%
21	Mississippi	429	1.87%
17	Missouri	475	2.07%
41	Montana	47	0.21%
37	Nebraska	67	0.29%
30	Nevada	171	0.75%
47	New Hampshire	17	0.07%
20	New Jersey	433	1.89%
31	New Mexico	170	0.74%
3	New York	1,582	6.91%
10	North Carolina	692	3.02%
50	North Dakota	13	0.06%
13	Ohio	538	2.35%
19	Oklahoma	441	1.93%
33	Oregon	149	0.65%
7	Pennsylvania	785	3.43%
44	Rhode Island	35	0.15%
22	South Carolina	328	1.43%
46	South Dakota	18	0.08%
12	Tennessee	585	2.56%
2	Texas	1,791	7.82%
36	Utah	76	0.33%
49	Vermont	14	0.06%
16	Virginia	519	2.27%
23	Washington	300	1.31%
35	West Virginia	100	0.44%
26	Wisconsin	242	1.06%
48	Wyoming	15	0.07%

RANK	STATE	HOMICIDES	% of USA
1	California	3,649	15.94%
2	Texas	1,791	7.82%
3	New York	1,582	6.91%
4	Illinois	1,296	5.66%
5	Florida	1,244	5.43%
6	Michigan	946	4.13%
7	Pennsylvania	785	3.43%
8	Louisiana	763	3.33%
9	Georgia	741	3.24%
10	North Carolina	692	3.02%
11	Maryland	640	2.80%
12	Tennessee	585	2.56%
13	Ohio	538	2.35%
14	Arizona	537	2.35%
15	Alabama	530	2.31%
16	Virginia	519	2.27%
17	Missouri	475	2.07%
18	Indiana	450	1.97%
19	Oklahoma	441	1.93%
20	New Jersey	433	1.89%
21	Mississippi	429	1.87%
22	South Carolina	328	1.43%
23	Washington	300	1.31%
24	Arkansas	287	1.25%
25	Kentucky	250	1.09%
26	Wisconsin	242	1.06%
27	Massachusetts	226	0.99%
28	Colorado	213	0.93%
29	Minnesota	177	0.77%
30	Nevada	171	0.75%
31	New Mexico	170	0.74%
32	Kansas	162	0.71%
33	Connecticut	149	0.65%
33	Oregon	149	0.65%
35	West Virginia	100	0.44%
36	Utah	76	0.33%
37	Nebraska	67	0.29%
38	Iowa	66	0.29%
39	Hawaii	58	0.25%
40	Alaska	54	0.24%
41	Idaho	47	0.21%
41	Montana	47	0.21%
43	Delaware	42	0.18%
44	Rhode Island	35	0.15%
45	Maine	21	0.09%
46	South Dakota	18	0.08%
47	New Hampshire	17	0.07%
48	Wyoming	15	0.07%
49	Vermont	14	0.06%
50	North Dakota	13	0.06%
	District of Columbia	315	1.38%

Source: U.S. Department of Health and Human Services, National Center for Health Statistics
     unpublished (http://wonder.cdc.gov/WONDER/)
*By state of residence. Includes legal intervention. Homicide data shown here are collected by the Centers for Disease Control and Prevention based on death certificates and differ from murder data collected by the F.B.I. from other sources.

Death Rate by Homicide in 1995

National Rate = 8.7 Deaths by Homicide per 100,000 Population*

ALPHA ORDER			RANK ORDER		
RANK	STATE	RATE	RANK	STATE	RATE
5	Alabama	12.5	1	Louisiana	17.6
17	Alaska	9.0	2	Mississippi	15.9
5	Arizona	12.5	3	Oklahoma	13.5
8	Arkansas	11.5	4	Maryland	12.7
7	California	11.6	5	Alabama	12.5
28	Colorado	5.7	5	Arizona	12.5
37	Connecticut	4.6	7	California	11.6
27	Delaware	5.9	8	Arkansas	11.5
20	Florida	8.8	9	Nevada	11.1
12	Georgia	10.3	9	Tennessee	11.1
33	Hawaii	4.9	11	Illinois	11.0
39	Idaho	4.0	12	Georgia	10.3
11	Illinois	11.0	13	New Mexico	10.1
22	Indiana	7.8	14	Michigan	9.9
47	Iowa	2.3	15	North Carolina	9.6
26	Kansas	6.3	16	Texas	9.5
24	Kentucky	6.5	17	Alaska	9.0
1	Louisiana	17.6	18	Missouri	8.9
49	Maine	1.7	18	South Carolina	8.9
4	Maryland	12.7	20	Florida	8.8
42	Massachusetts	3.7	21	New York	8.7
14	Michigan	9.9	22	Indiana	7.8
41	Minnesota	3.8	22	Virginia	7.8
2	Mississippi	15.9	24	Kentucky	6.5
18	Missouri	8.9	24	Pennsylvania	6.5
31	Montana	5.4	26	Kansas	6.3
38	Nebraska	4.1	27	Delaware	5.9
9	Nevada	11.1	28	Colorado	5.7
50	New Hampshire	1.5	29	Washington	5.5
31	New Jersey	5.4	29	West Virginia	5.5
13	New Mexico	10.1	31	Montana	5.4
21	New York	8.7	31	New Jersey	5.4
15	North Carolina	9.6	33	Hawaii	4.9
48	North Dakota	2.0	34	Ohio	4.8
34	Ohio	4.8	35	Oregon	4.7
3	Oklahoma	13.5	35	Wisconsin	4.7
35	Oregon	4.7	37	Connecticut	4.6
24	Pennsylvania	6.5	38	Nebraska	4.1
43	Rhode Island	3.5	39	Idaho	4.0
18	South Carolina	8.9	40	Utah	3.9
45	South Dakota	2.5	41	Minnesota	3.8
9	Tennessee	11.1	42	Massachusetts	3.7
16	Texas	9.5	43	Rhode Island	3.5
40	Utah	3.9	44	Wyoming	3.1
46	Vermont	2.4	45	South Dakota	2.5
22	Virginia	7.8	46	Vermont	2.4
29	Washington	5.5	47	Iowa	2.3
29	West Virginia	5.5	48	North Dakota	2.0
35	Wisconsin	4.7	49	Maine	1.7
44	Wyoming	3.1	50	New Hampshire	1.5
				District of Columbia	56.6

Source: U.S. Department of Health and Human Services, National Center for Health Statistics unpublished (http://wonder.cdc.gov/WONDER/)

By state of residence. Includes legal intervention. Homicide data shown here are collected by the Centers for Disease Control and Prevention based on death certificates and differ from murder data collected by the F.B.I. from other sources. Not age adjusted.

Deaths by Suicide in 1995

National Total = 31,284 Deaths*

ALPHA ORDER

RANK	STATE	DEATHS	% of USA
20	Alabama	563	1.80%
44	Alaska	103	0.33%
12	Arizona	805	2.57%
30	Arkansas	360	1.15%
1	California	3,694	11.81%
17	Colorado	654	2.09%
32	Connecticut	323	1.03%
49	Delaware	80	0.26%
3	Florida	2,165	6.92%
11	Georgia	825	2.64%
42	Hawaii	142	0.45%
40	Idaho	186	0.59%
6	Illinois	1,118	3.57%
15	Indiana	698	2.23%
31	Iowa	335	1.07%
35	Kansas	291	0.93%
27	Kentucky	480	1.53%
21	Louisiana	544	1.74%
41	Maine	161	0.51%
23	Maryland	509	1.63%
26	Massachusetts	489	1.56%
8	Michigan	980	3.13%
22	Minnesota	520	1.66%
33	Mississippi	319	1.02%
14	Missouri	721	2.30%
38	Montana	201	0.64%
39	Nebraska	187	0.60%
29	Nevada	395	1.26%
43	New Hampshire	137	0.44%
19	New Jersey	578	1.85%
34	New Mexico	297	0.95%
5	New York	1,370	4.38%
9	North Carolina	908	2.90%
45	North Dakota	94	0.30%
7	Ohio	1,077	3.44%
24	Oklahoma	502	1.60%
25	Oregon	497	1.59%
4	Pennsylvania	1,459	4.66%
46	Rhode Island	89	0.28%
28	South Carolina	436	1.39%
47	South Dakota	86	0.27%
16	Tennessee	681	2.18%
2	Texas	2,234	7.14%
36	Utah	288	0.92%
50	Vermont	76	0.24%
10	Virginia	827	2.64%
13	Washington	781	2.50%
37	West Virginia	276	0.88%
18	Wisconsin	622	1.99%
48	Wyoming	82	0.26%

RANK ORDER

RANK	STATE	DEATHS	% of USA
1	California	3,694	11.81%
2	Texas	2,234	7.14%
3	Florida	2,165	6.92%
4	Pennsylvania	1,459	4.66%
5	New York	1,370	4.38%
6	Illinois	1,118	3.57%
7	Ohio	1,077	3.44%
8	Michigan	980	3.13%
9	North Carolina	908	2.90%
10	Virginia	827	2.64%
11	Georgia	825	2.64%
12	Arizona	805	2.57%
13	Washington	781	2.50%
14	Missouri	721	2.30%
15	Indiana	698	2.23%
16	Tennessee	681	2.18%
17	Colorado	654	2.09%
18	Wisconsin	622	1.99%
19	New Jersey	578	1.85%
20	Alabama	563	1.80%
21	Louisiana	544	1.74%
22	Minnesota	520	1.66%
23	Maryland	509	1.63%
24	Oklahoma	502	1.60%
25	Oregon	497	1.59%
26	Massachusetts	489	1.56%
27	Kentucky	480	1.53%
28	South Carolina	436	1.39%
29	Nevada	395	1.26%
30	Arkansas	360	1.15%
31	Iowa	335	1.07%
32	Connecticut	323	1.03%
33	Mississippi	319	1.02%
34	New Mexico	297	0.95%
35	Kansas	291	0.93%
36	Utah	288	0.92%
37	West Virginia	276	0.88%
38	Montana	201	0.64%
39	Nebraska	187	0.60%
40	Idaho	186	0.59%
41	Maine	161	0.51%
42	Hawaii	142	0.45%
43	New Hampshire	137	0.44%
44	Alaska	103	0.33%
45	North Dakota	94	0.30%
46	Rhode Island	89	0.28%
47	South Dakota	86	0.27%
48	Wyoming	82	0.26%
49	Delaware	80	0.26%
50	Vermont	76	0.24%
	District of Columbia	39	0.12%

Source: U.S. Department of Health and Human Services, National Center for Health Statistics
"Monthly Vital Statistics Report" (Vol. 45, No. 11(S)2, June 12, 1997)
*Final data by state of residence.

Death Rate by Suicide in 1995

National Rate = 11.9 Suicides per 100,000 Population*

ALPHA ORDER

RANK	STATE	RATE
18	Alabama	13.2
6	Alaska	17.1
3	Arizona	19.1
15	Arkansas	14.5
36	California	11.7
5	Colorado	17.5
44	Connecticut	9.9
41	Delaware	11.2
10	Florida	15.3
37	Georgia	11.5
28	Hawaii	12.0
8	Idaho	16.0
46	Illinois	9.5
28	Indiana	12.0
33	Iowa	11.8
39	Kansas	11.3
25	Kentucky	12.4
23	Louisiana	12.5
19	Maine	13.0
43	Maryland	10.1
48	Massachusetts	8.1
42	Michigan	10.3
39	Minnesota	11.3
33	Mississippi	11.8
17	Missouri	13.5
2	Montana	23.1
38	Nebraska	11.4
1	Nevada	25.8
30	New Hampshire	11.9
50	New Jersey	7.3
4	New Mexico	17.6
49	New York	7.6
22	North Carolina	12.6
14	North Dakota	14.7
45	Ohio	9.7
10	Oklahoma	15.3
9	Oregon	15.8
26	Pennsylvania	12.1
47	Rhode Island	9.0
30	South Carolina	11.9
33	South Dakota	11.8
19	Tennessee	13.0
30	Texas	11.9
13	Utah	14.8
19	Vermont	13.0
23	Virginia	12.5
16	Washington	14.4
12	West Virginia	15.1
26	Wisconsin	12.1
6	Wyoming	17.1

RANK ORDER

RANK	STATE	RATE
1	Nevada	25.8
2	Montana	23.1
3	Arizona	19.1
4	New Mexico	17.6
5	Colorado	17.5
6	Alaska	17.1
6	Wyoming	17.1
8	Idaho	16.0
9	Oregon	15.8
10	Florida	15.3
10	Oklahoma	15.3
12	West Virginia	15.1
13	Utah	14.8
14	North Dakota	14.7
15	Arkansas	14.5
16	Washington	14.4
17	Missouri	13.5
18	Alabama	13.2
19	Maine	13.0
19	Tennessee	13.0
19	Vermont	13.0
22	North Carolina	12.6
23	Louisiana	12.5
23	Virginia	12.5
25	Kentucky	12.4
26	Pennsylvania	12.1
26	Wisconsin	12.1
28	Hawaii	12.0
28	Indiana	12.0
30	New Hampshire	11.9
30	South Carolina	11.9
30	Texas	11.9
33	Iowa	11.8
33	Mississippi	11.8
33	South Dakota	11.8
36	California	11.7
37	Georgia	11.5
38	Nebraska	11.4
39	Kansas	11.3
39	Minnesota	11.3
41	Delaware	11.2
42	Michigan	10.3
43	Maryland	10.1
44	Connecticut	9.9
45	Ohio	9.7
46	Illinois	9.5
47	Rhode Island	9.0
48	Massachusetts	8.1
49	New York	7.6
50	New Jersey	7.3
	District of Columbia	7.0

Source: U.S. Department of Health and Human Services, National Center for Health Statistics "Monthly Vital Statistics Report" (Vol. 45, No. 11(S)2, June 12, 1997)
Final data by state of residence. Not age adjusted.

Years Lost by Premature Death in 1994

National Average = 5,390.7 Years Lost per 100,000 Population*

ALPHA ORDER

RANK	STATE	YEARS
3	Alabama	6,665.2
23	Alaska	5,196.6
11	Arizona	5,949.7
4	Arkansas	6,417.7
24	California	5,127.4
36	Colorado	4,652.2
32	Connecticut	4,859.0
20	Delaware	5,372.1
7	Florida	6,065.2
6	Georgia	6,165.8
42	Hawaii	4,258.2
37	Idaho	4,528.7
16	Illinois	5,743.2
25	Indiana	5,118.1
41	Iowa	4,282.2
33	Kansas	4,766.7
21	Kentucky	5,328.5
2	Louisiana	7,053.4
47	Maine	4,132.3
14	Maryland	5,825.7
44	Massachusetts	4,178.0
19	Michigan	5,372.9
48	Minnesota	4,015.5
1	Mississippi	7,436.2
17	Missouri	5,675.6
35	Montana	4,726.4
38	Nebraska	4,479.0
9	Nevada	6,001.8
50	New Hampshire	3,718.0
22	New Jersey	5,243.3
15	New Mexico	5,752.4
12	New York	5,888.2
10	North Carolina	5,995.7
45	North Dakota	4,174.7
31	Ohio	4,864.0
13	Oklahoma	5,841.3
34	Oregon	4,763.7
26	Pennsylvania	5,067.0
46	Rhode Island	4,156.3
5	South Carolina	6,307.7
28	South Dakota	5,032.7
8	Tennessee	6,037.9
18	Texas	5,409.9
40	Utah	4,367.3
49	Vermont	3,794.1
30	Virginia	4,934.8
39	Washington	4,382.9
27	West Virginia	5,057.8
43	Wisconsin	4,242.1
29	Wyoming	4,995.7

RANK ORDER

RANK	STATE	YEARS
1	Mississippi	7,436.2
2	Louisiana	7,053.4
3	Alabama	6,665.2
4	Arkansas	6,417.7
5	South Carolina	6,307.7
6	Georgia	6,165.8
7	Florida	6,065.2
8	Tennessee	6,037.9
9	Nevada	6,001.8
10	North Carolina	5,995.7
11	Arizona	5,949.7
12	New York	5,888.2
13	Oklahoma	5,841.3
14	Maryland	5,825.7
15	New Mexico	5,752.4
16	Illinois	5,743.2
17	Missouri	5,675.6
18	Texas	5,409.9
19	Michigan	5,372.9
20	Delaware	5,372.1
21	Kentucky	5,328.5
22	New Jersey	5,243.3
23	Alaska	5,196.6
24	California	5,127.4
25	Indiana	5,118.1
26	Pennsylvania	5,067.0
27	West Virginia	5,057.8
28	South Dakota	5,032.7
29	Wyoming	4,995.7
30	Virginia	4,934.8
31	Ohio	4,864.0
32	Connecticut	4,859.0
33	Kansas	4,766.7
34	Oregon	4,763.7
35	Montana	4,726.4
36	Colorado	4,652.2
37	Idaho	4,528.7
38	Nebraska	4,479.0
39	Washington	4,382.9
40	Utah	4,367.3
41	Iowa	4,282.2
42	Hawaii	4,258.2
43	Wisconsin	4,242.1
44	Massachusetts	4,178.0
45	North Dakota	4,174.7
46	Rhode Island	4,156.3
47	Maine	4,132.3
48	Minnesota	4,015.5
49	Vermont	3,794.1
50	New Hampshire	3,718.0
	District of Columbia	14,095.1

Source: U.S. Department of Health and Human Services, National Center for Health Statistics
"State Health Profiles"
*Age-adjusted years of potential life lost due to death before age 65.

Years Lost by Premature Death from Cancer in 1994

National Average = 804.2 Years Lost per 100,000 Population*

ALPHA ORDER

RANK	STATE	YEARS
3	Alabama	936.4
49	Alaska	570.8
34	Arizona	744.8
2	Arkansas	943.1
36	California	739.2
44	Colorado	656.4
33	Connecticut	761.8
11	Delaware	883.4
12	Florida	878.9
22	Georgia	817.1
40	Hawaii	675.5
46	Idaho	617.8
24	Illinois	811.0
25	Indiana	802.2
30	Iowa	769.2
21	Kansas	818.4
5	Kentucky	916.1
4	Louisiana	922.7
6	Maine	907.8
23	Maryland	812.0
31	Massachusetts	767.9
18	Michigan	834.1
38	Minnesota	693.1
1	Mississippi	952.1
15	Missouri	851.4
50	Montana	564.1
31	Nebraska	767.9
26	Nevada	795.2
29	New Hampshire	773.4
14	New Jersey	853.3
45	New Mexico	625.6
17	New York	834.3
16	North Carolina	842.1
39	North Dakota	679.9
19	Ohio	833.4
13	Oklahoma	858.6
35	Oregon	742.4
20	Pennsylvania	820.6
9	Rhode Island	894.8
7	South Carolina	899.5
43	South Dakota	663.6
10	Tennessee	890.2
28	Texas	783.6
47	Utah	608.6
42	Vermont	668.9
27	Virginia	788.7
41	Washington	673.5
8	West Virginia	897.1
37	Wisconsin	714.3
48	Wyoming	608.3

RANK ORDER

RANK	STATE	YEARS
1	Mississippi	952.1
2	Arkansas	943.1
3	Alabama	936.4
4	Louisiana	922.7
5	Kentucky	916.1
6	Maine	907.8
7	South Carolina	899.5
8	West Virginia	897.1
9	Rhode Island	894.8
10	Tennessee	890.2
11	Delaware	883.4
12	Florida	878.9
13	Oklahoma	858.6
14	New Jersey	853.3
15	Missouri	851.4
16	North Carolina	842.1
17	New York	834.3
18	Michigan	834.1
19	Ohio	833.4
20	Pennsylvania	820.6
21	Kansas	818.4
22	Georgia	817.1
23	Maryland	812.0
24	Illinois	811.0
25	Indiana	802.2
26	Nevada	795.2
27	Virginia	788.7
28	Texas	783.6
29	New Hampshire	773.4
30	Iowa	769.2
31	Massachusetts	767.9
31	Nebraska	767.9
33	Connecticut	761.8
34	Arizona	744.8
35	Oregon	742.4
36	California	739.2
37	Wisconsin	714.3
38	Minnesota	693.1
39	North Dakota	679.9
40	Hawaii	675.5
41	Washington	673.5
42	Vermont	668.9
43	South Dakota	663.6
44	Colorado	656.4
45	New Mexico	625.6
46	Idaho	617.8
47	Utah	608.6
48	Wyoming	608.3
49	Alaska	570.8
50	Montana	564.1

District of Columbia	1,268.1

Source: U.S. Department of Health and Human Services, National Center for Health Statistics
"State Health Profiles"
Age-adjusted years of potential life lost due to death before age 65.

Years Lost by Premature Death from Heart Disease in 1994

National Average = 610.7 Years Lost per 100,000 Population*

ALPHA ORDER

RANK	STATE	YEARS
2	Alabama	869.1
42	Alaska	459.2
30	Arizona	543.6
8	Arkansas	768.0
39	California	477.4
46	Colorado	416.6
29	Connecticut	556.1
11	Delaware	726.4
26	Florida	584.2
10	Georgia	750.9
24	Hawaii	597.8
41	Idaho	467.9
15	Illinois	665.4
19	Indiana	639.3
36	Iowa	489.0
38	Kansas	480.2
9	Kentucky	755.8
3	Louisiana	862.1
33	Maine	504.4
16	Maryland	657.1
32	Massachusetts	504.7
14	Michigan	677.0
43	Minnesota	445.2
1	Mississippi	1,082.7
13	Missouri	702.5
47	Montana	406.8
34	Nebraska	501.6
17	Nevada	646.8
40	New Hampshire	473.4
28	New Jersey	570.1
49	New Mexico	393.0
23	New York	610.0
12	North Carolina	705.5
37	North Dakota	488.0
18	Ohio	642.3
5	Oklahoma	795.4
48	Oregon	401.8
20	Pennsylvania	636.5
31	Rhode Island	539.0
4	South Carolina	812.9
25	South Dakota	589.9
6	Tennessee	785.9
21	Texas	631.7
50	Utah	391.5
44	Vermont	441.2
22	Virginia	618.6
45	Washington	426.1
7	West Virginia	776.1
35	Wisconsin	494.0
27	Wyoming	576.5

RANK ORDER

RANK	STATE	YEARS
1	Mississippi	1,082.7
2	Alabama	869.1
3	Louisiana	862.1
4	South Carolina	812.9
5	Oklahoma	795.4
6	Tennessee	785.9
7	West Virginia	776.1
8	Arkansas	768.0
9	Kentucky	755.8
10	Georgia	750.9
11	Delaware	726.4
12	North Carolina	705.5
13	Missouri	702.5
14	Michigan	677.0
15	Illinois	665.4
16	Maryland	657.1
17	Nevada	646.8
18	Ohio	642.3
19	Indiana	639.3
20	Pennsylvania	636.5
21	Texas	631.7
22	Virginia	618.6
23	New York	610.0
24	Hawaii	597.8
25	South Dakota	589.9
26	Florida	584.2
27	Wyoming	576.5
28	New Jersey	570.1
29	Connecticut	556.1
30	Arizona	543.6
31	Rhode Island	539.0
32	Massachusetts	504.7
33	Maine	504.4
34	Nebraska	501.6
35	Wisconsin	494.0
36	Iowa	489.0
37	North Dakota	488.0
38	Kansas	480.2
39	California	477.4
40	New Hampshire	473.4
41	Idaho	467.9
42	Alaska	459.2
43	Minnesota	445.2
44	Vermont	441.2
45	Washington	426.1
46	Colorado	416.6
47	Montana	406.8
48	Oregon	401.8
49	New Mexico	393.0
50	Utah	391.5

District of Columbia 1,009.8

Source: U.S. Department of Health and Human Services, National Center for Health Statistics
"State Health Profiles"
*Age-adjusted years of potential life lost due to death before age 65.

Years Lost by Premature Death from HIV Infection in 1994

National Average = 432.8 Years Lost per 100,000 Population*

<table>
<tr><td colspan="3">ALPHA ORDER</td><td colspan="3">RANK ORDER</td></tr>
<tr><td>RANK</td><td>STATE</td><td>YEARS</td><td>RANK</td><td>STATE</td><td>YEARS</td></tr>
<tr><td>22</td><td>Alabama</td><td>280.3</td><td>1</td><td>New York</td><td>1,124.1</td></tr>
<tr><td>46</td><td>Alaska</td><td>82.2</td><td>2</td><td>Florida</td><td>861.4</td></tr>
<tr><td>17</td><td>Arizona</td><td>306.6</td><td>3</td><td>New Jersey</td><td>769.5</td></tr>
<tr><td>32</td><td>Arkansas</td><td>194.3</td><td>4</td><td>Maryland</td><td>611.5</td></tr>
<tr><td>6</td><td>California</td><td>527.6</td><td>5</td><td>Georgia</td><td>549.6</td></tr>
<tr><td>25</td><td>Colorado</td><td>264.4</td><td>6</td><td>California</td><td>527.6</td></tr>
<tr><td>8</td><td>Connecticut</td><td>448.0</td><td>7</td><td>Delaware</td><td>520.3</td></tr>
<tr><td>7</td><td>Delaware</td><td>520.3</td><td>8</td><td>Connecticut</td><td>448.0</td></tr>
<tr><td>2</td><td>Florida</td><td>861.4</td><td>9</td><td>Louisiana</td><td>441.9</td></tr>
<tr><td>5</td><td>Georgia</td><td>549.6</td><td>10</td><td>Texas</td><td>418.4</td></tr>
<tr><td>23</td><td>Hawaii</td><td>273.4</td><td>11</td><td>Massachusetts</td><td>405.3</td></tr>
<tr><td>47</td><td>Idaho</td><td>79.1</td><td>12</td><td>South Carolina</td><td>403.6</td></tr>
<tr><td>16</td><td>Illinois</td><td>325.6</td><td>13</td><td>North Carolina</td><td>380.0</td></tr>
<tr><td>36</td><td>Indiana</td><td>149.8</td><td>14</td><td>Nevada</td><td>376.8</td></tr>
<tr><td>45</td><td>Iowa</td><td>88.3</td><td>15</td><td>Mississippi</td><td>335.5</td></tr>
<tr><td>40</td><td>Kansas</td><td>125.7</td><td>16</td><td>Illinois</td><td>325.6</td></tr>
<tr><td>38</td><td>Kentucky</td><td>139.3</td><td>17</td><td>Arizona</td><td>306.6</td></tr>
<tr><td>9</td><td>Louisiana</td><td>441.9</td><td>18</td><td>Pennsylvania</td><td>306.4</td></tr>
<tr><td>33</td><td>Maine</td><td>156.6</td><td>19</td><td>Rhode Island</td><td>299.6</td></tr>
<tr><td>4</td><td>Maryland</td><td>611.5</td><td>20</td><td>Virginia</td><td>287.9</td></tr>
<tr><td>11</td><td>Massachusetts</td><td>405.3</td><td>21</td><td>Washington</td><td>284.1</td></tr>
<tr><td>30</td><td>Michigan</td><td>219.7</td><td>22</td><td>Alabama</td><td>280.3</td></tr>
<tr><td>34</td><td>Minnesota</td><td>154.5</td><td>23</td><td>Hawaii</td><td>273.4</td></tr>
<tr><td>15</td><td>Mississippi</td><td>335.5</td><td>24</td><td>Oregon</td><td>267.2</td></tr>
<tr><td>27</td><td>Missouri</td><td>248.6</td><td>25</td><td>Colorado</td><td>264.4</td></tr>
<tr><td>44</td><td>Montana</td><td>89.6</td><td>26</td><td>Tennessee</td><td>262.2</td></tr>
<tr><td>37</td><td>Nebraska</td><td>148.9</td><td>27</td><td>Missouri</td><td>248.6</td></tr>
<tr><td>14</td><td>Nevada</td><td>376.8</td><td>28</td><td>Oklahoma</td><td>244.8</td></tr>
<tr><td>43</td><td>New Hampshire</td><td>93.0</td><td>29</td><td>New Mexico</td><td>241.5</td></tr>
<tr><td>3</td><td>New Jersey</td><td>769.5</td><td>30</td><td>Michigan</td><td>219.7</td></tr>
<tr><td>29</td><td>New Mexico</td><td>241.5</td><td>31</td><td>Ohio</td><td>205.3</td></tr>
<tr><td>1</td><td>New York</td><td>1,124.1</td><td>32</td><td>Arkansas</td><td>194.3</td></tr>
<tr><td>13</td><td>North Carolina</td><td>380.0</td><td>33</td><td>Maine</td><td>156.6</td></tr>
<tr><td>NA</td><td>North Dakota**</td><td>NA</td><td>34</td><td>Minnesota</td><td>154.5</td></tr>
<tr><td>31</td><td>Ohio</td><td>205.3</td><td>34</td><td>Vermont</td><td>154.5</td></tr>
<tr><td>28</td><td>Oklahoma</td><td>244.8</td><td>36</td><td>Indiana</td><td>149.8</td></tr>
<tr><td>24</td><td>Oregon</td><td>267.2</td><td>37</td><td>Nebraska</td><td>148.9</td></tr>
<tr><td>18</td><td>Pennsylvania</td><td>306.4</td><td>38</td><td>Kentucky</td><td>139.3</td></tr>
<tr><td>19</td><td>Rhode Island</td><td>299.6</td><td>39</td><td>Utah</td><td>133.2</td></tr>
<tr><td>12</td><td>South Carolina</td><td>403.6</td><td>40</td><td>Kansas</td><td>125.7</td></tr>
<tr><td>NA</td><td>South Dakota**</td><td>NA</td><td>41</td><td>Wisconsin</td><td>113.1</td></tr>
<tr><td>26</td><td>Tennessee</td><td>262.2</td><td>42</td><td>West Virginia</td><td>99.1</td></tr>
<tr><td>10</td><td>Texas</td><td>418.4</td><td>43</td><td>New Hampshire</td><td>93.0</td></tr>
<tr><td>39</td><td>Utah</td><td>133.2</td><td>44</td><td>Montana</td><td>89.6</td></tr>
<tr><td>34</td><td>Vermont</td><td>154.5</td><td>45</td><td>Iowa</td><td>88.3</td></tr>
<tr><td>20</td><td>Virginia</td><td>287.9</td><td>46</td><td>Alaska</td><td>82.2</td></tr>
<tr><td>21</td><td>Washington</td><td>284.1</td><td>47</td><td>Idaho</td><td>79.1</td></tr>
<tr><td>42</td><td>West Virginia</td><td>99.1</td><td>NA</td><td>North Dakota**</td><td>NA</td></tr>
<tr><td>41</td><td>Wisconsin</td><td>113.1</td><td>NA</td><td>South Dakota**</td><td>NA</td></tr>
<tr><td>NA</td><td>Wyoming**</td><td>NA</td><td>NA</td><td>Wyoming**</td><td>NA</td></tr>
<tr><td></td><td></td><td></td><td></td><td>District of Columbia</td><td>2,790.6</td></tr>
</table>

Source: U.S. Department of Health and Human Services, National Center for Health Statistics "State Health Profiles"

*Age-adjusted years of potential life lost due to death before age 65.

**Data for states with fewer than 20 deaths from HIV infection for persons under 65 years of age are considered unreliable and are not shown.

Years Lost by Premature Death from Homicide and Suicide in 1994

National Average = 709.5 Years Lost per 100,000 Population*

ALPHA ORDER

RANK	STATE	YEARS
10	Alabama	864.4
9	Alaska	869.9
3	Arizona	1,009.1
6	Arkansas	903.5
13	California	808.8
23	Colorado	674.5
33	Connecticut	577.3
37	Delaware	508.9
16	Florida	765.4
20	Georgia	728.3
44	Hawaii	438.7
30	Idaho	622.8
12	Illinois	812.2
24	Indiana	667.9
46	Iowa	430.6
27	Kansas	653.6
34	Kentucky	566.3
1	Louisiana	1,213.8
45	Maine	437.3
11	Maryland	834.8
49	Massachusetts	383.4
17	Michigan	763.1
43	Minnesota	446.5
4	Mississippi	971.3
8	Missouri	876.6
26	Montana	661.7
41	Nebraska	463.3
2	Nevada	1,046.8
48	New Hampshire	391.7
47	New Jersey	419.6
5	New Mexico	952.2
22	New York	690.2
15	North Carolina	788.4
39	North Dakota	475.1
40	Ohio	468.3
18	Oklahoma	731.6
28	Oregon	648.5
35	Pennsylvania	562.5
42	Rhode Island	456.5
21	South Carolina	724.3
32	South Dakota	578.8
19	Tennessee	730.3
14	Texas	805.3
31	Utah	590.0
50	Vermont	287.4
25	Virginia	666.4
29	Washington	627.2
36	West Virginia	535.9
38	Wisconsin	503.2
7	Wyoming	890.5

RANK ORDER

RANK	STATE	YEARS
1	Louisiana	1,213.8
2	Nevada	1,046.8
3	Arizona	1,009.1
4	Mississippi	971.3
5	New Mexico	952.2
6	Arkansas	903.5
7	Wyoming	890.5
8	Missouri	876.6
9	Alaska	869.9
10	Alabama	864.4
11	Maryland	834.8
12	Illinois	812.2
13	California	808.8
14	Texas	805.3
15	North Carolina	788.4
16	Florida	765.4
17	Michigan	763.1
18	Oklahoma	731.6
19	Tennessee	730.3
20	Georgia	728.3
21	South Carolina	724.3
22	New York	690.2
23	Colorado	674.5
24	Indiana	667.9
25	Virginia	666.4
26	Montana	661.7
27	Kansas	653.6
28	Oregon	648.5
29	Washington	627.2
30	Idaho	622.8
31	Utah	590.0
32	South Dakota	578.8
33	Connecticut	577.3
34	Kentucky	566.3
35	Pennsylvania	562.5
36	West Virginia	535.9
37	Delaware	508.9
38	Wisconsin	503.2
39	North Dakota	475.1
40	Ohio	468.3
41	Nebraska	463.3
42	Rhode Island	456.5
43	Minnesota	446.5
44	Hawaii	438.7
45	Maine	437.3
46	Iowa	430.6
47	New Jersey	419.6
48	New Hampshire	391.7
49	Massachusetts	383.4
50	Vermont	287.4
	District of Columbia	3,062.7

Source: U.S. Department of Health and Human Services, National Center for Health Statistics
"State Health Profiles"
*Age-adjusted years of potential life lost due to death before age 65.

Years Lost by Premature Death from Unintentional Injuries in 1994

National Average = 928.2 Years Lost per 100,000 Population*

ALPHA ORDER

RANK	STATE	YEARS
7	Alabama	1,361.3
1	Alaska	1,645.5
9	Arizona	1,269.3
6	Arkansas	1,372.9
36	California	840.0
26	Colorado	973.1
41	Connecticut	731.3
30	Delaware	917.5
22	Florida	1,019.3
20	Georgia	1,043.5
42	Hawaii	713.4
14	Idaho	1,213.8
28	Illinois	945.3
31	Indiana	914.7
23	Iowa	1,012.3
24	Kansas	1,003.2
15	Kentucky	1,166.3
13	Louisiana	1,217.0
37	Maine	826.3
43	Maryland	704.5
50	Massachusetts	433.2
34	Michigan	855.9
40	Minnesota	797.4
2	Mississippi	1,599.5
16	Missouri	1,138.5
5	Montana	1,392.1
29	Nebraska	927.3
17	Nevada	1,131.0
48	New Hampshire	615.4
46	New Jersey	673.4
3	New Mexico	1,493.2
47	New York	673.2
18	North Carolina	1,104.4
32	North Dakota	879.3
44	Ohio	687.3
12	Oklahoma	1,236.9
19	Oregon	1,044.6
35	Pennsylvania	849.3
49	Rhode Island	468.1
8	South Carolina	1,282.3
11	South Dakota	1,253.7
10	Tennessee	1,268.4
25	Texas	974.7
27	Utah	947.2
45	Vermont	682.1
39	Virginia	818.1
33	Washington	861.0
21	West Virginia	1,028.5
38	Wisconsin	822.2
4	Wyoming	1,480.4

RANK ORDER

RANK	STATE	YEARS
1	Alaska	1,645.5
2	Mississippi	1,599.5
3	New Mexico	1,493.2
4	Wyoming	1,480.4
5	Montana	1,392.1
6	Arkansas	1,372.9
7	Alabama	1,361.3
8	South Carolina	1,282.3
9	Arizona	1,269.3
10	Tennessee	1,268.4
11	South Dakota	1,253.7
12	Oklahoma	1,236.9
13	Louisiana	1,217.0
14	Idaho	1,213.8
15	Kentucky	1,166.3
16	Missouri	1,138.5
17	Nevada	1,131.0
18	North Carolina	1,104.4
19	Oregon	1,044.6
20	Georgia	1,043.5
21	West Virginia	1,028.5
22	Florida	1,019.3
23	Iowa	1,012.3
24	Kansas	1,003.2
25	Texas	974.7
26	Colorado	973.1
27	Utah	947.2
28	Illinois	945.3
29	Nebraska	927.3
30	Delaware	917.5
31	Indiana	914.7
32	North Dakota	879.3
33	Washington	861.0
34	Michigan	855.9
35	Pennsylvania	849.3
36	California	840.0
37	Maine	826.3
38	Wisconsin	822.2
39	Virginia	818.1
40	Minnesota	797.4
41	Connecticut	731.3
42	Hawaii	713.4
43	Maryland	704.5
44	Ohio	687.3
45	Vermont	682.1
46	New Jersey	673.4
47	New York	673.2
48	New Hampshire	615.4
49	Rhode Island	468.1
50	Massachusetts	433.2

District of Columbia   721.4

Source: U.S. Department of Health and Human Services, National Center for Health Statistics
   "State Health Profiles"

*Age-adjusted years of potential life lost due to death before age 65. Includes such subcategories as falls, drowning, fires/burns, poisonings and motor vehicle injuries.

Estimated Years of Potential Life Lost Attributable to Smoking in 1990

National Estimated Total = 5,062,814 Years of Potential Life Lost*

ALPHA ORDER

RANK ORDER

RANK	STATE	YEARS	% of USA
20	Alabama	90,360	1.78%
50	Alaska	6,720	0.13%
26	Arizona	66,959	1.32%
29	Arkansas	58,742	1.16%
1	California	498,297	9.84%
33	Colorado	49,000	0.97%
27	Connecticut	60,535	1.20%
41	Delaware	15,248	0.30%
3	Florida	328,191	6.48%
11	Georgia	134,168	2.65%
42	Hawaii	15,222	0.30%
43	Idaho	14,708	0.29%
6	Illinois	235,933	4.66%
13	Indiana	123,584	2.44%
32	Iowa	50,521	1.00%
34	Kansas	42,540	0.84%
18	Kentucky	94,602	1.87%
17	Louisiana	94,886	1.87%
37	Maine	27,419	0.54%
19	Maryland	92,197	1.82%
16	Massachusetts	117,640	2.32%
8	Michigan	195,600	3.86%
25	Minnesota	67,835	1.34%
30	Mississippi	57,839	1.14%
14	Missouri	122,136	2.41%
45	Montana	14,491	0.29%
36	Nebraska	29,075	0.57%
35	Nevada	30,254	0.60%
40	New Hampshire	18,993	0.38%
9	New Jersey	151,773	3.00%
39	New Mexico	21,156	0.42%
2	New York	377,530	7.46%
10	North Carolina	147,810	2.92%
47	North Dakota	11,717	0.23%
7	Ohio	231,497	4.57%
24	Oklahoma	73,057	1.44%
28	Oregon	59,217	1.17%
5	Pennsylvania	271,839	5.37%
38	Rhode Island	21,541	0.43%
23	South Carolina	79,069	1.56%
46	South Dakota	12,684	0.25%
12	Tennessee	132,635	2.62%
4	Texas	317,631	6.27%
44	Utah	14,572	0.29%
48	Vermont	10,631	0.21%
15	Virginia	119,716	2.36%
21	Washington	89,222	1.76%
31	West Virginia	51,007	1.01%
22	Wisconsin	86,345	1.71%
49	Wyoming	7,298	0.14%

RANK	STATE	YEARS	% of USA
1	California	498,297	9.84%
2	New York	377,530	7.46%
3	Florida	328,191	6.48%
4	Texas	317,631	6.27%
5	Pennsylvania	271,839	5.37%
6	Illinois	235,933	4.66%
7	Ohio	231,497	4.57%
8	Michigan	195,600	3.86%
9	New Jersey	151,773	3.00%
10	North Carolina	147,810	2.92%
11	Georgia	134,168	2.65%
12	Tennessee	132,635	2.62%
13	Indiana	123,584	2.44%
14	Missouri	122,136	2.41%
15	Virginia	119,716	2.36%
16	Massachusetts	117,640	2.32%
17	Louisiana	94,886	1.87%
18	Kentucky	94,602	1.87%
19	Maryland	92,197	1.82%
20	Alabama	90,360	1.78%
21	Washington	89,222	1.76%
22	Wisconsin	86,345	1.71%
23	South Carolina	79,069	1.56%
24	Oklahoma	73,057	1.44%
25	Minnesota	67,835	1.34%
26	Arizona	66,959	1.32%
27	Connecticut	60,535	1.20%
28	Oregon	59,217	1.17%
29	Arkansas	58,742	1.16%
30	Mississippi	57,839	1.14%
31	West Virginia	51,007	1.01%
32	Iowa	50,521	1.00%
33	Colorado	49,000	0.97%
34	Kansas	42,540	0.84%
35	Nevada	30,254	0.60%
36	Nebraska	29,075	0.57%
37	Maine	27,419	0.54%
38	Rhode Island	21,541	0.43%
39	New Mexico	21,156	0.42%
40	New Hampshire	18,993	0.38%
41	Delaware	15,248	0.30%
42	Hawaii	15,222	0.30%
43	Idaho	14,708	0.29%
44	Utah	14,572	0.29%
45	Montana	14,491	0.29%
46	South Dakota	12,684	0.25%
47	North Dakota	11,717	0.23%
48	Vermont	10,631	0.21%
49	Wyoming	7,298	0.14%
50	Alaska	6,720	0.13%
	District of Columbia	21,172	0.42%

Source: U.S. Department of Health and Human Services, Centers for Disease Control and Prevention
"Surveillance for Smoking-Attributable Mortality, 1990" (MMWR, Vol. 43, No. SS-1, June 10, 1994)
*Calculated by using life expectancy at age of death.

Estimated Deaths Attributable to Smoking in 1990

National Estimated Total = 415,226 Deaths

ALPHA ORDER

RANK	STATE	DEATHS	% of USA
22	Alabama	6,801	1.64%
50	Alaska	402	0.10%
25	Arizona	5,697	1.37%
30	Arkansas	4,706	1.13%
1	California	42,574	10.25%
33	Colorado	4,171	1.00%
27	Connecticut	5,362	1.29%
44	Delaware	1,178	0.28%
3	Florida	28,596	6.89%
15	Georgia	9,694	2.33%
46	Hawaii	1,174	0.28%
42	Idaho	1,304	0.31%
6	Illinois	19,269	4.64%
12	Indiana	10,250	2.47%
29	Iowa	4,816	1.16%
34	Kansas	3,828	0.92%
19	Kentucky	7,449	1.79%
21	Louisiana	6,887	1.66%
36	Maine	2,376	0.57%
20	Maryland	7,370	1.77%
11	Massachusetts	10,430	2.51%
8	Michigan	15,454	3.72%
24	Minnesota	6,127	1.48%
31	Mississippi	4,458	1.07%
14	Missouri	10,177	2.45%
41	Montana	1,313	0.32%
35	Nebraska	2,675	0.64%
37	Nevada	2,234	0.54%
40	New Hampshire	1,655	0.40%
9	New Jersey	12,605	3.04%
39	New Mexico	1,741	0.42%
2	New York	30,992	7.46%
10	North Carolina	11,032	2.66%
47	North Dakota	1,031	0.25%
7	Ohio	18,114	4.36%
23	Oklahoma	6,138	1.48%
28	Oregon	5,226	1.26%
5	Pennsylvania	22,624	5.45%
38	Rhode Island	1,881	0.45%
26	South Carolina	5,619	1.35%
45	South Dakota	1,175	0.28%
13	Tennessee	10,214	2.46%
4	Texas	25,452	6.13%
43	Utah	1,228	0.30%
48	Vermont	913	0.22%
16	Virginia	9,237	2.22%
17	Washington	7,790	1.88%
32	West Virginia	4,221	1.02%
18	Wisconsin	7,620	1.84%
49	Wyoming	659	0.16%

RANK ORDER

RANK	STATE	DEATHS	% of USA
1	California	42,574	10.25%
2	New York	30,992	7.46%
3	Florida	28,596	6.89%
4	Texas	25,452	6.13%
5	Pennsylvania	22,624	5.45%
6	Illinois	19,269	4.64%
7	Ohio	18,114	4.36%
8	Michigan	15,454	3.72%
9	New Jersey	12,605	3.04%
10	North Carolina	11,032	2.66%
11	Massachusetts	10,430	2.51%
12	Indiana	10,250	2.47%
13	Tennessee	10,214	2.46%
14	Missouri	10,177	2.45%
15	Georgia	9,694	2.33%
16	Virginia	9,237	2.22%
17	Washington	7,790	1.88%
18	Wisconsin	7,620	1.84%
19	Kentucky	7,449	1.79%
20	Maryland	7,370	1.77%
21	Louisiana	6,887	1.66%
22	Alabama	6,801	1.64%
23	Oklahoma	6,138	1.48%
24	Minnesota	6,127	1.48%
25	Arizona	5,697	1.37%
26	South Carolina	5,619	1.35%
27	Connecticut	5,362	1.29%
28	Oregon	5,226	1.26%
29	Iowa	4,816	1.16%
30	Arkansas	4,706	1.13%
31	Mississippi	4,458	1.07%
32	West Virginia	4,221	1.02%
33	Colorado	4,171	1.00%
34	Kansas	3,828	0.92%
35	Nebraska	2,675	0.64%
36	Maine	2,376	0.57%
37	Nevada	2,234	0.54%
38	Rhode Island	1,881	0.45%
39	New Mexico	1,741	0.42%
40	New Hampshire	1,655	0.40%
41	Montana	1,313	0.32%
42	Idaho	1,304	0.31%
43	Utah	1,228	0.30%
44	Delaware	1,178	0.28%
45	South Dakota	1,175	0.28%
46	Hawaii	1,174	0.28%
47	North Dakota	1,031	0.25%
48	Vermont	913	0.22%
49	Wyoming	659	0.16%
50	Alaska	402	0.10%
	District of Columbia	1,287	0.31%

*Source: U.S. Department of Health and Human Services, Centers for Disease Control and Prevention
"Surveillance for Smoking-Attributable Mortality, 1990" (MMWR, Vol. 43, No. SS-1, June 10, 1994)*

Estimated Death Rate Attributable to Smoking in 1990

National Estimated Median Rate = 363.3 Deaths per 100,000 Population*

ALPHA ORDER

RANK ORDER

RANK	STATE	RATE		RANK	STATE	RATE
29	Alabama	350.4		1	Nevada	478.1
5	Alaska	398.2		2	Tennessee	442.1
35	Arizona	339.6		3	West Virginia	433.6
16	Arkansas	376.3		4	Kentucky	428.7
24	California	366.3		5	Alaska	398.2
38	Colorado	331.4		6	Indiana	394.3
39	Connecticut	325.7		7	Delaware	393.1
7	Delaware	393.1		8	Oklahoma	390.4
27	Florida	357.5		9	Maine	389.4
13	Georgia	383.5		10	Texas	389.1
49	Hawaii	257.2		11	Louisiana	388.2
47	Idaho	293.2		12	Missouri	383.8
26	Illinois	360.0		13	Georgia	383.5
6	Indiana	394.3		14	South Carolina	380.1
44	Iowa	304.2		15	Maryland	378.1
45	Kansas	300.8		16	Arkansas	376.3
4	Kentucky	428.7		17	Mississippi	375.1
11	Louisiana	388.2		18	Michigan	372.5
9	Maine	389.4		19	Wyoming	371.0
15	Maryland	378.1		20	Oregon	369.3
34	Massachusetts	345.3		21	North Carolina	367.6
18	Michigan	372.5		22	Washington	367.4
46	Minnesota	295.2		23	Virginia	366.6
17	Mississippi	375.1		24	California	366.3
12	Missouri	383.8		25	Vermont	363.3
36	Montana	334.2		26	Illinois	360.0
40	Nebraska	321.0		27	Florida	357.5
1	Nevada	478.1		28	New York	352.8
31	New Hampshire	349.3		29	Alabama	350.4
37	New Jersey	334.1		30	Rhode Island	350.3
48	New Mexico	287.7		31	New Hampshire	349.3
28	New York	352.8		32	Ohio	347.7
21	North Carolina	367.6		33	Pennsylvania	346.8
42	North Dakota	308.2		34	Massachusetts	345.3
32	Ohio	347.7		35	Arizona	339.6
8	Oklahoma	390.4		36	Montana	334.2
20	Oregon	369.3		37	New Jersey	334.1
33	Pennsylvania	346.8		38	Colorado	331.4
30	Rhode Island	350.3		39	Connecticut	325.7
14	South Carolina	380.1		40	Nebraska	321.0
43	South Dakota	307.9		41	Wisconsin	313.3
2	Tennessee	442.1		42	North Dakota	308.2
10	Texas	389.1		43	South Dakota	307.9
50	Utah	218.0		44	Iowa	304.2
25	Vermont	363.3		45	Kansas	300.8
23	Virginia	366.6		46	Minnesota	295.2
22	Washington	367.4		47	Idaho	293.2
3	West Virginia	433.6		48	New Mexico	287.7
41	Wisconsin	313.3		49	Hawaii	257.2
19	Wyoming	371.0		50	Utah	218.0

District of Columbia   444.7

Source: U.S. Department of Health and Human Services, Centers for Disease Control and Prevention
"Surveillance for Smoking-Attributable Mortality, 1990" (MMWR, Vol. 43, No. SS-1, June 10, 1994)
*Per 100,000 population of adults 35 years old or older in 1990. Deaths among infants and burn deaths among persons 1 to 34 years were excluded from rate calculations.

Alcohol-Induced Deaths in 1995

National Total = 20,231 Deaths*

ALPHA ORDER

RANK	STATE	DEATHS	% of USA
26	Alabama	282	1.39%
40	Alaska	93	0.46%
12	Arizona	437	2.16%
34	Arkansas	141	0.70%
1	California	3,476	17.18%
16	Colorado	393	1.94%
31	Connecticut	194	0.96%
50	Delaware	36	0.18%
4	Florida	1,159	5.73%
9	Georgia	569	2.81%
48	Hawaii	43	0.21%
42	Idaho	83	0.41%
6	Illinois	739	3.65%
22	Indiana	307	1.52%
35	Iowa	140	0.69%
37	Kansas	114	0.56%
28	Kentucky	250	1.24%
30	Louisiana	228	1.13%
40	Maine	93	0.46%
20	Maryland	343	1.70%
23	Massachusetts	303	1.50%
7	Michigan	724	3.58%
24	Minnesota	297	1.47%
32	Mississippi	185	0.91%
18	Missouri	346	1.71%
44	Montana	74	0.37%
39	Nebraska	96	0.47%
29	Nevada	235	1.16%
38	New Hampshire	105	0.52%
10	New Jersey	524	2.59%
27	New Mexico	256	1.27%
2	New York	1,690	8.35%
5	North Carolina	763	3.77%
47	North Dakota	46	0.23%
8	Ohio	615	3.04%
25	Oklahoma	294	1.45%
21	Oregon	312	1.54%
11	Pennsylvania	515	2.55%
43	Rhode Island	78	0.39%
13	South Carolina	434	2.15%
45	South Dakota	72	0.36%
15	Tennessee	397	1.96%
3	Texas	1,161	5.74%
36	Utah	134	0.66%
49	Vermont	42	0.21%
18	Virginia	346	1.71%
14	Washington	430	2.13%
33	West Virginia	147	0.73%
17	Wisconsin	358	1.77%
46	Wyoming	60	0.30%

RANK ORDER

RANK	STATE	DEATHS	% of USA
1	California	3,476	17.18%
2	New York	1,690	8.35%
3	Texas	1,161	5.74%
4	Florida	1,159	5.73%
5	North Carolina	763	3.77%
6	Illinois	739	3.65%
7	Michigan	724	3.58%
8	Ohio	615	3.04%
9	Georgia	569	2.81%
10	New Jersey	524	2.59%
11	Pennsylvania	515	2.55%
12	Arizona	437	2.16%
13	South Carolina	434	2.15%
14	Washington	430	2.13%
15	Tennessee	397	1.96%
16	Colorado	393	1.94%
17	Wisconsin	358	1.77%
18	Missouri	346	1.71%
18	Virginia	346	1.71%
20	Maryland	343	1.70%
21	Oregon	312	1.54%
22	Indiana	307	1.52%
23	Massachusetts	303	1.50%
24	Minnesota	297	1.47%
25	Oklahoma	294	1.45%
26	Alabama	282	1.39%
27	New Mexico	256	1.27%
28	Kentucky	250	1.24%
29	Nevada	235	1.16%
30	Louisiana	228	1.13%
31	Connecticut	194	0.96%
32	Mississippi	185	0.91%
33	West Virginia	147	0.73%
34	Arkansas	141	0.70%
35	Iowa	140	0.69%
36	Utah	134	0.66%
37	Kansas	114	0.56%
38	New Hampshire	105	0.52%
39	Nebraska	96	0.47%
40	Alaska	93	0.46%
40	Maine	93	0.46%
42	Idaho	83	0.41%
43	Rhode Island	78	0.39%
44	Montana	74	0.37%
45	South Dakota	72	0.36%
46	Wyoming	60	0.30%
47	North Dakota	46	0.23%
48	Hawaii	43	0.21%
49	Vermont	42	0.21%
50	Delaware	36	0.18%
	District of Columbia	72	0.36%

Source: U.S. Department of Health and Human Services, National Center for Health Statistics (http://wonder.cdc.gov/WONDER/)

By state of residence. Includes excessive blood level of alcohol, accidental poisoning by alcohol and the following alcohol-related causes: psychoses, dependence syndrome, polyneuropathy, cardiomyopathy, gastritis, chronic liver disease and cirrhosis. Excludes accidents, homicides and other causes indirectly related to alcohol use.

Death Rate from Alcohol-Induced Deaths in 1995

National Rate = 7.7 Deaths per 100,000 Population*

ALPHA ORDER

RANK	STATE	RATE
31	Alabama	6.6
1	Alaska	15.4
9	Arizona	10.1
40	Arkansas	5.7
6	California	11.0
8	Colorado	10.5
38	Connecticut	5.9
45	Delaware	5.0
16	Florida	8.2
18	Georgia	7.9
50	Hawaii	3.6
26	Idaho	7.1
36	Illinois	6.3
42	Indiana	5.3
47	Iowa	4.9
48	Kansas	4.4
33	Kentucky	6.5
42	Louisiana	5.3
23	Maine	7.5
29	Maryland	6.8
45	Massachusetts	5.0
21	Michigan	7.6
35	Minnesota	6.4
28	Mississippi	6.9
33	Missouri	6.5
15	Montana	8.5
38	Nebraska	5.9
2	Nevada	15.3
13	New Hampshire	9.1
31	New Jersey	6.6
3	New Mexico	15.1
12	New York	9.3
7	North Carolina	10.6
24	North Dakota	7.2
41	Ohio	5.5
14	Oklahoma	9.0
10	Oregon	9.9
49	Pennsylvania	4.3
18	Rhode Island	7.9
5	South Carolina	11.8
10	South Dakota	9.9
21	Tennessee	7.6
37	Texas	6.2
29	Utah	6.8
24	Vermont	7.2
44	Virginia	5.2
18	Washington	7.9
17	West Virginia	8.1
27	Wisconsin	7.0
4	Wyoming	12.5

RANK ORDER

RANK	STATE	RATE
1	Alaska	15.4
2	Nevada	15.3
3	New Mexico	15.1
4	Wyoming	12.5
5	South Carolina	11.8
6	California	11.0
7	North Carolina	10.6
8	Colorado	10.5
9	Arizona	10.1
10	Oregon	9.9
10	South Dakota	9.9
12	New York	9.3
13	New Hampshire	9.1
14	Oklahoma	9.0
15	Montana	8.5
16	Florida	8.2
17	West Virginia	8.1
18	Georgia	7.9
18	Rhode Island	7.9
18	Washington	7.9
21	Michigan	7.6
21	Tennessee	7.6
23	Maine	7.5
24	North Dakota	7.2
24	Vermont	7.2
26	Idaho	7.1
27	Wisconsin	7.0
28	Mississippi	6.9
29	Maryland	6.8
29	Utah	6.8
31	Alabama	6.6
31	New Jersey	6.6
33	Kentucky	6.5
33	Missouri	6.5
35	Minnesota	6.4
36	Illinois	6.3
37	Texas	6.2
38	Connecticut	5.9
38	Nebraska	5.9
40	Arkansas	5.7
41	Ohio	5.5
42	Indiana	5.3
42	Louisiana	5.3
44	Virginia	5.2
45	Delaware	5.0
45	Massachusetts	5.0
47	Iowa	4.9
48	Kansas	4.4
49	Pennsylvania	4.3
50	Hawaii	3.6

District of Columbia	12.9

Source: U.S. Department of Health and Human Services, National Center for Health Statistics
(http://wonder.cdc.gov/WONDER/)

*By state of residence. Includes excessive blood level of alcohol, accidental poisoning by alcohol and the following alcohol-related causes: psychoses, dependence syndrome, polyneuropathy, cardiomyopathy, gastritis, chronic liver disease and cirrhosis. Excludes accidents, homicides and other causes indirectly related to alcohol use. Not age adjusted.

Drug-Induced Deaths in 1995

National Total = 14,218 Deaths*

ALPHA ORDER

RANK	STATE	DEATHS	% of USA
31	Alabama	111	0.78%
46	Alaska	31	0.22%
12	Arizona	360	2.53%
34	Arkansas	75	0.53%
1	California	2,317	16.30%
14	Colorado	277	1.95%
17	Connecticut	250	1.76%
38	Delaware	47	0.33%
6	Florida	653	4.59%
20	Georgia	215	1.51%
33	Hawaii	83	0.58%
39	Idaho	46	0.32%
7	Illinois	590	4.15%
23	Indiana	177	1.24%
35	Iowa	67	0.47%
42	Kansas	38	0.27%
29	Kentucky	127	0.89%
24	Louisiana	161	1.13%
41	Maine	41	0.29%
8	Maryland	532	3.74%
11	Massachusetts	437	3.07%
9	Michigan	453	3.19%
32	Minnesota	96	0.68%
37	Mississippi	61	0.43%
22	Missouri	189	1.33%
45	Montana	32	0.23%
44	Nebraska	34	0.24%
24	Nevada	161	1.13%
40	New Hampshire	44	0.31%
5	New Jersey	755	5.31%
21	New Mexico	196	1.38%
2	New York	1,239	8.71%
16	North Carolina	254	1.79%
50	North Dakota	4	0.03%
13	Ohio	348	2.45%
28	Oklahoma	128	0.90%
18	Oregon	245	1.72%
3	Pennsylvania	977	6.87%
36	Rhode Island	63	0.44%
27	South Carolina	132	0.93%
48	South Dakota	13	0.09%
19	Tennessee	216	1.52%
4	Texas	869	6.11%
29	Utah	127	0.89%
47	Vermont	22	0.15%
15	Virginia	257	1.81%
10	Washington	447	3.14%
42	West Virginia	38	0.27%
26	Wisconsin	159	1.12%
49	Wyoming	9	0.06%

RANK ORDER

RANK	STATE	DEATHS	% of USA
1	California	2,317	16.30%
2	New York	1,239	8.71%
3	Pennsylvania	977	6.87%
4	Texas	869	6.11%
5	New Jersey	755	5.31%
6	Florida	653	4.59%
7	Illinois	590	4.15%
8	Maryland	532	3.74%
9	Michigan	453	3.19%
10	Washington	447	3.14%
11	Massachusetts	437	3.07%
12	Arizona	360	2.53%
13	Ohio	348	2.45%
14	Colorado	277	1.95%
15	Virginia	257	1.81%
16	North Carolina	254	1.79%
17	Connecticut	250	1.76%
18	Oregon	245	1.72%
19	Tennessee	216	1.52%
20	Georgia	215	1.51%
21	New Mexico	196	1.38%
22	Missouri	189	1.33%
23	Indiana	177	1.24%
24	Louisiana	161	1.13%
24	Nevada	161	1.13%
26	Wisconsin	159	1.12%
27	South Carolina	132	0.93%
28	Oklahoma	128	0.90%
29	Kentucky	127	0.89%
29	Utah	127	0.89%
31	Alabama	111	0.78%
32	Minnesota	96	0.68%
33	Hawaii	83	0.58%
34	Arkansas	75	0.53%
35	Iowa	67	0.47%
36	Rhode Island	63	0.44%
37	Mississippi	61	0.43%
38	Delaware	47	0.33%
39	Idaho	46	0.32%
40	New Hampshire	44	0.31%
41	Maine	41	0.29%
42	Kansas	38	0.27%
42	West Virginia	38	0.27%
44	Nebraska	34	0.24%
45	Montana	32	0.23%
46	Alaska	31	0.22%
47	Vermont	22	0.15%
48	South Dakota	13	0.09%
49	Wyoming	9	0.06%
50	North Dakota	4	0.03%
	District of Columbia	15	0.11%

Source: U.S. Department of Health and Human Services, National Center for Health Statistics (http://wonder.cdc.gov/WONDER/)

By state of residence. Includes drug psychoses, drug dependence, nondependent use excluding alcohol and tobacco, accidental poisoning or suicide by drugs, medicaments and biologicals. Excludes accidents, homicides and other causes indirectly related to drug use.

Death Rate from Drug-Induced Deaths in 1995

National Rate = 5.4 Deaths per 100,000 Population*

ALPHA ORDER

RANK	STATE	RATE
41	Alabama	2.6
18	Alaska	5.1
5	Arizona	8.4
39	Arkansas	3.0
11	California	7.3
10	Colorado	7.4
9	Connecticut	7.6
15	Delaware	6.6
21	Florida	4.6
39	Georgia	3.0
13	Hawaii	7.0
24	Idaho	3.9
19	Illinois	5.0
36	Indiana	3.1
42	Iowa	2.4
49	Kansas	1.5
34	Kentucky	3.3
29	Louisiana	3.7
34	Maine	3.3
2	Maryland	10.6
12	Massachusetts	7.2
20	Michigan	4.7
44	Minnesota	2.1
43	Mississippi	2.3
31	Missouri	3.6
29	Montana	3.7
44	Nebraska	2.1
3	Nevada	10.5
27	New Hampshire	3.8
4	New Jersey	9.5
1	New Mexico	11.6
14	New York	6.8
33	North Carolina	3.5
50	North Dakota	0.6
36	Ohio	3.1
24	Oklahoma	3.9
8	Oregon	7.8
7	Pennsylvania	8.1
17	Rhode Island	6.4
31	South Carolina	3.6
48	South Dakota	1.8
23	Tennessee	4.1
21	Texas	4.6
16	Utah	6.5
27	Vermont	3.8
24	Virginia	3.9
6	Washington	8.2
44	West Virginia	2.1
36	Wisconsin	3.1
47	Wyoming	1.9

RANK ORDER

RANK	STATE	RATE
1	New Mexico	11.6
2	Maryland	10.6
3	Nevada	10.5
4	New Jersey	9.5
5	Arizona	8.4
6	Washington	8.2
7	Pennsylvania	8.1
8	Oregon	7.8
9	Connecticut	7.6
10	Colorado	7.4
11	California	7.3
12	Massachusetts	7.2
13	Hawaii	7.0
14	New York	6.8
15	Delaware	6.6
16	Utah	6.5
17	Rhode Island	6.4
18	Alaska	5.1
19	Illinois	5.0
20	Michigan	4.7
21	Florida	4.6
21	Texas	4.6
23	Tennessee	4.1
24	Idaho	3.9
24	Oklahoma	3.9
24	Virginia	3.9
27	New Hampshire	3.8
27	Vermont	3.8
29	Louisiana	3.7
29	Montana	3.7
31	Missouri	3.6
31	South Carolina	3.6
33	North Carolina	3.5
34	Kentucky	3.3
34	Maine	3.3
36	Indiana	3.1
36	Ohio	3.1
36	Wisconsin	3.1
39	Arkansas	3.0
39	Georgia	3.0
41	Alabama	2.6
42	Iowa	2.4
43	Mississippi	2.3
44	Minnesota	2.1
44	Nebraska	2.1
44	West Virginia	2.1
47	Wyoming	1.9
48	South Dakota	1.8
49	Kansas	1.5
50	North Dakota	0.6

District of Columbia 2.7

Source: U.S. Department of Health and Human Services, National Center for Health Statistics
    (http://wonder.cdc.gov/WONDER/)
*By state of residence. Includes drug psychoses, drug dependence, nondependent use excluding alcohol and
tobacco, accidental poisoning or suicide by drugs, medicaments and biologicals. Excludes accidents, homicides
and other causes indirectly related to drug use. Not age adjusted.

Occupational Fatalities in 1996

National Total = 6,105 Deaths*

ALPHA ORDER

RANK	STATE	DEATHS	% of USA
11	Alabama	153	2.51%
34	Alaska	63	1.03%
30	Arizona	71	1.16%
25	Arkansas	88	1.44%
1	California	599	9.81%
24	Colorado	90	1.47%
41	Connecticut	35	0.57%
47	Delaware	18	0.29%
3	Florida	333	5.45%
7	Georgia	213	3.49%
44	Hawaii	27	0.44%
35	Idaho	62	1.02%
6	Illinois	262	4.29%
14	Indiana	143	2.34%
31	Iowa	70	1.15%
27	Kansas	85	1.39%
15	Kentucky	141	2.31%
19	Louisiana	103	1.69%
45	Maine	23	0.38%
29	Maryland	82	1.34%
35	Massachusetts	62	1.02%
10	Michigan	155	2.54%
23	Minnesota	92	1.51%
19	Mississippi	103	1.69%
16	Missouri	140	2.29%
40	Montana	50	0.82%
38	Nebraska	56	0.92%
39	Nevada	52	0.85%
48	New Hampshire	11	0.18%
22	New Jersey	99	1.62%
37	New Mexico	60	0.98%
4	New York	317	5.19%
9	North Carolina	191	3.13%
45	North Dakota	23	0.38%
8	Ohio	201	3.29%
26	Oklahoma	87	1.43%
27	Oregon	85	1.39%
5	Pennsylvania	282	4.62%
50	Rhode Island	6	0.10%
21	South Carolina	101	1.65%
42	South Dakota	32	0.52%
13	Tennessee	152	2.49%
2	Texas	514	8.42%
33	Utah	64	1.05%
49	Vermont	7	0.11%
11	Virginia	153	2.51%
17	Washington	128	2.10%
32	West Virginia	66	1.08%
18	Wisconsin	108	1.77%
43	Wyoming	28	0.46%

RANK ORDER

RANK	STATE	DEATHS	% of USA
1	California	599	9.81%
2	Texas	514	8.42%
3	Florida	333	5.45%
4	New York	317	5.19%
5	Pennsylvania	282	4.62%
6	Illinois	262	4.29%
7	Georgia	213	3.49%
8	Ohio	201	3.29%
9	North Carolina	191	3.13%
10	Michigan	155	2.54%
11	Alabama	153	2.51%
11	Virginia	153	2.51%
13	Tennessee	152	2.49%
14	Indiana	143	2.34%
15	Kentucky	141	2.31%
16	Missouri	140	2.29%
17	Washington	128	2.10%
18	Wisconsin	108	1.77%
19	Louisiana	103	1.69%
19	Mississippi	103	1.69%
21	South Carolina	101	1.65%
22	New Jersey	99	1.62%
23	Minnesota	92	1.51%
24	Colorado	90	1.47%
25	Arkansas	88	1.44%
26	Oklahoma	87	1.43%
27	Kansas	85	1.39%
27	Oregon	85	1.39%
29	Maryland	82	1.34%
30	Arizona	71	1.16%
31	Iowa	70	1.15%
32	West Virginia	66	1.08%
33	Utah	64	1.05%
34	Alaska	63	1.03%
35	Idaho	62	1.02%
35	Massachusetts	62	1.02%
37	New Mexico	60	0.98%
38	Nebraska	56	0.92%
39	Nevada	52	0.85%
40	Montana	50	0.82%
41	Connecticut	35	0.57%
42	South Dakota	32	0.52%
43	Wyoming	28	0.46%
44	Hawaii	27	0.44%
45	Maine	23	0.38%
45	North Dakota	23	0.38%
47	Delaware	18	0.29%
48	New Hampshire	11	0.18%
49	Vermont	7	0.11%
50	Rhode Island	6	0.10%
	District of Columbia	19	0.31%

Source: U.S. Department of Labor, Bureau of Labor Statistics
"National Census of Fatal Occupational Injuries, 1996" (press release, August 7, 1997)
*Does not include seven fatalities occurring outside the territorial boundaries of the 50 states.

Occupational Fatalities per 100,000 Workers in 1996

National Rate = 4.8 Deaths per 100,000 Workers*

ALPHA ORDER

RANK	STATE	RATE
10	Alabama	7.6
1	Alaska	21.8
42	Arizona	3.4
11	Arkansas	7.4
36	California	4.1
34	Colorado	4.5
47	Connecticut	2.1
28	Delaware	4.9
26	Florida	5.0
17	Georgia	5.8
29	Hawaii	4.8
4	Idaho	10.4
34	Illinois	4.5
29	Indiana	4.8
32	Iowa	4.6
13	Kansas	6.5
8	Kentucky	7.9
22	Louisiana	5.5
41	Maine	3.6
44	Maryland	3.0
48	Massachusetts	2.0
43	Michigan	3.3
39	Minnesota	3.7
6	Mississippi	8.6
25	Missouri	5.1
2	Montana	11.5
16	Nebraska	6.3
15	Nevada	6.4
49	New Hampshire	1.8
45	New Jersey	2.6
8	New Mexico	7.9
37	New York	3.9
23	North Carolina	5.3
12	North Dakota	6.9
39	Ohio	3.7
19	Oklahoma	5.7
24	Oregon	5.2
26	Pennsylvania	5.0
50	Rhode Island	1.3
19	South Carolina	5.7
7	South Dakota	8.4
17	Tennessee	5.8
21	Texas	5.6
13	Utah	6.5
46	Vermont	2.2
32	Virginia	4.6
31	Washington	4.7
5	West Virginia	8.8
38	Wisconsin	3.8
3	Wyoming	11.4

RANK ORDER

RANK	STATE	RATE
1	Alaska	21.8
2	Montana	11.5
3	Wyoming	11.4
4	Idaho	10.4
5	West Virginia	8.8
6	Mississippi	8.6
7	South Dakota	8.4
8	Kentucky	7.9
8	New Mexico	7.9
10	Alabama	7.6
11	Arkansas	7.4
12	North Dakota	6.9
13	Kansas	6.5
13	Utah	6.5
15	Nevada	6.4
16	Nebraska	6.3
17	Georgia	5.8
17	Tennessee	5.8
19	Oklahoma	5.7
19	South Carolina	5.7
21	Texas	5.6
22	Louisiana	5.5
23	North Carolina	5.3
24	Oregon	5.2
25	Missouri	5.1
26	Florida	5.0
26	Pennsylvania	5.0
28	Delaware	4.9
29	Hawaii	4.8
29	Indiana	4.8
31	Washington	4.7
32	Iowa	4.6
32	Virginia	4.6
34	Colorado	4.5
34	Illinois	4.5
36	California	4.1
37	New York	3.9
38	Wisconsin	3.8
39	Minnesota	3.7
39	Ohio	3.7
41	Maine	3.6
42	Arizona	3.4
43	Michigan	3.3
44	Maryland	3.0
45	New Jersey	2.6
46	Vermont	2.2
47	Connecticut	2.1
48	Massachusetts	2.0
49	New Hampshire	1.8
50	Rhode Island	1.3

District of Columbia — 7.7

Source: Morgan Quitno Press using data from U.S. Department of Labor, Bureau of Labor Statistics
"National Census of Fatal Occupational Injuries, 1996" (press release, August 7, 1997)
*Does not include seven fatalities occurring outside the territorial boundaries of the 50 states.

III. FACILITIES

Community Hospitals in 1996

National Total = 5,134 Hospitals*

<table>
<tr><td colspan="4"><u>ALPHA ORDER</u></td><td colspan="4"><u>RANK ORDER</u></td></tr>
<tr><td>RANK</td><td>STATE</td><td>HOSPITALS</td><td>% of USA</td><td>RANK</td><td>STATE</td><td>HOSPITALS</td><td>% of USA</td></tr>
<tr><td>19</td><td>Alabama</td><td>113</td><td>2.20%</td><td>1</td><td>California</td><td>420</td><td>8.18%</td></tr>
<tr><td>47</td><td>Alaska</td><td>17</td><td>0.33%</td><td>2</td><td>Texas</td><td>408</td><td>7.95%</td></tr>
<tr><td>32</td><td>Arizona</td><td>61</td><td>1.19%</td><td>3</td><td>New York</td><td>227</td><td>4.42%</td></tr>
<tr><td>28</td><td>Arkansas</td><td>84</td><td>1.64%</td><td>4</td><td>Pennsylvania</td><td>223</td><td>4.34%</td></tr>
<tr><td>1</td><td>California</td><td>420</td><td>8.18%</td><td>5</td><td>Florida</td><td>210</td><td>4.09%</td></tr>
<tr><td>29</td><td>Colorado</td><td>68</td><td>1.32%</td><td>6</td><td>Illinois</td><td>205</td><td>3.99%</td></tr>
<tr><td>42</td><td>Connecticut</td><td>33</td><td>0.64%</td><td>7</td><td>Ohio</td><td>178</td><td>3.47%</td></tr>
<tr><td>50</td><td>Delaware</td><td>6</td><td>0.12%</td><td>8</td><td>Michigan</td><td>164</td><td>3.19%</td></tr>
<tr><td>5</td><td>Florida</td><td>210</td><td>4.09%</td><td>9</td><td>Georgia</td><td>159</td><td>3.10%</td></tr>
<tr><td>9</td><td>Georgia</td><td>159</td><td>3.10%</td><td>10</td><td>Minnesota</td><td>142</td><td>2.77%</td></tr>
<tr><td>45</td><td>Hawaii</td><td>21</td><td>0.41%</td><td>11</td><td>Kansas</td><td>131</td><td>2.55%</td></tr>
<tr><td>38</td><td>Idaho</td><td>42</td><td>0.82%</td><td>12</td><td>Louisiana</td><td>129</td><td>2.51%</td></tr>
<tr><td>6</td><td>Illinois</td><td>205</td><td>3.99%</td><td>13</td><td>Missouri</td><td>125</td><td>2.43%</td></tr>
<tr><td>17</td><td>Indiana</td><td>115</td><td>2.24%</td><td>14</td><td>Tennessee</td><td>124</td><td>2.42%</td></tr>
<tr><td>17</td><td>Iowa</td><td>115</td><td>2.24%</td><td>14</td><td>Wisconsin</td><td>124</td><td>2.42%</td></tr>
<tr><td>11</td><td>Kansas</td><td>131</td><td>2.55%</td><td>16</td><td>North Carolina</td><td>119</td><td>2.32%</td></tr>
<tr><td>21</td><td>Kentucky</td><td>104</td><td>2.03%</td><td>17</td><td>Indiana</td><td>115</td><td>2.24%</td></tr>
<tr><td>12</td><td>Louisiana</td><td>129</td><td>2.51%</td><td>17</td><td>Iowa</td><td>115</td><td>2.24%</td></tr>
<tr><td>40</td><td>Maine</td><td>39</td><td>0.76%</td><td>19</td><td>Alabama</td><td>113</td><td>2.20%</td></tr>
<tr><td>35</td><td>Maryland</td><td>51</td><td>0.99%</td><td>20</td><td>Oklahoma</td><td>108</td><td>2.10%</td></tr>
<tr><td>27</td><td>Massachusetts</td><td>88</td><td>1.71%</td><td>21</td><td>Kentucky</td><td>104</td><td>2.03%</td></tr>
<tr><td>8</td><td>Michigan</td><td>164</td><td>3.19%</td><td>22</td><td>Mississippi</td><td>97</td><td>1.89%</td></tr>
<tr><td>10</td><td>Minnesota</td><td>142</td><td>2.77%</td><td>23</td><td>Virginia</td><td>95</td><td>1.85%</td></tr>
<tr><td>22</td><td>Mississippi</td><td>97</td><td>1.89%</td><td>24</td><td>Nebraska</td><td>90</td><td>1.75%</td></tr>
<tr><td>13</td><td>Missouri</td><td>125</td><td>2.43%</td><td>24</td><td>Washington</td><td>90</td><td>1.75%</td></tr>
<tr><td>34</td><td>Montana</td><td>53</td><td>1.03%</td><td>26</td><td>New Jersey</td><td>89</td><td>1.73%</td></tr>
<tr><td>24</td><td>Nebraska</td><td>90</td><td>1.75%</td><td>27</td><td>Massachusetts</td><td>88</td><td>1.71%</td></tr>
<tr><td>46</td><td>Nevada</td><td>20</td><td>0.39%</td><td>28</td><td>Arkansas</td><td>84</td><td>1.64%</td></tr>
<tr><td>43</td><td>New Hampshire</td><td>28</td><td>0.55%</td><td>29</td><td>Colorado</td><td>68</td><td>1.32%</td></tr>
<tr><td>26</td><td>New Jersey</td><td>89</td><td>1.73%</td><td>30</td><td>South Carolina</td><td>66</td><td>1.29%</td></tr>
<tr><td>41</td><td>New Mexico</td><td>36</td><td>0.70%</td><td>31</td><td>Oregon</td><td>63</td><td>1.23%</td></tr>
<tr><td>3</td><td>New York</td><td>227</td><td>4.42%</td><td>32</td><td>Arizona</td><td>61</td><td>1.19%</td></tr>
<tr><td>16</td><td>North Carolina</td><td>119</td><td>2.32%</td><td>33</td><td>West Virginia</td><td>59</td><td>1.15%</td></tr>
<tr><td>37</td><td>North Dakota</td><td>43</td><td>0.84%</td><td>34</td><td>Montana</td><td>53</td><td>1.03%</td></tr>
<tr><td>7</td><td>Ohio</td><td>178</td><td>3.47%</td><td>35</td><td>Maryland</td><td>51</td><td>0.99%</td></tr>
<tr><td>20</td><td>Oklahoma</td><td>108</td><td>2.10%</td><td>36</td><td>South Dakota</td><td>49</td><td>0.95%</td></tr>
<tr><td>31</td><td>Oregon</td><td>63</td><td>1.23%</td><td>37</td><td>North Dakota</td><td>43</td><td>0.84%</td></tr>
<tr><td>4</td><td>Pennsylvania</td><td>223</td><td>4.34%</td><td>38</td><td>Idaho</td><td>42</td><td>0.82%</td></tr>
<tr><td>49</td><td>Rhode Island</td><td>11</td><td>0.21%</td><td>39</td><td>Utah</td><td>41</td><td>0.80%</td></tr>
<tr><td>30</td><td>South Carolina</td><td>66</td><td>1.29%</td><td>40</td><td>Maine</td><td>39</td><td>0.76%</td></tr>
<tr><td>36</td><td>South Dakota</td><td>49</td><td>0.95%</td><td>41</td><td>New Mexico</td><td>36</td><td>0.70%</td></tr>
<tr><td>14</td><td>Tennessee</td><td>124</td><td>2.42%</td><td>42</td><td>Connecticut</td><td>33</td><td>0.64%</td></tr>
<tr><td>2</td><td>Texas</td><td>408</td><td>7.95%</td><td>43</td><td>New Hampshire</td><td>28</td><td>0.55%</td></tr>
<tr><td>39</td><td>Utah</td><td>41</td><td>0.80%</td><td>44</td><td>Wyoming</td><td>25</td><td>0.49%</td></tr>
<tr><td>48</td><td>Vermont</td><td>14</td><td>0.27%</td><td>45</td><td>Hawaii</td><td>21</td><td>0.41%</td></tr>
<tr><td>23</td><td>Virginia</td><td>95</td><td>1.85%</td><td>46</td><td>Nevada</td><td>20</td><td>0.39%</td></tr>
<tr><td>24</td><td>Washington</td><td>90</td><td>1.75%</td><td>47</td><td>Alaska</td><td>17</td><td>0.33%</td></tr>
<tr><td>33</td><td>West Virginia</td><td>59</td><td>1.15%</td><td>48</td><td>Vermont</td><td>14</td><td>0.27%</td></tr>
<tr><td>14</td><td>Wisconsin</td><td>124</td><td>2.42%</td><td>49</td><td>Rhode Island</td><td>11</td><td>0.21%</td></tr>
<tr><td>44</td><td>Wyoming</td><td>25</td><td>0.49%</td><td>50</td><td>Delaware</td><td>6</td><td>0.12%</td></tr>
<tr><td></td><td></td><td></td><td></td><td></td><td>District of Columbia</td><td>12</td><td>0.23%</td></tr>
</table>

Source: American Hospital Association (Chicago, IL)
   "Hospital Statistics" (1998 edition)
*Community hospitals are all nonfederal, short-term, general and special hospitals whose facilities and services are available to the public.

Community Hospitals per 100,000 Population in 1996

National Rate = 1.9 Community Hospitals per 100,000 Population*

ALPHA ORDER

RANK	STATE	RATE
18	Alabama	2.6
16	Alaska	2.8
40	Arizona	1.4
10	Arkansas	3.4
43	California	1.3
31	Colorado	1.8
48	Connecticut	1.0
50	Delaware	0.8
39	Florida	1.5
24	Georgia	2.2
31	Hawaii	1.8
9	Idaho	3.5
34	Illinois	1.7
27	Indiana	2.0
7	Iowa	4.0
6	Kansas	5.1
17	Kentucky	2.7
15	Louisiana	3.0
13	Maine	3.1
48	Maryland	1.0
40	Massachusetts	1.4
34	Michigan	1.7
13	Minnesota	3.1
8	Mississippi	3.6
22	Missouri	2.3
3	Montana	6.0
4	Nebraska	5.5
45	Nevada	1.2
19	New Hampshire	2.4
46	New Jersey	1.1
25	New Mexico	2.1
43	New York	1.3
36	North Carolina	1.6
1	North Dakota	6.7
36	Ohio	1.6
11	Oklahoma	3.3
27	Oregon	2.0
30	Pennsylvania	1.9
46	Rhode Island	1.1
31	South Carolina	1.8
2	South Dakota	6.6
22	Tennessee	2.3
25	Texas	2.1
27	Utah	2.0
19	Vermont	2.4
40	Virginia	1.4
36	Washington	1.6
12	West Virginia	3.2
19	Wisconsin	2.4
5	Wyoming	5.2

RANK ORDER

RANK	STATE	RATE
1	North Dakota	6.7
2	South Dakota	6.6
3	Montana	6.0
4	Nebraska	5.5
5	Wyoming	5.2
6	Kansas	5.1
7	Iowa	4.0
8	Mississippi	3.6
9	Idaho	3.5
10	Arkansas	3.4
11	Oklahoma	3.3
12	West Virginia	3.2
13	Maine	3.1
13	Minnesota	3.1
15	Louisiana	3.0
16	Alaska	2.8
17	Kentucky	2.7
18	Alabama	2.6
19	New Hampshire	2.4
19	Vermont	2.4
19	Wisconsin	2.4
22	Missouri	2.3
22	Tennessee	2.3
24	Georgia	2.2
25	New Mexico	2.1
25	Texas	2.1
27	Indiana	2.0
27	Oregon	2.0
27	Utah	2.0
30	Pennsylvania	1.9
31	Colorado	1.8
31	Hawaii	1.8
31	South Carolina	1.8
34	Illinois	1.7
34	Michigan	1.7
36	North Carolina	1.6
36	Ohio	1.6
36	Washington	1.6
39	Florida	1.5
40	Arizona	1.4
40	Massachusetts	1.4
40	Virginia	1.4
43	California	1.3
43	New York	1.3
45	Nevada	1.2
46	New Jersey	1.1
46	Rhode Island	1.1
48	Connecticut	1.0
48	Maryland	1.0
50	Delaware	0.8

District of Columbia	2.2

Source: Morgan Quitno Press using data from American Hospital Association (Chicago, IL)
"Hospital Statistics" (1998 edition)
*Community hospitals are all nonfederal, short-term, general and special hospitals whose facilities and services are available to the public.

Community Hospitals per 1,000 Square Miles in 1996

National Rate = 1.38 Community Hospitals*

ALPHA ORDER				RANK ORDER		
RANK	STATE	RATE		RANK	STATE	RATE
23	Alabama	2.16		1	New Jersey	10.83
50	Alaska	0.03		2	Massachusetts	9.52
43	Arizona	0.54		3	Rhode Island	8.94
32	Arkansas	1.58		4	Connecticut	5.95
16	California	2.64		5	Pennsylvania	4.84
39	Colorado	0.65		6	New York	4.20
4	Connecticut	5.95		7	Maryland	4.15
19	Delaware	2.50		8	Ohio	3.97
10	Florida	3.50		9	Illinois	3.54
15	Georgia	2.70		10	Florida	3.50
11	Hawaii	3.25		11	Hawaii	3.25
44	Idaho	0.50		12	Indiana	3.16
9	Illinois	3.54		13	New Hampshire	3.02
12	Indiana	3.16		14	Tennessee	2.94
25	Iowa	2.04		15	Georgia	2.70
31	Kansas	1.59		16	California	2.64
18	Kentucky	2.57		17	Louisiana	2.60
17	Louisiana	2.60		18	Kentucky	2.57
37	Maine	1.16		19	Delaware	2.50
7	Maryland	4.15		20	West Virginia	2.43
2	Massachusetts	9.52		21	North Carolina	2.26
29	Michigan	1.70		22	Virginia	2.24
30	Minnesota	1.63		23	Alabama	2.16
26	Mississippi	2.01		24	South Carolina	2.12
28	Missouri	1.79		25	Iowa	2.04
46	Montana	0.36		26	Mississippi	2.01
37	Nebraska	1.16		27	Wisconsin	1.89
49	Nevada	0.18		28	Missouri	1.79
13	New Hampshire	3.02		29	Michigan	1.70
1	New Jersey	10.83		30	Minnesota	1.63
47	New Mexico	0.30		31	Kansas	1.59
6	New York	4.20		32	Arkansas	1.58
21	North Carolina	2.26		33	Oklahoma	1.54
42	North Dakota	0.61		34	Texas	1.53
8	Ohio	3.97		35	Vermont	1.46
33	Oklahoma	1.54		36	Washington	1.27
39	Oregon	0.65		37	Maine	1.16
5	Pennsylvania	4.84		37	Nebraska	1.16
3	Rhode Island	8.94		39	Colorado	0.65
24	South Carolina	2.12		39	Oregon	0.65
41	South Dakota	0.64		41	South Dakota	0.64
14	Tennessee	2.94		42	North Dakota	0.61
34	Texas	1.53		43	Arizona	0.54
45	Utah	0.48		44	Idaho	0.50
35	Vermont	1.46		45	Utah	0.48
22	Virginia	2.24		46	Montana	0.36
36	Washington	1.27		47	New Mexico	0.30
20	West Virginia	2.43		48	Wyoming	0.26
27	Wisconsin	1.89		49	Nevada	0.18
48	Wyoming	0.26		50	Alaska	0.03
				District of Columbia**		NA

Source: Morgan Quitno Press using data from American Hospital Association (Chicago, IL)
"Hospital Statistics" (1998 edition)

*Based on revised 1990 Census land and water area figures. Community hospitals are nonfederal short-term general and other special hospitals, whose facilities and services are available to the public.

**The District of Columbia has 12 community hospitals for its 68 square miles.

Nongovernment Not-For-Profit Hospitals in 1996

National Total = 3,045 Hospitals*

ALPHA ORDER

RANK	STATE	HOSPITALS	% of USA
32	Alabama	36	1.18%
47	Alaska	7	0.23%
25	Arizona	43	1.41%
23	Arkansas	47	1.54%
1	California	228	7.49%
34	Colorado	34	1.12%
35	Connecticut	32	1.05%
48	Delaware	6	0.20%
9	Florida	92	3.02%
19	Georgia	53	1.74%
44	Hawaii	13	0.43%
45	Idaho	12	0.39%
4	Illinois	157	5.16%
17	Indiana	57	1.87%
19	Iowa	53	1.74%
18	Kansas	54	1.77%
15	Kentucky	68	2.23%
37	Louisiana	31	1.02%
33	Maine	35	1.15%
22	Maryland	49	1.61%
12	Massachusetts	76	2.50%
6	Michigan	138	4.53%
10	Minnesota	85	2.79%
38	Mississippi	29	0.95%
12	Missouri	76	2.50%
30	Montana	40	1.31%
24	Nebraska	44	1.44%
48	Nevada	6	0.20%
39	New Hampshire	24	0.79%
11	New Jersey	83	2.73%
40	New Mexico	20	0.66%
3	New York	191	6.27%
15	North Carolina	68	2.23%
27	North Dakota	42	1.38%
5	Ohio	150	4.93%
31	Oklahoma	37	1.22%
25	Oregon	43	1.41%
2	Pennsylvania	213	7.00%
46	Rhode Island	11	0.36%
40	South Carolina	20	0.66%
27	South Dakota	42	1.38%
21	Tennessee	50	1.64%
7	Texas	133	4.37%
40	Utah	20	0.66%
43	Vermont	14	0.46%
14	Virginia	74	2.43%
27	Washington	42	1.38%
35	West Virginia	32	1.05%
8	Wisconsin	119	3.91%
48	Wyoming	6	0.20%

RANK ORDER

RANK	STATE	HOSPITALS	% of USA
1	California	228	7.49%
2	Pennsylvania	213	7.00%
3	New York	191	6.27%
4	Illinois	157	5.16%
5	Ohio	150	4.93%
6	Michigan	138	4.53%
7	Texas	133	4.37%
8	Wisconsin	119	3.91%
9	Florida	92	3.02%
10	Minnesota	85	2.79%
11	New Jersey	83	2.73%
12	Massachusetts	76	2.50%
12	Missouri	76	2.50%
14	Virginia	74	2.43%
15	Kentucky	68	2.23%
15	North Carolina	68	2.23%
17	Indiana	57	1.87%
18	Kansas	54	1.77%
19	Georgia	53	1.74%
19	Iowa	53	1.74%
21	Tennessee	50	1.64%
22	Maryland	49	1.61%
23	Arkansas	47	1.54%
24	Nebraska	44	1.44%
25	Arizona	43	1.41%
25	Oregon	43	1.41%
27	North Dakota	42	1.38%
27	South Dakota	42	1.38%
27	Washington	42	1.38%
30	Montana	40	1.31%
31	Oklahoma	37	1.22%
32	Alabama	36	1.18%
33	Maine	35	1.15%
34	Colorado	34	1.12%
35	Connecticut	32	1.05%
35	West Virginia	32	1.05%
37	Louisiana	31	1.02%
38	Mississippi	29	0.95%
39	New Hampshire	24	0.79%
40	New Mexico	20	0.66%
40	South Carolina	20	0.66%
40	Utah	20	0.66%
43	Vermont	14	0.46%
44	Hawaii	13	0.43%
45	Idaho	12	0.39%
46	Rhode Island	11	0.36%
47	Alaska	7	0.23%
48	Delaware	6	0.20%
48	Nevada	6	0.20%
48	Wyoming	6	0.20%
	District of Columbia	10	0.33%

Source: American Hospital Association (Chicago, IL)
   "Hospital Statistics" (1998 edition)
*Nongovernment not-for-profit hospitals are a subset of community hospitals.

Investor-Owned (For-Profit) Hospitals in 1996

National Total = 759 Hospitals*

ALPHA ORDER

RANK	STATE	HOSPITALS	% of USA
7	Alabama	32	4.22%
38	Alaska	1	0.13%
16	Arizona	13	1.71%
10	Arkansas	19	2.50%
2	California	106	13.97%
23	Colorado	8	1.05%
44	Connecticut	0	0.00%
44	Delaware	0	0.00%
3	Florida	94	12.38%
6	Georgia	36	4.74%
38	Hawaii	1	0.13%
32	Idaho	3	0.40%
17	Illinois	12	1.58%
21	Indiana	9	1.19%
38	Iowa	1	0.13%
23	Kansas	8	1.05%
8	Kentucky	23	3.03%
5	Louisiana	39	5.14%
38	Maine	1	0.13%
33	Maryland	2	0.26%
26	Massachusetts	5	0.66%
33	Michigan	2	0.26%
44	Minnesota	0	0.00%
14	Mississippi	15	1.98%
19	Missouri	11	1.45%
44	Montana	0	0.00%
33	Nebraska	2	0.26%
26	Nevada	5	0.66%
28	New Hampshire	4	0.53%
33	New Jersey	2	0.26%
28	New Mexico	4	0.53%
20	New York	10	1.32%
14	North Carolina	15	1.98%
38	North Dakota	1	0.13%
28	Ohio	4	0.53%
11	Oklahoma	16	2.11%
28	Oregon	4	0.53%
21	Pennsylvania	9	1.19%
44	Rhode Island	0	0.00%
9	South Carolina	20	2.64%
44	South Dakota	0	0.00%
4	Tennessee	43	5.67%
1	Texas	126	16.60%
17	Utah	12	1.58%
44	Vermont	0	0.00%
11	Virginia	16	2.11%
25	Washington	6	0.79%
11	West Virginia	16	2.11%
38	Wisconsin	1	0.13%
33	Wyoming	2	0.26%

RANK ORDER

RANK	STATE	HOSPITALS	% of USA
1	Texas	126	16.60%
2	California	106	13.97%
3	Florida	94	12.38%
4	Tennessee	43	5.67%
5	Louisiana	39	5.14%
6	Georgia	36	4.74%
7	Alabama	32	4.22%
8	Kentucky	23	3.03%
9	South Carolina	20	2.64%
10	Arkansas	19	2.50%
11	Oklahoma	16	2.11%
11	Virginia	16	2.11%
11	West Virginia	16	2.11%
14	Mississippi	15	1.98%
14	North Carolina	15	1.98%
16	Arizona	13	1.71%
17	Illinois	12	1.58%
17	Utah	12	1.58%
19	Missouri	11	1.45%
20	New York	10	1.32%
21	Indiana	9	1.19%
21	Pennsylvania	9	1.19%
23	Colorado	8	1.05%
23	Kansas	8	1.05%
25	Washington	6	0.79%
26	Massachusetts	5	0.66%
26	Nevada	5	0.66%
28	New Hampshire	4	0.53%
28	New Mexico	4	0.53%
28	Ohio	4	0.53%
28	Oregon	4	0.53%
32	Idaho	3	0.40%
33	Maryland	2	0.26%
33	Michigan	2	0.26%
33	Nebraska	2	0.26%
33	New Jersey	2	0.26%
33	Wyoming	2	0.26%
38	Alaska	1	0.13%
38	Hawaii	1	0.13%
38	Iowa	1	0.13%
38	Maine	1	0.13%
38	North Dakota	1	0.13%
38	Wisconsin	1	0.13%
44	Connecticut	0	0.00%
44	Delaware	0	0.00%
44	Minnesota	0	0.00%
44	Montana	0	0.00%
44	Rhode Island	0	0.00%
44	South Dakota	0	0.00%
44	Vermont	0	0.00%
	District of Columbia	0	0.00%

Source: American Hospital Association (Chicago, IL)
   "Hospital Statistics" (1998 edition)
Investor-owned (for-profit) hospitals are a subset of community hospitals.

State and Local Government-Owned Hospitals in 1996

National Total = 1,330 Hospitals*

ALPHA ORDER					RANK ORDER			
RANK	STATE		HOSPITALS	% of USA	RANK	STATE	HOSPITALS	% of USA
11	Alabama		45	3.38%	1	Texas	149	11.20%
32	Alaska		9	0.68%	2	California	86	6.47%
38	Arizona		5	0.38%	3	Georgia	70	5.26%
25	Arkansas		18	1.35%	4	Kansas	69	5.19%
2	California		86	6.47%	5	Iowa	61	4.59%
19	Colorado		26	1.95%	6	Louisiana	59	4.44%
43	Connecticut		1	0.08%	7	Minnesota	57	4.29%
45	Delaware		0	0.00%	8	Oklahoma	55	4.14%
22	Florida		24	1.80%	9	Mississippi	53	3.98%
3	Georgia		70	5.26%	10	Indiana	49	3.68%
35	Hawaii		7	0.53%	11	Alabama	45	3.38%
18	Idaho		27	2.03%	12	Nebraska	44	3.31%
15	Illinois		36	2.71%	13	Washington	42	3.16%
10	Indiana		49	3.68%	14	Missouri	38	2.86%
5	Iowa		61	4.59%	15	Illinois	36	2.71%
4	Kansas		69	5.19%	15	North Carolina	36	2.71%
28	Kentucky		13	0.98%	17	Tennessee	31	2.33%
6	Louisiana		59	4.44%	18	Idaho	27	2.03%
42	Maine		3	0.23%	19	Colorado	26	1.95%
45	Maryland		0	0.00%	19	New York	26	1.95%
35	Massachusetts		7	0.53%	19	South Carolina	26	1.95%
22	Michigan		24	1.80%	22	Florida	24	1.80%
7	Minnesota		57	4.29%	22	Michigan	24	1.80%
9	Mississippi		53	3.98%	22	Ohio	24	1.80%
14	Missouri		38	2.86%	25	Arkansas	18	1.35%
28	Montana		13	0.98%	26	Wyoming	17	1.28%
12	Nebraska		44	3.31%	27	Oregon	16	1.20%
32	Nevada		9	0.68%	28	Kentucky	13	0.98%
45	New Hampshire		0	0.00%	28	Montana	13	0.98%
40	New Jersey		4	0.30%	30	New Mexico	12	0.90%
30	New Mexico		12	0.90%	31	West Virginia	11	0.83%
19	New York		26	1.95%	32	Alaska	9	0.68%
15	North Carolina		36	2.71%	32	Nevada	9	0.68%
45	North Dakota		0	0.00%	32	Utah	9	0.68%
22	Ohio		24	1.80%	35	Hawaii	7	0.53%
8	Oklahoma		55	4.14%	35	Massachusetts	7	0.53%
27	Oregon		16	1.20%	35	South Dakota	7	0.53%
43	Pennsylvania		1	0.08%	38	Arizona	5	0.38%
45	Rhode Island		0	0.00%	38	Virginia	5	0.38%
19	South Carolina		26	1.95%	40	New Jersey	4	0.30%
35	South Dakota		7	0.53%	40	Wisconsin	4	0.30%
17	Tennessee		31	2.33%	42	Maine	3	0.23%
1	Texas		149	11.20%	43	Connecticut	1	0.08%
32	Utah		9	0.68%	43	Pennsylvania	1	0.08%
45	Vermont		0	0.00%	45	Delaware	0	0.00%
38	Virginia		5	0.38%	45	Maryland	0	0.00%
13	Washington		42	3.16%	45	New Hampshire	0	0.00%
31	West Virginia		11	0.83%	45	North Dakota	0	0.00%
40	Wisconsin		4	0.30%	45	Rhode Island	0	0.00%
26	Wyoming		17	1.28%	45	Vermont	0	0.00%
						District of Columbia	2	0.15%

Source: American Hospital Association (Chicago, IL)
"Hospital Statistics" (1998 edition)
*State and local government-owned hospitals are a subset of community hospitals.

Beds in Community Hospitals in 1996

National Total = 862,352 Beds*

ALPHA ORDER

RANK	STATE	BEDS	% of USA
16	Alabama	18,675	2.17%
50	Alaska	1,138	0.13%
29	Arizona	10,312	1.20%
30	Arkansas	10,260	1.19%
1	California	75,696	8.78%
31	Colorado	9,140	1.06%
34	Connecticut	7,274	0.84%
49	Delaware	1,616	0.19%
4	Florida	50,033	5.80%
10	Georgia	25,897	3.00%
45	Hawaii	3,045	0.35%
43	Idaho	3,444	0.40%
6	Illinois	40,686	4.72%
14	Indiana	19,488	2.26%
24	Iowa	12,403	1.44%
27	Kansas	10,879	1.26%
21	Kentucky	14,996	1.74%
15	Louisiana	19,275	2.24%
40	Maine	3,856	0.45%
23	Maryland	12,455	1.44%
18	Massachusetts	17,990	2.09%
8	Michigan	28,849	3.35%
19	Minnesota	17,552	2.04%
22	Mississippi	13,260	1.54%
12	Missouri	21,544	2.50%
38	Montana	4,211	0.49%
32	Nebraska	8,167	0.95%
42	Nevada	3,571	0.41%
44	New Hampshire	3,238	0.38%
9	New Jersey	28,096	3.26%
41	New Mexico	3,692	0.43%
2	New York	72,061	8.36%
11	North Carolina	22,722	2.63%
39	North Dakota	4,191	0.49%
7	Ohio	36,909	4.28%
28	Oklahoma	10,838	1.26%
35	Oregon	7,147	0.83%
5	Pennsylvania	46,981	5.45%
46	Rhode Island	2,629	0.30%
26	South Carolina	11,020	1.28%
36	South Dakota	4,473	0.52%
13	Tennessee	20,636	2.39%
3	Texas	56,329	6.53%
37	Utah	4,316	0.50%
48	Vermont	1,632	0.19%
17	Virginia	18,498	2.15%
25	Washington	11,061	1.28%
33	West Virginia	8,023	0.93%
20	Wisconsin	16,457	1.91%
47	Wyoming	1,991	0.23%

RANK ORDER

RANK	STATE	BEDS	% of USA
1	California	75,696	8.78%
2	New York	72,061	8.36%
3	Texas	56,329	6.53%
4	Florida	50,033	5.80%
5	Pennsylvania	46,981	5.45%
6	Illinois	40,686	4.72%
7	Ohio	36,909	4.28%
8	Michigan	28,849	3.35%
9	New Jersey	28,096	3.26%
10	Georgia	25,897	3.00%
11	North Carolina	22,722	2.63%
12	Missouri	21,544	2.50%
13	Tennessee	20,636	2.39%
14	Indiana	19,488	2.26%
15	Louisiana	19,275	2.24%
16	Alabama	18,675	2.17%
17	Virginia	18,498	2.15%
18	Massachusetts	17,990	2.09%
19	Minnesota	17,552	2.04%
20	Wisconsin	16,457	1.91%
21	Kentucky	14,996	1.74%
22	Mississippi	13,260	1.54%
23	Maryland	12,455	1.44%
24	Iowa	12,403	1.44%
25	Washington	11,061	1.28%
26	South Carolina	11,020	1.28%
27	Kansas	10,879	1.26%
28	Oklahoma	10,838	1.26%
29	Arizona	10,312	1.20%
30	Arkansas	10,260	1.19%
31	Colorado	9,140	1.06%
32	Nebraska	8,167	0.95%
33	West Virginia	8,023	0.93%
34	Connecticut	7,274	0.84%
35	Oregon	7,147	0.83%
36	South Dakota	4,473	0.52%
37	Utah	4,316	0.50%
38	Montana	4,211	0.49%
39	North Dakota	4,191	0.49%
40	Maine	3,856	0.45%
41	New Mexico	3,692	0.43%
42	Nevada	3,571	0.41%
43	Idaho	3,444	0.40%
44	New Hampshire	3,238	0.38%
45	Hawaii	3,045	0.35%
46	Rhode Island	2,629	0.30%
47	Wyoming	1,991	0.23%
48	Vermont	1,632	0.19%
49	Delaware	1,616	0.19%
50	Alaska	1,138	0.13%
	District of Columbia	3,700	0.43%

Source: American Hospital Association (Chicago, IL)
"Hospital Statistics" (1998 edition)
All nonfederal short-term general and other special hospitals, whose facilities and services are available to the public.

Rate of Beds in Community Hospitals in 1996

National Rate = 325 Beds per 100,000 Population*

ALPHA ORDER RANK	STATE	RATE	RANK ORDER RANK	STATE	RATE
8	Alabama	436	1	North Dakota	652
50	Alaska	188	2	South Dakota	606
42	Arizona	233	3	Nebraska	495
12	Arkansas	409	4	Mississippi	489
41	California	238	5	Montana	480
40	Colorado	240	6	Louisiana	444
44	Connecticut	223	7	West Virginia	441
44	Delaware	223	8	Alabama	436
21	Florida	347	9	Iowa	435
19	Georgia	353	10	Kansas	422
38	Hawaii	257	11	Wyoming	415
33	Idaho	290	12	Arkansas	409
22	Illinois	343	13	Missouri	402
23	Indiana	334	14	New York	397
9	Iowa	435	15	Pennsylvania	390
10	Kansas	422	16	Tennessee	389
17	Kentucky	386	17	Kentucky	386
6	Louisiana	444	18	Minnesota	378
27	Maine	311	19	Georgia	353
39	Maryland	246	20	New Jersey	351
30	Massachusetts	296	21	Florida	347
30	Michigan	296	22	Illinois	343
18	Minnesota	378	23	Indiana	334
4	Mississippi	489	24	Ohio	331
13	Missouri	402	25	Oklahoma	329
5	Montana	480	26	Wisconsin	320
3	Nebraska	495	27	Maine	311
44	Nevada	223	27	North Carolina	311
34	New Hampshire	279	29	South Carolina	297
20	New Jersey	351	30	Massachusetts	296
47	New Mexico	216	30	Michigan	296
14	New York	397	32	Texas	295
27	North Carolina	311	33	Idaho	290
1	North Dakota	652	34	New Hampshire	279
24	Ohio	331	35	Vermont	278
25	Oklahoma	329	36	Virginia	277
43	Oregon	224	37	Rhode Island	266
15	Pennsylvania	390	38	Hawaii	257
37	Rhode Island	266	39	Maryland	246
29	South Carolina	297	40	Colorado	240
2	South Dakota	606	41	California	238
16	Tennessee	389	42	Arizona	233
32	Texas	295	43	Oregon	224
48	Utah	214	44	Connecticut	223
35	Vermont	278	44	Delaware	223
36	Virginia	277	44	Nevada	223
49	Washington	200	47	New Mexico	216
7	West Virginia	441	48	Utah	214
26	Wisconsin	320	49	Washington	200
11	Wyoming	415	50	Alaska	188
				District of Columbia	686

Source: Morgan Quitno Press using data from American Hospital Association (Chicago, IL)
    "Hospital Statistics" (1998 edition)
*All nonfederal short-term general and other special hospitals, whose facilities and services are available to the
public.

Average Number of Beds per Community Hospital in 1996

National Average = 168 Beds per Community Hospital*

ALPHA ORDER				RANK ORDER		
RANK	STATE	BEDS		RANK	STATE	BEDS
22	Alabama	165		1	New York	317
50	Alaska	67		2	New Jersey	316
18	Arizona	169		3	Delaware	269
34	Arkansas	122		4	Maryland	244
14	California	180		5	Rhode Island	239
30	Colorado	134		6	Florida	238
7	Connecticut	220		7	Connecticut	220
3	Delaware	269		8	Pennsylvania	211
6	Florida	238		9	Ohio	207
23	Georgia	163		10	Massachusetts	204
25	Hawaii	145		11	Illinois	198
47	Idaho	82		12	Virginia	195
11	Illinois	198		13	North Carolina	191
18	Indiana	169		14	California	180
38	Iowa	108		15	Nevada	179
46	Kansas	83		16	Michigan	176
26	Kentucky	144		17	Missouri	172
24	Louisiana	149		18	Arizona	169
42	Maine	99		18	Indiana	169
4	Maryland	244		20	South Carolina	167
10	Massachusetts	204		21	Tennessee	166
16	Michigan	176		22	Alabama	165
32	Minnesota	124		23	Georgia	163
28	Mississippi	137		24	Louisiana	149
17	Missouri	172		25	Hawaii	145
49	Montana	79		26	Kentucky	144
44	Nebraska	91		27	Texas	138
15	Nevada	179		28	Mississippi	137
36	New Hampshire	116		29	West Virginia	136
2	New Jersey	316		30	Colorado	134
40	New Mexico	103		31	Wisconsin	133
1	New York	317		32	Minnesota	124
13	North Carolina	191		33	Washington	123
43	North Dakota	97		34	Arkansas	122
9	Ohio	207		35	Vermont	117
41	Oklahoma	100		36	New Hampshire	116
37	Oregon	113		37	Oregon	113
8	Pennsylvania	211		38	Iowa	108
5	Rhode Island	239		39	Utah	105
20	South Carolina	167		40	New Mexico	103
44	South Dakota	91		41	Oklahoma	100
21	Tennessee	166		42	Maine	99
27	Texas	138		43	North Dakota	97
39	Utah	105		44	Nebraska	91
35	Vermont	117		44	South Dakota	91
12	Virginia	195		46	Kansas	83
33	Washington	123		47	Idaho	82
29	West Virginia	136		48	Wyoming	80
31	Wisconsin	133		49	Montana	79
48	Wyoming	80		50	Alaska	67
					District of Columbia	308

Source: Morgan Quitno Press using data from American Hospital Association (Chicago, IL)
"Hospital Statistics" (1998 edition)
*All nonfederal short-term general and other special hospitals, whose facilities and services are available to the public.

Admissions to Community Hospitals in 1996

National Total = 31,098,959 Admissions*

ALPHA ORDER

RANK	STATE	ADMISSIONS	% of USA
17	Alabama	672,932	2.16%
50	Alaska	38,079	0.12%
24	Arizona	452,495	1.46%
30	Arkansas	343,799	1.11%
1	California	3,071,570	9.88%
29	Colorado	351,195	1.13%
31	Connecticut	338,074	1.09%
47	Delaware	74,034	0.24%
4	Florida	1,816,083	5.84%
11	Georgia	837,832	2.69%
43	Hawaii	99,780	0.32%
41	Idaho	115,826	0.37%
6	Illinois	1,443,619	4.64%
16	Indiana	692,966	2.23%
28	Iowa	364,839	1.17%
33	Kansas	291,971	0.94%
21	Kentucky	528,870	1.70%
18	Louisiana	635,304	2.04%
39	Maine	145,923	0.47%
19	Maryland	570,477	1.83%
13	Massachusetts	729,703	2.35%
8	Michigan	1,115,658	3.59%
22	Minnesota	497,441	1.60%
25	Mississippi	416,065	1.34%
14	Missouri	728,282	2.34%
45	Montana	92,564	0.30%
35	Nebraska	187,467	0.60%
38	Nevada	152,475	0.49%
42	New Hampshire	108,340	0.35%
9	New Jersey	1,058,835	3.40%
37	New Mexico	158,989	0.51%
2	New York	2,385,375	7.67%
10	North Carolina	844,126	2.71%
46	North Dakota	88,025	0.28%
7	Ohio	1,372,878	4.41%
27	Oklahoma	368,113	1.18%
32	Oregon	301,603	0.97%
5	Pennsylvania	1,755,587	5.65%
40	Rhode Island	117,621	0.38%
26	South Carolina	411,965	1.32%
44	South Dakota	94,076	0.30%
12	Tennessee	754,254	2.43%
3	Texas	2,074,001	6.67%
36	Utah	173,707	0.56%
48	Vermont	54,505	0.18%
15	Virginia	699,754	2.25%
23	Washington	469,942	1.51%
34	West Virginia	271,320	0.87%
20	Wisconsin	541,370	1.74%
49	Wyoming	42,840	0.14%

RANK ORDER

RANK	STATE	ADMISSIONS	% of USA
1	California	3,071,570	9.88%
2	New York	2,385,375	7.67%
3	Texas	2,074,001	6.67%
4	Florida	1,816,083	5.84%
5	Pennsylvania	1,755,587	5.65%
6	Illinois	1,443,619	4.64%
7	Ohio	1,372,878	4.41%
8	Michigan	1,115,658	3.59%
9	New Jersey	1,058,835	3.40%
10	North Carolina	844,126	2.71%
11	Georgia	837,832	2.69%
12	Tennessee	754,254	2.43%
13	Massachusetts	729,703	2.35%
14	Missouri	728,282	2.34%
15	Virginia	699,754	2.25%
16	Indiana	692,966	2.23%
17	Alabama	672,932	2.16%
18	Louisiana	635,304	2.04%
19	Maryland	570,477	1.83%
20	Wisconsin	541,370	1.74%
21	Kentucky	528,870	1.70%
22	Minnesota	497,441	1.60%
23	Washington	469,942	1.51%
24	Arizona	452,495	1.46%
25	Mississippi	416,065	1.34%
26	South Carolina	411,965	1.32%
27	Oklahoma	368,113	1.18%
28	Iowa	364,839	1.17%
29	Colorado	351,195	1.13%
30	Arkansas	343,799	1.11%
31	Connecticut	338,074	1.09%
32	Oregon	301,603	0.97%
33	Kansas	291,971	0.94%
34	West Virginia	271,320	0.87%
35	Nebraska	187,467	0.60%
36	Utah	173,707	0.56%
37	New Mexico	158,989	0.51%
38	Nevada	152,475	0.49%
39	Maine	145,923	0.47%
40	Rhode Island	117,621	0.38%
41	Idaho	115,826	0.37%
42	New Hampshire	108,340	0.35%
43	Hawaii	99,780	0.32%
44	South Dakota	94,076	0.30%
45	Montana	92,564	0.30%
46	North Dakota	88,025	0.28%
47	Delaware	74,034	0.24%
48	Vermont	54,505	0.18%
49	Wyoming	42,840	0.14%
50	Alaska	38,079	0.12%
	District of Columbia	146,410	0.47%

Source: American Hospital Association (Chicago, IL)
"Hospital Statistics" (1998 edition)
*Admissions to all nonfederal short-term general and other special hospitals, whose facilities and services are available to the public.

Inpatient Days in Community Hospitals in 1996

National Total = 193,747,004 Inpatient Days*

ALPHA ORDER					RANK ORDER			
RANK	STATE		DAYS	% of USA	RANK	STATE	DAYS	% of USA
18	Alabama		3,939,546	2.03%	1	New York	20,153,194	10.40%
50	Alaska		235,569	0.12%	2	California	16,277,462	8.40%
26	Arizona		2,247,879	1.16%	3	Pennsylvania	11,544,652	5.96%
28	Arkansas		2,124,289	1.10%	4	Texas	11,218,158	5.79%
2	California		16,277,462	8.40%	5	Florida	10,514,353	5.43%
31	Colorado		1,903,038	0.98%	6	Illinois	8,710,238	4.50%
32	Connecticut		1,900,637	0.98%	7	Ohio	7,731,761	3.99%
47	Delaware		465,783	0.24%	8	New Jersey	7,210,932	3.72%
5	Florida		10,514,353	5.43%	9	Michigan	6,722,553	3.47%
10	Georgia		5,673,492	2.93%	10	Georgia	5,673,492	2.93%
40	Hawaii		855,086	0.44%	11	North Carolina	5,592,640	2.89%
45	Idaho		701,862	0.36%	12	Tennessee	4,538,765	2.34%
6	Illinois		8,710,238	4.50%	13	Massachusetts	4,427,909	2.29%
17	Indiana		4,034,618	2.08%	14	Missouri	4,424,710	2.28%
24	Iowa		2,581,278	1.33%	15	Virginia	4,217,893	2.18%
30	Kansas		2,050,618	1.06%	16	Minnesota	4,192,676	2.16%
21	Kentucky		3,148,033	1.62%	17	Indiana	4,034,618	2.08%
19	Louisiana		3,738,836	1.93%	18	Alabama	3,939,546	2.03%
39	Maine		908,456	0.47%	19	Louisiana	3,738,836	1.93%
22	Maryland		3,093,251	1.60%	20	Wisconsin	3,490,526	1.80%
13	Massachusetts		4,427,909	2.29%	21	Kentucky	3,148,033	1.62%
9	Michigan		6,722,553	3.47%	22	Maryland	3,093,251	1.60%
16	Minnesota		4,192,676	2.16%	23	Mississippi	2,980,732	1.54%
23	Mississippi		2,980,732	1.54%	24	Iowa	2,581,278	1.33%
14	Missouri		4,424,710	2.28%	25	South Carolina	2,540,887	1.31%
37	Montana		1,027,640	0.53%	26	Arizona	2,247,879	1.16%
34	Nebraska		1,651,868	0.85%	27	Washington	2,213,995	1.14%
41	Nevada		813,766	0.42%	28	Arkansas	2,124,289	1.10%
44	New Hampshire		706,396	0.36%	29	Oklahoma	2,086,766	1.08%
8	New Jersey		7,210,932	3.72%	30	Kansas	2,050,618	1.06%
43	New Mexico		778,795	0.40%	31	Colorado	1,903,038	0.98%
1	New York		20,153,194	10.40%	32	Connecticut	1,900,637	0.98%
11	North Carolina		5,592,640	2.89%	33	West Virginia	1,730,825	0.89%
38	North Dakota		953,928	0.49%	34	Nebraska	1,651,868	0.85%
7	Ohio		7,731,761	3.99%	35	Oregon	1,350,692	0.70%
29	Oklahoma		2,086,766	1.08%	36	South Dakota	1,055,897	0.54%
35	Oregon		1,350,692	0.70%	37	Montana	1,027,640	0.53%
3	Pennsylvania		11,544,652	5.96%	38	North Dakota	953,928	0.49%
46	Rhode Island		645,275	0.33%	39	Maine	908,456	0.47%
25	South Carolina		2,540,887	1.31%	40	Hawaii	855,086	0.44%
36	South Dakota		1,055,897	0.54%	41	Nevada	813,766	0.42%
12	Tennessee		4,538,765	2.34%	42	Utah	793,342	0.41%
4	Texas		11,218,158	5.79%	43	New Mexico	778,795	0.40%
42	Utah		793,342	0.41%	44	New Hampshire	706,396	0.36%
48	Vermont		440,539	0.23%	45	Idaho	701,862	0.36%
15	Virginia		4,217,893	2.18%	46	Rhode Island	645,275	0.33%
27	Washington		2,213,995	1.14%	47	Delaware	465,783	0.24%
33	West Virginia		1,730,825	0.89%	48	Vermont	440,539	0.23%
20	Wisconsin		3,490,526	1.80%	49	Wyoming	380,373	0.20%
49	Wyoming		380,373	0.20%	50	Alaska	235,569	0.12%
						District of Columbia	1,024,595	0.53%

Source: American Hospital Association (Chicago, IL)
  "Hospital Statistics" (1998 edition)
*Inpatient days in all nonfederal short-term general and other special hospitals, whose facilities and services are available to the public.

Average Daily Census in Community Hospitals in 1996

National Average = 529,363 Inpatients*

ALPHA ORDER

RANK ORDER

RANK	STATE	INPATIENTS
18	Alabama	10,764
50	Alaska	644
26	Arizona	6,142
28	Arkansas	5,804
2	California	44,474
31	Colorado	5,200
32	Connecticut	5,193
47	Delaware	1,273
5	Florida	28,728
10	Georgia	15,501
40	Hawaii	2,336
45	Idaho	1,918
6	Illinois	23,798
17	Indiana	11,024
24	Iowa	7,053
30	Kansas	5,603
21	Kentucky	8,601
19	Louisiana	10,215
39	Maine	2,482
22	Maryland	8,452
13	Massachusetts	12,098
9	Michigan	18,368
16	Minnesota	11,455
23	Mississippi	8,144
14	Missouri	12,089
37	Montana	2,808
34	Nebraska	4,513
41	Nevada	2,223
44	New Hampshire	1,930
8	New Jersey	19,702
43	New Mexico	2,128
1	New York	55,063
11	North Carolina	15,280
38	North Dakota	2,606
7	Ohio	21,125
29	Oklahoma	5,702
35	Oregon	3,690
3	Pennsylvania	31,543
46	Rhode Island	1,763
25	South Carolina	6,942
36	South Dakota	2,885
12	Tennessee	12,401
4	Texas	30,651
42	Utah	2,168
48	Vermont	1,204
15	Virginia	11,524
27	Washington	6,049
33	West Virginia	4,729
20	Wisconsin	9,537
49	Wyoming	1,039

RANK	STATE	INPATIENTS
1	New York	55,063
2	California	44,474
3	Pennsylvania	31,543
4	Texas	30,651
5	Florida	28,728
6	Illinois	23,798
7	Ohio	21,125
8	New Jersey	19,702
9	Michigan	18,368
10	Georgia	15,501
11	North Carolina	15,280
12	Tennessee	12,401
13	Massachusetts	12,098
14	Missouri	12,089
15	Virginia	11,524
16	Minnesota	11,455
17	Indiana	11,024
18	Alabama	10,764
19	Louisiana	10,215
20	Wisconsin	9,537
21	Kentucky	8,601
22	Maryland	8,452
23	Mississippi	8,144
24	Iowa	7,053
25	South Carolina	6,942
26	Arizona	6,142
27	Washington	6,049
28	Arkansas	5,804
29	Oklahoma	5,702
30	Kansas	5,603
31	Colorado	5,200
32	Connecticut	5,193
33	West Virginia	4,729
34	Nebraska	4,513
35	Oregon	3,690
36	South Dakota	2,885
37	Montana	2,808
38	North Dakota	2,606
39	Maine	2,482
40	Hawaii	2,336
41	Nevada	2,223
42	Utah	2,168
43	New Mexico	2,128
44	New Hampshire	1,930
45	Idaho	1,918
46	Rhode Island	1,763
47	Delaware	1,273
48	Vermont	1,204
49	Wyoming	1,039
50	Alaska	644
	District of Columbia	2,799

Source: Morgan Quitno Press using data from American Hospital Association (Chicago, IL)
    "Hospital Statistics" (1998 edition)
*Average total of inpatients receiving care in all nonfederal short-term general and other special hospitals, whose facilities and services are available to the public. Excludes newborns.

Average Stay in Community Hospitals in 1996

National Average = 6.2 Days*

ALPHA ORDER

RANK	STATE	DAYS
33	Alabama	5.9
21	Alaska	6.2
46	Arizona	5.0
21	Arkansas	6.2
44	California	5.3
41	Colorado	5.4
38	Connecticut	5.6
20	Delaware	6.3
35	Florida	5.8
13	Georgia	6.8
6	Hawaii	8.6
25	Idaho	6.1
28	Illinois	6.0
35	Indiana	5.8
11	Iowa	7.1
12	Kansas	7.0
28	Kentucky	6.0
33	Louisiana	5.9
21	Maine	6.2
41	Maryland	5.4
25	Massachusetts	6.1
28	Michigan	6.0
7	Minnesota	8.4
10	Mississippi	7.2
25	Missouri	6.1
2	Montana	11.1
5	Nebraska	8.8
44	Nevada	5.3
17	New Hampshire	6.5
13	New Jersey	6.8
47	New Mexico	4.9
7	New York	8.4
15	North Carolina	6.6
3	North Dakota	10.8
38	Ohio	5.6
37	Oklahoma	5.7
50	Oregon	4.5
15	Pennsylvania	6.6
40	Rhode Island	5.5
21	South Carolina	6.2
1	South Dakota	11.2
28	Tennessee	6.0
41	Texas	5.4
49	Utah	4.6
9	Vermont	8.1
28	Virginia	6.0
48	Washington	4.7
18	West Virginia	6.4
18	Wisconsin	6.4
4	Wyoming	8.9

RANK ORDER

RANK	STATE	DAYS
1	South Dakota	11.2
2	Montana	11.1
3	North Dakota	10.8
4	Wyoming	8.9
5	Nebraska	8.8
6	Hawaii	8.6
7	Minnesota	8.4
7	New York	8.4
9	Vermont	8.1
10	Mississippi	7.2
11	Iowa	7.1
12	Kansas	7.0
13	Georgia	6.8
13	New Jersey	6.8
15	North Carolina	6.6
15	Pennsylvania	6.6
17	New Hampshire	6.5
18	West Virginia	6.4
18	Wisconsin	6.4
20	Delaware	6.3
21	Alaska	6.2
21	Arkansas	6.2
21	Maine	6.2
21	South Carolina	6.2
25	Idaho	6.1
25	Massachusetts	6.1
25	Missouri	6.1
28	Illinois	6.0
28	Kentucky	6.0
28	Michigan	6.0
28	Tennessee	6.0
28	Virginia	6.0
33	Alabama	5.9
33	Louisiana	5.9
35	Florida	5.8
35	Indiana	5.8
37	Oklahoma	5.7
38	Connecticut	5.6
38	Ohio	5.6
40	Rhode Island	5.5
41	Colorado	5.4
41	Maryland	5.4
41	Texas	5.4
44	California	5.3
44	Nevada	5.3
46	Arizona	5.0
47	New Mexico	4.9
48	Washington	4.7
49	Utah	4.6
50	Oregon	4.5

District of Columbia	7.0

Source: American Hospital Association (Chicago, IL)
"Hospital Statistics" (1998 edition)
All nonfederal short-term general and other special hospitals, whose facilities and services are available to the public.

Occupancy Rate in Community Hospitals in 1996

National Rate = 61.4% of Community Hospital Beds Occupied*

ALPHA ORDER

RANK	STATE	PERCENT
30	Alabama	57.6
37	Alaska	56.6
24	Arizona	59.6
37	Arkansas	56.6
27	California	58.8
35	Colorado	56.9
5	Connecticut	71.4
1	Delaware	78.8
32	Florida	57.4
23	Georgia	59.9
2	Hawaii	76.7
41	Idaho	55.7
28	Illinois	58.5
37	Indiana	56.6
35	Iowa	56.9
49	Kansas	51.5
32	Kentucky	57.4
45	Louisiana	53.0
15	Maine	64.4
7	Maryland	67.9
8	Massachusetts	67.2
16	Michigan	63.7
13	Minnesota	65.3
21	Mississippi	61.4
40	Missouri	56.1
12	Montana	66.7
42	Nebraska	55.3
18	Nevada	62.3
24	New Hampshire	59.6
6	New Jersey	70.1
30	New Mexico	57.6
3	New York	76.4
8	North Carolina	67.2
20	North Dakota	62.2
34	Ohio	57.2
46	Oklahoma	52.6
48	Oregon	51.6
10	Pennsylvania	67.1
10	Rhode Island	67.1
17	South Carolina	63.0
14	South Dakota	64.5
22	Tennessee	60.1
44	Texas	54.4
50	Utah	50.2
4	Vermont	73.8
18	Virginia	62.3
43	Washington	54.7
26	West Virginia	58.9
29	Wisconsin	58.0
47	Wyoming	52.2

RANK ORDER

RANK	STATE	PERCENT
1	Delaware	78.8
2	Hawaii	76.7
3	New York	76.4
4	Vermont	73.8
5	Connecticut	71.4
6	New Jersey	70.1
7	Maryland	67.9
8	Massachusetts	67.2
8	North Carolina	67.2
10	Pennsylvania	67.1
10	Rhode Island	67.1
12	Montana	66.7
13	Minnesota	65.3
14	South Dakota	64.5
15	Maine	64.4
16	Michigan	63.7
17	South Carolina	63.0
18	Nevada	62.3
18	Virginia	62.3
20	North Dakota	62.2
21	Mississippi	61.4
22	Tennessee	60.1
23	Georgia	59.9
24	Arizona	59.6
24	New Hampshire	59.6
26	West Virginia	58.9
27	California	58.8
28	Illinois	58.5
29	Wisconsin	58.0
30	Alabama	57.6
30	New Mexico	57.6
32	Florida	57.4
32	Kentucky	57.4
34	Ohio	57.2
35	Colorado	56.9
35	Iowa	56.9
37	Alaska	56.6
37	Arkansas	56.6
37	Indiana	56.6
40	Missouri	56.1
41	Idaho	55.7
42	Nebraska	55.3
43	Washington	54.7
44	Texas	54.4
45	Louisiana	53.0
46	Oklahoma	52.6
47	Wyoming	52.2
48	Oregon	51.6
49	Kansas	51.5
50	Utah	50.2
	District of Columbia	75.6

Source: Morgan Quitno Press using data from American Hospital Association (Chicago, IL)
     "Hospital Statistics" (1998 edition)
*Average daily census compared to number of community hospital beds.

Outpatient Visits to Community Hospitals in 1996

National Total = 439,863,107 Visits*

ALPHA ORDER

RANK	STATE	VISITS	% of USA
20	Alabama	7,625,865	1.73%
50	Alaska	775,108	0.18%
33	Arizona	4,200,138	0.95%
34	Arkansas	4,090,671	0.93%
1	California	41,692,501	9.48%
24	Colorado	6,061,499	1.38%
23	Connecticut	6,083,836	1.38%
47	Delaware	1,198,704	0.27%
8	Florida	18,906,310	4.30%
13	Georgia	10,091,880	2.29%
39	Hawaii	2,261,933	0.51%
41	Idaho	1,961,976	0.45%
6	Illinois	21,592,348	4.91%
11	Indiana	12,294,241	2.80%
21	Iowa	6,963,523	1.58%
30	Kansas	4,398,277	1.00%
22	Kentucky	6,553,252	1.49%
16	Louisiana	8,416,510	1.91%
37	Maine	2,673,050	0.61%
27	Maryland	4,978,698	1.13%
9	Massachusetts	13,731,739	3.12%
7	Michigan	21,003,289	4.77%
26	Minnesota	5,357,924	1.22%
32	Mississippi	4,254,032	0.97%
12	Missouri	10,215,185	2.32%
44	Montana	1,458,560	0.33%
38	Nebraska	2,668,831	0.61%
45	Nevada	1,423,221	0.32%
40	New Hampshire	2,135,813	0.49%
10	New Jersey	13,464,532	3.06%
36	New Mexico	2,799,812	0.64%
2	New York	40,835,573	9.28%
14	North Carolina	9,621,226	2.19%
43	North Dakota	1,513,757	0.34%
5	Ohio	22,951,859	5.22%
31	Oklahoma	4,278,442	0.97%
25	Oregon	5,792,986	1.32%
3	Pennsylvania	27,073,090	6.15%
42	Rhode Island	1,806,387	0.41%
28	South Carolina	4,892,441	1.11%
46	South Dakota	1,240,570	0.28%
18	Tennessee	7,876,216	1.79%
4	Texas	24,423,910	5.55%
35	Utah	3,551,305	0.81%
48	Vermont	866,902	0.20%
19	Virginia	7,865,540	1.79%
17	Washington	8,378,107	1.90%
29	West Virginia	4,442,870	1.01%
15	Wisconsin	8,951,660	2.04%
49	Wyoming	790,822	0.18%

RANK ORDER

RANK	STATE	VISITS	% of USA
1	California	41,692,501	9.48%
2	New York	40,835,573	9.28%
3	Pennsylvania	27,073,090	6.15%
4	Texas	24,423,910	5.55%
5	Ohio	22,951,859	5.22%
6	Illinois	21,592,348	4.91%
7	Michigan	21,003,289	4.77%
8	Florida	18,906,310	4.30%
9	Massachusetts	13,731,739	3.12%
10	New Jersey	13,464,532	3.06%
11	Indiana	12,294,241	2.80%
12	Missouri	10,215,185	2.32%
13	Georgia	10,091,880	2.29%
14	North Carolina	9,621,226	2.19%
15	Wisconsin	8,951,660	2.04%
16	Louisiana	8,416,510	1.91%
17	Washington	8,378,107	1.90%
18	Tennessee	7,876,216	1.79%
19	Virginia	7,865,540	1.79%
20	Alabama	7,625,865	1.73%
21	Iowa	6,963,523	1.58%
22	Kentucky	6,553,252	1.49%
23	Connecticut	6,083,836	1.38%
24	Colorado	6,061,499	1.38%
25	Oregon	5,792,986	1.32%
26	Minnesota	5,357,924	1.22%
27	Maryland	4,978,698	1.13%
28	South Carolina	4,892,441	1.11%
29	West Virginia	4,442,870	1.01%
30	Kansas	4,398,277	1.00%
31	Oklahoma	4,278,442	0.97%
32	Mississippi	4,254,032	0.97%
33	Arizona	4,200,138	0.95%
34	Arkansas	4,090,671	0.93%
35	Utah	3,551,305	0.81%
36	New Mexico	2,799,812	0.64%
37	Maine	2,673,050	0.61%
38	Nebraska	2,668,831	0.61%
39	Hawaii	2,261,933	0.51%
40	New Hampshire	2,135,813	0.49%
41	Idaho	1,961,976	0.45%
42	Rhode Island	1,806,387	0.41%
43	North Dakota	1,513,757	0.34%
44	Montana	1,458,560	0.33%
45	Nevada	1,423,221	0.32%
46	South Dakota	1,240,570	0.28%
47	Delaware	1,198,704	0.27%
48	Vermont	866,902	0.20%
49	Wyoming	790,822	0.18%
50	Alaska	775,108	0.18%
	District of Columbia	1,376,186	0.31%

Source: American Hospital Association (Chicago, IL)
   "Hospital Statistics" (1998 edition)
*All nonfederal short-term general and other special hospitals, whose facilities and services are available to the public. Includes emergency and other visits.

Emergency Outpatient Visits to Community Hospitals in 1996

National Total = 93,111,592 Visits*

ALPHA ORDER

RANK	STATE	VISITS	% of USA
18	Alabama	2,057,139	2.21%
50	Alaska	146,222	0.16%
27	Arizona	1,170,796	1.26%
31	Arkansas	1,023,926	1.10%
1	California	8,938,655	9.60%
28	Colorado	1,062,079	1.14%
26	Connecticut	1,175,469	1.26%
44	Delaware	231,054	0.25%
4	Florida	4,872,099	5.23%
9	Georgia	2,798,491	3.01%
46	Hawaii	216,780	0.23%
42	Idaho	367,735	0.39%
7	Illinois	4,284,708	4.60%
17	Indiana	2,174,103	2.33%
32	Iowa	993,354	1.07%
34	Kansas	763,372	0.82%
20	Kentucky	1,639,912	1.76%
15	Louisiana	2,192,338	2.35%
36	Maine	621,554	0.67%
22	Maryland	1,567,626	1.68%
11	Massachusetts	2,581,076	2.77%
8	Michigan	3,427,334	3.68%
25	Minnesota	1,178,574	1.27%
24	Mississippi	1,397,406	1.50%
16	Missouri	2,192,111	2.35%
43	Montana	256,427	0.28%
39	Nebraska	441,082	0.47%
41	Nevada	392,108	0.42%
38	New Hampshire	443,088	0.48%
12	New Jersey	2,462,774	2.64%
37	New Mexico	507,493	0.55%
2	New York	6,714,141	7.21%
10	North Carolina	2,760,098	2.96%
45	North Dakota	225,676	0.24%
5	Ohio	4,753,046	5.10%
29	Oklahoma	1,039,358	1.12%
33	Oregon	941,568	1.01%
6	Pennsylvania	4,697,376	5.04%
40	Rhode Island	405,182	0.44%
23	South Carolina	1,420,940	1.53%
48	South Dakota	183,190	0.20%
13	Tennessee	2,272,839	2.44%
3	Texas	6,163,727	6.62%
35	Utah	625,238	0.67%
47	Vermont	213,421	0.23%
14	Virginia	2,256,233	2.42%
19	Washington	1,706,741	1.83%
30	West Virginia	1,032,809	1.11%
21	Wisconsin	1,592,044	1.71%
49	Wyoming	169,179	0.18%

RANK ORDER

RANK	STATE	VISITS	% of USA
1	California	8,938,655	9.60%
2	New York	6,714,141	7.21%
3	Texas	6,163,727	6.62%
4	Florida	4,872,099	5.23%
5	Ohio	4,753,046	5.10%
6	Pennsylvania	4,697,376	5.04%
7	Illinois	4,284,708	4.60%
8	Michigan	3,427,334	3.68%
9	Georgia	2,798,491	3.01%
10	North Carolina	2,760,098	2.96%
11	Massachusetts	2,581,076	2.77%
12	New Jersey	2,462,774	2.64%
13	Tennessee	2,272,839	2.44%
14	Virginia	2,256,233	2.42%
15	Louisiana	2,192,338	2.35%
16	Missouri	2,192,111	2.35%
17	Indiana	2,174,103	2.33%
18	Alabama	2,057,139	2.21%
19	Washington	1,706,741	1.83%
20	Kentucky	1,639,912	1.76%
21	Wisconsin	1,592,044	1.71%
22	Maryland	1,567,626	1.68%
23	South Carolina	1,420,940	1.53%
24	Mississippi	1,397,406	1.50%
25	Minnesota	1,178,574	1.27%
26	Connecticut	1,175,469	1.26%
27	Arizona	1,170,796	1.26%
28	Colorado	1,062,079	1.14%
29	Oklahoma	1,039,358	1.12%
30	West Virginia	1,032,809	1.11%
31	Arkansas	1,023,926	1.10%
32	Iowa	993,354	1.07%
33	Oregon	941,568	1.01%
34	Kansas	763,372	0.82%
35	Utah	625,238	0.67%
36	Maine	621,554	0.67%
37	New Mexico	507,493	0.55%
38	New Hampshire	443,088	0.48%
39	Nebraska	441,082	0.47%
40	Rhode Island	405,182	0.44%
41	Nevada	392,108	0.42%
42	Idaho	367,735	0.39%
43	Montana	256,427	0.28%
44	Delaware	231,054	0.25%
45	North Dakota	225,676	0.24%
46	Hawaii	216,780	0.23%
47	Vermont	213,421	0.23%
48	South Dakota	183,190	0.20%
49	Wyoming	169,179	0.18%
50	Alaska	146,222	0.16%
	District of Columbia	361,901	0.39%

Source: American Hospital Association (Chicago, IL)
    "Hospital Statistics" (1998 edition)
*All nonfederal short-term general and other special hospitals, whose facilities and services are available to the public.

Surgical Operations in Community Hospitals in 1996

National Total = 23,569,263 Surgical Operations*

ALPHA ORDER

RANK	STATE	OPERATIONS	% of USA
18	Alabama	468,141	1.99%
50	Alaska	29,143	0.12%
27	Arizona	286,793	1.22%
32	Arkansas	244,583	1.04%
1	California	2,012,052	8.54%
26	Colorado	307,310	1.30%
28	Connecticut	265,393	1.13%
45	Delaware	70,397	0.30%
5	Florida	1,263,459	5.36%
10	Georgia	653,197	2.77%
44	Hawaii	75,637	0.32%
41	Idaho	89,594	0.38%
7	Illinois	1,029,458	4.37%
12	Indiana	606,991	2.58%
24	Iowa	341,612	1.45%
33	Kansas	237,139	1.01%
21	Kentucky	401,102	1.70%
20	Louisiana	427,038	1.81%
38	Maine	119,348	0.51%
17	Maryland	479,871	2.04%
13	Massachusetts	603,588	2.56%
8	Michigan	950,501	4.03%
23	Minnesota	394,929	1.68%
31	Mississippi	250,054	1.06%
14	Missouri	552,323	2.34%
46	Montana	67,184	0.29%
35	Nebraska	190,768	0.81%
39	Nevada	107,662	0.46%
42	New Hampshire	83,814	0.36%
9	New Jersey	665,958	2.83%
36	New Mexico	160,000	0.68%
2	New York	1,747,234	7.41%
11	North Carolina	642,906	2.73%
43	North Dakota	80,667	0.34%
6	Ohio	1,195,831	5.07%
29	Oklahoma	262,777	1.11%
30	Oregon	259,069	1.10%
4	Pennsylvania	1,447,990	6.14%
40	Rhode Island	106,060	0.45%
25	South Carolina	317,810	1.35%
47	South Dakota	65,784	0.28%
15	Tennessee	545,845	2.32%
3	Texas	1,492,130	6.33%
37	Utah	153,354	0.65%
48	Vermont	44,532	0.19%
16	Virginia	538,874	2.29%
22	Washington	395,465	1.68%
34	West Virginia	232,016	0.98%
19	Wisconsin	463,095	1.96%
49	Wyoming	35,052	0.15%

RANK ORDER

RANK	STATE	OPERATIONS	% of USA
1	California	2,012,052	8.54%
2	New York	1,747,234	7.41%
3	Texas	1,492,130	6.33%
4	Pennsylvania	1,447,990	6.14%
5	Florida	1,263,459	5.36%
6	Ohio	1,195,831	5.07%
7	Illinois	1,029,458	4.37%
8	Michigan	950,501	4.03%
9	New Jersey	665,958	2.83%
10	Georgia	653,197	2.77%
11	North Carolina	642,906	2.73%
12	Indiana	606,991	2.58%
13	Massachusetts	603,588	2.56%
14	Missouri	552,323	2.34%
15	Tennessee	545,845	2.32%
16	Virginia	538,874	2.29%
17	Maryland	479,871	2.04%
18	Alabama	468,141	1.99%
19	Wisconsin	463,095	1.96%
20	Louisiana	427,038	1.81%
21	Kentucky	401,102	1.70%
22	Washington	395,465	1.68%
23	Minnesota	394,929	1.68%
24	Iowa	341,612	1.45%
25	South Carolina	317,810	1.35%
26	Colorado	307,310	1.30%
27	Arizona	286,793	1.22%
28	Connecticut	265,393	1.13%
29	Oklahoma	262,777	1.11%
30	Oregon	259,069	1.10%
31	Mississippi	250,054	1.06%
32	Arkansas	244,583	1.04%
33	Kansas	237,139	1.01%
34	West Virginia	232,016	0.98%
35	Nebraska	190,768	0.81%
36	New Mexico	160,000	0.68%
37	Utah	153,354	0.65%
38	Maine	119,348	0.51%
39	Nevada	107,662	0.46%
40	Rhode Island	106,060	0.45%
41	Idaho	89,594	0.38%
42	New Hampshire	83,814	0.36%
43	North Dakota	80,667	0.34%
44	Hawaii	75,637	0.32%
45	Delaware	70,397	0.30%
46	Montana	67,184	0.29%
47	South Dakota	65,784	0.28%
48	Vermont	44,532	0.19%
49	Wyoming	35,052	0.15%
50	Alaska	29,143	0.12%
	District of Columbia	107,733	0.46%

Source: American Hospital Association (Chicago, IL)
  "Hospital Statistics" (1998 edition)
*Includes inpatient and outpatient surgeries.

Medicare and Medicaid Certified Facilities in 1998

National Total = 225,216 Facilities*

ALPHA ORDER					RANK ORDER			
RANK	STATE	FACILITIES	% of USA		RANK	STATE	FACILITIES	% of USA
19	Alabama	3,940	1.75%		1	California	21,913	9.73%
50	Alaska	493	0.22%		2	Texas	19,875	8.82%
28	Arizona	3,202	1.42%		3	Florida	13,586	6.03%
31	Arkansas	2,653	1.18%		4	New York	12,223	5.43%
1	California	21,913	9.73%		5	Ohio	11,034	4.90%
30	Colorado	3,008	1.34%		6	Illinois	9,602	4.26%
29	Connecticut	3,138	1.39%		7	Pennsylvania	9,420	4.18%
47	Delaware	612	0.27%		8	Michigan	7,677	3.41%
3	Florida	13,586	6.03%		9	Georgia	6,085	2.70%
9	Georgia	6,085	2.70%		10	North Carolina	6,070	2.70%
45	Hawaii	882	0.39%		11	Indiana	6,036	2.68%
39	Idaho	1,045	0.46%		12	Missouri	5,619	2.49%
6	Illinois	9,602	4.26%		13	New Jersey	5,469	2.43%
11	Indiana	6,036	2.68%		14	Louisiana	5,364	2.38%
23	Iowa	3,435	1.53%		15	Virginia	4,979	2.21%
27	Kansas	3,218	1.43%		16	Tennessee	4,823	2.14%
26	Kentucky	3,233	1.44%		17	Massachusetts	4,777	2.12%
14	Louisiana	5,364	2.38%		18	Oklahoma	3,993	1.77%
38	Maine	1,306	0.58%		19	Alabama	3,940	1.75%
20	Maryland	3,927	1.74%		20	Maryland	3,927	1.74%
17	Massachusetts	4,777	2.12%		21	Minnesota	3,624	1.61%
8	Michigan	7,677	3.41%		22	Wisconsin	3,528	1.57%
21	Minnesota	3,624	1.61%		23	Iowa	3,435	1.53%
32	Mississippi	2,493	1.11%		24	Washington	3,425	1.52%
12	Missouri	5,619	2.49%		25	South Carolina	3,264	1.45%
42	Montana	920	0.41%		26	Kentucky	3,233	1.44%
35	Nebraska	1,722	0.76%		27	Kansas	3,218	1.43%
40	Nevada	1,034	0.46%		28	Arizona	3,202	1.42%
41	New Hampshire	1,032	0.46%		29	Connecticut	3,138	1.39%
13	New Jersey	5,469	2.43%		30	Colorado	3,008	1.34%
36	New Mexico	1,486	0.66%		31	Arkansas	2,653	1.18%
4	New York	12,223	5.43%		32	Mississippi	2,493	1.11%
10	North Carolina	6,070	2.70%		33	Oregon	2,341	1.04%
46	North Dakota	844	0.37%		34	West Virginia	2,014	0.89%
5	Ohio	11,034	4.90%		35	Nebraska	1,722	0.76%
18	Oklahoma	3,993	1.77%		36	New Mexico	1,486	0.66%
33	Oregon	2,341	1.04%		37	Utah	1,345	0.60%
7	Pennsylvania	9,420	4.18%		38	Maine	1,306	0.58%
44	Rhode Island	886	0.39%		39	Idaho	1,045	0.46%
25	South Carolina	3,264	1.45%		40	Nevada	1,034	0.46%
43	South Dakota	900	0.40%		41	New Hampshire	1,032	0.46%
16	Tennessee	4,823	2.14%		42	Montana	920	0.41%
2	Texas	19,875	8.82%		43	South Dakota	900	0.40%
37	Utah	1,345	0.60%		44	Rhode Island	886	0.39%
48	Vermont	514	0.23%		45	Hawaii	882	0.39%
15	Virginia	4,979	2.21%		46	North Dakota	844	0.37%
24	Washington	3,425	1.52%		47	Delaware	612	0.27%
34	West Virginia	2,014	0.89%		48	Vermont	514	0.23%
22	Wisconsin	3,528	1.57%		49	Wyoming	506	0.22%
49	Wyoming	506	0.22%		50	Alaska	493	0.22%
					District of Columbia		701	0.31%

Source: U.S. Department of Health and Human Services, Health Care Financing Administration
OSCAR Report 10 (March 18, 1998)

*Certified by HCFA to participate in the Medicare/Medicaid programs. All provider groups including hospitals, home health agencies, rural health centers, community mental health centers, nursing facilities, outpatient physical therapy facilities and hospices. Also includes 166,372 laboratories. National total does not include 1,183 certified facilities in U.S. territories.

Medicare and Medicaid Certified Hospitals in 1998

National Total = 6,143 Hospitals*

ALPHA ORDER					RANK ORDER			
RANK	STATE		HOSPITALS	% of USA	RANK	STATE	HOSPITALS	% of USA
20	Alabama		128	2.08%	1	California	496	8.07%
47	Alaska		25	0.41%	2	Texas	489	7.96%
29	Arizona		86	1.40%	3	New York	270	4.40%
28	Arkansas		95	1.55%	4	Florida	261	4.25%
1	California		496	8.07%	5	Pennsylvania	253	4.12%
30	Colorado		84	1.37%	6	Illinois	223	3.63%
40	Connecticut		48	0.78%	7	Ohio	206	3.35%
50	Delaware		10	0.16%	8	Georgia	198	3.22%
4	Florida		261	4.25%	9	Michigan	183	2.98%
8	Georgia		198	3.22%	10	Louisiana	178	2.90%
46	Hawaii		27	0.44%	11	Indiana	159	2.59%
40	Idaho		48	0.78%	12	Minnesota	152	2.47%
6	Illinois		223	3.63%	13	Missouri	149	2.43%
11	Indiana		159	2.59%	14	Oklahoma	148	2.41%
21	Iowa		121	1.97%	14	Tennessee	148	2.41%
18	Kansas		143	2.33%	16	North Carolina	147	2.39%
22	Kentucky		120	1.95%	17	Wisconsin	145	2.36%
10	Louisiana		178	2.90%	18	Kansas	143	2.33%
42	Maine		42	0.68%	19	Massachusetts	129	2.10%
32	Maryland		72	1.17%	20	Alabama	128	2.08%
19	Massachusetts		129	2.10%	21	Iowa	121	1.97%
9	Michigan		183	2.98%	22	Kentucky	120	1.95%
12	Minnesota		152	2.47%	22	Virginia	120	1.95%
25	Mississippi		108	1.76%	24	New Jersey	113	1.84%
13	Missouri		149	2.43%	25	Mississippi	108	1.76%
36	Montana		60	0.98%	26	Nebraska	98	1.60%
26	Nebraska		98	1.60%	26	Washington	98	1.60%
43	Nevada		39	0.63%	28	Arkansas	95	1.55%
44	New Hampshire		31	0.50%	29	Arizona	86	1.40%
24	New Jersey		113	1.84%	30	Colorado	84	1.37%
37	New Mexico		54	0.88%	31	South Carolina	74	1.20%
3	New York		270	4.40%	32	Maryland	72	1.17%
16	North Carolina		147	2.39%	33	Oregon	64	1.04%
39	North Dakota		49	0.80%	34	South Dakota	62	1.01%
7	Ohio		206	3.35%	35	West Virginia	61	0.99%
14	Oklahoma		148	2.41%	36	Montana	60	0.98%
33	Oregon		64	1.04%	37	New Mexico	54	0.88%
5	Pennsylvania		253	4.12%	38	Utah	51	0.83%
48	Rhode Island		17	0.28%	39	North Dakota	49	0.80%
31	South Carolina		74	1.20%	40	Connecticut	48	0.78%
34	South Dakota		62	1.01%	40	Idaho	48	0.78%
14	Tennessee		148	2.41%	42	Maine	42	0.68%
2	Texas		489	7.96%	43	Nevada	39	0.63%
38	Utah		51	0.83%	44	New Hampshire	31	0.50%
49	Vermont		16	0.26%	45	Wyoming	29	0.47%
22	Virginia		120	1.95%	46	Hawaii	27	0.44%
26	Washington		98	1.60%	47	Alaska	25	0.41%
35	West Virginia		61	0.99%	48	Rhode Island	17	0.28%
17	Wisconsin		145	2.36%	49	Vermont	16	0.26%
45	Wyoming		29	0.47%	50	Delaware	10	0.16%
						District of Columbia	16	0.26%

Source: U.S. Department of Health and Human Services, Health Care Financing Administration
   OSCAR Report 10 (March 18, 1998)
*Certified by HCFA to participate in the Medicare/Medicaid programs. Excludes licensed facilities that do not accept federal funding and facilities managed by the Department of Veterans Affairs. National total does not include 60 certified hospitals in U.S. territories.

Beds in Medicare and Medicaid Certified Hospitals in 1998

National Total = 1,078,702 Beds*

ALPHA ORDER				RANK ORDER			
RANK	STATE	BEDS	% of USA	RANK	STATE	BEDS	% of USA
17	Alabama	21,663	2.01%	1	California	99,484	9.22%
50	Alaska	1,743	0.16%	2	New York	84,223	7.81%
31	Arizona	11,056	1.02%	3	Texas	77,302	7.17%
29	Arkansas	12,270	1.14%	4	Florida	59,524	5.52%
1	California	99,484	9.22%	5	Pennsylvania	56,846	5.27%
30	Colorado	11,535	1.07%	6	Illinois	54,631	5.06%
32	Connecticut	10,277	0.95%	7	Ohio	53,035	4.92%
47	Delaware	2,563	0.24%	8	New Jersey	35,247	3.27%
4	Florida	59,524	5.52%	9	Michigan	34,724	3.22%
10	Georgia	29,715	2.75%	10	Georgia	29,715	2.75%
46	Hawaii	2,847	0.26%	11	Missouri	28,582	2.65%
45	Idaho	3,002	0.28%	12	North Carolina	27,733	2.57%
6	Illinois	54,631	5.06%	13	Tennessee	27,332	2.53%
15	Indiana	25,094	2.33%	14	Virginia	25,848	2.40%
25	Iowa	14,596	1.35%	15	Indiana	25,094	2.33%
27	Kansas	13,008	1.21%	16	Massachusetts	22,716	2.11%
20	Kentucky	18,848	1.75%	17	Alabama	21,663	2.01%
19	Louisiana	21,010	1.95%	18	Wisconsin	21,329	1.98%
39	Maine	4,592	0.43%	19	Louisiana	21,010	1.95%
21	Maryland	18,439	1.71%	20	Kentucky	18,848	1.75%
16	Massachusetts	22,716	2.11%	21	Maryland	18,439	1.71%
9	Michigan	34,724	3.22%	22	Minnesota	17,820	1.65%
22	Minnesota	17,820	1.65%	23	Oklahoma	16,992	1.58%
26	Mississippi	13,050	1.21%	24	Washington	14,758	1.37%
11	Missouri	28,582	2.65%	25	Iowa	14,596	1.35%
44	Montana	3,005	0.28%	26	Mississippi	13,050	1.21%
35	Nebraska	7,958	0.74%	27	Kansas	13,008	1.21%
36	Nevada	7,567	0.70%	28	South Carolina	12,672	1.17%
41	New Hampshire	4,031	0.37%	29	Arkansas	12,270	1.14%
8	New Jersey	35,247	3.27%	30	Colorado	11,535	1.07%
38	New Mexico	5,142	0.48%	31	Arizona	11,056	1.02%
2	New York	84,223	7.81%	32	Connecticut	10,277	0.95%
12	North Carolina	27,733	2.57%	33	West Virginia	9,786	0.91%
42	North Dakota	3,665	0.34%	34	Oregon	8,614	0.80%
7	Ohio	53,035	4.92%	35	Nebraska	7,958	0.74%
23	Oklahoma	16,992	1.58%	36	Nevada	7,567	0.70%
34	Oregon	8,614	0.80%	37	Utah	5,533	0.51%
5	Pennsylvania	56,846	5.27%	38	New Mexico	5,142	0.48%
40	Rhode Island	4,384	0.41%	39	Maine	4,592	0.43%
28	South Carolina	12,672	1.17%	40	Rhode Island	4,384	0.41%
43	South Dakota	3,475	0.32%	41	New Hampshire	4,031	0.37%
13	Tennessee	27,332	2.53%	42	North Dakota	3,665	0.34%
3	Texas	77,302	7.17%	43	South Dakota	3,475	0.32%
37	Utah	5,533	0.51%	44	Montana	3,005	0.28%
49	Vermont	2,008	0.19%	45	Idaho	3,002	0.28%
14	Virginia	25,848	2.40%	46	Hawaii	2,847	0.26%
24	Washington	14,758	1.37%	47	Delaware	2,563	0.24%
33	West Virginia	9,786	0.91%	48	Wyoming	2,087	0.19%
18	Wisconsin	21,329	1.98%	49	Vermont	2,008	0.19%
48	Wyoming	2,087	0.19%	50	Alaska	1,743	0.16%
					District of Columbia	5,341	0.50%

Source: U.S. Department of Health and Human Services, Health Care Financing Administration
   OSCAR Report 10 (March 18, 1998)

*Beds in hospitals certified by HCFA to participate in the Medicare/Medicaid programs. Excludes licensed facilities that do not accept federal funding and facilities managed by the Department of Veterans Affairs. National total does not include 11,192 beds in U.S. territories.

Medicare and Medicaid Certified Children's Hospitals in 1998

National Total = 70 Hospitals*

ALPHA ORDER				RANK ORDER			
RANK	STATE	HOSPITALS	% of USA	RANK	STATE	HOSPITALS	% of USA
18	Alabama	1	1.43%	1	Ohio	8	11.43%
33	Alaska	0	0.00%	2	California	7	10.00%
18	Arizona	1	1.43%	2	Texas	7	10.00%
18	Arkansas	1	1.43%	4	Pennsylvania	4	5.71%
2	California	7	10.00%	5	Minnesota	3	4.29%
18	Colorado	1	1.43%	5	Missouri	3	4.29%
18	Connecticut	1	1.43%	7	Florida	2	2.86%
18	Delaware	1	1.43%	7	Georgia	2	2.86%
7	Florida	2	2.86%	7	Illinois	2	2.86%
7	Georgia	2	2.86%	7	Maryland	2	2.86%
18	Hawaii	1	1.43%	7	Massachusetts	2	2.86%
33	Idaho	0	0.00%	7	Nebraska	2	2.86%
7	Illinois	2	2.86%	7	New York	2	2.86%
18	Indiana	1	1.43%	7	Oklahoma	2	2.86%
33	Iowa	0	0.00%	7	Tennessee	2	2.86%
18	Kansas	1	1.43%	7	Virginia	2	2.86%
33	Kentucky	0	0.00%	7	Washington	2	2.86%
18	Louisiana	1	1.43%	18	Alabama	1	1.43%
33	Maine	0	0.00%	18	Arizona	1	1.43%
7	Maryland	2	2.86%	18	Arkansas	1	1.43%
7	Massachusetts	2	2.86%	18	Colorado	1	1.43%
18	Michigan	1	1.43%	18	Connecticut	1	1.43%
5	Minnesota	3	4.29%	18	Delaware	1	1.43%
33	Mississippi	0	0.00%	18	Hawaii	1	1.43%
5	Missouri	3	4.29%	18	Indiana	1	1.43%
33	Montana	0	0.00%	18	Kansas	1	1.43%
7	Nebraska	2	2.86%	18	Louisiana	1	1.43%
33	Nevada	0	0.00%	18	Michigan	1	1.43%
33	New Hampshire	0	0.00%	18	New Jersey	1	1.43%
18	New Jersey	1	1.43%	18	New Mexico	1	1.43%
18	New Mexico	1	1.43%	18	Utah	1	1.43%
7	New York	2	2.86%	18	Wisconsin	1	1.43%
33	North Carolina	0	0.00%	33	Alaska	0	0.00%
33	North Dakota	0	0.00%	33	Idaho	0	0.00%
1	Ohio	8	11.43%	33	Iowa	0	0.00%
7	Oklahoma	2	2.86%	33	Kentucky	0	0.00%
33	Oregon	0	0.00%	33	Maine	0	0.00%
4	Pennsylvania	4	5.71%	33	Mississippi	0	0.00%
33	Rhode Island	0	0.00%	33	Montana	0	0.00%
33	South Carolina	0	0.00%	33	Nevada	0	0.00%
33	South Dakota	0	0.00%	33	New Hampshire	0	0.00%
7	Tennessee	2	2.86%	33	North Carolina	0	0.00%
2	Texas	7	10.00%	33	North Dakota	0	0.00%
18	Utah	1	1.43%	33	Oregon	0	0.00%
33	Vermont	0	0.00%	33	Rhode Island	0	0.00%
7	Virginia	2	2.86%	33	South Carolina	0	0.00%
7	Washington	2	2.86%	33	South Dakota	0	0.00%
33	West Virginia	0	0.00%	33	Vermont	0	0.00%
18	Wisconsin	1	1.43%	33	West Virginia	0	0.00%
33	Wyoming	0	0.00%	33	Wyoming	0	0.00%
					District of Columbia	1	1.43%

Source: U.S. Department of Health and Human Services, Health Care Financing Administration
   OSCAR Report 10 (March 18, 1998)
*Certified by HCFA to participate in the Medicare/Medicaid programs. National total does not include one facility in
U.S. territories. Excludes licensed facilities that do not accept federal funding and facilities managed by the
Department of Veterans Affairs.

Beds in Medicare and Medicaid Certified Children's Hospitals in 1998

National Total = 12,566 Beds*

ALPHA ORDER

RANK	STATE	BEDS	% of USA
18	Alabama	225	1.79%
33	Alaska	0	0.00%
32	Arizona	15	0.12%
12	Arkansas	280	2.23%
3	California	1,356	10.79%
14	Colorado	253	2.01%
26	Connecticut	97	0.77%
26	Delaware	97	0.77%
9	Florida	376	2.99%
8	Georgia	400	3.18%
17	Hawaii	232	1.85%
33	Idaho	0	0.00%
10	Illinois	351	2.79%
30	Indiana	35	0.28%
33	Iowa	0	0.00%
31	Kansas	34	0.27%
33	Kentucky	0	0.00%
20	Louisiana	188	1.50%
33	Maine	0	0.00%
24	Maryland	165	1.31%
6	Massachusetts	425	3.38%
16	Michigan	245	1.95%
11	Minnesota	329	2.62%
33	Mississippi	0	0.00%
5	Missouri	592	4.71%
33	Montana	0	0.00%
25	Nebraska	142	1.13%
33	Nevada	0	0.00%
33	New Hampshire	0	0.00%
28	New Jersey	60	0.48%
29	New Mexico	37	0.29%
7	New York	405	3.22%
33	North Carolina	0	0.00%
33	North Dakota	0	0.00%
1	Ohio	2,535	20.17%
23	Oklahoma	168	1.34%
33	Oregon	0	0.00%
4	Pennsylvania	681	5.42%
33	Rhode Island	0	0.00%
33	South Carolina	0	0.00%
33	South Dakota	0	0.00%
22	Tennessee	178	1.42%
2	Texas	1,480	11.78%
19	Utah	194	1.54%
33	Vermont	0	0.00%
15	Virginia	250	1.99%
13	Washington	276	2.20%
33	West Virginia	0	0.00%
21	Wisconsin	186	1.48%
33	Wyoming	0	0.00%

RANK ORDER

RANK	STATE	BEDS	% of USA
1	Ohio	2,535	20.17%
2	Texas	1,480	11.78%
3	California	1,356	10.79%
4	Pennsylvania	681	5.42%
5	Missouri	592	4.71%
6	Massachusetts	425	3.38%
7	New York	405	3.22%
8	Georgia	400	3.18%
9	Florida	376	2.99%
10	Illinois	351	2.79%
11	Minnesota	329	2.62%
12	Arkansas	280	2.23%
13	Washington	276	2.20%
14	Colorado	253	2.01%
15	Virginia	250	1.99%
16	Michigan	245	1.95%
17	Hawaii	232	1.85%
18	Alabama	225	1.79%
19	Utah	194	1.54%
20	Louisiana	188	1.50%
21	Wisconsin	186	1.48%
22	Tennessee	178	1.42%
23	Oklahoma	168	1.34%
24	Maryland	165	1.31%
25	Nebraska	142	1.13%
26	Connecticut	97	0.77%
26	Delaware	97	0.77%
28	New Jersey	60	0.48%
29	New Mexico	37	0.29%
30	Indiana	35	0.28%
31	Kansas	34	0.27%
32	Arizona	15	0.12%
33	Alaska	0	0.00%
33	Idaho	0	0.00%
33	Iowa	0	0.00%
33	Kentucky	0	0.00%
33	Maine	0	0.00%
33	Mississippi	0	0.00%
33	Montana	0	0.00%
33	Nevada	0	0.00%
33	New Hampshire	0	0.00%
33	North Carolina	0	0.00%
33	North Dakota	0	0.00%
33	Oregon	0	0.00%
33	Rhode Island	0	0.00%
33	South Carolina	0	0.00%
33	South Dakota	0	0.00%
33	Vermont	0	0.00%
33	West Virginia	0	0.00%
33	Wyoming	0	0.00%
	District of Columbia	279	2.22%

Source: U.S. Department of Health and Human Services, Health Care Financing Administration
OSCAR Report 10 (March 18, 1998)
*Beds in hospitals certified by HCFA to participate in the Medicare/Medicaid programs. Excludes licensed facilities that do not accept federal funding and facilities managed by the Department of Veterans Affairs. National total does not include 215 beds in U.S. territories.

Medicare and Medicaid Certified Rehabilitation Hospitals in 1998

National Total = 199 Hospitals*

ALPHA ORDER

RANK ORDER

RANK	STATE	HOSPITALS	% of USA
11	Alabama	5	2.51%
44	Alaska	0	0.00%
11	Arizona	5	2.51%
8	Arkansas	6	3.02%
4	California	12	6.03%
16	Colorado	4	2.01%
31	Connecticut	1	0.50%
31	Delaware	1	0.50%
3	Florida	14	7.04%
26	Georgia	2	1.01%
31	Hawaii	1	0.50%
31	Idaho	1	0.50%
22	Illinois	3	1.51%
11	Indiana	5	2.51%
44	Iowa	0	0.00%
11	Kansas	5	2.51%
16	Kentucky	4	2.01%
5	Louisiana	11	5.53%
31	Maine	1	0.50%
26	Maryland	2	1.01%
7	Massachusetts	7	3.52%
6	Michigan	8	4.02%
44	Minnesota	0	0.00%
31	Mississippi	1	0.50%
22	Missouri	3	1.51%
44	Montana	0	0.00%
31	Nebraska	1	0.50%
22	Nevada	3	1.51%
26	New Hampshire	2	1.01%
8	New Jersey	6	3.02%
16	New Mexico	4	2.01%
16	New York	4	2.01%
26	North Carolina	2	1.01%
44	North Dakota	0	0.00%
31	Ohio	1	0.50%
16	Oklahoma	4	2.01%
44	Oregon	0	0.00%
2	Pennsylvania	16	8.04%
31	Rhode Island	1	0.50%
22	South Carolina	3	1.51%
31	South Dakota	1	0.50%
11	Tennessee	5	2.51%
1	Texas	28	14.07%
31	Utah	1	0.50%
44	Vermont	0	0.00%
16	Virginia	4	2.01%
31	Washington	1	0.50%
8	West Virginia	6	3.02%
26	Wisconsin	2	1.01%
31	Wyoming	1	0.50%

RANK	STATE	HOSPITALS	% of USA
1	Texas	28	14.07%
2	Pennsylvania	16	8.04%
3	Florida	14	7.04%
4	California	12	6.03%
5	Louisiana	11	5.53%
6	Michigan	8	4.02%
7	Massachusetts	7	3.52%
8	Arkansas	6	3.02%
8	New Jersey	6	3.02%
8	West Virginia	6	3.02%
11	Alabama	5	2.51%
11	Arizona	5	2.51%
11	Indiana	5	2.51%
11	Kansas	5	2.51%
11	Tennessee	5	2.51%
16	Colorado	4	2.01%
16	Kentucky	4	2.01%
16	New Mexico	4	2.01%
16	New York	4	2.01%
16	Oklahoma	4	2.01%
16	Virginia	4	2.01%
22	Illinois	3	1.51%
22	Missouri	3	1.51%
22	Nevada	3	1.51%
22	South Carolina	3	1.51%
26	Georgia	2	1.01%
26	Maryland	2	1.01%
26	New Hampshire	2	1.01%
26	North Carolina	2	1.01%
26	Wisconsin	2	1.01%
31	Connecticut	1	0.50%
31	Delaware	1	0.50%
31	Hawaii	1	0.50%
31	Idaho	1	0.50%
31	Maine	1	0.50%
31	Mississippi	1	0.50%
31	Nebraska	1	0.50%
31	Ohio	1	0.50%
31	Rhode Island	1	0.50%
31	South Dakota	1	0.50%
31	Utah	1	0.50%
31	Washington	1	0.50%
31	Wyoming	1	0.50%
44	Alaska	0	0.00%
44	Iowa	0	0.00%
44	Minnesota	0	0.00%
44	Montana	0	0.00%
44	North Dakota	0	0.00%
44	Oregon	0	0.00%
44	Vermont	0	0.00%
	District of Columbia	1	0.50%

Source: U.S. Department of Health and Human Services, Health Care Financing Administration
    OSCAR Report 10 (March 18, 1998)
*Certified by HCFA to participate in the Medicare/Medicaid programs. Excludes licensed facilities that do not accept federal funding and facilities managed by the Department of Veterans Affairs.

Beds in Medicare and Medicaid Certified Rehabilitation Hospitals in 1998

National Total = 14,175 Beds*

ALPHA ORDER

RANK ORDER

RANK	STATE	BEDS	% of USA		RANK	STATE	BEDS	% of USA
14	Alabama	296	2.09%		1	Texas	1,835	12.95%
43	Alaska	0	0.00%		2	Pennsylvania	1,578	11.13%
17	Arizona	247	1.74%		3	Florida	893	6.30%
6	Arkansas	773	5.45%		4	California	786	5.54%
4	California	786	5.54%		5	Massachusetts	776	5.47%
15	Colorado	266	1.88%		6	Arkansas	773	5.45%
37	Connecticut	60	0.42%		7	New Jersey	728	5.14%
37	Delaware	60	0.42%		8	Louisiana	554	3.91%
3	Florida	893	6.30%		9	Michigan	442	3.12%
29	Georgia	108	0.76%		10	New York	428	3.02%
31	Hawaii	100	0.71%		11	Illinois	371	2.62%
40	Idaho	54	0.38%		12	Tennessee	350	2.47%
11	Illinois	371	2.62%		13	Indiana	307	2.17%
13	Indiana	307	2.17%		14	Alabama	296	2.09%
43	Iowa	0	0.00%		15	Colorado	266	1.88%
16	Kansas	252	1.78%		16	Kansas	252	1.78%
20	Kentucky	225	1.59%		17	Arizona	247	1.74%
8	Louisiana	554	3.91%		18	West Virginia	246	1.74%
35	Maine	80	0.56%		19	Virginia	231	1.63%
36	Maryland	66	0.47%		20	Kentucky	225	1.59%
5	Massachusetts	776	5.47%		21	North Carolina	223	1.57%
9	Michigan	442	3.12%		22	Oklahoma	214	1.51%
43	Minnesota	0	0.00%		23	South Carolina	213	1.50%
31	Mississippi	100	0.71%		24	New Mexico	182	1.28%
25	Missouri	180	1.27%		25	Missouri	180	1.27%
43	Montana	0	0.00%		26	New Hampshire	152	1.07%
37	Nebraska	60	0.42%		27	Nevada	129	0.91%
27	Nevada	129	0.91%		28	Ohio	120	0.85%
26	New Hampshire	152	1.07%		29	Georgia	108	0.76%
7	New Jersey	728	5.14%		30	Washington	102	0.72%
24	New Mexico	182	1.28%		31	Hawaii	100	0.71%
10	New York	428	3.02%		31	Mississippi	100	0.71%
21	North Carolina	223	1.57%		33	Rhode Island	82	0.58%
43	North Dakota	0	0.00%		34	Wisconsin	81	0.57%
28	Ohio	120	0.85%		35	Maine	80	0.56%
22	Oklahoma	214	1.51%		36	Maryland	66	0.47%
43	Oregon	0	0.00%		37	Connecticut	60	0.42%
2	Pennsylvania	1,578	11.13%		37	Delaware	60	0.42%
33	Rhode Island	82	0.58%		37	Nebraska	60	0.42%
23	South Carolina	213	1.50%		40	Idaho	54	0.38%
43	South Dakota	0	0.00%		41	Utah	50	0.35%
12	Tennessee	350	2.47%		42	Wyoming	15	0.11%
1	Texas	1,835	12.95%		43	Alaska	0	0.00%
41	Utah	50	0.35%		43	Iowa	0	0.00%
43	Vermont	0	0.00%		43	Minnesota	0	0.00%
19	Virginia	231	1.63%		43	Montana	0	0.00%
30	Washington	102	0.72%		43	North Dakota	0	0.00%
18	West Virginia	246	1.74%		43	Oregon	0	0.00%
34	Wisconsin	81	0.57%		43	South Dakota	0	0.00%
42	Wyoming	15	0.11%		43	Vermont	0	0.00%
						District of Columbia	160	1.13%

Source: U.S. Department of Health and Human Services, Health Care Financing Administration
   OSCAR Report 10 (March 18, 1998)
*Beds in hospitals certified by HCFA to participate in the Medicare/Medicaid programs. Excludes licensed facilities that do not accept federal funding and facilities managed by the Department of Veterans Affairs.

Medicare and Medicaid Certified Psychiatric Hospitals in 1998

National Total = 613 Psychiatric Hospitals*

ALPHA ORDER

RANK ORDER

RANK	STATE	HOSPITALS	% of USA
22	Alabama	10	1.63%
41	Alaska	3	0.49%
23	Arizona	9	1.47%
23	Arkansas	9	1.47%
1	California	51	8.32%
23	Colorado	9	1.47%
23	Connecticut	9	1.47%
41	Delaware	3	0.49%
4	Florida	34	5.55%
6	Georgia	27	4.40%
49	Hawaii	1	0.16%
35	Idaho	4	0.65%
12	Illinois	16	2.61%
6	Indiana	27	4.40%
35	Iowa	4	0.65%
23	Kansas	9	1.47%
20	Kentucky	13	2.12%
8	Louisiana	23	3.75%
35	Maine	4	0.65%
17	Maryland	14	2.28%
9	Massachusetts	19	3.10%
20	Michigan	13	2.12%
30	Minnesota	6	0.98%
35	Mississippi	4	0.65%
10	Missouri	17	2.77%
45	Montana	2	0.33%
35	Nebraska	4	0.65%
31	Nevada	5	0.82%
41	New Hampshire	3	0.49%
12	New Jersey	16	2.61%
31	New Mexico	5	0.82%
3	New York	36	5.87%
15	North Carolina	15	2.45%
45	North Dakota	2	0.33%
12	Ohio	16	2.61%
17	Oklahoma	14	2.28%
35	Oregon	4	0.65%
5	Pennsylvania	29	4.73%
41	Rhode Island	3	0.49%
28	South Carolina	8	1.31%
49	South Dakota	1	0.16%
17	Tennessee	14	2.28%
2	Texas	42	6.85%
29	Utah	7	1.14%
45	Vermont	2	0.33%
10	Virginia	17	2.77%
31	Washington	5	0.82%
31	West Virginia	5	0.82%
15	Wisconsin	15	2.45%
45	Wyoming	2	0.33%

RANK	STATE	HOSPITALS	% of USA
1	California	51	8.32%
2	Texas	42	6.85%
3	New York	36	5.87%
4	Florida	34	5.55%
5	Pennsylvania	29	4.73%
6	Georgia	27	4.40%
6	Indiana	27	4.40%
8	Louisiana	23	3.75%
9	Massachusetts	19	3.10%
10	Missouri	17	2.77%
10	Virginia	17	2.77%
12	Illinois	16	2.61%
12	New Jersey	16	2.61%
12	Ohio	16	2.61%
15	North Carolina	15	2.45%
15	Wisconsin	15	2.45%
17	Maryland	14	2.28%
17	Oklahoma	14	2.28%
17	Tennessee	14	2.28%
20	Kentucky	13	2.12%
20	Michigan	13	2.12%
22	Alabama	10	1.63%
23	Arizona	9	1.47%
23	Arkansas	9	1.47%
23	Colorado	9	1.47%
23	Connecticut	9	1.47%
23	Kansas	9	1.47%
28	South Carolina	8	1.31%
29	Utah	7	1.14%
30	Minnesota	6	0.98%
31	Nevada	5	0.82%
31	New Mexico	5	0.82%
31	Washington	5	0.82%
31	West Virginia	5	0.82%
35	Idaho	4	0.65%
35	Iowa	4	0.65%
35	Maine	4	0.65%
35	Mississippi	4	0.65%
35	Nebraska	4	0.65%
35	Oregon	4	0.65%
41	Alaska	3	0.49%
41	Delaware	3	0.49%
41	New Hampshire	3	0.49%
41	Rhode Island	3	0.49%
45	Montana	2	0.33%
45	North Dakota	2	0.33%
45	Vermont	2	0.33%
45	Wyoming	2	0.33%
49	Hawaii	1	0.16%
49	South Dakota	1	0.16%
	District of Columbia	3	0.49%

Source: U.S. Department of Health and Human Services, Health Care Financing Administration
OSCAR Report 10 (March 18, 1998)

*Certified by HCFA to participate in the Medicare/Medicaid programs. Excludes licensed facilities that do not accept federal funding and facilities managed by the Department of Veterans Affairs. National total does not include three certified psychiatric hospitals in U.S. territories.

Beds in Medicare and Medicaid Certified Psychiatric Hospitals in 1998

National Total = 97,686 Beds*

ALPHA ORDER

RANK	STATE	BEDS	% of USA
26	Alabama	1,319	1.35%
45	Alaska	228	0.23%
39	Arizona	420	0.43%
32	Arkansas	714	0.73%
3	California	6,100	6.24%
25	Colorado	1,385	1.42%
27	Connecticut	1,197	1.23%
37	Delaware	514	0.53%
5	Florida	4,555	4.66%
6	Georgia	4,182	4.28%
48	Hawaii	88	0.09%
47	Idaho	145	0.15%
13	Illinois	2,434	2.49%
17	Indiana	1,959	2.01%
36	Iowa	522	0.53%
24	Kansas	1,479	1.51%
16	Kentucky	2,079	2.13%
14	Louisiana	2,334	2.39%
35	Maine	551	0.56%
7	Maryland	3,812	3.90%
18	Massachusetts	1,779	1.82%
11	Michigan	2,662	2.73%
23	Minnesota	1,519	1.55%
43	Mississippi	316	0.32%
15	Missouri	2,141	2.19%
50	Montana	54	0.06%
31	Nebraska	727	0.74%
28	Nevada	1,193	1.22%
38	New Hampshire	495	0.51%
8	New Jersey	3,609	3.69%
40	New Mexico	373	0.38%
1	New York	13,963	14.29%
10	North Carolina	3,324	3.40%
42	North Dakota	354	0.36%
12	Ohio	2,462	2.52%
19	Oklahoma	1,716	1.76%
33	Oregon	610	0.62%
2	Pennsylvania	6,558	6.71%
41	Rhode Island	359	0.37%
29	South Carolina	931	0.95%
49	South Dakota	85	0.09%
22	Tennessee	1,560	1.60%
4	Texas	5,627	5.76%
30	Utah	759	0.78%
46	Vermont	184	0.19%
9	Virginia	3,500	3.58%
21	Washington	1,566	1.60%
34	West Virginia	564	0.58%
20	Wisconsin	1,680	1.72%
44	Wyoming	266	0.27%

RANK ORDER

RANK	STATE	BEDS	% of USA
1	New York	13,963	14.29%
2	Pennsylvania	6,558	6.71%
3	California	6,100	6.24%
4	Texas	5,627	5.76%
5	Florida	4,555	4.66%
6	Georgia	4,182	4.28%
7	Maryland	3,812	3.90%
8	New Jersey	3,609	3.69%
9	Virginia	3,500	3.58%
10	North Carolina	3,324	3.40%
11	Michigan	2,662	2.73%
12	Ohio	2,462	2.52%
13	Illinois	2,434	2.49%
14	Louisiana	2,334	2.39%
15	Missouri	2,141	2.19%
16	Kentucky	2,079	2.13%
17	Indiana	1,959	2.01%
18	Massachusetts	1,779	1.82%
19	Oklahoma	1,716	1.76%
20	Wisconsin	1,680	1.72%
21	Washington	1,566	1.60%
22	Tennessee	1,560	1.60%
23	Minnesota	1,519	1.55%
24	Kansas	1,479	1.51%
25	Colorado	1,385	1.42%
26	Alabama	1,319	1.35%
27	Connecticut	1,197	1.23%
28	Nevada	1,193	1.22%
29	South Carolina	931	0.95%
30	Utah	759	0.78%
31	Nebraska	727	0.74%
32	Arkansas	714	0.73%
33	Oregon	610	0.62%
34	West Virginia	564	0.58%
35	Maine	551	0.56%
36	Iowa	522	0.53%
37	Delaware	514	0.53%
38	New Hampshire	495	0.51%
39	Arizona	420	0.43%
40	New Mexico	373	0.38%
41	Rhode Island	359	0.37%
42	North Dakota	354	0.36%
43	Mississippi	316	0.32%
44	Wyoming	266	0.27%
45	Alaska	228	0.23%
46	Vermont	184	0.19%
47	Idaho	145	0.15%
48	Hawaii	88	0.09%
49	South Dakota	85	0.09%
50	Montana	54	0.06%
	District of Columbia	733	0.75%

Source: U.S. Department of Health and Human Services, Health Care Financing Administration OSCAR Report 10 (March 18, 1998)

*Beds in hospitals certified by HCFA to participate in the Medicare/Medicaid programs. Excludes licensed facilities that do not accept federal funding and facilities managed by the Department of Veterans Affairs. National total does not include 703 beds in U.S. territories.

Medicare and Medicaid Certified Community Mental Health Centers in 1998

National Total = 1,185 Centers*

ALPHA ORDER					RANK ORDER			
RANK	STATE		CENTERS	% of USA	RANK	STATE	CENTERS	% of USA
3	Alabama		111	9.37%	1	Florida	254	21.43%
46	Alaska		0	0.00%	2	Texas	146	12.32%
30	Arizona		9	0.76%	3	Alabama	111	9.37%
21	Arkansas		14	1.18%	4	Pennsylvania	70	5.91%
10	California		30	2.53%	5	Louisiana	49	4.14%
16	Colorado		17	1.43%	6	New Jersey	39	3.29%
31	Connecticut		8	0.68%	7	Washington	37	3.12%
46	Delaware		0	0.00%	8	Ohio	34	2.87%
1	Florida		254	21.43%	9	North Carolina	32	2.70%
21	Georgia		14	1.18%	10	California	30	2.53%
46	Hawaii		0	0.00%	11	Tennessee	29	2.45%
42	Idaho		1	0.08%	12	Illinois	23	1.94%
12	Illinois		23	1.94%	12	Missouri	23	1.94%
26	Indiana		13	1.10%	14	Kansas	20	1.69%
29	Iowa		11	0.93%	15	Michigan	19	1.60%
14	Kansas		20	1.69%	16	Colorado	17	1.43%
21	Kentucky		14	1.18%	16	New Mexico	17	1.43%
5	Louisiana		49	4.14%	16	Oregon	17	1.43%
36	Maine		4	0.34%	19	Massachusetts	16	1.35%
32	Maryland		7	0.59%	19	Minnesota	16	1.35%
19	Massachusetts		16	1.35%	21	Arkansas	14	1.18%
15	Michigan		19	1.60%	21	Georgia	14	1.18%
19	Minnesota		16	1.35%	21	Kentucky	14	1.18%
21	Mississippi		14	1.18%	21	Mississippi	14	1.18%
12	Missouri		23	1.94%	21	South Carolina	14	1.18%
36	Montana		4	0.34%	26	Indiana	13	1.10%
42	Nebraska		1	0.08%	26	New York	13	1.10%
41	Nevada		2	0.17%	26	Oklahoma	13	1.10%
35	New Hampshire		5	0.42%	29	Iowa	11	0.93%
6	New Jersey		39	3.29%	30	Arizona	9	0.76%
16	New Mexico		17	1.43%	31	Connecticut	8	0.68%
26	New York		13	1.10%	32	Maryland	7	0.59%
9	North Carolina		32	2.70%	32	Virginia	7	0.59%
46	North Dakota		0	0.00%	34	Utah	6	0.51%
8	Ohio		34	2.87%	35	New Hampshire	5	0.42%
26	Oklahoma		13	1.10%	36	Maine	4	0.34%
16	Oregon		17	1.43%	36	Montana	4	0.34%
4	Pennsylvania		70	5.91%	36	Wyoming	4	0.34%
42	Rhode Island		1	0.08%	39	South Dakota	3	0.25%
21	South Carolina		14	1.18%	39	West Virginia	3	0.25%
39	South Dakota		3	0.25%	41	Nevada	2	0.17%
11	Tennessee		29	2.45%	42	Idaho	1	0.08%
2	Texas		146	12.32%	42	Nebraska	1	0.08%
34	Utah		6	0.51%	42	Rhode Island	1	0.08%
46	Vermont		0	0.00%	42	Wisconsin	1	0.08%
32	Virginia		7	0.59%	46	Alaska	0	0.00%
7	Washington		37	3.12%	46	Delaware	0	0.00%
39	West Virginia		3	0.25%	46	Hawaii	0	0.00%
42	Wisconsin		1	0.08%	46	North Dakota	0	0.00%
36	Wyoming		4	0.34%	46	Vermont	0	0.00%
						District of Columbia	0	0.00%

Source: U.S. Department of Health and Human Services, Health Care Financing Administration
OSCAR Report 10 (March 18, 1998)

*Certified by HCFA to participate in the Medicare/Medicaid programs. Excludes licensed facilities that do not accept federal funding and facilities managed by the Department of Veterans Affairs. National total does not include 10 certified mental health centers in U.S. territories.

Medicare and Medicaid Certified Outpatient Physical Therapy Facilities in 1998

National Total = 2,802 Facilities*

ALPHA ORDER

RANK	STATE	FACILITIES	% of USA
32	Alabama	22	0.79%
36	Alaska	17	0.61%
22	Arizona	40	1.43%
30	Arkansas	24	0.86%
2	California	211	7.53%
20	Colorado	54	1.93%
24	Connecticut	39	1.39%
32	Delaware	22	0.79%
1	Florida	287	10.24%
5	Georgia	147	5.25%
45	Hawaii	7	0.25%
38	Idaho	15	0.54%
13	Illinois	71	2.53%
14	Indiana	66	2.36%
24	Iowa	39	1.39%
29	Kansas	30	1.07%
27	Kentucky	37	1.32%
17	Louisiana	57	2.03%
35	Maine	18	0.64%
11	Maryland	78	2.78%
37	Massachusetts	16	0.57%
4	Michigan	170	6.07%
15	Minnesota	59	2.11%
21	Mississippi	41	1.46%
12	Missouri	75	2.68%
43	Montana	8	0.29%
39	Nebraska	14	0.50%
41	Nevada	12	0.43%
40	New Hampshire	13	0.46%
9	New Jersey	109	3.89%
28	New Mexico	31	1.11%
31	New York	23	0.82%
18	North Carolina	55	1.96%
42	North Dakota	9	0.32%
7	Ohio	115	4.10%
26	Oklahoma	38	1.36%
34	Oregon	21	0.75%
6	Pennsylvania	134	4.78%
47	Rhode Island	4	0.14%
16	South Carolina	58	2.07%
49	South Dakota	2	0.07%
10	Tennessee	88	3.14%
3	Texas	197	7.03%
45	Utah	7	0.25%
49	Vermont	2	0.07%
8	Virginia	114	4.07%
22	Washington	40	1.43%
43	West Virginia	8	0.29%
18	Wisconsin	55	1.96%
48	Wyoming	3	0.11%

RANK ORDER

RANK	STATE	FACILITIES	% of USA
1	Florida	287	10.24%
2	California	211	7.53%
3	Texas	197	7.03%
4	Michigan	170	6.07%
5	Georgia	147	5.25%
6	Pennsylvania	134	4.78%
7	Ohio	115	4.10%
8	Virginia	114	4.07%
9	New Jersey	109	3.89%
10	Tennessee	88	3.14%
11	Maryland	78	2.78%
12	Missouri	75	2.68%
13	Illinois	71	2.53%
14	Indiana	66	2.36%
15	Minnesota	59	2.11%
16	South Carolina	58	2.07%
17	Louisiana	57	2.03%
18	North Carolina	55	1.96%
18	Wisconsin	55	1.96%
20	Colorado	54	1.93%
21	Mississippi	41	1.46%
22	Arizona	40	1.43%
22	Washington	40	1.43%
24	Connecticut	39	1.39%
24	Iowa	39	1.39%
26	Oklahoma	38	1.36%
27	Kentucky	37	1.32%
28	New Mexico	31	1.11%
29	Kansas	30	1.07%
30	Arkansas	24	0.86%
31	New York	23	0.82%
32	Alabama	22	0.79%
32	Delaware	22	0.79%
34	Oregon	21	0.75%
35	Maine	18	0.64%
36	Alaska	17	0.61%
37	Massachusetts	16	0.57%
38	Idaho	15	0.54%
39	Nebraska	14	0.50%
40	New Hampshire	13	0.46%
41	Nevada	12	0.43%
42	North Dakota	9	0.32%
43	Montana	8	0.29%
43	West Virginia	8	0.29%
45	Hawaii	7	0.25%
45	Utah	7	0.25%
47	Rhode Island	4	0.14%
48	Wyoming	3	0.11%
49	South Dakota	2	0.07%
49	Vermont	2	0.07%
	District of Columbia	0	0.00%

Source: U.S. Department of Health and Human Services, Health Care Financing Administration
    OSCAR Report 10 (March 18, 1998)
*Certified by HCFA to participate in the Medicare/Medicaid programs. Excludes licensed facilities that do not accept federal funding and facilities managed by the Department of Veterans Affairs. National total does not include three certified outpatient physical therapy facilities in U.S. territories.

Medicare and Medicaid Certified Rural Health Clinics in 1998

National Total = 3,549 Rural Health Clinics*

ALPHA ORDER

RANK ORDER

RANK	STATE	CLINICS	% of USA
18	Alabama	73	2.06%
40	Alaska	12	0.34%
39	Arizona	13	0.37%
12	Arkansas	97	2.73%
2	California	204	5.75%
30	Colorado	36	1.01%
46	Connecticut	0	0.00%
46	Delaware	0	0.00%
8	Florida	145	4.09%
7	Georgia	146	4.11%
44	Hawaii	1	0.03%
31	Idaho	26	0.73%
3	Illinois	181	5.10%
28	Indiana	49	1.38%
10	Iowa	134	3.78%
4	Kansas	180	5.07%
17	Kentucky	74	2.09%
19	Louisiana	68	1.92%
29	Maine	47	1.32%
46	Maryland	0	0.00%
46	Massachusetts	0	0.00%
11	Michigan	129	3.63%
22	Minnesota	58	1.63%
6	Mississippi	167	4.71%
5	Missouri	177	4.99%
32	Montana	24	0.68%
16	Nebraska	76	2.14%
43	Nevada	3	0.08%
35	New Hampshire	21	0.59%
46	New Jersey	0	0.00%
36	New Mexico	16	0.45%
42	New York	10	0.28%
9	North Carolina	135	3.80%
15	North Dakota	82	2.31%
41	Ohio	11	0.31%
14	Oklahoma	87	2.45%
34	Oregon	23	0.65%
26	Pennsylvania	55	1.55%
44	Rhode Island	1	0.03%
13	South Carolina	93	2.62%
24	South Dakota	57	1.61%
22	Tennessee	58	1.63%
1	Texas	489	13.78%
37	Utah	15	0.42%
32	Vermont	24	0.68%
21	Virginia	62	1.75%
27	Washington	54	1.52%
20	West Virginia	64	1.80%
24	Wisconsin	57	1.61%
37	Wyoming	15	0.42%

RANK	STATE	CLINICS	% of USA
1	Texas	489	13.78%
2	California	204	5.75%
3	Illinois	181	5.10%
4	Kansas	180	5.07%
5	Missouri	177	4.99%
6	Mississippi	167	4.71%
7	Georgia	146	4.11%
8	Florida	145	4.09%
9	North Carolina	135	3.80%
10	Iowa	134	3.78%
11	Michigan	129	3.63%
12	Arkansas	97	2.73%
13	South Carolina	93	2.62%
14	Oklahoma	87	2.45%
15	North Dakota	82	2.31%
16	Nebraska	76	2.14%
17	Kentucky	74	2.09%
18	Alabama	73	2.06%
19	Louisiana	68	1.92%
20	West Virginia	64	1.80%
21	Virginia	62	1.75%
22	Minnesota	58	1.63%
22	Tennessee	58	1.63%
24	South Dakota	57	1.61%
24	Wisconsin	57	1.61%
26	Pennsylvania	55	1.55%
27	Washington	54	1.52%
28	Indiana	49	1.38%
29	Maine	47	1.32%
30	Colorado	36	1.01%
31	Idaho	26	0.73%
32	Montana	24	0.68%
32	Vermont	24	0.68%
34	Oregon	23	0.65%
35	New Hampshire	21	0.59%
36	New Mexico	16	0.45%
37	Utah	15	0.42%
37	Wyoming	15	0.42%
39	Arizona	13	0.37%
40	Alaska	12	0.34%
41	Ohio	11	0.31%
42	New York	10	0.28%
43	Nevada	3	0.08%
44	Hawaii	1	0.03%
44	Rhode Island	1	0.03%
46	Connecticut	0	0.00%
46	Delaware	0	0.00%
46	Maryland	0	0.00%
46	Massachusetts	0	0.00%
46	New Jersey	0	0.00%
	District of Columbia	0	0.00%

Source: U.S. Department of Health and Human Services, Health Care Financing Administration
    OSCAR Report 10 (March 18, 1998)
*Certified by HCFA to participate in the Medicare/Medicaid programs. Excludes licensed facilities that do not accept federal funding and facilities managed by the Department of Veterans Affairs. There are no certified rural health centers in U.S. territories.

Medicare and Medicaid Certified Home Health Agencies in 1998

National Total = 10,414 Home Health Agencies*

ALPHA ORDER

RANK ORDER

RANK	STATE	AGENCIES	% of USA		RANK	STATE	AGENCIES	% of USA
21	Alabama	183	1.76%		1	Texas	1,893	18.18%
47	Alaska	27	0.26%		2	California	839	8.06%
24	Arizona	122	1.17%		3	Louisiana	505	4.85%
18	Arkansas	205	1.97%		4	Ohio	475	4.56%
2	California	839	8.06%		5	Florida	399	3.83%
19	Colorado	199	1.91%		6	Illinois	384	3.69%
25	Connecticut	115	1.10%		7	Pennsylvania	379	3.64%
49	Delaware	21	0.20%		8	Oklahoma	371	3.56%
5	Florida	399	3.83%		9	Indiana	296	2.84%
28	Georgia	98	0.94%		10	Missouri	270	2.59%
48	Hawaii	25	0.24%		11	Minnesota	265	2.54%
35	Idaho	77	0.74%		12	Tennessee	237	2.28%
6	Illinois	384	3.69%		13	Michigan	233	2.24%
9	Indiana	296	2.84%		14	Virginia	229	2.20%
17	Iowa	210	2.02%		15	New York	226	2.17%
16	Kansas	218	2.09%		16	Kansas	218	2.09%
27	Kentucky	110	1.06%		17	Iowa	210	2.02%
3	Louisiana	505	4.85%		18	Arkansas	205	1.97%
43	Maine	47	0.45%		19	Colorado	199	1.91%
34	Maryland	79	0.76%		19	Massachusetts	199	1.91%
19	Massachusetts	199	1.91%		21	Alabama	183	1.76%
13	Michigan	233	2.24%		22	Wisconsin	181	1.74%
11	Minnesota	265	2.54%		23	North Carolina	178	1.71%
36	Mississippi	70	0.67%		24	Arizona	122	1.17%
10	Missouri	270	2.59%		25	Connecticut	115	1.10%
39	Montana	62	0.60%		26	New Mexico	114	1.09%
32	Nebraska	84	0.81%		27	Kentucky	110	1.06%
42	Nevada	49	0.47%		28	Georgia	98	0.94%
44	New Hampshire	46	0.44%		29	Utah	91	0.87%
40	New Jersey	57	0.55%		29	West Virginia	91	0.87%
26	New Mexico	114	1.09%		31	Oregon	88	0.85%
15	New York	226	2.17%		32	Nebraska	84	0.81%
23	North Carolina	178	1.71%		33	South Carolina	81	0.78%
45	North Dakota	36	0.35%		34	Maryland	79	0.76%
4	Ohio	475	4.56%		35	Idaho	77	0.74%
8	Oklahoma	371	3.56%		36	Mississippi	70	0.67%
31	Oregon	88	0.85%		37	Washington	68	0.65%
7	Pennsylvania	379	3.64%		38	Wyoming	64	0.61%
46	Rhode Island	28	0.27%		39	Montana	62	0.60%
33	South Carolina	81	0.78%		40	New Jersey	57	0.55%
41	South Dakota	56	0.54%		41	South Dakota	56	0.54%
12	Tennessee	237	2.28%		42	Nevada	49	0.47%
1	Texas	1,893	18.18%		43	Maine	47	0.45%
29	Utah	91	0.87%		44	New Hampshire	46	0.44%
50	Vermont	13	0.12%		45	North Dakota	36	0.35%
14	Virginia	229	2.20%		46	Rhode Island	28	0.27%
37	Washington	68	0.65%		47	Alaska	27	0.26%
29	West Virginia	91	0.87%		48	Hawaii	25	0.24%
22	Wisconsin	181	1.74%		49	Delaware	21	0.20%
38	Wyoming	64	0.61%		50	Vermont	13	0.12%
						District of Columbia	21	0.20%

Source: U.S. Department of Health and Human Services, Health Care Financing Administration
    OSCAR Report 10 (March 18, 1998)

*Certified by HCFA to participate in the Medicare/Medicaid programs. Excludes agencies that do not accept federal funding. National total does not include 49 certified home health agencies in U.S. territories. A home health agency provides health services to individuals in their homes for the purpose of promoting, maintaining or restoring health or maximizing the level of independence, while minimizing the effects of disability and illness.

Medicare and Medicaid Certified Hospices in 1998

National Total = 2,248 Hospices*

ALPHA ORDER

RANK	STATE	HOSPICES	% of USA
9	Alabama	66	2.94%
50	Alaska	3	0.13%
22	Arizona	41	1.82%
14	Arkansas	59	2.62%
1	California	188	8.36%
23	Colorado	39	1.73%
32	Connecticut	29	1.29%
49	Delaware	5	0.22%
23	Florida	39	1.73%
13	Georgia	60	2.67%
46	Hawaii	8	0.36%
32	Idaho	29	1.29%
5	Illinois	84	3.74%
10	Indiana	62	2.76%
15	Iowa	57	2.54%
29	Kansas	32	1.42%
32	Kentucky	29	1.29%
23	Louisiana	39	1.73%
41	Maine	15	0.67%
29	Maryland	32	1.42%
21	Massachusetts	44	1.96%
7	Michigan	75	3.34%
11	Minnesota	61	2.71%
28	Mississippi	33	1.47%
6	Missouri	76	3.38%
40	Montana	17	0.76%
36	Nebraska	27	1.20%
48	Nevada	7	0.31%
37	New Hampshire	22	0.98%
19	New Jersey	45	2.00%
29	New Mexico	32	1.42%
16	New York	54	2.40%
8	North Carolina	71	3.16%
42	North Dakota	14	0.62%
4	Ohio	94	4.18%
18	Oklahoma	48	2.14%
23	Oregon	39	1.73%
3	Pennsylvania	118	5.25%
45	Rhode Island	9	0.40%
27	South Carolina	34	1.51%
42	South Dakota	14	0.62%
11	Tennessee	61	2.71%
2	Texas	148	6.58%
39	Utah	18	0.80%
46	Vermont	8	0.36%
19	Virginia	45	2.00%
35	Washington	28	1.25%
37	West Virginia	22	0.98%
17	Wisconsin	52	2.31%
44	Wyoming	12	0.53%

RANK ORDER

RANK	STATE	HOSPICES	% of USA
1	California	188	8.36%
2	Texas	148	6.58%
3	Pennsylvania	118	5.25%
4	Ohio	94	4.18%
5	Illinois	84	3.74%
6	Missouri	76	3.38%
7	Michigan	75	3.34%
8	North Carolina	71	3.16%
9	Alabama	66	2.94%
10	Indiana	62	2.76%
11	Minnesota	61	2.71%
11	Tennessee	61	2.71%
13	Georgia	60	2.67%
14	Arkansas	59	2.62%
15	Iowa	57	2.54%
16	New York	54	2.40%
17	Wisconsin	52	2.31%
18	Oklahoma	48	2.14%
19	New Jersey	45	2.00%
19	Virginia	45	2.00%
21	Massachusetts	44	1.96%
22	Arizona	41	1.82%
23	Colorado	39	1.73%
23	Florida	39	1.73%
23	Louisiana	39	1.73%
23	Oregon	39	1.73%
27	South Carolina	34	1.51%
28	Mississippi	33	1.47%
29	Kansas	32	1.42%
29	Maryland	32	1.42%
29	New Mexico	32	1.42%
32	Connecticut	29	1.29%
32	Idaho	29	1.29%
32	Kentucky	29	1.29%
35	Washington	28	1.25%
36	Nebraska	27	1.20%
37	New Hampshire	22	0.98%
37	West Virginia	22	0.98%
39	Utah	18	0.80%
40	Montana	17	0.76%
41	Maine	15	0.67%
42	North Dakota	14	0.62%
42	South Dakota	14	0.62%
44	Wyoming	12	0.53%
45	Rhode Island	9	0.40%
46	Hawaii	8	0.36%
46	Vermont	8	0.36%
48	Nevada	7	0.31%
49	Delaware	5	0.22%
50	Alaska	3	0.13%
	District of Columbia	4	0.18%

Source: U.S. Department of Health and Human Services, Health Care Financing Administration
   OSCAR Report 10 (March 18, 1998)
*Certified by HCFA to participate in the Medicare/Medicaid programs. Excludes licensed facilities that do not accept federal funding and facilities managed by the Department of Veterans Affairs. National total does not include 34 certified hospices in U.S. territories. An hospice provides specialized services for terminally ill people and their families.

Hospice Patients in Residential Facilities in 1998

National Total = 7,766 Patients*

ALPHA ORDER

RANK	STATE	PATIENTS	% of USA
35	Alabama	14	0.18%
47	Alaska	0	0.00%
25	Arizona	61	0.79%
19	Arkansas	107	1.38%
4	California	544	7.00%
12	Colorado	213	2.74%
28	Connecticut	42	0.54%
47	Delaware	0	0.00%
1	Florida	1,265	16.29%
23	Georgia	72	0.93%
47	Hawaii	0	0.00%
41	Idaho	5	0.06%
20	Illinois	95	1.22%
11	Indiana	247	3.18%
17	Iowa	135	1.74%
27	Kansas	49	0.63%
8	Kentucky	338	4.35%
34	Louisiana	17	0.22%
37	Maine	12	0.15%
32	Maryland	30	0.39%
16	Massachusetts	178	2.29%
31	Michigan	32	0.41%
18	Minnesota	114	1.47%
39	Mississippi	9	0.12%
9	Missouri	272	3.50%
29	Montana	41	0.53%
21	Nebraska	86	1.11%
22	Nevada	82	1.06%
47	New Hampshire	0	0.00%
10	New Jersey	258	3.32%
37	New Mexico	12	0.15%
12	New York	213	2.74%
15	North Carolina	180	2.32%
39	North Dakota	9	0.12%
14	Ohio	183	2.36%
5	Oklahoma	483	6.22%
6	Oregon	351	4.52%
2	Pennsylvania	793	10.21%
43	Rhode Island	3	0.04%
26	South Carolina	51	0.66%
42	South Dakota	4	0.05%
30	Tennessee	36	0.46%
3	Texas	658	8.47%
43	Utah	3	0.04%
36	Vermont	13	0.17%
33	Virginia	22	0.28%
7	Washington	343	4.42%
45	West Virginia	2	0.03%
24	Wisconsin	64	0.82%
45	Wyoming	2	0.03%

RANK ORDER

RANK	STATE	PATIENTS	% of USA
1	Florida	1,265	16.29%
2	Pennsylvania	793	10.21%
3	Texas	658	8.47%
4	California	544	7.00%
5	Oklahoma	483	6.22%
6	Oregon	351	4.52%
7	Washington	343	4.42%
8	Kentucky	338	4.35%
9	Missouri	272	3.50%
10	New Jersey	258	3.32%
11	Indiana	247	3.18%
12	Colorado	213	2.74%
12	New York	213	2.74%
14	Ohio	183	2.36%
15	North Carolina	180	2.32%
16	Massachusetts	178	2.29%
17	Iowa	135	1.74%
18	Minnesota	114	1.47%
19	Arkansas	107	1.38%
20	Illinois	95	1.22%
21	Nebraska	86	1.11%
22	Nevada	82	1.06%
23	Georgia	72	0.93%
24	Wisconsin	64	0.82%
25	Arizona	61	0.79%
26	South Carolina	51	0.66%
27	Kansas	49	0.63%
28	Connecticut	42	0.54%
29	Montana	41	0.53%
30	Tennessee	36	0.46%
31	Michigan	32	0.41%
32	Maryland	30	0.39%
33	Virginia	22	0.28%
34	Louisiana	17	0.22%
35	Alabama	14	0.18%
36	Vermont	13	0.17%
37	Maine	12	0.15%
37	New Mexico	12	0.15%
39	Mississippi	9	0.12%
39	North Dakota	9	0.12%
41	Idaho	5	0.06%
42	South Dakota	4	0.05%
43	Rhode Island	3	0.04%
43	Utah	3	0.04%
45	West Virginia	2	0.03%
45	Wyoming	2	0.03%
47	Alaska	0	0.00%
47	Delaware	0	0.00%
47	Hawaii	0	0.00%
47	New Hampshire	0	0.00%
	District of Columbia	23	0.30%

*Source: U.S. Department of Health and Human Services, Health Care Financing Administration
OSCAR Report 10 (March 18, 1998)*
*Patients in facilities certified by HCFA to participate in the Medicare/Medicaid programs. Excludes licensed
facilities that do not accept federal funding and facilities managed by the Department of Veterans Affairs. National
total does not include patients in U.S. territories. An hospice provides specialized services for terminally ill people
and their families.*

Medicare and Medicaid Certified Nursing Care Facilities in 1998

National Total = 17,360 Nursing Care Facilities*

ALPHA ORDER

RANK	STATE	FACILITIES	% of USA
30	Alabama	223	1.28%
50	Alaska	15	0.09%
33	Arizona	165	0.95%
25	Arkansas	272	1.57%
1	California	1,424	8.20%
29	Colorado	225	1.30%
27	Connecticut	260	1.50%
47	Delaware	44	0.25%
6	Florida	740	4.26%
18	Georgia	355	2.04%
47	Hawaii	44	0.25%
42	Idaho	85	0.49%
4	Illinois	873	5.03%
9	Indiana	579	3.34%
11	Iowa	473	2.72%
15	Kansas	417	2.40%
22	Kentucky	317	1.83%
20	Louisiana	347	2.00%
36	Maine	135	0.78%
26	Maryland	264	1.52%
10	Massachusetts	566	3.26%
13	Michigan	446	2.57%
12	Minnesota	451	2.60%
31	Mississippi	208	1.20%
8	Missouri	584	3.36%
38	Montana	104	0.60%
28	Nebraska	237	1.37%
45	Nevada	47	0.27%
44	New Hampshire	82	0.47%
21	New Jersey	345	1.99%
42	New Mexico	85	0.49%
7	New York	659	3.80%
17	North Carolina	404	2.33%
41	North Dakota	88	0.51%
3	Ohio	1,017	5.86%
16	Oklahoma	416	2.40%
34	Oregon	163	0.94%
5	Pennsylvania	802	4.62%
39	Rhode Island	100	0.58%
32	South Carolina	176	1.01%
37	South Dakota	114	0.66%
19	Tennessee	352	2.03%
2	Texas	1,313	7.56%
40	Utah	96	0.55%
46	Vermont	46	0.26%
24	Virginia	284	1.64%
23	Washington	285	1.64%
35	West Virginia	144	0.83%
14	Wisconsin	428	2.47%
49	Wyoming	39	0.22%

RANK ORDER

RANK	STATE	FACILITIES	% of USA
1	California	1,424	8.20%
2	Texas	1,313	7.56%
3	Ohio	1,017	5.86%
4	Illinois	873	5.03%
5	Pennsylvania	802	4.62%
6	Florida	740	4.26%
7	New York	659	3.80%
8	Missouri	584	3.36%
9	Indiana	579	3.34%
10	Massachusetts	566	3.26%
11	Iowa	473	2.72%
12	Minnesota	451	2.60%
13	Michigan	446	2.57%
14	Wisconsin	428	2.47%
15	Kansas	417	2.40%
16	Oklahoma	416	2.40%
17	North Carolina	404	2.33%
18	Georgia	355	2.04%
19	Tennessee	352	2.03%
20	Louisiana	347	2.00%
21	New Jersey	345	1.99%
22	Kentucky	317	1.83%
23	Washington	285	1.64%
24	Virginia	284	1.64%
25	Arkansas	272	1.57%
26	Maryland	264	1.52%
27	Connecticut	260	1.50%
28	Nebraska	237	1.37%
29	Colorado	225	1.30%
30	Alabama	223	1.28%
31	Mississippi	208	1.20%
32	South Carolina	176	1.01%
33	Arizona	165	0.95%
34	Oregon	163	0.94%
35	West Virginia	144	0.83%
36	Maine	135	0.78%
37	South Dakota	114	0.66%
38	Montana	104	0.60%
39	Rhode Island	100	0.58%
40	Utah	96	0.55%
41	North Dakota	88	0.51%
42	Idaho	85	0.49%
42	New Mexico	85	0.49%
44	New Hampshire	82	0.47%
45	Nevada	47	0.27%
46	Vermont	46	0.26%
47	Delaware	44	0.25%
47	Hawaii	44	0.25%
49	Wyoming	39	0.22%
50	Alaska	15	0.09%
	District of Columbia	22	0.13%

*Source: U.S. Department of Health and Human Services, Health Care Financing Administration
OSCAR Report 10 (March 18, 1998)*
*Certified by HCFA to participate in the Medicare/Medicaid programs. Excludes licensed facilities that do not accept federal funding and facilities managed by the Department of Veterans Affairs. National total does not include eight certified nursing facilities in U.S. territories.

Beds in Medicare and Medicaid Certified Nursing Care Facilities in 1998

National Total = 1,731,249 Beds*

ALPHA ORDER

RANK	STATE	BEDS	% of USA
27	Alabama	24,542	1.42%
50	Alaska	717	0.04%
32	Arizona	16,731	0.97%
26	Arkansas	25,393	1.47%
1	California	127,423	7.36%
29	Colorado	18,912	1.09%
21	Connecticut	31,654	1.83%
45	Delaware	4,525	0.26%
7	Florida	76,882	4.44%
17	Georgia	38,870	2.25%
47	Hawaii	3,896	0.23%
44	Idaho	5,309	0.31%
4	Illinois	99,465	5.75%
9	Indiana	55,144	3.19%
19	Iowa	35,099	2.03%
24	Kansas	27,020	1.56%
28	Kentucky	24,040	1.39%
18	Louisiana	37,186	2.15%
37	Maine	9,269	0.54%
22	Maryland	31,045	1.79%
8	Massachusetts	56,801	3.28%
12	Michigan	49,005	2.83%
14	Minnesota	44,611	2.58%
31	Mississippi	17,064	0.99%
10	Missouri	51,399	2.97%
40	Montana	7,514	0.43%
30	Nebraska	17,302	1.00%
46	Nevada	4,216	0.24%
39	New Hampshire	7,841	0.45%
11	New Jersey	50,486	2.92%
42	New Mexico	7,111	0.41%
2	New York	117,634	6.79%
15	North Carolina	39,354	2.27%
43	North Dakota	7,086	0.41%
6	Ohio	94,100	5.44%
20	Oklahoma	33,797	1.95%
34	Oregon	13,559	0.78%
5	Pennsylvania	95,721	5.53%
36	Rhode Island	10,119	0.58%
33	South Carolina	16,495	0.95%
38	South Dakota	8,070	0.47%
16	Tennessee	38,952	2.25%
3	Texas	115,689	6.68%
41	Utah	7,476	0.43%
48	Vermont	3,817	0.22%
23	Virginia	30,691	1.77%
25	Washington	26,472	1.53%
35	West Virginia	11,796	0.68%
13	Wisconsin	47,709	2.76%
49	Wyoming	3,131	0.18%

RANK ORDER

RANK	STATE	BEDS	% of USA
1	California	127,423	7.36%
2	New York	117,634	6.79%
3	Texas	115,689	6.68%
4	Illinois	99,465	5.75%
5	Pennsylvania	95,721	5.53%
6	Ohio	94,100	5.44%
7	Florida	76,882	4.44%
8	Massachusetts	56,801	3.28%
9	Indiana	55,144	3.19%
10	Missouri	51,399	2.97%
11	New Jersey	50,486	2.92%
12	Michigan	49,005	2.83%
13	Wisconsin	47,709	2.76%
14	Minnesota	44,611	2.58%
15	North Carolina	39,354	2.27%
16	Tennessee	38,952	2.25%
17	Georgia	38,870	2.25%
18	Louisiana	37,186	2.15%
19	Iowa	35,099	2.03%
20	Oklahoma	33,797	1.95%
21	Connecticut	31,654	1.83%
22	Maryland	31,045	1.79%
23	Virginia	30,691	1.77%
24	Kansas	27,020	1.56%
25	Washington	26,472	1.53%
26	Arkansas	25,393	1.47%
27	Alabama	24,542	1.42%
28	Kentucky	24,040	1.39%
29	Colorado	18,912	1.09%
30	Nebraska	17,302	1.00%
31	Mississippi	17,064	0.99%
32	Arizona	16,731	0.97%
33	South Carolina	16,495	0.95%
34	Oregon	13,559	0.78%
35	West Virginia	11,796	0.68%
36	Rhode Island	10,119	0.58%
37	Maine	9,269	0.54%
38	South Dakota	8,070	0.47%
39	New Hampshire	7,841	0.45%
40	Montana	7,514	0.43%
41	Utah	7,476	0.43%
42	New Mexico	7,111	0.41%
43	North Dakota	7,086	0.41%
44	Idaho	5,309	0.31%
45	Delaware	4,525	0.26%
46	Nevada	4,216	0.24%
47	Hawaii	3,896	0.23%
48	Vermont	3,817	0.22%
49	Wyoming	3,131	0.18%
50	Alaska	717	0.04%
	District of Columbia	3,109	0.18%

*Source: U.S. Department of Health and Human Services, Health Care Financing Administration
OSCAR Report 10 (March 18, 1998)*
*Beds in nursing care facilities certified by HCFA to participate in the Medicare/Medicaid programs. National total does not include 321 beds in U.S. territories.

Rate of Beds in Medicare and Medicaid Certified Nursing Care Facilities in 1998

National Rate = 460 Beds per 1,000 Population 85 Years Old and Older*

ALPHA ORDER

RANK	STATE	RATE
35	Alabama	407
43	Alaska	366
47	Arizona	301
4	Arkansas	605
45	California	339
27	Colorado	453
11	Connecticut	552
23	Delaware	517
49	Florida	274
24	Georgia	516
48	Hawaii	275
44	Idaho	347
6	Illinois	577
2	Indiana	671
7	Iowa	574
9	Kansas	563
28	Kentucky	446
1	Louisiana	712
29	Maine	443
20	Maryland	527
16	Massachusetts	535
40	Michigan	388
8	Minnesota	573
30	Mississippi	441
12	Missouri	551
10	Montana	554
19	Nebraska	529
46	Nevada	335
25	New Hampshire	483
33	New Jersey	426
41	New Mexico	376
34	New York	414
32	North Carolina	427
21	North Dakota	525
5	Ohio	583
3	Oklahoma	628
49	Oregon	274
26	Pennsylvania	460
18	Rhode Island	531
39	South Carolina	397
15	South Dakota	546
16	Tennessee	535
14	Texas	547
37	Utah	401
31	Vermont	431
36	Virginia	405
42	Washington	370
38	West Virginia	400
13	Wisconsin	549
22	Wyoming	524

RANK ORDER

RANK	STATE	RATE
1	Louisiana	712
2	Indiana	671
3	Oklahoma	628
4	Arkansas	605
5	Ohio	583
6	Illinois	577
7	Iowa	574
8	Minnesota	573
9	Kansas	563
10	Montana	554
11	Connecticut	552
12	Missouri	551
13	Wisconsin	549
14	Texas	547
15	South Dakota	546
16	Massachusetts	535
16	Tennessee	535
18	Rhode Island	531
19	Nebraska	529
20	Maryland	527
21	North Dakota	525
22	Wyoming	524
23	Delaware	517
24	Georgia	516
25	New Hampshire	483
26	Pennsylvania	460
27	Colorado	453
28	Kentucky	446
29	Maine	443
30	Mississippi	441
31	Vermont	431
32	North Carolina	427
33	New Jersey	426
34	New York	414
35	Alabama	407
36	Virginia	405
37	Utah	401
38	West Virginia	400
39	South Carolina	397
40	Michigan	388
41	New Mexico	376
42	Washington	370
43	Alaska	366
44	Idaho	347
45	California	339
46	Nevada	335
47	Arizona	301
48	Hawaii	275
49	Florida	274
49	Oregon	274

District of Columbia 353

Source: Morgan Quitno Press using data from U.S. Dept. of Health & Human Services, Health Care Financing Admin. OSCAR Report 10 (March 18, 1998)

Beds in nursing care facilities certified by HCFA to participate in the Medicare/Medicaid programs. National total does not include beds or population in U.S. territories. Calculated using 1996 Census population estimates.

Nursing Home Population in 1991

National Total = 1,478,903 Persons in Nursing Homes*

ALPHA ORDER

RANK	STATE	POPULATION	% of USA
27	Alabama	21,675	1.47%
50	Alaska	808	0.05%
34	Arizona	12,103	0.82%
28	Arkansas	20,298	1.37%
2	California	98,885	6.69%
30	Colorado	15,871	1.07%
20	Connecticut	27,921	1.89%
45	Delaware	4,308	0.29%
7	Florida	59,878	4.05%
15	Georgia	34,728	2.35%
48	Hawaii	2,840	0.19%
44	Idaho	4,871	0.33%
4	Illinois	87,540	5.92%
10	Indiana	46,231	3.13%
16	Iowa	33,214	2.25%
24	Kansas	25,304	1.71%
25	Kentucky	24,966	1.69%
17	Louisiana	32,367	2.19%
37	Maine	9,241	0.62%
22	Maryland	25,977	1.76%
8	Massachusetts	48,276	3.26%
11	Michigan	46,198	3.12%
13	Minnesota	43,298	2.93%
31	Mississippi	14,819	1.00%
12	Missouri	45,745	3.09%
41	Montana	6,297	0.43%
29	Nebraska	17,779	1.20%
47	Nevada	3,043	0.21%
39	New Hampshire	7,523	0.51%
14	New Jersey	40,068	2.71%
42	New Mexico	5,834	0.39%
1	New York	99,372	6.72%
19	North Carolina	28,546	1.93%
40	North Dakota	6,784	0.46%
6	Ohio	77,676	5.25%
21	Oklahoma	27,456	1.86%
32	Oregon	13,392	0.91%
5	Pennsylvania	83,107	5.62%
36	Rhode Island	9,440	0.64%
33	South Carolina	13,089	0.89%
38	South Dakota	8,192	0.55%
18	Tennessee	32,304	2.18%
3	Texas	90,405	6.11%
43	Utah	5,544	0.37%
46	Vermont	3,591	0.24%
23	Virginia	25,775	1.74%
26	Washington	24,525	1.66%
35	West Virginia	9,809	0.66%
9	Wisconsin	46,898	3.17%
49	Wyoming	2,211	0.15%

RANK ORDER

RANK	STATE	POPULATION	% of USA
1	New York	99,372	6.72%
2	California	98,885	6.69%
3	Texas	90,405	6.11%
4	Illinois	87,540	5.92%
5	Pennsylvania	83,107	5.62%
6	Ohio	77,676	5.25%
7	Florida	59,878	4.05%
8	Massachusetts	48,276	3.26%
9	Wisconsin	46,898	3.17%
10	Indiana	46,231	3.13%
11	Michigan	46,198	3.12%
12	Missouri	45,745	3.09%
13	Minnesota	43,298	2.93%
14	New Jersey	40,068	2.71%
15	Georgia	34,728	2.35%
16	Iowa	33,214	2.25%
17	Louisiana	32,367	2.19%
18	Tennessee	32,304	2.18%
19	North Carolina	28,546	1.93%
20	Connecticut	27,921	1.89%
21	Oklahoma	27,456	1.86%
22	Maryland	25,977	1.76%
23	Virginia	25,775	1.74%
24	Kansas	25,304	1.71%
25	Kentucky	24,966	1.69%
26	Washington	24,525	1.66%
27	Alabama	21,675	1.47%
28	Arkansas	20,298	1.37%
29	Nebraska	17,779	1.20%
30	Colorado	15,871	1.07%
31	Mississippi	14,819	1.00%
32	Oregon	13,392	0.91%
33	South Carolina	13,089	0.89%
34	Arizona	12,103	0.82%
35	West Virginia	9,809	0.66%
36	Rhode Island	9,440	0.64%
37	Maine	9,241	0.62%
38	South Dakota	8,192	0.55%
39	New Hampshire	7,523	0.51%
40	North Dakota	6,784	0.46%
41	Montana	6,297	0.43%
42	New Mexico	5,834	0.39%
43	Utah	5,544	0.37%
44	Idaho	4,871	0.33%
45	Delaware	4,308	0.29%
46	Vermont	3,591	0.24%
47	Nevada	3,043	0.21%
48	Hawaii	2,840	0.19%
49	Wyoming	2,211	0.15%
50	Alaska	808	0.05%
	District of Columbia	2,881	0.19%

*Source: U.S. Department of Health and Human Services, National Center for Health Statistics
"National Health Provider Inventory" (Advance Data, No. 266, September 19, 1995)*
A nursing home is facility with three or more beds that is either licensed as a nursing home, certified as a nursing facility under Medicare or Medicaid, identified as a nursing care unit of a retirement center or determined to provide nursing or medical care.

Percent of Nursing Home Population 65 Years Old or Older in 1991

National Percent = 92.3% of Nursing Home Population*

ALPHA ORDER

RANK	STATE	PERCENT
25	Alabama	92.5
50	Alaska	78.7
36	Arizona	91.9
44	Arkansas	90.5
47	California	88.8
41	Colorado	90.9
28	Connecticut	92.3
28	Delaware	92.3
7	Florida	94.9
42	Georgia	90.7
33	Hawaii	92.0
42	Idaho	90.7
46	Illinois	89.0
40	Indiana	91.1
5	Iowa	95.2
22	Kansas	92.7
31	Kentucky	92.1
45	Louisiana	89.1
3	Maine	95.6
33	Maryland	92.0
15	Massachusetts	93.5
39	Michigan	91.5
9	Minnesota	94.3
20	Mississippi	92.9
17	Missouri	93.1
25	Montana	92.5
13	Nebraska	93.9
48	Nevada	88.0
6	New Hampshire	95.1
16	New Jersey	93.4
33	New Mexico	92.0
11	New York	94.1
28	North Carolina	92.3
4	North Dakota	95.4
37	Ohio	91.7
21	Oklahoma	92.8
18	Oregon	93.0
12	Pennsylvania	94.0
1	Rhode Island	96.5
24	South Carolina	92.6
2	South Dakota	95.7
22	Tennessee	92.7
18	Texas	93.0
49	Utah	86.5
8	Vermont	94.5
27	Virginia	92.4
31	Washington	92.1
10	West Virginia	94.2
38	Wisconsin	91.6
14	Wyoming	93.6

RANK ORDER

RANK	STATE	PERCENT
1	Rhode Island	96.5
2	South Dakota	95.7
3	Maine	95.6
4	North Dakota	95.4
5	Iowa	95.2
6	New Hampshire	95.1
7	Florida	94.9
8	Vermont	94.5
9	Minnesota	94.3
10	West Virginia	94.2
11	New York	94.1
12	Pennsylvania	94.0
13	Nebraska	93.9
14	Wyoming	93.6
15	Massachusetts	93.5
16	New Jersey	93.4
17	Missouri	93.1
18	Oregon	93.0
18	Texas	93.0
20	Mississippi	92.9
21	Oklahoma	92.8
22	Kansas	92.7
22	Tennessee	92.7
24	South Carolina	92.6
25	Alabama	92.5
25	Montana	92.5
27	Virginia	92.4
28	Connecticut	92.3
28	Delaware	92.3
28	North Carolina	92.3
31	Kentucky	92.1
31	Washington	92.1
33	Hawaii	92.0
33	Maryland	92.0
33	New Mexico	92.0
36	Arizona	91.9
37	Ohio	91.7
38	Wisconsin	91.6
39	Michigan	91.5
40	Indiana	91.1
41	Colorado	90.9
42	Georgia	90.7
42	Idaho	90.7
44	Arkansas	90.5
45	Louisiana	89.1
46	Illinois	89.0
47	California	88.8
48	Nevada	88.0
49	Utah	86.5
50	Alaska	78.7

District of Columbia	93.3

Source: U.S. Department of Health and Human Services, National Center for Health Statistics
    "National Health Provider Inventory" (Advance Data, No. 266, September 19, 1995)
*A nursing home is facility with three or more beds that is either licensed as a nursing home, certified as a nursing facility under Medicare or Medicaid, identified as a nursing care unit of a retirement center or determined to provide nursing or medical care.

Percent of Nursing Home Population 85 Years Old or Older in 1991

National Percent = 33.7% of Nursing Home Population*

<table>
<tr><td colspan="3">ALPHA ORDER</td><td colspan="3">RANK ORDER</td></tr>
<tr><td>RANK</td><td>STATE</td><td>PERCENT</td><td>RANK</td><td>STATE</td><td>PERCENT</td></tr>
<tr><td>43</td><td>Alabama</td><td>28.6</td><td>1</td><td>New Hampshire</td><td>49.0</td></tr>
<tr><td>48</td><td>Alaska</td><td>24.9</td><td>2</td><td>Hawaii</td><td>46.8</td></tr>
<tr><td>20</td><td>Arizona</td><td>34.8</td><td>3</td><td>South Dakota</td><td>45.5</td></tr>
<tr><td>44</td><td>Arkansas</td><td>28.5</td><td>4</td><td>Nebraska</td><td>43.8</td></tr>
<tr><td>34</td><td>California</td><td>31.3</td><td>5</td><td>Iowa</td><td>42.8</td></tr>
<tr><td>15</td><td>Colorado</td><td>37.3</td><td>6</td><td>Maine</td><td>41.4</td></tr>
<tr><td>37</td><td>Connecticut</td><td>31.1</td><td>7</td><td>North Dakota</td><td>41.3</td></tr>
<tr><td>15</td><td>Delaware</td><td>37.3</td><td>8</td><td>Kansas</td><td>40.0</td></tr>
<tr><td>22</td><td>Florida</td><td>34.6</td><td>8</td><td>Vermont</td><td>40.0</td></tr>
<tr><td>37</td><td>Georgia</td><td>31.1</td><td>10</td><td>Rhode Island</td><td>39.9</td></tr>
<tr><td>2</td><td>Hawaii</td><td>46.8</td><td>11</td><td>Massachusetts</td><td>38.5</td></tr>
<tr><td>29</td><td>Idaho</td><td>32.6</td><td>12</td><td>Minnesota</td><td>38.4</td></tr>
<tr><td>32</td><td>Illinois</td><td>31.8</td><td>13</td><td>New York</td><td>38.3</td></tr>
<tr><td>31</td><td>Indiana</td><td>32.1</td><td>14</td><td>Wisconsin</td><td>37.7</td></tr>
<tr><td>5</td><td>Iowa</td><td>42.8</td><td>15</td><td>Colorado</td><td>37.3</td></tr>
<tr><td>8</td><td>Kansas</td><td>40.0</td><td>15</td><td>Delaware</td><td>37.3</td></tr>
<tr><td>39</td><td>Kentucky</td><td>30.8</td><td>17</td><td>Montana</td><td>37.1</td></tr>
<tr><td>50</td><td>Louisiana</td><td>23.8</td><td>18</td><td>New Jersey</td><td>35.6</td></tr>
<tr><td>6</td><td>Maine</td><td>41.4</td><td>19</td><td>Wyoming</td><td>35.2</td></tr>
<tr><td>46</td><td>Maryland</td><td>27.8</td><td>20</td><td>Arizona</td><td>34.8</td></tr>
<tr><td>11</td><td>Massachusetts</td><td>38.5</td><td>20</td><td>New Mexico</td><td>34.8</td></tr>
<tr><td>26</td><td>Michigan</td><td>33.4</td><td>22</td><td>Florida</td><td>34.6</td></tr>
<tr><td>12</td><td>Minnesota</td><td>38.4</td><td>23</td><td>Missouri</td><td>33.9</td></tr>
<tr><td>47</td><td>Mississippi</td><td>27.5</td><td>23</td><td>South Carolina</td><td>33.9</td></tr>
<tr><td>23</td><td>Missouri</td><td>33.9</td><td>23</td><td>Virginia</td><td>33.9</td></tr>
<tr><td>17</td><td>Montana</td><td>37.1</td><td>26</td><td>Michigan</td><td>33.4</td></tr>
<tr><td>4</td><td>Nebraska</td><td>43.8</td><td>27</td><td>Oklahoma</td><td>33.2</td></tr>
<tr><td>49</td><td>Nevada</td><td>24.2</td><td>28</td><td>Pennsylvania</td><td>33.0</td></tr>
<tr><td>1</td><td>New Hampshire</td><td>49.0</td><td>29</td><td>Idaho</td><td>32.6</td></tr>
<tr><td>18</td><td>New Jersey</td><td>35.6</td><td>29</td><td>Oregon</td><td>32.6</td></tr>
<tr><td>20</td><td>New Mexico</td><td>34.8</td><td>31</td><td>Indiana</td><td>32.1</td></tr>
<tr><td>13</td><td>New York</td><td>38.3</td><td>32</td><td>Illinois</td><td>31.8</td></tr>
<tr><td>45</td><td>North Carolina</td><td>28.4</td><td>32</td><td>Ohio</td><td>31.8</td></tr>
<tr><td>7</td><td>North Dakota</td><td>41.3</td><td>34</td><td>California</td><td>31.3</td></tr>
<tr><td>32</td><td>Ohio</td><td>31.8</td><td>34</td><td>Texas</td><td>31.3</td></tr>
<tr><td>27</td><td>Oklahoma</td><td>33.2</td><td>36</td><td>Tennessee</td><td>31.2</td></tr>
<tr><td>29</td><td>Oregon</td><td>32.6</td><td>37</td><td>Connecticut</td><td>31.1</td></tr>
<tr><td>28</td><td>Pennsylvania</td><td>33.0</td><td>37</td><td>Georgia</td><td>31.1</td></tr>
<tr><td>10</td><td>Rhode Island</td><td>39.9</td><td>39</td><td>Kentucky</td><td>30.8</td></tr>
<tr><td>23</td><td>South Carolina</td><td>33.9</td><td>40</td><td>West Virginia</td><td>30.5</td></tr>
<tr><td>3</td><td>South Dakota</td><td>45.5</td><td>41</td><td>Washington</td><td>30.4</td></tr>
<tr><td>36</td><td>Tennessee</td><td>31.2</td><td>42</td><td>Utah</td><td>29.3</td></tr>
<tr><td>34</td><td>Texas</td><td>31.3</td><td>43</td><td>Alabama</td><td>28.6</td></tr>
<tr><td>42</td><td>Utah</td><td>29.3</td><td>44</td><td>Arkansas</td><td>28.5</td></tr>
<tr><td>8</td><td>Vermont</td><td>40.0</td><td>45</td><td>North Carolina</td><td>28.4</td></tr>
<tr><td>23</td><td>Virginia</td><td>33.9</td><td>46</td><td>Maryland</td><td>27.8</td></tr>
<tr><td>41</td><td>Washington</td><td>30.4</td><td>47</td><td>Mississippi</td><td>27.5</td></tr>
<tr><td>40</td><td>West Virginia</td><td>30.5</td><td>48</td><td>Alaska</td><td>24.9</td></tr>
<tr><td>14</td><td>Wisconsin</td><td>37.7</td><td>49</td><td>Nevada</td><td>24.2</td></tr>
<tr><td>19</td><td>Wyoming</td><td>35.2</td><td>50</td><td>Louisiana</td><td>23.8</td></tr>
<tr><td></td><td></td><td></td><td></td><td>District of Columbia</td><td>26.5</td></tr>
</table>

Source: Morgan Quitno Press using data from U.S. Dept of Health & Human Serv's, Nat'l Center for Health Statistics
     "National Health Provider Inventory" (unpublished data)
*A nursing home is facility with three or more beds that is either licensed as a nursing home, certified as a nursing
facility under Medicare or Medicaid, identified as a nursing care unit of a retirement center or determined to provide
nursing or medical care.

Percent of Population in Nursing Homes in 1991

National Percent = 0.59% of Population*

RANK	STATE	PERCENT
29	Alabama	0.53
50	Alaska	0.14
46	Arizona	0.32
11	Arkansas	0.86
45	California	0.33
37	Colorado	0.47
12	Connecticut	0.85
24	Delaware	0.63
40	Florida	0.45
31	Georgia	0.52
48	Hawaii	0.25
37	Idaho	0.47
16	Illinois	0.76
13	Indiana	0.82
1	Iowa	1.19
5	Kansas	1.02
22	Kentucky	0.67
16	Louisiana	0.76
18	Maine	0.75
29	Maryland	0.53
14	Massachusetts	0.80
34	Michigan	0.49
6	Minnesota	0.98
26	Mississippi	0.57
9	Missouri	0.89
15	Montana	0.78
3	Nebraska	1.12
49	Nevada	0.24
21	New Hampshire	0.68
31	New Jersey	0.52
43	New Mexico	0.38
27	New York	0.55
41	North Carolina	0.42
4	North Dakota	1.07
19	Ohio	0.71
10	Oklahoma	0.87
39	Oregon	0.46
20	Pennsylvania	0.70
8	Rhode Island	0.94
44	South Carolina	0.37
2	South Dakota	1.17
23	Tennessee	0.65
31	Texas	0.52
47	Utah	0.31
24	Vermont	0.63
42	Virginia	0.41
34	Washington	0.49
27	West Virginia	0.55
7	Wisconsin	0.95
36	Wyoming	0.48

RANK	STATE	PERCENT
1	Iowa	1.19
2	South Dakota	1.17
3	Nebraska	1.12
4	North Dakota	1.07
5	Kansas	1.02
6	Minnesota	0.98
7	Wisconsin	0.95
8	Rhode Island	0.94
9	Missouri	0.89
10	Oklahoma	0.87
11	Arkansas	0.86
12	Connecticut	0.85
13	Indiana	0.82
14	Massachusetts	0.80
15	Montana	0.78
16	Illinois	0.76
16	Louisiana	0.76
18	Maine	0.75
19	Ohio	0.71
20	Pennsylvania	0.70
21	New Hampshire	0.68
22	Kentucky	0.67
23	Tennessee	0.65
24	Delaware	0.63
24	Vermont	0.63
26	Mississippi	0.57
27	New York	0.55
27	West Virginia	0.55
29	Alabama	0.53
29	Maryland	0.53
31	Georgia	0.52
31	New Jersey	0.52
31	Texas	0.52
34	Michigan	0.49
34	Washington	0.49
36	Wyoming	0.48
37	Colorado	0.47
37	Idaho	0.47
39	Oregon	0.46
40	Florida	0.45
41	North Carolina	0.42
42	Virginia	0.41
43	New Mexico	0.38
44	South Carolina	0.37
45	California	0.33
46	Arizona	0.32
47	Utah	0.31
48	Hawaii	0.25
49	Nevada	0.24
50	Alaska	0.14
	District of Columbia	0.49

Source: Morgan Quitno Press using data from U.S. Dept of Health & Human Serv's, Nat'l Center for Health Statistics "National Health Provider Inventory" (Advance Data, No. 266, September 19, 1995)

*A nursing home is facility with three or more beds that is either licensed as a nursing home, certified as a nursing facility under Medicare or Medicaid, identified as a nursing care unit of a retirement center or determined to provide nursing or medical care.

Nursing Home Population in 1980

National Total = 1,426,371 Persons in Nursing Homes

ALPHA ORDER

RANK	STATE	POPULATION	% of USA
27	Alabama	18,702	1.31%
50	Alaska	854	0.06%
35	Arizona	8,424	0.59%
28	Arkansas	18,631	1.31%
1	California	134,756	9.45%
30	Colorado	16,109	1.13%
19	Connecticut	27,873	1.95%
46	Delaware	2,771	0.19%
13	Florida	36,306	2.55%
17	Georgia	29,376	2.06%
45	Hawaii	3,159	0.22%
42	Idaho	5,084	0.36%
4	Illinois	80,410	5.64%
11	Indiana	40,112	2.81%
14	Iowa	36,217	2.54%
21	Kansas	24,545	1.72%
23	Kentucky	23,591	1.65%
24	Louisiana	22,776	1.60%
34	Maine	9,570	0.67%
26	Maryland	19,821	1.39%
8	Massachusetts	49,728	3.49%
7	Michigan	55,805	3.91%
10	Minnesota	44,553	3.12%
32	Mississippi	12,753	0.89%
12	Missouri	37,942	2.66%
41	Montana	5,479	0.38%
29	Nebraska	17,650	1.24%
48	Nevada	2,339	0.16%
39	New Hampshire	6,673	0.47%
15	New Jersey	34,414	2.41%
47	New Mexico	2,585	0.18%
2	New York	114,276	8.01%
16	North Carolina	29,596	2.07%
38	North Dakota	7,486	0.52%
6	Ohio	71,479	5.01%
20	Oklahoma	25,732	1.80%
31	Oregon	16,052	1.13%
5	Pennsylvania	72,285	5.07%
36	Rhode Island	8,146	0.57%
33	South Carolina	11,666	0.82%
37	South Dakota	8,087	0.57%
25	Tennessee	22,014	1.54%
3	Texas	89,275	6.26%
43	Utah	4,921	0.35%
44	Vermont	4,354	0.31%
22	Virginia	24,323	1.71%
18	Washington	27,970	1.96%
40	West Virginia	6,355	0.45%
9	Wisconsin	48,282	3.38%
49	Wyoming	2,198	0.15%

RANK ORDER

RANK	STATE	POPULATION	% of USA
1	California	134,756	9.45%
2	New York	114,276	8.01%
3	Texas	89,275	6.26%
4	Illinois	80,410	5.64%
5	Pennsylvania	72,285	5.07%
6	Ohio	71,479	5.01%
7	Michigan	55,805	3.91%
8	Massachusetts	49,728	3.49%
9	Wisconsin	48,282	3.38%
10	Minnesota	44,553	3.12%
11	Indiana	40,112	2.81%
12	Missouri	37,942	2.66%
13	Florida	36,306	2.55%
14	Iowa	36,217	2.54%
15	New Jersey	34,414	2.41%
16	North Carolina	29,596	2.07%
17	Georgia	29,376	2.06%
18	Washington	27,970	1.96%
19	Connecticut	27,873	1.95%
20	Oklahoma	25,732	1.80%
21	Kansas	24,545	1.72%
22	Virginia	24,323	1.71%
23	Kentucky	23,591	1.65%
24	Louisiana	22,776	1.60%
25	Tennessee	22,014	1.54%
26	Maryland	19,821	1.39%
27	Alabama	18,702	1.31%
28	Arkansas	18,631	1.31%
29	Nebraska	17,650	1.24%
30	Colorado	16,109	1.13%
31	Oregon	16,052	1.13%
32	Mississippi	12,753	0.89%
33	South Carolina	11,666	0.82%
34	Maine	9,570	0.67%
35	Arizona	8,424	0.59%
36	Rhode Island	8,146	0.57%
37	South Dakota	8,087	0.57%
38	North Dakota	7,486	0.52%
39	New Hampshire	6,673	0.47%
40	West Virginia	6,355	0.45%
41	Montana	5,479	0.38%
42	Idaho	5,084	0.36%
43	Utah	4,921	0.35%
44	Vermont	4,354	0.31%
45	Hawaii	3,159	0.22%
46	Delaware	2,771	0.19%
47	New Mexico	2,585	0.18%
48	Nevada	2,339	0.16%
49	Wyoming	2,198	0.15%
50	Alaska	854	0.06%
	District of Columbia	2,866	0.20%

Source: U.S. Bureau of the Census
"Nursing Homes Persons in Institutions and Other Group Quarters" (PC80-2-4D)

Percent of Population in Nursing Homes in 1980

National Percent = 0.63% of Population in Nursing Homes

ALPHA ORDER				RANK ORDER		
RANK	STATE	PERCENT		RANK	STATE	PERCENT
35	Alabama	0.48		1	Iowa	1.24
49	Alaska	0.21		2	South Dakota	1.17
47	Arizona	0.31		3	North Dakota	1.15
14	Arkansas	0.81		4	Nebraska	1.12
28	California	0.57		5	Minnesota	1.09
29	Colorado	0.56		6	Kansas	1.04
8	Connecticut	0.90		7	Wisconsin	1.03
37	Delaware	0.47		8	Connecticut	0.90
42	Florida	0.37		9	Massachusetts	0.87
30	Georgia	0.54		10	Rhode Island	0.86
45	Hawaii	0.33		11	Maine	0.85
30	Idaho	0.54		11	Oklahoma	0.85
18	Illinois	0.70		11	Vermont	0.85
16	Indiana	0.73		14	Arkansas	0.81
1	Iowa	1.24		15	Missouri	0.77
6	Kansas	1.04		16	Indiana	0.73
23	Kentucky	0.64		17	New Hampshire	0.72
30	Louisiana	0.54		18	Illinois	0.70
11	Maine	0.85		18	Montana	0.70
37	Maryland	0.47		20	Washington	0.68
9	Massachusetts	0.87		21	Ohio	0.66
27	Michigan	0.60		22	New York	0.65
5	Minnesota	1.09		23	Kentucky	0.64
33	Mississippi	0.51		24	Texas	0.63
15	Missouri	0.77		25	Oregon	0.61
18	Montana	0.70		25	Pennsylvania	0.61
4	Nebraska	1.12		27	Michigan	0.60
48	Nevada	0.29		28	California	0.57
17	New Hampshire	0.72		29	Colorado	0.56
37	New Jersey	0.47		30	Georgia	0.54
50	New Mexico	0.20		30	Idaho	0.54
22	New York	0.65		30	Louisiana	0.54
34	North Carolina	0.50		33	Mississippi	0.51
3	North Dakota	1.15		34	North Carolina	0.50
21	Ohio	0.66		35	Alabama	0.48
11	Oklahoma	0.85		35	Tennessee	0.48
25	Oregon	0.61		37	Delaware	0.47
25	Pennsylvania	0.61		37	Maryland	0.47
10	Rhode Island	0.86		37	New Jersey	0.47
42	South Carolina	0.37		37	Wyoming	0.47
2	South Dakota	1.17		41	Virginia	0.45
35	Tennessee	0.48		42	Florida	0.37
24	Texas	0.63		42	South Carolina	0.37
44	Utah	0.34		44	Utah	0.34
11	Vermont	0.85		45	Hawaii	0.33
41	Virginia	0.45		45	West Virginia	0.33
20	Washington	0.68		47	Arizona	0.31
45	West Virginia	0.33		48	Nevada	0.29
7	Wisconsin	1.03		49	Alaska	0.21
37	Wyoming	0.47		50	New Mexico	0.20
					District of Columbia	0.45

Source: Morgan Quitno Press using data from U.S. Bureau of the Census
"Nursing Homes Persons in Institutions and Other Group Quarters" (PC80-2-4D)

Change in Nursing Home Population: 1980 to 1990

National Change = 345,661 Increase in Nursing Home Population

ALPHA ORDER

RANK ORDER

RANK	STATE	INCREASE	% of USA	RANK	STATE	INCREASE	% of USA
21	Alabama	5,329	1.54%	1	Florida	43,992	12.73%
47	Alaska	348	0.10%	2	Pennsylvania	34,169	9.89%
19	Arizona	6,048	1.75%	3	Ohio	22,290	6.45%
26	Arkansas	3,178	0.92%	4	North Carolina	17,418	5.04%
6	California	13,606	3.94%	5	Missouri	14,118	4.08%
30	Colorado	2,397	0.69%	6	California	13,606	3.94%
27	Connecticut	3,089	0.89%	7	Virginia	13,439	3.89%
35	Delaware	1,825	0.53%	8	Illinois	13,252	3.83%
1	Florida	43,992	12.73%	9	Tennessee	13,178	3.81%
15	Georgia	7,173	2.08%	10	New Jersey	12,640	3.66%
50	Hawaii	66	0.02%	11	New York	11,899	3.44%
43	Idaho	1,234	0.36%	12	Texas	11,730	3.39%
8	Illinois	13,252	3.83%	13	Indiana	10,733	3.11%
13	Indiana	10,733	3.11%	14	Louisiana	9,296	2.69%
49	Iowa	238	0.07%	15	Georgia	7,173	2.08%
37	Kansas	1,610	0.47%	16	Maryland	7,063	2.04%
23	Kentucky	4,283	1.24%	17	South Carolina	6,562	1.90%
14	Louisiana	9,296	2.69%	18	West Virginia	6,236	1.80%
48	Maine	285	0.08%	19	Arizona	6,048	1.75%
16	Maryland	7,063	2.04%	20	Massachusetts	5,934	1.72%
20	Massachusetts	5,934	1.72%	21	Alabama	5,329	1.54%
36	Michigan	1,817	0.53%	22	Washington	4,870	1.41%
29	Minnesota	2,498	0.72%	23	Kentucky	4,283	1.24%
28	Mississippi	3,050	0.88%	24	Oklahoma	3,934	1.14%
5	Missouri	14,118	4.08%	25	New Mexico	3,691	1.07%
31	Montana	2,285	0.66%	26	Arkansas	3,178	0.92%
39	Nebraska	1,521	0.44%	27	Connecticut	3,089	0.89%
42	Nevada	1,266	0.37%	28	Mississippi	3,050	0.88%
38	New Hampshire	1,529	0.44%	29	Minnesota	2,498	0.72%
10	New Jersey	12,640	3.66%	30	Colorado	2,397	0.69%
25	New Mexico	3,691	1.07%	31	Montana	2,285	0.66%
11	New York	11,899	3.44%	32	Oregon	2,148	0.62%
4	North Carolina	17,418	5.04%	33	Wisconsin	2,063	0.60%
44	North Dakota	673	0.19%	34	Rhode Island	2,010	0.58%
3	Ohio	22,290	6.45%	35	Delaware	1,825	0.53%
24	Oklahoma	3,934	1.14%	36	Michigan	1,817	0.53%
32	Oregon	2,148	0.62%	37	Kansas	1,610	0.47%
2	Pennsylvania	34,169	9.89%	38	New Hampshire	1,529	0.44%
34	Rhode Island	2,010	0.58%	39	Nebraska	1,521	0.44%
17	South Carolina	6,562	1.90%	40	Utah	1,301	0.38%
41	South Dakota	1,269	0.37%	41	South Dakota	1,269	0.37%
9	Tennessee	13,178	3.81%	42	Nevada	1,266	0.37%
12	Texas	11,730	3.39%	43	Idaho	1,234	0.36%
40	Utah	1,301	0.38%	44	North Dakota	673	0.19%
46	Vermont	455	0.13%	45	Wyoming	481	0.14%
7	Virginia	13,439	3.89%	46	Vermont	455	0.13%
22	Washington	4,870	1.41%	47	Alaska	348	0.10%
18	West Virginia	6,236	1.80%	48	Maine	285	0.08%
33	Wisconsin	2,063	0.60%	49	Iowa	238	0.07%
45	Wyoming	481	0.14%	50	Hawaii	66	0.02%
					District of Columbia	4,142	1.20%

Source: Morgan Quitno Press using data from U.S. Bureau of the Census
"Nursing Homes Persons in Institutions and Other Group Quarters" (PC80-2-4D) and
"Nursing Home Population 1990" (CPH-L-137)

Percent Change in Nursing Home Population: 1980 to 1990

National Percent Change = 24.2% Increase

ALPHA ORDER				RANK ORDER		
RANK	STATE	PERCENT		RANK	STATE	PERCENT
19	Alabama	28.5		1	New Mexico	142.8
14	Alaska	40.7		2	Florida	121.2
4	Arizona	71.8		3	West Virginia	98.1
30	Arkansas	17.1		4	Arizona	71.8
41	California	10.1		5	Delaware	65.9
34	Colorado	14.9		6	Tennessee	59.9
38	Connecticut	11.1		7	North Carolina	58.9
5	Delaware	65.9		8	South Carolina	56.2
2	Florida	121.2		9	Virginia	55.3
23	Georgia	24.4		10	Nevada	54.1
49	Hawaii	2.1		11	Pennsylvania	47.3
24	Idaho	24.3		12	Montana	41.7
31	Illinois	16.5		13	Louisiana	40.8
20	Indiana	26.8		14	Alaska	40.7
50	Iowa	0.7		15	Missouri	37.2
44	Kansas	6.6		16	New Jersey	36.7
28	Kentucky	18.2		17	Maryland	35.6
13	Louisiana	40.8		18	Ohio	31.2
48	Maine	3.0		19	Alabama	28.5
17	Maryland	35.6		20	Indiana	26.8
37	Massachusetts	11.9		21	Utah	26.4
47	Michigan	3.3		22	Rhode Island	24.7
45	Minnesota	5.6		23	Georgia	24.4
25	Mississippi	23.9		24	Idaho	24.3
15	Missouri	37.2		25	Mississippi	23.9
12	Montana	41.7		26	New Hampshire	22.9
43	Nebraska	8.6		27	Wyoming	21.9
10	Nevada	54.1		28	Kentucky	18.2
26	New Hampshire	22.9		29	Washington	17.4
16	New Jersey	36.7		30	Arkansas	17.1
1	New Mexico	142.8		31	Illinois	16.5
40	New York	10.4		32	South Dakota	15.7
7	North Carolina	58.9		33	Oklahoma	15.3
42	North Dakota	9.0		34	Colorado	14.9
18	Ohio	31.2		35	Oregon	13.4
33	Oklahoma	15.3		36	Texas	13.1
35	Oregon	13.4		37	Massachusetts	11.9
11	Pennsylvania	47.3		38	Connecticut	11.1
22	Rhode Island	24.7		39	Vermont	10.5
8	South Carolina	56.2		40	New York	10.4
32	South Dakota	15.7		41	California	10.1
6	Tennessee	59.9		42	North Dakota	9.0
36	Texas	13.1		43	Nebraska	8.6
21	Utah	26.4		44	Kansas	6.6
39	Vermont	10.5		45	Minnesota	5.6
9	Virginia	55.3		46	Wisconsin	4.3
29	Washington	17.4		47	Michigan	3.3
3	West Virginia	98.1		48	Maine	3.0
46	Wisconsin	4.3		49	Hawaii	2.1
27	Wyoming	21.9		50	Iowa	0.7
					District of Columbia	144.5

Source: Morgan Quitno Press using data from U.S. Bureau of the Census
  "Nursing Homes Persons in Institutions and Other Group Quarters" (PC80-2-4D) and
  "Nursing Home Population 1990" (CPH-L-137)

Health Service Establishments in 1995

National Total = 478,286 Establishments*

ALPHA ORDER					RANK ORDER			
RANK	STATE	ESTABLISH'S	% of USA		RANK	STATE	ESTABLISH'S	% of USA
25	Alabama	6,250	1.31%		1	California	62,797	13.13%
48	Alaska	997	0.21%		2	New York	35,180	7.36%
19	Arizona	7,855	1.64%		3	Texas	32,805	6.86%
32	Arkansas	4,074	0.85%		4	Florida	32,309	6.76%
1	California	62,797	13.13%		5	Pennsylvania	23,591	4.93%
21	Colorado	7,796	1.63%		6	Illinois	20,243	4.23%
23	Connecticut	7,049	1.47%		7	Ohio	19,939	4.17%
45	Delaware	1,318	0.28%		8	New Jersey	17,741	3.71%
4	Florida	32,309	6.76%		9	Michigan	16,819	3.52%
10	Georgia	12,231	2.56%		10	Georgia	12,231	2.56%
39	Hawaii	2,420	0.51%		11	Massachusetts	11,340	2.37%
43	Idaho	1,998	0.42%		12	Virginia	10,484	2.19%
6	Illinois	20,243	4.23%		13	North Carolina	10,018	2.09%
16	Indiana	9,401	1.97%		14	Maryland	9,944	2.08%
30	Iowa	4,625	0.97%		15	Washington	9,919	2.07%
31	Kansas	4,417	0.92%		16	Indiana	9,401	1.97%
26	Kentucky	6,210	1.30%		17	Tennessee	8,924	1.87%
22	Louisiana	7,528	1.57%		18	Missouri	8,861	1.85%
40	Maine	2,384	0.50%		19	Arizona	7,855	1.64%
14	Maryland	9,944	2.08%		20	Wisconsin	7,842	1.64%
11	Massachusetts	11,340	2.37%		21	Colorado	7,796	1.63%
9	Michigan	16,819	3.52%		22	Louisiana	7,528	1.57%
24	Minnesota	6,861	1.43%		23	Connecticut	7,049	1.47%
33	Mississippi	3,401	0.71%		24	Minnesota	6,861	1.43%
18	Missouri	8,861	1.85%		25	Alabama	6,250	1.31%
44	Montana	1,749	0.37%		26	Kentucky	6,210	1.30%
38	Nebraska	2,643	0.55%		27	Oregon	5,913	1.24%
37	Nevada	2,669	0.56%		28	Oklahoma	5,877	1.23%
42	New Hampshire	2,019	0.42%		29	South Carolina	5,156	1.08%
8	New Jersey	17,741	3.71%		30	Iowa	4,625	0.97%
36	New Mexico	2,734	0.57%		31	Kansas	4,417	0.92%
2	New York	35,180	7.36%		32	Arkansas	4,074	0.85%
13	North Carolina	10,018	2.09%		33	Mississippi	3,401	0.71%
49	North Dakota	953	0.20%		34	Utah	3,396	0.71%
7	Ohio	19,939	4.17%		35	West Virginia	3,036	0.63%
28	Oklahoma	5,877	1.23%		36	New Mexico	2,734	0.57%
27	Oregon	5,913	1.24%		37	Nevada	2,669	0.56%
5	Pennsylvania	23,591	4.93%		38	Nebraska	2,643	0.55%
41	Rhode Island	2,046	0.43%		39	Hawaii	2,420	0.51%
29	South Carolina	5,156	1.08%		40	Maine	2,384	0.50%
46	South Dakota	1,189	0.25%		41	Rhode Island	2,046	0.43%
17	Tennessee	8,924	1.87%		42	New Hampshire	2,019	0.42%
3	Texas	32,805	6.86%		43	Idaho	1,998	0.42%
34	Utah	3,396	0.71%		44	Montana	1,749	0.37%
47	Vermont	1,055	0.22%		45	Delaware	1,318	0.28%
12	Virginia	10,484	2.19%		46	South Dakota	1,189	0.25%
15	Washington	9,919	2.07%		47	Vermont	1,055	0.22%
35	West Virginia	3,036	0.63%		48	Alaska	997	0.21%
20	Wisconsin	7,842	1.64%		49	North Dakota	953	0.20%
50	Wyoming	863	0.18%		50	Wyoming	863	0.18%
						District of Columbia	1,417	0.30%

*Source: U.S. Bureau of the Census
"1995 County Business Patterns"*
Includes establishments exempt from, as well as subject to, the federal income tax. Includes those establishments within the Standard Industry Classification (SIC) 8000. These include those primarily engaged in furnishing medical, surgical and other health services to persons.

Offices and Clinics of Doctors of Medicine in 1992

National Total = 197,701 Establishments*

ALPHA ORDER

RANK	STATE	ESTABLISH'S	% of USA
23	Alabama	2,611	1.32%
47	Alaska	349	0.18%
20	Arizona	3,150	1.59%
29	Arkansas	1,664	0.84%
1	California	28,494	14.41%
22	Colorado	2,698	1.36%
21	Connecticut	3,039	1.54%
45	Delaware	587	0.30%
3	Florida	14,487	7.33%
10	Georgia	5,214	2.64%
37	Hawaii	1,066	0.54%
43	Idaho	728	0.37%
6	Illinois	8,424	4.26%
16	Indiana	3,744	1.89%
33	Iowa	1,349	0.68%
32	Kansas	1,382	0.70%
24	Kentucky	2,565	1.30%
18	Louisiana	3,293	1.67%
39	Maine	914	0.46%
11	Maryland	4,760	2.41%
13	Massachusetts	4,524	2.29%
9	Michigan	5,935	3.00%
30	Minnesota	1,480	0.75%
31	Mississippi	1,458	0.74%
19	Missouri	3,280	1.66%
44	Montana	599	0.30%
41	Nebraska	886	0.45%
36	Nevada	1,096	0.55%
42	New Hampshire	754	0.38%
8	New Jersey	7,718	3.90%
38	New Mexico	1,033	0.52%
2	New York	16,226	8.21%
15	North Carolina	3,826	1.94%
50	North Dakota	243	0.12%
7	Ohio	8,004	4.05%
28	Oklahoma	2,052	1.04%
26	Oregon	2,263	1.14%
5	Pennsylvania	9,347	4.73%
40	Rhode Island	889	0.45%
27	South Carolina	2,219	1.12%
47	South Dakota	349	0.18%
14	Tennessee	3,840	1.94%
4	Texas	14,367	7.27%
35	Utah	1,261	0.64%
46	Vermont	393	0.20%
12	Virginia	4,724	2.39%
17	Washington	3,464	1.75%
34	West Virginia	1,340	0.68%
25	Wisconsin	2,546	1.29%
49	Wyoming	294	0.15%

RANK ORDER

RANK	STATE	ESTABLISH'S	% of USA
1	California	28,494	14.41%
2	New York	16,226	8.21%
3	Florida	14,487	7.33%
4	Texas	14,367	7.27%
5	Pennsylvania	9,347	4.73%
6	Illinois	8,424	4.26%
7	Ohio	8,004	4.05%
8	New Jersey	7,718	3.90%
9	Michigan	5,935	3.00%
10	Georgia	5,214	2.64%
11	Maryland	4,760	2.41%
12	Virginia	4,724	2.39%
13	Massachusetts	4,524	2.29%
14	Tennessee	3,840	1.94%
15	North Carolina	3,826	1.94%
16	Indiana	3,744	1.89%
17	Washington	3,464	1.75%
18	Louisiana	3,293	1.67%
19	Missouri	3,280	1.66%
20	Arizona	3,150	1.59%
21	Connecticut	3,039	1.54%
22	Colorado	2,698	1.36%
23	Alabama	2,611	1.32%
24	Kentucky	2,565	1.30%
25	Wisconsin	2,546	1.29%
26	Oregon	2,263	1.14%
27	South Carolina	2,219	1.12%
28	Oklahoma	2,052	1.04%
29	Arkansas	1,664	0.84%
30	Minnesota	1,480	0.75%
31	Mississippi	1,458	0.74%
32	Kansas	1,382	0.70%
33	Iowa	1,349	0.68%
34	West Virginia	1,340	0.68%
35	Utah	1,261	0.64%
36	Nevada	1,096	0.55%
37	Hawaii	1,066	0.54%
38	New Mexico	1,033	0.52%
39	Maine	914	0.46%
40	Rhode Island	889	0.45%
41	Nebraska	886	0.45%
42	New Hampshire	754	0.38%
43	Idaho	728	0.37%
44	Montana	599	0.30%
45	Delaware	587	0.30%
46	Vermont	393	0.20%
47	Alaska	349	0.18%
47	South Dakota	349	0.18%
49	Wyoming	294	0.15%
50	North Dakota	243	0.12%
	District of Columbia	773	0.39%

Source: U.S. Bureau of the Census
   "1992 Census of Service Industries, Geographic Area Series, United States" (SC92-A-52)
*Includes only establishments subject to the federal income tax.

Offices and Clinics of Dentists in 1992

National Total = 108,804 Establishments*

ALPHA ORDER

RANK	STATE	ESTABLISH'S	% of USA
27	Alabama	1,331	1.22%
45	Alaska	262	0.24%
25	Arizona	1,522	1.40%
33	Arkansas	822	0.76%
1	California	14,806	13.61%
21	Colorado	1,911	1.76%
22	Connecticut	1,740	1.60%
49	Delaware	215	0.20%
4	Florida	5,374	4.94%
13	Georgia	2,346	2.16%
36	Hawaii	640	0.59%
42	Idaho	455	0.42%
6	Illinois	5,156	4.74%
16	Indiana	2,177	2.00%
30	Iowa	1,149	1.06%
31	Kansas	1,003	0.92%
26	Kentucky	1,462	1.34%
24	Louisiana	1,548	1.42%
41	Maine	458	0.42%
15	Maryland	2,195	2.02%
10	Massachusetts	2,941	2.70%
8	Michigan	4,348	4.00%
19	Minnesota	2,010	1.85%
34	Mississippi	784	0.72%
18	Missouri	2,047	1.88%
44	Montana	397	0.36%
35	Nebraska	747	0.69%
40	Nevada	478	0.44%
39	New Hampshire	514	0.47%
9	New Jersey	4,033	3.71%
38	New Mexico	532	0.49%
2	New York	8,560	7.87%
17	North Carolina	2,162	1.99%
47	North Dakota	250	0.23%
7	Ohio	4,497	4.13%
28	Oklahoma	1,229	1.13%
23	Oregon	1,587	1.46%
5	Pennsylvania	5,316	4.89%
43	Rhode Island	406	0.37%
29	South Carolina	1,153	1.06%
46	South Dakota	260	0.24%
20	Tennessee	1,984	1.82%
3	Texas	6,233	5.73%
32	Utah	974	0.90%
48	Vermont	245	0.23%
12	Virginia	2,524	2.32%
11	Washington	2,674	2.46%
37	West Virginia	563	0.52%
14	Wisconsin	2,235	2.05%
50	Wyoming	202	0.19%

RANK ORDER

RANK	STATE	ESTABLISH'S	% of USA
1	California	14,806	13.61%
2	New York	8,560	7.87%
3	Texas	6,233	5.73%
4	Florida	5,374	4.94%
5	Pennsylvania	5,316	4.89%
6	Illinois	5,156	4.74%
7	Ohio	4,497	4.13%
8	Michigan	4,348	4.00%
9	New Jersey	4,033	3.71%
10	Massachusetts	2,941	2.70%
11	Washington	2,674	2.46%
12	Virginia	2,524	2.32%
13	Georgia	2,346	2.16%
14	Wisconsin	2,235	2.05%
15	Maryland	2,195	2.02%
16	Indiana	2,177	2.00%
17	North Carolina	2,162	1.99%
18	Missouri	2,047	1.88%
19	Minnesota	2,010	1.85%
20	Tennessee	1,984	1.82%
21	Colorado	1,911	1.76%
22	Connecticut	1,740	1.60%
23	Oregon	1,587	1.46%
24	Louisiana	1,548	1.42%
25	Arizona	1,522	1.40%
26	Kentucky	1,462	1.34%
27	Alabama	1,331	1.22%
28	Oklahoma	1,229	1.13%
29	South Carolina	1,153	1.06%
30	Iowa	1,149	1.06%
31	Kansas	1,003	0.92%
32	Utah	974	0.90%
33	Arkansas	822	0.76%
34	Mississippi	784	0.72%
35	Nebraska	747	0.69%
36	Hawaii	640	0.59%
37	West Virginia	563	0.52%
38	New Mexico	532	0.49%
39	New Hampshire	514	0.47%
40	Nevada	478	0.44%
41	Maine	458	0.42%
42	Idaho	455	0.42%
43	Rhode Island	406	0.37%
44	Montana	397	0.36%
45	Alaska	262	0.24%
46	South Dakota	260	0.24%
47	North Dakota	250	0.23%
48	Vermont	245	0.23%
49	Delaware	215	0.20%
50	Wyoming	202	0.19%
	District of Columbia	347	0.32%

Source: U.S. Bureau of the Census
"1992 Census of Service Industries, Geographic Area Series, United States" (SC92-A-52)
*Includes only establishments subject to the federal income tax.

Offices and Clinics of Doctors of Osteopathy in 1992

National Total = 8,708 Establishments*

ALPHA ORDER

RANK	STATE	ESTABLISH'S	% of USA
31	Alabama	32	0.37%
41	Alaska	11	0.13%
10	Arizona	317	3.64%
32	Arkansas	26	0.30%
9	California	322	3.70%
11	Colorado	207	2.38%
38	Connecticut	14	0.16%
26	Delaware	50	0.57%
4	Florida	762	8.75%
17	Georgia	124	1.42%
41	Hawaii	11	0.13%
39	Idaho	13	0.15%
14	Illinois	173	1.99%
16	Indiana	142	1.63%
13	Iowa	193	2.22%
20	Kansas	97	1.11%
30	Kentucky	38	0.44%
47	Louisiana	6	0.07%
18	Maine	120	1.38%
36	Maryland	16	0.18%
28	Massachusetts	40	0.46%
1	Michigan	1,201	13.79%
36	Minnesota	16	0.18%
34	Mississippi	20	0.23%
6	Missouri	446	5.12%
40	Montana	12	0.14%
49	Nebraska	2	0.02%
27	Nevada	41	0.47%
45	New Hampshire	9	0.10%
7	New Jersey	399	4.58%
23	New Mexico	57	0.65%
12	New York	201	2.31%
35	North Carolina	19	0.22%
49	North Dakota	2	0.02%
3	Ohio	821	9.43%
8	Oklahoma	328	3.77%
19	Oregon	112	1.29%
2	Pennsylvania	1,062	12.20%
24	Rhode Island	55	0.63%
33	South Carolina	21	0.24%
45	South Dakota	9	0.10%
25	Tennessee	52	0.60%
5	Texas	707	8.12%
43	Utah	10	0.11%
47	Vermont	6	0.07%
29	Virginia	39	0.45%
15	Washington	149	1.71%
22	West Virginia	90	1.03%
21	Wisconsin	96	1.10%
43	Wyoming	10	0.11%

RANK ORDER

RANK	STATE	ESTABLISH'S	% of USA
1	Michigan	1,201	13.79%
2	Pennsylvania	1,062	12.20%
3	Ohio	821	9.43%
4	Florida	762	8.75%
5	Texas	707	8.12%
6	Missouri	446	5.12%
7	New Jersey	399	4.58%
8	Oklahoma	328	3.77%
9	California	322	3.70%
10	Arizona	317	3.64%
11	Colorado	207	2.38%
12	New York	201	2.31%
13	Iowa	193	2.22%
14	Illinois	173	1.99%
15	Washington	149	1.71%
16	Indiana	142	1.63%
17	Georgia	124	1.42%
18	Maine	120	1.38%
19	Oregon	112	1.29%
20	Kansas	97	1.11%
21	Wisconsin	96	1.10%
22	West Virginia	90	1.03%
23	New Mexico	57	0.65%
24	Rhode Island	55	0.63%
25	Tennessee	52	0.60%
26	Delaware	50	0.57%
27	Nevada	41	0.47%
28	Massachusetts	40	0.46%
29	Virginia	39	0.45%
30	Kentucky	38	0.44%
31	Alabama	32	0.37%
32	Arkansas	26	0.30%
33	South Carolina	21	0.24%
34	Mississippi	20	0.23%
35	North Carolina	19	0.22%
36	Maryland	16	0.18%
36	Minnesota	16	0.18%
38	Connecticut	14	0.16%
39	Idaho	13	0.15%
40	Montana	12	0.14%
41	Alaska	11	0.13%
41	Hawaii	11	0.13%
43	Utah	10	0.11%
43	Wyoming	10	0.11%
45	New Hampshire	9	0.10%
45	South Dakota	9	0.10%
47	Louisiana	6	0.07%
47	Vermont	6	0.07%
49	Nebraska	2	0.02%
49	North Dakota	2	0.02%
	District of Columbia	2	0.02%

Source: U.S. Bureau of the Census
   "1992 Census of Service Industries, Geographic Area Series, United States" (SC92-A-52)
*Includes only establishments subject to the federal income tax.

Offices and Clinics of Chiropractors in 1992

National Total = 27,329 Establishments*

<u>ALPHA ORDER</u>

RANK	STATE	ESTABLISH'S	% of USA
29	Alabama	282	1.03%
47	Alaska	71	0.26%
14	Arizona	622	2.28%
31	Arkansas	237	0.87%
1	California	4,364	15.97%
16	Colorado	589	2.16%
24	Connecticut	347	1.27%
49	Delaware	50	0.18%
2	Florida	1,847	6.76%
12	Georgia	760	2.78%
39	Hawaii	119	0.44%
37	Idaho	134	0.49%
7	Illinois	1,068	3.91%
20	Indiana	436	1.60%
18	Iowa	446	1.63%
25	Kansas	321	1.17%
30	Kentucky	269	0.98%
28	Louisiana	284	1.04%
38	Maine	126	0.46%
32	Maryland	231	0.85%
17	Massachusetts	575	2.10%
8	Michigan	938	3.43%
10	Minnesota	824	3.02%
42	Mississippi	113	0.41%
15	Missouri	598	2.19%
41	Montana	117	0.43%
35	Nebraska	163	0.60%
34	Nevada	166	0.61%
43	New Hampshire	108	0.40%
6	New Jersey	1,245	4.56%
33	New Mexico	185	0.68%
3	New York	1,741	6.37%
19	North Carolina	439	1.61%
45	North Dakota	90	0.33%
9	Ohio	871	3.19%
27	Oklahoma	316	1.16%
21	Oregon	428	1.57%
5	Pennsylvania	1,310	4.79%
46	Rhode Island	79	0.29%
26	South Carolina	319	1.17%
40	South Dakota	118	0.43%
22	Tennessee	356	1.30%
4	Texas	1,426	5.22%
36	Utah	153	0.56%
48	Vermont	65	0.24%
23	Virginia	355	1.30%
11	Washington	804	2.94%
44	West Virginia	105	0.38%
13	Wisconsin	665	2.43%
50	Wyoming	41	0.15%

<u>RANK ORDER</u>

RANK	STATE	ESTABLISH'S	% of USA
1	California	4,364	15.97%
2	Florida	1,847	6.76%
3	New York	1,741	6.37%
4	Texas	1,426	5.22%
5	Pennsylvania	1,310	4.79%
6	New Jersey	1,245	4.56%
7	Illinois	1,068	3.91%
8	Michigan	938	3.43%
9	Ohio	871	3.19%
10	Minnesota	824	3.02%
11	Washington	804	2.94%
12	Georgia	760	2.78%
13	Wisconsin	665	2.43%
14	Arizona	622	2.28%
15	Missouri	598	2.19%
16	Colorado	589	2.16%
17	Massachusetts	575	2.10%
18	Iowa	446	1.63%
19	North Carolina	439	1.61%
20	Indiana	436	1.60%
21	Oregon	428	1.57%
22	Tennessee	356	1.30%
23	Virginia	355	1.30%
24	Connecticut	347	1.27%
25	Kansas	321	1.17%
26	South Carolina	319	1.17%
27	Oklahoma	316	1.16%
28	Louisiana	284	1.04%
29	Alabama	282	1.03%
30	Kentucky	269	0.98%
31	Arkansas	237	0.87%
32	Maryland	231	0.85%
33	New Mexico	185	0.68%
34	Nevada	166	0.61%
35	Nebraska	163	0.60%
36	Utah	153	0.56%
37	Idaho	134	0.49%
38	Maine	126	0.46%
39	Hawaii	119	0.44%
40	South Dakota	118	0.43%
41	Montana	117	0.43%
42	Mississippi	113	0.41%
43	New Hampshire	108	0.40%
44	West Virginia	105	0.38%
45	North Dakota	90	0.33%
46	Rhode Island	79	0.29%
47	Alaska	71	0.26%
48	Vermont	65	0.24%
49	Delaware	50	0.18%
50	Wyoming	41	0.15%
	District of Columbia	13	0.05%

Source: U.S. Bureau of the Census
"1992 Census of Service Industries, Geographic Area Series, United States" (SC92-A-52)
*Includes only establishments subject to the federal income tax.

Offices and Clinics of Optometrists in 1992

National Total = 17,135 Establishments*

ALPHA ORDER

RANK	STATE	ESTABLISH'S	% of USA
26	Alabama	229	1.34%
49	Alaska	44	0.26%
32	Arizona	189	1.10%
29	Arkansas	202	1.18%
1	California	2,382	13.90%
22	Colorado	257	1.50%
27	Connecticut	228	1.33%
50	Delaware	40	0.23%
4	Florida	854	4.98%
13	Georgia	373	2.18%
40	Hawaii	99	0.58%
41	Idaho	94	0.55%
7	Illinois	698	4.07%
11	Indiana	463	2.70%
21	Iowa	270	1.58%
24	Kansas	247	1.44%
23	Kentucky	248	1.45%
31	Louisiana	196	1.14%
35	Maine	123	0.72%
25	Maryland	235	1.37%
14	Massachusetts	370	2.16%
8	Michigan	607	3.54%
20	Minnesota	281	1.64%
34	Mississippi	148	0.86%
19	Missouri	301	1.76%
39	Montana	103	0.60%
36	Nebraska	121	0.71%
37	Nevada	110	0.64%
44	New Hampshire	74	0.43%
9	New Jersey	550	3.21%
38	New Mexico	104	0.61%
6	New York	791	4.62%
10	North Carolina	498	2.91%
46	North Dakota	64	0.37%
5	Ohio	836	4.88%
18	Oklahoma	317	1.85%
28	Oregon	222	1.30%
3	Pennsylvania	869	5.07%
45	Rhode Island	72	0.42%
30	South Carolina	198	1.16%
43	South Dakota	80	0.47%
15	Tennessee	364	2.12%
2	Texas	1,100	6.42%
42	Utah	81	0.47%
48	Vermont	50	0.29%
12	Virginia	436	2.54%
17	Washington	341	1.99%
33	West Virginia	151	0.88%
16	Wisconsin	347	2.03%
47	Wyoming	54	0.32%

RANK ORDER

RANK	STATE	ESTABLISH'S	% of USA
1	California	2,382	13.90%
2	Texas	1,100	6.42%
3	Pennsylvania	869	5.07%
4	Florida	854	4.98%
5	Ohio	836	4.88%
6	New York	791	4.62%
7	Illinois	698	4.07%
8	Michigan	607	3.54%
9	New Jersey	550	3.21%
10	North Carolina	498	2.91%
11	Indiana	463	2.70%
12	Virginia	436	2.54%
13	Georgia	373	2.18%
14	Massachusetts	370	2.16%
15	Tennessee	364	2.12%
16	Wisconsin	347	2.03%
17	Washington	341	1.99%
18	Oklahoma	317	1.85%
19	Missouri	301	1.76%
20	Minnesota	281	1.64%
21	Iowa	270	1.58%
22	Colorado	257	1.50%
23	Kentucky	248	1.45%
24	Kansas	247	1.44%
25	Maryland	235	1.37%
26	Alabama	229	1.34%
27	Connecticut	228	1.33%
28	Oregon	222	1.30%
29	Arkansas	202	1.18%
30	South Carolina	198	1.16%
31	Louisiana	196	1.14%
32	Arizona	189	1.10%
33	West Virginia	151	0.88%
34	Mississippi	148	0.86%
35	Maine	123	0.72%
36	Nebraska	121	0.71%
37	Nevada	110	0.64%
38	New Mexico	104	0.61%
39	Montana	103	0.60%
40	Hawaii	99	0.58%
41	Idaho	94	0.55%
42	Utah	81	0.47%
43	South Dakota	80	0.47%
44	New Hampshire	74	0.43%
45	Rhode Island	72	0.42%
46	North Dakota	64	0.37%
47	Wyoming	54	0.32%
48	Vermont	50	0.29%
49	Alaska	44	0.26%
50	Delaware	40	0.23%
	District of Columbia	24	0.14%

Source: U.S. Bureau of the Census
"1992 Census of Service Industries, Geographic Area Series, United States" (SC92-A-52)
*Includes only establishments subject to the federal income tax.

Offices and Clinics of Podiatrists in 1992

National Total = 7,948 Establishments*

ALPHA ORDER

RANK	STATE	ESTABLISH'S	% of USA
29	Alabama	49	0.62%
49	Alaska	5	0.06%
18	Arizona	121	1.52%
41	Arkansas	20	0.25%
2	California	930	11.70%
22	Colorado	88	1.11%
14	Connecticut	152	1.91%
39	Delaware	25	0.31%
4	Florida	564	7.10%
17	Georgia	139	1.75%
44	Hawaii	16	0.20%
43	Idaho	17	0.21%
7	Illinois	419	5.27%
12	Indiana	166	2.09%
23	Iowa	75	0.94%
26	Kansas	55	0.69%
31	Kentucky	46	0.58%
30	Louisiana	48	0.60%
34	Maine	36	0.45%
10	Maryland	211	2.65%
11	Massachusetts	208	2.62%
8	Michigan	400	5.03%
25	Minnesota	60	0.75%
42	Mississippi	18	0.23%
20	Missouri	98	1.23%
44	Montana	16	0.20%
35	Nebraska	34	0.43%
37	Nevada	28	0.35%
40	New Hampshire	24	0.30%
6	New Jersey	449	5.65%
36	New Mexico	33	0.42%
1	New York	938	11.80%
16	North Carolina	140	1.76%
48	North Dakota	7	0.09%
5	Ohio	490	6.17%
27	Oklahoma	52	0.65%
24	Oregon	61	0.77%
3	Pennsylvania	589	7.41%
28	Rhode Island	50	0.63%
33	South Carolina	40	0.50%
46	South Dakota	14	0.18%
21	Tennessee	90	1.13%
9	Texas	382	4.81%
32	Utah	44	0.55%
47	Vermont	9	0.11%
13	Virginia	164	2.06%
15	Washington	146	1.84%
38	West Virginia	26	0.33%
19	Wisconsin	119	1.50%
49	Wyoming	5	0.06%

RANK ORDER

RANK	STATE	ESTABLISH'S	% of USA
1	New York	938	11.80%
2	California	930	11.70%
3	Pennsylvania	589	7.41%
4	Florida	564	7.10%
5	Ohio	490	6.17%
6	New Jersey	449	5.65%
7	Illinois	419	5.27%
8	Michigan	400	5.03%
9	Texas	382	4.81%
10	Maryland	211	2.65%
11	Massachusetts	208	2.62%
12	Indiana	166	2.09%
13	Virginia	164	2.06%
14	Connecticut	152	1.91%
15	Washington	146	1.84%
16	North Carolina	140	1.76%
17	Georgia	139	1.75%
18	Arizona	121	1.52%
19	Wisconsin	119	1.50%
20	Missouri	98	1.23%
21	Tennessee	90	1.13%
22	Colorado	88	1.11%
23	Iowa	75	0.94%
24	Oregon	61	0.77%
25	Minnesota	60	0.75%
26	Kansas	55	0.69%
27	Oklahoma	52	0.65%
28	Rhode Island	50	0.63%
29	Alabama	49	0.62%
30	Louisiana	48	0.60%
31	Kentucky	46	0.58%
32	Utah	44	0.55%
33	South Carolina	40	0.50%
34	Maine	36	0.45%
35	Nebraska	34	0.43%
36	New Mexico	33	0.42%
37	Nevada	28	0.35%
38	West Virginia	26	0.33%
39	Delaware	25	0.31%
40	New Hampshire	24	0.30%
41	Arkansas	20	0.25%
42	Mississippi	18	0.23%
43	Idaho	17	0.21%
44	Hawaii	16	0.20%
44	Montana	16	0.20%
46	South Dakota	14	0.18%
47	Vermont	9	0.11%
48	North Dakota	7	0.09%
49	Alaska	5	0.06%
49	Wyoming	5	0.06%
	District of Columbia	32	0.40%

Source: U.S. Bureau of the Census
   "1992 Census of Service Industries, Geographic Area Series, United States" (SC92-A-52)
*Includes only establishments subject to the federal income tax.

Offices and Clinics of Other Health Practitioners in 1992

National Total = 22,260 Establishments*

ALPHA ORDER

RANK	STATE	ESTABLISH'S	% of USA
28	Alabama	174	0.78%
47	Alaska	60	0.27%
17	Arizona	447	2.01%
33	Arkansas	156	0.70%
1	California	3,954	17.76%
14	Colorado	515	2.31%
24	Connecticut	312	1.40%
43	Delaware	76	0.34%
2	Florida	1,644	7.39%
12	Georgia	544	2.44%
37	Hawaii	120	0.54%
42	Idaho	79	0.35%
7	Illinois	722	3.24%
25	Indiana	275	1.24%
33	Iowa	156	0.70%
32	Kansas	158	0.71%
27	Kentucky	212	0.95%
23	Louisiana	324	1.46%
38	Maine	112	0.50%
11	Maryland	592	2.66%
13	Massachusetts	526	2.36%
8	Michigan	669	3.01%
19	Minnesota	361	1.62%
40	Mississippi	102	0.46%
18	Missouri	374	1.68%
41	Montana	86	0.39%
39	Nebraska	107	0.48%
35	Nevada	130	0.58%
36	New Hampshire	128	0.58%
9	New Jersey	666	2.99%
30	New Mexico	167	0.75%
4	New York	1,344	6.04%
15	North Carolina	497	2.23%
50	North Dakota	31	0.14%
6	Ohio	860	3.86%
26	Oklahoma	228	1.02%
19	Oregon	361	1.62%
5	Pennsylvania	899	4.04%
46	Rhode Island	66	0.30%
29	South Carolina	169	0.76%
48	South Dakota	37	0.17%
22	Tennessee	330	1.48%
3	Texas	1,636	7.35%
31	Utah	166	0.75%
44	Vermont	69	0.31%
16	Virginia	485	2.18%
10	Washington	620	2.79%
44	West Virginia	69	0.31%
21	Wisconsin	340	1.53%
48	Wyoming	37	0.17%

RANK ORDER

RANK	STATE	ESTABLISH'S	% of USA
1	California	3,954	17.76%
2	Florida	1,644	7.39%
3	Texas	1,636	7.35%
4	New York	1,344	6.04%
5	Pennsylvania	899	4.04%
6	Ohio	860	3.86%
7	Illinois	722	3.24%
8	Michigan	669	3.01%
9	New Jersey	666	2.99%
10	Washington	620	2.79%
11	Maryland	592	2.66%
12	Georgia	544	2.44%
13	Massachusetts	526	2.36%
14	Colorado	515	2.31%
15	North Carolina	497	2.23%
16	Virginia	485	2.18%
17	Arizona	447	2.01%
18	Missouri	374	1.68%
19	Minnesota	361	1.62%
19	Oregon	361	1.62%
21	Wisconsin	340	1.53%
22	Tennessee	330	1.48%
23	Louisiana	324	1.46%
24	Connecticut	312	1.40%
25	Indiana	275	1.24%
26	Oklahoma	228	1.02%
27	Kentucky	212	0.95%
28	Alabama	174	0.78%
29	South Carolina	169	0.76%
30	New Mexico	167	0.75%
31	Utah	166	0.75%
32	Kansas	158	0.71%
33	Arkansas	156	0.70%
33	Iowa	156	0.70%
35	Nevada	130	0.58%
36	New Hampshire	128	0.58%
37	Hawaii	120	0.54%
38	Maine	112	0.50%
39	Nebraska	107	0.48%
40	Mississippi	102	0.46%
41	Montana	86	0.39%
42	Idaho	79	0.35%
43	Delaware	76	0.34%
44	Vermont	69	0.31%
44	West Virginia	69	0.31%
46	Rhode Island	66	0.30%
47	Alaska	60	0.27%
48	South Dakota	37	0.17%
48	Wyoming	37	0.17%
50	North Dakota	31	0.14%
	District of Columbia	68	0.31%

Source: U.S. Bureau of the Census
"1992 Census of Service Industries, Geographic Area Series, United States" (SC92-A-52)
*Includes only establishments subject to the federal income tax. Includes health practitioners not otherwise classified such as acupuncturists, midwives, nutritionists, physical and occupational therapists and psychologists.

IV. FINANCE

IV. FINANCE (Continued)

National Health Care Finance Data 1996

Total Health Care Expenditures = $1,035,100,000,000*

The 1993 health care expenditures broken down to the state level and shown in this book were released in the fall of 1995. The Health Care Financing Administration (HCFA) is committed to updating these numbers. Updates were expected in the summer of 1997 but difficulties inherent in allocating more than one trillion dollars in expenditures among the states have delayed the release of any updates a number of times. As we go to press in May of 1998, no updates for the 1993 numbers at the state level are yet available.

Given the high level of interest in health care finance data, we have assembled a table showing the most recent national level health care expenditure data. We will continue to monitor HCFA data releases and will include the state expenditure updates in forthcoming editions.

	EXPENDITURES IN 1996	PERCENT CHANGE: 1995 TO 1996
Total Health Care Expenditures	$1,035,100,000,000	4.4
Per Capita Total Health Care Expenditures	$3,903	
Personal Health Care Expenditures	$907,200,000,000	4.4
Per Capita Personal Health Care Expenditures	$3,421	
Hospital Care Expenditures	$358,500,000,000	3.4
Per Capita Hospital Care Expenditures	$1,352	
Physician Services Expenditures	$202,100,000,000	2.9
Per Capita Physician Services Expenditures	$762	
Dental Services Expenditures	$47,600,000,000	6.4
Per Capita Dental Services Expenditures	$180	
Other Professional Services	$58,000,000,000	6.8
Per Capita Other Professional Services	$219	
Home Health Care Expenditures	$30,200,000,000	6.2
Per Capita Home Health Care Expenditures	$114	
Drugs and Other Medical Nondurables	$91,400,000,000	7.7
Per Capita Drugs and Other Medical Nondurables	$345	
Vision Products and Other Medical Durables	$13,300,000,000	1.4
Per Capita Vision Products and Other Medical Durables	$50	
Nursing Home Care	$78,500,000,000	4.3
Per Capita Nursing Home Care	$296	
Other Personal Care Expenditures	$27,600,000,000	9.4
Per Capita Other Personal Care Expenditures	$104	

Source: U.S. Department of Health and Human Services, Health Care Financing Administration
  "National Health Expenditures Aggregate Amounts and Average Annual Percent Change, by Type of Expenditure"
    (www.hcfa.gov/stats/nhe-oact/tables/t10.htm)
*Per Capita figures calculated by Morgan Quitno Press. For definitions see the corresponding 1993 state tables in this chapter.

Personal Health Care Expenditures in 1993

National Total = $778,510,000,000*

ALPHA ORDER

RANK	STATE	EXPENDITURES	% of USA
23	Alabama	$12,060,000,000	1.55%
48	Alaska	1,573,000,000	0.20%
24	Arizona	10,635,000,000	1.37%
33	Arkansas	6,111,000,000	0.78%
1	California	94,178,000,000	12.10%
26	Colorado	10,066,000,000	1.29%
22	Connecticut	12,216,000,000	1.57%
44	Delaware	2,260,000,000	0.29%
4	Florida	44,811,000,000	5.76%
11	Georgia	20,104,000,000	2.58%
39	Hawaii	3,485,000,000	0.45%
43	Idaho	2,277,000,000	0.29%
6	Illinois	34,747,000,000	4.46%
14	Indiana	16,401,000,000	2.11%
30	Iowa	7,341,000,000	0.94%
31	Kansas	6,903,000,000	0.89%
25	Kentucky	10,384,000,000	1.33%
21	Louisiana	13,014,000,000	1.67%
41	Maine	3,433,000,000	0.44%
17	Maryland	15,154,000,000	1.95%
10	Massachusetts	23,421,000,000	3.01%
8	Michigan	27,136,000,000	3.49%
20	Minnesota	14,194,000,000	1.82%
32	Mississippi	6,187,000,000	0.79%
16	Missouri	15,949,000,000	2.05%
45	Montana	2,103,000,000	0.27%
35	Nebraska	4,400,000,000	0.57%
38	Nevada	3,747,000,000	0.48%
40	New Hampshire	3,452,000,000	0.44%
9	New Jersey	25,741,000,000	3.31%
37	New Mexico	3,878,000,000	0.50%
2	New York	67,033,000,000	8.61%
12	North Carolina	18,241,000,000	2.34%
46	North Dakota	2,021,000,000	0.26%
7	Ohio	33,456,000,000	4.30%
28	Oklahoma	8,041,000,000	1.03%
29	Oregon	7,999,000,000	1.03%
5	Pennsylvania	41,521,000,000	5.33%
42	Rhode Island	3,428,000,000	0.44%
27	South Carolina	9,029,000,000	1.16%
47	South Dakota	1,953,000,000	0.25%
15	Tennessee	16,203,000,000	2.08%
3	Texas	49,816,000,000	6.40%
36	Utah	4,118,000,000	0.53%
49	Vermont	1,499,000,000	0.19%
13	Virginia	16,682,000,000	2.14%
18	Washington	15,129,000,000	1.94%
34	West Virginia	5,197,000,000	0.67%
19	Wisconsin	14,502,000,000	1.86%
50	Wyoming	998,000,000	0.13%

RANK ORDER

RANK	STATE	EXPENDITURES	% of USA
1	California	$94,178,000,000	12.10%
2	New York	67,033,000,000	8.61%
3	Texas	49,816,000,000	6.40%
4	Florida	44,811,000,000	5.76%
5	Pennsylvania	41,521,000,000	5.33%
6	Illinois	34,747,000,000	4.46%
7	Ohio	33,456,000,000	4.30%
8	Michigan	27,136,000,000	3.49%
9	New Jersey	25,741,000,000	3.31%
10	Massachusetts	23,421,000,000	3.01%
11	Georgia	20,104,000,000	2.58%
12	North Carolina	18,241,000,000	2.34%
13	Virginia	16,682,000,000	2.14%
14	Indiana	16,401,000,000	2.11%
15	Tennessee	16,203,000,000	2.08%
16	Missouri	15,949,000,000	2.05%
17	Maryland	15,154,000,000	1.95%
18	Washington	15,129,000,000	1.94%
19	Wisconsin	14,502,000,000	1.86%
20	Minnesota	14,194,000,000	1.82%
21	Louisiana	13,014,000,000	1.67%
22	Connecticut	12,216,000,000	1.57%
23	Alabama	12,060,000,000	1.55%
24	Arizona	10,635,000,000	1.37%
25	Kentucky	10,384,000,000	1.33%
26	Colorado	10,066,000,000	1.29%
27	South Carolina	9,029,000,000	1.16%
28	Oklahoma	8,041,000,000	1.03%
29	Oregon	7,999,000,000	1.03%
30	Iowa	7,341,000,000	0.94%
31	Kansas	6,903,000,000	0.89%
32	Mississippi	6,187,000,000	0.79%
33	Arkansas	6,111,000,000	0.78%
34	West Virginia	5,197,000,000	0.67%
35	Nebraska	4,400,000,000	0.57%
36	Utah	4,118,000,000	0.53%
37	New Mexico	3,878,000,000	0.50%
38	Nevada	3,747,000,000	0.48%
39	Hawaii	3,485,000,000	0.45%
40	New Hampshire	3,452,000,000	0.44%
41	Maine	3,433,000,000	0.44%
42	Rhode Island	3,428,000,000	0.44%
43	Idaho	2,277,000,000	0.29%
44	Delaware	2,260,000,000	0.29%
45	Montana	2,103,000,000	0.27%
46	North Dakota	2,021,000,000	0.26%
47	South Dakota	1,953,000,000	0.25%
48	Alaska	1,573,000,000	0.20%
49	Vermont	1,499,000,000	0.19%
50	Wyoming	998,000,000	0.13%
	District of Columbia	4,285,000,000	0.55%

Source: U.S. Department of Health and Human Services, Health Care Financing Administration
"State Health Expenditure Accounts" (Health Care Financing Review, Fall 1995, Volume 17, Number 1)
*By state of provider. Includes hospital care, physician services, dental services, home health care, drugs, vision products and other personal health care services and products.

Health Care Expenditures as a Percent of Gross State Product in 1993

National Percent = 12.1% of Total Gross State Product*

<table>
<tr><td colspan="3">ALPHA ORDER</td><td colspan="3">RANK ORDER</td></tr>
<tr><td>RANK</td><td>STATE</td><td>PERCENT</td><td>RANK</td><td>STATE</td><td>PERCENT</td></tr>
<tr><td>6</td><td>Alabama</td><td>14.6</td><td>1</td><td>West Virginia</td><td>16.2</td></tr>
<tr><td>50</td><td>Alaska</td><td>6.3</td><td>2</td><td>North Dakota</td><td>16.0</td></tr>
<tr><td>19</td><td>Arizona</td><td>12.6</td><td>3</td><td>Florida</td><td>15.0</td></tr>
<tr><td>13</td><td>Arkansas</td><td>13.1</td><td>4</td><td>Pennsylvania</td><td>14.7</td></tr>
<tr><td>36</td><td>California</td><td>11.2</td><td>4</td><td>Rhode Island</td><td>14.7</td></tr>
<tr><td>40</td><td>Colorado</td><td>10.8</td><td>6</td><td>Alabama</td><td>14.6</td></tr>
<tr><td>33</td><td>Connecticut</td><td>11.5</td><td>7</td><td>Tennessee</td><td>14.0</td></tr>
<tr><td>48</td><td>Delaware</td><td>9.3</td><td>8</td><td>Louisiana</td><td>13.8</td></tr>
<tr><td>3</td><td>Florida</td><td>15.0</td><td>9</td><td>Maine</td><td>13.7</td></tr>
<tr><td>30</td><td>Georgia</td><td>11.8</td><td>10</td><td>Massachusetts</td><td>13.4</td></tr>
<tr><td>46</td><td>Hawaii</td><td>9.6</td><td>10</td><td>Mississippi</td><td>13.4</td></tr>
<tr><td>44</td><td>Idaho</td><td>10.2</td><td>10</td><td>Missouri</td><td>13.4</td></tr>
<tr><td>37</td><td>Illinois</td><td>11.1</td><td>13</td><td>Arkansas</td><td>13.1</td></tr>
<tr><td>16</td><td>Indiana</td><td>12.9</td><td>13</td><td>Ohio</td><td>13.1</td></tr>
<tr><td>28</td><td>Iowa</td><td>11.9</td><td>15</td><td>Montana</td><td>13.0</td></tr>
<tr><td>28</td><td>Kansas</td><td>11.9</td><td>16</td><td>Indiana</td><td>12.9</td></tr>
<tr><td>16</td><td>Kentucky</td><td>12.9</td><td>16</td><td>Kentucky</td><td>12.9</td></tr>
<tr><td>8</td><td>Louisiana</td><td>13.8</td><td>18</td><td>New Hampshire</td><td>12.7</td></tr>
<tr><td>9</td><td>Maine</td><td>13.7</td><td>19</td><td>Arizona</td><td>12.6</td></tr>
<tr><td>25</td><td>Maryland</td><td>12.2</td><td>19</td><td>Oklahoma</td><td>12.6</td></tr>
<tr><td>10</td><td>Massachusetts</td><td>13.4</td><td>21</td><td>Michigan</td><td>12.5</td></tr>
<tr><td>21</td><td>Michigan</td><td>12.5</td><td>22</td><td>Minnesota</td><td>12.3</td></tr>
<tr><td>22</td><td>Minnesota</td><td>12.3</td><td>22</td><td>New York</td><td>12.3</td></tr>
<tr><td>10</td><td>Mississippi</td><td>13.4</td><td>22</td><td>Wisconsin</td><td>12.3</td></tr>
<tr><td>10</td><td>Missouri</td><td>13.4</td><td>25</td><td>Maryland</td><td>12.2</td></tr>
<tr><td>15</td><td>Montana</td><td>13.0</td><td>26</td><td>South Dakota</td><td>12.1</td></tr>
<tr><td>33</td><td>Nebraska</td><td>11.5</td><td>27</td><td>South Carolina</td><td>12.0</td></tr>
<tr><td>47</td><td>Nevada</td><td>9.5</td><td>28</td><td>Iowa</td><td>11.9</td></tr>
<tr><td>18</td><td>New Hampshire</td><td>12.7</td><td>28</td><td>Kansas</td><td>11.9</td></tr>
<tr><td>43</td><td>New Jersey</td><td>10.5</td><td>30</td><td>Georgia</td><td>11.8</td></tr>
<tr><td>35</td><td>New Mexico</td><td>11.3</td><td>30</td><td>Vermont</td><td>11.8</td></tr>
<tr><td>22</td><td>New York</td><td>12.3</td><td>32</td><td>Oregon</td><td>11.6</td></tr>
<tr><td>40</td><td>North Carolina</td><td>10.8</td><td>33</td><td>Connecticut</td><td>11.5</td></tr>
<tr><td>2</td><td>North Dakota</td><td>16.0</td><td>33</td><td>Nebraska</td><td>11.5</td></tr>
<tr><td>13</td><td>Ohio</td><td>13.1</td><td>35</td><td>New Mexico</td><td>11.3</td></tr>
<tr><td>19</td><td>Oklahoma</td><td>12.6</td><td>36</td><td>California</td><td>11.2</td></tr>
<tr><td>32</td><td>Oregon</td><td>11.6</td><td>37</td><td>Illinois</td><td>11.1</td></tr>
<tr><td>4</td><td>Pennsylvania</td><td>14.7</td><td>37</td><td>Texas</td><td>11.1</td></tr>
<tr><td>4</td><td>Rhode Island</td><td>14.7</td><td>37</td><td>Washington</td><td>11.1</td></tr>
<tr><td>27</td><td>South Carolina</td><td>12.0</td><td>40</td><td>Colorado</td><td>10.8</td></tr>
<tr><td>26</td><td>South Dakota</td><td>12.1</td><td>40</td><td>North Carolina</td><td>10.8</td></tr>
<tr><td>7</td><td>Tennessee</td><td>14.0</td><td>40</td><td>Utah</td><td>10.8</td></tr>
<tr><td>37</td><td>Texas</td><td>11.1</td><td>43</td><td>New Jersey</td><td>10.5</td></tr>
<tr><td>40</td><td>Utah</td><td>10.8</td><td>44</td><td>Idaho</td><td>10.2</td></tr>
<tr><td>30</td><td>Vermont</td><td>11.8</td><td>45</td><td>Virginia</td><td>9.8</td></tr>
<tr><td>45</td><td>Virginia</td><td>9.8</td><td>46</td><td>Hawaii</td><td>9.6</td></tr>
<tr><td>37</td><td>Washington</td><td>11.1</td><td>47</td><td>Nevada</td><td>9.5</td></tr>
<tr><td>1</td><td>West Virginia</td><td>16.2</td><td>48</td><td>Delaware</td><td>9.3</td></tr>
<tr><td>22</td><td>Wisconsin</td><td>12.3</td><td>49</td><td>Wyoming</td><td>6.7</td></tr>
<tr><td>49</td><td>Wyoming</td><td>6.7</td><td>50</td><td>Alaska</td><td>6.3</td></tr>
<tr><td></td><td></td><td></td><td></td><td>District of Columbia</td><td>9.1</td></tr>
</table>

Source: Morgan Quitno Press using data from U.S. Dept of Health & Human Services, Health Care Financing Admin.
"State Health Expenditure Accounts" (Health Care Financing Review, Fall 1995, Volume 17, Number 1)
*By state of provider. Includes hospital care, physician services, dental services, home health care, drugs, vision products and other personal health care services and products.

Per Capita Personal Health Care Expenditures in 1993

National Per Capita = $3,020*

ALPHA ORDER

RANK	STATE	PER CAPITA
21	Alabama	$2,884
37	Alaska	2,630
35	Arizona	2,697
42	Arkansas	2,520
17	California	3,017
27	Colorado	2,821
2	Connecticut	3,727
8	Delaware	3,233
7	Florida	3,266
20	Georgia	2,913
18	Hawaii	2,989
50	Idaho	2,068
19	Illinois	2,972
24	Indiana	2,874
40	Iowa	2,601
31	Kansas	2,726
30	Kentucky	2,738
15	Louisiana	3,034
28	Maine	2,771
13	Maryland	3,060
1	Massachusetts	3,892
25	Michigan	2,869
11	Minnesota	3,137
47	Mississippi	2,344
14	Missouri	3,047
43	Montana	2,501
31	Nebraska	2,726
34	Nevada	2,705
12	New Hampshire	3,074
6	New Jersey	3,275
46	New Mexico	2,400
3	New York	3,693
38	North Carolina	2,623
10	North Dakota	3,173
16	Ohio	3,025
45	Oklahoma	2,488
36	Oregon	2,636
4	Pennsylvania	3,451
5	Rhode Island	3,431
44	South Carolina	2,489
33	South Dakota	2,724
9	Tennessee	3,181
29	Texas	2,760
48	Utah	2,214
39	Vermont	2,602
41	Virginia	2,576
22	Washington	2,879
26	West Virginia	2,859
23	Wisconsin	2,875
49	Wyoming	2,123

RANK ORDER

RANK	STATE	PER CAPITA
1	Massachusetts	$3,892
2	Connecticut	3,727
3	New York	3,693
4	Pennsylvania	3,451
5	Rhode Island	3,431
6	New Jersey	3,275
7	Florida	3,266
8	Delaware	3,233
9	Tennessee	3,181
10	North Dakota	3,173
11	Minnesota	3,137
12	New Hampshire	3,074
13	Maryland	3,060
14	Missouri	3,047
15	Louisiana	3,034
16	Ohio	3,025
17	California	3,017
18	Hawaii	2,989
19	Illinois	2,972
20	Georgia	2,913
21	Alabama	2,884
22	Washington	2,879
23	Wisconsin	2,875
24	Indiana	2,874
25	Michigan	2,869
26	West Virginia	2,859
27	Colorado	2,821
28	Maine	2,771
29	Texas	2,760
30	Kentucky	2,738
31	Kansas	2,726
31	Nebraska	2,726
33	South Dakota	2,724
34	Nevada	2,705
35	Arizona	2,697
36	Oregon	2,636
37	Alaska	2,630
38	North Carolina	2,623
39	Vermont	2,602
40	Iowa	2,601
41	Virginia	2,576
42	Arkansas	2,520
43	Montana	2,501
44	South Carolina	2,489
45	Oklahoma	2,488
46	New Mexico	2,400
47	Mississippi	2,344
48	Utah	2,214
49	Wyoming	2,123
50	Idaho	2,068

District of Columbia   7,413

Source: Morgan Quitno Press using data from U.S. Dept of Health & Human Services, Health Care Financing Admin. "State Health Expenditure Accounts" (Health Care Financing Review, Fall 1995, Volume 17, Number 1)
*By state of provider. Includes hospital care, physician services, dental services, home health care, drugs, vision products and other personal health care services and products.

Percent Change in Personal Health Care Expenditures: 1990 to 1993

National Percent Change = 28.0% Increase*

ALPHA ORDER

RANK ORDER

RANK	STATE	PERCENT CHANGE		RANK	STATE	PERCENT CHANGE
13	Alabama	31.7		1	Idaho	37.4
32	Alaska	27.0		2	New Hampshire	36.9
41	Arizona	25.4		3	Nevada	35.4
37	Arkansas	26.1		3	Washington	35.4
30	California	27.1		5	South Carolina	34.8
20	Colorado	30.3		6	New Mexico	34.0
48	Connecticut	22.5		7	Texas	33.7
12	Delaware	32.2		8	North Carolina	33.1
28	Florida	27.6		8	Tennessee	33.1
15	Georgia	31.5		8	West Virginia	33.1
29	Hawaii	27.5		11	Kentucky	32.7
1	Idaho	37.4		12	Delaware	32.2
34	Illinois	26.7		13	Alabama	31.7
19	Indiana	30.7		14	Louisiana	31.6
50	Iowa	21.9		15	Georgia	31.5
43	Kansas	25.3		16	Mississippi	31.2
11	Kentucky	32.7		17	Montana	30.9
14	Louisiana	31.6		18	South Dakota	30.8
30	Maine	27.1		19	Indiana	30.7
27	Maryland	28.0		20	Colorado	30.3
49	Massachusetts	22.2		20	Oregon	30.3
46	Michigan	23.5		22	Utah	29.9
47	Minnesota	23.3		23	New Jersey	29.0
16	Mississippi	31.2		24	Oklahoma	28.1
34	Missouri	26.7		24	Pennsylvania	28.1
17	Montana	30.9		24	Wisconsin	28.1
36	Nebraska	26.5		27	Maryland	28.0
3	Nevada	35.4		28	Florida	27.6
2	New Hampshire	36.9		29	Hawaii	27.5
23	New Jersey	29.0		30	California	27.1
6	New Mexico	34.0		30	Maine	27.1
44	New York	24.8		32	Alaska	27.0
8	North Carolina	33.1		33	Vermont	26.8
44	North Dakota	24.8		34	Illinois	26.7
41	Ohio	25.4		34	Missouri	26.7
24	Oklahoma	28.1		36	Nebraska	26.5
20	Oregon	30.3		37	Arkansas	26.1
24	Pennsylvania	28.1		38	Virginia	25.9
40	Rhode Island	25.5		39	Wyoming	25.7
5	South Carolina	34.8		40	Rhode Island	25.5
18	South Dakota	30.8		41	Arizona	25.4
8	Tennessee	33.1		41	Ohio	25.4
7	Texas	33.7		43	Kansas	25.3
22	Utah	29.9		44	New York	24.8
33	Vermont	26.8		44	North Dakota	24.8
38	Virginia	25.9		46	Michigan	23.5
3	Washington	35.4		47	Minnesota	23.3
8	West Virginia	33.1		48	Connecticut	22.5
24	Wisconsin	28.1		49	Massachusetts	22.2
39	Wyoming	25.7		50	Iowa	21.9
					District of Columbia	21.2

Source: Morgan Quitno Press using data from U.S. Dept of Health & Human Services, Health Care Financing Admin. "State Health Expenditure Accounts" (Health Care Financing Review, Fall 1995, Volume 17, Number 1)
*By state of provider. Includes hospital care, physician services, dental services, home health care, drugs, vision products and other personal health care services and products.

Percent Change in Per Capita Expenditures for
Personal Health Care: 1990 to 1993
National Percent Change = 23.5% Increase*

ALPHA ORDER				RANK ORDER		
RANK	STATE	PERCENT CHANGE		RANK	STATE	PERCENT CHANGE
8	Alabama	27.2		1	New Hampshire	35.2
49	Alaska	16.7		2	West Virginia	31.3
50	Arizona	16.6		3	Louisiana	29.5
35	Arkansas	22.2		3	South Carolina	29.5
41	California	21.1		5	Kentucky	29.0
42	Colorado	20.3		6	Mississippi	28.0
33	Connecticut	22.8		7	Tennessee	27.4
16	Delaware	25.9		8	Alabama	27.2
42	Florida	20.3		9	North Carolina	27.0
31	Georgia	23.4		9	South Dakota	27.0
40	Hawaii	21.2		11	Indiana	26.9
18	Idaho	25.7		11	New Jersey	26.9
26	Illinois	23.9		13	Pennsylvania	26.5
11	Indiana	26.9		14	Maine	26.0
46	Iowa	20.0		14	Rhode Island	26.0
34	Kansas	22.6		16	Delaware	25.9
5	Kentucky	29.0		17	Texas	25.8
3	Louisiana	29.5		18	Idaho	25.7
14	Maine	26.0		19	New Mexico	25.6
30	Maryland	23.6		20	Washington	25.4
36	Massachusetts	22.1		21	North Dakota	25.2
38	Michigan	21.4		22	Oklahoma	24.6
47	Minnesota	19.3		23	Montana	24.4
6	Mississippi	28.0		24	Wisconsin	24.2
27	Missouri	23.8		25	Vermont	24.0
23	Montana	24.4		26	Illinois	23.9
28	Nebraska	23.7		27	Missouri	23.8
48	Nevada	17.5		28	Nebraska	23.7
1	New Hampshire	35.2		28	New York	23.7
11	New Jersey	26.9		30	Maryland	23.6
19	New Mexico	25.6		31	Georgia	23.4
28	New York	23.7		32	Ohio	23.0
9	North Carolina	27.0		33	Connecticut	22.8
21	North Dakota	25.2		34	Kansas	22.6
32	Ohio	23.0		35	Arkansas	22.2
22	Oklahoma	24.6		36	Massachusetts	22.1
36	Oregon	22.1		36	Oregon	22.1
13	Pennsylvania	26.5		38	Michigan	21.4
14	Rhode Island	26.0		38	Wyoming	21.4
3	South Carolina	29.5		40	Hawaii	21.2
9	South Dakota	27.0		41	California	21.1
7	Tennessee	27.4		42	Colorado	20.3
17	Texas	25.8		42	Florida	20.3
42	Utah	20.3		42	Utah	20.3
25	Vermont	24.0		42	Virginia	20.3
42	Virginia	20.3		46	Iowa	20.0
20	Washington	25.4		47	Minnesota	19.3
2	West Virginia	31.3		48	Nevada	17.5
24	Wisconsin	24.2		49	Alaska	16.7
38	Wyoming	21.4		50	Arizona	16.6
					District of Columbia	27.3

Source: Morgan Quitno Press using data from U.S. Dept of Health & Human Services, Health Care Financing Admin.
"State Health Expenditure Accounts" (Health Care Financing Review, Fall 1995, Volume 17, Number 1)
*By state of provider. Includes hospital care, physician services, dental services, home health care, drugs, vision products and other personal health care services and products.

Average Annual Change in Expenditures for Personal Health Care: 1980 to 1993
National Percent = 10.3% Average Annual Growth*

<u>ALPHA ORDER</u>

RANK	STATE	PERCENT
16	Alabama	10.9
27	Alaska	10.2
5	Arizona	11.9
32	Arkansas	10.1
27	California	10.2
23	Colorado	10.5
15	Connecticut	11.0
9	Delaware	11.3
2	Florida	12.4
4	Georgia	12.1
19	Hawaii	10.8
24	Idaho	10.4
47	Illinois	8.7
26	Indiana	10.3
50	Iowa	8.3
45	Kansas	9.0
16	Kentucky	10.9
24	Louisiana	10.4
21	Maine	10.6
21	Maryland	10.6
27	Massachusetts	10.2
49	Michigan	8.5
37	Minnesota	9.7
32	Mississippi	10.1
39	Missouri	9.6
35	Montana	9.8
46	Nebraska	8.9
3	Nevada	12.2
1	New Hampshire	13.0
10	New Jersey	11.2
8	New Mexico	11.7
37	New York	9.7
5	North Carolina	11.9
43	North Dakota	9.4
39	Ohio	9.6
44	Oklahoma	9.1
34	Oregon	9.9
27	Pennsylvania	10.2
27	Rhode Island	10.2
5	South Carolina	11.9
35	South Dakota	9.8
10	Tennessee	11.2
12	Texas	11.1
12	Utah	11.1
19	Vermont	10.8
16	Virginia	10.9
12	Washington	11.1
39	West Virginia	9.6
42	Wisconsin	9.5
47	Wyoming	8.7

<u>RANK ORDER</u>

RANK	STATE	PERCENT
1	New Hampshire	13.0
2	Florida	12.4
3	Nevada	12.2
4	Georgia	12.1
5	Arizona	11.9
5	North Carolina	11.9
5	South Carolina	11.9
8	New Mexico	11.7
9	Delaware	11.3
10	New Jersey	11.2
10	Tennessee	11.2
12	Texas	11.1
12	Utah	11.1
12	Washington	11.1
15	Connecticut	11.0
16	Alabama	10.9
16	Kentucky	10.9
16	Virginia	10.9
19	Hawaii	10.8
19	Vermont	10.8
21	Maine	10.6
21	Maryland	10.6
23	Colorado	10.5
24	Idaho	10.4
24	Louisiana	10.4
26	Indiana	10.3
27	Alaska	10.2
27	California	10.2
27	Massachusetts	10.2
27	Pennsylvania	10.2
27	Rhode Island	10.2
32	Arkansas	10.1
32	Mississippi	10.1
34	Oregon	9.9
35	Montana	9.8
35	South Dakota	9.8
37	Minnesota	9.7
37	New York	9.7
39	Missouri	9.6
39	Ohio	9.6
39	West Virginia	9.6
42	Wisconsin	9.5
43	North Dakota	9.4
44	Oklahoma	9.1
45	Kansas	9.0
46	Nebraska	8.9
47	Illinois	8.7
47	Wyoming	8.7
49	Michigan	8.5
50	Iowa	8.3
	District of Columbia	9.1

Source: U.S. Department of Health and Human Services, Health Care Financing Administration
"State Health Expenditure Accounts" (Health Care Financing Review, Fall 1995, Volume 17, Number 1)
*By state of provider. Includes hospital care, physician services, dental services, home health care, drugs, vision products and other personal health care services and products.

Average Annual Change in Per Capita Expenditures For Personal Health Care: 1980 to 1993 National Percent = 9.3% Average Annual Increase*

ALPHA ORDER

ALPHA ORDER

RANK ORDER

RANK	STATE	PERCENT		RANK	STATE	PERCENT
7	Alabama	10.3		1	New Hampshire	11.3
50	Alaska	6.8		2	New Jersey	10.7
38	Arizona	8.8		3	Kentucky	10.6
21	Arkansas	9.6		3	South Carolina	10.6
48	California	7.9		5	Connecticut	10.5
38	Colorado	8.8		5	North Carolina	10.5
5	Connecticut	10.5		7	Alabama	10.3
13	Delaware	10.0		7	Louisiana	10.3
23	Florida	9.5		7	Tennessee	10.3
11	Georgia	10.1		10	West Virginia	10.2
30	Hawaii	9.2		11	Georgia	10.1
31	Idaho	9.1		11	Pennsylvania	10.1
45	Illinois	8.5		13	Delaware	10.0
13	Indiana	10.0		13	Indiana	10.0
42	Iowa	8.6		15	New Mexico	9.9
46	Kansas	8.4		16	Maine	9.8
3	Kentucky	10.6		16	Massachusetts	9.8
7	Louisiana	10.3		16	Vermont	9.8
16	Maine	9.8		19	Mississippi	9.7
27	Maryland	9.3		19	Rhode Island	9.7
16	Massachusetts	9.8		21	Arkansas	9.6
46	Michigan	8.4		21	North Dakota	9.6
37	Minnesota	8.9		23	Florida	9.5
19	Mississippi	9.7		23	South Dakota	9.5
31	Missouri	9.1		25	New York	9.4
27	Montana	9.3		25	Ohio	9.4
42	Nebraska	8.6		27	Maryland	9.3
49	Nevada	7.6		27	Montana	9.3
1	New Hampshire	11.3		27	Virginia	9.3
2	New Jersey	10.7		30	Hawaii	9.2
15	New Mexico	9.9		31	Idaho	9.1
25	New York	9.4		31	Missouri	9.1
5	North Carolina	10.5		31	Texas	9.1
21	North Dakota	9.6		31	Washington	9.1
25	Ohio	9.4		35	Utah	9.0
42	Oklahoma	8.6		35	Wisconsin	9.0
40	Oregon	8.7		37	Minnesota	8.9
11	Pennsylvania	10.1		38	Arizona	8.8
19	Rhode Island	9.7		38	Colorado	8.8
3	South Carolina	10.6		40	Oregon	8.7
23	South Dakota	9.5		40	Wyoming	8.7
7	Tennessee	10.3		42	Iowa	8.6
31	Texas	9.1		42	Nebraska	8.6
35	Utah	9.0		42	Oklahoma	8.6
16	Vermont	9.8		45	Illinois	8.5
27	Virginia	9.3		46	Kansas	8.4
31	Washington	9.1		46	Michigan	8.4
10	West Virginia	10.2		48	California	7.9
35	Wisconsin	9.0		49	Nevada	7.6
40	Wyoming	8.7		50	Alaska	6.8
					District of Columbia	9.9

Source: Morgan Quitno Press using data from U.S. Dept of Health & Human Services, Health Care Financing Admin.
"State Health Expenditure Accounts" (Health Care Financing Review, Fall 1995, Volume 17, Number 1)
*By state of provider. Includes hospital care, physician services, dental services, home health care, drugs, vision products and other personal health care services and products.

Expenditures for Hospital Care in 1993

National Total = $323,919,000,000*

ALPHA ORDER

RANK	STATE	EXPENDITURES	% of USA
21	Alabama	$5,301,000,000	1.64%
48	Alaska	701,000,000	0.22%
26	Arizona	3,999,000,000	1.24%
33	Arkansas	2,723,000,000	0.84%
1	California	34,827,000,000	10.77%
27	Colorado	3,932,000,000	1.22%
24	Connecticut	4,380,000,000	1.35%
43	Delaware	937,000,000	0.29%
5	Florida	17,131,000,000	5.30%
11	Georgia	8,704,000,000	2.69%
38	Hawaii	1,460,000,000	0.45%
46	Idaho	900,000,000	0.28%
6	Illinois	15,621,000,000	4.83%
16	Indiana	6,998,000,000	2.16%
29	Iowa	3,111,000,000	0.96%
32	Kansas	2,868,000,000	0.89%
23	Kentucky	4,515,000,000	1.40%
17	Louisiana	5,956,000,000	1.84%
40	Maine	1,376,000,000	0.43%
18	Maryland	5,926,000,000	1.83%
10	Massachusetts	10,034,000,000	3.10%
8	Michigan	11,711,000,000	3.62%
22	Minnesota	4,796,000,000	1.48%
31	Mississippi	2,897,000,000	0.90%
13	Missouri	7,652,000,000	2.37%
47	Montana	894,000,000	0.28%
35	Nebraska	2,003,000,000	0.62%
41	Nevada	1,362,000,000	0.42%
39	New Hampshire	1,388,000,000	0.43%
9	New Jersey	10,312,000,000	3.19%
36	New Mexico	1,848,000,000	0.57%
2	New York	28,001,000,000	8.66%
12	North Carolina	7,801,000,000	2.41%
45	North Dakota	903,000,000	0.28%
7	Ohio	14,305,000,000	4.42%
28	Oklahoma	3,329,000,000	1.03%
30	Oregon	2,966,000,000	0.92%
4	Pennsylvania	19,540,000,000	6.04%
42	Rhode Island	1,314,000,000	0.41%
25	South Carolina	4,221,000,000	1.30%
44	South Dakota	920,000,000	0.28%
14	Tennessee	7,208,000,000	2.23%
3	Texas	21,592,000,000	6.68%
37	Utah	1,743,000,000	0.54%
49	Vermont	562,000,000	0.17%
15	Virginia	7,031,000,000	2.17%
20	Washington	5,305,000,000	1.64%
34	West Virginia	2,346,000,000	0.73%
19	Wisconsin	5,537,000,000	1.71%
50	Wyoming	417,000,000	0.13%

RANK ORDER

RANK	STATE	EXPENDITURES	% of USA
1	California	$34,827,000,000	10.77%
2	New York	28,001,000,000	8.66%
3	Texas	21,592,000,000	6.68%
4	Pennsylvania	19,540,000,000	6.04%
5	Florida	17,131,000,000	5.30%
6	Illinois	15,621,000,000	4.83%
7	Ohio	14,305,000,000	4.42%
8	Michigan	11,711,000,000	3.62%
9	New Jersey	10,312,000,000	3.19%
10	Massachusetts	10,034,000,000	3.10%
11	Georgia	8,704,000,000	2.69%
12	North Carolina	7,801,000,000	2.41%
13	Missouri	7,652,000,000	2.37%
14	Tennessee	7,208,000,000	2.23%
15	Virginia	7,031,000,000	2.17%
16	Indiana	6,998,000,000	2.16%
17	Louisiana	5,956,000,000	1.84%
18	Maryland	5,926,000,000	1.83%
19	Wisconsin	5,537,000,000	1.71%
20	Washington	5,305,000,000	1.64%
21	Alabama	5,301,000,000	1.64%
22	Minnesota	4,796,000,000	1.48%
23	Kentucky	4,515,000,000	1.40%
24	Connecticut	4,380,000,000	1.35%
25	South Carolina	4,221,000,000	1.30%
26	Arizona	3,999,000,000	1.24%
27	Colorado	3,932,000,000	1.22%
28	Oklahoma	3,329,000,000	1.03%
29	Iowa	3,111,000,000	0.96%
30	Oregon	2,966,000,000	0.92%
31	Mississippi	2,897,000,000	0.90%
32	Kansas	2,868,000,000	0.89%
33	Arkansas	2,723,000,000	0.84%
34	West Virginia	2,346,000,000	0.73%
35	Nebraska	2,003,000,000	0.62%
36	New Mexico	1,848,000,000	0.57%
37	Utah	1,743,000,000	0.54%
38	Hawaii	1,460,000,000	0.45%
39	New Hampshire	1,388,000,000	0.43%
40	Maine	1,376,000,000	0.43%
41	Nevada	1,362,000,000	0.42%
42	Rhode Island	1,314,000,000	0.41%
43	Delaware	937,000,000	0.29%
44	South Dakota	920,000,000	0.28%
45	North Dakota	903,000,000	0.28%
46	Idaho	900,000,000	0.28%
47	Montana	894,000,000	0.28%
48	Alaska	701,000,000	0.22%
49	Vermont	562,000,000	0.17%
50	Wyoming	417,000,000	0.13%
	District of Columbia	2,612,000,000	0.81%

Source: U.S. Department of Health and Human Services, Health Care Financing Administration
   "State Health Expenditure Accounts" (Health Care Financing Review, Fall 1995, Volume 17, Number 1)
*By state of provider.

Percent of Total Personal Health Care Expenditures
Spent on Hospital Care in 1993
National Percent = 41.6%*

ALPHA ORDER

RANK	STATE	PERCENT
15	Alabama	44.0
12	Alaska	44.6
43	Arizona	37.6
12	Arkansas	44.6
46	California	37.0
38	Colorado	39.1
48	Connecticut	35.9
31	Delaware	41.5
41	Florida	38.2
17	Georgia	43.3
28	Hawaii	41.9
37	Idaho	39.5
10	Illinois	45.0
23	Indiana	42.7
25	Iowa	42.4
31	Kansas	41.5
16	Kentucky	43.5
7	Louisiana	45.8
35	Maine	40.1
38	Maryland	39.1
20	Massachusetts	42.8
19	Michigan	43.2
50	Minnesota	33.8
5	Mississippi	46.8
1	Missouri	48.0
24	Montana	42.5
8	Nebraska	45.5
47	Nevada	36.3
34	New Hampshire	40.2
35	New Jersey	40.1
2	New Mexico	47.7
29	New York	41.8
20	North Carolina	42.8
11	North Dakota	44.7
20	Ohio	42.8
33	Oklahoma	41.4
45	Oregon	37.1
3	Pennsylvania	47.1
40	Rhode Island	38.3
6	South Carolina	46.7
3	South Dakota	47.1
14	Tennessee	44.5
17	Texas	43.3
26	Utah	42.3
44	Vermont	37.5
27	Virginia	42.1
49	Washington	35.1
9	West Virginia	45.1
41	Wisconsin	38.2
29	Wyoming	41.8

RANK ORDER

RANK	STATE	PERCENT
1	Missouri	48.0
2	New Mexico	47.7
3	Pennsylvania	47.1
3	South Dakota	47.1
5	Mississippi	46.8
6	South Carolina	46.7
7	Louisiana	45.8
8	Nebraska	45.5
9	West Virginia	45.1
10	Illinois	45.0
11	North Dakota	44.7
12	Alaska	44.6
12	Arkansas	44.6
14	Tennessee	44.5
15	Alabama	44.0
16	Kentucky	43.5
17	Georgia	43.3
17	Texas	43.3
19	Michigan	43.2
20	Massachusetts	42.8
20	North Carolina	42.8
20	Ohio	42.8
23	Indiana	42.7
24	Montana	42.5
25	Iowa	42.4
26	Utah	42.3
27	Virginia	42.1
28	Hawaii	41.9
29	New York	41.8
29	Wyoming	41.8
31	Delaware	41.5
31	Kansas	41.5
33	Oklahoma	41.4
34	New Hampshire	40.2
35	Maine	40.1
35	New Jersey	40.1
37	Idaho	39.5
38	Colorado	39.1
38	Maryland	39.1
40	Rhode Island	38.3
41	Florida	38.2
41	Wisconsin	38.2
43	Arizona	37.6
44	Vermont	37.5
45	Oregon	37.1
46	California	37.0
47	Nevada	36.3
48	Connecticut	35.9
49	Washington	35.1
50	Minnesota	33.8
	District of Columbia	61.0

Source: Morgan Quitno Press using data from U.S. Dept of Health & Human Services, Health Care Financing Admin.
"State Health Expenditure Accounts" (Health Care Financing Review, Fall 1995, Volume 17, Number 1)
*By state of provider.

Per Capita Expenditures for Hospital Care in 1993

National Per Capita = $1,256*

ALPHA ORDER

RANK	STATE	PER CAPITA
16	Alabama	$1,268
27	Alaska	1,172
43	Arizona	1,014
31	Arkansas	1,123
33	California	1,116
35	Colorado	1,102
9	Connecticut	1,336
8	Delaware	1,340
19	Florida	1,248
17	Georgia	1,261
18	Hawaii	1,252
50	Idaho	817
9	Illinois	1,336
23	Indiana	1,226
35	Iowa	1,102
30	Kansas	1,133
26	Kentucky	1,190
7	Louisiana	1,389
34	Maine	1,111
24	Maryland	1,197
1	Massachusetts	1,667
21	Michigan	1,238
41	Minnesota	1,060
37	Mississippi	1,098
4	Missouri	1,462
40	Montana	1,063
20	Nebraska	1,241
45	Nevada	983
22	New Hampshire	1,236
12	New Jersey	1,312
29	New Mexico	1,144
3	New York	1,542
32	North Carolina	1,122
5	North Dakota	1,418
13	Ohio	1,293
42	Oklahoma	1,030
46	Oregon	977
2	Pennsylvania	1,624
11	Rhode Island	1,315
28	South Carolina	1,164
15	South Dakota	1,283
6	Tennessee	1,415
25	Texas	1,196
48	Utah	937
47	Vermont	976
39	Virginia	1,086
44	Washington	1,010
14	West Virginia	1,290
37	Wisconsin	1,098
49	Wyoming	887

RANK ORDER

RANK	STATE	PER CAPITA
1	Massachusetts	$1,667
2	Pennsylvania	1,624
3	New York	1,542
4	Missouri	1,462
5	North Dakota	1,418
6	Tennessee	1,415
7	Louisiana	1,389
8	Delaware	1,340
9	Connecticut	1,336
9	Illinois	1,336
11	Rhode Island	1,315
12	New Jersey	1,312
13	Ohio	1,293
14	West Virginia	1,290
15	South Dakota	1,283
16	Alabama	1,268
17	Georgia	1,261
18	Hawaii	1,252
19	Florida	1,248
20	Nebraska	1,241
21	Michigan	1,238
22	New Hampshire	1,236
23	Indiana	1,226
24	Maryland	1,197
25	Texas	1,196
26	Kentucky	1,190
27	Alaska	1,172
28	South Carolina	1,164
29	New Mexico	1,144
30	Kansas	1,133
31	Arkansas	1,123
32	North Carolina	1,122
33	California	1,116
34	Maine	1,111
35	Colorado	1,102
35	Iowa	1,102
37	Mississippi	1,098
37	Wisconsin	1,098
39	Virginia	1,086
40	Montana	1,063
41	Minnesota	1,060
42	Oklahoma	1,030
43	Arizona	1,014
44	Washington	1,010
45	Nevada	983
46	Oregon	977
47	Vermont	976
48	Utah	937
49	Wyoming	887
50	Idaho	817

District of Columbia**   4,519

Source: Morgan Quitno Press using data from U.S. Dept of Health & Human Services, Health Care Financing Admin.
"State Health Expenditure Accounts" (Health Care Financing Review, Fall 1995, Volume 17, Number 1)
*By state of provider.
**The District of Columbia's per capita is greatly affected by residents of Maryland and Virginia receiving services.

Percent Change in Expenditures for Hospital Care: 1990 to 1993

National Percent Change = 27.4% Increase*

<table>
<tr><td colspan="3">ALPHA ORDER</td><td colspan="3">RANK ORDER</td></tr>
<tr><td>RANK</td><td>STATE</td><td>PERCENT</td><td>RANK</td><td>STATE</td><td>PERCENT</td></tr>
<tr><td>12</td><td>Alabama</td><td>32.0</td><td>1</td><td>South Carolina</td><td>35.8</td></tr>
<tr><td>33</td><td>Alaska</td><td>25.9</td><td>2</td><td>New Mexico</td><td>35.5</td></tr>
<tr><td>40</td><td>Arizona</td><td>24.3</td><td>2</td><td>Texas</td><td>35.5</td></tr>
<tr><td>22</td><td>Arkansas</td><td>29.1</td><td>4</td><td>Idaho</td><td>35.3</td></tr>
<tr><td>38</td><td>California</td><td>24.6</td><td>5</td><td>Washington</td><td>33.9</td></tr>
<tr><td>29</td><td>Colorado</td><td>26.8</td><td>6</td><td>West Virginia</td><td>33.1</td></tr>
<tr><td>47</td><td>Connecticut</td><td>19.5</td><td>7</td><td>South Dakota</td><td>32.6</td></tr>
<tr><td>10</td><td>Delaware</td><td>32.2</td><td>8</td><td>Mississippi</td><td>32.5</td></tr>
<tr><td>26</td><td>Florida</td><td>27.3</td><td>9</td><td>Indiana</td><td>32.3</td></tr>
<tr><td>21</td><td>Georgia</td><td>30.2</td><td>10</td><td>Delaware</td><td>32.2</td></tr>
<tr><td>28</td><td>Hawaii</td><td>27.2</td><td>10</td><td>North Carolina</td><td>32.2</td></tr>
<tr><td>4</td><td>Idaho</td><td>35.3</td><td>12</td><td>Alabama</td><td>32.0</td></tr>
<tr><td>32</td><td>Illinois</td><td>26.0</td><td>13</td><td>Montana</td><td>31.7</td></tr>
<tr><td>9</td><td>Indiana</td><td>32.3</td><td>14</td><td>Utah</td><td>31.5</td></tr>
<tr><td>48</td><td>Iowa</td><td>18.1</td><td>15</td><td>Kentucky</td><td>31.4</td></tr>
<tr><td>37</td><td>Kansas</td><td>24.7</td><td>15</td><td>New Hampshire</td><td>31.4</td></tr>
<tr><td>15</td><td>Kentucky</td><td>31.4</td><td>15</td><td>Pennsylvania</td><td>31.4</td></tr>
<tr><td>24</td><td>Louisiana</td><td>28.7</td><td>18</td><td>New Jersey</td><td>31.2</td></tr>
<tr><td>44</td><td>Maine</td><td>23.0</td><td>19</td><td>Tennessee</td><td>30.8</td></tr>
<tr><td>26</td><td>Maryland</td><td>27.3</td><td>20</td><td>Nevada</td><td>30.6</td></tr>
<tr><td>44</td><td>Massachusetts</td><td>23.0</td><td>21</td><td>Georgia</td><td>30.2</td></tr>
<tr><td>42</td><td>Michigan</td><td>23.3</td><td>22</td><td>Arkansas</td><td>29.1</td></tr>
<tr><td>50</td><td>Minnesota</td><td>17.1</td><td>22</td><td>Oregon</td><td>29.1</td></tr>
<tr><td>8</td><td>Mississippi</td><td>32.5</td><td>24</td><td>Louisiana</td><td>28.7</td></tr>
<tr><td>25</td><td>Missouri</td><td>27.8</td><td>25</td><td>Missouri</td><td>27.8</td></tr>
<tr><td>13</td><td>Montana</td><td>31.7</td><td>26</td><td>Florida</td><td>27.3</td></tr>
<tr><td>31</td><td>Nebraska</td><td>26.2</td><td>26</td><td>Maryland</td><td>27.3</td></tr>
<tr><td>20</td><td>Nevada</td><td>30.6</td><td>28</td><td>Hawaii</td><td>27.2</td></tr>
<tr><td>15</td><td>New Hampshire</td><td>31.4</td><td>29</td><td>Colorado</td><td>26.8</td></tr>
<tr><td>18</td><td>New Jersey</td><td>31.2</td><td>30</td><td>Wisconsin</td><td>26.5</td></tr>
<tr><td>2</td><td>New Mexico</td><td>35.5</td><td>31</td><td>Nebraska</td><td>26.2</td></tr>
<tr><td>43</td><td>New York</td><td>23.1</td><td>32</td><td>Illinois</td><td>26.0</td></tr>
<tr><td>10</td><td>North Carolina</td><td>32.2</td><td>33</td><td>Alaska</td><td>25.9</td></tr>
<tr><td>33</td><td>North Dakota</td><td>25.9</td><td>33</td><td>North Dakota</td><td>25.9</td></tr>
<tr><td>36</td><td>Ohio</td><td>25.3</td><td>35</td><td>Vermont</td><td>25.7</td></tr>
<tr><td>39</td><td>Oklahoma</td><td>24.5</td><td>36</td><td>Ohio</td><td>25.3</td></tr>
<tr><td>22</td><td>Oregon</td><td>29.1</td><td>37</td><td>Kansas</td><td>24.7</td></tr>
<tr><td>15</td><td>Pennsylvania</td><td>31.4</td><td>38</td><td>California</td><td>24.6</td></tr>
<tr><td>46</td><td>Rhode Island</td><td>20.0</td><td>39</td><td>Oklahoma</td><td>24.5</td></tr>
<tr><td>1</td><td>South Carolina</td><td>35.8</td><td>40</td><td>Arizona</td><td>24.3</td></tr>
<tr><td>7</td><td>South Dakota</td><td>32.6</td><td>41</td><td>Virginia</td><td>24.2</td></tr>
<tr><td>19</td><td>Tennessee</td><td>30.8</td><td>42</td><td>Michigan</td><td>23.3</td></tr>
<tr><td>2</td><td>Texas</td><td>35.5</td><td>43</td><td>New York</td><td>23.1</td></tr>
<tr><td>14</td><td>Utah</td><td>31.5</td><td>44</td><td>Maine</td><td>23.0</td></tr>
<tr><td>35</td><td>Vermont</td><td>25.7</td><td>44</td><td>Massachusetts</td><td>23.0</td></tr>
<tr><td>41</td><td>Virginia</td><td>24.2</td><td>46</td><td>Rhode Island</td><td>20.0</td></tr>
<tr><td>5</td><td>Washington</td><td>33.9</td><td>47</td><td>Connecticut</td><td>19.5</td></tr>
<tr><td>6</td><td>West Virginia</td><td>33.1</td><td>48</td><td>Iowa</td><td>18.1</td></tr>
<tr><td>30</td><td>Wisconsin</td><td>26.5</td><td>48</td><td>Wyoming</td><td>18.1</td></tr>
<tr><td>48</td><td>Wyoming</td><td>18.1</td><td>50</td><td>Minnesota</td><td>17.1</td></tr>
<tr><td></td><td></td><td></td><td></td><td>District of Columbia</td><td>22.5</td></tr>
</table>

Source: Morgan Quitno Press using data from U.S. Dept of Health & Human Services, Health Care Financing Admin.
"State Health Expenditure Accounts" (Health Care Financing Review, Fall 1995, Volume 17, Number 1)
*By state of provider.

Percent Change in Per Capita Expenditures for Hospital Care: 1990 to 1993

National Percent Change = 22.9% Increase*

<table>
<tr><td colspan="3"><u>ALPHA ORDER</u></td><td colspan="3"><u>RANK ORDER</u></td></tr>
<tr><th>RANK</th><th>STATE</th><th>PERCENT CHANGE</th><th>RANK</th><th>STATE</th><th>PERCENT CHANGE</th></tr>
<tr><td>10</td><td>Alabama</td><td>27.6</td><td>1</td><td>West Virginia</td><td>31.2</td></tr>
<tr><td>46</td><td>Alaska</td><td>15.7</td><td>2</td><td>South Carolina</td><td>30.5</td></tr>
<tr><td>47</td><td>Arizona</td><td>15.5</td><td>3</td><td>New Hampshire</td><td>29.8</td></tr>
<tr><td>17</td><td>Arkansas</td><td>25.2</td><td>4</td><td>Pennsylvania</td><td>29.7</td></tr>
<tr><td>42</td><td>California</td><td>18.8</td><td>5</td><td>Mississippi</td><td>29.3</td></tr>
<tr><td>44</td><td>Colorado</td><td>17.1</td><td>6</td><td>New Jersey</td><td>29.1</td></tr>
<tr><td>41</td><td>Connecticut</td><td>19.8</td><td>7</td><td>South Dakota</td><td>28.7</td></tr>
<tr><td>16</td><td>Delaware</td><td>25.8</td><td>8</td><td>Indiana</td><td>28.5</td></tr>
<tr><td>40</td><td>Florida</td><td>19.9</td><td>9</td><td>Kentucky</td><td>27.7</td></tr>
<tr><td>30</td><td>Georgia</td><td>22.2</td><td>10</td><td>Alabama</td><td>27.6</td></tr>
<tr><td>38</td><td>Hawaii</td><td>20.8</td><td>11</td><td>Texas</td><td>27.5</td></tr>
<tr><td>22</td><td>Idaho</td><td>23.8</td><td>12</td><td>New Mexico</td><td>27.1</td></tr>
<tr><td>24</td><td>Illinois</td><td>23.1</td><td>13</td><td>Louisiana</td><td>26.7</td></tr>
<tr><td>8</td><td>Indiana</td><td>28.5</td><td>14</td><td>North Dakota</td><td>26.4</td></tr>
<tr><td>45</td><td>Iowa</td><td>16.1</td><td>15</td><td>North Carolina</td><td>26.1</td></tr>
<tr><td>31</td><td>Kansas</td><td>22.1</td><td>16</td><td>Delaware</td><td>25.8</td></tr>
<tr><td>9</td><td>Kentucky</td><td>27.7</td><td>17</td><td>Arkansas</td><td>25.2</td></tr>
<tr><td>13</td><td>Louisiana</td><td>26.7</td><td>17</td><td>Tennessee</td><td>25.2</td></tr>
<tr><td>32</td><td>Maine</td><td>22.0</td><td>19</td><td>Montana</td><td>25.1</td></tr>
<tr><td>25</td><td>Maryland</td><td>22.9</td><td>20</td><td>Missouri</td><td>25.0</td></tr>
<tr><td>25</td><td>Massachusetts</td><td>22.9</td><td>21</td><td>Washington</td><td>24.1</td></tr>
<tr><td>36</td><td>Michigan</td><td>21.1</td><td>22</td><td>Idaho</td><td>23.8</td></tr>
<tr><td>49</td><td>Minnesota</td><td>13.2</td><td>23</td><td>Nebraska</td><td>23.4</td></tr>
<tr><td>5</td><td>Mississippi</td><td>29.3</td><td>24</td><td>Illinois</td><td>23.1</td></tr>
<tr><td>20</td><td>Missouri</td><td>25.0</td><td>25</td><td>Maryland</td><td>22.9</td></tr>
<tr><td>19</td><td>Montana</td><td>25.1</td><td>25</td><td>Massachusetts</td><td>22.9</td></tr>
<tr><td>23</td><td>Nebraska</td><td>23.4</td><td>25</td><td>Vermont</td><td>22.9</td></tr>
<tr><td>49</td><td>Nevada</td><td>13.2</td><td>28</td><td>Ohio</td><td>22.8</td></tr>
<tr><td>3</td><td>New Hampshire</td><td>29.8</td><td>29</td><td>Wisconsin</td><td>22.7</td></tr>
<tr><td>6</td><td>New Jersey</td><td>29.1</td><td>30</td><td>Georgia</td><td>22.2</td></tr>
<tr><td>12</td><td>New Mexico</td><td>27.1</td><td>31</td><td>Kansas</td><td>22.1</td></tr>
<tr><td>32</td><td>New York</td><td>22.0</td><td>32</td><td>Maine</td><td>22.0</td></tr>
<tr><td>15</td><td>North Carolina</td><td>26.1</td><td>32</td><td>New York</td><td>22.0</td></tr>
<tr><td>14</td><td>North Dakota</td><td>26.4</td><td>34</td><td>Utah</td><td>21.8</td></tr>
<tr><td>28</td><td>Ohio</td><td>22.8</td><td>35</td><td>Oklahoma</td><td>21.2</td></tr>
<tr><td>35</td><td>Oklahoma</td><td>21.2</td><td>36</td><td>Michigan</td><td>21.1</td></tr>
<tr><td>37</td><td>Oregon</td><td>20.9</td><td>37</td><td>Oregon</td><td>20.9</td></tr>
<tr><td>4</td><td>Pennsylvania</td><td>29.7</td><td>38</td><td>Hawaii</td><td>20.8</td></tr>
<tr><td>39</td><td>Rhode Island</td><td>20.4</td><td>39</td><td>Rhode Island</td><td>20.4</td></tr>
<tr><td>2</td><td>South Carolina</td><td>30.5</td><td>40</td><td>Florida</td><td>19.9</td></tr>
<tr><td>7</td><td>South Dakota</td><td>28.7</td><td>41</td><td>Connecticut</td><td>19.8</td></tr>
<tr><td>17</td><td>Tennessee</td><td>25.2</td><td>42</td><td>California</td><td>18.8</td></tr>
<tr><td>11</td><td>Texas</td><td>27.5</td><td>43</td><td>Virginia</td><td>18.7</td></tr>
<tr><td>34</td><td>Utah</td><td>21.8</td><td>44</td><td>Colorado</td><td>17.1</td></tr>
<tr><td>25</td><td>Vermont</td><td>22.9</td><td>45</td><td>Iowa</td><td>16.1</td></tr>
<tr><td>43</td><td>Virginia</td><td>18.7</td><td>46</td><td>Alaska</td><td>15.7</td></tr>
<tr><td>21</td><td>Washington</td><td>24.1</td><td>47</td><td>Arizona</td><td>15.5</td></tr>
<tr><td>1</td><td>West Virginia</td><td>31.2</td><td>48</td><td>Wyoming</td><td>14.0</td></tr>
<tr><td>29</td><td>Wisconsin</td><td>22.7</td><td>49</td><td>Minnesota</td><td>13.2</td></tr>
<tr><td>48</td><td>Wyoming</td><td>14.0</td><td>49</td><td>Nevada</td><td>13.2</td></tr>
<tr><td></td><td></td><td></td><td></td><td>District of Columbia</td><td>28.6</td></tr>
</table>

Source: Morgan Quitno Press using data from U.S. Dept of Health & Human Services, Health Care Financing Admin.
"State Health Expenditure Accounts" (Health Care Financing Review, Fall 1995, Volume 17, Number 1)
*By state of provider.

Average Annual Change in Expenditures for Hospital Care: 1980 to 1993

National Percent = 9.4% Average Annual Growth*

ALPHA ORDER				RANK ORDER		
RANK	STATE	PERCENT		RANK	STATE	PERCENT
23	Alabama	9.8		1	New Hampshire	12.2
19	Alaska	10.2		2	South Carolina	12.0
15	Arizona	10.5		3	Hawaii	11.5
13	Arkansas	10.6		3	New Mexico	11.5
33	California	8.8		5	Georgia	11.4
27	Colorado	9.5		6	North Carolina	11.3
31	Connecticut	9.2		7	Florida	11.1
16	Delaware	10.4		7	Texas	11.1
7	Florida	11.1		9	Utah	11.0
5	Georgia	11.4		10	Washington	10.9
3	Hawaii	11.5		11	Idaho	10.7
11	Idaho	10.7		11	New Jersey	10.7
50	Illinois	7.4		13	Arkansas	10.6
26	Indiana	9.7		13	Kentucky	10.6
47	Iowa	7.8		15	Arizona	10.5
47	Kansas	7.8		16	Delaware	10.4
13	Kentucky	10.6		17	Nevada	10.3
20	Louisiana	10.0		17	Tennessee	10.3
33	Maine	8.8		19	Alaska	10.2
37	Maryland	8.6		20	Louisiana	10.0
45	Massachusetts	8.1		21	Montana	9.9
49	Michigan	7.7		21	Virginia	9.9
44	Minnesota	8.2		23	Alabama	9.8
23	Mississippi	9.8		23	Mississippi	9.8
32	Missouri	8.9		23	South Dakota	9.8
21	Montana	9.9		26	Indiana	9.7
33	Nebraska	8.8		27	Colorado	9.5
17	Nevada	10.3		27	Pennsylvania	9.5
1	New Hampshire	12.2		27	Vermont	9.5
11	New Jersey	10.7		30	Oregon	9.4
3	New Mexico	11.5		31	Connecticut	9.2
37	New York	8.6		32	Missouri	8.9
6	North Carolina	11.3		33	California	8.8
39	North Dakota	8.5		33	Maine	8.8
33	Ohio	8.8		33	Nebraska	8.8
39	Oklahoma	8.5		33	Ohio	8.8
30	Oregon	9.4		37	Maryland	8.6
27	Pennsylvania	9.5		37	New York	8.6
45	Rhode Island	8.1		39	North Dakota	8.5
2	South Carolina	12.0		39	Oklahoma	8.5
23	South Dakota	9.8		39	Wyoming	8.5
17	Tennessee	10.3		42	West Virginia	8.4
7	Texas	11.1		42	Wisconsin	8.4
9	Utah	11.0		44	Minnesota	8.2
27	Vermont	9.5		45	Massachusetts	8.1
21	Virginia	9.9		45	Rhode Island	8.1
10	Washington	10.9		47	Iowa	7.8
42	West Virginia	8.4		47	Kansas	7.8
42	Wisconsin	8.4		49	Michigan	7.7
39	Wyoming	8.5		50	Illinois	7.4
					District of Columbia	8.4

Source: U.S. Department of Health and Human Services, Health Care Financing Administration
    "State Health Expenditure Accounts" (Health Care Financing Review, Fall 1995, Volume 17, Number 1)
*By state of provider.

Average Annual Change in Per Capita Expenditures
For Hospital Care: 1980 to 1993
National Percent = 8.3% Average Annual Increase*

ALPHA ORDER

RANK	STATE	PERCENT
18	Alabama	9.1
48	Alaska	6.9
43	Arizona	7.4
5	Arkansas	10.0
49	California	6.5
39	Colorado	7.7
24	Connecticut	8.7
19	Delaware	9.0
32	Florida	8.2
10	Georgia	9.4
6	Hawaii	9.8
14	Idaho	9.3
44	Illinois	7.2
14	Indiana	9.3
35	Iowa	8.0
44	Kansas	7.2
3	Kentucky	10.2
8	Louisiana	9.7
35	Maine	8.0
44	Maryland	7.2
39	Massachusetts	7.7
42	Michigan	7.5
44	Minnesota	7.2
14	Mississippi	9.3
27	Missouri	8.4
14	Montana	9.3
27	Nebraska	8.4
50	Nevada	5.6
2	New Hampshire	10.4
4	New Jersey	10.1
9	New Mexico	9.6
31	New York	8.3
6	North Carolina	9.8
24	North Dakota	8.7
26	Ohio	8.6
37	Oklahoma	7.8
32	Oregon	8.2
10	Pennsylvania	9.4
41	Rhode Island	7.6
1	South Carolina	10.6
10	South Dakota	9.4
10	Tennessee	9.4
19	Texas	9.0
21	Utah	8.9
27	Vermont	8.4
32	Virginia	8.2
23	Washington	8.8
21	West Virginia	8.9
37	Wisconsin	7.8
27	Wyoming	8.4

RANK ORDER

RANK	STATE	PERCENT
1	South Carolina	10.6
2	New Hampshire	10.4
3	Kentucky	10.2
4	New Jersey	10.1
5	Arkansas	10.0
6	Hawaii	9.8
6	North Carolina	9.8
8	Louisiana	9.7
9	New Mexico	9.6
10	Georgia	9.4
10	Pennsylvania	9.4
10	South Dakota	9.4
10	Tennessee	9.4
14	Idaho	9.3
14	Indiana	9.3
14	Mississippi	9.3
14	Montana	9.3
18	Alabama	9.1
19	Delaware	9.0
19	Texas	9.0
21	Utah	8.9
21	West Virginia	8.9
23	Washington	8.8
24	Connecticut	8.7
24	North Dakota	8.7
26	Ohio	8.6
27	Missouri	8.4
27	Nebraska	8.4
27	Vermont	8.4
27	Wyoming	8.4
31	New York	8.3
32	Florida	8.2
32	Oregon	8.2
32	Virginia	8.2
35	Iowa	8.0
35	Maine	8.0
37	Oklahoma	7.8
37	Wisconsin	7.8
39	Colorado	7.7
39	Massachusetts	7.7
41	Rhode Island	7.6
42	Michigan	7.5
43	Arizona	7.4
44	Illinois	7.2
44	Kansas	7.2
44	Maryland	7.2
44	Minnesota	7.2
48	Alaska	6.9
49	California	6.5
50	Nevada	5.6

| | District of Columbia | 9.3 |

Source: Morgan Quitno Press using data from U.S. Dept of Health & Human Services, Health Care Financing Admin.
"State Health Expenditure Accounts" (Health Care Financing Review, Fall 1995, Volume 17, Number 1)
*By state of provider.

Central Lakes College
Brainerd Campus
Brainerd, MN 56401

Expenditures for Physician Services in 1993

National Total = $171,226,000,000*

ALPHA ORDER

RANK	STATE	EXPENDITURES	% of USA
22	Alabama	$2,631,000,000	1.54%
48	Alaska	301,000,000	0.18%
21	Arizona	2,799,000,000	1.63%
32	Arkansas	1,244,000,000	0.73%
1	California	28,981,000,000	16.93%
25	Colorado	2,452,000,000	1.43%
23	Connecticut	2,587,000,000	1.51%
44	Delaware	466,000,000	0.27%
4	Florida	10,498,000,000	6.13%
10	Georgia	4,543,000,000	2.65%
39	Hawaii	771,000,000	0.45%
43	Idaho	486,000,000	0.28%
7	Illinois	6,970,000,000	4.07%
18	Indiana	3,263,000,000	1.91%
31	Iowa	1,376,000,000	0.80%
30	Kansas	1,425,000,000	0.83%
26	Kentucky	2,038,000,000	1.19%
24	Louisiana	2,537,000,000	1.48%
41	Maine	601,000,000	0.35%
15	Maryland	3,704,000,000	2.16%
11	Massachusetts	4,442,000,000	2.59%
9	Michigan	5,562,000,000	3.25%
16	Minnesota	3,617,000,000	2.11%
33	Mississippi	1,107,000,000	0.65%
20	Missouri	2,958,000,000	1.73%
46	Montana	392,000,000	0.23%
37	Nebraska	825,000,000	0.48%
34	Nevada	1,029,000,000	0.60%
38	New Hampshire	780,000,000	0.46%
8	New Jersey	5,776,000,000	3.37%
40	New Mexico	716,000,000	0.42%
2	New York	12,003,000,000	7.01%
14	North Carolina	3,717,000,000	2.17%
45	North Dakota	445,000,000	0.26%
6	Ohio	7,118,000,000	4.16%
29	Oklahoma	1,640,000,000	0.96%
27	Oregon	1,904,000,000	1.11%
5	Pennsylvania	7,460,000,000	4.36%
42	Rhode Island	575,000,000	0.34%
28	South Carolina	1,685,000,000	0.98%
47	South Dakota	342,000,000	0.20%
19	Tennessee	3,137,000,000	1.83%
3	Texas	10,526,000,000	6.15%
36	Utah	864,000,000	0.50%
49	Vermont	265,000,000	0.15%
12	Virginia	3,769,000,000	2.20%
13	Washington	3,720,000,000	2.17%
35	West Virginia	988,000,000	0.58%
17	Wisconsin	3,362,000,000	1.96%
50	Wyoming	160,000,000	0.09%

RANK ORDER

RANK	STATE	EXPENDITURES	% of USA
1	California	$28,981,000,000	16.93%
2	New York	12,003,000,000	7.01%
3	Texas	10,526,000,000	6.15%
4	Florida	10,498,000,000	6.13%
5	Pennsylvania	7,460,000,000	4.36%
6	Ohio	7,118,000,000	4.16%
7	Illinois	6,970,000,000	4.07%
8	New Jersey	5,776,000,000	3.37%
9	Michigan	5,562,000,000	3.25%
10	Georgia	4,543,000,000	2.65%
11	Massachusetts	4,442,000,000	2.59%
12	Virginia	3,769,000,000	2.20%
13	Washington	3,720,000,000	2.17%
14	North Carolina	3,717,000,000	2.17%
15	Maryland	3,704,000,000	2.16%
16	Minnesota	3,617,000,000	2.11%
17	Wisconsin	3,362,000,000	1.96%
18	Indiana	3,263,000,000	1.91%
19	Tennessee	3,137,000,000	1.83%
20	Missouri	2,958,000,000	1.73%
21	Arizona	2,799,000,000	1.63%
22	Alabama	2,631,000,000	1.54%
23	Connecticut	2,587,000,000	1.51%
24	Louisiana	2,537,000,000	1.48%
25	Colorado	2,452,000,000	1.43%
26	Kentucky	2,038,000,000	1.19%
27	Oregon	1,904,000,000	1.11%
28	South Carolina	1,685,000,000	0.98%
29	Oklahoma	1,640,000,000	0.96%
30	Kansas	1,425,000,000	0.83%
31	Iowa	1,376,000,000	0.80%
32	Arkansas	1,244,000,000	0.73%
33	Mississippi	1,107,000,000	0.65%
34	Nevada	1,029,000,000	0.60%
35	West Virginia	988,000,000	0.58%
36	Utah	864,000,000	0.50%
37	Nebraska	825,000,000	0.48%
38	New Hampshire	780,000,000	0.46%
39	Hawaii	771,000,000	0.45%
40	New Mexico	716,000,000	0.42%
41	Maine	601,000,000	0.35%
42	Rhode Island	575,000,000	0.34%
43	Idaho	486,000,000	0.28%
44	Delaware	466,000,000	0.27%
45	North Dakota	445,000,000	0.26%
46	Montana	392,000,000	0.23%
47	South Dakota	342,000,000	0.20%
48	Alaska	301,000,000	0.18%
49	Vermont	265,000,000	0.15%
50	Wyoming	160,000,000	0.09%
	District of Columbia	672,000,000	0.39%

Source: U.S. Department of Health and Human Services, Health Care Financing Administration
    "State Health Expenditure Accounts" (Health Care Financing Review, Fall 1995, Volume 17, Number 1)
*By state of provider.

Percent of Total Personal Health Care Expenditures
Spent on Physician Services in 1993
National Percent = 22.0%*

ALPHA ORDER

RANK ORDER

RANK	STATE	PERCENT		RANK	STATE	PERCENT
17	Alabama	21.8		1	California	30.8
34	Alaska	19.1		2	Nevada	27.5
3	Arizona	26.3		3	Arizona	26.3
26	Arkansas	20.4		4	Minnesota	25.5
1	California	30.8		5	Washington	24.6
6	Colorado	24.4		6	Colorado	24.4
20	Connecticut	21.2		6	Maryland	24.4
23	Delaware	20.6		8	Oregon	23.8
9	Florida	23.4		9	Florida	23.4
11	Georgia	22.6		10	Wisconsin	23.2
15	Hawaii	22.1		11	Georgia	22.6
18	Idaho	21.3		11	New Hampshire	22.6
29	Illinois	20.1		11	Virginia	22.6
30	Indiana	19.9		14	New Jersey	22.4
38	Iowa	18.7		15	Hawaii	22.1
23	Kansas	20.6		16	North Dakota	22.0
31	Kentucky	19.6		17	Alabama	21.8
32	Louisiana	19.5		18	Idaho	21.3
47	Maine	17.5		18	Ohio	21.3
6	Maryland	24.4		20	Connecticut	21.2
35	Massachusetts	19.0		21	Texas	21.1
25	Michigan	20.5		22	Utah	21.0
4	Minnesota	25.5		23	Delaware	20.6
44	Mississippi	17.9		23	Kansas	20.6
41	Missouri	18.5		25	Michigan	20.5
40	Montana	18.6		26	Arkansas	20.4
37	Nebraska	18.8		26	North Carolina	20.4
2	Nevada	27.5		26	Oklahoma	20.4
11	New Hampshire	22.6		29	Illinois	20.1
14	New Jersey	22.4		30	Indiana	19.9
41	New Mexico	18.5		31	Kentucky	19.6
44	New York	17.9		32	Louisiana	19.5
26	North Carolina	20.4		33	Tennessee	19.4
16	North Dakota	22.0		34	Alaska	19.1
18	Ohio	21.3		35	Massachusetts	19.0
26	Oklahoma	20.4		35	West Virginia	19.0
8	Oregon	23.8		37	Nebraska	18.8
43	Pennsylvania	18.0		38	Iowa	18.7
49	Rhode Island	16.8		38	South Carolina	18.7
38	South Carolina	18.7		40	Montana	18.6
47	South Dakota	17.5		41	Missouri	18.5
33	Tennessee	19.4		41	New Mexico	18.5
21	Texas	21.1		43	Pennsylvania	18.0
22	Utah	21.0		44	Mississippi	17.9
46	Vermont	17.7		44	New York	17.9
11	Virginia	22.6		46	Vermont	17.7
5	Washington	24.6		47	Maine	17.5
35	West Virginia	19.0		47	South Dakota	17.5
10	Wisconsin	23.2		49	Rhode Island	16.8
50	Wyoming	16.0		50	Wyoming	16.0
					District of Columbia	15.7

Source: Morgan Quitno Press using data from U.S. Dept of Health & Human Services, Health Care Financing Admin.
"State Health Expenditure Accounts" (Health Care Financing Review, Fall 1995, Volume 17, Number 1)
*By state of provider.

Per Capita Expenditures for Physician Services in 1993

National Per Capita = $664*

ALPHA ORDER				RANK ORDER		
RANK	STATE	PER CAPITA		RANK	STATE	PER CAPITA
20	Alabama	$629		1	California	$928
39	Alaska	503		2	Minnesota	800
9	Arizona	710		3	Connecticut	789
36	Arkansas	513		4	Florida	765
1	California	928		5	Maryland	748
13	Colorado	687		6	Nevada	743
3	Connecticut	789		7	Massachusetts	738
14	Delaware	667		8	New Jersey	735
4	Florida	765		9	Arizona	710
18	Georgia	658		10	Washington	708
16	Hawaii	661		11	North Dakota	699
48	Idaho	441		12	New Hampshire	695
24	Illinois	596		13	Colorado	687
30	Indiana	572		14	Delaware	667
40	Iowa	488		14	Wisconsin	667
32	Kansas	563		16	Hawaii	661
34	Kentucky	537		16	New York	661
25	Louisiana	592		18	Georgia	658
41	Maine	485		19	Ohio	644
5	Maryland	748		20	Alabama	629
7	Massachusetts	738		21	Oregon	627
26	Michigan	588		22	Pennsylvania	620
2	Minnesota	800		23	Tennessee	616
49	Mississippi	419		24	Illinois	596
31	Missouri	565		25	Louisiana	592
43	Montana	466		26	Michigan	588
37	Nebraska	511		27	Texas	583
6	Nevada	743		28	Virginia	582
12	New Hampshire	695		29	Rhode Island	576
8	New Jersey	735		30	Indiana	572
47	New Mexico	443		31	Missouri	565
16	New York	661		32	Kansas	563
35	North Carolina	535		33	West Virginia	543
11	North Dakota	699		34	Kentucky	537
19	Ohio	644		35	North Carolina	535
38	Oklahoma	507		36	Arkansas	513
21	Oregon	627		37	Nebraska	511
22	Pennsylvania	620		38	Oklahoma	507
29	Rhode Island	576		39	Alaska	503
44	South Carolina	465		40	Iowa	488
42	South Dakota	477		41	Maine	485
23	Tennessee	616		42	South Dakota	477
27	Texas	583		43	Montana	466
44	Utah	465		44	South Carolina	465
46	Vermont	460		44	Utah	465
28	Virginia	582		46	Vermont	460
10	Washington	708		47	New Mexico	443
33	West Virginia	543		48	Idaho	441
14	Wisconsin	667		49	Mississippi	419
50	Wyoming	340		50	Wyoming	340
					District of Columbia**	1,163

Source: Morgan Quitno Press using data from U.S. Dept of Health & Human Services, Health Care Financing Admin.
   "State Health Expenditure Accounts" (Health Care Financing Review, Fall 1995, Volume 17, Number 1)
*By state of provider.
**The District of Columbia's per capita is greatly affected by residents of Maryland and Virginia receiving services.

Percent Change in Expenditures for Physician Services: 1990 to 1993

National Percent Change = 21.9% Increase*

ALPHA ORDER				RANK ORDER		
RANK	STATE	PERCENT CHANGE		RANK	STATE	PERCENT CHANGE
42	Alabama	17.1		1	New Hampshire	58.9
44	Alaska	16.7		2	Washington	31.3
46	Arizona	12.0		3	Wisconsin	31.1
49	Arkansas	9.7		4	Idaho	29.9
6	California	29.6		5	Colorado	29.7
5	Colorado	29.7		6	California	29.6
37	Connecticut	18.4		7	New Jersey	27.8
19	Delaware	23.6		8	South Carolina	27.2
48	Florida	11.2		9	Nevada	26.7
15	Georgia	24.6		10	Montana	26.0
20	Hawaii	22.6		11	Maine	25.2
4	Idaho	29.9		12	Maryland	24.8
34	Illinois	18.9		12	South Dakota	24.8
23	Indiana	21.8		14	New Mexico	24.7
25	Iowa	20.5		15	Georgia	24.6
40	Kansas	17.7		16	Kentucky	24.3
16	Kentucky	24.3		17	New York	23.8
30	Louisiana	19.2		18	North Carolina	23.7
11	Maine	25.2		19	Delaware	23.6
12	Maryland	24.8		20	Hawaii	22.6
38	Massachusetts	18.0		21	Minnesota	22.3
30	Michigan	19.2		22	Tennessee	22.1
21	Minnesota	22.3		23	Indiana	21.8
28	Mississippi	19.7		24	North Dakota	20.9
33	Missouri	19.0		25	Iowa	20.5
10	Montana	26.0		26	Nebraska	19.9
26	Nebraska	19.9		26	Vermont	19.9
9	Nevada	26.7		28	Mississippi	19.7
1	New Hampshire	58.9		29	Pennsylvania	19.3
7	New Jersey	27.8		30	Louisiana	19.2
14	New Mexico	24.7		30	Michigan	19.2
17	New York	23.8		30	Oregon	19.2
18	North Carolina	23.7		33	Missouri	19.0
24	North Dakota	20.9		34	Illinois	18.9
40	Ohio	17.7		35	Virginia	18.8
36	Oklahoma	18.7		36	Oklahoma	18.7
30	Oregon	19.2		37	Connecticut	18.4
29	Pennsylvania	19.3		38	Massachusetts	18.0
47	Rhode Island	11.9		38	Texas	18.0
8	South Carolina	27.2		40	Kansas	17.7
12	South Dakota	24.8		40	Ohio	17.7
22	Tennessee	22.1		42	Alabama	17.1
38	Texas	18.0		43	Utah	16.9
43	Utah	16.9		44	Alaska	16.7
26	Vermont	19.9		45	West Virginia	15.4
35	Virginia	18.8		46	Arizona	12.0
2	Washington	31.3		47	Rhode Island	11.9
45	West Virginia	15.4		48	Florida	11.2
3	Wisconsin	31.1		49	Arkansas	9.7
50	Wyoming	9.6		50	Wyoming	9.6
					District of Columbia	2.3

Source: Morgan Quitno Press using data from U.S. Dept of Health & Human Services, Health Care Financing Admin.
"State Health Expenditure Accounts" (Health Care Financing Review, Fall 1995, Volume 17, Number 1)
*By state of provider.

Percent Change in Per Capita Expenditures for Physician Services: 1990 to 1993

National Percent Change = 17.5% Increase*

ALPHA ORDER				RANK ORDER		
RANK	STATE	PERCENT CHANGE		RANK	STATE	PERCENT CHANGE
40	Alabama	13.1		1	New Hampshire	56.9
46	Alaska	7.2		2	Wisconsin	27.3
50	Arizona	4.1		3	New Jersey	25.6
47	Arkansas	6.4		4	Maine	24.0
5	California	23.4		5	California	23.4
14	Colorado	19.7		6	New York	22.6
17	Connecticut	18.6		7	South Carolina	22.4
23	Delaware	17.8		8	Washington	21.6
49	Florida	4.8		9	North Dakota	21.4
28	Georgia	16.9		10	South Dakota	21.1
32	Hawaii	16.4		11	Kentucky	20.7
15	Idaho	18.9		12	Maryland	20.5
34	Illinois	16.2		13	Montana	19.8
18	Indiana	18.4		14	Colorado	19.7
16	Iowa	18.7		15	Idaho	18.9
37	Kansas	15.1		16	Iowa	18.7
11	Kentucky	20.7		17	Connecticut	18.6
24	Louisiana	17.2		18	Indiana	18.4
4	Maine	24.0		19	Minnesota	18.3
12	Maryland	20.5		20	North Carolina	18.1
21	Massachusetts	17.9		21	Massachusetts	17.9
26	Michigan	17.1		21	Pennsylvania	17.9
19	Minnesota	18.3		23	Delaware	17.8
31	Mississippi	16.7		24	Louisiana	17.2
33	Missouri	16.3		24	Nebraska	17.2
13	Montana	19.8		26	Michigan	17.1
24	Nebraska	17.2		27	Vermont	17.0
44	Nevada	9.9		28	Georgia	16.9
1	New Hampshire	56.9		28	New Mexico	16.9
3	New Jersey	25.6		28	Tennessee	16.9
28	New Mexico	16.9		31	Mississippi	16.7
6	New York	22.6		32	Hawaii	16.4
20	North Carolina	18.1		33	Missouri	16.3
9	North Dakota	21.4		34	Illinois	16.2
36	Ohio	15.4		35	Oklahoma	15.5
35	Oklahoma	15.5		36	Ohio	15.4
42	Oregon	11.6		37	Kansas	15.1
21	Pennsylvania	17.9		38	West Virginia	13.8
41	Rhode Island	12.5		39	Virginia	13.5
7	South Carolina	22.4		40	Alabama	13.1
10	South Dakota	21.1		41	Rhode Island	12.5
28	Tennessee	16.9		42	Oregon	11.6
43	Texas	11.0		43	Texas	11.0
45	Utah	8.4		44	Nevada	9.9
27	Vermont	17.0		45	Utah	8.4
39	Virginia	13.5		46	Alaska	7.2
8	Washington	21.6		47	Arkansas	6.4
38	West Virginia	13.8		48	Wyoming	5.6
2	Wisconsin	27.3		49	Florida	4.8
48	Wyoming	5.6		50	Arizona	4.1
					District of Columbia	7.5

Source: Morgan Quitno Press using data from U.S. Dept of Health & Human Services, Health Care Financing Admin. "State Health Expenditure Accounts" (Health Care Financing Review, Fall 1995, Volume 17, Number 1)
*By state of provider.

Average Annual Change in Expenditures for Physician Services: 1980 to 1993

National Percent = 10.8% Average Annual Increase*

ALPHA ORDER				RANK ORDER		
RANK	STATE	PERCENT CHANGE		RANK	STATE	PERCENT CHANGE
14	Alabama	11.6		1	New Hampshire	14.8
41	Alaska	9.1		2	Nevada	13.1
5	Arizona	12.1		3	Georgia	12.5
36	Arkansas	9.7		4	Massachusetts	12.3
14	California	11.6		5	Arizona	12.1
16	Colorado	11.4		5	Connecticut	12.1
5	Connecticut	12.1		5	Maryland	12.1
20	Delaware	11.0		8	North Carolina	11.9
11	Florida	11.7		9	New Jersey	11.8
3	Georgia	12.5		9	Virginia	11.8
41	Hawaii	9.1		11	Florida	11.7
29	Idaho	10.1		11	Maine	11.7
38	Illinois	9.6		11	South Carolina	11.7
24	Indiana	10.5		14	Alabama	11.6
48	Iowa	8.3		14	California	11.6
41	Kansas	9.1		16	Colorado	11.4
25	Kentucky	10.4		16	Washington	11.4
32	Louisiana	9.9		18	New Mexico	11.1
11	Maine	11.7		18	Vermont	11.1
5	Maryland	12.1		20	Delaware	11.0
4	Massachusetts	12.3		21	Minnesota	10.9
49	Michigan	8.2		21	Pennsylvania	10.9
21	Minnesota	10.9		23	Tennessee	10.7
33	Mississippi	9.8		24	Indiana	10.5
33	Missouri	9.8		25	Kentucky	10.4
47	Montana	8.4		25	New York	10.4
45	Nebraska	8.8		27	Wisconsin	10.3
2	Nevada	13.1		28	Utah	10.2
1	New Hampshire	14.8		29	Idaho	10.1
9	New Jersey	11.8		29	Texas	10.1
18	New Mexico	11.1		31	Rhode Island	10.0
25	New York	10.4		32	Louisiana	9.9
8	North Carolina	11.9		33	Mississippi	9.8
39	North Dakota	9.4		33	Missouri	9.8
36	Ohio	9.7		33	South Dakota	9.8
44	Oklahoma	9.0		36	Arkansas	9.7
40	Oregon	9.3		36	Ohio	9.7
21	Pennsylvania	10.9		38	Illinois	9.6
31	Rhode Island	10.0		39	North Dakota	9.4
11	South Carolina	11.7		40	Oregon	9.3
33	South Dakota	9.8		41	Alaska	9.1
23	Tennessee	10.7		41	Hawaii	9.1
29	Texas	10.1		41	Kansas	9.1
28	Utah	10.2		44	Oklahoma	9.0
18	Vermont	11.1		45	Nebraska	8.8
9	Virginia	11.8		45	West Virginia	8.8
16	Washington	11.4		47	Montana	8.4
45	West Virginia	8.8		48	Iowa	8.3
27	Wisconsin	10.3		49	Michigan	8.2
50	Wyoming	7.3		50	Wyoming	7.3
					District of Columbia	8.4

Source: U.S. Department of Health and Human Services, Health Care Financing Administration
"State Health Expenditure Accounts" (Health Care Financing Review, Fall 1995, Volume 17, Number 1)
*By state of provider.

Average Annual Change in Per Capita Expenditures
For Physician Services: 1980 to 1993
National Percent = 9.7% Average Annual Increase*

ALPHA ORDER

RANK	STATE	PERCENT
5	Alabama	11.0
50	Alaska	5.8
35	Arizona	8.9
33	Arkansas	9.2
33	California	9.2
21	Colorado	9.6
3	Connecticut	11.6
21	Delaware	9.6
36	Florida	8.8
9	Georgia	10.4
48	Hawaii	7.5
36	Idaho	8.8
26	Illinois	9.4
12	Indiana	10.2
38	Iowa	8.6
39	Kansas	8.5
13	Kentucky	10.1
20	Louisiana	9.7
6	Maine	10.9
7	Maryland	10.8
2	Massachusetts	12.0
46	Michigan	8.0
16	Minnesota	10.0
26	Mississippi	9.4
31	Missouri	9.3
47	Montana	7.8
39	Nebraska	8.5
41	Nevada	8.4
1	New Hampshire	13.1
4	New Jersey	11.2
31	New Mexico	9.3
13	New York	10.1
9	North Carolina	10.4
21	North Dakota	9.6
25	Ohio	9.5
41	Oklahoma	8.4
43	Oregon	8.2
7	Pennsylvania	10.8
21	Rhode Island	9.6
9	South Carolina	10.4
26	South Dakota	9.4
18	Tennessee	9.8
45	Texas	8.1
43	Utah	8.2
16	Vermont	10.0
13	Virginia	10.1
26	Washington	9.4
26	West Virginia	9.4
18	Wisconsin	9.8
49	Wyoming	7.3

RANK ORDER

RANK	STATE	PERCENT
1	New Hampshire	13.1
2	Massachusetts	12.0
3	Connecticut	11.6
4	New Jersey	11.2
5	Alabama	11.0
6	Maine	10.9
7	Maryland	10.8
7	Pennsylvania	10.8
9	Georgia	10.4
9	North Carolina	10.4
9	South Carolina	10.4
12	Indiana	10.2
13	Kentucky	10.1
13	New York	10.1
13	Virginia	10.1
16	Minnesota	10.0
16	Vermont	10.0
18	Tennessee	9.8
18	Wisconsin	9.8
20	Louisiana	9.7
21	Colorado	9.6
21	Delaware	9.6
21	North Dakota	9.6
21	Rhode Island	9.6
25	Ohio	9.5
26	Illinois	9.4
26	Mississippi	9.4
26	South Dakota	9.4
26	Washington	9.4
26	West Virginia	9.4
31	Missouri	9.3
31	New Mexico	9.3
33	Arkansas	9.2
33	California	9.2
35	Arizona	8.9
36	Florida	8.8
36	Idaho	8.8
38	Iowa	8.6
39	Kansas	8.5
39	Nebraska	8.5
41	Nevada	8.4
41	Oklahoma	8.4
43	Oregon	8.2
43	Utah	8.2
45	Texas	8.1
46	Michigan	8.0
47	Montana	7.8
48	Hawaii	7.5
49	Wyoming	7.3
50	Alaska	5.8

District of Columbia   9.2

Source: Morgan Quitno Press using data from U.S. Dept of Health & Human Services, Health Care Financing Admin.
"State Health Expenditure Accounts" (Health Care Financing Review, Fall 1995, Volume 17, Number 1)
*By state of provider.

Expenditures for Dental Service in 1993

National Total = $37,383,000,000*

ALPHA ORDER

RANK	STATE	EXPENDITURES	% of USA
25	Alabama	$456,000,000	1.22%
44	Alaska	124,000,000	0.33%
24	Arizona	551,000,000	1.47%
33	Arkansas	242,000,000	0.65%
1	California	5,664,000,000	15.15%
21	Colorado	605,000,000	1.62%
19	Connecticut	685,000,000	1.83%
45	Delaware	104,000,000	0.28%
4	Florida	2,029,000,000	5.43%
12	Georgia	898,000,000	2.40%
34	Hawaii	235,000,000	0.63%
41	Idaho	163,000,000	0.44%
6	Illinois	1,588,000,000	4.25%
18	Indiana	692,000,000	1.85%
30	Iowa	341,000,000	0.91%
31	Kansas	325,000,000	0.87%
28	Kentucky	369,000,000	0.99%
26	Louisiana	432,000,000	1.16%
42	Maine	157,000,000	0.42%
16	Maryland	749,000,000	2.00%
11	Massachusetts	1,022,000,000	2.73%
7	Michigan	1,531,000,000	4.10%
17	Minnesota	741,000,000	1.98%
36	Mississippi	214,000,000	0.57%
22	Missouri	602,000,000	1.61%
46	Montana	103,000,000	0.28%
37	Nebraska	191,000,000	0.51%
35	Nevada	215,000,000	0.58%
39	New Hampshire	177,000,000	0.47%
8	New Jersey	1,460,000,000	3.91%
40	New Mexico	175,000,000	0.47%
2	New York	2,837,000,000	7.59%
14	North Carolina	810,000,000	2.17%
49	North Dakota	78,000,000	0.21%
9	Ohio	1,398,000,000	3.74%
29	Oklahoma	356,000,000	0.95%
23	Oregon	578,000,000	1.55%
5	Pennsylvania	1,634,000,000	4.37%
43	Rhode Island	150,000,000	0.40%
27	South Carolina	387,000,000	1.04%
47	South Dakota	87,000,000	0.23%
20	Tennessee	609,000,000	1.63%
3	Texas	2,081,000,000	5.57%
32	Utah	276,000,000	0.74%
48	Vermont	84,000,000	0.22%
13	Virginia	863,000,000	2.31%
10	Washington	1,189,000,000	3.18%
38	West Virginia	182,000,000	0.49%
15	Wisconsin	765,000,000	2.05%
50	Wyoming	57,000,000	0.15%

RANK ORDER

RANK	STATE	EXPENDITURES	% of USA
1	California	$5,664,000,000	15.15%
2	New York	2,837,000,000	7.59%
3	Texas	2,081,000,000	5.57%
4	Florida	2,029,000,000	5.43%
5	Pennsylvania	1,634,000,000	4.37%
6	Illinois	1,588,000,000	4.25%
7	Michigan	1,531,000,000	4.10%
8	New Jersey	1,460,000,000	3.91%
9	Ohio	1,398,000,000	3.74%
10	Washington	1,189,000,000	3.18%
11	Massachusetts	1,022,000,000	2.73%
12	Georgia	898,000,000	2.40%
13	Virginia	863,000,000	2.31%
14	North Carolina	810,000,000	2.17%
15	Wisconsin	765,000,000	2.05%
16	Maryland	749,000,000	2.00%
17	Minnesota	741,000,000	1.98%
18	Indiana	692,000,000	1.85%
19	Connecticut	685,000,000	1.83%
20	Tennessee	609,000,000	1.63%
21	Colorado	605,000,000	1.62%
22	Missouri	602,000,000	1.61%
23	Oregon	578,000,000	1.55%
24	Arizona	551,000,000	1.47%
25	Alabama	456,000,000	1.22%
26	Louisiana	432,000,000	1.16%
27	South Carolina	387,000,000	1.04%
28	Kentucky	369,000,000	0.99%
29	Oklahoma	356,000,000	0.95%
30	Iowa	341,000,000	0.91%
31	Kansas	325,000,000	0.87%
32	Utah	276,000,000	0.74%
33	Arkansas	242,000,000	0.65%
34	Hawaii	235,000,000	0.63%
35	Nevada	215,000,000	0.58%
36	Mississippi	214,000,000	0.57%
37	Nebraska	191,000,000	0.51%
38	West Virginia	182,000,000	0.49%
39	New Hampshire	177,000,000	0.47%
40	New Mexico	175,000,000	0.47%
41	Idaho	163,000,000	0.44%
42	Maine	157,000,000	0.42%
43	Rhode Island	150,000,000	0.40%
44	Alaska	124,000,000	0.33%
45	Delaware	104,000,000	0.28%
46	Montana	103,000,000	0.28%
47	South Dakota	87,000,000	0.23%
48	Vermont	84,000,000	0.22%
49	North Dakota	78,000,000	0.21%
50	Wyoming	57,000,000	0.15%
	District of Columbia	119,000,000	0.32%

Source: U.S. Department of Health and Human Services, Health Care Financing Administration
   "State Health Expenditure Accounts" (Health Care Financing Review, Fall 1995, Volume 17, Number 1)
*By state of provider.

Percent of Total Personal Health Care Expenditures
Spent on Dental Service in 1993
National Percent = 4.8%*

ALPHA ORDER				RANK ORDER		
RANK	STATE	PERCENT		RANK	STATE	PERCENT
44	Alabama	3.8		1	Alaska	7.9
1	Alaska	7.9		1	Washington	7.9
16	Arizona	5.2		3	Idaho	7.2
41	Arkansas	4.0		3	Oregon	7.2
7	California	6.0		5	Hawaii	6.7
7	Colorado	6.0		5	Utah	6.7
12	Connecticut	5.6		7	California	6.0
23	Delaware	4.6		7	Colorado	6.0
27	Florida	4.5		9	Nevada	5.7
27	Georgia	4.5		9	New Jersey	5.7
5	Hawaii	6.7		9	Wyoming	5.7
3	Idaho	7.2		12	Connecticut	5.6
23	Illinois	4.6		12	Michigan	5.6
37	Indiana	4.2		12	Vermont	5.6
23	Iowa	4.6		15	Wisconsin	5.3
22	Kansas	4.7		16	Arizona	5.2
47	Kentucky	3.6		16	Minnesota	5.2
50	Louisiana	3.3		16	Virginia	5.2
23	Maine	4.6		19	New Hampshire	5.1
20	Maryland	4.9		20	Maryland	4.9
31	Massachusetts	4.4		20	Montana	4.9
12	Michigan	5.6		22	Kansas	4.7
16	Minnesota	5.2		23	Delaware	4.6
48	Mississippi	3.5		23	Illinois	4.6
44	Missouri	3.8		23	Iowa	4.6
20	Montana	4.9		23	Maine	4.6
35	Nebraska	4.3		27	Florida	4.5
9	Nevada	5.7		27	Georgia	4.5
19	New Hampshire	5.1		27	New Mexico	4.5
9	New Jersey	5.7		27	South Dakota	4.5
27	New Mexico	4.5		31	Massachusetts	4.4
37	New York	4.2		31	North Carolina	4.4
31	North Carolina	4.4		31	Oklahoma	4.4
42	North Dakota	3.9		31	Rhode Island	4.4
37	Ohio	4.2		35	Nebraska	4.3
31	Oklahoma	4.4		35	South Carolina	4.3
3	Oregon	7.2		37	Indiana	4.2
42	Pennsylvania	3.9		37	New York	4.2
31	Rhode Island	4.4		37	Ohio	4.2
35	South Carolina	4.3		37	Texas	4.2
27	South Dakota	4.5		41	Arkansas	4.0
44	Tennessee	3.8		42	North Dakota	3.9
37	Texas	4.2		42	Pennsylvania	3.9
5	Utah	6.7		44	Alabama	3.8
12	Vermont	5.6		44	Missouri	3.8
16	Virginia	5.2		44	Tennessee	3.8
1	Washington	7.9		47	Kentucky	3.6
48	West Virginia	3.5		48	Mississippi	3.5
15	Wisconsin	5.3		48	West Virginia	3.5
9	Wyoming	5.7		50	Louisiana	3.3
					District of Columbia	2.8

Source: Morgan Quitno Press using data from U.S. Dept of Health & Human Services, Health Care Financing Admin.
"State Health Expenditure Accounts" (Health Care Financing Review, Fall 1995, Volume 17, Number 1)
*By state of provider.

Per Capita Expenditures for Dental Service in 1993

National Per Capita = $145*

ALPHA ORDER

RANK	STATE	PER CAPITA
43	Alabama	$109
3	Alaska	207
23	Arizona	140
47	Arkansas	100
7	California	181
8	Colorado	170
2	Connecticut	209
18	Delaware	149
19	Florida	148
27	Georgia	130
4	Hawaii	202
19	Idaho	148
24	Illinois	136
33	Indiana	121
33	Iowa	121
28	Kansas	128
49	Kentucky	97
46	Louisiana	101
29	Maine	127
16	Maryland	151
8	Massachusetts	170
11	Michigan	162
10	Minnesota	164
50	Mississippi	81
40	Missouri	115
31	Montana	122
38	Nebraska	118
14	Nevada	155
12	New Hampshire	158
6	New Jersey	186
44	New Mexico	108
13	New York	156
39	North Carolina	116
31	North Dakota	122
30	Ohio	126
42	Oklahoma	110
5	Oregon	190
24	Pennsylvania	136
17	Rhode Island	150
45	South Carolina	107
33	South Dakota	121
37	Tennessee	120
40	Texas	115
19	Utah	148
22	Vermont	146
26	Virginia	133
1	Washington	226
47	West Virginia	100
15	Wisconsin	152
33	Wyoming	121

RANK ORDER

RANK	STATE	PER CAPITA
1	Washington	$226
2	Connecticut	209
3	Alaska	207
4	Hawaii	202
5	Oregon	190
6	New Jersey	186
7	California	181
8	Colorado	170
8	Massachusetts	170
10	Minnesota	164
11	Michigan	162
12	New Hampshire	158
13	New York	156
14	Nevada	155
15	Wisconsin	152
16	Maryland	151
17	Rhode Island	150
18	Delaware	149
19	Florida	148
19	Idaho	148
19	Utah	148
22	Vermont	146
23	Arizona	140
24	Illinois	136
24	Pennsylvania	136
26	Virginia	133
27	Georgia	130
28	Kansas	128
29	Maine	127
30	Ohio	126
31	Montana	122
31	North Dakota	122
33	Indiana	121
33	Iowa	121
33	South Dakota	121
33	Wyoming	121
37	Tennessee	120
38	Nebraska	118
39	North Carolina	116
40	Missouri	115
40	Texas	115
42	Oklahoma	110
43	Alabama	109
44	New Mexico	108
45	South Carolina	107
46	Louisiana	101
47	Arkansas	100
47	West Virginia	100
49	Kentucky	97
50	Mississippi	81

District of Columbia 206

Source: Morgan Quitno Press using data from U.S. Dept of Health & Human Services, Health Care Financing Admin.
"State Health Expenditure Accounts" (Health Care Financing Review, Fall 1995, Volume 17, Number 1)
By state of provider.

Average Annual Change in Expenditures for Dental Service: 1980 to 1993

National Percent = 8.3% Average Annual Growth*

ALPHA ORDER				RANK ORDER		
RANK	STATE	PERCENT		RANK	STATE	PERCENT
29	Alabama	8.3		1	Alaska	10.6
1	Alaska	10.6		2	New Hampshire	10.4
8	Arizona	9.7		3	Maine	10.1
26	Arkansas	8.5		3	Utah	10.1
31	California	8.1		5	Florida	10.0
14	Colorado	9.2		5	Nevada	10.0
19	Connecticut	8.8		7	South Carolina	9.8
19	Delaware	8.8		8	Arizona	9.7
5	Florida	10.0		8	Georgia	9.7
8	Georgia	9.7		10	Vermont	9.5
24	Hawaii	8.6		11	Virginia	9.4
14	Idaho	9.2		12	Rhode Island	9.3
44	Illinois	7.0		12	Washington	9.3
32	Indiana	7.9		14	Colorado	9.2
49	Iowa	6.5		14	Idaho	9.2
37	Kansas	7.7		16	Maryland	9.1
26	Kentucky	8.5		16	North Carolina	9.1
44	Louisiana	7.0		16	South Dakota	9.1
3	Maine	10.1		19	Connecticut	8.8
16	Maryland	9.1		19	Delaware	8.8
29	Massachusetts	8.3		19	Texas	8.8
50	Michigan	6.4		22	New Jersey	8.7
32	Minnesota	7.9		22	New Mexico	8.7
32	Mississippi	7.9		24	Hawaii	8.6
37	Missouri	7.7		24	Tennessee	8.6
48	Montana	6.8		26	Arkansas	8.5
44	Nebraska	7.0		26	Kentucky	8.5
5	Nevada	10.0		26	Oregon	8.5
2	New Hampshire	10.4		29	Alabama	8.3
22	New Jersey	8.7		29	Massachusetts	8.3
22	New Mexico	8.7		31	California	8.1
37	New York	7.7		32	Indiana	7.9
16	North Carolina	9.1		32	Minnesota	7.9
40	North Dakota	7.4		32	Mississippi	7.9
43	Ohio	7.2		32	Pennsylvania	7.9
41	Oklahoma	7.3		32	West Virginia	7.9
26	Oregon	8.5		37	Kansas	7.7
32	Pennsylvania	7.9		37	Missouri	7.7
12	Rhode Island	9.3		37	New York	7.7
7	South Carolina	9.8		40	North Dakota	7.4
16	South Dakota	9.1		41	Oklahoma	7.3
24	Tennessee	8.6		41	Wisconsin	7.3
19	Texas	8.8		43	Ohio	7.2
3	Utah	10.1		44	Illinois	7.0
10	Vermont	9.5		44	Louisiana	7.0
11	Virginia	9.4		44	Nebraska	7.0
12	Washington	9.3		44	Wyoming	7.0
32	West Virginia	7.9		48	Montana	6.8
41	Wisconsin	7.3		49	Iowa	6.5
44	Wyoming	7.0		50	Michigan	6.4
					District of Columbia	8.4

Source: U.S. Department of Health and Human Services, Health Care Financing Administration
   "State Health Expenditure Accounts" (Health Care Financing Review, Fall 1995, Volume 17, Number 1)
*By state of provider.

Expenditures for Other Professional Health Care Services in 1993

National Total = $51,200,000,000*

ALPHA ORDER

RANK	STATE	EXPENDITURES	% of USA
26	Alabama	$641,000,000	1.25%
45	Alaska	127,000,000	0.25%
21	Arizona	821,000,000	1.60%
32	Arkansas	332,000,000	0.65%
1	California	6,859,000,000	13.39%
23	Colorado	751,000,000	1.47%
22	Connecticut	769,000,000	1.50%
44	Delaware	156,000,000	0.30%
4	Florida	3,505,000,000	6.84%
11	Georgia	1,226,000,000	2.39%
40	Hawaii	222,000,000	0.43%
46	Idaho	126,000,000	0.25%
6	Illinois	2,063,000,000	4.03%
16	Indiana	993,000,000	1.94%
31	Iowa	431,000,000	0.84%
30	Kansas	470,000,000	0.92%
25	Kentucky	691,000,000	1.35%
24	Louisiana	736,000,000	1.44%
42	Maine	210,000,000	0.41%
18	Maryland	942,000,000	1.84%
10	Massachusetts	1,524,000,000	2.98%
9	Michigan	1,844,000,000	3.60%
19	Minnesota	933,000,000	1.82%
35	Mississippi	288,000,000	0.56%
15	Missouri	1,013,000,000	1.98%
43	Montana	166,000,000	0.32%
39	Nebraska	225,000,000	0.44%
34	Nevada	307,000,000	0.60%
36	New Hampshire	269,000,000	0.53%
8	New Jersey	1,870,000,000	3.65%
37	New Mexico	254,000,000	0.50%
2	New York	3,717,000,000	7.26%
13	North Carolina	1,102,000,000	2.15%
49	North Dakota	93,000,000	0.18%
7	Ohio	1,969,000,000	3.84%
28	Oklahoma	504,000,000	0.98%
27	Oregon	530,000,000	1.03%
5	Pennsylvania	3,005,000,000	5.87%
38	Rhode Island	239,000,000	0.47%
29	South Carolina	472,000,000	0.92%
48	South Dakota	117,000,000	0.23%
12	Tennessee	1,166,000,000	2.28%
3	Texas	3,591,000,000	7.01%
41	Utah	220,000,000	0.43%
47	Vermont	122,000,000	0.24%
17	Virginia	970,000,000	1.89%
13	Washington	1,102,000,000	2.15%
33	West Virginia	326,000,000	0.64%
20	Wisconsin	875,000,000	1.71%
50	Wyoming	68,000,000	0.13%

RANK ORDER

RANK	STATE	EXPENDITURES	% of USA
1	California	$6,859,000,000	13.39%
2	New York	3,717,000,000	7.26%
3	Texas	3,591,000,000	7.01%
4	Florida	3,505,000,000	6.84%
5	Pennsylvania	3,005,000,000	5.87%
6	Illinois	2,063,000,000	4.03%
7	Ohio	1,969,000,000	3.84%
8	New Jersey	1,870,000,000	3.65%
9	Michigan	1,844,000,000	3.60%
10	Massachusetts	1,524,000,000	2.98%
11	Georgia	1,226,000,000	2.39%
12	Tennessee	1,166,000,000	2.28%
13	North Carolina	1,102,000,000	2.15%
13	Washington	1,102,000,000	2.15%
15	Missouri	1,013,000,000	1.98%
16	Indiana	993,000,000	1.94%
17	Virginia	970,000,000	1.89%
18	Maryland	942,000,000	1.84%
19	Minnesota	933,000,000	1.82%
20	Wisconsin	875,000,000	1.71%
21	Arizona	821,000,000	1.60%
22	Connecticut	769,000,000	1.50%
23	Colorado	751,000,000	1.47%
24	Louisiana	736,000,000	1.44%
25	Kentucky	691,000,000	1.35%
26	Alabama	641,000,000	1.25%
27	Oregon	530,000,000	1.03%
28	Oklahoma	504,000,000	0.98%
29	South Carolina	472,000,000	0.92%
30	Kansas	470,000,000	0.92%
31	Iowa	431,000,000	0.84%
32	Arkansas	332,000,000	0.65%
33	West Virginia	326,000,000	0.64%
34	Nevada	307,000,000	0.60%
35	Mississippi	288,000,000	0.56%
36	New Hampshire	269,000,000	0.53%
37	New Mexico	254,000,000	0.50%
38	Rhode Island	239,000,000	0.47%
39	Nebraska	225,000,000	0.44%
40	Hawaii	222,000,000	0.43%
41	Utah	220,000,000	0.43%
42	Maine	210,000,000	0.41%
43	Montana	166,000,000	0.32%
44	Delaware	156,000,000	0.30%
45	Alaska	127,000,000	0.25%
46	Idaho	126,000,000	0.25%
47	Vermont	122,000,000	0.24%
48	South Dakota	117,000,000	0.23%
49	North Dakota	93,000,000	0.18%
50	Wyoming	68,000,000	0.13%
	District of Columbia	267,000,000	0.52%

Source: U.S. Department of Health and Human Services, Health Care Financing Administration
"State Health Expenditure Accounts" (Health Care Financing Review, Fall 1995, Volume 17, Number 1)
*By state of provider. Includes services by chiropractors, optometrists and podiatrists. Also includes spending in kidney dialysis clinics, alcohol treatment centers, rehabilitation clinics and other health care establishments not elsewhere classified. Medicare ambulance expenditures are also included.

Percent of Total Personal Health Care Expenditures
Spent on Other Professional Services in 1993
National Percent = 6.6%*

ALPHA ORDER

 RANK STATE / PERCENT (Alpha Order) and RANK ORDER combined:

ALPHA ORDER RANK	STATE	PERCENT		RANK ORDER RANK	STATE	PERCENT
45	Alabama	5.3		1	Nevada	8.2
2	Alaska	8.1		2	Alaska	8.1
7	Arizona	7.7		2	Vermont	8.1
44	Arkansas	5.4		4	Montana	7.9
9	California	7.3		5	Florida	7.8
8	Colorado	7.5		5	New Hampshire	7.8
27	Connecticut	6.3		7	Arizona	7.7
16	Delaware	6.9		8	Colorado	7.5
5	Florida	7.8		9	California	7.3
31	Georgia	6.1		9	New Jersey	7.3
25	Hawaii	6.4		9	Washington	7.3
42	Idaho	5.5		12	Pennsylvania	7.2
37	Illinois	5.9		12	Tennessee	7.2
31	Indiana	6.1		12	Texas	7.2
37	Iowa	5.9		15	Rhode Island	7.0
17	Kansas	6.8		16	Delaware	6.9
20	Kentucky	6.7		17	Kansas	6.8
41	Louisiana	5.7		17	Michigan	6.8
31	Maine	6.1		17	Wyoming	6.8
30	Maryland	6.2		20	Kentucky	6.7
23	Massachusetts	6.5		21	Minnesota	6.6
17	Michigan	6.8		21	Oregon	6.6
21	Minnesota	6.6		23	Massachusetts	6.5
49	Mississippi	4.7		23	New Mexico	6.5
25	Missouri	6.4		25	Hawaii	6.4
4	Montana	7.9		25	Missouri	6.4
48	Nebraska	5.1		27	Connecticut	6.3
1	Nevada	8.2		27	Oklahoma	6.3
5	New Hampshire	7.8		27	West Virginia	6.3
9	New Jersey	7.3		30	Maryland	6.2
23	New Mexico	6.5		31	Georgia	6.1
42	New York	5.5		31	Indiana	6.1
34	North Carolina	6.0		31	Maine	6.1
50	North Dakota	4.6		34	North Carolina	6.0
37	Ohio	5.9		34	South Dakota	6.0
27	Oklahoma	6.3		34	Wisconsin	6.0
21	Oregon	6.6		37	Illinois	5.9
12	Pennsylvania	7.2		37	Iowa	5.9
15	Rhode Island	7.0		37	Ohio	5.9
47	South Carolina	5.2		40	Virginia	5.8
34	South Dakota	6.0		41	Louisiana	5.7
12	Tennessee	7.2		42	Idaho	5.5
12	Texas	7.2		42	New York	5.5
45	Utah	5.3		44	Arkansas	5.4
2	Vermont	8.1		45	Alabama	5.3
40	Virginia	5.8		45	Utah	5.3
9	Washington	7.3		47	South Carolina	5.2
27	West Virginia	6.3		48	Nebraska	5.1
34	Wisconsin	6.0		49	Mississippi	4.7
17	Wyoming	6.8		50	North Dakota	4.6

District of Columbia   6.2

Source: Morgan Quitno Press using data from U.S. Dept of Health & Human Services, Health Care Financing Admin.
"State Health Expenditure Accounts" (Health Care Financing Review, Fall 1995, Volume 17, Number 1)
*By state of provider. Includes services by chiropractors, optometrists and podiatrists. Also includes spending in kidney dialysis clinics, alcohol treatment centers, rehabilitation clinics and other health care establishments not elsewhere classified. Medicare ambulance expenditures are also included.

Per Capita Expenditures for Other Professional Health Care Services in 1993

National Per Capita = $199*

ALPHA ORDER

RANK	STATE	PER CAPITA
40	Alabama	$153
12	Alaska	212
16	Arizona	208
46	Arkansas	137
11	California	220
14	Colorado	210
7	Connecticut	235
9	Delaware	223
1	Florida	255
28	Georgia	178
23	Hawaii	190
49	Idaho	114
30	Illinois	176
32	Indiana	174
40	Iowa	153
25	Kansas	186
26	Kentucky	182
34	Louisiana	172
35	Maine	169
23	Maryland	190
2	Massachusetts	253
21	Michigan	195
17	Minnesota	206
50	Mississippi	109
22	Missouri	194
20	Montana	197
45	Nebraska	139
10	Nevada	222
4	New Hampshire	240
6	New Jersey	238
38	New Mexico	157
18	New York	205
37	North Carolina	158
43	North Dakota	146
28	Ohio	178
39	Oklahoma	156
31	Oregon	175
3	Pennsylvania	250
5	Rhode Island	239
47	South Carolina	130
36	South Dakota	163
8	Tennessee	229
19	Texas	199
48	Utah	118
12	Vermont	212
42	Virginia	150
14	Washington	210
27	West Virginia	179
33	Wisconsin	173
44	Wyoming	145

RANK ORDER

RANK	STATE	PER CAPITA
1	Florida	$255
2	Massachusetts	253
3	Pennsylvania	250
4	New Hampshire	240
5	Rhode Island	239
6	New Jersey	238
7	Connecticut	235
8	Tennessee	229
9	Delaware	223
10	Nevada	222
11	California	220
12	Alaska	212
12	Vermont	212
14	Colorado	210
14	Washington	210
16	Arizona	208
17	Minnesota	206
18	New York	205
19	Texas	199
20	Montana	197
21	Michigan	195
22	Missouri	194
23	Hawaii	190
23	Maryland	190
25	Kansas	186
26	Kentucky	182
27	West Virginia	179
28	Georgia	178
28	Ohio	178
30	Illinois	176
31	Oregon	175
32	Indiana	174
33	Wisconsin	173
34	Louisiana	172
35	Maine	169
36	South Dakota	163
37	North Carolina	158
38	New Mexico	157
39	Oklahoma	156
40	Alabama	153
40	Iowa	153
42	Virginia	150
43	North Dakota	146
44	Wyoming	145
45	Nebraska	139
46	Arkansas	137
47	South Carolina	130
48	Utah	118
49	Idaho	114
50	Mississippi	109

District of Columbia 462

Source: Morgan Quitno Press using data from U.S. Dept of Health & Human Services, Health Care Financing Admin.
"State Health Expenditure Accounts" (Health Care Financing Review, Fall 1995, Volume 17, Number 1)
*By state of provider. Includes services by chiropractors, optometrists and podiatrists. Also includes spending in kidney dialysis clinics, alcohol treatment centers, rehabilitation clinics and other health care establishments not elsewhere classified. Medicare ambulance expenditures are also included.

Average Annual Change in Expenditures for Other Professional Health Care Services: 1980 to 1993
National Percent = 17.4% Average Annual Increase*

ALPHA ORDER

RANK	STATE	PERCENT
17	Alabama	18.6
30	Alaska	16.3
12	Arizona	19.1
44	Arkansas	15.3
34	California	16.2
14	Colorado	18.7
14	Connecticut	18.7
2	Delaware	20.6
7	Florida	19.6
3	Georgia	20.3
9	Hawaii	19.4
49	Idaho	13.1
45	Illinois	15.2
36	Indiana	15.7
50	Iowa	13.0
41	Kansas	15.5
22	Kentucky	17.5
18	Louisiana	18.4
29	Maine	16.4
4	Maryland	19.8
14	Massachusetts	18.7
43	Michigan	15.4
46	Minnesota	15.0
35	Mississippi	16.0
23	Missouri	17.4
37	Montana	15.6
41	Nebraska	15.5
1	Nevada	21.3
13	New Hampshire	18.9
9	New Jersey	19.4
30	New Mexico	16.3
25	New York	17.2
4	North Carolina	19.8
47	North Dakota	14.9
37	Ohio	15.6
37	Oklahoma	15.6
28	Oregon	16.9
19	Pennsylvania	18.2
24	Rhode Island	17.3
21	South Carolina	17.8
37	South Dakota	15.6
7	Tennessee	19.6
6	Texas	19.7
20	Utah	18.1
25	Vermont	17.2
11	Virginia	19.2
30	Washington	16.3
30	West Virginia	16.3
27	Wisconsin	17.0
48	Wyoming	13.2

RANK ORDER

RANK	STATE	PERCENT
1	Nevada	21.3
2	Delaware	20.6
3	Georgia	20.3
4	Maryland	19.8
4	North Carolina	19.8
6	Texas	19.7
7	Florida	19.6
7	Tennessee	19.6
9	Hawaii	19.4
9	New Jersey	19.4
11	Virginia	19.2
12	Arizona	19.1
13	New Hampshire	18.9
14	Colorado	18.7
14	Connecticut	18.7
14	Massachusetts	18.7
17	Alabama	18.6
18	Louisiana	18.4
19	Pennsylvania	18.2
20	Utah	18.1
21	South Carolina	17.8
22	Kentucky	17.5
23	Missouri	17.4
24	Rhode Island	17.3
25	New York	17.2
25	Vermont	17.2
27	Wisconsin	17.0
28	Oregon	16.9
29	Maine	16.4
30	Alaska	16.3
30	New Mexico	16.3
30	Washington	16.3
30	West Virginia	16.3
34	California	16.2
35	Mississippi	16.0
36	Indiana	15.7
37	Montana	15.6
37	Ohio	15.6
37	Oklahoma	15.6
37	South Dakota	15.6
41	Kansas	15.5
41	Nebraska	15.5
43	Michigan	15.4
44	Arkansas	15.3
45	Illinois	15.2
46	Minnesota	15.0
47	North Dakota	14.9
48	Wyoming	13.2
49	Idaho	13.1
50	Iowa	13.0

| | District of Columbia | 15.9 |

Source: U.S. Department of Health and Human Services, Health Care Financing Administration
"State Health Expenditure Accounts" (Health Care Financing Review, Fall 1995, Volume 17, Number 1)
By state of provider. Includes services by chiropractors, optometrists and podiatrists. Also includes spending in kidney dialysis clinics, alcohol treatment centers, rehabilitation clinics and other health care establishments not elsewhere classified. Medicare ambulance expenditures are also included.

Expenditures for Home Health Care in 1993

National Total = $22,982,000,000*

ALPHA ORDER

RANK	STATE	EXPENDITURES	% of USA
13	Alabama	$602,000,000	2.62%
50	Alaska	5,000,000	0.02%
22	Arizona	317,000,000	1.38%
32	Arkansas	145,000,000	0.63%
3	California	1,640,000,000	7.14%
29	Colorado	195,000,000	0.85%
17	Connecticut	391,000,000	1.70%
43	Delaware	51,000,000	0.22%
2	Florida	2,323,000,000	10.11%
9	Georgia	729,000,000	3.17%
46	Hawaii	32,000,000	0.14%
45	Idaho	49,000,000	0.21%
6	Illinois	853,000,000	3.71%
24	Indiana	308,000,000	1.34%
33	Iowa	137,000,000	0.60%
30	Kansas	152,000,000	0.66%
20	Kentucky	357,000,000	1.55%
16	Louisiana	410,000,000	1.78%
36	Maine	104,000,000	0.45%
23	Maryland	314,000,000	1.37%
7	Massachusetts	835,000,000	3.63%
11	Michigan	714,000,000	3.11%
15	Minnesota	414,000,000	1.80%
25	Mississippi	300,000,000	1.31%
21	Missouri	347,000,000	1.51%
44	Montana	50,000,000	0.22%
39	Nebraska	74,000,000	0.32%
35	Nevada	120,000,000	0.52%
40	New Hampshire	71,000,000	0.31%
10	New Jersey	718,000,000	3.12%
41	New Mexico	62,000,000	0.27%
1	New York	3,562,000,000	15.50%
14	North Carolina	541,000,000	2.35%
48	North Dakota	16,000,000	0.07%
12	Ohio	649,000,000	2.82%
26	Oklahoma	273,000,000	1.19%
34	Oregon	122,000,000	0.53%
8	Pennsylvania	796,000,000	3.46%
37	Rhode Island	103,000,000	0.45%
28	South Carolina	216,000,000	0.94%
48	South Dakota	16,000,000	0.07%
5	Tennessee	899,000,000	3.91%
4	Texas	1,583,000,000	6.89%
38	Utah	100,000,000	0.44%
42	Vermont	52,000,000	0.23%
19	Virginia	368,000,000	1.60%
18	Washington	380,000,000	1.65%
31	West Virginia	150,000,000	0.65%
27	Wisconsin	265,000,000	1.15%
47	Wyoming	29,000,000	0.13%

RANK ORDER

RANK	STATE	EXPENDITURES	% of USA
1	New York	$3,562,000,000	15.50%
2	Florida	2,323,000,000	10.11%
3	California	1,640,000,000	7.14%
4	Texas	1,583,000,000	6.89%
5	Tennessee	899,000,000	3.91%
6	Illinois	853,000,000	3.71%
7	Massachusetts	835,000,000	3.63%
8	Pennsylvania	796,000,000	3.46%
9	Georgia	729,000,000	3.17%
10	New Jersey	718,000,000	3.12%
11	Michigan	714,000,000	3.11%
12	Ohio	649,000,000	2.82%
13	Alabama	602,000,000	2.62%
14	North Carolina	541,000,000	2.35%
15	Minnesota	414,000,000	1.80%
16	Louisiana	410,000,000	1.78%
17	Connecticut	391,000,000	1.70%
18	Washington	380,000,000	1.65%
19	Virginia	368,000,000	1.60%
20	Kentucky	357,000,000	1.55%
21	Missouri	347,000,000	1.51%
22	Arizona	317,000,000	1.38%
23	Maryland	314,000,000	1.37%
24	Indiana	308,000,000	1.34%
25	Mississippi	300,000,000	1.31%
26	Oklahoma	273,000,000	1.19%
27	Wisconsin	265,000,000	1.15%
28	South Carolina	216,000,000	0.94%
29	Colorado	195,000,000	0.85%
30	Kansas	152,000,000	0.66%
31	West Virginia	150,000,000	0.65%
32	Arkansas	145,000,000	0.63%
33	Iowa	137,000,000	0.60%
34	Oregon	122,000,000	0.53%
35	Nevada	120,000,000	0.52%
36	Maine	104,000,000	0.45%
37	Rhode Island	103,000,000	0.45%
38	Utah	100,000,000	0.44%
39	Nebraska	74,000,000	0.32%
40	New Hampshire	71,000,000	0.31%
41	New Mexico	62,000,000	0.27%
42	Vermont	52,000,000	0.23%
43	Delaware	51,000,000	0.22%
44	Montana	50,000,000	0.22%
45	Idaho	49,000,000	0.21%
46	Hawaii	32,000,000	0.14%
47	Wyoming	29,000,000	0.13%
48	North Dakota	16,000,000	0.07%
48	South Dakota	16,000,000	0.07%
50	Alaska	5,000,000	0.02%
	District of Columbia	45,000,000	0.20%

Source: U.S. Department of Health and Human Services, Health Care Financing Administration
"State Health Expenditure Accounts" (Health Care Financing Review, Fall 1995, Volume 17, Number 1)
By state of provider. Includes spending for services and products by public and private freestanding home health agencies. Excludes home health care services provided by hospital-based agencies which are included in hospital expenditures.

Percent of Total Personal Health Care Expenditures
Spent on Home Health Care in 1993
National Percent = 3.0%*

ALPHA ORDER

RANK ORDER

RANK	STATE	PERCENT		RANK	STATE	PERCENT
4	Alabama	5.0		1	Tennessee	5.5
50	Alaska	0.3		2	New York	5.3
15	Arizona	3.0		3	Florida	5.2
26	Arkansas	2.4		4	Alabama	5.0
43	California	1.7		5	Mississippi	4.8
37	Colorado	1.9		6	Georgia	3.6
11	Connecticut	3.2		6	Massachusetts	3.6
30	Delaware	2.3		8	Vermont	3.5
3	Florida	5.2		9	Kentucky	3.4
6	Georgia	3.6		9	Oklahoma	3.4
47	Hawaii	0.9		11	Connecticut	3.2
31	Idaho	2.2		11	Louisiana	3.2
24	Illinois	2.5		11	Nevada	3.2
37	Indiana	1.9		11	Texas	3.2
37	Iowa	1.9		15	Arizona	3.0
31	Kansas	2.2		15	Maine	3.0
9	Kentucky	3.4		15	North Carolina	3.0
11	Louisiana	3.2		15	Rhode Island	3.0
15	Maine	3.0		19	Minnesota	2.9
35	Maryland	2.1		19	West Virginia	2.9
6	Massachusetts	3.6		19	Wyoming	2.9
23	Michigan	2.6		22	New Jersey	2.8
19	Minnesota	2.9		23	Michigan	2.6
5	Mississippi	4.8		24	Illinois	2.5
31	Missouri	2.2		24	Washington	2.5
26	Montana	2.4		26	Arkansas	2.4
43	Nebraska	1.7		26	Montana	2.4
11	Nevada	3.2		26	South Carolina	2.4
35	New Hampshire	2.1		26	Utah	2.4
22	New Jersey	2.8		30	Delaware	2.3
45	New Mexico	1.6		31	Idaho	2.2
2	New York	5.3		31	Kansas	2.2
15	North Carolina	3.0		31	Missouri	2.2
48	North Dakota	0.8		31	Virginia	2.2
37	Ohio	1.9		35	Maryland	2.1
9	Oklahoma	3.4		35	New Hampshire	2.1
46	Oregon	1.5		37	Colorado	1.9
37	Pennsylvania	1.9		37	Indiana	1.9
15	Rhode Island	3.0		37	Iowa	1.9
26	South Carolina	2.4		37	Ohio	1.9
48	South Dakota	0.8		37	Pennsylvania	1.9
1	Tennessee	5.5		42	Wisconsin	1.8
11	Texas	3.2		43	California	1.7
26	Utah	2.4		43	Nebraska	1.7
8	Vermont	3.5		45	New Mexico	1.6
31	Virginia	2.2		46	Oregon	1.5
24	Washington	2.5		47	Hawaii	0.9
19	West Virginia	2.9		48	North Dakota	0.8
42	Wisconsin	1.8		48	South Dakota	0.8
19	Wyoming	2.9		50	Alaska	0.3
					District of Columbia	1.1

Source: Morgan Quitno Press using data from U.S. Dept of Health & Human Services, Health Care Financing Admin.
"State Health Expenditure Accounts" (Health Care Financing Review, Fall 1995, Volume 17, Number 1)
By state of provider. Includes spending for services and products by public and private freestanding home health agencies. Excludes home health care services provided by hospital-based agencies which are included in hospital expenditures.

Per Capita Expenditures for Home Health Care in 1993

National Per Capita = $89*

ALPHA ORDER

RANK	STATE	PER CAPITA
4	Alabama	$144
50	Alaska	8
20	Arizona	80
31	Arkansas	60
40	California	53
37	Colorado	55
6	Connecticut	119
23	Delaware	73
3	Florida	169
8	Georgia	106
47	Hawaii	27
44	Idaho	45
23	Illinois	73
38	Indiana	54
42	Iowa	49
31	Kansas	60
11	Kentucky	94
10	Louisiana	96
17	Maine	84
28	Maryland	63
5	Massachusetts	139
22	Michigan	75
12	Minnesota	92
7	Mississippi	114
26	Missouri	66
34	Montana	59
43	Nebraska	46
16	Nevada	87
28	New Hampshire	63
13	New Jersey	91
46	New Mexico	38
1	New York	196
21	North Carolina	78
48	North Dakota	25
34	Ohio	59
17	Oklahoma	84
45	Oregon	40
26	Pennsylvania	66
9	Rhode Island	103
31	South Carolina	60
49	South Dakota	22
2	Tennessee	177
15	Texas	88
38	Utah	54
14	Vermont	90
36	Virginia	57
25	Washington	72
19	West Virginia	83
40	Wisconsin	53
30	Wyoming	62

RANK ORDER

RANK	STATE	PER CAPITA
1	New York	$196
2	Tennessee	177
3	Florida	169
4	Alabama	144
5	Massachusetts	139
6	Connecticut	119
7	Mississippi	114
8	Georgia	106
9	Rhode Island	103
10	Louisiana	96
11	Kentucky	94
12	Minnesota	92
13	New Jersey	91
14	Vermont	90
15	Texas	88
16	Nevada	87
17	Maine	84
17	Oklahoma	84
19	West Virginia	83
20	Arizona	80
21	North Carolina	78
22	Michigan	75
23	Delaware	73
23	Illinois	73
25	Washington	72
26	Missouri	66
26	Pennsylvania	66
28	Maryland	63
28	New Hampshire	63
30	Wyoming	62
31	Arkansas	60
31	Kansas	60
31	South Carolina	60
34	Montana	59
34	Ohio	59
36	Virginia	57
37	Colorado	55
38	Indiana	54
38	Utah	54
40	California	53
40	Wisconsin	53
42	Iowa	49
43	Nebraska	46
44	Idaho	45
45	Oregon	40
46	New Mexico	38
47	Hawaii	27
48	North Dakota	25
49	South Dakota	22
50	Alaska	8
	District of Columbia	78

Source: Morgan Quitno Press using data from U.S. Dept of Health & Human Services, Health Care Financing Admin.
"State Health Expenditure Accounts" (Health Care Financing Review, Fall 1995, Volume 17, Number 1)
*By state of provider. Includes spending for services and products by public and private freestanding home health agencies. Excludes home health care services provided by hospital-based agencies which are included in hospital expenditures.

Average Annual Change in Expenditures for Home Health Care: 1980 to 1993

National Percent = 19.1% Average Annual Increase*

ALPHA ORDER				RANK ORDER		
RANK	STATE	PERCENT		RANK	STATE	PERCENT
9	Alabama	26.0		1	Nevada	35.2
3	Alaska	31.8		2	Utah	33.9
5	Arizona	30.5		3	Alaska	31.8
25	Arkansas	20.4		4	Tennessee	31.2
33	California	17.6		5	Arizona	30.5
37	Colorado	17.0		6	North Carolina	29.1
30	Connecticut	18.7		7	Louisiana	27.7
24	Delaware	20.7		8	Kentucky	26.8
18	Florida	22.3		9	Alabama	26.0
11	Georgia	25.2		10	Wyoming	25.7
39	Hawaii	16.7		11	Georgia	25.2
42	Idaho	16.0		12	West Virginia	24.4
38	Illinois	16.9		13	Texas	24.3
19	Indiana	21.5		14	Minnesota	23.5
30	Iowa	18.7		15	Kansas	23.3
15	Kansas	23.3		16	Mississippi	22.8
8	Kentucky	26.8		16	Nebraska	22.8
7	Louisiana	27.7		18	Florida	22.3
36	Maine	17.3		19	Indiana	21.5
34	Maryland	17.5		19	North Dakota	21.5
28	Massachusetts	19.2		21	South Carolina	21.2
28	Michigan	19.2		21	Virginia	21.2
14	Minnesota	23.5		23	Montana	20.9
16	Mississippi	22.8		24	Delaware	20.7
48	Missouri	15.2		25	Arkansas	20.4
23	Montana	20.9		26	New Mexico	20.2
16	Nebraska	22.8		26	South Dakota	20.2
1	Nevada	35.2		28	Massachusetts	19.2
44	New Hampshire	15.7		28	Michigan	19.2
50	New Jersey	11.1		30	Connecticut	18.7
26	New Mexico	20.2		30	Iowa	18.7
44	New York	15.7		30	Oklahoma	18.7
6	North Carolina	29.1		33	California	17.6
19	North Dakota	21.5		34	Maryland	17.5
34	Ohio	17.5		34	Ohio	17.5
30	Oklahoma	18.7		36	Maine	17.3
47	Oregon	15.3		37	Colorado	17.0
46	Pennsylvania	15.4		38	Illinois	16.9
48	Rhode Island	15.2		39	Hawaii	16.7
21	South Carolina	21.2		40	Washington	16.6
26	South Dakota	20.2		41	Wisconsin	16.3
4	Tennessee	31.2		42	Idaho	16.0
13	Texas	24.3		42	Vermont	16.0
2	Utah	33.9		44	New Hampshire	15.7
42	Vermont	16.0		44	New York	15.7
21	Virginia	21.2		46	Pennsylvania	15.4
40	Washington	16.6		47	Oregon	15.3
12	West Virginia	24.4		48	Missouri	15.2
41	Wisconsin	16.3		48	Rhode Island	15.2
10	Wyoming	25.7		50	New Jersey	11.1
					District of Columbia	11.7

Source: U.S. Department of Health and Human Services, Health Care Financing Administration
"State Health Expenditure Accounts" (Health Care Financing Review, Fall 1995, Volume 17, Number 1)
*By state of provider. Includes spending for services and products by public and private freestanding home health agencies. Excludes home health care services provided by hospital-based agencies which are included in hospital expenditures.

Expenditures for Drug and Other Medical Non-Durables in 1993

National Total = $74,956,000,000*

ALPHA ORDER

RANK	STATE	EXPENDITURES	% of USA
21	Alabama	$1,247,000,000	1.66%
46	Alaska	165,000,000	0.22%
24	Arizona	1,124,000,000	1.50%
33	Arkansas	684,000,000	0.91%
1	California	9,017,000,000	12.03%
27	Colorado	919,000,000	1.23%
25	Connecticut	996,000,000	1.33%
44	Delaware	214,000,000	0.29%
4	Florida	4,450,000,000	5.94%
10	Georgia	2,117,000,000	2.82%
37	Hawaii	416,000,000	0.55%
43	Idaho	265,000,000	0.35%
6	Illinois	3,263,000,000	4.35%
16	Indiana	1,594,000,000	2.13%
30	Iowa	743,000,000	0.99%
32	Kansas	695,000,000	0.93%
22	Kentucky	1,196,000,000	1.60%
20	Louisiana	1,269,000,000	1.69%
40	Maine	333,000,000	0.44%
14	Maryland	1,749,000,000	2.33%
13	Massachusetts	1,961,000,000	2.62%
8	Michigan	2,937,000,000	3.92%
23	Minnesota	1,146,000,000	1.53%
31	Mississippi	720,000,000	0.96%
18	Missouri	1,420,000,000	1.89%
45	Montana	209,000,000	0.28%
36	Nebraska	421,000,000	0.56%
39	Nevada	408,000,000	0.54%
41	New Hampshire	319,000,000	0.43%
9	New Jersey	2,452,000,000	3.27%
38	New Mexico	409,000,000	0.55%
3	New York	5,081,000,000	6.78%
11	North Carolina	2,027,000,000	2.70%
49	North Dakota	160,000,000	0.21%
7	Ohio	3,218,000,000	4.29%
28	Oklahoma	874,000,000	1.17%
29	Oregon	762,000,000	1.02%
5	Pennsylvania	3,519,000,000	4.69%
42	Rhode Island	310,000,000	0.41%
26	South Carolina	978,000,000	1.30%
47	South Dakota	163,000,000	0.22%
15	Tennessee	1,635,000,000	2.18%
2	Texas	5,131,000,000	6.85%
35	Utah	439,000,000	0.59%
48	Vermont	161,000,000	0.21%
12	Virginia	2,015,000,000	2.69%
17	Washington	1,474,000,000	1.97%
34	West Virginia	574,000,000	0.77%
19	Wisconsin	1,290,000,000	1.72%
50	Wyoming	113,000,000	0.15%

RANK ORDER

RANK	STATE	EXPENDITURES	% of USA
1	California	$9,017,000,000	12.03%
2	Texas	5,131,000,000	6.85%
3	New York	5,081,000,000	6.78%
4	Florida	4,450,000,000	5.94%
5	Pennsylvania	3,519,000,000	4.69%
6	Illinois	3,263,000,000	4.35%
7	Ohio	3,218,000,000	4.29%
8	Michigan	2,937,000,000	3.92%
9	New Jersey	2,452,000,000	3.27%
10	Georgia	2,117,000,000	2.82%
11	North Carolina	2,027,000,000	2.70%
12	Virginia	2,015,000,000	2.69%
13	Massachusetts	1,961,000,000	2.62%
14	Maryland	1,749,000,000	2.33%
15	Tennessee	1,635,000,000	2.18%
16	Indiana	1,594,000,000	2.13%
17	Washington	1,474,000,000	1.97%
18	Missouri	1,420,000,000	1.89%
19	Wisconsin	1,290,000,000	1.72%
20	Louisiana	1,269,000,000	1.69%
21	Alabama	1,247,000,000	1.66%
22	Kentucky	1,196,000,000	1.60%
23	Minnesota	1,146,000,000	1.53%
24	Arizona	1,124,000,000	1.50%
25	Connecticut	996,000,000	1.33%
26	South Carolina	978,000,000	1.30%
27	Colorado	919,000,000	1.23%
28	Oklahoma	874,000,000	1.17%
29	Oregon	762,000,000	1.02%
30	Iowa	743,000,000	0.99%
31	Mississippi	720,000,000	0.96%
32	Kansas	695,000,000	0.93%
33	Arkansas	684,000,000	0.91%
34	West Virginia	574,000,000	0.77%
35	Utah	439,000,000	0.59%
36	Nebraska	421,000,000	0.56%
37	Hawaii	416,000,000	0.55%
38	New Mexico	409,000,000	0.55%
39	Nevada	408,000,000	0.54%
40	Maine	333,000,000	0.44%
41	New Hampshire	319,000,000	0.43%
42	Rhode Island	310,000,000	0.41%
43	Idaho	265,000,000	0.35%
44	Delaware	214,000,000	0.29%
45	Montana	209,000,000	0.28%
46	Alaska	165,000,000	0.22%
47	South Dakota	163,000,000	0.22%
48	Vermont	161,000,000	0.21%
49	North Dakota	160,000,000	0.21%
50	Wyoming	113,000,000	0.15%
	District of Columbia	175,000,000	0.23%

Source: U.S. Department of Health and Human Services, Health Care Financing Administration
"State Health Expenditure Accounts" (Health Care Financing Review, Fall 1995, Volume 17, Number 1)
*By state of provider. Includes prescription and over-the-counter drugs and sundries. Limited to spending that occurs in retail outlets such as food stores, drug stores, HMO pharmacies or through mail-order pharmacies.

Percent of Total Personal Health Care Expenditures
Spent on Drugs and Other Medical Non-Durables in 1993
National Percent = 9.6%*

ALPHA ORDER

RANK	STATE	PERCENT
21	Alabama	10.3
18	Alaska	10.5
17	Arizona	10.6
8	Arkansas	11.2
32	California	9.6
40	Colorado	9.1
47	Connecticut	8.2
35	Delaware	9.5
26	Florida	9.9
18	Georgia	10.5
2	Hawaii	11.9
3	Idaho	11.6
38	Illinois	9.4
29	Indiana	9.7
23	Iowa	10.1
23	Kansas	10.1
5	Kentucky	11.5
28	Louisiana	9.8
29	Maine	9.7
5	Maryland	11.5
45	Massachusetts	8.4
13	Michigan	10.8
48	Minnesota	8.1
3	Mississippi	11.6
42	Missouri	8.9
26	Montana	9.9
32	Nebraska	9.6
11	Nevada	10.9
39	New Hampshire	9.2
35	New Jersey	9.5
18	New Mexico	10.5
50	New York	7.6
9	North Carolina	11.1
49	North Dakota	7.9
32	Ohio	9.6
11	Oklahoma	10.9
35	Oregon	9.5
44	Pennsylvania	8.5
41	Rhode Island	9.0
13	South Carolina	10.8
46	South Dakota	8.3
23	Tennessee	10.1
21	Texas	10.3
15	Utah	10.7
15	Vermont	10.7
1	Virginia	12.1
29	Washington	9.7
10	West Virginia	11.0
42	Wisconsin	8.9
7	Wyoming	11.3

RANK ORDER

RANK	STATE	PERCENT
1	Virginia	12.1
2	Hawaii	11.9
3	Idaho	11.6
3	Mississippi	11.6
5	Kentucky	11.5
5	Maryland	11.5
7	Wyoming	11.3
8	Arkansas	11.2
9	North Carolina	11.1
10	West Virginia	11.0
11	Nevada	10.9
11	Oklahoma	10.9
13	Michigan	10.8
13	South Carolina	10.8
15	Utah	10.7
15	Vermont	10.7
17	Arizona	10.6
18	Alaska	10.5
18	Georgia	10.5
18	New Mexico	10.5
21	Alabama	10.3
21	Texas	10.3
23	Iowa	10.1
23	Kansas	10.1
23	Tennessee	10.1
26	Florida	9.9
26	Montana	9.9
28	Louisiana	9.8
29	Indiana	9.7
29	Maine	9.7
29	Washington	9.7
32	California	9.6
32	Nebraska	9.6
32	Ohio	9.6
35	Delaware	9.5
35	New Jersey	9.5
35	Oregon	9.5
38	Illinois	9.4
39	New Hampshire	9.2
40	Colorado	9.1
41	Rhode Island	9.0
42	Missouri	8.9
42	Wisconsin	8.9
44	Pennsylvania	8.5
45	Massachusetts	8.4
46	South Dakota	8.3
47	Connecticut	8.2
48	Minnesota	8.1
49	North Dakota	7.9
50	New York	7.6

District of Columbia 4.1

Source: Morgan Quitno Press using data from U.S. Dept of Health & Human Services, Health Care Financing Admin. "State Health Expenditure Accounts" (Health Care Financing Review, Fall 1995, Volume 17, Number 1)
By state of provider. Includes prescription and over-the-counter drugs and sundries. Limited to spending that occurs in retail outlets such as food stores, drug stores, HMO pharmacies or through mail-order pharmacies.

Per Capita Expenditures for Drugs and Other Medical Non-Durables in 1993

National Per Capita = $291*

ALPHA ORDER

RANK	STATE	PER CAPITA
15	Alabama	$298
31	Alaska	276
22	Arizona	285
25	Arkansas	282
21	California	289
40	Colorado	258
14	Connecticut	304
13	Delaware	306
4	Florida	324
12	Georgia	307
1	Hawaii	357
47	Idaho	241
29	Illinois	279
29	Indiana	279
38	Iowa	263
32	Kansas	274
7	Kentucky	315
16	Louisiana	296
37	Maine	269
2	Maryland	353
3	Massachusetts	326
9	Michigan	311
42	Minnesota	253
33	Mississippi	273
34	Missouri	271
46	Montana	249
39	Nebraska	261
17	Nevada	295
23	New Hampshire	284
8	New Jersey	312
42	New Mexico	253
26	New York	280
18	North Carolina	292
44	North Dakota	251
20	Ohio	291
35	Oklahoma	270
44	Oregon	251
18	Pennsylvania	292
11	Rhode Island	310
35	South Carolina	270
50	South Dakota	227
5	Tennessee	321
23	Texas	284
49	Utah	236
26	Vermont	280
9	Virginia	311
26	Washington	280
6	West Virginia	316
41	Wisconsin	256
48	Wyoming	240

RANK ORDER

RANK	STATE	PER CAPITA
1	Hawaii	$357
2	Maryland	353
3	Massachusetts	326
4	Florida	324
5	Tennessee	321
6	West Virginia	316
7	Kentucky	315
8	New Jersey	312
9	Michigan	311
9	Virginia	311
11	Rhode Island	310
12	Georgia	307
13	Delaware	306
14	Connecticut	304
15	Alabama	298
16	Louisiana	296
17	Nevada	295
18	North Carolina	292
18	Pennsylvania	292
20	Ohio	291
21	California	289
22	Arizona	285
23	New Hampshire	284
23	Texas	284
25	Arkansas	282
26	New York	280
26	Vermont	280
26	Washington	280
29	Illinois	279
29	Indiana	279
31	Alaska	276
32	Kansas	274
33	Mississippi	273
34	Missouri	271
35	Oklahoma	270
35	South Carolina	270
37	Maine	269
38	Iowa	263
39	Nebraska	261
40	Colorado	258
41	Wisconsin	256
42	Minnesota	253
42	New Mexico	253
44	North Dakota	251
44	Oregon	251
46	Montana	249
47	Idaho	241
48	Wyoming	240
49	Utah	236
50	South Dakota	227

| District of Columbia | 303 |

Source: Morgan Quitno Press using data from U.S. Dept of Health & Human Services, Health Care Financing Admin.
"State Health Expenditure Accounts" (Health Care Financing Review, Fall 1995, Volume 17, Number 1)
*By state of provider. Includes prescription and over-the-counter drugs and sundries. Limited to spending that
occurs in retail outlets such as food stores, drug stores, HMO pharmacies or through mail-order pharmacies.

Average Annual Change in Expenditures for Drugs and Other Medical Non-Durables: 1980 to 1993
National Percent = 10.0% Average Annual Growth*

RANK	STATE	PERCENT
25	Alabama	9.9
14	Alaska	10.8
3	Arizona	11.9
45	Arkansas	8.7
19	California	10.3
17	Colorado	10.4
26	Connecticut	9.8
11	Delaware	10.9
2	Florida	12.1
7	Georgia	11.4
11	Hawaii	10.9
34	Idaho	9.3
37	Illinois	9.2
42	Indiana	9.0
45	Iowa	8.7
37	Kansas	9.2
30	Kentucky	9.7
47	Louisiana	8.6
8	Maine	11.3
4	Maryland	11.7
15	Massachusetts	10.7
31	Michigan	9.5
26	Minnesota	9.8
34	Mississippi	9.3
44	Missouri	8.8
31	Montana	9.5
42	Nebraska	9.0
1	Nevada	12.6
4	New Hampshire	11.7
22	New Jersey	10.2
10	New Mexico	11.2
26	New York	9.8
19	North Carolina	10.3
37	North Dakota	9.2
40	Ohio	9.1
49	Oklahoma	8.4
48	Oregon	8.5
31	Pennsylvania	9.5
11	Rhode Island	10.9
19	South Carolina	10.3
34	South Dakota	9.3
22	Tennessee	10.2
26	Texas	9.8
15	Utah	10.7
6	Vermont	11.6
8	Virginia	11.3
17	Washington	10.4
40	West Virginia	9.1
24	Wisconsin	10.1
50	Wyoming	7.8

RANK	STATE	PERCENT
1	Nevada	12.6
2	Florida	12.1
3	Arizona	11.9
4	Maryland	11.7
4	New Hampshire	11.7
6	Vermont	11.6
7	Georgia	11.4
8	Maine	11.3
8	Virginia	11.3
10	New Mexico	11.2
11	Delaware	10.9
11	Hawaii	10.9
11	Rhode Island	10.9
14	Alaska	10.8
15	Massachusetts	10.7
15	Utah	10.7
17	Colorado	10.4
17	Washington	10.4
19	California	10.3
19	North Carolina	10.3
19	South Carolina	10.3
22	New Jersey	10.2
22	Tennessee	10.2
24	Wisconsin	10.1
25	Alabama	9.9
26	Connecticut	9.8
26	Minnesota	9.8
26	New York	9.8
26	Texas	9.8
30	Kentucky	9.7
31	Michigan	9.5
31	Montana	9.5
31	Pennsylvania	9.5
34	Idaho	9.3
34	Mississippi	9.3
34	South Dakota	9.3
37	Illinois	9.2
37	Kansas	9.2
37	North Dakota	9.2
40	Ohio	9.1
40	West Virginia	9.1
42	Indiana	9.0
42	Nebraska	9.0
44	Missouri	8.8
45	Arkansas	8.7
45	Iowa	8.7
47	Louisiana	8.6
48	Oregon	8.5
49	Oklahoma	8.4
50	Wyoming	7.8
	District of Columbia	8.6

Source: U.S. Department of Health and Human Services, Health Care Financing Administration
   "State Health Expenditure Accounts" (Health Care Financing Review, Fall 1995, Volume 17, Number 1)
*By state of provider. Includes prescription and over-the-counter drugs and sundries. Limited to spending that occurs in retail outlets such as food stores, drug stores, HMO pharmacies or through mail-order pharmacies.

Expenditures for Prescription Drugs in 1993

National Total = $48,840,000,000*

ALPHA ORDER					RANK ORDER			

RANK	STATE	EXPENDITURES	% of USA	RANK	STATE	EXPENDITURES	% of USA
18	Alabama	$904,000,000	1.85%	1	California	$5,501,000,000	11.26%
49	Alaska	85,000,000	0.17%	2	New York	3,232,000,000	6.62%
24	Arizona	728,000,000	1.49%	3	Texas	3,153,000,000	6.46%
31	Arkansas	484,000,000	0.99%	4	Florida	2,832,000,000	5.80%
1	California	5,501,000,000	11.26%	5	Pennsylvania	2,386,000,000	4.89%
28	Colorado	534,000,000	1.09%	6	Illinois	2,206,000,000	4.52%
26	Connecticut	650,000,000	1.33%	7	Ohio	2,095,000,000	4.29%
44	Delaware	129,000,000	0.26%	8	Michigan	2,054,000,000	4.21%
4	Florida	2,832,000,000	5.80%	9	New Jersey	1,601,000,000	3.28%
10	Georgia	1,397,000,000	2.86%	10	Georgia	1,397,000,000	2.86%
41	Hawaii	197,000,000	0.40%	11	North Carolina	1,392,000,000	2.85%
43	Idaho	182,000,000	0.37%	12	Virginia	1,343,000,000	2.75%
6	Illinois	2,206,000,000	4.52%	13	Massachusetts	1,337,000,000	2.74%
16	Indiana	1,106,000,000	2.26%	14	Tennessee	1,153,000,000	2.36%
29	Iowa	516,000,000	1.06%	15	Maryland	1,140,000,000	2.33%
32	Kansas	465,000,000	0.95%	16	Indiana	1,106,000,000	2.26%
21	Kentucky	846,000,000	1.73%	17	Missouri	975,000,000	2.00%
22	Louisiana	832,000,000	1.70%	18	Alabama	904,000,000	1.85%
39	Maine	213,000,000	0.44%	19	Wisconsin	899,000,000	1.84%
15	Maryland	1,140,000,000	2.33%	20	Washington	853,000,000	1.75%
13	Massachusetts	1,337,000,000	2.74%	21	Kentucky	846,000,000	1.73%
8	Michigan	2,054,000,000	4.21%	22	Louisiana	832,000,000	1.70%
23	Minnesota	739,000,000	1.51%	23	Minnesota	739,000,000	1.51%
30	Mississippi	499,000,000	1.02%	24	Arizona	728,000,000	1.49%
17	Missouri	975,000,000	2.00%	25	South Carolina	665,000,000	1.36%
45	Montana	120,000,000	0.25%	26	Connecticut	650,000,000	1.33%
36	Nebraska	293,000,000	0.60%	27	Oklahoma	569,000,000	1.17%
38	Nevada	246,000,000	0.50%	28	Colorado	534,000,000	1.09%
41	New Hampshire	197,000,000	0.40%	29	Iowa	516,000,000	1.06%
9	New Jersey	1,601,000,000	3.28%	30	Mississippi	499,000,000	1.02%
37	New Mexico	259,000,000	0.53%	31	Arkansas	484,000,000	0.99%
2	New York	3,232,000,000	6.62%	32	Kansas	465,000,000	0.95%
11	North Carolina	1,392,000,000	2.85%	33	Oregon	431,000,000	0.88%
48	North Dakota	103,000,000	0.21%	34	West Virginia	412,000,000	0.84%
7	Ohio	2,095,000,000	4.29%	35	Utah	302,000,000	0.62%
27	Oklahoma	569,000,000	1.17%	36	Nebraska	293,000,000	0.60%
33	Oregon	431,000,000	0.88%	37	New Mexico	259,000,000	0.53%
5	Pennsylvania	2,386,000,000	4.89%	38	Nevada	246,000,000	0.50%
40	Rhode Island	206,000,000	0.42%	39	Maine	213,000,000	0.44%
25	South Carolina	665,000,000	1.36%	40	Rhode Island	206,000,000	0.42%
47	South Dakota	104,000,000	0.21%	41	Hawaii	197,000,000	0.40%
14	Tennessee	1,153,000,000	2.36%	41	New Hampshire	197,000,000	0.40%
3	Texas	3,153,000,000	6.46%	43	Idaho	182,000,000	0.37%
35	Utah	302,000,000	0.62%	44	Delaware	129,000,000	0.26%
46	Vermont	108,000,000	0.22%	45	Montana	120,000,000	0.25%
12	Virginia	1,343,000,000	2.75%	46	Vermont	108,000,000	0.22%
20	Washington	853,000,000	1.75%	47	South Dakota	104,000,000	0.21%
34	West Virginia	412,000,000	0.84%	48	North Dakota	103,000,000	0.21%
19	Wisconsin	899,000,000	1.84%	49	Alaska	85,000,000	0.17%
50	Wyoming	64,000,000	0.13%	50	Wyoming	64,000,000	0.13%
					District of Columbia	103,000,000	0.21%

Source: U.S. Department of Health and Human Services, Health Care Financing Administration
"State Health Expenditure Accounts" (Health Care Financing Review, Fall 1995, Volume 17, Number 1)
*Purchases in retail outlets. By state of outlet. This is a subset of overall "Drug and Other Medical Non-Durable Expenditures" shown elsewhere in this book.

Percent of Total Personal Health Care Expenditures
Spent on Prescription Drugs in 1993
National Percent = 6.3%*

ALPHA ORDER

RANK	STATE	PERCENT
9	Alabama	7.5
43	Alaska	5.4
18	Arizona	6.8
5	Arkansas	7.9
35	California	5.8
45	Colorado	5.3
45	Connecticut	5.3
36	Delaware	5.7
26	Florida	6.3
17	Georgia	6.9
36	Hawaii	5.7
4	Idaho	8.0
26	Illinois	6.3
19	Indiana	6.7
16	Iowa	7.0
19	Kansas	6.7
1	Kentucky	8.1
24	Louisiana	6.4
30	Maine	6.2
9	Maryland	7.5
36	Massachusetts	5.7
7	Michigan	7.6
48	Minnesota	5.2
1	Mississippi	8.1
33	Missouri	6.1
36	Montana	5.7
19	Nebraska	6.7
23	Nevada	6.6
36	New Hampshire	5.7
30	New Jersey	6.2
19	New Mexico	6.7
50	New York	4.8
7	North Carolina	7.6
49	North Dakota	5.1
26	Ohio	6.3
14	Oklahoma	7.1
43	Oregon	5.4
36	Pennsylvania	5.7
34	Rhode Island	6.0
11	South Carolina	7.4
45	South Dakota	5.3
14	Tennessee	7.1
26	Texas	6.3
12	Utah	7.3
13	Vermont	7.2
1	Virginia	8.1
42	Washington	5.6
5	West Virginia	7.9
30	Wisconsin	6.2
24	Wyoming	6.4

RANK ORDER

RANK	STATE	PERCENT
1	Kentucky	8.1
1	Mississippi	8.1
1	Virginia	8.1
4	Idaho	8.0
5	Arkansas	7.9
5	West Virginia	7.9
7	Michigan	7.6
7	North Carolina	7.6
9	Alabama	7.5
9	Maryland	7.5
11	South Carolina	7.4
12	Utah	7.3
13	Vermont	7.2
14	Oklahoma	7.1
14	Tennessee	7.1
16	Iowa	7.0
17	Georgia	6.9
18	Arizona	6.8
19	Indiana	6.7
19	Kansas	6.7
19	Nebraska	6.7
19	New Mexico	6.7
23	Nevada	6.6
24	Louisiana	6.4
24	Wyoming	6.4
26	Florida	6.3
26	Illinois	6.3
26	Ohio	6.3
26	Texas	6.3
30	Maine	6.2
30	New Jersey	6.2
30	Wisconsin	6.2
33	Missouri	6.1
34	Rhode Island	6.0
35	California	5.8
36	Delaware	5.7
36	Hawaii	5.7
36	Massachusetts	5.7
36	Montana	5.7
36	New Hampshire	5.7
36	Pennsylvania	5.7
42	Washington	5.6
43	Alaska	5.4
43	Oregon	5.4
45	Colorado	5.3
45	Connecticut	5.3
45	South Dakota	5.3
48	Minnesota	5.2
49	North Dakota	5.1
50	New York	4.8

District of Columbia	2.4

*Source: Morgan Quitno Press using data from U.S. Dept of Health & Human Services, Health Care Financing Admin.
"State Health Expenditure Accounts" (Health Care Financing Review, Fall 1995, Volume 17, Number 1)
Purchases in retail outlets. By state of outlet. This is a subset of overall "Drug and Other Medical Non-Durable Expenditures" shown elsewhere in this book.

Per Capita Expenditures for Prescription Drugs in 1993

National Per Capita = $189*

ALPHA ORDER				RANK ORDER		
RANK	STATE	PER CAPITA		RANK	STATE	PER CAPITA
7	Alabama	$216		1	Maryland	$230
48	Alaska	142		2	West Virginia	227
24	Arizona	185		3	Tennessee	226
13	Arkansas	200		4	Kentucky	223
33	California	176		5	Massachusetts	222
45	Colorado	150		6	Michigan	217
15	Connecticut	198		7	Alabama	216
24	Delaware	185		8	Virginia	207
9	Florida	206		9	Florida	206
12	Georgia	202		9	Rhode Island	206
38	Hawaii	169		11	New Jersey	204
39	Idaho	165		12	Georgia	202
19	Illinois	189		13	Arkansas	200
17	Indiana	194		13	North Carolina	200
27	Iowa	183		15	Connecticut	198
26	Kansas	184		15	Pennsylvania	198
4	Kentucky	223		17	Indiana	194
17	Louisiana	194		17	Louisiana	194
37	Maine	172		19	Illinois	189
1	Maryland	230		19	Mississippi	189
5	Massachusetts	222		19	Ohio	189
6	Michigan	217		22	Vermont	188
40	Minnesota	163		23	Missouri	186
19	Mississippi	189		24	Arizona	185
23	Missouri	186		24	Delaware	185
47	Montana	143		26	Kansas	184
29	Nebraska	182		27	Iowa	183
30	Nevada	178		27	South Carolina	183
35	New Hampshire	175		29	Nebraska	182
11	New Jersey	204		30	Nevada	178
44	New Mexico	160		30	New York	178
30	New York	178		30	Wisconsin	178
13	North Carolina	200		33	California	176
41	North Dakota	162		33	Oklahoma	176
19	Ohio	189		35	New Hampshire	175
33	Oklahoma	176		35	Texas	175
48	Oregon	142		37	Maine	172
15	Pennsylvania	198		38	Hawaii	169
9	Rhode Island	206		39	Idaho	165
27	South Carolina	183		40	Minnesota	163
46	South Dakota	145		41	North Dakota	162
3	Tennessee	226		41	Utah	162
35	Texas	175		41	Washington	162
41	Utah	162		44	New Mexico	160
22	Vermont	188		45	Colorado	150
8	Virginia	207		46	South Dakota	145
41	Washington	162		47	Montana	143
2	West Virginia	227		48	Alaska	142
30	Wisconsin	178		48	Oregon	142
50	Wyoming	136		50	Wyoming	136
					District of Columbia	178

Source: Morgan Quitno Press using data from U.S. Dept of Health & Human Services, Health Care Financing Admin.
"State Health Expenditure Accounts" (Health Care Financing Review, Fall 1995, Volume 17, Number 1)
*Purchases in retail outlets. By state of outlet. This is a subset of overall "Drug and Other Medical Non-Durable Expenditures" shown elsewhere in this book.

Percent Change in Expenditures for Prescription Drugs: 1990 to 1993

National Percent Change = 27.9% Increase*

ALPHA ORDER				RANK ORDER		
RANK	**STATE**	**PERCENT CHANGE**		**RANK**	**STATE**	**PERCENT CHANGE**
23	Alabama	27.9		1	Nevada	55.7
2	Alaska	46.6		2	Alaska	46.6
6	Arizona	38.4		3	Idaho	41.1
28	Arkansas	26.7		4	Colorado	40.9
19	California	30.3		5	Utah	38.5
4	Colorado	40.9		6	Arizona	38.4
49	Connecticut	19.5		7	Washington	38.0
15	Delaware	31.6		8	New Mexico	36.3
14	Florida	32.6		9	Oregon	35.5
10	Georgia	35.0		10	Georgia	35.0
13	Hawaii	33.1		11	Texas	34.4
3	Idaho	41.1		12	Montana	33.3
35	Illinois	24.6		13	Hawaii	33.1
29	Indiana	26.5		14	Florida	32.6
42	Iowa	23.2		15	Delaware	31.6
33	Kansas	24.7		16	North Carolina	31.2
26	Kentucky	26.8		17	Virginia	30.9
35	Louisiana	24.6		18	Wyoming	30.6
45	Maine	22.4		19	California	30.3
22	Maryland	28.4		20	South Carolina	30.1
47	Massachusetts	20.1		20	Tennessee	30.1
39	Michigan	24.2		22	Maryland	28.4
24	Minnesota	27.4		23	Alabama	27.9
32	Mississippi	25.1		24	Minnesota	27.4
37	Missouri	24.5		25	Wisconsin	27.0
12	Montana	33.3		26	Kentucky	26.8
33	Nebraska	24.7		26	South Dakota	26.8
1	Nevada	55.7		28	Arkansas	26.7
43	New Hampshire	23.1		29	Indiana	26.5
41	New Jersey	23.3		30	Oklahoma	26.4
8	New Mexico	36.3		31	Vermont	25.6
46	New York	21.3		32	Mississippi	25.1
16	North Carolina	31.2		33	Kansas	24.7
48	North Dakota	19.8		33	Nebraska	24.7
38	Ohio	24.4		35	Illinois	24.6
30	Oklahoma	26.4		35	Louisiana	24.6
9	Oregon	35.5		37	Missouri	24.5
44	Pennsylvania	22.5		38	Ohio	24.4
50	Rhode Island	18.4		39	Michigan	24.2
20	South Carolina	30.1		40	West Virginia	23.7
26	South Dakota	26.8		41	New Jersey	23.3
20	Tennessee	30.1		42	Iowa	23.2
11	Texas	34.4		43	New Hampshire	23.1
5	Utah	38.5		44	Pennsylvania	22.5
31	Vermont	25.6		45	Maine	22.4
17	Virginia	30.9		46	New York	21.3
7	Washington	38.0		47	Massachusetts	20.1
40	West Virginia	23.7		48	North Dakota	19.8
25	Wisconsin	27.0		49	Connecticut	19.5
18	Wyoming	30.6		50	Rhode Island	18.4
					District of Columbia	10.8

Source: Morgan Quitno Press using data from U.S. Dept of Health & Human Services, Health Care Financing Admin.
"State Health Expenditure Accounts" (Health Care Financing Review, Fall 1995, Volume 17, Number 1)
*Purchases in retail outlets. By state of outlet. This is a subset of overall "Drug and Other Medical Non-Durable Expenditures" shown elsewhere in this book.

Percent Change in Per Capita Expenditures for Prescription Drugs: 1990 to 1993

National Percent Change = 22.7% Increase*

ALPHA ORDER			RANK ORDER		
RANK	STATE	PERCENT CHANGE	RANK	STATE	PERCENT CHANGE
24	Alabama	23.4	1	Nevada	35.9
2	Alaska	35.2	2	Alaska	35.2
5	Arizona	28.5	3	Colorado	30.4
23	Arkansas	23.5	4	Idaho	28.9
21	California	23.9	5	Arizona	28.5
3	Colorado	30.4	6	New Mexico	28.0
49	Connecticut	19.3	7	Utah	27.6
14	Delaware	25.9	7	Washington	27.6
17	Florida	24.8	9	Oregon	26.8
12	Georgia	26.3	9	Texas	26.8
13	Hawaii	26.1	11	Montana	26.5
4	Idaho	28.9	12	Georgia	26.3
35	Illinois	21.9	13	Hawaii	26.1
29	Indiana	22.8	14	Delaware	25.9
43	Iowa	21.2	14	Wyoming	25.9
35	Kansas	21.9	16	North Carolina	25.0
25	Kentucky	23.2	17	Florida	24.8
29	Louisiana	22.8	18	Virginia	24.7
44	Maine	21.1	19	South Carolina	24.5
22	Maryland	23.7	20	Tennessee	24.2
47	Massachusetts	20.0	21	California	23.9
35	Michigan	21.9	22	Maryland	23.7
32	Minnesota	22.6	23	Arkansas	23.5
35	Mississippi	21.9	24	Alabama	23.4
40	Missouri	21.6	25	Kentucky	23.2
11	Montana	26.5	26	Oklahoma	23.1
33	Nebraska	22.1	27	South Dakota	22.9
1	Nevada	35.9	27	Vermont	22.9
41	New Hampshire	21.5	29	Indiana	22.8
42	New Jersey	21.4	29	Louisiana	22.8
6	New Mexico	28.0	29	Wisconsin	22.8
46	New York	20.3	32	Minnesota	22.6
16	North Carolina	25.0	33	Nebraska	22.1
47	North Dakota	20.0	34	West Virginia	22.0
35	Ohio	21.9	35	Illinois	21.9
26	Oklahoma	23.1	35	Kansas	21.9
9	Oregon	26.8	35	Michigan	21.9
45	Pennsylvania	20.7	35	Mississippi	21.9
50	Rhode Island	19.1	35	Ohio	21.9
19	South Carolina	24.5	40	Missouri	21.6
27	South Dakota	22.9	41	New Hampshire	21.5
20	Tennessee	24.2	42	New Jersey	21.4
9	Texas	26.8	43	Iowa	21.2
7	Utah	27.6	44	Maine	21.1
27	Vermont	22.9	45	Pennsylvania	20.7
18	Virginia	24.7	46	New York	20.3
7	Washington	27.6	47	Massachusetts	20.0
34	West Virginia	22.0	47	North Dakota	20.0
29	Wisconsin	22.8	49	Connecticut	19.3
14	Wyoming	25.9	50	Rhode Island	19.1
				District of Columbia	16.3

Source: Morgan Quitno Press using data from U.S. Dept of Health & Human Services, Health Care Financing Admin.
"State Health Expenditure Accounts" (Health Care Financing Review, Fall 1995, Volume 17, Number 1)
*Purchases in retail outlets. By state of outlet. This is a subset of overall "Drug and Other Medical Non-Durable
Expenditures" shown elsewhere in this book.

Average Annual Change in Expenditures for Prescription Drugs: 1980 to 1993

National Percent = 11.4% Average Annual Increase*

ALPHA ORDER			RANK ORDER		
RANK	STATE	PERCENT	RANK	STATE	PERCENT
32	Alabama	10.9	1	Nevada	15.8
4	Alaska	13.7	2	Arizona	14.7
2	Arizona	14.7	3	Utah	14.2
49	Arkansas	9.3	4	Alaska	13.7
16	California	11.8	4	Florida	13.7
18	Colorado	11.7	6	Delaware	13.3
33	Connecticut	10.7	6	Maryland	13.3
6	Delaware	13.3	6	New Hampshire	13.3
4	Florida	13.7	9	New Mexico	13.2
12	Georgia	12.7	10	Vermont	13.0
14	Hawaii	12.2	10	Virginia	13.0
20	Idaho	11.6	12	Georgia	12.7
26	Illinois	11.1	13	Massachusetts	12.5
39	Indiana	10.4	14	Hawaii	12.2
46	Iowa	9.6	15	South Carolina	11.9
37	Kansas	10.5	16	California	11.8
33	Kentucky	10.7	16	Rhode Island	11.8
47	Louisiana	9.5	18	Colorado	11.7
20	Maine	11.6	18	New Jersey	11.7
6	Maryland	13.3	20	Idaho	11.6
13	Massachusetts	12.5	20	Maine	11.6
28	Michigan	11.0	22	North Carolina	11.5
28	Minnesota	11.0	22	Wisconsin	11.5
42	Mississippi	10.1	24	Washington	11.3
41	Missouri	10.2	25	Tennessee	11.2
28	Montana	11.0	26	Illinois	11.1
37	Nebraska	10.5	26	New York	11.1
1	Nevada	15.8	28	Michigan	11.0
6	New Hampshire	13.3	28	Minnesota	11.0
18	New Jersey	11.7	28	Montana	11.0
9	New Mexico	13.2	28	Pennsylvania	11.0
26	New York	11.1	32	Alabama	10.9
22	North Carolina	11.5	33	Connecticut	10.7
35	North Dakota	10.6	33	Kentucky	10.7
43	Ohio	10.0	35	North Dakota	10.6
47	Oklahoma	9.5	35	Texas	10.6
43	Oregon	10.0	37	Kansas	10.5
28	Pennsylvania	11.0	37	Nebraska	10.5
16	Rhode Island	11.8	39	Indiana	10.4
15	South Carolina	11.9	40	West Virginia	10.3
43	South Dakota	10.0	41	Missouri	10.2
25	Tennessee	11.2	42	Mississippi	10.1
35	Texas	10.6	43	Ohio	10.0
3	Utah	14.2	43	Oregon	10.0
10	Vermont	13.0	43	South Dakota	10.0
10	Virginia	13.0	46	Iowa	9.6
24	Washington	11.3	47	Louisiana	9.5
40	West Virginia	10.3	47	Oklahoma	9.5
22	Wisconsin	11.5	49	Arkansas	9.3
50	Wyoming	8.2	50	Wyoming	8.2
				District of Columbia	9.5

Source: U.S. Department of Health and Human Services, Health Care Financing Administration
   "State Health Expenditure Accounts" (Health Care Financing Review, Fall 1995, Volume 17, Number 1)
*Purchases in retail outlets. By state of outlet. This is a subset of overall "Drug and Other Medical Non-Durable
Expenditures" shown elsewhere in this book.

Average Annual Change in Per Capita Expenditures
For Prescription Drugs: 1980 to 1993
National Percent = 10.3% Average Annual Increase*

ALPHA ORDER

RANK	STATE	PERCENT
27	Alabama	10.4
30	Alaska	10.2
7	Arizona	11.5
48	Arkansas	8.8
43	California	9.4
36	Colorado	9.9
30	Connecticut	10.2
1	Delaware	12.1
20	Florida	10.7
20	Georgia	10.7
24	Hawaii	10.5
32	Idaho	10.1
14	Illinois	10.9
33	Indiana	10.0
38	Iowa	9.8
36	Kansas	9.9
24	Kentucky	10.5
43	Louisiana	9.4
14	Maine	10.9
5	Maryland	11.8
2	Massachusetts	12.0
17	Michigan	10.8
33	Minnesota	10.0
38	Mississippi	9.8
42	Missouri	9.7
24	Montana	10.5
28	Nebraska	10.3
11	Nevada	11.2
6	New Hampshire	11.6
12	New Jersey	11.1
9	New Mexico	11.3
17	New York	10.8
33	North Carolina	10.0
20	North Dakota	10.7
38	Ohio	9.8
46	Oklahoma	8.9
46	Oregon	8.9
17	Pennsylvania	10.8
9	Rhode Island	11.3
20	South Carolina	10.7
38	South Dakota	9.8
28	Tennessee	10.3
49	Texas	8.6
2	Utah	12.0
2	Vermont	12.0
8	Virginia	11.4
45	Washington	9.3
14	West Virginia	10.9
13	Wisconsin	11.0
50	Wyoming	8.2

RANK ORDER

RANK	STATE	PERCENT
1	Delaware	12.1
2	Massachusetts	12.0
2	Utah	12.0
2	Vermont	12.0
5	Maryland	11.8
6	New Hampshire	11.6
7	Arizona	11.5
8	Virginia	11.4
9	New Mexico	11.3
9	Rhode Island	11.3
11	Nevada	11.2
12	New Jersey	11.1
13	Wisconsin	11.0
14	Illinois	10.9
14	Maine	10.9
14	West Virginia	10.9
17	Michigan	10.8
17	New York	10.8
17	Pennsylvania	10.8
20	Florida	10.7
20	Georgia	10.7
20	North Dakota	10.7
20	South Carolina	10.7
24	Hawaii	10.5
24	Kentucky	10.5
24	Montana	10.5
27	Alabama	10.4
28	Nebraska	10.3
28	Tennessee	10.3
30	Alaska	10.2
30	Connecticut	10.2
32	Idaho	10.1
33	Indiana	10.0
33	Minnesota	10.0
33	North Carolina	10.0
36	Colorado	9.9
36	Kansas	9.9
38	Iowa	9.8
38	Mississippi	9.8
38	Ohio	9.8
38	South Dakota	9.8
42	Missouri	9.7
43	California	9.4
43	Louisiana	9.4
45	Washington	9.3
46	Oklahoma	8.9
46	Oregon	8.9
48	Arkansas	8.8
49	Texas	8.6
50	Wyoming	8.2

| | District of Columbia | 10.3 |

Source: Morgan Quitno Press using data from U.S. Dept of Health & Human Services, Health Care Financing Admin.
"State Health Expenditure Accounts" (Health Care Financing Review, Fall 1995, Volume 17, Number 1)
*Purchases in retail outlets. By state of outlet. This is a subset of overall "Drug and Other Medical Non-Durable Expenditures" shown elsewhere in this book.

Expenditures for Vision Products and Other Medical Durables in 1993

National Total = $12,636,000,000*

ALPHA ORDER				RANK ORDER			
RANK	STATE	EXPENDITURES	% of USA	RANK	STATE	EXPENDITURES	% of USA
25	Alabama	$155,000,000	1.23%	1	California	$1,522,000,000	12.04%
48	Alaska	26,000,000	0.21%	2	New York	1,090,000,000	8.63%
21	Arizona	227,000,000	1.80%	3	Texas	883,000,000	6.99%
39	Arkansas	56,000,000	0.44%	4	Florida	872,000,000	6.90%
1	California	1,522,000,000	12.04%	5	Pennsylvania	617,000,000	4.88%
22	Colorado	226,000,000	1.79%	6	Illinois	604,000,000	4.78%
23	Connecticut	192,000,000	1.52%	7	Ohio	531,000,000	4.20%
43	Delaware	35,000,000	0.28%	8	Michigan	457,000,000	3.62%
4	Florida	872,000,000	6.90%	8	New Jersey	457,000,000	3.62%
10	Georgia	331,000,000	2.62%	10	Georgia	331,000,000	2.62%
37	Hawaii	64,000,000	0.51%	11	Virginia	295,000,000	2.33%
43	Idaho	35,000,000	0.28%	12	Minnesota	277,000,000	2.19%
6	Illinois	604,000,000	4.78%	13	Maryland	272,000,000	2.15%
14	Indiana	270,000,000	2.14%	14	Indiana	270,000,000	2.14%
26	Iowa	148,000,000	1.17%	15	Massachusetts	269,000,000	2.13%
31	Kansas	107,000,000	0.85%	16	North Carolina	268,000,000	2.12%
27	Kentucky	141,000,000	1.12%	17	Missouri	244,000,000	1.93%
24	Louisiana	160,000,000	1.27%	18	Washington	242,000,000	1.92%
40	Maine	46,000,000	0.36%	19	Wisconsin	240,000,000	1.90%
13	Maryland	272,000,000	2.15%	20	Tennessee	228,000,000	1.80%
15	Massachusetts	269,000,000	2.13%	21	Arizona	227,000,000	1.80%
8	Michigan	457,000,000	3.62%	22	Colorado	226,000,000	1.79%
12	Minnesota	277,000,000	2.19%	23	Connecticut	192,000,000	1.52%
38	Mississippi	60,000,000	0.47%	24	Louisiana	160,000,000	1.27%
17	Missouri	244,000,000	1.93%	25	Alabama	155,000,000	1.23%
42	Montana	36,000,000	0.28%	26	Iowa	148,000,000	1.17%
33	Nebraska	80,000,000	0.63%	27	Kentucky	141,000,000	1.12%
34	Nevada	76,000,000	0.60%	28	Oklahoma	121,000,000	0.96%
41	New Hampshire	43,000,000	0.34%	29	Utah	117,000,000	0.93%
8	New Jersey	457,000,000	3.62%	30	South Carolina	115,000,000	0.91%
36	New Mexico	69,000,000	0.55%	31	Kansas	107,000,000	0.85%
2	New York	1,090,000,000	8.63%	32	Oregon	91,000,000	0.72%
16	North Carolina	268,000,000	2.12%	33	Nebraska	80,000,000	0.63%
47	North Dakota	28,000,000	0.22%	34	Nevada	76,000,000	0.60%
7	Ohio	531,000,000	4.20%	35	West Virginia	74,000,000	0.59%
28	Oklahoma	121,000,000	0.96%	36	New Mexico	69,000,000	0.55%
32	Oregon	91,000,000	0.72%	37	Hawaii	64,000,000	0.51%
5	Pennsylvania	617,000,000	4.88%	38	Mississippi	60,000,000	0.47%
45	Rhode Island	33,000,000	0.26%	39	Arkansas	56,000,000	0.44%
30	South Carolina	115,000,000	0.91%	40	Maine	46,000,000	0.36%
46	South Dakota	30,000,000	0.24%	41	New Hampshire	43,000,000	0.34%
20	Tennessee	228,000,000	1.80%	42	Montana	36,000,000	0.28%
3	Texas	883,000,000	6.99%	43	Delaware	35,000,000	0.28%
29	Utah	117,000,000	0.93%	43	Idaho	35,000,000	0.28%
49	Vermont	24,000,000	0.19%	45	Rhode Island	33,000,000	0.26%
11	Virginia	295,000,000	2.33%	46	South Dakota	30,000,000	0.24%
18	Washington	242,000,000	1.92%	47	North Dakota	28,000,000	0.22%
35	West Virginia	74,000,000	0.59%	48	Alaska	26,000,000	0.21%
19	Wisconsin	240,000,000	1.90%	49	Vermont	24,000,000	0.19%
50	Wyoming	17,000,000	0.13%	50	Wyoming	17,000,000	0.13%
					District of Columbia	34,000,000	0.27%

Source: U.S. Department of Health and Human Services, Health Care Financing Administration
"State Health Expenditure Accounts" (Health Care Financing Review, Fall 1995, Volume 17, Number 1)
*By state of provider. Includes eyeglasses, hearing aids, surgical appliances and supplies, bulk and cylinder oxygen and medical equipment rentals.

Percent of Total Personal Health Care Expenditures
Spent on Vision Products and Other Medical Durables in 1993
National Percent = 1.6%*

<table>
<tr><td colspan="3">ALPHA ORDER</td><td colspan="3">RANK ORDER</td></tr>
<tr><td>RANK</td><td>STATE</td><td>PERCENT</td><td>RANK</td><td>STATE</td><td>PERCENT</td></tr>
<tr><td>41</td><td>Alabama</td><td>1.3</td><td>1</td><td>Utah</td><td>2.8</td></tr>
<tr><td>15</td><td>Alaska</td><td>1.7</td><td>2</td><td>Colorado</td><td>2.2</td></tr>
<tr><td>3</td><td>Arizona</td><td>2.1</td><td>3</td><td>Arizona</td><td>2.1</td></tr>
<tr><td>50</td><td>Arkansas</td><td>0.9</td><td>4</td><td>Iowa</td><td>2.0</td></tr>
<tr><td>21</td><td>California</td><td>1.6</td><td>4</td><td>Minnesota</td><td>2.0</td></tr>
<tr><td>2</td><td>Colorado</td><td>2.2</td><td>4</td><td>Nevada</td><td>2.0</td></tr>
<tr><td>21</td><td>Connecticut</td><td>1.6</td><td>7</td><td>Florida</td><td>1.9</td></tr>
<tr><td>30</td><td>Delaware</td><td>1.5</td><td>8</td><td>Hawaii</td><td>1.8</td></tr>
<tr><td>7</td><td>Florida</td><td>1.9</td><td>8</td><td>Maryland</td><td>1.8</td></tr>
<tr><td>21</td><td>Georgia</td><td>1.6</td><td>8</td><td>Nebraska</td><td>1.8</td></tr>
<tr><td>8</td><td>Hawaii</td><td>1.8</td><td>8</td><td>New Jersey</td><td>1.8</td></tr>
<tr><td>30</td><td>Idaho</td><td>1.5</td><td>8</td><td>New Mexico</td><td>1.8</td></tr>
<tr><td>15</td><td>Illinois</td><td>1.7</td><td>8</td><td>Texas</td><td>1.8</td></tr>
<tr><td>21</td><td>Indiana</td><td>1.6</td><td>8</td><td>Virginia</td><td>1.8</td></tr>
<tr><td>4</td><td>Iowa</td><td>2.0</td><td>15</td><td>Alaska</td><td>1.7</td></tr>
<tr><td>21</td><td>Kansas</td><td>1.6</td><td>15</td><td>Illinois</td><td>1.7</td></tr>
<tr><td>37</td><td>Kentucky</td><td>1.4</td><td>15</td><td>Michigan</td><td>1.7</td></tr>
<tr><td>44</td><td>Louisiana</td><td>1.2</td><td>15</td><td>Montana</td><td>1.7</td></tr>
<tr><td>41</td><td>Maine</td><td>1.3</td><td>15</td><td>Wisconsin</td><td>1.7</td></tr>
<tr><td>8</td><td>Maryland</td><td>1.8</td><td>15</td><td>Wyoming</td><td>1.7</td></tr>
<tr><td>46</td><td>Massachusetts</td><td>1.1</td><td>21</td><td>California</td><td>1.6</td></tr>
<tr><td>15</td><td>Michigan</td><td>1.7</td><td>21</td><td>Connecticut</td><td>1.6</td></tr>
<tr><td>4</td><td>Minnesota</td><td>2.0</td><td>21</td><td>Georgia</td><td>1.6</td></tr>
<tr><td>48</td><td>Mississippi</td><td>1.0</td><td>21</td><td>Indiana</td><td>1.6</td></tr>
<tr><td>30</td><td>Missouri</td><td>1.5</td><td>21</td><td>Kansas</td><td>1.6</td></tr>
<tr><td>15</td><td>Montana</td><td>1.7</td><td>21</td><td>New York</td><td>1.6</td></tr>
<tr><td>8</td><td>Nebraska</td><td>1.8</td><td>21</td><td>Ohio</td><td>1.6</td></tr>
<tr><td>4</td><td>Nevada</td><td>2.0</td><td>21</td><td>Vermont</td><td>1.6</td></tr>
<tr><td>44</td><td>New Hampshire</td><td>1.2</td><td>21</td><td>Washington</td><td>1.6</td></tr>
<tr><td>8</td><td>New Jersey</td><td>1.8</td><td>30</td><td>Delaware</td><td>1.5</td></tr>
<tr><td>8</td><td>New Mexico</td><td>1.8</td><td>30</td><td>Idaho</td><td>1.5</td></tr>
<tr><td>21</td><td>New York</td><td>1.6</td><td>30</td><td>Missouri</td><td>1.5</td></tr>
<tr><td>30</td><td>North Carolina</td><td>1.5</td><td>30</td><td>North Carolina</td><td>1.5</td></tr>
<tr><td>37</td><td>North Dakota</td><td>1.4</td><td>30</td><td>Oklahoma</td><td>1.5</td></tr>
<tr><td>21</td><td>Ohio</td><td>1.6</td><td>30</td><td>Pennsylvania</td><td>1.5</td></tr>
<tr><td>30</td><td>Oklahoma</td><td>1.5</td><td>30</td><td>South Dakota</td><td>1.5</td></tr>
<tr><td>46</td><td>Oregon</td><td>1.1</td><td>37</td><td>Kentucky</td><td>1.4</td></tr>
<tr><td>30</td><td>Pennsylvania</td><td>1.5</td><td>37</td><td>North Dakota</td><td>1.4</td></tr>
<tr><td>48</td><td>Rhode Island</td><td>1.0</td><td>37</td><td>Tennessee</td><td>1.4</td></tr>
<tr><td>41</td><td>South Carolina</td><td>1.3</td><td>37</td><td>West Virginia</td><td>1.4</td></tr>
<tr><td>30</td><td>South Dakota</td><td>1.5</td><td>41</td><td>Alabama</td><td>1.3</td></tr>
<tr><td>37</td><td>Tennessee</td><td>1.4</td><td>41</td><td>Maine</td><td>1.3</td></tr>
<tr><td>8</td><td>Texas</td><td>1.8</td><td>41</td><td>South Carolina</td><td>1.3</td></tr>
<tr><td>1</td><td>Utah</td><td>2.8</td><td>44</td><td>Louisiana</td><td>1.2</td></tr>
<tr><td>21</td><td>Vermont</td><td>1.6</td><td>44</td><td>New Hampshire</td><td>1.2</td></tr>
<tr><td>8</td><td>Virginia</td><td>1.8</td><td>46</td><td>Massachusetts</td><td>1.1</td></tr>
<tr><td>21</td><td>Washington</td><td>1.6</td><td>46</td><td>Oregon</td><td>1.1</td></tr>
<tr><td>37</td><td>West Virginia</td><td>1.4</td><td>48</td><td>Mississippi</td><td>1.0</td></tr>
<tr><td>15</td><td>Wisconsin</td><td>1.7</td><td>48</td><td>Rhode Island</td><td>1.0</td></tr>
<tr><td>15</td><td>Wyoming</td><td>1.7</td><td>50</td><td>Arkansas</td><td>0.9</td></tr>
<tr><td></td><td></td><td></td><td></td><td>District of Columbia</td><td>0.8</td></tr>
</table>

Source: Morgan Quitno Press using data from U.S. Dept of Health & Human Services, Health Care Financing Admin.
"State Health Expenditure Accounts" (Health Care Financing Review, Fall 1995, Volume 17, Number 1)
*By state of provider. Includes eyeglasses, hearing aids, surgical appliances and supplies, bulk and cylinder oxygen and medical equipment rentals.

Per Capita Expenditures for Vision Products and Other Medical Durables in 1993

National Per Capita = $49*

ALPHA ORDER

RANK	STATE	PER CAPITA
39	Alabama	$37
30	Alaska	43
7	Arizona	58
49	Arkansas	23
17	California	49
2	Colorado	63
6	Connecticut	59
15	Delaware	50
1	Florida	64
19	Georgia	48
9	Hawaii	55
46	Idaho	32
12	Illinois	52
23	Indiana	47
12	Iowa	52
33	Kansas	42
39	Kentucky	37
39	Louisiana	37
39	Maine	37
9	Maryland	55
27	Massachusetts	45
19	Michigan	48
4	Minnesota	61
49	Mississippi	23
23	Missouri	47
30	Montana	43
15	Nebraska	50
9	Nevada	55
38	New Hampshire	38
7	New Jersey	58
30	New Mexico	43
5	New York	60
37	North Carolina	39
29	North Dakota	44
19	Ohio	48
39	Oklahoma	37
48	Oregon	30
14	Pennsylvania	51
45	Rhode Island	33
46	South Carolina	32
33	South Dakota	42
27	Tennessee	45
17	Texas	49
2	Utah	63
33	Vermont	42
25	Virginia	46
25	Washington	46
36	West Virginia	41
19	Wisconsin	48
44	Wyoming	36

RANK ORDER

RANK	STATE	PER CAPITA
1	Florida	$64
2	Colorado	63
2	Utah	63
4	Minnesota	61
5	New York	60
6	Connecticut	59
7	Arizona	58
7	New Jersey	58
9	Hawaii	55
9	Maryland	55
9	Nevada	55
12	Illinois	52
12	Iowa	52
14	Pennsylvania	51
15	Delaware	50
15	Nebraska	50
17	California	49
17	Texas	49
19	Georgia	48
19	Michigan	48
19	Ohio	48
19	Wisconsin	48
23	Indiana	47
23	Missouri	47
25	Virginia	46
25	Washington	46
27	Massachusetts	45
27	Tennessee	45
29	North Dakota	44
30	Alaska	43
30	Montana	43
30	New Mexico	43
33	Kansas	42
33	South Dakota	42
33	Vermont	42
36	West Virginia	41
37	North Carolina	39
38	New Hampshire	38
39	Alabama	37
39	Kentucky	37
39	Louisiana	37
39	Maine	37
39	Oklahoma	37
44	Wyoming	36
45	Rhode Island	33
46	Idaho	32
46	South Carolina	32
48	Oregon	30
49	Arkansas	23
49	Mississippi	23
	District of Columbia	59

Source: Morgan Quitno Press using data from U.S. Dept of Health & Human Services, Health Care Financing Admin. "State Health Expenditure Accounts" (Health Care Financing Review, Fall 1995, Volume 17, Number 1)

*By state of provider. Includes eyeglasses, hearing aids, surgical appliances and supplies, bulk and cylinder oxygen and medical equipment rentals.

Average Annual Change in Expenditures for
Vision Products and Other Medical Durables: 1980 to 1993
National Percent = 8.3% Average Annual Growth*

ALPHA ORDER

RANK	STATE	PERCENT
15	Alabama	8.7
49	Alaska	5.3
1	Arizona	10.5
26	Arkansas	8.0
8	California	9.4
12	Colorado	8.9
18	Connecticut	8.5
33	Delaware	7.4
6	Florida	9.9
8	Georgia	9.4
23	Hawaii	8.1
36	Idaho	7.1
30	Illinois	7.8
29	Indiana	7.9
39	Iowa	7.0
39	Kansas	7.0
21	Kentucky	8.3
46	Louisiana	6.7
19	Maine	8.4
19	Maryland	8.4
15	Massachusetts	8.7
33	Michigan	7.4
30	Minnesota	7.8
44	Mississippi	6.8
36	Missouri	7.1
44	Montana	6.8
48	Nebraska	5.7
3	Nevada	10.2
2	New Hampshire	10.3
15	New Jersey	8.7
11	New Mexico	9.3
23	New York	8.1
5	North Carolina	10.1
36	North Dakota	7.1
43	Ohio	6.9
39	Oklahoma	7.0
47	Oregon	6.4
32	Pennsylvania	7.7
22	Rhode Island	8.2
3	South Carolina	10.2
39	South Dakota	7.0
7	Tennessee	9.6
35	Texas	7.2
8	Utah	9.4
12	Vermont	8.9
14	Virginia	8.8
26	Washington	8.0
23	West Virginia	8.1
26	Wisconsin	8.0
50	Wyoming	5.1

RANK ORDER

RANK	STATE	PERCENT
1	Arizona	10.5
2	New Hampshire	10.3
3	Nevada	10.2
3	South Carolina	10.2
5	North Carolina	10.1
6	Florida	9.9
7	Tennessee	9.6
8	California	9.4
8	Georgia	9.4
8	Utah	9.4
11	New Mexico	9.3
12	Colorado	8.9
12	Vermont	8.9
14	Virginia	8.8
15	Alabama	8.7
15	Massachusetts	8.7
15	New Jersey	8.7
18	Connecticut	8.5
19	Maine	8.4
19	Maryland	8.4
21	Kentucky	8.3
22	Rhode Island	8.2
23	Hawaii	8.1
23	New York	8.1
23	West Virginia	8.1
26	Arkansas	8.0
26	Washington	8.0
26	Wisconsin	8.0
29	Indiana	7.9
30	Illinois	7.8
30	Minnesota	7.8
32	Pennsylvania	7.7
33	Delaware	7.4
33	Michigan	7.4
35	Texas	7.2
36	Idaho	7.1
36	Missouri	7.1
36	North Dakota	7.1
39	Iowa	7.0
39	Kansas	7.0
39	Oklahoma	7.0
39	South Dakota	7.0
43	Ohio	6.9
44	Mississippi	6.8
44	Montana	6.8
46	Louisiana	6.7
47	Oregon	6.4
48	Nebraska	5.7
49	Alaska	5.3
50	Wyoming	5.1
	District of Columbia	4.6

Source: U.S. Department of Health and Human Services, Health Care Financing Administration
    "State Health Expenditure Accounts" (Health Care Financing Review, Fall 1995, Volume 17, Number 1)
*By state of provider. Includes eyeglasses, hearing aids, surgical appliances and supplies, bulk and cylinder oxygen and medical equipment rentals.

Expenditures for Nursing Home Care in 1993

National Total = $66,201,000,000*

ALPHA ORDER

RANK	STATE	EXPENDITURES	% of USA
27	Alabama	$703,000,000	1.06%
50	Alaska	56,000,000	0.08%
31	Arizona	567,000,000	0.86%
32	Arkansas	558,000,000	0.84%
3	California	4,103,000,000	6.20%
28	Colorado	661,000,000	1.00%
14	Connecticut	1,749,000,000	2.64%
41	Delaware	217,000,000	0.33%
7	Florida	3,089,000,000	4.67%
21	Georgia	1,038,000,000	1.57%
45	Hawaii	181,000,000	0.27%
44	Idaho	197,000,000	0.30%
5	Illinois	3,148,000,000	4.76%
10	Indiana	2,018,000,000	3.05%
23	Iowa	927,000,000	1.40%
26	Kansas	721,000,000	1.09%
24	Kentucky	850,000,000	1.28%
18	Louisiana	1,186,000,000	1.79%
36	Maine	453,000,000	0.68%
19	Maryland	1,185,000,000	1.79%
8	Massachusetts	2,737,000,000	4.13%
12	Michigan	1,849,000,000	2.79%
11	Minnesota	1,884,000,000	2.85%
35	Mississippi	460,000,000	0.69%
16	Missouri	1,368,000,000	2.07%
46	Montana	178,000,000	0.27%
34	Nebraska	482,000,000	0.73%
47	Nevada	164,000,000	0.25%
38	New Hampshire	268,000,000	0.40%
9	New Jersey	2,128,000,000	3.21%
43	New Mexico	215,000,000	0.32%
1	New York	9,106,000,000	13.76%
15	North Carolina	1,562,000,000	2.36%
40	North Dakota	246,000,000	0.37%
4	Ohio	3,758,000,000	5.68%
25	Oklahoma	748,000,000	1.13%
29	Oregon	656,000,000	0.99%
2	Pennsylvania	4,153,000,000	6.27%
33	Rhode Island	485,000,000	0.73%
30	South Carolina	638,000,000	0.96%
42	South Dakota	216,000,000	0.33%
20	Tennessee	1,085,000,000	1.64%
6	Texas	3,104,000,000	4.69%
39	Utah	260,000,000	0.39%
48	Vermont	148,000,000	0.22%
22	Virginia	976,000,000	1.47%
17	Washington	1,291,000,000	1.95%
37	West Virginia	365,000,000	0.55%
13	Wisconsin	1,752,000,000	2.65%
49	Wyoming	83,000,000	0.13%

RANK ORDER

RANK	STATE	EXPENDITURES	% of USA
1	New York	$9,106,000,000	13.76%
2	Pennsylvania	4,153,000,000	6.27%
3	California	4,103,000,000	6.20%
4	Ohio	3,758,000,000	5.68%
5	Illinois	3,148,000,000	4.76%
6	Texas	3,104,000,000	4.69%
7	Florida	3,089,000,000	4.67%
8	Massachusetts	2,737,000,000	4.13%
9	New Jersey	2,128,000,000	3.21%
10	Indiana	2,018,000,000	3.05%
11	Minnesota	1,884,000,000	2.85%
12	Michigan	1,849,000,000	2.79%
13	Wisconsin	1,752,000,000	2.65%
14	Connecticut	1,749,000,000	2.64%
15	North Carolina	1,562,000,000	2.36%
16	Missouri	1,368,000,000	2.07%
17	Washington	1,291,000,000	1.95%
18	Louisiana	1,186,000,000	1.79%
19	Maryland	1,185,000,000	1.79%
20	Tennessee	1,085,000,000	1.64%
21	Georgia	1,038,000,000	1.57%
22	Virginia	976,000,000	1.47%
23	Iowa	927,000,000	1.40%
24	Kentucky	850,000,000	1.28%
25	Oklahoma	748,000,000	1.13%
26	Kansas	721,000,000	1.09%
27	Alabama	703,000,000	1.06%
28	Colorado	661,000,000	1.00%
29	Oregon	656,000,000	0.99%
30	South Carolina	638,000,000	0.96%
31	Arizona	567,000,000	0.86%
32	Arkansas	558,000,000	0.84%
33	Rhode Island	485,000,000	0.73%
34	Nebraska	482,000,000	0.73%
35	Mississippi	460,000,000	0.69%
36	Maine	453,000,000	0.68%
37	West Virginia	365,000,000	0.55%
38	New Hampshire	268,000,000	0.40%
39	Utah	260,000,000	0.39%
40	North Dakota	246,000,000	0.37%
41	Delaware	217,000,000	0.33%
42	South Dakota	216,000,000	0.33%
43	New Mexico	215,000,000	0.32%
44	Idaho	197,000,000	0.30%
45	Hawaii	181,000,000	0.27%
46	Montana	178,000,000	0.27%
47	Nevada	164,000,000	0.25%
48	Vermont	148,000,000	0.22%
49	Wyoming	83,000,000	0.13%
50	Alaska	56,000,000	0.08%
	District of Columbia	231,000,000	0.35%

Source: U.S. Department of Health and Human Services, Health Care Financing Administration
"State Health Expenditure Accounts" (Health Care Financing Review, Fall 1995, Volume 17, Number 1)
By state of provider. Includes freestanding nursing and personal-care facilities. Includes Medicare- and Medicaid-certified skilled nursing and intermediate care facilities as well as facilities that are not certified. Excludes hospital-based facilities as they are counted in hospital care expenditures.

Percent of Total Personal Health Care Expenditures
Spent on Nursing Home Care in 1993
National Percent = 8.5%*

ALPHA ORDER

RANK	STATE	PERCENT
43	Alabama	5.8
50	Alaska	3.6
45	Arizona	5.3
19	Arkansas	9.1
48	California	4.4
39	Colorado	6.6
1	Connecticut	14.3
17	Delaware	9.6
36	Florida	6.9
46	Georgia	5.2
46	Hawaii	5.2
22	Idaho	8.7
19	Illinois	9.1
7	Indiana	12.3
6	Iowa	12.6
14	Kansas	10.4
29	Kentucky	8.2
19	Louisiana	9.1
5	Maine	13.2
31	Maryland	7.8
10	Massachusetts	11.7
37	Michigan	6.8
4	Minnesota	13.3
33	Mississippi	7.4
23	Missouri	8.6
25	Montana	8.5
13	Nebraska	11.0
48	Nevada	4.4
31	New Hampshire	7.8
27	New Jersey	8.3
44	New Mexico	5.5
3	New York	13.6
23	North Carolina	8.6
8	North Dakota	12.2
11	Ohio	11.2
18	Oklahoma	9.3
29	Oregon	8.2
15	Pennsylvania	10.0
2	Rhode Island	14.1
34	South Carolina	7.1
12	South Dakota	11.1
38	Tennessee	6.7
41	Texas	6.2
40	Utah	6.3
16	Vermont	9.9
42	Virginia	5.9
25	Washington	8.5
35	West Virginia	7.0
9	Wisconsin	12.1
27	Wyoming	8.3

RANK ORDER

RANK	STATE	PERCENT
1	Connecticut	14.3
2	Rhode Island	14.1
3	New York	13.6
4	Minnesota	13.3
5	Maine	13.2
6	Iowa	12.6
7	Indiana	12.3
8	North Dakota	12.2
9	Wisconsin	12.1
10	Massachusetts	11.7
11	Ohio	11.2
12	South Dakota	11.1
13	Nebraska	11.0
14	Kansas	10.4
15	Pennsylvania	10.0
16	Vermont	9.9
17	Delaware	9.6
18	Oklahoma	9.3
19	Arkansas	9.1
19	Illinois	9.1
19	Louisiana	9.1
22	Idaho	8.7
23	Missouri	8.6
23	North Carolina	8.6
25	Montana	8.5
25	Washington	8.5
27	New Jersey	8.3
27	Wyoming	8.3
29	Kentucky	8.2
29	Oregon	8.2
31	Maryland	7.8
31	New Hampshire	7.8
33	Mississippi	7.4
34	South Carolina	7.1
35	West Virginia	7.0
36	Florida	6.9
37	Michigan	6.8
38	Tennessee	6.7
39	Colorado	6.6
40	Utah	6.3
41	Texas	6.2
42	Virginia	5.9
43	Alabama	5.8
44	New Mexico	5.5
45	Arizona	5.3
46	Georgia	5.2
46	Hawaii	5.2
48	California	4.4
48	Nevada	4.4
50	Alaska	3.6

District of Columbia   5.4

Source: Morgan Quitno Press using data from U.S. Dept of Health & Human Services, Health Care Financing Admin.
"State Health Expenditure Accounts" (Health Care Financing Review, Fall 1995, Volume 17, Number 1)
*By state of provider. Includes freestanding nursing and personal-care facilities. Includes Medicare- and
Medicaid-certified skilled nursing and intermediate care facilities as well as facilities that are not certified.
Excludes hospital-based facilities as they are counted in hospital care expenditures.

Per Capita Expenditures for Nursing Home Care in 1993

National Per Capita = $257*

ALPHA ORDER

RANK	STATE	PER CAPITA
41	Alabama	$168
50	Alaska	94
45	Arizona	144
26	Arkansas	230
48	California	131
35	Colorado	185
1	Connecticut	534
13	Delaware	310
27	Florida	225
44	Georgia	150
42	Hawaii	155
36	Idaho	179
19	Illinois	269
8	Indiana	354
12	Iowa	328
16	Kansas	285
29	Kentucky	224
17	Louisiana	277
7	Maine	366
23	Maryland	239
4	Massachusetts	455
34	Michigan	196
5	Minnesota	416
39	Mississippi	174
20	Missouri	261
32	Montana	212
15	Nebraska	299
49	Nevada	118
23	New Hampshire	239
18	New Jersey	271
47	New Mexico	133
2	New York	502
27	North Carolina	225
6	North Dakota	386
11	Ohio	340
25	Oklahoma	231
30	Oregon	216
10	Pennsylvania	345
3	Rhode Island	485
38	South Carolina	176
14	South Dakota	301
31	Tennessee	213
40	Texas	172
46	Utah	140
21	Vermont	257
43	Virginia	151
22	Washington	246
33	West Virginia	201
9	Wisconsin	347
37	Wyoming	177

RANK ORDER

RANK	STATE	PER CAPITA
1	Connecticut	$534
2	New York	502
3	Rhode Island	485
4	Massachusetts	455
5	Minnesota	416
6	North Dakota	386
7	Maine	366
8	Indiana	354
9	Wisconsin	347
10	Pennsylvania	345
11	Ohio	340
12	Iowa	328
13	Delaware	310
14	South Dakota	301
15	Nebraska	299
16	Kansas	285
17	Louisiana	277
18	New Jersey	271
19	Illinois	269
20	Missouri	261
21	Vermont	257
22	Washington	246
23	Maryland	239
23	New Hampshire	239
25	Oklahoma	231
26	Arkansas	230
27	Florida	225
27	North Carolina	225
29	Kentucky	224
30	Oregon	216
31	Tennessee	213
32	Montana	212
33	West Virginia	201
34	Michigan	196
35	Colorado	185
36	Idaho	179
37	Wyoming	177
38	South Carolina	176
39	Mississippi	174
40	Texas	172
41	Alabama	168
42	Hawaii	155
43	Virginia	151
44	Georgia	150
45	Arizona	144
46	Utah	140
47	New Mexico	133
48	California	131
49	Nevada	118
50	Alaska	94
	District of Columbia	400

Source: Morgan Quitno Press using data from U.S. Dept of Health & Human Services, Health Care Financing Admin. "State Health Expenditure Accounts" (Health Care Financing Review, Fall 1995, Volume 17, Number 1)
By state of provider. Includes freestanding nursing and personal-care facilities. Includes Medicare- and Medicaid-certified skilled nursing and intermediate care facilities as well as facilities that are not certified. Excludes hospital-based facilities as they are counted in hospital care expenditures.

Average Annual Change in Expenditures for Nursing Home Care: 1980 to 1993

National Percent = 10.7% Average Annual Increase*

ALPHA ORDER				RANK ORDER		
RANK	STATE	PERCENT		RANK	STATE	PERCENT
23	Alabama	10.8		1	Florida	16.7
50	Alaska	7.3		2	Arizona	15.9
2	Arizona	15.9		3	New Mexico	15.6
46	Arkansas	8.5		4	West Virginia	14.7
43	California	9.0		5	North Carolina	14.4
42	Colorado	9.2		6	Nevada	13.7
11	Connecticut	12.6		7	Indiana	13.1
9	Delaware	12.8		8	Louisiana	12.9
1	Florida	16.7		9	Delaware	12.8
27	Georgia	10.5		10	Ohio	12.7
19	Hawaii	11.2		11	Connecticut	12.6
22	Idaho	10.9		11	Maryland	12.6
23	Illinois	10.8		13	New Jersey	11.8
7	Indiana	13.1		13	North Dakota	11.8
47	Iowa	8.2		15	Tennessee	11.7
35	Kansas	9.8		16	Massachusetts	11.4
29	Kentucky	10.1		16	New Hampshire	11.4
8	Louisiana	12.9		18	Wyoming	11.3
23	Maine	10.8		19	Hawaii	11.2
11	Maryland	12.6		19	South Carolina	11.2
16	Massachusetts	11.4		21	Rhode Island	11.1
44	Michigan	8.9		22	Idaho	10.9
40	Minnesota	9.4		23	Alabama	10.8
31	Mississippi	10.0		23	Illinois	10.8
23	Missouri	10.8		23	Maine	10.8
27	Montana	10.5		23	Missouri	10.8
49	Nebraska	7.7		27	Georgia	10.5
6	Nevada	13.7		27	Montana	10.5
16	New Hampshire	11.4		29	Kentucky	10.1
13	New Jersey	11.8		29	Washington	10.1
3	New Mexico	15.6		31	Mississippi	10.0
39	New York	9.5		31	Oklahoma	10.0
5	North Carolina	14.4		31	Pennsylvania	10.0
13	North Dakota	11.8		31	Utah	10.0
10	Ohio	12.7		35	Kansas	9.8
31	Oklahoma	10.0		36	Oregon	9.7
36	Oregon	9.7		36	Texas	9.7
31	Pennsylvania	10.0		36	Virginia	9.7
21	Rhode Island	11.1		39	New York	9.5
19	South Carolina	11.2		40	Minnesota	9.4
47	South Dakota	8.2		40	Wisconsin	9.4
15	Tennessee	11.7		42	Colorado	9.2
36	Texas	9.7		43	California	9.0
31	Utah	10.0		44	Michigan	8.9
44	Vermont	8.9		44	Vermont	8.9
36	Virginia	9.7		46	Arkansas	8.5
29	Washington	10.1		47	Iowa	8.2
4	West Virginia	14.7		47	South Dakota	8.2
40	Wisconsin	9.4		49	Nebraska	7.7
18	Wyoming	11.3		50	Alaska	7.3
					District of Columbia	18.3

Source: U.S. Department of Health and Human Services, Health Care Financing Administration
"State Health Expenditure Accounts" (Health Care Financing Review, Fall 1995, Volume 17, Number 1)
*By state of provider. Includes freestanding nursing and personal-care facilities. Includes Medicare- and Medicaid-certified skilled nursing and intermediate care facilities as well as facilities that are not certified. Excludes hospital-based facilities as they are counted in hospital care expenditures.

Other Personal Health Care Expenditures in 1993

National Total = $17,988,000,000*

RANK	STATE	EXPENDITURES	% of USA		RANK	STATE	EXPENDITURES	% of USA
22	Alabama	$323,000,000	1.80%		1	New York	$1,635,000,000	9.09%
45	Alaska	68,000,000	0.38%		2	California	1,565,000,000	8.70%
27	Arizona	230,000,000	1.28%		3	Texas	1,325,000,000	7.37%
37	Arkansas	127,000,000	0.71%		4	Florida	912,000,000	5.07%
2	California	1,565,000,000	8.70%		5	Pennsylvania	798,000,000	4.44%
21	Colorado	327,000,000	1.82%		6	Illinois	636,000,000	3.54%
12	Connecticut	467,000,000	2.60%		7	Massachusetts	597,000,000	3.32%
43	Delaware	79,000,000	0.44%		8	New Jersey	570,000,000	3.17%
4	Florida	912,000,000	5.07%		9	Michigan	532,000,000	2.96%
10	Georgia	516,000,000	2.87%		10	Georgia	516,000,000	2.87%
39	Hawaii	104,000,000	0.58%		11	Ohio	511,000,000	2.84%
48	Idaho	55,000,000	0.31%		12	Connecticut	467,000,000	2.60%
6	Illinois	636,000,000	3.54%		13	Washington	425,000,000	2.36%
25	Indiana	264,000,000	1.47%		14	Wisconsin	415,000,000	2.31%
37	Iowa	127,000,000	0.71%		15	North Carolina	413,000,000	2.30%
34	Kansas	140,000,000	0.78%		16	Virginia	395,000,000	2.20%
28	Kentucky	228,000,000	1.27%		17	Oregon	391,000,000	2.17%
20	Louisiana	328,000,000	1.82%		18	Minnesota	386,000,000	2.15%
32	Maine	153,000,000	0.85%		19	Missouri	346,000,000	1.92%
24	Maryland	312,000,000	1.73%		20	Louisiana	328,000,000	1.82%
7	Massachusetts	597,000,000	3.32%		21	Colorado	327,000,000	1.82%
9	Michigan	532,000,000	2.96%		22	Alabama	323,000,000	1.80%
18	Minnesota	386,000,000	2.15%		23	South Carolina	317,000,000	1.76%
33	Mississippi	141,000,000	0.78%		24	Maryland	312,000,000	1.73%
19	Missouri	346,000,000	1.92%		25	Indiana	264,000,000	1.47%
44	Montana	74,000,000	0.41%		26	Tennessee	235,000,000	1.31%
40	Nebraska	99,000,000	0.55%		27	Arizona	230,000,000	1.28%
46	Nevada	67,000,000	0.37%		28	Kentucky	228,000,000	1.27%
35	New Hampshire	136,000,000	0.76%		29	Rhode Island	219,000,000	1.22%
8	New Jersey	570,000,000	3.17%		30	Oklahoma	196,000,000	1.09%
36	New Mexico	131,000,000	0.73%		31	West Virginia	192,000,000	1.07%
1	New York	1,635,000,000	9.09%		32	Maine	153,000,000	0.85%
15	North Carolina	413,000,000	2.30%		33	Mississippi	141,000,000	0.78%
50	North Dakota	52,000,000	0.29%		34	Kansas	140,000,000	0.78%
11	Ohio	511,000,000	2.84%		35	New Hampshire	136,000,000	0.76%
30	Oklahoma	196,000,000	1.09%		36	New Mexico	131,000,000	0.73%
17	Oregon	391,000,000	2.17%		37	Arkansas	127,000,000	0.71%
5	Pennsylvania	798,000,000	4.44%		37	Iowa	127,000,000	0.71%
29	Rhode Island	219,000,000	1.22%		39	Hawaii	104,000,000	0.58%
23	South Carolina	317,000,000	1.76%		40	Nebraska	99,000,000	0.55%
47	South Dakota	63,000,000	0.35%		40	Utah	99,000,000	0.55%
26	Tennessee	235,000,000	1.31%		42	Vermont	82,000,000	0.46%
3	Texas	1,325,000,000	7.37%		43	Delaware	79,000,000	0.44%
40	Utah	99,000,000	0.55%		44	Montana	74,000,000	0.41%
42	Vermont	82,000,000	0.46%		45	Alaska	68,000,000	0.38%
16	Virginia	395,000,000	2.20%		46	Nevada	67,000,000	0.37%
13	Washington	425,000,000	2.36%		47	South Dakota	63,000,000	0.35%
31	West Virginia	192,000,000	1.07%		48	Idaho	55,000,000	0.31%
14	Wisconsin	415,000,000	2.31%		48	Wyoming	55,000,000	0.31%
48	Wyoming	55,000,000	0.31%		50	North Dakota	52,000,000	0.29%
						District of Columbia	130,000,000	0.72%

Source: U.S. Department of Health and Human Services, Health Care Financing Administration
"State Health Expenditure Accounts" (Health Care Financing Review, Fall 1995, Volume 17, Number 1)
*By state of provider. "Other" covers spending for health care that is not provided through health care establishments. Services in this category are provided through non-medical locations such as job sites, schools, military field-stations or community centers where delivery of medical services is incidental to the function of the site.

Percent of Total Personal Health Care Expenditures
Spent on Other Personal Health Care in 1993
National Percent = 2.3%*

ALPHA ORDER

RANK	STATE	PERCENT
19	Alabama	2.7
6	Alaska	4.3
34	Arizona	2.2
38	Arkansas	2.1
46	California	1.7
14	Colorado	3.2
8	Connecticut	3.8
10	Delaware	3.5
40	Florida	2.0
22	Georgia	2.6
16	Hawaii	3.0
26	Idaho	2.4
44	Illinois	1.8
48	Indiana	1.6
46	Iowa	1.7
40	Kansas	2.0
34	Kentucky	2.2
24	Louisiana	2.5
5	Maine	4.5
38	Maryland	2.1
24	Massachusetts	2.5
40	Michigan	2.0
19	Minnesota	2.7
31	Mississippi	2.3
34	Missouri	2.2
10	Montana	3.5
31	Nebraska	2.3
44	Nevada	1.8
7	New Hampshire	3.9
34	New Jersey	2.2
13	New Mexico	3.4
26	New York	2.4
31	North Carolina	2.3
22	North Dakota	2.6
49	Ohio	1.5
26	Oklahoma	2.4
4	Oregon	4.9
43	Pennsylvania	1.9
1	Rhode Island	6.4
10	South Carolina	3.5
14	South Dakota	3.2
49	Tennessee	1.5
19	Texas	2.7
26	Utah	2.4
2	Vermont	5.5
26	Virginia	2.4
18	Washington	2.8
9	West Virginia	3.7
17	Wisconsin	2.9
2	Wyoming	5.5

RANK ORDER

RANK	STATE	PERCENT
1	Rhode Island	6.4
2	Vermont	5.5
2	Wyoming	5.5
4	Oregon	4.9
5	Maine	4.5
6	Alaska	4.3
7	New Hampshire	3.9
8	Connecticut	3.8
9	West Virginia	3.7
10	Delaware	3.5
10	Montana	3.5
10	South Carolina	3.5
13	New Mexico	3.4
14	Colorado	3.2
14	South Dakota	3.2
16	Hawaii	3.0
17	Wisconsin	2.9
18	Washington	2.8
19	Alabama	2.7
19	Minnesota	2.7
19	Texas	2.7
22	Georgia	2.6
22	North Dakota	2.6
24	Louisiana	2.5
24	Massachusetts	2.5
26	Idaho	2.4
26	New York	2.4
26	Oklahoma	2.4
26	Utah	2.4
26	Virginia	2.4
31	Mississippi	2.3
31	Nebraska	2.3
31	North Carolina	2.3
34	Arizona	2.2
34	Kentucky	2.2
34	Missouri	2.2
34	New Jersey	2.2
38	Arkansas	2.1
38	Maryland	2.1
40	Florida	2.0
40	Kansas	2.0
40	Michigan	2.0
43	Pennsylvania	1.9
44	Illinois	1.8
44	Nevada	1.8
46	California	1.7
46	Iowa	1.7
48	Indiana	1.6
49	Ohio	1.5
49	Tennessee	1.5

| | District of Columbia | 3.0 |

Source: Morgan Quitno Press using data from U.S. Dept of Health & Human Services, Health Care Financing Admin. "State Health Expenditure Accounts" (Health Care Financing Review, Fall 1995, Volume 17, Number 1)
*By state of provider. "Other" covers spending for health care that is not provided through health care establishments. Services in this category are provided through non-medical locations such as job sites, schools, military field-stations or community centers where delivery of medical services is incidental to the function of the site.

Per Capita Other Personal Health Care Expenditures in 1993

National Per Capita = $69.78*

ALPHA ORDER				RANK ORDER		
RANK	STATE	PER CAPITA		RANK	STATE	PER CAPITA
23	Alabama	$77.25		1	Rhode Island	$219.22
8	Alaska	113.71		2	Connecticut	142.46
37	Arizona	58.32		3	Vermont	142.36
43	Arkansas	52.37		4	Oregon	128.83
44	California	50.13		5	Maine	123.49
12	Colorado	91.65		6	New Hampshire	121.10
2	Connecticut	142.46		7	Wyoming	117.02
9	Delaware	113.02		8	Alaska	113.71
28	Florida	66.46		9	Delaware	113.02
25	Georgia	74.77		10	West Virginia	105.61
14	Hawaii	89.19		11	Massachusetts	99.20
45	Idaho	49.95		12	Colorado	91.65
40	Illinois	54.41		13	New York	90.07
47	Indiana	46.26		14	Hawaii	89.19
50	Iowa	45.00		15	Montana	87.99
39	Kansas	55.29		16	South Dakota	87.87
35	Kentucky	60.11		17	South Carolina	87.40
24	Louisiana	76.47		18	Minnesota	85.32
5	Maine	123.49		19	Wisconsin	82.28
31	Maryland	63.00		20	North Dakota	81.63
11	Massachusetts	99.20		21	New Mexico	81.06
38	Michigan	56.25		22	Washington	80.88
18	Minnesota	85.32		23	Alabama	77.25
41	Mississippi	53.43		24	Louisiana	76.47
30	Missouri	66.09		25	Georgia	74.77
15	Montana	87.99		26	Texas	73.41
32	Nebraska	61.34		27	New Jersey	72.53
46	Nevada	48.38		28	Florida	66.46
6	New Hampshire	121.10		29	Pennsylvania	66.33
27	New Jersey	72.53		30	Missouri	66.09
21	New Mexico	81.06		31	Maryland	63.00
13	New York	90.07		32	Nebraska	61.34
36	North Carolina	59.40		33	Virginia	61.00
20	North Dakota	81.63		34	Oklahoma	60.64
48	Ohio	46.20		35	Kentucky	60.11
34	Oklahoma	60.64		36	North Carolina	59.40
4	Oregon	128.83		37	Arizona	58.32
29	Pennsylvania	66.33		38	Michigan	56.25
1	Rhode Island	219.22		39	Kansas	55.29
17	South Carolina	87.40		40	Illinois	54.41
16	South Dakota	87.87		41	Mississippi	53.43
49	Tennessee	46.14		42	Utah	53.23
26	Texas	73.41		43	Arkansas	52.37
42	Utah	53.23		44	California	50.13
3	Vermont	142.36		45	Idaho	49.95
33	Virginia	61.00		46	Nevada	48.38
22	Washington	80.88		47	Indiana	46.26
10	West Virginia	105.61		48	Ohio	46.20
19	Wisconsin	82.28		49	Tennessee	46.14
7	Wyoming	117.02		50	Iowa	45.00
					District of Columbia	224.91

Source: Morgan Quitno Press using data from U.S. Dept of Health & Human Services, Health Care Financing Admin. "State Health Expenditure Accounts" (Health Care Financing Review, Fall 1995, Volume 17, Number 1)
*By state of provider. "Other" covers spending for health care that is not provided through health care establishments. Services in this category are provided through non-medical locations such as job sites, schools, military field-stations or community centers where delivery of medical services is incidental to the function of the site.

Average Annual Change in
Other Personal Health Care Expenditures: 1980 to 1993
National Percent = 12.4% Average Annual Increase*

ALPHA ORDER			RANK ORDER		
RANK	**STATE**	**PERCENT**	**RANK**	**STATE**	**PERCENT**
25	Alabama	12.4	1	Rhode Island	21.2
47	Alaska	9.9	2	Oregon	19.4
38	Arizona	11.4	3	New Hampshire	17.4
36	Arkansas	11.5	4	Maine	16.7
33	California	11.7	5	Vermont	15.9
36	Colorado	11.5	6	Texas	15.5
10	Connecticut	14.7	7	Delaware	15.2
7	Delaware	15.2	8	Florida	15.1
8	Florida	15.1	9	West Virginia	15.0
22	Georgia	13.1	10	Connecticut	14.7
39	Hawaii	11.3	11	Washington	14.3
20	Idaho	13.2	12	Minnesota	14.0
44	Illinois	10.5	13	Wisconsin	13.9
49	Indiana	8.5	14	Louisiana	13.8
39	Iowa	11.3	14	South Carolina	13.8
19	Kansas	13.5	14	Utah	13.8
20	Kentucky	13.2	17	Missouri	13.6
14	Louisiana	13.8	17	North Dakota	13.6
4	Maine	16.7	19	Kansas	13.5
31	Maryland	11.9	20	Idaho	13.2
25	Massachusetts	12.4	20	Kentucky	13.2
41	Michigan	10.8	22	Georgia	13.1
12	Minnesota	14.0	23	Nevada	12.9
48	Mississippi	9.0	23	North Carolina	12.9
17	Missouri	13.6	25	Alabama	12.4
33	Montana	11.7	25	Massachusetts	12.4
29	Nebraska	12.2	25	New Mexico	12.4
23	Nevada	12.9	25	Oklahoma	12.4
3	New Hampshire	17.4	29	Nebraska	12.2
35	New Jersey	11.6	30	Virginia	12.0
25	New Mexico	12.4	31	Maryland	11.9
43	New York	10.6	32	South Dakota	11.8
23	North Carolina	12.9	33	California	11.7
17	North Dakota	13.6	33	Montana	11.7
50	Ohio	8.2	35	New Jersey	11.6
25	Oklahoma	12.4	36	Arkansas	11.5
2	Oregon	19.4	36	Colorado	11.5
41	Pennsylvania	10.8	38	Arizona	11.4
1	Rhode Island	21.2	39	Hawaii	11.3
14	South Carolina	13.8	39	Iowa	11.3
32	South Dakota	11.8	41	Michigan	10.8
45	Tennessee	10.2	41	Pennsylvania	10.8
6	Texas	15.5	43	New York	10.6
14	Utah	13.8	44	Illinois	10.5
5	Vermont	15.9	45	Tennessee	10.2
30	Virginia	12.0	45	Wyoming	10.2
11	Washington	14.3	47	Alaska	9.9
9	West Virginia	15.0	48	Mississippi	9.0
13	Wisconsin	13.9	49	Indiana	8.5
45	Wyoming	10.2	50	Ohio	8.2

District of Columbia		8.9

Source: U.S. Department of Health and Human Services, Health Care Financing Administration
   "State Health Expenditure Accounts" (Health Care Financing Review, Fall 1995, Volume 17, Number 1)
By state of provider. "Other" covers spending for health care that is not provided through health care
establishments. Services in this category are provided through non-medical locations such as job sites, schools,
military field-stations or community centers where delivery of medical services is incidental to the function of the
site.

Persons Not Covered by Health Insurance in 1996

National Total = 41,716,000 Uninsured*

ALPHA ORDER

RANK	STATE	UNINSURED	% of USA
26	Alabama	550,000	1.32%
46	Alaska	89,000	0.21%
10	Arizona	1,159,000	2.78%
25	Arkansas	566,000	1.36%
1	California	6,514,000	15.62%
19	Colorado	644,000	1.54%
32	Connecticut	368,000	0.88%
44	Delaware	98,000	0.23%
4	Florida	2,722,000	6.53%
6	Georgia	1,319,000	3.16%
43	Hawaii	101,000	0.24%
38	Idaho	196,000	0.47%
5	Illinois	1,337,000	3.21%
22	Indiana	600,000	1.44%
33	Iowa	335,000	0.80%
34	Kansas	292,000	0.70%
21	Kentucky	601,000	1.44%
12	Louisiana	890,000	2.13%
40	Maine	146,000	0.35%
23	Maryland	581,000	1.39%
16	Massachusetts	766,000	1.84%
13	Michigan	857,000	2.05%
29	Minnesota	480,000	1.15%
27	Mississippi	518,000	1.24%
18	Missouri	700,000	1.68%
41	Montana	124,000	0.30%
39	Nebraska	190,000	0.46%
36	Nevada	255,000	0.61%
42	New Hampshire	109,000	0.26%
7	New Jersey	1,317,000	3.16%
31	New Mexico	412,000	0.99%
3	New York	3,132,000	7.51%
9	North Carolina	1,160,000	2.78%
50	North Dakota	62,000	0.15%
8	Ohio	1,292,000	3.10%
24	Oklahoma	570,000	1.37%
28	Oregon	496,000	1.19%
11	Pennsylvania	1,133,000	2.72%
45	Rhode Island	93,000	0.22%
20	South Carolina	634,000	1.52%
47	South Dakota	67,000	0.16%
14	Tennessee	841,000	2.02%
2	Texas	4,680,000	11.22%
37	Utah	240,000	0.58%
49	Vermont	65,000	0.16%
15	Virginia	811,000	1.94%
17	Washington	761,000	1.82%
35	West Virginia	261,000	0.63%
30	Wisconsin	438,000	1.05%
48	Wyoming	66,000	0.16%

RANK ORDER

RANK	STATE	UNINSURED	% of USA
1	California	6,514,000	15.62%
2	Texas	4,680,000	11.22%
3	New York	3,132,000	7.51%
4	Florida	2,722,000	6.53%
5	Illinois	1,337,000	3.21%
6	Georgia	1,319,000	3.16%
7	New Jersey	1,317,000	3.16%
8	Ohio	1,292,000	3.10%
9	North Carolina	1,160,000	2.78%
10	Arizona	1,159,000	2.78%
11	Pennsylvania	1,133,000	2.72%
12	Louisiana	890,000	2.13%
13	Michigan	857,000	2.05%
14	Tennessee	841,000	2.02%
15	Virginia	811,000	1.94%
16	Massachusetts	766,000	1.84%
17	Washington	761,000	1.82%
18	Missouri	700,000	1.68%
19	Colorado	644,000	1.54%
20	South Carolina	634,000	1.52%
21	Kentucky	601,000	1.44%
22	Indiana	600,000	1.44%
23	Maryland	581,000	1.39%
24	Oklahoma	570,000	1.37%
25	Arkansas	566,000	1.36%
26	Alabama	550,000	1.32%
27	Mississippi	518,000	1.24%
28	Oregon	496,000	1.19%
29	Minnesota	480,000	1.15%
30	Wisconsin	438,000	1.05%
31	New Mexico	412,000	0.99%
32	Connecticut	368,000	0.88%
33	Iowa	335,000	0.80%
34	Kansas	292,000	0.70%
35	West Virginia	261,000	0.63%
36	Nevada	255,000	0.61%
37	Utah	240,000	0.58%
38	Idaho	196,000	0.47%
39	Nebraska	190,000	0.46%
40	Maine	146,000	0.35%
41	Montana	124,000	0.30%
42	New Hampshire	109,000	0.26%
43	Hawaii	101,000	0.24%
44	Delaware	98,000	0.23%
45	Rhode Island	93,000	0.22%
46	Alaska	89,000	0.21%
47	South Dakota	67,000	0.16%
48	Wyoming	66,000	0.16%
49	Vermont	65,000	0.16%
50	North Dakota	62,000	0.15%
	District of Columbia	80,000	0.19%

Source: U.S. Bureau of the Census
"Health Insurance Coverage: 1996" (http://www.census.gov/hhes/hlthins/cover96/c96tabf.html)

Percent of Population Not Covered by Health Insurance in 1996

National Percent = 15.6% Not Covered by Health Insurance

<table>
<tr><td colspan="3">ALPHA ORDER</td><td colspan="3">RANK ORDER</td></tr>
<tr><td>RANK</td><td>STATE</td><td>PERCENT</td><td>RANK</td><td>STATE</td><td>PERCENT</td></tr>
<tr><td>28</td><td>Alabama</td><td>12.9</td><td>1</td><td>Texas</td><td>24.3</td></tr>
<tr><td>23</td><td>Alaska</td><td>13.5</td><td>2</td><td>Arizona</td><td>24.1</td></tr>
<tr><td>2</td><td>Arizona</td><td>24.1</td><td>3</td><td>New Mexico</td><td>22.3</td></tr>
<tr><td>4</td><td>Arkansas</td><td>21.7</td><td>4</td><td>Arkansas</td><td>21.7</td></tr>
<tr><td>6</td><td>California</td><td>20.1</td><td>5</td><td>Louisiana</td><td>20.9</td></tr>
<tr><td>14</td><td>Colorado</td><td>16.6</td><td>6</td><td>California</td><td>20.1</td></tr>
<tr><td>40</td><td>Connecticut</td><td>11.0</td><td>7</td><td>Florida</td><td>18.9</td></tr>
<tr><td>26</td><td>Delaware</td><td>13.4</td><td>8</td><td>Mississippi</td><td>18.5</td></tr>
<tr><td>7</td><td>Florida</td><td>18.9</td><td>9</td><td>Georgia</td><td>17.8</td></tr>
<tr><td>9</td><td>Georgia</td><td>17.8</td><td>10</td><td>South Carolina</td><td>17.1</td></tr>
<tr><td>49</td><td>Hawaii</td><td>8.6</td><td>11</td><td>New York</td><td>17.0</td></tr>
<tr><td>15</td><td>Idaho</td><td>16.5</td><td>11</td><td>Oklahoma</td><td>17.0</td></tr>
<tr><td>38</td><td>Illinois</td><td>11.3</td><td>13</td><td>New Jersey</td><td>16.7</td></tr>
<tr><td>41</td><td>Indiana</td><td>10.6</td><td>14</td><td>Colorado</td><td>16.6</td></tr>
<tr><td>33</td><td>Iowa</td><td>11.6</td><td>15</td><td>Idaho</td><td>16.5</td></tr>
<tr><td>35</td><td>Kansas</td><td>11.4</td><td>16</td><td>North Carolina</td><td>16.0</td></tr>
<tr><td>18</td><td>Kentucky</td><td>15.4</td><td>17</td><td>Nevada</td><td>15.6</td></tr>
<tr><td>5</td><td>Louisiana</td><td>20.9</td><td>18</td><td>Kentucky</td><td>15.4</td></tr>
<tr><td>31</td><td>Maine</td><td>12.1</td><td>19</td><td>Oregon</td><td>15.3</td></tr>
<tr><td>35</td><td>Maryland</td><td>11.4</td><td>20</td><td>Tennessee</td><td>15.2</td></tr>
<tr><td>30</td><td>Massachusetts</td><td>12.4</td><td>21</td><td>West Virginia</td><td>14.9</td></tr>
<tr><td>48</td><td>Michigan</td><td>8.9</td><td>22</td><td>Montana</td><td>13.6</td></tr>
<tr><td>42</td><td>Minnesota</td><td>10.2</td><td>23</td><td>Alaska</td><td>13.5</td></tr>
<tr><td>8</td><td>Mississippi</td><td>18.5</td><td>23</td><td>Washington</td><td>13.5</td></tr>
<tr><td>27</td><td>Missouri</td><td>13.2</td><td>23</td><td>Wyoming</td><td>13.5</td></tr>
<tr><td>22</td><td>Montana</td><td>13.6</td><td>26</td><td>Delaware</td><td>13.4</td></tr>
<tr><td>35</td><td>Nebraska</td><td>11.4</td><td>27</td><td>Missouri</td><td>13.2</td></tr>
<tr><td>17</td><td>Nevada</td><td>15.6</td><td>28</td><td>Alabama</td><td>12.9</td></tr>
<tr><td>45</td><td>New Hampshire</td><td>9.5</td><td>29</td><td>Virginia</td><td>12.5</td></tr>
<tr><td>13</td><td>New Jersey</td><td>16.7</td><td>30</td><td>Massachusetts</td><td>12.4</td></tr>
<tr><td>3</td><td>New Mexico</td><td>22.3</td><td>31</td><td>Maine</td><td>12.1</td></tr>
<tr><td>11</td><td>New York</td><td>17.0</td><td>32</td><td>Utah</td><td>12.0</td></tr>
<tr><td>16</td><td>North Carolina</td><td>16.0</td><td>33</td><td>Iowa</td><td>11.6</td></tr>
<tr><td>44</td><td>North Dakota</td><td>9.8</td><td>34</td><td>Ohio</td><td>11.5</td></tr>
<tr><td>34</td><td>Ohio</td><td>11.5</td><td>35</td><td>Kansas</td><td>11.4</td></tr>
<tr><td>11</td><td>Oklahoma</td><td>17.0</td><td>35</td><td>Maryland</td><td>11.4</td></tr>
<tr><td>19</td><td>Oregon</td><td>15.3</td><td>35</td><td>Nebraska</td><td>11.4</td></tr>
<tr><td>45</td><td>Pennsylvania</td><td>9.5</td><td>38</td><td>Illinois</td><td>11.3</td></tr>
<tr><td>43</td><td>Rhode Island</td><td>9.9</td><td>39</td><td>Vermont</td><td>11.1</td></tr>
<tr><td>10</td><td>South Carolina</td><td>17.1</td><td>40</td><td>Connecticut</td><td>11.0</td></tr>
<tr><td>45</td><td>South Dakota</td><td>9.5</td><td>41</td><td>Indiana</td><td>10.6</td></tr>
<tr><td>20</td><td>Tennessee</td><td>15.2</td><td>42</td><td>Minnesota</td><td>10.2</td></tr>
<tr><td>1</td><td>Texas</td><td>24.3</td><td>43</td><td>Rhode Island</td><td>9.9</td></tr>
<tr><td>32</td><td>Utah</td><td>12.0</td><td>44</td><td>North Dakota</td><td>9.8</td></tr>
<tr><td>39</td><td>Vermont</td><td>11.1</td><td>45</td><td>New Hampshire</td><td>9.5</td></tr>
<tr><td>29</td><td>Virginia</td><td>12.5</td><td>45</td><td>Pennsylvania</td><td>9.5</td></tr>
<tr><td>23</td><td>Washington</td><td>13.5</td><td>45</td><td>South Dakota</td><td>9.5</td></tr>
<tr><td>21</td><td>West Virginia</td><td>14.9</td><td>48</td><td>Michigan</td><td>8.9</td></tr>
<tr><td>50</td><td>Wisconsin</td><td>8.4</td><td>49</td><td>Hawaii</td><td>8.6</td></tr>
<tr><td>23</td><td>Wyoming</td><td>13.5</td><td>50</td><td>Wisconsin</td><td>8.4</td></tr>
<tr><td></td><td></td><td></td><td></td><td>District of Columbia</td><td>14.8</td></tr>
</table>

Source: U.S. Bureau of the Census
  "Health Insurance Coverage: 1996" (http://www.census.gov/hhes/hlthins/cover96/c96tabf.html)

Persons Covered by Health Insurance in 1996

National Total = 223,463,411 Insured*

ALPHA ORDER

RANK	STATE	INSURED	% of USA
21	Alabama	3,737,178	1.67%
49	Alaska	515,966	0.23%
24	Arizona	3,275,340	1.47%
33	Arkansas	1,940,293	0.87%
1	California	25,343,646	11.34%
25	Colorado	3,172,179	1.42%
27	Connecticut	2,899,293	1.30%
46	Delaware	625,475	0.28%
4	Florida	11,696,917	5.23%
11	Georgia	6,015,274	2.69%
40	Hawaii	1,081,948	0.48%
42	Idaho	991,597	0.44%
6	Illinois	10,508,316	4.70%
14	Indiana	5,228,090	2.34%
30	Iowa	2,513,033	1.12%
31	Kansas	2,287,149	1.02%
23	Kentucky	3,281,071	1.47%
22	Louisiana	3,450,818	1.54%
39	Maine	1,092,566	0.49%
18	Maryland	4,479,296	2.00%
13	Massachusetts	5,319,395	2.38%
8	Michigan	8,873,925	3.97%
20	Minnesota	4,168,596	1.87%
32	Mississippi	2,192,750	0.98%
17	Missouri	4,663,669	2.09%
44	Montana	752,684	0.34%
36	Nebraska	1,458,696	0.65%
37	Nevada	1,345,810	0.60%
41	New Hampshire	1,051,213	0.47%
9	New Jersey	6,684,850	2.99%
38	New Mexico	1,299,256	0.58%
2	New York	15,002,226	6.71%
10	North Carolina	6,149,055	2.75%
47	North Dakota	580,633	0.26%
7	Ohio	9,870,797	4.42%
28	Oklahoma	2,725,315	1.22%
29	Oregon	2,700,313	1.21%
5	Pennsylvania	10,907,084	4.88%
43	Rhode Island	895,283	0.40%
26	South Carolina	3,082,645	1.38%
45	South Dakota	670,561	0.30%
19	Tennessee	4,466,381	2.00%
3	Texas	14,411,207	6.45%
34	Utah	1,777,573	0.80%
48	Vermont	521,461	0.23%
12	Virginia	5,855,167	2.62%
15	Washington	4,758,525	2.13%
35	West Virginia	1,559,407	0.70%
16	Wisconsin	4,708,199	2.11%
50	Wyoming	414,011	0.19%

RANK ORDER

RANK	STATE	INSURED	% of USA
1	California	25,343,646	11.34%
2	New York	15,002,226	6.71%
3	Texas	14,411,207	6.45%
4	Florida	11,696,917	5.23%
5	Pennsylvania	10,907,084	4.88%
6	Illinois	10,508,316	4.70%
7	Ohio	9,870,797	4.42%
8	Michigan	8,873,925	3.97%
9	New Jersey	6,684,850	2.99%
10	North Carolina	6,149,055	2.75%
11	Georgia	6,015,274	2.69%
12	Virginia	5,855,167	2.62%
13	Massachusetts	5,319,395	2.38%
14	Indiana	5,228,090	2.34%
15	Washington	4,758,525	2.13%
16	Wisconsin	4,708,199	2.11%
17	Missouri	4,663,669	2.09%
18	Maryland	4,479,296	2.00%
19	Tennessee	4,466,381	2.00%
20	Minnesota	4,168,596	1.87%
21	Alabama	3,737,178	1.67%
22	Louisiana	3,450,818	1.54%
23	Kentucky	3,281,071	1.47%
24	Arizona	3,275,340	1.47%
25	Colorado	3,172,179	1.42%
26	South Carolina	3,082,645	1.38%
27	Connecticut	2,899,293	1.30%
28	Oklahoma	2,725,315	1.22%
29	Oregon	2,700,313	1.21%
30	Iowa	2,513,033	1.12%
31	Kansas	2,287,149	1.02%
32	Mississippi	2,192,750	0.98%
33	Arkansas	1,940,293	0.87%
34	Utah	1,777,573	0.80%
35	West Virginia	1,559,407	0.70%
36	Nebraska	1,458,696	0.65%
37	Nevada	1,345,810	0.60%
38	New Mexico	1,299,256	0.58%
39	Maine	1,092,566	0.49%
40	Hawaii	1,081,948	0.48%
41	New Hampshire	1,051,213	0.47%
42	Idaho	991,597	0.44%
43	Rhode Island	895,283	0.40%
44	Montana	752,684	0.34%
45	South Dakota	670,561	0.30%
46	Delaware	625,475	0.28%
47	North Dakota	580,633	0.26%
48	Vermont	521,461	0.23%
49	Alaska	515,966	0.23%
50	Wyoming	414,011	0.19%
	District of Columbia	459,279	0.21%

Source: Morgan Quitno Press using data from U.S. Bureau of the Census
"Health Insurance Coverage: 1996" (http://www.census.gov/hhes/hlthins/cover96/c96tabf.html)
*Calculated by the editors by subtracting number of uninsured reported by Census from latest 1996 Census population estimates.

Percent of Population Covered by Health Insurance in 1996

National Percent = 84.4% of Population Covered by Health Insurance*

ALPHA ORDER

RANK	STATE	PERCENT
23	Alabama	87.1
26	Alaska	86.5
49	Arizona	75.9
47	Arkansas	78.3
45	California	79.9
37	Colorado	83.4
11	Connecticut	89.0
25	Delaware	86.6
44	Florida	81.1
42	Georgia	82.2
2	Hawaii	91.4
36	Idaho	83.5
13	Illinois	88.7
10	Indiana	89.4
18	Iowa	88.4
14	Kansas	88.6
33	Kentucky	84.6
46	Louisiana	79.1
20	Maine	87.9
14	Maryland	88.6
21	Massachusetts	87.6
3	Michigan	91.1
9	Minnesota	89.8
43	Mississippi	81.5
24	Missouri	86.8
29	Montana	86.4
14	Nebraska	88.6
34	Nevada	84.4
4	New Hampshire	90.5
38	New Jersey	83.3
48	New Mexico	77.7
39	New York	83.0
35	North Carolina	84.0
7	North Dakota	90.2
17	Ohio	88.5
39	Oklahoma	83.0
32	Oregon	84.7
4	Pennsylvania	90.5
8	Rhode Island	90.1
41	South Carolina	82.9
4	South Dakota	90.5
31	Tennessee	84.8
50	Texas	75.7
19	Utah	88.0
12	Vermont	88.9
22	Virginia	87.5
26	Washington	86.5
30	West Virginia	85.1
1	Wisconsin	91.6
26	Wyoming	86.5

RANK ORDER

RANK	STATE	PERCENT
1	Wisconsin	91.6
2	Hawaii	91.4
3	Michigan	91.1
4	New Hampshire	90.5
4	Pennsylvania	90.5
4	South Dakota	90.5
7	North Dakota	90.2
8	Rhode Island	90.1
9	Minnesota	89.8
10	Indiana	89.4
11	Connecticut	89.0
12	Vermont	88.9
13	Illinois	88.7
14	Kansas	88.6
14	Maryland	88.6
14	Nebraska	88.6
17	Ohio	88.5
18	Iowa	88.4
19	Utah	88.0
20	Maine	87.9
21	Massachusetts	87.6
22	Virginia	87.5
23	Alabama	87.1
24	Missouri	86.8
25	Delaware	86.6
26	Alaska	86.5
26	Washington	86.5
26	Wyoming	86.5
29	Montana	86.4
30	West Virginia	85.1
31	Tennessee	84.8
32	Oregon	84.7
33	Kentucky	84.6
34	Nevada	84.4
35	North Carolina	84.0
36	Idaho	83.5
37	Colorado	83.4
38	New Jersey	83.3
39	New York	83.0
39	Oklahoma	83.0
41	South Carolina	82.9
42	Georgia	82.2
43	Mississippi	81.5
44	Florida	81.1
45	California	79.9
46	Louisiana	79.1
47	Arkansas	78.3
48	New Mexico	77.7
49	Arizona	75.9
50	Texas	75.7

District of Columbia	85.2

Source: Morgan Quitno Press using data from U.S. Bureau of the Census
  "Health Insurance Coverage: 1996" (http://www.census.gov/hhes/hlthins/cover96/c96tabf.html)
*This is the reverse of percent of population not covered in each state issued by Census.

Persons Not Covered by Health Insurance in 1991

National Total = 36,306,864 Uninsured*

ALPHA ORDER

RANK	STATE	UNINSURED	% of USA
14	Alabama	739,747	2.04%
46	Alaska	77,953	0.21%
18	Arizona	659,472	1.82%
29	Arkansas	374,618	1.03%
1	California	5,900,704	16.25%
30	Colorado	347,110	0.96%
35	Connecticut	250,116	0.69%
44	Delaware	92,480	0.25%
3	Florida	2,511,432	6.92%
10	Georgia	940,608	2.59%
45	Hawaii	80,514	0.22%
38	Idaho	187,020	0.52%
5	Illinois	1,359,950	3.75%
15	Indiana	733,993	2.02%
34	Iowa	251,280	0.69%
32	Kansas	286,580	0.79%
24	Kentucky	486,665	1.34%
11	Louisiana	886,369	2.44%
39	Maine	137,307	0.38%
19	Maryland	641,388	1.77%
16	Massachusetts	666,222	1.83%
13	Michigan	852,670	2.35%
27	Minnesota	411,897	1.13%
23	Mississippi	495,454	1.36%
20	Missouri	634,434	1.75%
42	Montana	103,424	0.28%
40	Nebraska	132,136	0.36%
37	Nevada	242,865	0.67%
41	New Hampshire	111,908	0.31%
12	New Jersey	854,370	2.35%
31	New Mexico	341,887	0.94%
4	New York	2,291,207	6.31%
8	North Carolina	1,012,800	2.79%
50	North Dakota	47,550	0.13%
6	Ohio	1,125,996	3.10%
21	Oklahoma	586,080	1.61%
26	Oregon	426,320	1.17%
9	Pennsylvania	955,760	2.63%
43	Rhode Island	103,412	0.28%
25	South Carolina	473,081	1.30%
48	South Dakota	70,200	0.19%
17	Tennessee	663,300	1.83%
2	Texas	3,954,432	10.89%
36	Utah	247,380	0.68%
47	Vermont	72,704	0.20%
7	Virginia	1,031,068	2.84%
22	Washington	531,908	1.47%
33	West Virginia	282,443	0.78%
28	Wisconsin	400,869	1.10%
49	Wyoming	51,296	0.14%

RANK ORDER

RANK	STATE	UNINSURED	% of USA
1	California	5,900,704	16.25%
2	Texas	3,954,432	10.89%
3	Florida	2,511,432	6.92%
4	New York	2,291,207	6.31%
5	Illinois	1,359,950	3.75%
6	Ohio	1,125,996	3.10%
7	Virginia	1,031,068	2.84%
8	North Carolina	1,012,800	2.79%
9	Pennsylvania	955,760	2.63%
10	Georgia	940,608	2.59%
11	Louisiana	886,369	2.44%
12	New Jersey	854,370	2.35%
13	Michigan	852,670	2.35%
14	Alabama	739,747	2.04%
15	Indiana	733,993	2.02%
16	Massachusetts	666,222	1.83%
17	Tennessee	663,300	1.83%
18	Arizona	659,472	1.82%
19	Maryland	641,388	1.77%
20	Missouri	634,434	1.75%
21	Oklahoma	586,080	1.61%
22	Washington	531,908	1.47%
23	Mississippi	495,454	1.36%
24	Kentucky	486,665	1.34%
25	South Carolina	473,081	1.30%
26	Oregon	426,320	1.17%
27	Minnesota	411,897	1.13%
28	Wisconsin	400,869	1.10%
29	Arkansas	374,618	1.03%
30	Colorado	347,110	0.96%
31	New Mexico	341,887	0.94%
32	Kansas	286,580	0.79%
33	West Virginia	282,443	0.78%
34	Iowa	251,280	0.69%
35	Connecticut	250,116	0.69%
36	Utah	247,380	0.68%
37	Nevada	242,865	0.67%
38	Idaho	187,020	0.52%
39	Maine	137,307	0.38%
40	Nebraska	132,136	0.36%
41	New Hampshire	111,908	0.31%
42	Montana	103,424	0.28%
43	Rhode Island	103,412	0.28%
44	Delaware	92,480	0.25%
45	Hawaii	80,514	0.22%
46	Alaska	77,953	0.21%
47	Vermont	72,704	0.20%
48	South Dakota	70,200	0.19%
49	Wyoming	51,296	0.14%
50	North Dakota	47,550	0.13%

District of Columbia	155,628	0.43%

*Source: Morgan Quitno Press using data from U.S. Bureau of the Census
"Health Insurance Coverage - 1993" (Statistical Brief, SB/94-28, October 1994)*
**Based on percent of uninsured in each state issued by Census and 1991 state population estimates. National
total calculated using 1991 national population estimate multiplied by Census national uninsured figure of 14.4%.*

Percent of Persons Not Covered by Health Insurance in 1991

National Percent = 14.4% Uninsured

ALPHA ORDER				RANK ORDER		
RANK	STATE	PERCENT		RANK	STATE	PERCENT
9	Alabama	18.1		1	Texas	22.8
19	Alaska	13.7		2	New Mexico	22.1
11	Arizona	17.6		3	Louisiana	20.9
13	Arkansas	15.8		4	California	19.4
4	California	19.4		5	Mississippi	19.1
37	Colorado	10.3		6	Florida	18.9
48	Connecticut	7.6		6	Nevada	18.9
20	Delaware	13.6		8	Oklahoma	18.5
6	Florida	18.9		9	Alabama	18.1
17	Georgia	14.2		10	Idaho	18.0
50	Hawaii	7.1		11	Arizona	17.6
10	Idaho	18.0		12	Virginia	16.4
30	Illinois	11.8		13	Arkansas	15.8
24	Indiana	13.1		14	West Virginia	15.7
44	Iowa	9.0		15	North Carolina	15.0
31	Kansas	11.5		16	Oregon	14.6
24	Kentucky	13.1		17	Georgia	14.2
3	Louisiana	20.9		18	Utah	14.0
33	Maine	11.1		19	Alaska	13.7
23	Maryland	13.2		20	Delaware	13.6
33	Massachusetts	11.1		21	Tennessee	13.4
43	Michigan	9.1		22	South Carolina	13.3
42	Minnesota	9.3		23	Maryland	13.2
5	Mississippi	19.1		24	Indiana	13.1
29	Missouri	12.3		24	Kentucky	13.1
26	Montana	12.8		26	Montana	12.8
45	Nebraska	8.3		26	Vermont	12.8
6	Nevada	18.9		28	New York	12.7
40	New Hampshire	10.1		29	Missouri	12.3
35	New Jersey	11.0		30	Illinois	11.8
2	New Mexico	22.1		31	Kansas	11.5
28	New York	12.7		32	Wyoming	11.2
15	North Carolina	15.0		33	Maine	11.1
49	North Dakota	7.5		33	Massachusetts	11.1
37	Ohio	10.3		35	New Jersey	11.0
8	Oklahoma	18.5		36	Washington	10.6
16	Oregon	14.6		37	Colorado	10.3
47	Pennsylvania	8.0		37	Ohio	10.3
37	Rhode Island	10.3		37	Rhode Island	10.3
22	South Carolina	13.3		40	New Hampshire	10.1
41	South Dakota	10.0		41	South Dakota	10.0
21	Tennessee	13.4		42	Minnesota	9.3
1	Texas	22.8		43	Michigan	9.1
18	Utah	14.0		44	Iowa	9.0
26	Vermont	12.8		45	Nebraska	8.3
12	Virginia	16.4		46	Wisconsin	8.1
36	Washington	10.6		47	Pennsylvania	8.0
14	West Virginia	15.7		48	Connecticut	7.6
46	Wisconsin	8.1		49	North Dakota	7.5
32	Wyoming	11.2		50	Hawaii	7.1
					District of Columbia	26.2

Source: U.S. Bureau of the Census
   "Health Insurance Coverage - 1993" (Statistical Brief, SB/94-28, October 1994)

Change in Number of Persons Uninsured: 1991 to 1996

National Change = 5,409,136 Increase

ALPHA ORDER		
RANK	STATE	CHANGE
49	Alabama	(189,747)
32	Alaska	11,047
4	Arizona	499,528
10	Arkansas	191,382
3	California	613,296
7	Colorado	296,890
16	Connecticut	117,884
35	Delaware	5,520
9	Florida	210,568
6	Georgia	378,392
28	Hawaii	20,486
33	Idaho	8,980
46	Illinois	(22,950)
48	Indiana	(133,993)
19	Iowa	83,720
36	Kansas	5,420
17	Kentucky	114,335
38	Louisiana	3,631
34	Maine	8,693
47	Maryland	(60,388)
18	Massachusetts	99,778
37	Michigan	4,330
22	Minnesota	68,103
26	Mississippi	22,546
23	Missouri	65,566
27	Montana	20,576
24	Nebraska	57,864
31	Nevada	12,135
39	New Hampshire	(2,908)
5	New Jersey	462,630
20	New Mexico	70,113
1	New York	840,793
15	North Carolina	147,200
30	North Dakota	14,450
13	Ohio	166,004
44	Oklahoma	(16,080)
21	Oregon	69,680
12	Pennsylvania	177,240
43	Rhode Island	(10,412)
14	South Carolina	160,919
40	South Dakota	(3,200)
11	Tennessee	177,700
2	Texas	725,568
41	Utah	(7,380)
42	Vermont	(7,704)
50	Virginia	(220,068)
8	Washington	229,092
45	West Virginia	(21,443)
25	Wisconsin	37,131
29	Wyoming	14,704

RANK ORDER		
RANK	STATE	CHANGE
1	New York	840,793
2	Texas	725,568
3	California	613,296
4	Arizona	499,528
5	New Jersey	462,630
6	Georgia	378,392
7	Colorado	296,890
8	Washington	229,092
9	Florida	210,568
10	Arkansas	191,382
11	Tennessee	177,700
12	Pennsylvania	177,240
13	Ohio	166,004
14	South Carolina	160,919
15	North Carolina	147,200
16	Connecticut	117,884
17	Kentucky	114,335
18	Massachusetts	99,778
19	Iowa	83,720
20	New Mexico	70,113
21	Oregon	69,680
22	Minnesota	68,103
23	Missouri	65,566
24	Nebraska	57,864
25	Wisconsin	37,131
26	Mississippi	22,546
27	Montana	20,576
28	Hawaii	20,486
29	Wyoming	14,704
30	North Dakota	14,450
31	Nevada	12,135
32	Alaska	11,047
33	Idaho	8,980
34	Maine	8,693
35	Delaware	5,520
36	Kansas	5,420
37	Michigan	4,330
38	Louisiana	3,631
39	New Hampshire	(2,908)
40	South Dakota	(3,200)
41	Utah	(7,380)
42	Vermont	(7,704)
43	Rhode Island	(10,412)
44	Oklahoma	(16,080)
45	West Virginia	(21,443)
46	Illinois	(22,950)
47	Maryland	(60,388)
48	Indiana	(133,993)
49	Alabama	(189,747)
50	Virginia	(220,068)
	District of Columbia	(75,628)

Source: Morgan Quitno Press using data from U.S. Bureau of the Census
"Health Insurance Coverage: 1996" (http://www.census.gov/hhes/hlthins/cover96/c96tabf.html)
"Health Insurance Coverage: 1993" (Statistical Brief, SB/94-28, October 1994)

Percent Change in Number of Uninsured: 1991 to 1996

National Percent Change = 14.9% Increase

ALPHA ORDER

RANK	STATE	PERCENT CHANGE
50	Alabama	(25.7)
26	Alaska	14.2
2	Arizona	75.7
4	Arkansas	51.1
27	California	10.4
1	Colorado	85.5
5	Connecticut	47.1
32	Delaware	6.0
30	Florida	8.4
8	Georgia	40.2
15	Hawaii	25.4
34	Idaho	4.8
39	Illinois	(1.7)
48	Indiana	(18.3)
11	Iowa	33.3
36	Kansas	1.9
16	Kentucky	23.5
38	Louisiana	0.4
31	Maine	6.3
45	Maryland	(9.4)
23	Massachusetts	15.0
37	Michigan	0.5
21	Minnesota	16.5
35	Mississippi	4.6
28	Missouri	10.3
18	Montana	19.9
6	Nebraska	43.8
33	Nevada	5.0
40	New Hampshire	(2.6)
3	New Jersey	54.1
17	New Mexico	20.5
9	New York	36.7
25	North Carolina	14.5
12	North Dakota	30.4
24	Ohio	14.7
41	Oklahoma	(2.7)
22	Oregon	16.3
19	Pennsylvania	18.5
46	Rhode Island	(10.1)
10	South Carolina	34.0
43	South Dakota	(4.6)
14	Tennessee	26.8
20	Texas	18.3
42	Utah	(3.0)
47	Vermont	(10.6)
49	Virginia	(21.3)
7	Washington	43.1
44	West Virginia	(7.6)
29	Wisconsin	9.3
13	Wyoming	28.7

RANK ORDER

RANK	STATE	PERCENT CHANGE
1	Colorado	85.5
2	Arizona	75.7
3	New Jersey	54.1
4	Arkansas	51.1
5	Connecticut	47.1
6	Nebraska	43.8
7	Washington	43.1
8	Georgia	40.2
9	New York	36.7
10	South Carolina	34.0
11	Iowa	33.3
12	North Dakota	30.4
13	Wyoming	28.7
14	Tennessee	26.8
15	Hawaii	25.4
16	Kentucky	23.5
17	New Mexico	20.5
18	Montana	19.9
19	Pennsylvania	18.5
20	Texas	18.3
21	Minnesota	16.5
22	Oregon	16.3
23	Massachusetts	15.0
24	Ohio	14.7
25	North Carolina	14.5
26	Alaska	14.2
27	California	10.4
28	Missouri	10.3
29	Wisconsin	9.3
30	Florida	8.4
31	Maine	6.3
32	Delaware	6.0
33	Nevada	5.0
34	Idaho	4.8
35	Mississippi	4.6
36	Kansas	1.9
37	Michigan	0.5
38	Louisiana	0.4
39	Illinois	(1.7)
40	New Hampshire	(2.6)
41	Oklahoma	(2.7)
42	Utah	(3.0)
43	South Dakota	(4.6)
44	West Virginia	(7.6)
45	Maryland	(9.4)
46	Rhode Island	(10.1)
47	Vermont	(10.6)
48	Indiana	(18.3)
49	Virginia	(21.3)
50	Alabama	(25.7)

District of Columbia   (48.6)

Source: Morgan Quitno Press using data from U.S. Bureau of the Census
"Health Insurance Coverage: 1996" (http://www.census.gov/hhes/hlthins/cover96/c96tabf.html)
"Health Insurance Coverage: 1993" (Statistical Brief, SB/94-28, October 1994)

Change in Percent of Population Uninsured: 1991 to 1996

National Percent Change = 8.3% Increase

ALPHA ORDER

RANK	STATE	PERCENT CHANGE
50	Alabama	(28.7)
33	Alaska	(1.5)
6	Arizona	36.9
4	Arkansas	37.3
28	California	3.6
1	Colorado	61.2
3	Connecticut	44.7
33	Delaware	(1.5)
30	Florida	0.0
12	Georgia	25.4
13	Hawaii	21.1
43	Idaho	(8.3)
38	Illinois	(4.2)
48	Indiana	(19.1)
9	Iowa	28.9
32	Kansas	(0.9)
16	Kentucky	17.6
30	Louisiana	0.0
21	Maine	9.0
45	Maryland	(13.6)
18	Massachusetts	11.7
35	Michigan	(2.2)
20	Minnesota	9.7
36	Mississippi	(3.1)
22	Missouri	7.3
25	Montana	6.3
4	Nebraska	37.3
47	Nevada	(17.5)
41	New Hampshire	(5.9)
2	New Jersey	51.8
29	New Mexico	0.9
7	New York	33.9
23	North Carolina	6.7
8	North Dakota	30.7
18	Ohio	11.7
42	Oklahoma	(8.1)
26	Oregon	4.8
15	Pennsylvania	18.8
37	Rhode Island	(3.9)
10	South Carolina	28.6
39	South Dakota	(5.0)
17	Tennessee	13.4
24	Texas	6.6
46	Utah	(14.3)
44	Vermont	(13.3)
49	Virginia	(23.8)
11	Washington	27.4
40	West Virginia	(5.1)
27	Wisconsin	3.7
14	Wyoming	20.5

RANK ORDER

RANK	STATE	PERCENT CHANGE
1	Colorado	61.2
2	New Jersey	51.8
3	Connecticut	44.7
4	Arkansas	37.3
4	Nebraska	37.3
6	Arizona	36.9
7	New York	33.9
8	North Dakota	30.7
9	Iowa	28.9
10	South Carolina	28.6
11	Washington	27.4
12	Georgia	25.4
13	Hawaii	21.1
14	Wyoming	20.5
15	Pennsylvania	18.8
16	Kentucky	17.6
17	Tennessee	13.4
18	Massachusetts	11.7
18	Ohio	11.7
20	Minnesota	9.7
21	Maine	9.0
22	Missouri	7.3
23	North Carolina	6.7
24	Texas	6.6
25	Montana	6.3
26	Oregon	4.8
27	Wisconsin	3.7
28	California	3.6
29	New Mexico	0.9
30	Florida	0.0
30	Louisiana	0.0
32	Kansas	(0.9)
33	Alaska	(1.5)
33	Delaware	(1.5)
35	Michigan	(2.2)
36	Mississippi	(3.1)
37	Rhode Island	(3.9)
38	Illinois	(4.2)
39	South Dakota	(5.0)
40	West Virginia	(5.1)
41	New Hampshire	(5.9)
42	Oklahoma	(8.1)
43	Idaho	(8.3)
44	Vermont	(13.3)
45	Maryland	(13.6)
46	Utah	(14.3)
47	Nevada	(17.5)
48	Indiana	(19.1)
49	Virginia	(23.8)
50	Alabama	(28.7)
	District of Columbia	(43.5)

Source: Morgan Quitno Press using data from U.S. Bureau of the Census
"Health Insurance Coverage: 1996" (http://www.census.gov/hhes/hlthins/cover96/c96tabf.html)
"Health Insurance Coverage: 1993" (Statistical Brief, SB/94-28, October 1994)

Managed Care Organizations (MCOs) in 1995

National Total = 1,691 MCOs*

ALPHA ORDER

RANK ORDER

RANK	STATE	MCOs	% of USA		RANK	STATE	MCOs	% of USA
21	Alabama	35	2.07%		1	Florida	118	6.98%
46	Alaska	3	0.18%		2	California	114	6.74%
12	Arizona	47	2.78%		3	Texas	105	6.21%
36	Arkansas	15	0.89%		4	Ohio	82	4.85%
2	California	114	6.74%		5	Pennsylvania	76	4.49%
15	Colorado	40	2.37%		6	Illinois	72	4.26%
26	Connecticut	27	1.60%		7	New York	57	3.37%
38	Delaware	12	0.71%		7	Tennessee	57	3.37%
1	Florida	118	6.98%		9	Wisconsin	53	3.13%
10	Georgia	52	3.08%		10	Georgia	52	3.08%
37	Hawaii	13	0.77%		11	Missouri	48	2.84%
46	Idaho	3	0.18%		12	Arizona	47	2.78%
6	Illinois	72	4.26%		13	Michigan	46	2.72%
14	Indiana	45	2.66%		14	Indiana	45	2.66%
33	Iowa	18	1.06%		15	Colorado	40	2.37%
28	Kansas	26	1.54%		15	Louisiana	40	2.37%
30	Kentucky	22	1.30%		17	North Carolina	39	2.31%
15	Louisiana	40	2.37%		18	Maryland	37	2.19%
39	Maine	11	0.65%		19	Massachusetts	36	2.13%
18	Maryland	37	2.19%		19	Virginia	36	2.13%
19	Massachusetts	36	2.13%		21	Alabama	35	2.07%
13	Michigan	46	2.72%		22	Washington	34	2.01%
25	Minnesota	28	1.66%		23	Nevada	33	1.95%
40	Mississippi	8	0.47%		24	New Jersey	32	1.89%
11	Missouri	48	2.84%		25	Minnesota	28	1.66%
49	Montana	2	0.12%		26	Connecticut	27	1.60%
34	Nebraska	17	1.01%		26	Oklahoma	27	1.60%
23	Nevada	33	1.95%		28	Kansas	26	1.54%
40	New Hampshire	8	0.47%		29	South Carolina	23	1.36%
24	New Jersey	32	1.89%		30	Kentucky	22	1.30%
35	New Mexico	16	0.95%		31	Utah	21	1.24%
7	New York	57	3.37%		32	Oregon	19	1.12%
17	North Carolina	39	2.31%		33	Iowa	18	1.06%
45	North Dakota	4	0.24%		34	Nebraska	17	1.01%
4	Ohio	82	4.85%		35	New Mexico	16	0.95%
26	Oklahoma	27	1.60%		36	Arkansas	15	0.89%
32	Oregon	19	1.12%		37	Hawaii	13	0.77%
5	Pennsylvania	76	4.49%		38	Delaware	12	0.71%
43	Rhode Island	6	0.35%		39	Maine	11	0.65%
29	South Carolina	23	1.36%		40	Mississippi	8	0.47%
44	South Dakota	5	0.30%		40	New Hampshire	8	0.47%
7	Tennessee	57	3.37%		40	West Virginia	8	0.47%
3	Texas	105	6.21%		43	Rhode Island	6	0.35%
31	Utah	21	1.24%		44	South Dakota	5	0.30%
46	Vermont	3	0.18%		45	North Dakota	4	0.24%
19	Virginia	36	2.13%		46	Alaska	3	0.18%
22	Washington	34	2.01%		46	Idaho	3	0.18%
40	West Virginia	8	0.47%		46	Vermont	3	0.18%
9	Wisconsin	53	3.13%		49	Montana	2	0.12%
50	Wyoming	0	0.00%		50	Wyoming	0	0.00%
						District of Columbia	9	0.53%

Source: Morgan Quitno Press using data from American Association of Health Plans
   "1995-1996 Managed Health Care Overview"
*As of October 1995. Managed Care Organizations (MCOs) are a combination of Health Maintenance
Organizations (HMOs) and Preferred Provider Organizations (PPOs). Total does not include MCOs in Guam or
Puerto Rico. Health plans are allocated to states based upon their primary service areas. This means each plan is
counted once. However, many plans serve more than one state.

Enrollment in Managed Care Organizations (MCOs) in 1994

National Total = 136,092,671 Enrollees*

ALPHA ORDER

RANK	STATE	ENROLLEES	% of USA
28	Alabama	1,201,925	0.88%
49	Alaska	135,764	0.10%
20	Arizona	2,419,360	1.78%
36	Arkansas	662,168	0.49%
1	California	19,776,089	14.53%
25	Colorado	2,035,070	1.50%
24	Connecticut	2,043,761	1.50%
43	Delaware	260,781	0.19%
5	Florida	7,276,214	5.35%
15	Georgia	3,199,759	2.35%
35	Hawaii*	753,942	0.55%
44	Idaho	238,108	0.17%
6	Illinois	6,840,835	5.03%
19	Indiana	2,551,244	1.87%
27	Iowa	1,399,578	1.03%
31	Kansas	988,869	0.73%
26	Kentucky	1,417,466	1.04%
21	Louisiana	2,336,434	1.72%
42	Maine	327,029	0.24%
9	Maryland	3,975,222	2.92%
11	Massachusetts	3,795,701	2.79%
8	Michigan	4,876,209	3.58%
10	Minnesota	3,833,657	2.82%
38	Mississippi	603,075	0.44%
16	Missouri	2,939,247	2.16%
46	Montana	182,542	0.13%
37	Nebraska	621,263	0.46%
33	Nevada	843,816	0.62%
40	New Hampshire	432,635	0.32%
12	New Jersey	3,769,843	2.77%
34	New Mexico	779,386	0.57%
3	New York	8,398,596	6.17%
14	North Carolina	3,240,256	2.38%
45	North Dakota	185,217	0.14%
7	Ohio	6,057,577	4.45%
29	Oklahoma	1,144,255	0.84%
23	Oregon	2,077,673	1.53%
4	Pennsylvania	7,299,494	5.36%
41	Rhode Island	412,425	0.30%
30	South Carolina	1,027,572	0.76%
47	South Dakota	179,752	0.13%
13	Tennessee	3,500,036	2.57%
2	Texas	10,296,211	7.57%
32	Utah	966,574	0.71%
48	Vermont	164,127	0.12%
22	Virginia	2,226,008	1.64%
18	Washington	2,710,393	1.99%
39	West Virginia	442,034	0.32%
17	Wisconsin	2,773,074	2.04%
50	Wyoming	92,969	0.07%

RANK ORDER

RANK	STATE	ENROLLEES	% of USA
1	California	19,776,089	14.53%
2	Texas	10,296,211	7.57%
3	New York	8,398,596	6.17%
4	Pennsylvania	7,299,494	5.36%
5	Florida	7,276,214	5.35%
6	Illinois	6,840,835	5.03%
7	Ohio	6,057,577	4.45%
8	Michigan	4,876,209	3.58%
9	Maryland	3,975,222	2.92%
10	Minnesota	3,833,657	2.82%
11	Massachusetts	3,795,701	2.79%
12	New Jersey	3,769,843	2.77%
13	Tennessee	3,500,036	2.57%
14	North Carolina	3,240,256	2.38%
15	Georgia	3,199,759	2.35%
16	Missouri	2,939,247	2.16%
17	Wisconsin	2,773,074	2.04%
18	Washington	2,710,393	1.99%
19	Indiana	2,551,244	1.87%
20	Arizona	2,419,360	1.78%
21	Louisiana	2,336,434	1.72%
22	Virginia	2,226,008	1.64%
23	Oregon	2,077,673	1.53%
24	Connecticut	2,043,761	1.50%
25	Colorado	2,035,070	1.50%
26	Kentucky	1,417,466	1.04%
27	Iowa	1,399,578	1.03%
28	Alabama	1,201,925	0.88%
29	Oklahoma	1,144,255	0.84%
30	South Carolina	1,027,572	0.76%
31	Kansas	988,869	0.73%
32	Utah	966,574	0.71%
33	Nevada	843,816	0.62%
34	New Mexico	779,386	0.57%
35	Hawaii*	753,942	0.55%
36	Arkansas	662,168	0.49%
37	Nebraska	621,263	0.46%
38	Mississippi	603,075	0.44%
39	West Virginia	442,034	0.32%
40	New Hampshire	432,635	0.32%
41	Rhode Island	412,425	0.30%
42	Maine	327,029	0.24%
43	Delaware	260,781	0.19%
44	Idaho	238,108	0.17%
45	North Dakota	185,217	0.14%
46	Montana	182,542	0.13%
47	South Dakota	179,752	0.13%
48	Vermont	164,127	0.12%
49	Alaska	135,764	0.10%
50	Wyoming	92,969	0.07%
	District of Columbia	381,436	0.28%

*Source: American Association of Health Plans (formerly American Managed Care and Review Association)
"Managed Care Covered Lives, Year-end 1994"*

As of December 31, 1994 except Hawaii is December 31, 1993. Managed Care Organizations (MCOs) are a combination of Health Maintenance Organizations (HMOs) and Preferred Provider Organizations (PPOs). Total excludes 234,768 enrollees in Puerto Rico and 81,087 enrollees in Guam. Includes dependents.

Percent of Population Enrolled in a
Managed Care Organization (MCO) in 1994
National Percent = 52.2% of Population*

ALPHA ORDER

RANK	STATE	PERCENT
39	Alabama	28.5
47	Alaska	22.4
10	Arizona	59.4
42	Arkansas	27.0
6	California	62.9
14	Colorado	55.7
8	Connecticut	62.4
35	Delaware	36.9
19	Florida	52.1
28	Georgia	45.4
5	Hawaii*	63.9
49	Idaho	21.0
11	Illinois	58.2
29	Indiana	44.4
23	Iowa	49.5
31	Kansas	38.7
34	Kentucky	37.0
18	Louisiana	54.1
43	Maine	26.4
2	Maryland	79.4
7	Massachusetts	62.8
20	Michigan	51.4
1	Minnesota	83.9
46	Mississippi	22.6
14	Missouri	55.7
48	Montana	21.3
32	Nebraska	38.3
12	Nevada	57.9
33	New Hampshire	38.1
24	New Jersey	47.7
25	New Mexico	47.1
26	New York	46.2
27	North Carolina	45.8
38	North Dakota	29.0
16	Ohio	54.6
36	Oklahoma	35.1
4	Oregon	67.3
9	Pennsylvania	60.6
30	Rhode Island	41.4
41	South Carolina	28.0
44	South Dakota	24.9
3	Tennessee	67.6
13	Texas	56.0
21	Utah	50.7
40	Vermont	28.3
37	Virginia	34.0
21	Washington	50.7
45	West Virginia	24.3
16	Wisconsin	54.6
50	Wyoming	19.5

RANK ORDER

RANK	STATE	PERCENT
1	Minnesota	83.9
2	Maryland	79.4
3	Tennessee	67.6
4	Oregon	67.3
5	Hawaii*	63.9
6	California	62.9
7	Massachusetts	62.8
8	Connecticut	62.4
9	Pennsylvania	60.6
10	Arizona	59.4
11	Illinois	58.2
12	Nevada	57.9
13	Texas	56.0
14	Colorado	55.7
14	Missouri	55.7
16	Ohio	54.6
16	Wisconsin	54.6
18	Louisiana	54.1
19	Florida	52.1
20	Michigan	51.4
21	Utah	50.7
21	Washington	50.7
23	Iowa	49.5
24	New Jersey	47.7
25	New Mexico	47.1
26	New York	46.2
27	North Carolina	45.8
28	Georgia	45.4
29	Indiana	44.4
30	Rhode Island	41.4
31	Kansas	38.7
32	Nebraska	38.3
33	New Hampshire	38.1
34	Kentucky	37.0
35	Delaware	36.9
36	Oklahoma	35.1
37	Virginia	34.0
38	North Dakota	29.0
39	Alabama	28.5
40	Vermont	28.3
41	South Carolina	28.0
42	Arkansas	27.0
43	Maine	26.4
44	South Dakota	24.9
45	West Virginia	24.3
46	Mississippi	22.6
47	Alaska	22.4
48	Montana	21.3
49	Idaho	21.0
50	Wyoming	19.5

| | District of Columbia | 66.9 |

Source: American Association of Health Plans (formerly American Managed Care and Review Association)
  "Managed Care Covered Lives, Year-end 1994"
As of December 31, 1994 except Hawaii is December 31, 1993. Managed Care Organizations (MCOs) are a combination of Health Maintenance Organizations (HMOs) and Preferred Provider Organizations (PPOs). Includes dependents.

Health Maintenance Organizations (HMOs) in 1997

National Total = 648 HMOs*

RANK	STATE	HMOs	% of USA
21	Alabama	11	1.70%
49	Alaska	0	0.00%
24	Arizona	10	1.54%
39	Arkansas	4	0.62%
4	California	38	5.86%
13	Colorado	17	2.62%
17	Connecticut	14	2.16%
34	Delaware	6	0.93%
1	Florida	41	6.33%
15	Georgia	15	2.31%
33	Hawaii	7	1.08%
40	Idaho	3	0.46%
6	Illinois	28	4.32%
15	Indiana	15	2.31%
40	Iowa	3	0.46%
21	Kansas	11	1.70%
24	Kentucky	10	1.54%
18	Louisiana	13	2.01%
40	Maine	3	0.46%
20	Maryland	12	1.85%
21	Massachusetts	11	1.70%
7	Michigan	23	3.55%
27	Minnesota	9	1.39%
27	Mississippi	9	1.39%
7	Missouri	23	3.55%
44	Montana	2	0.31%
38	Nebraska	5	0.77%
27	Nevada	9	1.39%
40	New Hampshire	3	0.46%
11	New Jersey	20	3.09%
34	New Mexico	6	0.93%
5	New York	36	5.56%
11	North Carolina	20	3.09%
44	North Dakota	2	0.31%
3	Ohio	40	6.17%
24	Oklahoma	10	1.54%
31	Oregon	8	1.23%
10	Pennsylvania	21	3.24%
44	Rhode Island	2	0.31%
34	South Carolina	6	0.93%
44	South Dakota	2	0.31%
14	Tennessee	16	2.47%
1	Texas	41	6.33%
31	Utah	8	1.23%
49	Vermont	0	0.00%
18	Virginia	13	2.01%
27	Washington	9	1.39%
34	West Virginia	6	0.93%
7	Wisconsin	23	3.55%
48	Wyoming	1	0.15%

RANK	STATE	HMOs	% of USA
1	Florida	41	6.33%
1	Texas	41	6.33%
3	Ohio	40	6.17%
4	California	38	5.86%
5	New York	36	5.56%
6	Illinois	28	4.32%
7	Michigan	23	3.55%
7	Missouri	23	3.55%
7	Wisconsin	23	3.55%
10	Pennsylvania	21	3.24%
11	New Jersey	20	3.09%
11	North Carolina	20	3.09%
13	Colorado	17	2.62%
14	Tennessee	16	2.47%
15	Georgia	15	2.31%
15	Indiana	15	2.31%
17	Connecticut	14	2.16%
18	Louisiana	13	2.01%
18	Virginia	13	2.01%
20	Maryland	12	1.85%
21	Alabama	11	1.70%
21	Kansas	11	1.70%
21	Massachusetts	11	1.70%
24	Arizona	10	1.54%
24	Kentucky	10	1.54%
24	Oklahoma	10	1.54%
27	Minnesota	9	1.39%
27	Mississippi	9	1.39%
27	Nevada	9	1.39%
27	Washington	9	1.39%
31	Oregon	8	1.23%
31	Utah	8	1.23%
33	Hawaii	7	1.08%
34	Delaware	6	0.93%
34	New Mexico	6	0.93%
34	South Carolina	6	0.93%
34	West Virginia	6	0.93%
38	Nebraska	5	0.77%
39	Arkansas	4	0.62%
40	Idaho	3	0.46%
40	Iowa	3	0.46%
40	Maine	3	0.46%
40	New Hampshire	3	0.46%
44	Montana	2	0.31%
44	North Dakota	2	0.31%
44	Rhode Island	2	0.31%
44	South Dakota	2	0.31%
48	Wyoming	1	0.15%
49	Alaska	0	0.00%
49	Vermont	0	0.00%
	District of Columbia	3	0.46%

Source: InterStudy Publications (Minneapolis, MN)
   "The Competitive Edge Industry Report 7.2" (October 1997)

As of January 1, 1997. Total does not include two HMOs in Guam. Health plans are allocated to states based upon their primary service areas. This means each plan is counted once. However, many plans serve more than one state.

Enrollees in Health Maintenance Organizations (HMOs) in 1997

National Total = 66,710,393 Enrollees*

ALPHA ORDER

RANK ORDER

RANK	STATE	ENROLLEES	% of USA		RANK	STATE	ENROLLEES	% of USA
28	Alabama	418,987	0.63%		1	California	13,965,660	20.93%
49	Alaska	0	0.00%		2	New York	6,483,993	9.72%
17	Arizona	1,275,330	1.91%		3	Florida	4,177,083	6.26%
38	Arkansas	219,162	0.33%		4	Pennsylvania	3,599,848	5.40%
1	California	13,965,660	20.93%		5	Texas	2,929,684	4.39%
18	Colorado	1,189,392	1.78%		6	Massachusetts	2,715,893	4.07%
19	Connecticut	1,137,504	1.71%		7	Michigan	2,252,061	3.38%
35	Delaware	281,027	0.42%		8	New Jersey	2,192,810	3.29%
3	Florida	4,177,083	6.26%		9	Illinois	2,028,769	3.04%
23	Georgia	934,729	1.40%		10	Ohio	1,965,376	2.95%
33	Hawaii	296,214	0.44%		11	Maryland	1,925,992	2.89%
44	Idaho	51,333	0.08%		12	Missouri	1,618,886	2.43%
9	Illinois	2,028,769	3.04%		13	Minnesota	1,525,155	2.29%
26	Indiana	697,020	1.04%		14	Oregon	1,510,992	2.27%
41	Iowa	130,735	0.20%		15	Washington	1,386,139	2.08%
34	Kansas	294,860	0.44%		16	Wisconsin	1,284,893	1.93%
21	Kentucky	1,065,836	1.60%		17	Arizona	1,275,330	1.91%
27	Louisiana	640,530	0.96%		18	Colorado	1,189,392	1.78%
39	Maine	197,814	0.30%		19	Connecticut	1,137,504	1.71%
11	Maryland	1,925,992	2.89%		20	North Carolina	1,070,293	1.60%
6	Massachusetts	2,715,893	4.07%		21	Kentucky	1,065,836	1.60%
7	Michigan	2,252,061	3.38%		22	Virginia	1,049,404	1.57%
13	Minnesota	1,525,155	2.29%		23	Georgia	934,729	1.40%
43	Mississippi	64,672	0.10%		24	Tennessee	832,059	1.25%
12	Missouri	1,618,886	2.43%		25	Utah	813,861	1.22%
45	Montana	26,851	0.04%		26	Indiana	697,020	1.04%
37	Nebraska	253,615	0.38%		27	Louisiana	640,530	0.96%
31	Nevada	333,539	0.50%		28	Alabama	418,987	0.63%
36	New Hampshire	277,412	0.42%		29	Oklahoma	410,473	0.62%
8	New Jersey	2,192,810	3.29%		30	New Mexico	360,186	0.54%
30	New Mexico	360,186	0.54%		31	Nevada	333,539	0.50%
2	New York	6,483,993	9.72%		32	South Carolina	311,942	0.47%
20	North Carolina	1,070,293	1.60%		33	Hawaii	296,214	0.44%
47	North Dakota	10,891	0.02%		34	Kansas	294,860	0.44%
10	Ohio	1,965,376	2.95%		35	Delaware	281,027	0.42%
29	Oklahoma	410,473	0.62%		36	New Hampshire	277,412	0.42%
14	Oregon	1,510,992	2.27%		37	Nebraska	253,615	0.38%
4	Pennsylvania	3,599,848	5.40%		38	Arkansas	219,162	0.33%
42	Rhode Island	116,372	0.17%		39	Maine	197,814	0.30%
32	South Carolina	311,942	0.47%		40	West Virginia	171,943	0.26%
46	South Dakota	25,947	0.04%		41	Iowa	130,735	0.20%
24	Tennessee	832,059	1.25%		42	Rhode Island	116,372	0.17%
5	Texas	2,929,684	4.39%		43	Mississippi	64,672	0.10%
25	Utah	813,861	1.22%		44	Idaho	51,333	0.08%
49	Vermont	0	0.00%		45	Montana	26,851	0.04%
22	Virginia	1,049,404	1.57%		46	South Dakota	25,947	0.04%
15	Washington	1,386,139	2.08%		47	North Dakota	10,891	0.02%
40	West Virginia	171,943	0.26%		48	Wyoming	1,990	0.00%
16	Wisconsin	1,284,893	1.93%		49	Alaska	0	0.00%
48	Wyoming	1,990	0.00%		49	Vermont	0	0.00%
						District of Columbia	185,236	0.28%

Source: InterStudy Publications (Minneapolis, MN)
   "The Competitive Edge Industry Report 7.2" (October 1997)
*As of January 1, 1997. Total does not include 90,749 enrollees in Guam.

Percent Change in Enrollees in Health Maintenance Organizations (HMOs): 1996 to 1997
National Percent Change = 13.9% Increase*

ALPHA ORDER

RANK	STATE	PERCENT CHANGE
21	Alabama	23.1
NA	Alaska**	NA
40	Arizona	5.7
5	Arkansas	61.4
36	California	7.5
23	Colorado	21.3
29	Connecticut	15.2
13	Delaware	32.2
26	Florida	19.3
14	Georgia	32.1
32	Hawaii	12.8
28	Idaho	15.4
45	Illinois	(7.8)
22	Indiana	22.0
38	Iowa	7.2
2	Kansas	76.3
3	Kentucky	68.2
12	Louisiana	34.1
4	Maine	65.9
36	Maryland	7.5
30	Massachusetts	14.6
39	Michigan	6.2
16	Minnesota	28.2
1	Mississippi	103.5
18	Missouri	25.4
42	Montana	2.9
6	Nebraska	45.0
27	Nevada	16.2
35	New Hampshire	9.3
33	New Jersey	12.3
7	New Mexico	38.5
20	New York	23.6
11	North Carolina	34.8
8	North Dakota	38.1
43	Ohio	(4.3)
24	Oklahoma	20.9
41	Oregon	5.3
34	Pennsylvania	9.4
47	Rhode Island	(46.6)
44	South Carolina	(7.4)
17	South Dakota	27.1
31	Tennessee	13.4
19	Texas	24.8
9	Utah	35.1
48	Vermont	(100.0)
15	Virginia	31.6
25	Washington	20.3
10	West Virginia	35.0
46	Wisconsin	(9.4)
NA	Wyoming**	NA

RANK ORDER

RANK	STATE	PERCENT CHANGE
1	Mississippi	103.5
2	Kansas	76.3
3	Kentucky	68.2
4	Maine	65.9
5	Arkansas	61.4
6	Nebraska	45.0
7	New Mexico	38.5
8	North Dakota	38.1
9	Utah	35.1
10	West Virginia	35.0
11	North Carolina	34.8
12	Louisiana	34.1
13	Delaware	32.2
14	Georgia	32.1
15	Virginia	31.6
16	Minnesota	28.2
17	South Dakota	27.1
18	Missouri	25.4
19	Texas	24.8
20	New York	23.6
21	Alabama	23.1
22	Indiana	22.0
23	Colorado	21.3
24	Oklahoma	20.9
25	Washington	20.3
26	Florida	19.3
27	Nevada	16.2
28	Idaho	15.4
29	Connecticut	15.2
30	Massachusetts	14.6
31	Tennessee	13.4
32	Hawaii	12.8
33	New Jersey	12.3
34	Pennsylvania	9.4
35	New Hampshire	9.3
36	California	7.5
36	Maryland	7.5
38	Iowa	7.2
39	Michigan	6.2
40	Arizona	5.7
41	Oregon	5.3
42	Montana	2.9
43	Ohio	(4.3)
44	South Carolina	(7.4)
45	Illinois	(7.8)
46	Wisconsin	(9.4)
47	Rhode Island	(46.6)
48	Vermont	(100.0)
NA	Alaska**	NA
NA	Wyoming**	NA

District of Columbia 18.8

Source: Morgan Quitno Press using data from InterStudy Publications (Minneapolis, MN)
   "The Competitive Edge Industry Report 7.2" (October 1997)
As of January 1, 1997.
**Not applicable.*

Percent of Population Enrolled in Health Maintenance Organizations (HMOs) in 1997
National Total = 26.7% Enrolled in HMOs*

ALPHA ORDER

RANK	STATE	PERCENT
38	Alabama	9.8
49	Alaska	0.0
14	Arizona	28.8
40	Arkansas	8.7
3	California	43.8
10	Colorado	31.1
8	Connecticut	34.7
5	Delaware	38.8
13	Florida	29.0
33	Georgia	12.7
18	Hawaii	25.0
43	Idaho	4.3
25	Illinois	17.1
35	Indiana	11.9
42	Iowa	4.6
37	Kansas	11.5
16	Kentucky	27.4
31	Louisiana	14.7
26	Maine	15.9
6	Maryland	38.0
2	Massachusetts	44.6
21	Michigan	23.5
9	Minnesota	32.7
46	Mississippi	2.4
11	Missouri	30.2
45	Montana	3.1
28	Nebraska	15.4
23	Nevada	20.8
20	New Hampshire	23.9
15	New Jersey	27.5
22	New Mexico	21.0
7	New York	35.7
32	North Carolina	14.6
47	North Dakota	1.7
24	Ohio	17.6
34	Oklahoma	12.4
1	Oregon	47.2
12	Pennsylvania	29.9
36	Rhode Island	11.8
41	South Carolina	8.4
44	South Dakota	3.5
29	Tennessee	15.3
29	Texas	15.3
4	Utah	40.7
49	Vermont	0.0
27	Virginia	15.7
17	Washington	25.1
39	West Virginia	9.4
19	Wisconsin	24.9
48	Wyoming	0.4

RANK ORDER

RANK	STATE	PERCENT
1	Oregon	47.2
2	Massachusetts	44.6
3	California	43.8
4	Utah	40.7
5	Delaware	38.8
6	Maryland	38.0
7	New York	35.7
8	Connecticut	34.7
9	Minnesota	32.7
10	Colorado	31.1
11	Missouri	30.2
12	Pennsylvania	29.9
13	Florida	29.0
14	Arizona	28.8
15	New Jersey	27.5
16	Kentucky	27.4
17	Washington	25.1
18	Hawaii	25.0
19	Wisconsin	24.9
20	New Hampshire	23.9
21	Michigan	23.5
22	New Mexico	21.0
23	Nevada	20.8
24	Ohio	17.6
25	Illinois	17.1
26	Maine	15.9
27	Virginia	15.7
28	Nebraska	15.4
29	Tennessee	15.3
29	Texas	15.3
31	Louisiana	14.7
32	North Carolina	14.6
33	Georgia	12.7
34	Oklahoma	12.4
35	Indiana	11.9
36	Rhode Island	11.8
37	Kansas	11.5
38	Alabama	9.8
39	West Virginia	9.4
40	Arkansas	8.7
41	South Carolina	8.4
42	Iowa	4.6
43	Idaho	4.3
44	South Dakota	3.5
45	Montana	3.1
46	Mississippi	2.4
47	North Dakota	1.7
48	Wyoming	0.4
49	Alaska	0.0
49	Vermont	0.0

District of Columbia   34.1

Source: InterStudy Publications (Minneapolis, MN)
"The Competitive Edge Industry Report 7.2" (October 1997)
*As of January 1, 1997.

Percent of Insured Population
Enrolled in Health Maintenance Organizations (HMOs) in 1997
National Percent = 29.9% of Insured are Enrolled in HMOs*

ALPHA ORDER

RANK ORDER

RANK	STATE	PERCENT		RANK	STATE	PERCENT
39	Alabama	11.2		1	Oregon	56.0
49	Alaska	0.0		2	California	55.1
9	Arizona	38.9		3	Massachusetts	51.1
38	Arkansas	11.3		4	Utah	45.8
2	California	55.1		5	Delaware	44.9
10	Colorado	37.5		6	New York	43.2
8	Connecticut	39.2		7	Maryland	43.0
5	Delaware	44.9		8	Connecticut	39.2
12	Florida	35.7		9	Arizona	38.9
33	Georgia	15.5		10	Colorado	37.5
19	Hawaii	27.4		11	Minnesota	36.6
42	Idaho	5.2		12	Florida	35.7
26	Illinois	19.3		13	Missouri	34.7
35	Indiana	13.3		14	Pennsylvania	33.0
42	Iowa	5.2		15	New Jersey	32.8
37	Kansas	12.9		16	Kentucky	32.5
16	Kentucky	32.5		17	Washington	29.1
27	Louisiana	18.6		18	New Mexico	27.7
29	Maine	18.1		19	Hawaii	27.4
7	Maryland	43.0		20	Wisconsin	27.3
3	Massachusetts	51.1		21	New Hampshire	26.4
22	Michigan	25.4		22	Michigan	25.4
11	Minnesota	36.6		23	Nevada	24.8
46	Mississippi	2.9		24	Texas	20.3
13	Missouri	34.7		25	Ohio	19.9
45	Montana	3.6		26	Illinois	19.3
31	Nebraska	17.4		27	Louisiana	18.6
23	Nevada	24.8		27	Tennessee	18.6
21	New Hampshire	26.4		29	Maine	18.1
15	New Jersey	32.8		30	Virginia	17.9
18	New Mexico	27.7		31	Nebraska	17.4
6	New York	43.2		31	North Carolina	17.4
31	North Carolina	17.4		33	Georgia	15.5
47	North Dakota	1.9		34	Oklahoma	15.1
25	Ohio	19.9		35	Indiana	13.3
34	Oklahoma	15.1		36	Rhode Island	13.0
1	Oregon	56.0		37	Kansas	12.9
14	Pennsylvania	33.0		38	Arkansas	11.3
36	Rhode Island	13.0		39	Alabama	11.2
41	South Carolina	10.1		40	West Virginia	11.0
44	South Dakota	3.9		41	South Carolina	10.1
27	Tennessee	18.6		42	Idaho	5.2
24	Texas	20.3		42	Iowa	5.2
4	Utah	45.8		44	South Dakota	3.9
49	Vermont	0.0		45	Montana	3.6
30	Virginia	17.9		46	Mississippi	2.9
17	Washington	29.1		47	North Dakota	1.9
40	West Virginia	11.0		48	Wyoming	0.5
20	Wisconsin	27.3		49	Alaska	0.0
48	Wyoming	0.5		49	Vermont	0.0
					District of Columbia	40.3

Source: Morgan Quitno Press using data from InterStudy Publications (Minneapolis, MN)
"The Competitive Edge Industry Report 7.2" (October 1997)
As of January 1, 1997. Calculated using estimated number of insured as of 1996.

Preferred Provider Organizations (PPOs) in 1995

National Total = 1,023 PPOs*

RANK	STATE	PPOs	% of USA
15	Alabama	25	2.44%
45	Alaska	3	0.29%
11	Arizona	27	2.64%
36	Arkansas	8	0.78%
1	California	72	7.04%
10	Colorado	28	2.74%
31	Connecticut	11	1.08%
40	Delaware	5	0.49%
1	Florida	72	7.04%
7	Georgia	37	3.62%
40	Hawaii	5	0.49%
47	Idaho	1	0.10%
5	Illinois	46	4.50%
9	Indiana	30	2.93%
30	Iowa	13	1.27%
26	Kansas	17	1.66%
28	Kentucky	16	1.56%
13	Louisiana	26	2.54%
37	Maine	7	0.68%
23	Maryland	18	1.76%
21	Massachusetts	19	1.86%
11	Michigan	27	2.64%
28	Minnesota	16	1.56%
37	Mississippi	7	0.68%
15	Missouri	25	2.44%
49	Montana	0	0.00%
31	Nebraska	11	1.08%
17	Nevada	24	2.35%
42	New Hampshire	4	0.39%
21	New Jersey	19	1.86%
34	New Mexico	9	0.88%
19	New York	22	2.15%
18	North Carolina	23	2.25%
47	North Dakota	1	0.10%
6	Ohio	44	4.30%
23	Oklahoma	18	1.76%
33	Oregon	10	0.98%
4	Pennsylvania	54	5.28%
42	Rhode Island	4	0.39%
26	South Carolina	17	1.66%
42	South Dakota	4	0.39%
7	Tennessee	37	3.62%
3	Texas	71	6.94%
34	Utah	9	0.88%
46	Vermont	2	0.20%
23	Virginia	18	1.76%
20	Washington	21	2.05%
39	West Virginia	6	0.59%
13	Wisconsin	26	2.54%
49	Wyoming	0	0.00%

RANK	STATE	PPOs	% of USA
1	California	72	7.04%
1	Florida	72	7.04%
3	Texas	71	6.94%
4	Pennsylvania	54	5.28%
5	Illinois	46	4.50%
6	Ohio	44	4.30%
7	Georgia	37	3.62%
7	Tennessee	37	3.62%
9	Indiana	30	2.93%
10	Colorado	28	2.74%
11	Arizona	27	2.64%
11	Michigan	27	2.64%
13	Louisiana	26	2.54%
13	Wisconsin	26	2.54%
15	Alabama	25	2.44%
15	Missouri	25	2.44%
17	Nevada	24	2.35%
18	North Carolina	23	2.25%
19	New York	22	2.15%
20	Washington	21	2.05%
21	Massachusetts	19	1.86%
21	New Jersey	19	1.86%
23	Maryland	18	1.76%
23	Oklahoma	18	1.76%
23	Virginia	18	1.76%
26	Kansas	17	1.66%
26	South Carolina	17	1.66%
28	Kentucky	16	1.56%
28	Minnesota	16	1.56%
30	Iowa	13	1.27%
31	Connecticut	11	1.08%
31	Nebraska	11	1.08%
33	Oregon	10	0.98%
34	New Mexico	9	0.88%
34	Utah	9	0.88%
36	Arkansas	8	0.78%
37	Maine	7	0.68%
37	Mississippi	7	0.68%
39	West Virginia	6	0.59%
40	Delaware	5	0.49%
40	Hawaii	5	0.49%
42	New Hampshire	4	0.39%
42	Rhode Island	4	0.39%
42	South Dakota	4	0.39%
45	Alaska	3	0.29%
46	Vermont	2	0.20%
47	Idaho	1	0.10%
47	North Dakota	1	0.10%
49	Montana	0	0.00%
49	Wyoming	0	0.00%
	District of Columbia	6	0.59%

Source: American Association of Health Plans (formerly American Managed Care and Review Association)
    "1995-1996 Managed Health Care Overview"
*As of October 1995. Total does not include two PPOs in Puerto Rico. Health plans are allocated to states based upon their primary service areas. This means each plan is counted once. However, many plans serve more than one state.

Enrollment in Preferred Provider Organizations (PPOs) in 1994

National Total = 82,718,223 Enrollees*

ALPHA ORDER

RANK	STATE	ENROLLEES	% of USA
28	Alabama	894,189	1.08%
48	Alaska	135,764	0.16%
24	Arizona	1,139,211	1.38%
34	Arkansas	543,067	0.66%
1	California	8,158,166	9.86%
25	Colorado	1,047,306	1.27%
22	Connecticut	1,216,321	1.47%
47	Delaware	142,408	0.17%
5	Florida	4,441,239	5.37%
12	Georgia	2,548,488	3.08%
36	Hawaii*	476,921	0.58%
42	Idaho	223,436	0.27%
3	Illinois	4,492,062	5.43%
15	Indiana	2,019,924	2.44%
21	Iowa	1,273,853	1.54%
30	Kansas	828,451	1.00%
26	Kentucky	997,952	1.21%
16	Louisiana	1,905,941	2.30%
41	Maine	237,285	0.29%
14	Maryland	2,030,314	2.45%
23	Massachusetts	1,212,304	1.47%
8	Michigan	2,993,934	3.62%
11	Minnesota	2,551,797	3.08%
33	Mississippi	595,775	0.72%
17	Missouri	1,765,073	2.13%
45	Montana	164,302	0.20%
39	Nebraska	429,040	0.52%
32	Nevada	758,716	0.92%
40	New Hampshire	247,763	0.30%
13	New Jersey	2,473,101	2.99%
35	New Mexico	502,898	0.61%
7	New York	3,736,986	4.52%
10	North Carolina	2,653,587	3.21%
44	North Dakota	175,524	0.21%
6	Ohio	3,834,255	4.64%
31	Oklahoma	797,987	0.96%
27	Oregon	944,388	1.14%
4	Pennsylvania	4,477,910	5.41%
43	Rhode Island	206,880	0.25%
29	South Carolina	846,363	1.02%
46	South Dakota	158,904	0.19%
9	Tennessee	2,758,071	3.33%
2	Texas	7,695,401	9.30%
37	Utah	471,422	0.57%
49	Vermont	116,900	0.14%
19	Virginia	1,640,166	1.98%
18	Washington	1,674,736	2.02%
38	West Virginia	442,034	0.53%
20	Wisconsin	1,402,472	1.70%
50	Wyoming	92,969	0.11%

RANK ORDER

RANK	STATE	ENROLLEES	% of USA
1	California	8,158,166	9.86%
2	Texas	7,695,401	9.30%
3	Illinois	4,492,062	5.43%
4	Pennsylvania	4,477,910	5.41%
5	Florida	4,441,239	5.37%
6	Ohio	3,834,255	4.64%
7	New York	3,736,986	4.52%
8	Michigan	2,993,934	3.62%
9	Tennessee	2,758,071	3.33%
10	North Carolina	2,653,587	3.21%
11	Minnesota	2,551,797	3.08%
12	Georgia	2,548,488	3.08%
13	New Jersey	2,473,101	2.99%
14	Maryland	2,030,314	2.45%
15	Indiana	2,019,924	2.44%
16	Louisiana	1,905,941	2.30%
17	Missouri	1,765,073	2.13%
18	Washington	1,674,736	2.02%
19	Virginia	1,640,166	1.98%
20	Wisconsin	1,402,472	1.70%
21	Iowa	1,273,853	1.54%
22	Connecticut	1,216,321	1.47%
23	Massachusetts	1,212,304	1.47%
24	Arizona	1,139,211	1.38%
25	Colorado	1,047,306	1.27%
26	Kentucky	997,952	1.21%
27	Oregon	944,388	1.14%
28	Alabama	894,189	1.08%
29	South Carolina	846,363	1.02%
30	Kansas	828,451	1.00%
31	Oklahoma	797,987	0.96%
32	Nevada	758,716	0.92%
33	Mississippi	595,775	0.72%
34	Arkansas	543,067	0.66%
35	New Mexico	502,898	0.61%
36	Hawaii*	476,921	0.58%
37	Utah	471,422	0.57%
38	West Virginia	442,034	0.53%
39	Nebraska	429,040	0.52%
40	New Hampshire	247,763	0.30%
41	Maine	237,285	0.29%
42	Idaho	223,436	0.27%
43	Rhode Island	206,880	0.25%
44	North Dakota	175,524	0.21%
45	Montana	164,302	0.20%
46	South Dakota	158,904	0.19%
47	Delaware	142,408	0.17%
48	Alaska	135,764	0.16%
49	Vermont	116,900	0.14%
50	Wyoming	92,969	0.11%
	District of Columbia	144,267	0.17%

Source: American Association of Health Plans (formerly American Managed Care and Review Association)
"Managed Care Covered Lives, Year-end 1994"
*As of December 31, 1994 except Hawaii is December 31, 1993. Total excludes 234,768 enrollees in Puerto Rico.
Includes dependents.

Percent of Population Enrolled in a
Preferred Provider Organization (PPO) in 1994
National Percent = 31.7% of Population*

RANK	STATE	PERCENT
41	Alabama	21.2
36	Alaska	22.4
25	Arizona	28.0
38	Arkansas	22.1
30	California	26.0
24	Colorado	28.6
12	Connecticut	37.1
44	Delaware	20.2
18	Florida	31.8
13	Georgia	36.1
8	Hawaii*	40.5
47	Idaho	19.7
9	Illinois	38.2
14	Indiana	35.1
4	Iowa	45.0
17	Kansas	32.4
29	Kentucky	26.1
5	Louisiana	44.2
50	Maine	19.1
7	Maryland	40.6
46	Massachusetts	20.1
19	Michigan	31.5
1	Minnesota	55.9
37	Mississippi	22.3
16	Missouri	33.4
49	Montana	19.2
28	Nebraska	26.4
3	Nevada	52.1
40	New Hampshire	21.8
20	New Jersey	31.3
23	New Mexico	30.4
43	New York	20.6
10	North Carolina	37.5
27	North Dakota	27.5
15	Ohio	34.5
33	Oklahoma	24.5
22	Oregon	30.6
11	Pennsylvania	37.2
42	Rhode Island	20.8
35	South Carolina	23.1
39	South Dakota	22.0
2	Tennessee	53.3
6	Texas	41.9
32	Utah	24.7
44	Vermont	20.2
31	Virginia	25.0
20	Washington	31.3
34	West Virginia	24.3
26	Wisconsin	27.6
48	Wyoming	19.5

RANK	STATE	PERCENT
1	Minnesota	55.9
2	Tennessee	53.3
3	Nevada	52.1
4	Iowa	45.0
5	Louisiana	44.2
6	Texas	41.9
7	Maryland	40.6
8	Hawaii*	40.5
9	Illinois	38.2
10	North Carolina	37.5
11	Pennsylvania	37.2
12	Connecticut	37.1
13	Georgia	36.1
14	Indiana	35.1
15	Ohio	34.5
16	Missouri	33.4
17	Kansas	32.4
18	Florida	31.8
19	Michigan	31.5
20	New Jersey	31.3
20	Washington	31.3
22	Oregon	30.6
23	New Mexico	30.4
24	Colorado	28.6
25	Arizona	28.0
26	Wisconsin	27.6
27	North Dakota	27.5
28	Nebraska	26.4
29	Kentucky	26.1
30	California	26.0
31	Virginia	25.0
32	Utah	24.7
33	Oklahoma	24.5
34	West Virginia	24.3
35	South Carolina	23.1
36	Alaska	22.4
37	Mississippi	22.3
38	Arkansas	22.1
39	South Dakota	22.0
40	New Hampshire	21.8
41	Alabama	21.2
42	Rhode Island	20.8
43	New York	20.6
44	Delaware	20.2
44	Vermont	20.2
46	Massachusetts	20.1
47	Idaho	19.7
48	Wyoming	19.5
49	Montana	19.2
50	Maine	19.1

| | District of Columbia | 25.3 |

Source: American Association of Health Plans (formerly American Managed Care and Review Association)
   "Managed Care Covered Lives, Year-end 1994"
*As of December 31, 1994 except Hawaii is December 31, 1993. National rate excludes enrollees in Puerto Rico.
Includes dependents.

Percent of Insured Population in a Preferred Provider Organization (PPO) in 1994
National Percent = 37.20% of Insured Population*

ALPHA ORDER

RANK	STATE	PERCENT
39	Alabama	25.70
38	Alaska	26.46
24	Arizona	33.71
36	Arkansas	27.22
25	California	32.61
26	Colorado	31.93
11	Connecticut	42.51
42	Delaware	24.18
19	Florida	37.59
12	Georgia	42.01
7	Hawaii	47.45
46	Idaho	22.80
10	Illinois	42.82
17	Indiana	37.72
6	Iowa	50.05
18	Kansas	37.64
28	Kentucky	30.54
4	Louisiana	54.07
47	Maine	22.71
8	Maryland	46.00
45	Massachusetts	23.05
22	Michigan	35.24
1	Minnesota	62.74
34	Mississippi	27.97
14	Missouri	39.33
49	Montana	22.51
32	Nebraska	29.15
2	Nevada	59.09
40	New Hampshire	24.85
21	New Jersey	35.87
15	New Mexico	38.74
41	New York	24.38
9	North Carolina	44.32
29	North Dakota	30.47
16	Ohio	38.61
30	Oklahoma	30.03
23	Oregon	34.34
13	Pennsylvania	41.74
43	Rhode Island	24.14
37	South Carolina	26.98
44	South Dakota	23.86
3	Tennessee	57.40
5	Texas	53.62
35	Utah	27.62
50	Vermont	21.57
33	Virginia	28.12
20	Washington	36.45
31	West Virginia	29.24
27	Wisconsin	30.75
48	Wyoming	22.62

RANK ORDER

RANK	STATE	PERCENT
1	Minnesota	62.74
2	Nevada	59.09
3	Tennessee	57.40
4	Louisiana	54.07
5	Texas	53.62
6	Iowa	50.05
7	Hawaii	47.45
8	Maryland	46.00
9	North Carolina	44.32
10	Illinois	42.82
11	Connecticut	42.51
12	Georgia	42.01
13	Pennsylvania	41.74
14	Missouri	39.33
15	New Mexico	38.74
16	Ohio	38.61
17	Indiana	37.72
18	Kansas	37.64
19	Florida	37.59
20	Washington	36.45
21	New Jersey	35.87
22	Michigan	35.24
23	Oregon	34.34
24	Arizona	33.71
25	California	32.61
26	Colorado	31.93
27	Wisconsin	30.75
28	Kentucky	30.54
29	North Dakota	30.47
30	Oklahoma	30.03
31	West Virginia	29.24
32	Nebraska	29.15
33	Virginia	28.12
34	Mississippi	27.97
35	Utah	27.62
36	Arkansas	27.22
37	South Carolina	26.98
38	Alaska	26.46
39	Alabama	25.70
40	New Hampshire	24.85
41	New York	24.38
42	Delaware	24.18
43	Rhode Island	24.14
44	South Dakota	23.86
45	Massachusetts	23.05
46	Idaho	22.80
47	Maine	22.71
48	Wyoming	22.62
49	Montana	22.51
50	Vermont	21.57

District of Columbia 28.23

Source: MQ Press using data from American Assn. of Health Plans (formerly American Managed Care & Review Assn.) "Managed Care Covered Lives, Year-end 1994"

*As of December 31, 1994. National rate includes enrollees for whom state of resident is not known but excludes enrollees in Puerto Rico. Includes dependents.

Persons Eligible for the Civilian Health and Medical Program
National Of the Uniformed Services (CHAMPUS) in 1997
National Total = 5,103,419 Eligible to Enroll*

ALPHA ORDER

RANK ORDER

RANK	STATE	ELIGIBLE	% of USA		RANK	STATE	ELIGIBLE	% of USA
11	Alabama	126,924	2.49%		1	California	567,182	11.11%
30	Alaska	47,275	0.93%		2	Texas	471,290	9.23%
12	Arizona	117,700	2.31%		3	Virginia	445,972	8.74%
27	Arkansas	51,777	1.01%		4	Florida	424,309	8.31%
1	California	567,182	11.11%		5	Georgia	257,438	5.04%
10	Colorado	134,281	2.63%		6	North Carolina	247,018	4.84%
36	Connecticut	27,955	0.55%		7	Washington	220,149	4.31%
43	Delaware	18,564	0.36%		8	South Carolina	143,861	2.82%
4	Florida	424,309	8.31%		9	Maryland	140,215	2.75%
5	Georgia	257,438	5.04%		10	Colorado	134,281	2.63%
15	Hawaii	93,265	1.83%		11	Alabama	126,924	2.49%
38	Idaho	27,327	0.54%		12	Arizona	117,700	2.31%
18	Illinois	81,534	1.60%		13	Tennessee	102,713	2.01%
32	Indiana	41,088	0.81%		14	Oklahoma	100,283	1.97%
44	Iowa	17,905	0.35%		15	Hawaii	93,265	1.83%
23	Kansas	70,436	1.38%		16	Ohio	91,133	1.79%
22	Kentucky	73,565	1.44%		17	Louisiana	82,508	1.62%
17	Louisiana	82,508	1.62%		18	Illinois	81,534	1.60%
37	Maine	27,619	0.54%		19	New York	80,828	1.58%
9	Maryland	140,215	2.75%		20	Missouri	80,172	1.57%
33	Massachusetts	35,311	0.69%		21	Pennsylvania	77,985	1.53%
29	Michigan	48,113	0.94%		22	Kentucky	73,565	1.44%
40	Minnesota	24,477	0.48%		23	Kansas	70,436	1.38%
24	Mississippi	66,919	1.31%		24	Mississippi	66,919	1.31%
20	Missouri	80,172	1.57%		25	New Mexico	63,772	1.25%
42	Montana	19,662	0.39%		26	Nevada	56,534	1.11%
31	Nebraska	43,333	0.85%		27	Arkansas	51,777	1.01%
26	Nevada	56,534	1.11%		28	New Jersey	49,341	0.97%
47	New Hampshire	15,489	0.30%		29	Michigan	48,113	0.94%
28	New Jersey	49,341	0.97%		30	Alaska	47,275	0.93%
25	New Mexico	63,772	1.25%		31	Nebraska	43,333	0.85%
19	New York	80,828	1.58%		32	Indiana	41,088	0.81%
6	North Carolina	247,018	4.84%		33	Massachusetts	35,311	0.69%
41	North Dakota	23,179	0.45%		34	Oregon	34,609	0.68%
16	Ohio	91,133	1.79%		35	Utah	33,349	0.65%
14	Oklahoma	100,283	1.97%		36	Connecticut	27,955	0.55%
34	Oregon	34,609	0.68%		37	Maine	27,619	0.54%
21	Pennsylvania	77,985	1.53%		38	Idaho	27,327	0.54%
49	Rhode Island	13,082	0.26%		39	Wisconsin	27,148	0.53%
8	South Carolina	143,861	2.82%		40	Minnesota	24,477	0.48%
46	South Dakota	17,654	0.35%		41	North Dakota	23,179	0.45%
13	Tennessee	102,713	2.01%		42	Montana	19,662	0.39%
2	Texas	471,290	9.23%		43	Delaware	18,564	0.36%
35	Utah	33,349	0.65%		44	Iowa	17,905	0.35%
50	Vermont	4,933	0.10%		45	West Virginia	17,730	0.35%
3	Virginia	445,972	8.74%		46	South Dakota	17,654	0.35%
7	Washington	220,149	4.31%		47	New Hampshire	15,489	0.30%
45	West Virginia	17,730	0.35%		48	Wyoming	13,639	0.27%
39	Wisconsin	27,148	0.53%		49	Rhode Island	13,082	0.26%
48	Wyoming	13,639	0.27%		50	Vermont	4,933	0.10%
					District of Columbia		4,874	0.10%

Source: U.S. Department of Defense, Office of CHAMPUS
   "Defense Enrollment Eligibility Reporting System (DEERS) Report" (November 4, 1997)
As of November 4, 1997. National total does not include 29,445 eligible in U.S. territories and possessions.
CHAMPUS provides health care coverage for current or former U.S. military personnel and their dependents.

Percent of Population Eligible for CHAMPUS in 1997

National Percent = 1.9% of Population Eligible*

ALPHA ORDER

RANK	STATE	PERCENT
13	Alabama	2.9
2	Alaska	7.8
18	Arizona	2.6
27	Arkansas	2.1
31	California	1.8
8	Colorado	3.4
38	Connecticut	0.9
20	Delaware	2.5
13	Florida	2.9
8	Georgia	3.4
1	Hawaii	7.9
24	Idaho	2.3
41	Illinois	0.7
41	Indiana	0.7
43	Iowa	0.6
17	Kansas	2.7
28	Kentucky	1.9
28	Louisiana	1.9
25	Maine	2.2
15	Maryland	2.8
43	Massachusetts	0.6
47	Michigan	0.5
47	Minnesota	0.5
20	Mississippi	2.5
33	Missouri	1.5
25	Montana	2.2
18	Nebraska	2.6
8	Nevada	3.4
34	New Hampshire	1.3
43	New Jersey	0.6
6	New Mexico	3.7
50	New York	0.4
11	North Carolina	3.3
7	North Dakota	3.6
39	Ohio	0.8
12	Oklahoma	3.0
36	Oregon	1.1
43	Pennsylvania	0.6
34	Rhode Island	1.3
5	South Carolina	3.8
22	South Dakota	2.4
28	Tennessee	1.9
22	Texas	2.4
32	Utah	1.6
39	Vermont	0.8
3	Virginia	6.6
4	Washington	3.9
37	West Virginia	1.0
47	Wisconsin	0.5
15	Wyoming	2.8

RANK ORDER

RANK	STATE	PERCENT
1	Hawaii	7.9
2	Alaska	7.8
3	Virginia	6.6
4	Washington	3.9
5	South Carolina	3.8
6	New Mexico	3.7
7	North Dakota	3.6
8	Colorado	3.4
8	Georgia	3.4
8	Nevada	3.4
11	North Carolina	3.3
12	Oklahoma	3.0
13	Alabama	2.9
13	Florida	2.9
15	Maryland	2.8
15	Wyoming	2.8
17	Kansas	2.7
18	Arizona	2.6
18	Nebraska	2.6
20	Delaware	2.5
20	Mississippi	2.5
22	South Dakota	2.4
22	Texas	2.4
24	Idaho	2.3
25	Maine	2.2
25	Montana	2.2
27	Arkansas	2.1
28	Kentucky	1.9
28	Louisiana	1.9
28	Tennessee	1.9
31	California	1.8
32	Utah	1.6
33	Missouri	1.5
34	New Hampshire	1.3
34	Rhode Island	1.3
36	Oregon	1.1
37	West Virginia	1.0
38	Connecticut	0.9
39	Ohio	0.8
39	Vermont	0.8
41	Illinois	0.7
41	Indiana	0.7
43	Iowa	0.6
43	Massachusetts	0.6
43	New Jersey	0.6
43	Pennsylvania	0.6
47	Michigan	0.5
47	Minnesota	0.5
47	Wisconsin	0.5
50	New York	0.4

District of Columbia	0.9

Source: U.S. Department of Defense, Office of CHAMPUS
    "Defense Enrollment Eligibility Reporting System (DEERS) Report" (November 4, 1997)
*As of November 4, 1997. National rate does not include those eligible in U.S. territories and possessions.
CHAMPUS provides health care coverage for current or former U.S. military personnel and their dependents.
Percentages calculated using Census estimates as of July 1, 1997.

Medicare Benefit Payments in 1997

National Total = $207,123,498,023*

ALPHA ORDER

RANK	STATE	BENEFITS	% of USA
18	Alabama	$3,583,456,605	1.73%
50	Alaska	162,659,047	0.08%
20	Arizona	3,210,752,245	1.55%
30	Arkansas	1,905,935,489	0.92%
1	California	22,088,410,238	10.66%
28	Colorado	2,215,951,443	1.07%
22	Connecticut	3,082,139,428	1.49%
46	Delaware	471,068,715	0.23%
2	Florida	17,525,291,927	8.46%
12	Georgia	4,724,810,788	2.28%
42	Hawaii	655,491,278	0.32%
43	Idaho	565,126,263	0.27%
7	Illinois	8,313,616,485	4.01%
16	Indiana	4,080,167,054	1.97%
32	Iowa	1,737,545,562	0.84%
33	Kansas	1,690,755,072	0.82%
24	Kentucky	2,889,228,058	1.39%
15	Louisiana	4,285,657,035	2.07%
39	Maine	879,433,409	0.42%
19	Maryland	3,437,762,756	1.66%
10	Massachusetts	6,454,553,073	3.12%
8	Michigan	7,400,601,066	3.57%
25	Minnesota	2,733,427,992	1.32%
29	Mississippi	2,213,773,234	1.07%
14	Missouri	4,579,394,498	2.21%
44	Montana	495,858,384	0.24%
36	Nebraska	1,029,591,464	0.50%
35	Nevada	1,123,421,035	0.54%
41	New Hampshire	713,662,332	0.34%
9	New Jersey	6,572,769,568	3.17%
40	New Mexico	873,159,349	0.42%
3	New York	16,450,524,694	7.94%
11	North Carolina	5,079,024,248	2.45%
47	North Dakota	468,312,800	0.23%
6	Ohio	8,556,050,777	4.13%
26	Oklahoma	2,677,076,692	1.29%
31	Oregon	1,887,052,049	0.91%
5	Pennsylvania	12,445,285,235	6.01%
37	Rhode Island	988,768,239	0.48%
27	South Carolina	2,366,411,982	1.14%
45	South Dakota	476,377,705	0.23%
13	Tennessee	4,721,533,262	2.28%
4	Texas	14,275,435,805	6.89%
38	Utah	886,569,445	0.43%
48	Vermont	328,060,306	0.16%
17	Virginia	3,635,662,436	1.76%
23	Washington	3,033,372,291	1.46%
34	West Virginia	1,503,805,090	0.73%
21	Wisconsin	3,109,141,278	1.50%
49	Wyoming	215,531,347	0.10%

RANK ORDER

RANK	STATE	BENEFITS	% of USA
1	California	$22,088,410,238	10.66%
2	Florida	17,525,291,927	8.46%
3	New York	16,450,524,694	7.94%
4	Texas	14,275,435,805	6.89%
5	Pennsylvania	12,445,285,235	6.01%
6	Ohio	8,556,050,777	4.13%
7	Illinois	8,313,616,485	4.01%
8	Michigan	7,400,601,066	3.57%
9	New Jersey	6,572,769,568	3.17%
10	Massachusetts	6,454,553,073	3.12%
11	North Carolina	5,079,024,248	2.45%
12	Georgia	4,724,810,788	2.28%
13	Tennessee	4,721,533,262	2.28%
14	Missouri	4,579,394,498	2.21%
15	Louisiana	4,285,657,035	2.07%
16	Indiana	4,080,167,054	1.97%
17	Virginia	3,635,662,436	1.76%
18	Alabama	3,583,456,605	1.73%
19	Maryland	3,437,762,756	1.66%
20	Arizona	3,210,752,245	1.55%
21	Wisconsin	3,109,141,278	1.50%
22	Connecticut	3,082,139,428	1.49%
23	Washington	3,033,372,291	1.46%
24	Kentucky	2,889,228,058	1.39%
25	Minnesota	2,733,427,992	1.32%
26	Oklahoma	2,677,076,692	1.29%
27	South Carolina	2,366,411,982	1.14%
28	Colorado	2,215,951,443	1.07%
29	Mississippi	2,213,773,234	1.07%
30	Arkansas	1,905,935,489	0.92%
31	Oregon	1,887,052,049	0.91%
32	Iowa	1,737,545,562	0.84%
33	Kansas	1,690,755,072	0.82%
34	West Virginia	1,503,805,090	0.73%
35	Nevada	1,123,421,035	0.54%
36	Nebraska	1,029,591,464	0.50%
37	Rhode Island	988,768,239	0.48%
38	Utah	886,569,445	0.43%
39	Maine	879,433,409	0.42%
40	New Mexico	873,159,349	0.42%
41	New Hampshire	713,662,332	0.34%
42	Hawaii	655,491,278	0.32%
43	Idaho	565,126,263	0.27%
44	Montana	495,858,384	0.24%
45	South Dakota	476,377,705	0.23%
46	Delaware	471,068,715	0.23%
47	North Dakota	468,312,800	0.23%
48	Vermont	328,060,306	0.16%
49	Wyoming	215,531,347	0.10%
50	Alaska	162,659,047	0.08%
	District of Columbia	1,264,092,575	0.61%

Source: U.S. Department of Health and Human Services, Health Care Financing Administration unpublished data

*For fiscal year 1997. Includes payments to aged and disabled enrollees. Total includes $1,025,150,312 in payments to enrollees in Puerto Rico and $34,788,565 to enrollees in all other areas.

Percent of Personal Health Care Expenditures Paid by Medicare in 1993

National Percent = 19.3%*

<table>
<tr><th colspan="3">ALPHA ORDER</th><th colspan="3">RANK ORDER</th></tr>
<tr><th>RANK</th><th>STATE</th><th>PERCENT</th><th>RANK</th><th>STATE</th><th>PERCENT</th></tr>
<tr><td>6</td><td>Alabama</td><td>21.8</td><td>1</td><td>Florida</td><td>27.9</td></tr>
<tr><td>50</td><td>Alaska</td><td>6.4</td><td>2</td><td>Pennsylvania</td><td>24.2</td></tr>
<tr><td>8</td><td>Arizona</td><td>21.4</td><td>3</td><td>Arkansas</td><td>23.3</td></tr>
<tr><td>3</td><td>Arkansas</td><td>23.3</td><td>4</td><td>Mississippi</td><td>22.1</td></tr>
<tr><td>27</td><td>California</td><td>18.4</td><td>5</td><td>Tennessee</td><td>21.9</td></tr>
<tr><td>43</td><td>Colorado</td><td>15.5</td><td>6</td><td>Alabama</td><td>21.8</td></tr>
<tr><td>34</td><td>Connecticut</td><td>17.5</td><td>7</td><td>Missouri</td><td>21.6</td></tr>
<tr><td>38</td><td>Delaware</td><td>16.7</td><td>8</td><td>Arizona</td><td>21.4</td></tr>
<tr><td>1</td><td>Florida</td><td>27.9</td><td>9</td><td>West Virginia</td><td>21.3</td></tr>
<tr><td>30</td><td>Georgia</td><td>17.7</td><td>10</td><td>Louisiana</td><td>21.0</td></tr>
<tr><td>48</td><td>Hawaii</td><td>14.2</td><td>11</td><td>Oklahoma</td><td>20.7</td></tr>
<tr><td>37</td><td>Idaho</td><td>16.9</td><td>12</td><td>Kentucky</td><td>20.6</td></tr>
<tr><td>27</td><td>Illinois</td><td>18.4</td><td>13</td><td>Massachusetts</td><td>20.1</td></tr>
<tr><td>20</td><td>Indiana</td><td>19.1</td><td>14</td><td>Michigan</td><td>19.9</td></tr>
<tr><td>15</td><td>Iowa</td><td>19.7</td><td>15</td><td>Iowa</td><td>19.7</td></tr>
<tr><td>19</td><td>Kansas</td><td>19.2</td><td>16</td><td>Nevada</td><td>19.5</td></tr>
<tr><td>12</td><td>Kentucky</td><td>20.6</td><td>16</td><td>North Carolina</td><td>19.5</td></tr>
<tr><td>10</td><td>Louisiana</td><td>21.0</td><td>18</td><td>Rhode Island</td><td>19.4</td></tr>
<tr><td>32</td><td>Maine</td><td>17.6</td><td>19</td><td>Kansas</td><td>19.2</td></tr>
<tr><td>29</td><td>Maryland</td><td>17.8</td><td>20</td><td>Indiana</td><td>19.1</td></tr>
<tr><td>13</td><td>Massachusetts</td><td>20.1</td><td>21</td><td>Oregon</td><td>19.0</td></tr>
<tr><td>14</td><td>Michigan</td><td>19.9</td><td>22</td><td>New Jersey</td><td>18.8</td></tr>
<tr><td>44</td><td>Minnesota</td><td>15.2</td><td>23</td><td>Montana</td><td>18.6</td></tr>
<tr><td>4</td><td>Mississippi</td><td>22.1</td><td>23</td><td>South Dakota</td><td>18.6</td></tr>
<tr><td>7</td><td>Missouri</td><td>21.6</td><td>25</td><td>North Dakota</td><td>18.5</td></tr>
<tr><td>23</td><td>Montana</td><td>18.6</td><td>25</td><td>Ohio</td><td>18.5</td></tr>
<tr><td>36</td><td>Nebraska</td><td>17.0</td><td>27</td><td>California</td><td>18.4</td></tr>
<tr><td>16</td><td>Nevada</td><td>19.5</td><td>27</td><td>Illinois</td><td>18.4</td></tr>
<tr><td>49</td><td>New Hampshire</td><td>13.7</td><td>29</td><td>Maryland</td><td>17.8</td></tr>
<tr><td>22</td><td>New Jersey</td><td>18.8</td><td>30</td><td>Georgia</td><td>17.7</td></tr>
<tr><td>47</td><td>New Mexico</td><td>14.6</td><td>30</td><td>New York</td><td>17.7</td></tr>
<tr><td>30</td><td>New York</td><td>17.7</td><td>32</td><td>Maine</td><td>17.6</td></tr>
<tr><td>16</td><td>North Carolina</td><td>19.5</td><td>32</td><td>Texas</td><td>17.6</td></tr>
<tr><td>25</td><td>North Dakota</td><td>18.5</td><td>34</td><td>Connecticut</td><td>17.5</td></tr>
<tr><td>25</td><td>Ohio</td><td>18.5</td><td>35</td><td>South Carolina</td><td>17.1</td></tr>
<tr><td>11</td><td>Oklahoma</td><td>20.7</td><td>36</td><td>Nebraska</td><td>17.0</td></tr>
<tr><td>21</td><td>Oregon</td><td>19.0</td><td>37</td><td>Idaho</td><td>16.9</td></tr>
<tr><td>2</td><td>Pennsylvania</td><td>24.2</td><td>38</td><td>Delaware</td><td>16.7</td></tr>
<tr><td>18</td><td>Rhode Island</td><td>19.4</td><td>39</td><td>Wisconsin</td><td>16.5</td></tr>
<tr><td>35</td><td>South Carolina</td><td>17.1</td><td>40</td><td>Virginia</td><td>16.4</td></tr>
<tr><td>23</td><td>South Dakota</td><td>18.6</td><td>41</td><td>Vermont</td><td>16.1</td></tr>
<tr><td>5</td><td>Tennessee</td><td>21.9</td><td>42</td><td>Washington</td><td>15.6</td></tr>
<tr><td>32</td><td>Texas</td><td>17.6</td><td>43</td><td>Colorado</td><td>15.5</td></tr>
<tr><td>44</td><td>Utah</td><td>15.2</td><td>44</td><td>Minnesota</td><td>15.2</td></tr>
<tr><td>41</td><td>Vermont</td><td>16.1</td><td>44</td><td>Utah</td><td>15.2</td></tr>
<tr><td>40</td><td>Virginia</td><td>16.4</td><td>46</td><td>Wyoming</td><td>15.0</td></tr>
<tr><td>42</td><td>Washington</td><td>15.6</td><td>47</td><td>New Mexico</td><td>14.6</td></tr>
<tr><td>9</td><td>West Virginia</td><td>21.3</td><td>48</td><td>Hawaii</td><td>14.2</td></tr>
<tr><td>39</td><td>Wisconsin</td><td>16.5</td><td>49</td><td>New Hampshire</td><td>13.7</td></tr>
<tr><td>46</td><td>Wyoming</td><td>15.0</td><td>50</td><td>Alaska</td><td>6.4</td></tr>
<tr><td></td><td></td><td></td><td></td><td>District of Columbia</td><td>14.1</td></tr>
</table>

Source: U.S. Department of Health and Human Services, Health Care Financing Administration
   "State Health Expenditure Accounts" (Health Care Financing Review, Fall 1995, Volume 17, Number 1)
*By state of provider.

Medicare Enrollees in 1997

National Total = 38,341,718 Enrollees*

ALPHA ORDER

RANK	STATE	ENROLLEES	% of USA
19	Alabama	660,276	1.72%
50	Alaska	36,803	0.10%
21	Arizona	632,333	1.65%
31	Arkansas	429,183	1.12%
1	California	3,726,572	9.72%
30	Colorado	442,371	1.15%
26	Connecticut	507,699	1.32%
46	Delaware	105,345	0.27%
2	Florida	2,702,987	7.05%
12	Georgia	865,747	2.26%
42	Hawaii	155,906	0.41%
43	Idaho	155,419	0.41%
7	Illinois	1,619,637	4.22%
15	Indiana	833,061	2.17%
29	Iowa	475,150	1.24%
33	Kansas	386,470	1.01%
23	Kentucky	601,139	1.57%
24	Louisiana	590,641	1.54%
38	Maine	208,086	0.54%
22	Maryland	617,521	1.61%
11	Massachusetts	944,858	2.46%
8	Michigan	1,368,299	3.57%
20	Minnesota	638,828	1.67%
32	Mississippi	406,245	1.06%
14	Missouri	842,960	2.20%
44	Montana	132,937	0.35%
35	Nebraska	250,685	0.65%
37	Nevada	212,071	0.55%
41	New Hampshire	161,679	0.42%
9	New Jersey	1,180,814	3.08%
36	New Mexico	220,711	0.58%
3	New York	2,657,451	6.93%
10	North Carolina	1,071,266	2.79%
47	North Dakota	102,899	0.27%
6	Ohio	1,679,362	4.38%
27	Oklahoma	495,022	1.29%
28	Oregon	475,298	1.24%
5	Pennsylvania	2,078,507	5.42%
40	Rhode Island	169,060	0.44%
25	South Carolina	532,914	1.39%
45	South Dakota	117,721	0.31%
16	Tennessee	793,801	2.07%
4	Texas	2,153,357	5.62%
39	Utah	194,889	0.51%
48	Vermont	85,600	0.22%
13	Virginia	846,877	2.21%
18	Washington	707,094	1.84%
34	West Virginia	332,169	0.87%
17	Wisconsin	769,699	2.01%
49	Wyoming	62,654	0.16%

RANK ORDER

RANK	STATE	ENROLLEES	% of USA
1	California	3,726,572	9.72%
2	Florida	2,702,987	7.05%
3	New York	2,657,451	6.93%
4	Texas	2,153,357	5.62%
5	Pennsylvania	2,078,507	5.42%
6	Ohio	1,679,362	4.38%
7	Illinois	1,619,637	4.22%
8	Michigan	1,368,299	3.57%
9	New Jersey	1,180,814	3.08%
10	North Carolina	1,071,266	2.79%
11	Massachusetts	944,858	2.46%
12	Georgia	865,747	2.26%
13	Virginia	846,877	2.21%
14	Missouri	842,960	2.20%
15	Indiana	833,061	2.17%
16	Tennessee	793,801	2.07%
17	Wisconsin	769,699	2.01%
18	Washington	707,094	1.84%
19	Alabama	660,276	1.72%
20	Minnesota	638,828	1.67%
21	Arizona	632,333	1.65%
22	Maryland	617,521	1.61%
23	Kentucky	601,139	1.57%
24	Louisiana	590,641	1.54%
25	South Carolina	532,914	1.39%
26	Connecticut	507,699	1.32%
27	Oklahoma	495,022	1.29%
28	Oregon	475,298	1.24%
29	Iowa	475,150	1.24%
30	Colorado	442,371	1.15%
31	Arkansas	429,183	1.12%
32	Mississippi	406,245	1.06%
33	Kansas	386,470	1.01%
34	West Virginia	332,169	0.87%
35	Nebraska	250,685	0.65%
36	New Mexico	220,711	0.58%
37	Nevada	212,071	0.55%
38	Maine	208,086	0.54%
39	Utah	194,889	0.51%
40	Rhode Island	169,060	0.44%
41	New Hampshire	161,679	0.42%
42	Hawaii	155,906	0.41%
43	Idaho	155,419	0.41%
44	Montana	132,937	0.35%
45	South Dakota	117,721	0.31%
46	Delaware	105,345	0.27%
47	North Dakota	102,899	0.27%
48	Vermont	85,600	0.22%
49	Wyoming	62,654	0.16%
50	Alaska	36,803	0.10%
	District of Columbia	76,172	0.20%

Source: U.S. Department of Health and Human Services, Health Care Financing Administration unpublished data

*For fiscal year 1997. Includes aged and disabled enrollees. Total includes 502,463 enrollees in Puerto Rico and 325,000 enrollees in "other outlying areas."

Medicare Payments per Enrollee in 1997

National Rate = $5,402*

ALPHA ORDER				RANK ORDER		
RANK	STATE	PER ENROLLEE		RANK	STATE	PER ENROLLEE
16	Alabama	$5,427		1	Louisiana	$7,256
33	Alaska	4,420		2	Massachusetts	6,831
22	Arizona	5,078		3	Texas	6,629
31	Arkansas	4,441		4	Florida	6,484
9	California	5,927		5	New York	6,190
23	Colorado	5,009		6	Connecticut	6,071
6	Connecticut	6,071		7	Pennsylvania	5,988
30	Delaware	4,472		8	Tennessee	5,948
4	Florida	6,484		9	California	5,927
13	Georgia	5,457		10	Rhode Island	5,849
40	Hawaii	4,204		11	Maryland	5,567
49	Idaho	3,636		12	New Jersey	5,566
20	Illinois	5,133		13	Georgia	5,457
24	Indiana	4,898		14	Mississippi	5,449
48	Iowa	3,657		15	Missouri	5,433
35	Kansas	4,375		16	Alabama	5,427
25	Kentucky	4,806		17	Michigan	5,409
1	Louisiana	7,256		18	Oklahoma	5,408
39	Maine	4,226		19	Nevada	5,297
11	Maryland	5,567		20	Illinois	5,133
2	Massachusetts	6,831		21	Ohio	5,095
17	Michigan	5,409		22	Arizona	5,078
38	Minnesota	4,279		23	Colorado	5,009
14	Mississippi	5,449		24	Indiana	4,898
15	Missouri	5,433		25	Kentucky	4,806
47	Montana	3,730		26	North Carolina	4,741
41	Nebraska	4,107		27	North Dakota	4,551
19	Nevada	5,297		28	Utah	4,549
34	New Hampshire	4,414		29	West Virginia	4,527
12	New Jersey	5,566		30	Delaware	4,472
45	New Mexico	3,956		31	Arkansas	4,441
5	New York	6,190		31	South Carolina	4,441
26	North Carolina	4,741		33	Alaska	4,420
27	North Dakota	4,551		34	New Hampshire	4,414
21	Ohio	5,095		35	Kansas	4,375
18	Oklahoma	5,408		36	Virginia	4,293
44	Oregon	3,970		37	Washington	4,290
7	Pennsylvania	5,988		38	Minnesota	4,279
10	Rhode Island	5,849		39	Maine	4,226
31	South Carolina	4,441		40	Hawaii	4,204
42	South Dakota	4,047		41	Nebraska	4,107
8	Tennessee	5,948		42	South Dakota	4,047
3	Texas	6,629		43	Wisconsin	4,039
28	Utah	4,549		44	Oregon	3,970
46	Vermont	3,832		45	New Mexico	3,956
36	Virginia	4,293		46	Vermont	3,832
37	Washington	4,290		47	Montana	3,730
29	West Virginia	4,527		48	Iowa	3,657
43	Wisconsin	4,039		49	Idaho	3,636
50	Wyoming	3,440		50	Wyoming	3,440
					District of Columbia	16,595

Source: Morgan Quitno Press using data from U.S. Dept. of Health and Human Services, Health Care Financing Admn
    unpublished data

*For fiscal year 1997. Includes aged and disabled enrollees. National rate includes payments to enrollees in
Puerto Rico and in "other outlying areas."

Percent of Population Enrolled in Medicare in 1997

National Percent = 14.0% of Population*

ALPHA ORDER

RANK	STATE	PERCENT
14	Alabama	15.3
50	Alaska	6.0
32	Arizona	13.9
5	Arkansas	17.0
46	California	11.5
47	Colorado	11.4
11	Connecticut	15.5
27	Delaware	14.4
1	Florida	18.4
45	Georgia	11.6
37	Hawaii	13.1
39	Idaho	12.8
34	Illinois	13.6
29	Indiana	14.2
7	Iowa	16.7
18	Kansas	14.9
12	Kentucky	15.4
34	Louisiana	13.6
6	Maine	16.8
44	Maryland	12.1
12	Massachusetts	15.4
31	Michigan	14.0
34	Minnesota	13.6
18	Mississippi	14.9
10	Missouri	15.6
15	Montana	15.1
15	Nebraska	15.1
41	Nevada	12.6
33	New Hampshire	13.8
23	New Jersey	14.7
39	New Mexico	12.8
23	New York	14.7
27	North Carolina	14.4
8	North Dakota	16.1
17	Ohio	15.0
18	Oklahoma	14.9
23	Oregon	14.7
3	Pennsylvania	17.3
4	Rhode Island	17.1
29	South Carolina	14.2
9	South Dakota	16.0
22	Tennessee	14.8
48	Texas	11.1
49	Utah	9.5
26	Vermont	14.5
41	Virginia	12.6
41	Washington	12.6
2	West Virginia	18.3
18	Wisconsin	14.9
37	Wyoming	13.1

RANK ORDER

RANK	STATE	PERCENT
1	Florida	18.4
2	West Virginia	18.3
3	Pennsylvania	17.3
4	Rhode Island	17.1
5	Arkansas	17.0
6	Maine	16.8
7	Iowa	16.7
8	North Dakota	16.1
9	South Dakota	16.0
10	Missouri	15.6
11	Connecticut	15.5
12	Kentucky	15.4
12	Massachusetts	15.4
14	Alabama	15.3
15	Montana	15.1
15	Nebraska	15.1
17	Ohio	15.0
18	Kansas	14.9
18	Mississippi	14.9
18	Oklahoma	14.9
18	Wisconsin	14.9
22	Tennessee	14.8
23	New Jersey	14.7
23	New York	14.7
23	Oregon	14.7
26	Vermont	14.5
27	Delaware	14.4
27	North Carolina	14.4
29	Indiana	14.2
29	South Carolina	14.2
31	Michigan	14.0
32	Arizona	13.9
33	New Hampshire	13.8
34	Illinois	13.6
34	Louisiana	13.6
34	Minnesota	13.6
37	Hawaii	13.1
37	Wyoming	13.1
39	Idaho	12.8
39	New Mexico	12.8
41	Nevada	12.6
41	Virginia	12.6
41	Washington	12.6
44	Maryland	12.1
45	Georgia	11.6
46	California	11.5
47	Colorado	11.4
48	Texas	11.1
49	Utah	9.5
50	Alaska	6.0

District of Columbia 14.4

Source: Morgan Quitno Press using data from U.S. Dept. of Health and Human Services, Health Care Financing Admn
    unpublished data

*For fiscal year 1997. Includes aged and disabled enrollees. National rate includes only residents of the 50 states
and the District of Columbia.

Medicare Health Maintenance Organizations (HMOs) in 1997

National Total = 237 Medicare HMOs*

ALPHA ORDER

RANK	STATE	HMOs	% of USA
24	Alabama	3	1.27%
43	Alaska	0	0.00%
8	Arizona	8	3.38%
32	Arkansas	2	0.84%
1	California	22	9.28%
8	Colorado	8	3.38%
15	Connecticut	5	2.11%
32	Delaware	2	0.84%
3	Florida	19	8.02%
19	Georgia	4	1.69%
37	Hawaii	1	0.42%
43	Idaho	0	0.00%
8	Illinois	8	3.38%
15	Indiana	5	2.11%
24	Iowa	3	1.27%
24	Kansas	3	1.27%
37	Kentucky	1	0.42%
19	Louisiana	4	1.69%
43	Maine	0	0.00%
19	Maryland	4	1.69%
15	Massachusetts	5	2.11%
24	Michigan	3	1.27%
15	Minnesota	5	2.11%
43	Mississippi	0	0.00%
11	Missouri	7	2.95%
43	Montana	0	0.00%
32	Nebraska	2	0.84%
24	Nevada	3	1.27%
32	New Hampshire	2	0.84%
6	New Jersey	10	4.22%
19	New Mexico	4	1.69%
2	New York	20	8.44%
24	North Carolina	3	1.27%
37	North Dakota	1	0.42%
4	Ohio	14	5.91%
19	Oklahoma	4	1.69%
12	Oregon	6	2.53%
5	Pennsylvania	11	4.64%
37	Rhode Island	1	0.42%
37	South Carolina	1	0.42%
43	South Dakota	0	0.00%
32	Tennessee	2	0.84%
6	Texas	10	4.22%
24	Utah	3	1.27%
43	Vermont	0	0.00%
24	Virginia	3	1.27%
12	Washington	6	2.53%
37	West Virginia	1	0.42%
12	Wisconsin	6	2.53%
43	Wyoming	0	0.00%

RANK ORDER

RANK	STATE	HMOs	% of USA
1	California	22	9.28%
2	New York	20	8.44%
3	Florida	19	8.02%
4	Ohio	14	5.91%
5	Pennsylvania	11	4.64%
6	New Jersey	10	4.22%
6	Texas	10	4.22%
8	Arizona	8	3.38%
8	Colorado	8	3.38%
8	Illinois	8	3.38%
11	Missouri	7	2.95%
12	Oregon	6	2.53%
12	Washington	6	2.53%
12	Wisconsin	6	2.53%
15	Connecticut	5	2.11%
15	Indiana	5	2.11%
15	Massachusetts	5	2.11%
15	Minnesota	5	2.11%
19	Georgia	4	1.69%
19	Louisiana	4	1.69%
19	Maryland	4	1.69%
19	New Mexico	4	1.69%
19	Oklahoma	4	1.69%
24	Alabama	3	1.27%
24	Iowa	3	1.27%
24	Kansas	3	1.27%
24	Michigan	3	1.27%
24	Nevada	3	1.27%
24	North Carolina	3	1.27%
24	Utah	3	1.27%
24	Virginia	3	1.27%
32	Arkansas	2	0.84%
32	Delaware	2	0.84%
32	Nebraska	2	0.84%
32	New Hampshire	2	0.84%
32	Tennessee	2	0.84%
37	Hawaii	1	0.42%
37	Kentucky	1	0.42%
37	North Dakota	1	0.42%
37	Rhode Island	1	0.42%
37	South Carolina	1	0.42%
37	West Virginia	1	0.42%
43	Alaska	0	0.00%
43	Idaho	0	0.00%
43	Maine	0	0.00%
43	Mississippi	0	0.00%
43	Montana	0	0.00%
43	South Dakota	0	0.00%
43	Vermont	0	0.00%
43	Wyoming	0	0.00%
	District of Columbia	2	0.84%

Source: InterStudy Publications (Minneapolis, MN)
    "The Competitive Edge Industry Report 7.2" (October 1997)
*As of January 1, 1997. Health plans are allocated to states based upon their primary service areas. This means each plan is counted once. However, many plans serve more than one state.

Medicare Managed Care Enrollees in 1998

National Total = 6,255,919 Enrollees*

ALPHA ORDER

RANK	STATE	ENROLLEES	% of USA
26	Alabama	37,574	0.60%
45	Alaska	0	0.00%
7	Arizona	244,053	3.90%
35	Arkansas	11,667	0.19%
1	California	1,523,767	24.36%
12	Colorado	143,240	2.29%
18	Connecticut	86,233	1.38%
45	Delaware	0	0.00%
2	Florida	741,102	11.85%
27	Georgia	32,986	0.53%
20	Hawaii	52,966	0.85%
39	Idaho	6,130	0.10%
11	Illinois	166,999	2.67%
30	Indiana	22,038	0.35%
37	Iowa	8,136	0.13%
40	Kansas	5,289	0.08%
34	Kentucky	11,816	0.19%
17	Louisiana	94,130	1.50%
45	Maine	0	0.00%
16	Maryland	101,541	1.62%
8	Massachusetts	203,309	3.25%
22	Michigan	46,464	0.74%
15	Minnesota	108,322	1.73%
45	Mississippi	0	0.00%
14	Missouri	124,466	1.99%
42	Montana	1,310	0.02%
33	Nebraska	12,592	0.20%
19	Nevada	74,212	1.19%
36	New Hampshire	11,456	0.18%
13	New Jersey	133,865	2.14%
23	New Mexico	41,384	0.66%
4	New York	487,549	7.79%
29	North Carolina	25,562	0.41%
44	North Dakota	733	0.01%
6	Ohio	248,338	3.97%
25	Oklahoma	37,827	0.60%
9	Oregon	190,205	3.04%
3	Pennsylvania	499,582	7.99%
21	Rhode Island	48,636	0.78%
43	South Carolina	1,131	0.02%
45	South Dakota	0	0.00%
32	Tennessee	14,116	0.23%
5	Texas	314,334	5.02%
24	Utah	40,261	0.64%
41	Vermont	1,495	0.02%
31	Virginia	14,537	0.23%
10	Washington	173,177	2.77%
38	West Virginia	7,601	0.12%
28	Wisconsin	31,506	0.50%
45	Wyoming	0	0.00%

RANK ORDER

RANK	STATE	ENROLLEES	% of USA
1	California	1,523,767	24.36%
2	Florida	741,102	11.85%
3	Pennsylvania	499,582	7.99%
4	New York	487,549	7.79%
5	Texas	314,334	5.02%
6	Ohio	248,338	3.97%
7	Arizona	244,053	3.90%
8	Massachusetts	203,309	3.25%
9	Oregon	190,205	3.04%
10	Washington	173,177	2.77%
11	Illinois	166,999	2.67%
12	Colorado	143,240	2.29%
13	New Jersey	133,865	2.14%
14	Missouri	124,466	1.99%
15	Minnesota	108,322	1.73%
16	Maryland	101,541	1.62%
17	Louisiana	94,130	1.50%
18	Connecticut	86,233	1.38%
19	Nevada	74,212	1.19%
20	Hawaii	52,966	0.85%
21	Rhode Island	48,636	0.78%
22	Michigan	46,464	0.74%
23	New Mexico	41,384	0.66%
24	Utah	40,261	0.64%
25	Oklahoma	37,827	0.60%
26	Alabama	37,574	0.60%
27	Georgia	32,986	0.53%
28	Wisconsin	31,506	0.50%
29	North Carolina	25,562	0.41%
30	Indiana	22,038	0.35%
31	Virginia	14,537	0.23%
32	Tennessee	14,116	0.23%
33	Nebraska	12,592	0.20%
34	Kentucky	11,816	0.19%
35	Arkansas	11,667	0.19%
36	New Hampshire	11,456	0.18%
37	Iowa	8,136	0.13%
38	West Virginia	7,601	0.12%
39	Idaho	6,130	0.10%
40	Kansas	5,289	0.08%
41	Vermont	1,495	0.02%
42	Montana	1,310	0.02%
43	South Carolina	1,131	0.02%
44	North Dakota	733	0.01%
45	Alaska	0	0.00%
45	Delaware	0	0.00%
45	Maine	0	0.00%
45	Mississippi	0	0.00%
45	South Dakota	0	0.00%
45	Wyoming	0	0.00%
	District of Columbia	0	0.00%

Source: U.S. Department of Health and Human Services, Health Care Financing Administration
"Medicare Managed Care Contract Report" (April 1, 1998, http://www.hcfa.gov/stats/mmcc0498.txt)
*As of April 1st. Includes TEFRA, Cost, and Health Care Prepayment Plans (HCCP). National total includes 112,642 enrollees in "Other Demonstration" plans. National total includes 72,282 enrollees in the United Mine Workers' plan not shown separately by state.

Percent of Medicare Enrollees in Managed Care Programs in 1997

National Percent = 15.0% of Medicare Enrollees*

ALPHA ORDER RANK	STATE	PERCENT
25	Alabama	4.5
45	Alaska	0.0
3	Arizona	36.3
35	Arkansas	1.8
1	California	39.9
6	Colorado	29.5
21	Connecticut	9.9
45	Delaware	0.0
7	Florida	24.8
30	Georgia	2.5
4	Hawaii	32.5
33	Idaho	2.1
23	Illinois	9.7
34	Indiana	1.9
35	Iowa	1.8
29	Kansas	3.1
37	Kentucky	1.7
19	Louisiana	11.9
45	Maine	0.0
16	Maryland	12.8
12	Massachusetts	19.3
32	Michigan	2.2
14	Minnesota	17.6
45	Mississippi	0.0
17	Missouri	12.5
44	Montana	0.2
26	Nebraska	4.3
4	Nevada	32.5
27	New Hampshire	3.8
21	New Jersey	9.9
13	New Mexico	17.9
15	New York	16.2
39	North Carolina	1.4
43	North Dakota	0.7
20	Ohio	11.0
24	Oklahoma	6.9
2	Oregon	39.6
10	Pennsylvania	20.9
11	Rhode Island	20.8
42	South Carolina	0.8
45	South Dakota	0.0
41	Tennessee	1.0
18	Texas	12.3
9	Utah	21.1
38	Vermont	1.6
40	Virginia	1.2
8	Washington	22.9
31	West Virginia	2.3
28	Wisconsin	3.3
45	Wyoming	0.0

RANK ORDER RANK	STATE	PERCENT
1	California	39.9
2	Oregon	39.6
3	Arizona	36.3
4	Hawaii	32.5
4	Nevada	32.5
6	Colorado	29.5
7	Florida	24.8
8	Washington	22.9
9	Utah	21.1
10	Pennsylvania	20.9
11	Rhode Island	20.8
12	Massachusetts	19.3
13	New Mexico	17.9
14	Minnesota	17.6
15	New York	16.2
16	Maryland	12.8
17	Missouri	12.5
18	Texas	12.3
19	Louisiana	11.9
20	Ohio	11.0
21	Connecticut	9.9
21	New Jersey	9.9
23	Illinois	9.7
24	Oklahoma	6.9
25	Alabama	4.5
26	Nebraska	4.3
27	New Hampshire	3.8
28	Wisconsin	3.3
29	Kansas	3.1
30	Georgia	2.5
31	West Virginia	2.3
32	Michigan	2.2
33	Idaho	2.1
34	Indiana	1.9
35	Arkansas	1.8
35	Iowa	1.8
37	Kentucky	1.7
38	Vermont	1.6
39	North Carolina	1.4
40	Virginia	1.2
41	Tennessee	1.0
42	South Carolina	0.8
43	North Dakota	0.7
44	Montana	0.2
45	Alaska	0.0
45	Delaware	0.0
45	Maine	0.0
45	Mississippi	0.0
45	South Dakota	0.0
45	Wyoming	0.0
	District of Columbia	14.6

Source: Morgan Quitno Press using data from U.S. Dept. of Health and Human Services, Health Care Financing Admin. Medicare Managed Care Contract Report as of 9/1/97 (www.hcfa.gov/stats/mmcc0997.txt)
*For fiscal year 1997. Includes aged and disabled enrollees. National percent does not include enrollees in Puerto Rico and other outlying areas."

Medicare Physicians in 1997

National Total = 782,887 Physicians*

<u>ALPHA ORDER</u>

<u>RANK ORDER</u>

RANK	STATE	PHYSICIANS	% of USA		RANK	STATE	PHYSICIANS	% of USA
25	Alabama	10,018	1.28%		1	California	92,309	11.79%
49	Alaska	1,209	0.15%		2	North Dakota	73,200	9.35%
24	Arizona	10,535	1.35%		3	Pennsylvania	46,509	5.94%
32	Arkansas	6,876	0.88%		4	Texas	45,629	5.83%
1	California	92,309	11.79%		5	Florida	38,979	4.98%
22	Colorado	11,874	1.52%		6	Indiana	31,346	4.00%
23	Connecticut	11,509	1.47%		7	Ohio	30,067	3.84%
47	Delaware	2,055	0.26%		8	Michigan	29,566	3.78%
5	Florida	38,979	4.98%		9	Maine	27,784	3.55%
13	Georgia	16,725	2.14%		10	New Mexico	25,061	3.20%
40	Hawaii**	3,543	0.45%		11	Nebraska	21,112	2.70%
28	Idaho	8,205	1.05%		12	Maryland	17,263	2.21%
43	Illinois	2,576	0.33%		13	Georgia	16,725	2.14%
6	Indiana	31,346	4.00%		14	Mississippi	16,109	2.06%
20	Iowa	14,763	1.89%		15	Tennessee	15,953	2.04%
31	Kansas	6,895	0.88%		16	Vermont	15,728	2.01%
26	Kentucky	9,603	1.23%		17	Washington	15,179	1.94%
21	Louisiana	12,502	1.60%		18	West Virginia	15,168	1.94%
9	Maine	27,784	3.55%		19	Minnesota	15,045	1.92%
12	Maryland	17,263	2.21%		20	Iowa	14,763	1.89%
36	Massachusetts	4,257	0.54%		21	Louisiana	12,502	1.60%
8	Michigan	29,566	3.78%		22	Colorado	11,874	1.52%
19	Minnesota	15,045	1.92%		23	Connecticut	11,509	1.47%
14	Mississippi	16,109	2.06%		24	Arizona	10,535	1.35%
33	Missouri	4,856	0.62%		25	Alabama	10,018	1.28%
44	Montana	2,490	0.32%		26	Kentucky	9,603	1.23%
11	Nebraska	21,112	2.70%		27	Oregon	8,848	1.13%
45	Nevada	2,186	0.28%		28	Idaho	8,205	1.05%
37	New Hampshire	4,248	0.54%		29	South Carolina	7,889	1.01%
39	New Jersey	3,965	0.51%		30	Oklahoma	7,530	0.96%
10	New Mexico	25,061	3.20%		31	Kansas	6,895	0.88%
38	New York	4,076	0.52%		32	Arkansas	6,876	0.88%
42	North Carolina	3,093	0.40%		33	Missouri	4,856	0.62%
2	North Dakota	73,200	9.35%		34	Utah	4,545	0.58%
7	Ohio	30,067	3.84%		35	Wisconsin	4,337	0.55%
30	Oklahoma	7,530	0.96%		36	Massachusetts	4,257	0.54%
27	Oregon	8,848	1.13%		37	New Hampshire	4,248	0.54%
3	Pennsylvania	46,509	5.94%		38	New York	4,076	0.52%
41	Rhode Island	3,362	0.43%		39	New Jersey	3,965	0.51%
29	South Carolina	7,889	1.01%		40	Hawaii**	3,543	0.45%
48	South Dakota	1,992	0.25%		41	Rhode Island	3,362	0.43%
15	Tennessee	15,953	2.04%		42	North Carolina	3,093	0.40%
4	Texas	45,629	5.83%		43	Illinois	2,576	0.33%
34	Utah	4,545	0.58%		44	Montana	2,490	0.32%
16	Vermont	15,728	2.01%		45	Nevada	2,186	0.28%
46	Virginia	2,085	0.27%		46	Virginia	2,085	0.27%
17	Washington	15,179	1.94%		47	Delaware	2,055	0.26%
18	West Virginia	15,168	1.94%		48	South Dakota	1,992	0.25%
35	Wisconsin	4,337	0.55%		49	Alaska	1,209	0.15%
50	Wyoming	1,107	0.14%		50	Wyoming	1,107	0.14%
						District of Columbia	3,950	0.50%

Source: U.S. Department of Health and Human Services, Health Care Financing Administration
  "1997 Data Compendium" (March 1997)
Medicare Part B. "Physicians" include MD, DO, DDM, DDS, DPM, OD and CH. National total includes 7,174 physicians in Puerto Rico and the Virgin Islands.
***Physicians for Guam are included in Hawaii's total.*

Percent of Physicians Participating in Medicare in 1996

National Percent = 72.3% of Physicians Participate in Medicare*

ALPHA ORDER

ALPHA ORDER

RANK ORDER

RANK	STATE	PERCENT		RANK	STATE	PERCENT
2	Alabama	91.8		1	North Dakota	92.2
40	Alaska	73.5		2	Alabama	91.8
14	Arizona	85.2		2	Ohio	91.8
32	Arkansas	77.2		4	Kansas	91.1
26	California	80.5		5	Nevada	90.8
29	Colorado	79.5		6	Maryland	89.9
15	Connecticut	84.3		7	West Virginia	89.3
41	Delaware	72.3		8	Georgia	87.2
43	Florida	70.9		9	Missouri	86.8
8	Georgia	87.2		9	Utah	86.8
18	Hawaii	83.6		11	Washington	86.4
50	Idaho	60.1		12	Nebraska	86.3
38	Illinois	75.6		13	Kentucky	85.8
37	Indiana	75.7		14	Arizona	85.2
18	Iowa	83.6		15	Connecticut	84.3
4	Kansas	91.1		15	Virginia	84.3
13	Kentucky	85.8		17	Wisconsin	83.9
48	Louisiana	61.0		18	Hawaii	83.6
32	Maine	77.2		18	Iowa	83.6
6	Maryland	89.9		20	Tennessee	83.1
39	Massachusetts	74.9		21	South Carolina	82.7
28	Michigan	80.2		22	Oregon	82.1
44	Minnesota	70.6		23	Wyoming	81.2
31	Mississippi	77.3		24	North Carolina	81.0
9	Missouri	86.8		25	New Mexico	80.7
30	Montana	77.4		26	California	80.5
12	Nebraska	86.3		27	Texas	80.3
5	Nevada	90.8		28	Michigan	80.2
34	New Hampshire	77.0		29	Colorado	79.5
49	New Jersey	60.6		30	Montana	77.4
25	New Mexico	80.7		31	Mississippi	77.3
47	New York	64.2		32	Arkansas	77.2
24	North Carolina	81.0		32	Maine	77.2
1	North Dakota	92.2		34	New Hampshire	77.0
2	Ohio	91.8		35	Oklahoma	76.1
35	Oklahoma	76.1		35	Vermont	76.1
22	Oregon	82.1		37	Indiana	75.7
45	Pennsylvania	69.3		38	Illinois	75.6
46	Rhode Island	66.8		39	Massachusetts	74.9
21	South Carolina	82.7		40	Alaska	73.5
42	South Dakota	71.4		41	Delaware	72.3
20	Tennessee	83.1		42	South Dakota	71.4
27	Texas	80.3		43	Florida	70.9
9	Utah	86.8		44	Minnesota	70.6
35	Vermont	76.1		45	Pennsylvania	69.3
15	Virginia	84.3		46	Rhode Island	66.8
11	Washington	86.4		47	New York	64.2
7	West Virginia	89.3		48	Louisiana	61.0
17	Wisconsin	83.9		49	New Jersey	60.6
23	Wyoming	81.2		50	Idaho	60.1
					District of Columbia	65.3

Source: U.S. Department of Health and Human Services, Health Care Financing Administration
    "1997 Data Compendium" (March 1997)
*Medicare Part B. Physicians include MD's, DO's, limited license practitioners and non-physician practitioners.
National percent is for 1995.

Medicaid Expenditures in 1996

National Total = $121,684,650,271*

ALPHA ORDER

RANK	STATE	EXPENDITURES	% of USA
24	Alabama	$1,461,101,085	1.20%
47	Alaska	278,454,890	0.23%
49	Arizona	210,981,689	0.17%
28	Arkansas	1,223,839,204	1.01%
2	California	11,123,655,013	9.14%
31	Colorado	1,032,388,114	0.85%
18	Connecticut	2,030,311,861	1.67%
44	Delaware	308,470,254	0.25%
6	Florida	4,670,085,277	3.84%
12	Georgia	3,085,207,931	2.54%
48	Hawaii	266,356,069	0.22%
40	Idaho	405,316,064	0.33%
5	Illinois	5,365,025,893	4.41%
15	Indiana	2,451,592,642	2.01%
30	Iowa	1,088,441,757	0.89%
34	Kansas	860,281,872	0.71%
20	Kentucky	1,930,812,385	1.59%
14	Louisiana	2,452,543,946	2.02%
35	Maine	722,718,672	0.59%
17	Maryland	2,047,492,180	1.68%
8	Massachusetts	3,776,967,216	3.10%
11	Michigan	3,359,306,651	2.76%
16	Minnesota	2,430,408,222	2.00%
26	Mississippi	1,341,660,815	1.10%
19	Missouri	2,017,609,226	1.66%
42	Montana	352,221,184	0.29%
37	Nebraska	678,268,020	0.56%
41	Nevada	365,239,732	0.30%
38	New Hampshire	547,355,844	0.45%
9	New Jersey	3,726,087,488	3.06%
33	New Mexico	877,576,545	0.72%
1	New York	22,347,344,824	18.36%
10	North Carolina	3,677,756,007	3.02%
46	North Dakota	298,086,305	0.24%
4	Ohio	5,511,943,301	4.53%
32	Oklahoma	1,021,231,344	0.84%
27	Oregon	1,313,198,803	1.08%
7	Pennsylvania	4,663,428,976	3.83%
36	Rhode Island	684,030,676	0.56%
23	South Carolina	1,522,740,572	1.25%
43	South Dakota	315,836,128	0.26%
13	Tennessee	2,886,334,809	2.37%
3	Texas	6,871,224,596	5.65%
39	Utah	422,065,108	0.35%
45	Vermont	301,954,836	0.25%
22	Virginia	1,776,068,416	1.46%
25	Washington	1,393,317,886	1.15%
29	West Virginia	1,127,715,335	0.93%
21	Wisconsin	1,904,143,232	1.56%
50	Wyoming	182,928,368	0.15%

RANK ORDER

RANK	STATE	EXPENDITURES	% of USA
1	New York	$22,347,344,824	18.36%
2	California	11,123,655,013	9.14%
3	Texas	6,871,224,596	5.65%
4	Ohio	5,511,943,301	4.53%
5	Illinois	5,365,025,893	4.41%
6	Florida	4,670,085,277	3.84%
7	Pennsylvania	4,663,428,976	3.83%
8	Massachusetts	3,776,967,216	3.10%
9	New Jersey	3,726,087,488	3.06%
10	North Carolina	3,677,756,007	3.02%
11	Michigan	3,359,306,651	2.76%
12	Georgia	3,085,207,931	2.54%
13	Tennessee	2,886,334,809	2.37%
14	Louisiana	2,452,543,946	2.02%
15	Indiana	2,451,592,642	2.01%
16	Minnesota	2,430,408,222	2.00%
17	Maryland	2,047,492,180	1.68%
18	Connecticut	2,030,311,861	1.67%
19	Missouri	2,017,609,226	1.66%
20	Kentucky	1,930,812,385	1.59%
21	Wisconsin	1,904,143,232	1.56%
22	Virginia	1,776,068,416	1.46%
23	South Carolina	1,522,740,572	1.25%
24	Alabama	1,461,101,085	1.20%
25	Washington	1,393,317,886	1.15%
26	Mississippi	1,341,660,815	1.10%
27	Oregon	1,313,198,803	1.08%
28	Arkansas	1,223,839,204	1.01%
29	West Virginia	1,127,715,335	0.93%
30	Iowa	1,088,441,757	0.89%
31	Colorado	1,032,388,114	0.85%
32	Oklahoma	1,021,231,344	0.84%
33	New Mexico	877,576,545	0.72%
34	Kansas	860,281,872	0.71%
35	Maine	722,718,672	0.59%
36	Rhode Island	684,030,676	0.56%
37	Nebraska	678,268,020	0.56%
38	New Hampshire	547,355,844	0.45%
39	Utah	422,065,108	0.35%
40	Idaho	405,316,064	0.33%
41	Nevada	365,239,732	0.30%
42	Montana	352,221,184	0.29%
43	South Dakota	315,836,128	0.26%
44	Delaware	308,470,254	0.25%
45	Vermont	301,954,836	0.25%
46	North Dakota	298,086,305	0.24%
47	Alaska	278,454,890	0.23%
48	Hawaii	266,356,069	0.22%
49	Arizona	210,981,689	0.17%
50	Wyoming	182,928,368	0.15%
	District of Columbia	710,155,666	0.58%

Source: U.S. Department of Health and Human Services, Health Care Financing Administration
   "Medicaid Medical Vendor Payments by Type of Service, Region and State: FY 1996" (HCFA-2082)
*For fiscal year ending September 30, 1996. National total includes $256,200,000 for Puerto Rico and $9,167,342 for the Virgin Islands.

Percent Change in Medicaid Expenditures: 1990 to 1996

National Percent Change = 87.6% Increase*

ALPHA ORDER				RANK ORDER		
RANK	STATE	PERCENT CHANGE		RANK	STATE	PERCENT CHANGE
11	Alabama	139.8		1	New Mexico	218.8
20	Alaska	100.2		2	West Virginia	212.3
NA	Arizona**	NA		3	Wyoming	210.4
19	Arkansas	104.2		4	North Carolina	157.9
36	California	71.0		5	Oregon	153.1
20	Colorado	100.2		6	Delaware	150.4
37	Connecticut	68.5		7	Idaho	149.9
6	Delaware	150.4		8	Tennessee	148.2
22	Florida	97.8		9	Texas	147.1
45	Georgia	48.6		10	Nevada	145.8
48	Hawaii	39.2		11	Alabama	139.8
7	Idaho	149.9		12	Mississippi	128.9
15	Illinois	121.3		13	New Hampshire	125.2
29	Indiana	82.6		14	Missouri	124.9
32	Iowa	75.5		15	Illinois	121.3
33	Kansas	75.4		16	Nebraska	119.3
23	Kentucky	97.7		17	Montana	106.5
28	Louisiana	86.5		18	South Carolina	104.9
38	Maine	67.3		19	Arkansas	104.2
27	Maryland	87.8		20	Alaska	100.2
49	Massachusetts	38.3		20	Colorado	100.2
43	Michigan	53.1		22	Florida	97.8
34	Minnesota	72.3		23	Kentucky	97.7
12	Mississippi	128.9		24	Vermont	97.5
14	Missouri	124.9		25	South Dakota	90.2
17	Montana	106.5		26	New York	88.2
16	Nebraska	119.3		27	Maryland	87.8
10	Nevada	145.8		28	Louisiana	86.5
13	New Hampshire	125.2		29	Indiana	82.6
39	New Jersey	62.1		30	Virginia	80.3
1	New Mexico	218.8		31	Ohio	76.0
26	New York	88.2		32	Iowa	75.5
4	North Carolina	157.9		33	Kansas	75.4
42	North Dakota	53.8		34	Minnesota	72.3
31	Ohio	76.0		35	Utah	71.1
46	Oklahoma	48.5		36	California	71.0
5	Oregon	153.1		37	Connecticut	68.5
40	Pennsylvania	61.8		38	Maine	67.3
41	Rhode Island	54.7		39	New Jersey	62.1
18	South Carolina	104.9		40	Pennsylvania	61.8
25	South Dakota	90.2		41	Rhode Island	54.7
8	Tennessee	148.2		42	North Dakota	53.8
9	Texas	147.1		43	Michigan	53.1
35	Utah	71.1		44	Wisconsin	52.5
24	Vermont	97.5		45	Georgia	48.6
30	Virginia	80.3		46	Oklahoma	48.5
47	Washington	46.3		47	Washington	46.3
2	West Virginia	212.3		48	Hawaii	39.2
44	Wisconsin	52.5		49	Massachusetts	38.3
3	Wyoming	210.4		NA	Arizona**	NA
					District of Columbia	189.0

Source: Morgan Quitno Press using data from U.S. Dept. of Health & Human Services, Health Care Financing Admin.
    "Medicaid Recipients, Vendor Payments and Average Cost per Recipient by State: FY 1996" (HCFA-2082)
*For fiscal year ending September 30, 1996.
**Not available.

Percent of Personal Health Care Expenditures Paid by Medicaid in 1993

National Percent = 14.5%*

ALPHA ORDER				RANK ORDER		
RANK	STATE	PERCENT		RANK	STATE	PERCENT
44	Alabama	10.6		1	New York	26.9
6	Alaska	17.4		2	Rhode Island	23.1
38	Arizona	11.9		3	Maine	21.0
9	Arkansas	16.5		4	West Virginia	20.7
37	California	12.0		5	Louisiana	20.5
49	Colorado	9.6		6	Alaska	17.4
10	Connecticut	16.4		7	Indiana	16.9
43	Delaware	11.0		8	Mississippi	16.8
45	Florida	10.5		9	Arkansas	16.5
24	Georgia	13.7		10	Connecticut	16.4
47	Hawaii	10.2		11	Kentucky	16.2
32	Idaho	12.7		12	Massachusetts	15.8
28	Illinois	13.3		13	Minnesota	15.7
7	Indiana	16.9		14	Vermont	15.5
30	Iowa	13.1		15	Montana	15.3
42	Kansas	11.1		16	New Jersey	15.0
11	Kentucky	16.2		17	New Mexico	14.9
5	Louisiana	20.5		18	South Carolina	14.7
3	Maine	21.0		18	Wisconsin	14.7
32	Maryland	12.7		20	Washington	14.3
12	Massachusetts	15.8		21	Michigan	14.2
21	Michigan	14.2		22	North Carolina	14.1
13	Minnesota	15.7		23	Ohio	13.9
8	Mississippi	16.8		24	Georgia	13.7
46	Missouri	10.3		24	Wyoming	13.7
15	Montana	15.3		26	South Dakota	13.5
32	Nebraska	12.7		26	Tennessee	13.5
50	Nevada	9.2		28	Illinois	13.3
31	New Hampshire	12.9		28	North Dakota	13.3
16	New Jersey	15.0		30	Iowa	13.1
17	New Mexico	14.9		31	New Hampshire	12.9
1	New York	26.9		32	Idaho	12.7
22	North Carolina	14.1		32	Maryland	12.7
28	North Dakota	13.3		32	Nebraska	12.7
23	Ohio	13.9		35	Oklahoma	12.6
35	Oklahoma	12.6		36	Pennsylvania	12.3
38	Oregon	11.9		37	California	12.0
36	Pennsylvania	12.3		38	Arizona	11.9
2	Rhode Island	23.1		38	Oregon	11.9
18	South Carolina	14.7		38	Texas	11.9
26	South Dakota	13.5		41	Utah	11.6
26	Tennessee	13.5		42	Kansas	11.1
38	Texas	11.9		43	Delaware	11.0
41	Utah	11.6		44	Alabama	10.6
14	Vermont	15.5		45	Florida	10.5
48	Virginia	9.7		46	Missouri	10.3
20	Washington	14.3		47	Hawaii	10.2
4	West Virginia	20.7		48	Virginia	9.7
18	Wisconsin	14.7		49	Colorado	9.6
24	Wyoming	13.7		50	Nevada	9.2
				District of Columbia		15.8

Source: U.S. Department of Health and Human Services, Health Care Financing Administration
    "State Health Expenditure Accounts" (Health Care Financing Review, Fall 1995, Volume 17, Number 1)
*By state of provider.

Medicaid Recipients in 1996

National Total = 36,117,956 Recipients*

ALPHA ORDER

RANK	STATE	RECIPIENTS	% of USA
20	Alabama	546,272	1.51%
47	Alaska	69,146	0.19%
21	Arizona	528,321	1.46%
29	Arkansas	362,635	1.00%
1	California	5,106,746	14.14%
34	Colorado	270,580	0.75%
31	Connecticut	328,585	0.91%
45	Delaware	81,766	0.23%
4	Florida	1,638,049	4.54%
8	Georgia	1,184,833	3.28%
50	Hawaii	40,514	0.11%
40	Idaho	119,150	0.33%
6	Illinois	1,454,152	4.03%
19	Indiana	593,625	1.64%
33	Iowa	307,974	0.85%
35	Kansas	251,171	0.70%
15	Kentucky	640,541	1.77%
12	Louisiana	777,708	2.15%
37	Maine	167,238	0.46%
27	Maryland	398,537	1.10%
13	Massachusetts	714,639	1.98%
9	Michigan	1,171,622	3.24%
24	Minnesota	454,944	1.26%
22	Mississippi	509,581	1.41%
16	Missouri	636,176	1.76%
43	Montana	101,271	0.28%
36	Nebraska	191,155	0.53%
41	Nevada	108,662	0.30%
44	New Hampshire	99,594	0.28%
14	New Jersey	714,180	1.98%
32	New Mexico	318,356	0.88%
2	New York	3,281,016	9.08%
11	North Carolina	1,130,024	3.13%
48	North Dakota	60,971	0.17%
5	Ohio	1,478,183	4.09%
30	Oklahoma	358,121	0.99%
25	Oregon	450,466	1.25%
10	Pennsylvania	1,168,022	3.23%
39	Rhode Island	129,542	0.36%
23	South Carolina	503,295	1.39%
46	South Dakota	76,776	0.21%
7	Tennessee	1,408,918	3.90%
3	Texas	2,571,547	7.12%
38	Utah	152,076	0.42%
42	Vermont	102,220	0.28%
17	Virginia	623,315	1.73%
18	Washington	621,462	1.72%
28	West Virginia	394,963	1.09%
26	Wisconsin	434,314	1.20%
49	Wyoming	51,231	0.14%

RANK ORDER

RANK	STATE	RECIPIENTS	% of USA
1	California	5,106,746	14.14%
2	New York	3,281,016	9.08%
3	Texas	2,571,547	7.12%
4	Florida	1,638,049	4.54%
5	Ohio	1,478,183	4.09%
6	Illinois	1,454,152	4.03%
7	Tennessee	1,408,918	3.90%
8	Georgia	1,184,833	3.28%
9	Michigan	1,171,622	3.24%
10	Pennsylvania	1,168,022	3.23%
11	North Carolina	1,130,024	3.13%
12	Louisiana	777,708	2.15%
13	Massachusetts	714,639	1.98%
14	New Jersey	714,180	1.98%
15	Kentucky	640,541	1.77%
16	Missouri	636,176	1.76%
17	Virginia	623,315	1.73%
18	Washington	621,462	1.72%
19	Indiana	593,625	1.64%
20	Alabama	546,272	1.51%
21	Arizona	528,321	1.46%
22	Mississippi	509,581	1.41%
23	South Carolina	503,295	1.39%
24	Minnesota	454,944	1.26%
25	Oregon	450,466	1.25%
26	Wisconsin	434,314	1.20%
27	Maryland	398,537	1.10%
28	West Virginia	394,963	1.09%
29	Arkansas	362,635	1.00%
30	Oklahoma	358,121	0.99%
31	Connecticut	328,585	0.91%
32	New Mexico	318,356	0.88%
33	Iowa	307,974	0.85%
34	Colorado	270,580	0.75%
35	Kansas	251,171	0.70%
36	Nebraska	191,155	0.53%
37	Maine	167,238	0.46%
38	Utah	152,076	0.42%
39	Rhode Island	129,542	0.36%
40	Idaho	119,150	0.33%
41	Nevada	108,662	0.30%
42	Vermont	102,220	0.28%
43	Montana	101,271	0.28%
44	New Hampshire	99,594	0.28%
45	Delaware	81,766	0.23%
46	South Dakota	76,776	0.21%
47	Alaska	69,146	0.19%
48	North Dakota	60,971	0.17%
49	Wyoming	51,231	0.14%
50	Hawaii	40,514	0.11%
	District of Columbia	143,325	0.40%

Source: U.S. Department of Health and Human Services, Health Care Financing Administration
    "Medicaid Recipients by Maintenance Assistance Status, Region and State: FY 1996" (HCFA-2082)
*For fiscal year ending September 30, 1996. National total includes 1,073,792 recipients Puerto Rico and 16,654 recipients in the Virgin Islands.

Percent Change In Number of Medicaid Recipients: 1990 to 1996

National Percent Change = 43.0% Increase*

RANK	STATE	PERCENT CHANGE
22	Alabama	55.2
11	Alaska	77.1
NA	Arizona**	NA
29	Arkansas	37.2
25	California	40.9
23	Colorado	41.9
33	Connecticut	31.7
7	Delaware	99.4
20	Florida	57.7
9	Georgia	82.0
NA	Hawaii**	NA
5	Idaho	118.4
31	Illinois	36.2
13	Indiana	70.6
36	Iowa	28.5
35	Kansas	29.2
30	Kentucky	37.0
32	Louisiana	32.9
38	Maine	25.7
42	Maryland	20.6
41	Massachusetts	21.0
45	Michigan	11.8
43	Minnesota	19.6
44	Mississippi	17.7
23	Missouri	41.9
15	Montana	65.9
17	Nebraska	60.4
2	Nevada	131.2
4	New Hampshire	122.2
37	New Jersey	26.0
1	New Mexico	145.2
26	New York	40.8
6	North Carolina	100.6
39	North Dakota	24.4
40	Ohio	21.1
34	Oklahoma	31.1
8	Oregon	98.3
48	Pennsylvania	(0.8)
46	Rhode Island	10.7
18	South Carolina	58.7
21	South Dakota	55.7
3	Tennessee	129.7
10	Texas	78.3
27	Utah	40.5
14	Vermont	69.2
16	Virginia	64.3
28	Washington	38.8
19	West Virginia	57.8
47	Wisconsin	10.6
12	Wyoming	77.0

RANK	STATE	PERCENT CHANGE
1	New Mexico	145.2
2	Nevada	131.2
3	Tennessee	129.7
4	New Hampshire	122.2
5	Idaho	118.4
6	North Carolina	100.6
7	Delaware	99.4
8	Oregon	98.3
9	Georgia	82.0
10	Texas	78.3
11	Alaska	77.1
12	Wyoming	77.0
13	Indiana	70.6
14	Vermont	69.2
15	Montana	65.9
16	Virginia	64.3
17	Nebraska	60.4
18	South Carolina	58.7
19	West Virginia	57.8
20	Florida	57.7
21	South Dakota	55.7
22	Alabama	55.2
23	Colorado	41.9
23	Missouri	41.9
25	California	40.9
26	New York	40.8
27	Utah	40.5
28	Washington	38.8
29	Arkansas	37.2
30	Kentucky	37.0
31	Illinois	36.2
32	Louisiana	32.9
33	Connecticut	31.7
34	Oklahoma	31.1
35	Kansas	29.2
36	Iowa	28.5
37	New Jersey	26.0
38	Maine	25.7
39	North Dakota	24.4
40	Ohio	21.1
41	Massachusetts	21.0
42	Maryland	20.6
43	Minnesota	19.6
44	Mississippi	17.7
45	Michigan	11.8
46	Rhode Island	10.7
47	Wisconsin	10.6
48	Pennsylvania	(0.8)
NA	Arizona**	NA
NA	Hawaii**	NA
	District of Columbia	53.3

Source: Morgan Quitno Press using data from U.S. Dept. of Health & Human Services, Health Care Financing Admin. "Medicaid Recipients, Vendor Payments and Average Cost per Recipient by State: FY 1996" (HCFA-2082)
For fiscal year ending September 30, 1996. National rate includes recipients Puerto Rico and the Virgin Islands.
**Not available.*

Medicaid Cost per Recipient in 1996

National Per Capita = $3,369 per Recipient*

ALPHA ORDER

RANK ORDER

RANK	STATE	PER CAPITA		RANK	STATE	PER CAPITA
43	Alabama	$2,675		1	New York	$6,811
15	Alaska	4,027		2	Hawaii	6,574
50	Arizona	399		3	Connecticut	6,179
27	Arkansas	3,375		4	New Hampshire	5,496
48	California	2,178		5	Minnesota	5,342
17	Colorado	3,815		6	Massachusetts	5,285
3	Connecticut	6,179		7	Rhode Island	5,280
18	Delaware	3,773		8	New Jersey	5,217
39	Florida	2,851		9	Maryland	5,138
46	Georgia	2,604		10	North Dakota	4,889
2	Hawaii	6,574		11	Wisconsin	4,384
26	Idaho	3,402		12	Maine	4,321
20	Illinois	3,689		13	Indiana	4,130
13	Indiana	4,130		14	South Dakota	4,114
23	Iowa	3,534		15	Alaska	4,027
25	Kansas	3,425		16	Pennsylvania	3,993
33	Kentucky	3,014		17	Colorado	3,815
31	Louisiana	3,154		18	Delaware	3,773
12	Maine	4,321		19	Ohio	3,729
9	Maryland	5,138		20	Illinois	3,689
6	Massachusetts	5,285		21	Wyoming	3,571
36	Michigan	2,867		22	Nebraska	3,548
5	Minnesota	5,342		23	Iowa	3,534
45	Mississippi	2,633		24	Montana	3,478
30	Missouri	3,171		25	Kansas	3,425
24	Montana	3,478		26	Idaho	3,402
22	Nebraska	3,548		27	Arkansas	3,375
28	Nevada	3,361		28	Nevada	3,361
4	New Hampshire	5,496		29	North Carolina	3,255
8	New Jersey	5,217		30	Missouri	3,171
42	New Mexico	2,757		31	Louisiana	3,154
1	New York	6,811		32	South Carolina	3,026
29	North Carolina	3,255		33	Kentucky	3,014
10	North Dakota	4,889		34	Vermont	2,954
19	Ohio	3,729		35	Oregon	2,915
38	Oklahoma	2,852		36	Michigan	2,867
35	Oregon	2,915		37	West Virginia	2,855
16	Pennsylvania	3,993		38	Oklahoma	2,852
7	Rhode Island	5,280		39	Florida	2,851
32	South Carolina	3,026		40	Virginia	2,849
14	South Dakota	4,114		41	Utah	2,775
49	Tennessee	2,049		42	New Mexico	2,757
44	Texas	2,672		43	Alabama	2,675
41	Utah	2,775		44	Texas	2,672
34	Vermont	2,954		45	Mississippi	2,633
40	Virginia	2,849		46	Georgia	2,604
47	Washington	2,242		47	Washington	2,242
37	West Virginia	2,855		48	California	2,178
11	Wisconsin	4,384		49	Tennessee	2,049
21	Wyoming	3,571		50	Arizona	399
					District of Columbia	4,955

Source: U.S. Department of Health and Human Services, Health Care Financing Administration
"Medicaid Recipients, Vendor Payments and Average Cost per Recipient by State: FY 1996" (HCFA-2082)
*For fiscal year ending September 30, 1996. The cost per recipient is $239 in Puerto Rico and $550 in the Virgin Islands.

Percent Change in Cost per Medicaid Recipient: 1990 to 1996

National Percent Change = 31.2% Increase*

ALPHA ORDER

RANK	STATE	PERCENT CHANGE
8	Alabama	54.5
41	Alaska	13.1
NA	Arizona**	NA
9	Arkansas	48.9
36	California	21.3
13	Colorado	41.0
28	Connecticut	28.0
30	Delaware	25.6
31	Florida	25.4
48	Georgia	(18.4)
NA	Hawaii**	NA
38	Idaho	14.4
5	Illinois	62.4
44	Indiana	7.0
20	Iowa	36.5
21	Kansas	35.7
11	Kentucky	44.3
14	Louisiana	40.4
23	Maine	33.0
7	Maryland	55.7
39	Massachusetts	14.3
18	Michigan	36.9
12	Minnesota	44.0
2	Mississippi	94.5
6	Missouri	58.4
32	Montana	24.5
19	Nebraska	36.7
45	Nevada	6.3
47	New Hampshire	1.3
26	New Jersey	28.7
24	New Mexico	30.0
22	New York	33.6
27	North Carolina	28.6
33	North Dakota	23.6
10	Ohio	45.3
40	Oklahoma	13.4
29	Oregon	27.7
4	Pennsylvania	63.0
15	Rhode Island	39.8
25	South Carolina	29.2
34	South Dakota	22.1
43	Tennessee	8.1
16	Texas	38.6
35	Utah	21.8
37	Vermont	16.8
42	Virginia	9.7
46	Washington	5.4
1	West Virginia	97.9
17	Wisconsin	37.9
3	Wyoming	75.4

RANK ORDER

RANK	STATE	PERCENT CHANGE
1	West Virginia	97.9
2	Mississippi	94.5
3	Wyoming	75.4
4	Pennsylvania	63.0
5	Illinois	62.4
6	Missouri	58.4
7	Maryland	55.7
8	Alabama	54.5
9	Arkansas	48.9
10	Ohio	45.3
11	Kentucky	44.3
12	Minnesota	44.0
13	Colorado	41.0
14	Louisiana	40.4
15	Rhode Island	39.8
16	Texas	38.6
17	Wisconsin	37.9
18	Michigan	36.9
19	Nebraska	36.7
20	Iowa	36.5
21	Kansas	35.7
22	New York	33.6
23	Maine	33.0
24	New Mexico	30.0
25	South Carolina	29.2
26	New Jersey	28.7
27	North Carolina	28.6
28	Connecticut	28.0
29	Oregon	27.7
30	Delaware	25.6
31	Florida	25.4
32	Montana	24.5
33	North Dakota	23.6
34	South Dakota	22.1
35	Utah	21.8
36	California	21.3
37	Vermont	16.8
38	Idaho	14.4
39	Massachusetts	14.3
40	Oklahoma	13.4
41	Alaska	13.1
42	Virginia	9.7
43	Tennessee	8.1
44	Indiana	7.0
45	Nevada	6.3
46	Washington	5.4
47	New Hampshire	1.3
48	Georgia	(18.4)
NA	Arizona**	NA
NA	Hawaii**	NA

District of Columbia 88.5

Source: Morgan Quitno Press using data from U.S. Dept. of Health & Human Services, Health Care Financing Admin.
"Medicaid Recipients, Vendor Payments and Average Cost per Recipient by State: FY 1996" (HCFA-2082)
*For fiscal year ending September 30, 1996. National rate includes recipients Puerto Rico and the Virgin Islands.
**Not available.

Federal Medicaid Matching Fund Rate for 1998

National Average = 72.46% of States' Fund Matched by Federal Government*

ALPHA ORDER

RANK	STATE	RATE
13	Alabama	78.52
28	Alaska	71.86
16	Arizona	75.73
3	Arkansas	80.99
40	California	65.86
38	Colorado	66.38
41	Connecticut	65.00
41	Delaware	65.00
32	Florida	68.96
26	Georgia	72.59
41	Hawaii	65.00
12	Idaho	78.71
41	Illinois	65.00
24	Indiana	72.99
17	Iowa	74.63
29	Kansas	71.80
9	Kentucky	79.26
11	Louisiana	79.02
15	Maine	76.23
41	Maryland	65.00
41	Massachusetts	65.00
33	Michigan	67.51
37	Minnesota	66.50
1	Mississippi	83.96
27	Missouri	72.48
6	Montana	79.39
25	Nebraska	72.82
41	Nevada	65.00
41	New Hampshire	65.00
41	New Jersey	65.00
4	New Mexico	80.83
41	New York	65.00
19	North Carolina	74.16
8	North Dakota	79.30
31	Ohio	70.70
7	Oklahoma	79.36
23	Oregon	73.02
34	Pennsylvania	67.37
35	Rhode Island	67.22
10	South Carolina	79.16
14	South Dakota	77.43
18	Tennessee	74.35
21	Texas	73.60
5	Utah	80.81
22	Vermont	73.53
39	Virginia	66.04
36	Washington	66.51
2	West Virginia	81.57
30	Wisconsin	71.19
20	Wyoming	74.11

RANK ORDER

RANK	STATE	RATE
1	Mississippi	83.96
2	West Virginia	81.57
3	Arkansas	80.99
4	New Mexico	80.83
5	Utah	80.81
6	Montana	79.39
7	Oklahoma	79.36
8	North Dakota	79.30
9	Kentucky	79.26
10	South Carolina	79.16
11	Louisiana	79.02
12	Idaho	78.71
13	Alabama	78.52
14	South Dakota	77.43
15	Maine	76.23
16	Arizona	75.73
17	Iowa	74.63
18	Tennessee	74.35
19	North Carolina	74.16
20	Wyoming	74.11
21	Texas	73.60
22	Vermont	73.53
23	Oregon	73.02
24	Indiana	72.99
25	Nebraska	72.82
26	Georgia	72.59
27	Missouri	72.48
28	Alaska	71.86
29	Kansas	71.80
30	Wisconsin	71.19
31	Ohio	70.70
32	Florida	68.96
33	Michigan	67.51
34	Pennsylvania	67.37
35	Rhode Island	67.22
36	Washington	66.51
37	Minnesota	66.50
38	Colorado	66.38
39	Virginia	66.04
40	California	65.86
41	Connecticut	65.00
41	Delaware	65.00
41	Hawaii	65.00
41	Illinois	65.00
41	Maryland	65.00
41	Massachusetts	65.00
41	Nevada	65.00
41	New Hampshire	65.00
41	New Jersey	65.00
41	New York	65.00
	District of Columbia	79.00

Source: U.S. Department of Health and Human Services, Health Care Financing Administration
    "Enhanced Federal Medical Assistance Percentages" (Federal Register, 9/9/97, www.hcfa.gov/init/1mb115.htm)
*For fiscal year 1998. These are "enhanced" matching rates established by the Children's Health Insurance
Program, singed into law in August 1997. Sixty-five percent is the minimum. National average is a simple average of
the 51 individual rates and is not weighted for population or funds.

Percent of Population Receiving Medicaid in 1996

National Percent = 13.2% of Population*

ALPHA ORDER

RANK	STATE	PERCENT
19	Alabama	12.7
27	Alaska	11.4
22	Arizona	11.9
12	Arkansas	14.5
10	California	16.0
48	Colorado	7.1
36	Connecticut	10.1
29	Delaware	11.3
27	Florida	11.4
9	Georgia	16.2
50	Hawaii	3.4
37	Idaho	10.0
20	Illinois	12.3
35	Indiana	10.2
32	Iowa	10.8
39	Kansas	9.7
8	Kentucky	16.5
6	Louisiana	17.9
14	Maine	13.5
46	Maryland	7.9
24	Massachusetts	11.7
21	Michigan	12.0
38	Minnesota	9.8
3	Mississippi	18.8
22	Missouri	11.9
25	Montana	11.6
25	Nebraska	11.6
49	Nevada	6.8
44	New Hampshire	8.6
43	New Jersey	8.9
4	New Mexico	18.6
5	New York	18.1
11	North Carolina	15.5
41	North Dakota	9.5
17	Ohio	13.2
31	Oklahoma	10.9
13	Oregon	14.1
39	Pennsylvania	9.7
18	Rhode Island	13.1
14	South Carolina	13.5
34	South Dakota	10.4
1	Tennessee	26.5
14	Texas	13.5
47	Utah	7.5
7	Vermont	17.4
42	Virginia	9.4
29	Washington	11.3
2	West Virginia	21.7
45	Wisconsin	8.4
33	Wyoming	10.7

RANK ORDER

RANK	STATE	PERCENT
1	Tennessee	26.5
2	West Virginia	21.7
3	Mississippi	18.8
4	New Mexico	18.6
5	New York	18.1
6	Louisiana	17.9
7	Vermont	17.4
8	Kentucky	16.5
9	Georgia	16.2
10	California	16.0
11	North Carolina	15.5
12	Arkansas	14.5
13	Oregon	14.1
14	Maine	13.5
14	South Carolina	13.5
14	Texas	13.5
17	Ohio	13.2
18	Rhode Island	13.1
19	Alabama	12.7
20	Illinois	12.3
21	Michigan	12.0
22	Arizona	11.9
22	Missouri	11.9
24	Massachusetts	11.7
25	Montana	11.6
25	Nebraska	11.6
27	Alaska	11.4
27	Florida	11.4
29	Delaware	11.3
29	Washington	11.3
31	Oklahoma	10.9
32	Iowa	10.8
33	Wyoming	10.7
34	South Dakota	10.4
35	Indiana	10.2
36	Connecticut	10.1
37	Idaho	10.0
38	Minnesota	9.8
39	Kansas	9.7
39	Pennsylvania	9.7
41	North Dakota	9.5
42	Virginia	9.4
43	New Jersey	8.9
44	New Hampshire	8.6
45	Wisconsin	8.4
46	Maryland	7.9
47	Utah	7.5
48	Colorado	7.1
49	Nevada	6.8
50	Hawaii	3.4

District of Columbia 26.6

Source: Morgan Quitno Press using data from US Dept. of Health & Human Services, Health Care Financing Admin.
"Medicaid Recipients by Maintenance Assistance Status, Region and State: FY 1996" (HCFA-2082)
For fiscal year ending September 30, 1996. National percent does not include recipients Puerto Rico and the Virgin Islands.

Medicaid Health Maintenance Organizations (HMOs) in 1997

National Total = 266 Medicaid HMOs*

ALPHA ORDER

RANK	STATE	HMOs	% of USA
40	Alabama	0	0.00%
40	Alaska	0	0.00%
15	Arizona	5	1.88%
40	Arkansas	0	0.00%
2	California	19	7.14%
15	Colorado	5	1.88%
15	Connecticut	5	1.88%
23	Delaware	4	1.50%
7	Florida	11	4.14%
23	Georgia	4	1.50%
27	Hawaii	3	1.13%
37	Idaho	1	0.38%
10	Illinois	9	3.38%
30	Indiana	2	0.75%
40	Iowa	0	0.00%
30	Kansas	2	0.75%
37	Kentucky	1	0.38%
40	Louisiana	0	0.00%
40	Maine	0	0.00%
23	Maryland	4	1.50%
15	Massachusetts	5	1.88%
5	Michigan	16	6.02%
12	Minnesota	8	3.01%
23	Mississippi	4	1.50%
7	Missouri	11	4.14%
37	Montana	1	0.38%
27	Nebraska	3	1.13%
30	Nevada	2	0.75%
30	New Hampshire	2	0.75%
6	New Jersey	15	5.64%
40	New Mexico	0	0.00%
1	New York	26	9.77%
15	North Carolina	5	1.88%
40	North Dakota	0	0.00%
4	Ohio	17	6.39%
27	Oklahoma	3	1.13%
15	Oregon	5	1.88%
9	Pennsylvania	10	3.76%
30	Rhode Island	2	0.75%
30	South Carolina	2	0.75%
40	South Dakota	0	0.00%
13	Tennessee	6	2.26%
10	Texas	9	3.38%
15	Utah	5	1.88%
40	Vermont	0	0.00%
13	Virginia	6	2.26%
15	Washington	5	1.88%
30	West Virginia	2	0.75%
2	Wisconsin	19	7.14%
40	Wyoming	0	0.00%

RANK ORDER

RANK	STATE	HMOs	% of USA
1	New York	26	9.77%
2	California	19	7.14%
2	Wisconsin	19	7.14%
4	Ohio	17	6.39%
5	Michigan	16	6.02%
6	New Jersey	15	5.64%
7	Florida	11	4.14%
7	Missouri	11	4.14%
9	Pennsylvania	10	3.76%
10	Illinois	9	3.38%
10	Texas	9	3.38%
12	Minnesota	8	3.01%
13	Tennessee	6	2.26%
13	Virginia	6	2.26%
15	Arizona	5	1.88%
15	Colorado	5	1.88%
15	Connecticut	5	1.88%
15	Massachusetts	5	1.88%
15	North Carolina	5	1.88%
15	Oregon	5	1.88%
15	Utah	5	1.88%
15	Washington	5	1.88%
23	Delaware	4	1.50%
23	Georgia	4	1.50%
23	Maryland	4	1.50%
23	Mississippi	4	1.50%
27	Hawaii	3	1.13%
27	Nebraska	3	1.13%
27	Oklahoma	3	1.13%
30	Indiana	2	0.75%
30	Kansas	2	0.75%
30	Nevada	2	0.75%
30	New Hampshire	2	0.75%
30	Rhode Island	2	0.75%
30	South Carolina	2	0.75%
30	West Virginia	2	0.75%
37	Idaho	1	0.38%
37	Kentucky	1	0.38%
37	Montana	1	0.38%
40	Alabama	0	0.00%
40	Alaska	0	0.00%
40	Arkansas	0	0.00%
40	Iowa	0	0.00%
40	Louisiana	0	0.00%
40	Maine	0	0.00%
40	New Mexico	0	0.00%
40	North Dakota	0	0.00%
40	South Dakota	0	0.00%
40	Vermont	0	0.00%
40	Wyoming	0	0.00%
	District of Columbia	2	0.75%

Source: InterStudy Publications (Minneapolis, MN)
    "The Competitive Edge Industry Report 7.2" (October 1997)
*As of January 1, 1997. Health plans are allocated to states based upon their primary service areas. This means each plan is counted once. However, many plans serve more than one state.

Medicaid Managed Care Enrollment in 1997

National Total = 15,345,502 Medicaid Enrollees*

ALPHA ORDER

RANK	STATE	ENROLLEES	% of USA
10	Alabama	407,643	2.66%
NA	Alaska**	NA	NA
14	Arizona	349,142	2.28%
28	Arkansas	159,458	1.04%
1	California	1,854,294	12.08%
26	Colorado	184,000	1.20%
21	Connecticut	231,966	1.51%
38	Delaware	65,061	0.42%
3	Florida	896,559	5.84%
8	Georgia	560,771	3.65%
30	Hawaii	135,200	0.88%
42	Idaho	32,428	0.21%
25	Illinois	187,048	1.22%
23	Indiana	220,000	1.43%
35	Iowa	88,282	0.58%
32	Kansas	94,430	0.62%
19	Kentucky	268,205	1.75%
41	Louisiana	40,469	0.26%
47	Maine	12,511	0.08%
15	Maryland	347,640	2.27%
9	Massachusetts	461,989	3.01%
5	Michigan	865,434	5.64%
27	Minnesota	169,329	1.10%
36	Mississippi	81,255	0.53%
20	Missouri	264,496	1.72%
39	Montana	62,004	0.40%
34	Nebraska	93,085	0.61%
43	Nevada	26,376	0.17%
48	New Hampshire	9,102	0.06%
11	New Jersey	384,644	2.51%
29	New Mexico	139,337	0.91%
7	New York	660,725	4.31%
13	North Carolina	351,043	2.29%
44	North Dakota	24,295	0.16%
12	Ohio	352,833	2.30%
22	Oklahoma	222,818	1.45%
16	Oregon	312,345	2.04%
4	Pennsylvania	870,365	5.67%
37	Rhode Island	70,944	0.46%
46	South Carolina	14,311	0.09%
40	South Dakota	41,542	0.27%
2	Tennessee	1,188,570	7.75%
18	Texas	275,951	1.80%
33	Utah	93,785	0.61%
45	Vermont	22,946	0.15%
17	Virginia	306,804	2.00%
6	Washington	730,052	4.76%
31	West Virginia	125,521	0.82%
24	Wisconsin	205,523	1.34%
NA	Wyoming**	NA	NA

RANK ORDER

RANK	STATE	ENROLLEES	% of USA
1	California	1,854,294	12.08%
2	Tennessee	1,188,570	7.75%
3	Florida	896,559	5.84%
4	Pennsylvania	870,365	5.67%
5	Michigan	865,434	5.64%
6	Washington	730,052	4.76%
7	New York	660,725	4.31%
8	Georgia	560,771	3.65%
9	Massachusetts	461,989	3.01%
10	Alabama	407,643	2.66%
11	New Jersey	384,644	2.51%
12	Ohio	352,833	2.30%
13	North Carolina	351,043	2.29%
14	Arizona	349,142	2.28%
15	Maryland	347,640	2.27%
16	Oregon	312,345	2.04%
17	Virginia	306,804	2.00%
18	Texas	275,951	1.80%
19	Kentucky	268,205	1.75%
20	Missouri	264,496	1.72%
21	Connecticut	231,966	1.51%
22	Oklahoma	222,818	1.45%
23	Indiana	220,000	1.43%
24	Wisconsin	205,523	1.34%
25	Illinois	187,048	1.22%
26	Colorado	184,000	1.20%
27	Minnesota	169,329	1.10%
28	Arkansas	159,458	1.04%
29	New Mexico	139,337	0.91%
30	Hawaii	135,200	0.88%
31	West Virginia	125,521	0.82%
32	Kansas	94,430	0.62%
33	Utah	93,785	0.61%
34	Nebraska	93,085	0.61%
35	Iowa	88,282	0.58%
36	Mississippi	81,255	0.53%
37	Rhode Island	70,944	0.46%
38	Delaware	65,061	0.42%
39	Montana	62,004	0.40%
40	South Dakota	41,542	0.27%
41	Louisiana	40,469	0.26%
42	Idaho	32,428	0.21%
43	Nevada	26,376	0.17%
44	North Dakota	24,295	0.16%
45	Vermont	22,946	0.15%
46	South Carolina	14,311	0.09%
47	Maine	12,511	0.08%
48	New Hampshire	9,102	0.06%
NA	Alaska**	NA	NA
NA	Wyoming**	NA	NA
	District of Columbia	80,721	0.53%

Source: U.S. Department of Health and Human Services, Health Care Financing Administration
"Medicaid Managed Care State Enrollment" (http://www.hcfa.gov/medicaid/plantyp7.htm)
*As of June 30, 1997. National total includes 702,250 Medicaid enrollees in Puerto Rico.
**None or not available.

State Government Expenditures for Health Programs in 1996

National Total = $32,612,198,000*

ALPHA ORDER

RANK	STATE	EXPENDITURES	% of USA
21	Alabama	$514,380,000	1.63%
39	Alaska	159,218,000	0.50%
18	Arizona	543,341,000	1.72%
31	Arkansas	246,981,000	0.78%
1	California	5,564,254,000	17.60%
35	Colorado	235,366,000	0.74%
25	Connecticut	365,838,000	1.16%
41	Delaware	152,191,000	0.48%
3	Florida	2,079,149,000	6.58%
14	Georgia	637,639,000	2.02%
28	Hawaii	305,725,000	0.97%
47	Idaho	68,235,000	0.22%
5	Illinois	1,512,257,000	4.78%
23	Indiana	401,790,000	1.27%
37	Iowa	178,610,000	0.57%
32	Kansas	242,856,000	0.77%
29	Kentucky	272,247,000	0.86%
24	Louisiana	387,843,000	1.23%
38	Maine	175,768,000	0.56%
12	Maryland	760,690,000	2.41%
7	Massachusetts	1,285,098,000	4.07%
4	Michigan	1,957,679,000	6.19%
22	Minnesota	511,199,000	1.62%
33	Mississippi	242,541,000	0.77%
16	Missouri	551,261,000	1.74%
42	Montana	135,250,000	0.43%
36	Nebraska	215,763,000	0.68%
46	Nevada	78,560,000	0.25%
44	New Hampshire	106,147,000	0.34%
15	New Jersey	593,636,000	1.88%
30	New Mexico	268,229,000	0.85%
2	New York	2,699,015,000	8.54%
11	North Carolina	827,710,000	2.62%
50	North Dakota	40,496,000	0.13%
6	Ohio	1,304,288,000	4.13%
27	Oklahoma	309,846,000	0.98%
26	Oregon	365,736,000	1.16%
8	Pennsylvania	1,255,006,000	3.97%
34	Rhode Island	241,935,000	0.77%
13	South Carolina	710,015,000	2.25%
48	South Dakota	58,578,000	0.19%
17	Tennessee	545,985,000	1.73%
9	Texas	1,179,941,000	3.73%
40	Utah	158,471,000	0.50%
49	Vermont	51,296,000	0.16%
20	Virginia	522,502,000	1.65%
10	Washington	853,254,000	2.70%
43	West Virginia	121,639,000	0.38%
19	Wisconsin	530,720,000	1.68%
45	Wyoming	86,024,000	0.27%

RANK ORDER

RANK	STATE	EXPENDITURES	% of USA
1	California	$5,564,254,000	17.60%
2	New York	2,699,015,000	8.54%
3	Florida	2,079,149,000	6.58%
4	Michigan	1,957,679,000	6.19%
5	Illinois	1,512,257,000	4.78%
6	Ohio	1,304,288,000	4.13%
7	Massachusetts	1,285,098,000	4.07%
8	Pennsylvania	1,255,006,000	3.97%
9	Texas	1,179,941,000	3.73%
10	Washington	853,254,000	2.70%
11	North Carolina	827,710,000	2.62%
12	Maryland	760,690,000	2.41%
13	South Carolina	710,015,000	2.25%
14	Georgia	637,639,000	2.02%
15	New Jersey	593,636,000	1.88%
16	Missouri	551,261,000	1.74%
17	Tennessee	545,985,000	1.73%
18	Arizona	543,341,000	1.72%
19	Wisconsin	530,720,000	1.68%
20	Virginia	522,502,000	1.65%
21	Alabama	514,380,000	1.63%
22	Minnesota	511,199,000	1.62%
23	Indiana	401,790,000	1.27%
24	Louisiana	387,843,000	1.23%
25	Connecticut	365,838,000	1.16%
26	Oregon	365,736,000	1.16%
27	Oklahoma	309,846,000	0.98%
28	Hawaii	305,725,000	0.97%
29	Kentucky	272,247,000	0.86%
30	New Mexico	268,229,000	0.85%
31	Arkansas	246,981,000	0.78%
32	Kansas	242,856,000	0.77%
33	Mississippi	242,541,000	0.77%
34	Rhode Island	241,935,000	0.77%
35	Colorado	235,366,000	0.74%
36	Nebraska	215,763,000	0.68%
37	Iowa	178,610,000	0.57%
38	Maine	175,768,000	0.56%
39	Alaska	159,218,000	0.50%
40	Utah	158,471,000	0.50%
41	Delaware	152,191,000	0.48%
42	Montana	135,250,000	0.43%
43	West Virginia	121,639,000	0.38%
44	New Hampshire	106,147,000	0.34%
45	Wyoming	86,024,000	0.27%
46	Nevada	78,560,000	0.25%
47	Idaho	68,235,000	0.22%
48	South Dakota	58,578,000	0.19%
49	Vermont	51,296,000	0.16%
50	North Dakota	40,496,000	0.13%
	District of Columbia**	NA	NA

Source: U.S. Bureau of the Census, Governments Division
"1996 State Government Finance Data" (http://www.census.gov/govs/www/st96.html)
*Includes outpatient health services other than hospital care, research and education, categorical health programs, treatment and immunization clinics, nursing and environmental health activities. Includes capital expenditures.
**Not applicable.

Per Capita State Government Expenditures for Health Programs in 1996

National Per Capita = $122.98*

ALPHA ORDER

RANK	STATE	PER CAPITA
20	Alabama	$119.98
1	Alaska	263.19
19	Arizona	122.53
30	Arkansas	98.54
9	California	174.66
48	Colorado	61.68
24	Connecticut	111.97
5	Delaware	210.36
15	Florida	144.20
37	Georgia	86.94
2	Hawaii	258.44
49	Idaho	57.46
18	Illinois	127.67
43	Indiana	68.94
46	Iowa	62.71
31	Kansas	94.16
42	Kentucky	70.13
35	Louisiana	89.35
16	Maine	141.91
13	Maryland	150.33
4	Massachusetts	211.18
6	Michigan	201.18
25	Minnesota	109.97
34	Mississippi	89.47
29	Missouri	102.78
12	Montana	154.27
17	Nebraska	130.87
50	Nevada	49.08
33	New Hampshire	91.49
41	New Jersey	74.19
10	New Mexico	156.74
14	New York	148.84
23	North Carolina	113.24
45	North Dakota	63.02
21	Ohio	116.84
32	Oklahoma	94.03
22	Oregon	114.42
26	Pennsylvania	104.24
3	Rhode Island	244.80
7	South Carolina	191.04
38	South Dakota	79.42
28	Tennessee	102.87
47	Texas	61.81
39	Utah	78.55
36	Vermont	87.47
40	Virginia	78.38
11	Washington	154.59
44	West Virginia	66.82
27	Wisconsin	103.13
8	Wyoming	179.21

RANK ORDER

RANK	STATE	PER CAPITA
1	Alaska	$263.19
2	Hawaii	258.44
3	Rhode Island	244.80
4	Massachusetts	211.18
5	Delaware	210.36
6	Michigan	201.18
7	South Carolina	191.04
8	Wyoming	179.21
9	California	174.66
10	New Mexico	156.74
11	Washington	154.59
12	Montana	154.27
13	Maryland	150.33
14	New York	148.84
15	Florida	144.20
16	Maine	141.91
17	Nebraska	130.87
18	Illinois	127.67
19	Arizona	122.53
20	Alabama	119.98
21	Ohio	116.84
22	Oregon	114.42
23	North Carolina	113.24
24	Connecticut	111.97
25	Minnesota	109.97
26	Pennsylvania	104.24
27	Wisconsin	103.13
28	Tennessee	102.87
29	Missouri	102.78
30	Arkansas	98.54
31	Kansas	94.16
32	Oklahoma	94.03
33	New Hampshire	91.49
34	Mississippi	89.47
35	Louisiana	89.35
36	Vermont	87.47
37	Georgia	86.94
38	South Dakota	79.42
39	Utah	78.55
40	Virginia	78.38
41	New Jersey	74.19
42	Kentucky	70.13
43	Indiana	68.94
44	West Virginia	66.82
45	North Dakota	63.02
46	Iowa	62.71
47	Texas	61.81
48	Colorado	61.68
49	Idaho	57.46
50	Nevada	49.08

District of Columbia**   NA

Source: Morgan Quitno Press using data from U.S. Bureau of the Census, Governments Division
"1996 State Government Finance Data" (http://www.census.gov/govs/www/st96.html)
*Includes outpatient health services other than hospital care, research and education, categorical health programs, treatment and immunization clinics, nursing and environmental health activities. Includes capital expenditures.
**Not applicable.

State Government Expenditures for Hospitals in 1996

National Total = $29,421,119,000*

ALPHA ORDER

RANK	STATE	EXPENDITURES	% of USA
12	Alabama	$815,698,000	2.77%
49	Alaska	31,317,000	0.11%
42	Arizona	56,490,000	0.19%
27	Arkansas	341,661,000	1.16%
2	California	2,779,960,000	9.45%
36	Colorado	145,831,000	0.50%
9	Connecticut	974,436,000	3.31%
41	Delaware	58,416,000	0.20%
19	Florida	526,928,000	1.79%
15	Georgia	651,520,000	2.21%
35	Hawaii	181,127,000	0.62%
46	Idaho	37,358,000	0.13%
13	Illinois	797,307,000	2.71%
34	Indiana	206,466,000	0.70%
20	Iowa	518,934,000	1.76%
28	Kansas	321,986,000	1.09%
26	Kentucky	365,802,000	1.24%
6	Louisiana	1,106,628,000	3.76%
40	Maine	58,821,000	0.20%
29	Maryland	311,714,000	1.06%
11	Massachusetts	896,689,000	3.05%
5	Michigan	1,448,596,000	4.92%
16	Minnesota	605,893,000	2.06%
25	Mississippi	380,099,000	1.29%
22	Missouri	480,455,000	1.63%
47	Montana	32,655,000	0.11%
31	Nebraska	286,905,000	0.98%
39	Nevada	61,659,000	0.21%
45	New Hampshire	39,522,000	0.13%
8	New Jersey	993,930,000	3.38%
30	New Mexico	308,578,000	1.05%
1	New York	3,734,213,000	12.69%
14	North Carolina	748,896,000	2.55%
44	North Dakota	43,076,000	0.15%
10	Ohio	964,128,000	3.28%
32	Oklahoma	283,127,000	0.96%
23	Oregon	443,076,000	1.51%
4	Pennsylvania	1,749,499,000	5.95%
37	Rhode Island	89,839,000	0.31%
17	South Carolina	597,611,000	2.03%
43	South Dakota	48,410,000	0.16%
21	Tennessee	512,404,000	1.74%
3	Texas	1,899,361,000	6.46%
33	Utah	281,063,000	0.96%
50	Vermont	9,146,000	0.03%
7	Virginia	1,090,825,000	3.71%
18	Washington	551,833,000	1.88%
38	West Virginia	81,311,000	0.28%
24	Wisconsin	438,162,000	1.49%
48	Wyoming	31,758,000	0.11%

RANK ORDER

RANK	STATE	EXPENDITURES	% of USA
1	New York	$3,734,213,000	12.69%
2	California	2,779,960,000	9.45%
3	Texas	1,899,361,000	6.46%
4	Pennsylvania	1,749,499,000	5.95%
5	Michigan	1,448,596,000	4.92%
6	Louisiana	1,106,628,000	3.76%
7	Virginia	1,090,825,000	3.71%
8	New Jersey	993,930,000	3.38%
9	Connecticut	974,436,000	3.31%
10	Ohio	964,128,000	3.28%
11	Massachusetts	896,689,000	3.05%
12	Alabama	815,698,000	2.77%
13	Illinois	797,307,000	2.71%
14	North Carolina	748,896,000	2.55%
15	Georgia	651,520,000	2.21%
16	Minnesota	605,893,000	2.06%
17	South Carolina	597,611,000	2.03%
18	Washington	551,833,000	1.88%
19	Florida	526,928,000	1.79%
20	Iowa	518,934,000	1.76%
21	Tennessee	512,404,000	1.74%
22	Missouri	480,455,000	1.63%
23	Oregon	443,076,000	1.51%
24	Wisconsin	438,162,000	1.49%
25	Mississippi	380,099,000	1.29%
26	Kentucky	365,802,000	1.24%
27	Arkansas	341,661,000	1.16%
28	Kansas	321,986,000	1.09%
29	Maryland	311,714,000	1.06%
30	New Mexico	308,578,000	1.05%
31	Nebraska	286,905,000	0.98%
32	Oklahoma	283,127,000	0.96%
33	Utah	281,063,000	0.96%
34	Indiana	206,466,000	0.70%
35	Hawaii	181,127,000	0.62%
36	Colorado	145,831,000	0.50%
37	Rhode Island	89,839,000	0.31%
38	West Virginia	81,311,000	0.28%
39	Nevada	61,659,000	0.21%
40	Maine	58,821,000	0.20%
41	Delaware	58,416,000	0.20%
42	Arizona	56,490,000	0.19%
43	South Dakota	48,410,000	0.16%
44	North Dakota	43,076,000	0.15%
45	New Hampshire	39,522,000	0.13%
46	Idaho	37,358,000	0.13%
47	Montana	32,655,000	0.11%
48	Wyoming	31,758,000	0.11%
49	Alaska	31,317,000	0.11%
50	Vermont	9,146,000	0.03%
	District of Columbia**	NA	NA

Source: U.S. Bureau of the Census, Governments Division
"1996 State Government Finance Data" (http://www.census.gov/govs/www/st96.html)
*Financing, construction, acquisition, maintenance or operation of hospital facilities, provision of hospital care and support of public or private hospitals.
**Not applicable.

Per Capita State Government Expenditures for Hospitals in 1996

National Per Capita = $110.95*

<table>
<tr><td colspan="3">ALPHA ORDER</td><td colspan="3">RANK ORDER</td></tr>
<tr><th>RANK</th><th>STATE</th><th>PER CAPITA</th><th>RANK</th><th>STATE</th><th>PER CAPITA</th></tr>
<tr><td>4</td><td>Alabama</td><td>$190.26</td><td>1</td><td>Connecticut</td><td>$298.24</td></tr>
<tr><td>39</td><td>Alaska</td><td>51.77</td><td>2</td><td>Louisiana</td><td>254.94</td></tr>
<tr><td>50</td><td>Arizona</td><td>12.74</td><td>3</td><td>New York</td><td>205.92</td></tr>
<tr><td>17</td><td>Arkansas</td><td>136.32</td><td>4</td><td>Alabama</td><td>190.26</td></tr>
<tr><td>29</td><td>California</td><td>87.26</td><td>5</td><td>Iowa</td><td>182.21</td></tr>
<tr><td>43</td><td>Colorado</td><td>38.21</td><td>6</td><td>New Mexico</td><td>180.32</td></tr>
<tr><td>1</td><td>Connecticut</td><td>298.24</td><td>7</td><td>Nebraska</td><td>174.02</td></tr>
<tr><td>33</td><td>Delaware</td><td>80.74</td><td>8</td><td>Virginia</td><td>163.64</td></tr>
<tr><td>45</td><td>Florida</td><td>36.54</td><td>9</td><td>South Carolina</td><td>160.79</td></tr>
<tr><td>28</td><td>Georgia</td><td>88.83</td><td>10</td><td>Hawaii</td><td>153.11</td></tr>
<tr><td>10</td><td>Hawaii</td><td>153.11</td><td>11</td><td>Michigan</td><td>148.87</td></tr>
<tr><td>48</td><td>Idaho</td><td>31.46</td><td>12</td><td>Massachusetts</td><td>147.35</td></tr>
<tr><td>34</td><td>Illinois</td><td>67.31</td><td>13</td><td>Pennsylvania</td><td>145.31</td></tr>
<tr><td>46</td><td>Indiana</td><td>35.43</td><td>14</td><td>Mississippi</td><td>140.22</td></tr>
<tr><td>5</td><td>Iowa</td><td>182.21</td><td>15</td><td>Utah</td><td>139.31</td></tr>
<tr><td>19</td><td>Kansas</td><td>124.84</td><td>16</td><td>Oregon</td><td>138.62</td></tr>
<tr><td>25</td><td>Kentucky</td><td>94.23</td><td>17</td><td>Arkansas</td><td>136.32</td></tr>
<tr><td>2</td><td>Louisiana</td><td>254.94</td><td>18</td><td>Minnesota</td><td>130.34</td></tr>
<tr><td>40</td><td>Maine</td><td>47.49</td><td>19</td><td>Kansas</td><td>124.84</td></tr>
<tr><td>38</td><td>Maryland</td><td>61.60</td><td>20</td><td>New Jersey</td><td>124.21</td></tr>
<tr><td>12</td><td>Massachusetts</td><td>147.35</td><td>21</td><td>North Carolina</td><td>102.46</td></tr>
<tr><td>11</td><td>Michigan</td><td>148.87</td><td>22</td><td>Washington</td><td>99.98</td></tr>
<tr><td>18</td><td>Minnesota</td><td>130.34</td><td>23</td><td>Texas</td><td>99.49</td></tr>
<tr><td>14</td><td>Mississippi</td><td>140.22</td><td>24</td><td>Tennessee</td><td>96.55</td></tr>
<tr><td>27</td><td>Missouri</td><td>89.58</td><td>25</td><td>Kentucky</td><td>94.23</td></tr>
<tr><td>44</td><td>Montana</td><td>37.25</td><td>26</td><td>Rhode Island</td><td>90.90</td></tr>
<tr><td>7</td><td>Nebraska</td><td>174.02</td><td>27</td><td>Missouri</td><td>89.58</td></tr>
<tr><td>42</td><td>Nevada</td><td>38.52</td><td>28</td><td>Georgia</td><td>88.83</td></tr>
<tr><td>47</td><td>New Hampshire</td><td>34.06</td><td>29</td><td>California</td><td>87.26</td></tr>
<tr><td>20</td><td>New Jersey</td><td>124.21</td><td>30</td><td>Ohio</td><td>86.37</td></tr>
<tr><td>6</td><td>New Mexico</td><td>180.32</td><td>31</td><td>Oklahoma</td><td>85.92</td></tr>
<tr><td>3</td><td>New York</td><td>205.92</td><td>32</td><td>Wisconsin</td><td>85.14</td></tr>
<tr><td>21</td><td>North Carolina</td><td>102.46</td><td>33</td><td>Delaware</td><td>80.74</td></tr>
<tr><td>35</td><td>North Dakota</td><td>67.03</td><td>34</td><td>Illinois</td><td>67.31</td></tr>
<tr><td>30</td><td>Ohio</td><td>86.37</td><td>35</td><td>North Dakota</td><td>67.03</td></tr>
<tr><td>31</td><td>Oklahoma</td><td>85.92</td><td>36</td><td>Wyoming</td><td>66.16</td></tr>
<tr><td>16</td><td>Oregon</td><td>138.62</td><td>37</td><td>South Dakota</td><td>65.64</td></tr>
<tr><td>13</td><td>Pennsylvania</td><td>145.31</td><td>38</td><td>Maryland</td><td>61.60</td></tr>
<tr><td>26</td><td>Rhode Island</td><td>90.90</td><td>39</td><td>Alaska</td><td>51.77</td></tr>
<tr><td>9</td><td>South Carolina</td><td>160.79</td><td>40</td><td>Maine</td><td>47.49</td></tr>
<tr><td>37</td><td>South Dakota</td><td>65.64</td><td>41</td><td>West Virginia</td><td>44.67</td></tr>
<tr><td>24</td><td>Tennessee</td><td>96.55</td><td>42</td><td>Nevada</td><td>38.52</td></tr>
<tr><td>23</td><td>Texas</td><td>99.49</td><td>43</td><td>Colorado</td><td>38.21</td></tr>
<tr><td>15</td><td>Utah</td><td>139.31</td><td>44</td><td>Montana</td><td>37.25</td></tr>
<tr><td>49</td><td>Vermont</td><td>15.60</td><td>45</td><td>Florida</td><td>36.54</td></tr>
<tr><td>8</td><td>Virginia</td><td>163.64</td><td>46</td><td>Indiana</td><td>35.43</td></tr>
<tr><td>22</td><td>Washington</td><td>99.98</td><td>47</td><td>New Hampshire</td><td>34.06</td></tr>
<tr><td>41</td><td>West Virginia</td><td>44.67</td><td>48</td><td>Idaho</td><td>31.46</td></tr>
<tr><td>32</td><td>Wisconsin</td><td>85.14</td><td>49</td><td>Vermont</td><td>15.60</td></tr>
<tr><td>36</td><td>Wyoming</td><td>66.16</td><td>50</td><td>Arizona</td><td>12.74</td></tr>
<tr><td></td><td></td><td></td><td></td><td>District of Columbia**</td><td>NA</td></tr>
</table>

Source: Morgan Quitno Press using data from U.S. Bureau of the Census, Governments Division
"1996 State Government Finance Data" (http://www.census.gov/govs/www/st96.html)
*Financing, construction, acquisition, maintenance or operation of hospital facilities, provision of hospital care and support of public or private hospitals.
**Not applicable.

Receipts of Health Services Establishments in 1992

National Total = $623,480,434,000*

RANK	STATE	RECEIPTS	% of USA
23	Alabama	$9,400,816,000	1.51%
48	Alaska	1,225,327,000	0.20%
24	Arizona	8,624,782,000	1.38%
32	Arkansas	4,791,668,000	0.77%
1	California	79,130,980,000	12.69%
25	Colorado	8,000,876,000	1.28%
22	Connecticut	9,932,092,000	1.59%
43	Delaware	1,780,075,000	0.29%
4	Florida	36,667,132,000	5.88%
11	Georgia	15,774,705,000	2.53%
39	Hawaii	2,757,575,000	0.44%
44	Idaho	1,775,447,000	0.28%
6	Illinois	27,961,997,000	4.48%
14	Indiana	13,010,617,000	2.09%
30	Iowa	5,852,492,000	0.94%
31	Kansas	5,763,990,000	0.92%
26	Kentucky	7,923,070,000	1.27%
21	Louisiana	10,204,980,000	1.64%
40	Maine	2,666,876,000	0.43%
18	Maryland	11,824,018,000	1.90%
10	Massachusetts	19,296,743,000	3.10%
8	Michigan	21,891,285,000	3.51%
20	Minnesota	11,199,561,000	1.80%
33	Mississippi	4,605,036,000	0.74%
15	Missouri	12,918,009,000	2.07%
46	Montana	1,589,295,000	0.25%
35	Nebraska	3,483,096,000	0.56%
37	Nevada	3,016,118,000	0.48%
41	New Hampshire	2,642,095,000	0.42%
9	New Jersey	21,102,821,000	3.38%
38	New Mexico	2,881,524,000	0.46%
2	New York	53,091,018,000	8.52%
12	North Carolina	14,227,452,000	2.28%
45	North Dakota	1,651,634,000	0.26%
7	Ohio	27,492,361,000	4.41%
28	Oklahoma	6,268,749,000	1.01%
29	Oregon	6,137,525,000	0.98%
5	Pennsylvania	33,155,698,000	5.32%
42	Rhode Island	2,617,386,000	0.42%
27	South Carolina	6,612,570,000	1.06%
47	South Dakota	1,543,627,000	0.25%
16	Tennessee	12,807,220,000	2.05%
3	Texas	38,769,630,000	6.22%
36	Utah	3,216,121,000	0.52%
49	Vermont	1,121,735,000	0.18%
13	Virginia	13,140,339,000	2.11%
17	Washington	12,022,436,000	1.93%
34	West Virginia	4,040,621,000	0.65%
19	Wisconsin	11,288,091,000	1.81%
50	Wyoming	708,286,000	0.11%

RANK	STATE	RECEIPTS	% of USA
1	California	$79,130,980,000	12.69%
2	New York	53,091,018,000	8.52%
3	Texas	38,769,630,000	6.22%
4	Florida	36,667,132,000	5.88%
5	Pennsylvania	33,155,698,000	5.32%
6	Illinois	27,961,997,000	4.48%
7	Ohio	27,492,361,000	4.41%
8	Michigan	21,891,285,000	3.51%
9	New Jersey	21,102,821,000	3.38%
10	Massachusetts	19,296,743,000	3.10%
11	Georgia	15,774,705,000	2.53%
12	North Carolina	14,227,452,000	2.28%
13	Virginia	13,140,339,000	2.11%
14	Indiana	13,010,617,000	2.09%
15	Missouri	12,918,009,000	2.07%
16	Tennessee	12,807,220,000	2.05%
17	Washington	12,022,436,000	1.93%
18	Maryland	11,824,018,000	1.90%
19	Wisconsin	11,288,091,000	1.81%
20	Minnesota	11,199,561,000	1.80%
21	Louisiana	10,204,980,000	1.64%
22	Connecticut	9,932,092,000	1.59%
23	Alabama	9,400,816,000	1.51%
24	Arizona	8,624,782,000	1.38%
25	Colorado	8,000,876,000	1.28%
26	Kentucky	7,923,070,000	1.27%
27	South Carolina	6,612,570,000	1.06%
28	Oklahoma	6,268,749,000	1.01%
29	Oregon	6,137,525,000	0.98%
30	Iowa	5,852,492,000	0.94%
31	Kansas	5,763,990,000	0.92%
32	Arkansas	4,791,668,000	0.77%
33	Mississippi	4,605,036,000	0.74%
34	West Virginia	4,040,621,000	0.65%
35	Nebraska	3,483,096,000	0.56%
36	Utah	3,216,121,000	0.52%
37	Nevada	3,016,118,000	0.48%
38	New Mexico	2,881,524,000	0.46%
39	Hawaii	2,757,575,000	0.44%
40	Maine	2,666,876,000	0.43%
41	New Hampshire	2,642,095,000	0.42%
42	Rhode Island	2,617,386,000	0.42%
43	Delaware	1,780,075,000	0.29%
44	Idaho	1,775,447,000	0.28%
45	North Dakota	1,651,634,000	0.26%
46	Montana	1,589,295,000	0.25%
47	South Dakota	1,543,627,000	0.25%
48	Alaska	1,225,327,000	0.20%
49	Vermont	1,121,735,000	0.18%
50	Wyoming	708,286,000	0.11%
	District of Columbia	3,872,837,000	0.62%

Source: Morgan Quitno Press using data from U.S. Bureau of the Census
"1992 Census of Service Industries, Geographic Area Series, United States" (SC92-A-52)
*Includes establishments exempt from as well as subject to the federal income tax. Includes those establishments within the Standard Industry Classification (SIC) 80. These include those primarily engaged in furnishing medical, surgical and other health services to persons. See Facilities Chapter for establishments.

Receipts per Health Service Establishment in 1992

National Rate = $1,339,792 per Establishment*

ALPHA ORDER

RANK ORDER

RANK	STATE	PER ESTABLISHMENT
4	Alabama	$1,606,428
27	Alaska	1,304,928
40	Arizona	1,155,517
31	Arkansas	1,261,297
33	California	1,251,696
44	Colorado	1,081,199
10	Connecticut	1,430,931
13	Delaware	1,419,518
38	Florida	1,201,768
19	Georgia	1,375,541
39	Hawaii	1,183,509
48	Idaho	966,493
14	Illinois	1,415,296
15	Indiana	1,392,701
32	Iowa	1,252,942
20	Kansas	1,360,073
24	Kentucky	1,322,495
11	Louisiana	1,430,872
42	Maine	1,114,449
35	Maryland	1,244,110
2	Massachusetts	1,700,753
26	Michigan	1,307,333
3	Minnesota	1,676,581
16	Mississippi	1,391,670
8	Missouri	1,452,768
49	Montana	944,323
22	Nebraska	1,348,469
29	Nevada	1,274,237
25	New Hampshire	1,312,516
36	New Jersey	1,239,884
43	New Mexico	1,109,132
5	New York	1,549,922
6	North Carolina	1,520,839
1	North Dakota	1,736,734
17	Ohio	1,388,854
41	Oklahoma	1,116,032
45	Oregon	1,041,317
12	Pennsylvania	1,420,492
30	Rhode Island	1,265,661
21	South Carolina	1,357,817
23	South Dakota	1,348,146
7	Tennessee	1,478,040
34	Texas	1,249,666
47	Utah	1,021,964
46	Vermont	1,040,571
28	Virginia	1,298,581
37	Washington	1,237,003
18	West Virginia	1,378,111
9	Wisconsin	1,438,340
50	Wyoming	897,701

RANK	STATE	PER ESTABLISHMENT
1	North Dakota	$1,736,734
2	Massachusetts	1,700,753
3	Minnesota	1,676,581
4	Alabama	1,606,428
5	New York	1,549,922
6	North Carolina	1,520,839
7	Tennessee	1,478,040
8	Missouri	1,452,768
9	Wisconsin	1,438,340
10	Connecticut	1,430,931
11	Louisiana	1,430,872
12	Pennsylvania	1,420,492
13	Delaware	1,419,518
14	Illinois	1,415,296
15	Indiana	1,392,701
16	Mississippi	1,391,670
17	Ohio	1,388,854
18	West Virginia	1,378,111
19	Georgia	1,375,541
20	Kansas	1,360,073
21	South Carolina	1,357,817
22	Nebraska	1,348,469
23	South Dakota	1,348,146
24	Kentucky	1,322,495
25	New Hampshire	1,312,516
26	Michigan	1,307,333
27	Alaska	1,304,928
28	Virginia	1,298,581
29	Nevada	1,274,237
30	Rhode Island	1,265,661
31	Arkansas	1,261,297
32	Iowa	1,252,942
33	California	1,251,696
34	Texas	1,249,666
35	Maryland	1,244,110
36	New Jersey	1,239,884
37	Washington	1,237,003
38	Florida	1,201,768
39	Hawaii	1,183,509
40	Arizona	1,155,517
41	Oklahoma	1,116,032
42	Maine	1,114,449
43	New Mexico	1,109,132
44	Colorado	1,081,199
45	Oregon	1,041,317
46	Vermont	1,040,571
47	Utah	1,021,964
48	Idaho	966,493
49	Montana	944,323
50	Wyoming	897,701

District of Columbia   2,639,971

Source: Morgan Quitno Press using data from U.S. Bureau of the Census
  "1992 Census of Service Industries, Geographic Area Series, United States" (SC92-A-52)
*Includes establishments exempt from as well as subject to the federal income tax. Includes those establishments
within the Standard Industry Classification (SIC) 80. These include those primarily engaged in furnishing medical,
surgical and other health services to persons. See Facilities Chapter for establishments.

Receipts of Offices and Clinics of Doctors of Medicine in 1992

National Total = $141,429,109,000*

ALPHA ORDER

RANK	STATE	RECEIPTS	% of USA
23	Alabama	$2,194,200,000	1.55%
48	Alaska	257,847,000	0.18%
21	Arizona	2,358,063,000	1.67%
31	Arkansas	1,184,434,000	0.84%
1	California	21,969,551,000	15.53%
26	Colorado	1,823,874,000	1.29%
22	Connecticut	2,264,576,000	1.60%
45	Delaware	402,076,000	0.28%
2	Florida	10,360,884,000	7.33%
9	Georgia	4,096,050,000	2.90%
38	Hawaii	621,177,000	0.44%
43	Idaho	435,493,000	0.31%
5	Illinois	6,252,042,000	4.42%
16	Indiana	2,829,577,000	2.00%
32	Iowa	1,169,464,000	0.83%
30	Kansas	1,269,708,000	0.90%
25	Kentucky	1,867,177,000	1.32%
20	Louisiana	2,411,609,000	1.71%
41	Maine	493,897,000	0.35%
14	Maryland	3,054,253,000	2.16%
13	Massachusetts	3,103,826,000	2.19%
10	Michigan	3,899,622,000	2.76%
24	Minnesota	1,964,322,000	1.39%
33	Mississippi	968,510,000	0.68%
17	Missouri	2,562,807,000	1.81%
46	Montana	336,865,000	0.24%
37	Nebraska	750,417,000	0.53%
34	Nevada	947,372,000	0.67%
40	New Hampshire	495,024,000	0.35%
8	New Jersey	5,079,647,000	3.59%
39	New Mexico	620,805,000	0.44%
3	New York	9,895,040,000	7.00%
12	North Carolina	3,170,587,000	2.24%
44	North Dakota	422,058,000	0.30%
7	Ohio	5,703,695,000	4.03%
29	Oklahoma	1,366,055,000	0.97%
27	Oregon	1,491,857,000	1.05%
6	Pennsylvania	6,183,845,000	4.37%
42	Rhode Island	458,399,000	0.32%
28	South Carolina	1,491,246,000	1.05%
47	South Dakota	305,158,000	0.22%
15	Tennessee	2,927,905,000	2.07%
4	Texas	9,488,688,000	6.71%
36	Utah	816,997,000	0.58%
49	Vermont	187,557,000	0.13%
11	Virginia	3,207,044,000	2.27%
19	Washington	2,415,635,000	1.71%
35	West Virginia	848,606,000	0.60%
18	Wisconsin	2,415,679,000	1.71%
50	Wyoming	148,221,000	0.10%

RANK ORDER

RANK	STATE	RECEIPTS	% of USA
1	California	$21,969,551,000	15.53%
2	Florida	10,360,884,000	7.33%
3	New York	9,895,040,000	7.00%
4	Texas	9,488,688,000	6.71%
5	Illinois	6,252,042,000	4.42%
6	Pennsylvania	6,183,845,000	4.37%
7	Ohio	5,703,695,000	4.03%
8	New Jersey	5,079,647,000	3.59%
9	Georgia	4,096,050,000	2.90%
10	Michigan	3,899,622,000	2.76%
11	Virginia	3,207,044,000	2.27%
12	North Carolina	3,170,587,000	2.24%
13	Massachusetts	3,103,826,000	2.19%
14	Maryland	3,054,253,000	2.16%
15	Tennessee	2,927,905,000	2.07%
16	Indiana	2,829,577,000	2.00%
17	Missouri	2,562,807,000	1.81%
18	Wisconsin	2,415,679,000	1.71%
19	Washington	2,415,635,000	1.71%
20	Louisiana	2,411,609,000	1.71%
21	Arizona	2,358,063,000	1.67%
22	Connecticut	2,264,576,000	1.60%
23	Alabama	2,194,200,000	1.55%
24	Minnesota	1,964,322,000	1.39%
25	Kentucky	1,867,177,000	1.32%
26	Colorado	1,823,874,000	1.29%
27	Oregon	1,491,857,000	1.05%
28	South Carolina	1,491,246,000	1.05%
29	Oklahoma	1,366,055,000	0.97%
30	Kansas	1,269,708,000	0.90%
31	Arkansas	1,184,434,000	0.84%
32	Iowa	1,169,464,000	0.83%
33	Mississippi	968,510,000	0.68%
34	Nevada	947,372,000	0.67%
35	West Virginia	848,606,000	0.60%
36	Utah	816,997,000	0.58%
37	Nebraska	750,417,000	0.53%
38	Hawaii	621,177,000	0.44%
39	New Mexico	620,805,000	0.44%
40	New Hampshire	495,024,000	0.35%
41	Maine	493,897,000	0.35%
42	Rhode Island	458,399,000	0.32%
43	Idaho	435,493,000	0.31%
44	North Dakota	422,058,000	0.30%
45	Delaware	402,076,000	0.28%
46	Montana	336,865,000	0.24%
47	South Dakota	305,158,000	0.22%
48	Alaska	257,847,000	0.18%
49	Vermont	187,557,000	0.13%
50	Wyoming	148,221,000	0.10%
	District of Columbia	439,668,000	0.31%

Source: U.S. Bureau of the Census
"1992 Census of Service Industries, Geographic Area Series, United States" (SC92-A-52)
*Includes only establishments subject to the federal income tax. See Facilities Chapter for establishments.

Receipts per Office or Clinic of Doctors of Medicine in 1992

National Rate = $715,369 per Establishment*

ALPHA ORDER

RANK	STATE	PER ESTABLISHMENT
9	Alabama	$840,368
19	Alaska	738,817
16	Arizona	748,591
24	Arkansas	711,799
13	California	771,024
29	Colorado	676,010
17	Connecticut	745,171
27	Delaware	684,968
22	Florida	715,185
11	Georgia	785,587
45	Hawaii	582,718
44	Idaho	598,205
18	Illinois	742,170
15	Indiana	755,763
6	Iowa	866,912
4	Kansas	918,747
21	Kentucky	727,944
20	Louisiana	732,344
47	Maine	540,369
40	Maryland	641,650
26	Massachusetts	686,080
37	Michigan	657,055
2	Minnesota	1,327,245
32	Mississippi	664,273
12	Missouri	781,344
46	Montana	562,379
8	Nebraska	846,972
7	Nevada	864,391
38	New Hampshire	656,531
36	New Jersey	658,156
43	New Mexico	600,973
42	New York	609,826
10	North Carolina	828,695
1	North Dakota	1,736,864
23	Ohio	712,606
31	Oklahoma	665,719
35	Oregon	659,239
33	Pennsylvania	661,586
48	Rhode Island	515,634
30	South Carolina	672,035
5	South Dakota	874,378
14	Tennessee	762,475
34	Texas	660,450
39	Utah	647,896
50	Vermont	477,244
28	Virginia	678,883
25	Washington	697,354
41	West Virginia	633,288
3	Wisconsin	948,813
49	Wyoming	504,153

RANK ORDER

RANK	STATE	PER ESTABLISHMENT
1	North Dakota	$1,736,864
2	Minnesota	1,327,245
3	Wisconsin	948,813
4	Kansas	918,747
5	South Dakota	874,378
6	Iowa	866,912
7	Nevada	864,391
8	Nebraska	846,972
9	Alabama	840,368
10	North Carolina	828,695
11	Georgia	785,587
12	Missouri	781,344
13	California	771,024
14	Tennessee	762,475
15	Indiana	755,763
16	Arizona	748,591
17	Connecticut	745,171
18	Illinois	742,170
19	Alaska	738,817
20	Louisiana	732,344
21	Kentucky	727,944
22	Florida	715,185
23	Ohio	712,606
24	Arkansas	711,799
25	Washington	697,354
26	Massachusetts	686,080
27	Delaware	684,968
28	Virginia	678,883
29	Colorado	676,010
30	South Carolina	672,035
31	Oklahoma	665,719
32	Mississippi	664,273
33	Pennsylvania	661,586
34	Texas	660,450
35	Oregon	659,239
36	New Jersey	658,156
37	Michigan	657,055
38	New Hampshire	656,531
39	Utah	647,896
40	Maryland	641,650
41	West Virginia	633,288
42	New York	609,826
43	New Mexico	600,973
44	Idaho	598,205
45	Hawaii	582,718
46	Montana	562,379
47	Maine	540,369
48	Rhode Island	515,634
49	Wyoming	504,153
50	Vermont	477,244
	District of Columbia	568,781

Source: Morgan Quitno Press using data from U.S. Bureau of the Census
   "1992 Census of Service Industries, Geographic Area Series, United States" (SC92-A-52)
*Includes only establishments subject to the federal income tax. See Facilities Chapter for establishments.

Receipts of Offices and Clinics of Dentists in 1992

National Total = $35,522,953,000*

ALPHA ORDER

RANK	STATE	RECEIPTS	% of USA
25	Alabama	$423,367,000	1.30%
44	Alaska	114,760,000	0.35%
24	Arizona	506,268,000	1.56%
33	Arkansas	226,609,000	0.70%
1	California	5,523,663,000	16.98%
22	Colorado	555,652,000	1.71%
18	Connecticut	669,243,000	2.06%
45	Delaware	102,416,000	0.31%
4	Florida	1,893,179,000	5.82%
19	Georgia	644,777,000	1.98%
34	Hawaii	219,683,000	0.68%
42	Idaho	150,221,000	0.46%
6	Illinois	1,510,700,000	4.65%
12	Indiana	840,283,000	2.58%
30	Iowa	320,371,000	0.99%
31	Kansas	306,171,000	0.94%
28	Kentucky	338,975,000	1.04%
26	Louisiana	409,110,000	1.26%
41	Maine	150,904,000	0.46%
16	Maryland	713,076,000	2.19%
11	Massachusetts	992,382,000	3.05%
7	Michigan	1,475,023,000	4.54%
17	Minnesota	686,914,000	2.11%
36	Mississippi	198,070,000	0.61%
21	Missouri	569,399,000	1.75%
46	Montana	96,335,000	0.30%
37	Nebraska	185,366,000	0.57%
35	Nevada	204,068,000	0.63%
39	New Hampshire	167,595,000	0.52%
8	New Jersey	1,415,884,000	4.35%
40	New Mexico	160,064,000	0.49%
2	New York	2,770,069,000	8.52%
14	North Carolina	760,910,000	2.34%
49	North Dakota	70,632,000	0.22%
9	Ohio	1,337,215,000	4.11%
29	Oklahoma	338,025,000	1.04%
23	Oregon	526,242,000	1.62%
5	Pennsylvania	1,571,424,000	4.83%
43	Rhode Island	148,838,000	0.46%
27	South Carolina	364,380,000	1.12%
47	South Dakota	79,410,000	0.24%
20	Tennessee	572,138,000	1.76%
3	Texas	1,919,816,000	5.90%
32	Utah	257,633,000	0.79%
48	Vermont	78,673,000	0.24%
13	Virginia	811,992,000	2.50%
10	Washington	1,088,396,000	3.35%
38	West Virginia	174,028,000	0.54%
15	Wisconsin	718,189,000	2.21%
50	Wyoming	52,712,000	0.16%

RANK ORDER

RANK	STATE	RECEIPTS	% of USA
1	California	$5,523,663,000	16.98%
2	New York	2,770,069,000	8.52%
3	Texas	1,919,816,000	5.90%
4	Florida	1,893,179,000	5.82%
5	Pennsylvania	1,571,424,000	4.83%
6	Illinois	1,510,700,000	4.65%
7	Michigan	1,475,023,000	4.54%
8	New Jersey	1,415,884,000	4.35%
9	Ohio	1,337,215,000	4.11%
10	Washington	1,088,396,000	3.35%
11	Massachusetts	992,382,000	3.05%
12	Indiana	840,283,000	2.58%
13	Virginia	811,992,000	2.50%
14	North Carolina	760,910,000	2.34%
15	Wisconsin	718,189,000	2.21%
16	Maryland	713,076,000	2.19%
17	Minnesota	686,914,000	2.11%
18	Connecticut	669,243,000	2.06%
19	Georgia	644,777,000	1.98%
20	Tennessee	572,138,000	1.76%
21	Missouri	569,399,000	1.75%
22	Colorado	555,652,000	1.71%
23	Oregon	526,242,000	1.62%
24	Arizona	506,268,000	1.56%
25	Alabama	423,367,000	1.30%
26	Louisiana	409,110,000	1.26%
27	South Carolina	364,380,000	1.12%
28	Kentucky	338,975,000	1.04%
29	Oklahoma	338,025,000	1.04%
30	Iowa	320,371,000	0.99%
31	Kansas	306,171,000	0.94%
32	Utah	257,633,000	0.79%
33	Arkansas	226,609,000	0.70%
34	Hawaii	219,683,000	0.68%
35	Nevada	204,068,000	0.63%
36	Mississippi	198,070,000	0.61%
37	Nebraska	185,366,000	0.57%
38	West Virginia	174,028,000	0.54%
39	New Hampshire	167,595,000	0.52%
40	New Mexico	160,064,000	0.49%
41	Maine	150,904,000	0.46%
42	Idaho	150,221,000	0.46%
43	Rhode Island	148,838,000	0.46%
44	Alaska	114,760,000	0.35%
45	Delaware	102,416,000	0.31%
46	Montana	96,335,000	0.30%
47	South Dakota	79,410,000	0.24%
48	Vermont	78,673,000	0.24%
49	North Dakota	70,632,000	0.22%
50	Wyoming	52,712,000	0.16%
	District of Columbia	111,703,000	0.34%

Source: U.S. Bureau of the Census
"1992 Census of Service Industries, Geographic Area Series, United States" (SC92-A-52)
*Includes only establishments subject to the federal income tax. See Facilities Chapter for establishments.

Receipts per Office or Clinic of Dentists in 1992

National Rate = $326,486 per Establishment*

ALPHA ORDER

RANK	STATE	PER ESTABLISHMENT
26	Alabama	$318,082
2	Alaska	438,015
16	Arizona	332,633
41	Arkansas	275,680
7	California	373,069
36	Colorado	290,765
6	Connecticut	384,622
1	Delaware	476,353
9	Florida	352,285
43	Georgia	274,841
12	Hawaii	343,255
18	Idaho	330,156
35	Illinois	292,998
5	Indiana	385,982
39	Iowa	278,826
31	Kansas	305,255
50	Kentucky	231,857
45	Louisiana	264,283
19	Maine	329,485
21	Maryland	324,864
15	Massachusetts	337,430
14	Michigan	339,242
13	Minnesota	341,748
47	Mississippi	252,640
40	Missouri	278,163
49	Montana	242,657
48	Nebraska	248,147
3	Nevada	426,921
20	New Hampshire	326,060
11	New Jersey	351,075
32	New Mexico	300,872
22	New York	323,606
10	North Carolina	351,947
38	North Dakota	282,528
33	Ohio	297,357
42	Oklahoma	275,041
17	Oregon	331,595
34	Pennsylvania	295,603
8	Rhode Island	366,596
27	South Carolina	316,028
30	South Dakota	305,423
37	Tennessee	288,376
29	Texas	308,008
44	Utah	264,510
25	Vermont	321,114
23	Virginia	321,708
4	Washington	407,029
28	West Virginia	309,108
24	Wisconsin	321,337
46	Wyoming	260,950

RANK ORDER

RANK	STATE	PER ESTABLISHMENT
1	Delaware	$476,353
2	Alaska	438,015
3	Nevada	426,921
4	Washington	407,029
5	Indiana	385,982
6	Connecticut	384,622
7	California	373,069
8	Rhode Island	366,596
9	Florida	352,285
10	North Carolina	351,947
11	New Jersey	351,075
12	Hawaii	343,255
13	Minnesota	341,748
14	Michigan	339,242
15	Massachusetts	337,430
16	Arizona	332,633
17	Oregon	331,595
18	Idaho	330,156
19	Maine	329,485
20	New Hampshire	326,060
21	Maryland	324,864
22	New York	323,606
23	Virginia	321,708
24	Wisconsin	321,337
25	Vermont	321,114
26	Alabama	318,082
27	South Carolina	316,028
28	West Virginia	309,108
29	Texas	308,008
30	South Dakota	305,423
31	Kansas	305,255
32	New Mexico	300,872
33	Ohio	297,357
34	Pennsylvania	295,603
35	Illinois	292,998
36	Colorado	290,765
37	Tennessee	288,376
38	North Dakota	282,528
39	Iowa	278,826
40	Missouri	278,163
41	Arkansas	275,680
42	Oklahoma	275,041
43	Georgia	274,841
44	Utah	264,510
45	Louisiana	264,283
46	Wyoming	260,950
47	Mississippi	252,640
48	Nebraska	248,147
49	Montana	242,657
50	Kentucky	231,857
	District of Columbia	321,911

Source: Morgan Quitno Press using data from U.S. Bureau of the Census
"1992 Census of Service Industries, Geographic Area Series, United States" (SC92-A-52)
*Includes only establishments subject to the federal income tax. See Facilities Chapter for establishments.

Receipts of Offices and Clinics of Doctors of Osteopathy in 1992

National Total = $3,638,144,000*

RANK	STATE	RECEIPTS	% of USA
31	Alabama	$10,073,000	0.28%
36	Alaska	5,757,000	0.16%
8	Arizona	141,382,000	3.89%
33	Arkansas	7,486,000	0.21%
9	California	128,791,000	3.54%
13	Colorado	68,206,000	1.87%
NA	Connecticut**	NA	NA
23	Delaware	23,457,000	0.64%
4	Florida	325,522,000	8.95%
17	Georgia	42,184,000	1.16%
NA	Hawaii**	NA	NA
37	Idaho	4,797,000	0.13%
14	Illinois	62,781,000	1.73%
15	Indiana	54,594,000	1.50%
11	Iowa	77,485,000	2.13%
18	Kansas	39,828,000	1.09%
30	Kentucky	10,275,000	0.28%
44	Louisiana	1,804,000	0.05%
20	Maine	36,670,000	1.01%
38	Maryland	4,765,000	0.13%
29	Massachusetts	10,746,000	0.30%
1	Michigan	593,339,000	16.31%
NA	Minnesota**	NA	NA
32	Mississippi	8,865,000	0.24%
7	Missouri	160,312,000	4.41%
41	Montana	3,003,000	0.08%
NA	Nebraska**	NA	NA
27	Nevada	16,329,000	0.45%
42	New Hampshire	2,867,000	0.08%
6	New Jersey	213,199,000	5.86%
25	New Mexico	18,596,000	0.51%
12	New York	74,955,000	2.06%
35	North Carolina	6,445,000	0.18%
NA	North Dakota**	NA	NA
3	Ohio	386,003,000	10.61%
10	Oklahoma	127,260,000	3.50%
22	Oregon	32,862,000	0.90%
2	Pennsylvania	447,326,000	12.30%
26	Rhode Island	16,940,000	0.47%
34	South Carolina	6,489,000	0.18%
39	South Dakota	3,914,000	0.11%
24	Tennessee	22,588,000	0.62%
5	Texas	286,680,000	7.88%
40	Utah	3,446,000	0.09%
45	Vermont	1,074,000	0.03%
28	Virginia	13,366,000	0.37%
16	Washington	46,322,000	1.27%
19	West Virginia	37,666,000	1.04%
21	Wisconsin	36,056,000	0.99%
43	Wyoming	2,617,000	0.07%

RANK	STATE	RECEIPTS	% of USA
1	Michigan	$593,339,000	16.31%
2	Pennsylvania	447,326,000	12.30%
3	Ohio	386,003,000	10.61%
4	Florida	325,522,000	8.95%
5	Texas	286,680,000	7.88%
6	New Jersey	213,199,000	5.86%
7	Missouri	160,312,000	4.41%
8	Arizona	141,382,000	3.89%
9	California	128,791,000	3.54%
10	Oklahoma	127,260,000	3.50%
11	Iowa	77,485,000	2.13%
12	New York	74,955,000	2.06%
13	Colorado	68,206,000	1.87%
14	Illinois	62,781,000	1.73%
15	Indiana	54,594,000	1.50%
16	Washington	46,322,000	1.27%
17	Georgia	42,184,000	1.16%
18	Kansas	39,828,000	1.09%
19	West Virginia	37,666,000	1.04%
20	Maine	36,670,000	1.01%
21	Wisconsin	36,056,000	0.99%
22	Oregon	32,862,000	0.90%
23	Delaware	23,457,000	0.64%
24	Tennessee	22,588,000	0.62%
25	New Mexico	18,596,000	0.51%
26	Rhode Island	16,940,000	0.47%
27	Nevada	16,329,000	0.45%
28	Virginia	13,366,000	0.37%
29	Massachusetts	10,746,000	0.30%
30	Kentucky	10,275,000	0.28%
31	Alabama	10,073,000	0.28%
32	Mississippi	8,865,000	0.24%
33	Arkansas	7,486,000	0.21%
34	South Carolina	6,489,000	0.18%
35	North Carolina	6,445,000	0.18%
36	Alaska	5,757,000	0.16%
37	Idaho	4,797,000	0.13%
38	Maryland	4,765,000	0.13%
39	South Dakota	3,914,000	0.11%
40	Utah	3,446,000	0.09%
41	Montana	3,003,000	0.08%
42	New Hampshire	2,867,000	0.08%
43	Wyoming	2,617,000	0.07%
44	Louisiana	1,804,000	0.05%
45	Vermont	1,074,000	0.03%
NA	Connecticut**	NA	NA
NA	Hawaii**	NA	NA
NA	Minnesota**	NA	NA
NA	Nebraska**	NA	NA
NA	North Dakota**	NA	NA
	District of Columbia**	NA	NA

Source: U.S. Bureau of the Census
"1992 Census of Service Industries, Geographic Area Series, United States" (SC92-A-52)
*Includes only establishments subject to the federal income tax. See Facilities Chapter for establishments.
**Not available.

Receipts per Office or Clinic of Doctors of Osteopathy in 1992

National Rate = $417,793 per Establishment*

RANK	STATE	PER ESTABLISHMENT
32	Alabama	$314,781
2	Alaska	523,364
6	Arizona	446,000
40	Arkansas	287,923
16	California	399,972
29	Colorado	329,498
NA	Connecticut**	NA
5	Delaware	469,140
10	Florida	427,194
27	Georgia	340,194
NA	Hawaii**	NA
22	Idaho	369,000
23	Illinois	362,896
19	Indiana	384,465
15	Iowa	401,477
13	Kansas	410,598
41	Kentucky	270,395
37	Louisiana	300,667
36	Maine	305,583
38	Maryland	297,813
42	Massachusetts	268,650
3	Michigan	494,037
NA	Minnesota**	NA
7	Mississippi	443,250
24	Missouri	359,444
44	Montana	250,250
NA	Nebraska**	NA
17	Nevada	398,268
31	New Hampshire	318,556
1	New Jersey	534,333
30	New Mexico	326,246
21	New York	372,910
28	North Carolina	339,211
NA	North Dakota**	NA
4	Ohio	470,162
18	Oklahoma	387,988
39	Oregon	293,411
11	Pennsylvania	421,211
35	Rhode Island	308,000
34	South Carolina	309,000
8	South Dakota	434,889
9	Tennessee	434,385
14	Texas	405,488
25	Utah	344,600
45	Vermont	179,000
26	Virginia	342,718
33	Washington	310,886
12	West Virginia	418,511
20	Wisconsin	375,583
43	Wyoming	261,700

RANK	STATE	PER ESTABLISHMENT
1	New Jersey	$534,333
2	Alaska	523,364
3	Michigan	494,037
4	Ohio	470,162
5	Delaware	469,140
6	Arizona	446,000
7	Mississippi	443,250
8	South Dakota	434,889
9	Tennessee	434,385
10	Florida	427,194
11	Pennsylvania	421,211
12	West Virginia	418,511
13	Kansas	410,598
14	Texas	405,488
15	Iowa	401,477
16	California	399,972
17	Nevada	398,268
18	Oklahoma	387,988
19	Indiana	384,465
20	Wisconsin	375,583
21	New York	372,910
22	Idaho	369,000
23	Illinois	362,896
24	Missouri	359,444
25	Utah	344,600
26	Virginia	342,718
27	Georgia	340,194
28	North Carolina	339,211
29	Colorado	329,498
30	New Mexico	326,246
31	New Hampshire	318,556
32	Alabama	314,781
33	Washington	310,886
34	South Carolina	309,000
35	Rhode Island	308,000
36	Maine	305,583
37	Louisiana	300,667
38	Maryland	297,813
39	Oregon	293,411
40	Arkansas	287,923
41	Kentucky	270,395
42	Massachusetts	268,650
43	Wyoming	261,700
44	Montana	250,250
45	Vermont	179,000
NA	Connecticut**	NA
NA	Hawaii**	NA
NA	Minnesota**	NA
NA	Nebraska**	NA
NA	North Dakota**	NA
	District of Columbia**	NA

Source: Morgan Quitno Press using data from U.S. Bureau of the Census
"1992 Census of Service Industries, Geographic Area Series, United States" (SC92-A-52)
Includes only establishments subject to the federal income tax. See Facilities Chapter for establishments.
**Not available.*

Receipts of Offices and Clinics of Chiropractors in 1992

National Total = $5,917,909,000*

ALPHA ORDER

RANK	STATE	RECEIPTS	% of USA
31	Alabama	$50,995,000	0.86%
41	Alaska	21,901,000	0.37%
15	Arizona	123,169,000	2.08%
33	Arkansas	39,365,000	0.67%
1	California	972,152,000	16.43%
17	Colorado	100,648,000	1.70%
16	Connecticut	101,975,000	1.72%
48	Delaware	13,666,000	0.23%
2	Florida	444,248,000	7.51%
12	Georgia	154,081,000	2.60%
34	Hawaii	38,828,000	0.66%
40	Idaho	22,470,000	0.38%
8	Illinois	216,560,000	3.66%
19	Indiana	98,161,000	1.66%
24	Iowa	68,192,000	1.15%
28	Kansas	58,992,000	1.00%
30	Kentucky	51,115,000	0.86%
29	Louisiana	58,506,000	0.99%
38	Maine	26,779,000	0.45%
22	Maryland	76,300,000	1.29%
9	Massachusetts	163,870,000	2.77%
11	Michigan	155,693,000	2.63%
10	Minnesota	160,994,000	2.72%
44	Mississippi	19,203,000	0.32%
20	Missouri	89,333,000	1.51%
46	Montana	16,310,000	0.28%
36	Nebraska	30,074,000	0.51%
32	Nevada	47,657,000	0.81%
42	New Hampshire	21,688,000	0.37%
5	New Jersey	326,710,000	5.52%
35	New Mexico	34,298,000	0.58%
3	New York	388,348,000	6.56%
18	North Carolina	99,116,000	1.67%
47	North Dakota	14,992,000	0.25%
7	Ohio	237,979,000	4.02%
25	Oklahoma	66,456,000	1.12%
27	Oregon	60,225,000	1.02%
6	Pennsylvania	293,051,000	4.95%
45	Rhode Island	17,967,000	0.30%
26	South Carolina	60,285,000	1.02%
43	South Dakota	20,907,000	0.35%
23	Tennessee	74,113,000	1.25%
4	Texas	331,418,000	5.60%
37	Utah	27,714,000	0.47%
49	Vermont	10,566,000	0.18%
21	Virginia	85,384,000	1.44%
13	Washington	147,177,000	2.49%
39	West Virginia	24,442,000	0.41%
14	Wisconsin	142,761,000	2.41%
50	Wyoming	6,966,000	0.12%

RANK ORDER

RANK	STATE	RECEIPTS	% of USA
1	California	$972,152,000	16.43%
2	Florida	444,248,000	7.51%
3	New York	388,348,000	6.56%
4	Texas	331,418,000	5.60%
5	New Jersey	326,710,000	5.52%
6	Pennsylvania	293,051,000	4.95%
7	Ohio	237,979,000	4.02%
8	Illinois	216,560,000	3.66%
9	Massachusetts	163,870,000	2.77%
10	Minnesota	160,994,000	2.72%
11	Michigan	155,693,000	2.63%
12	Georgia	154,081,000	2.60%
13	Washington	147,177,000	2.49%
14	Wisconsin	142,761,000	2.41%
15	Arizona	123,169,000	2.08%
16	Connecticut	101,975,000	1.72%
17	Colorado	100,648,000	1.70%
18	North Carolina	99,116,000	1.67%
19	Indiana	98,161,000	1.66%
20	Missouri	89,333,000	1.51%
21	Virginia	85,384,000	1.44%
22	Maryland	76,300,000	1.29%
23	Tennessee	74,113,000	1.25%
24	Iowa	68,192,000	1.15%
25	Oklahoma	66,456,000	1.12%
26	South Carolina	60,285,000	1.02%
27	Oregon	60,225,000	1.02%
28	Kansas	58,992,000	1.00%
29	Louisiana	58,506,000	0.99%
30	Kentucky	51,115,000	0.86%
31	Alabama	50,995,000	0.86%
32	Nevada	47,657,000	0.81%
33	Arkansas	39,365,000	0.67%
34	Hawaii	38,828,000	0.66%
35	New Mexico	34,298,000	0.58%
36	Nebraska	30,074,000	0.51%
37	Utah	27,714,000	0.47%
38	Maine	26,779,000	0.45%
39	West Virginia	24,442,000	0.41%
40	Idaho	22,470,000	0.38%
41	Alaska	21,901,000	0.37%
42	New Hampshire	21,688,000	0.37%
43	South Dakota	20,907,000	0.35%
44	Mississippi	19,203,000	0.32%
45	Rhode Island	17,967,000	0.30%
46	Montana	16,310,000	0.28%
47	North Dakota	14,992,000	0.25%
48	Delaware	13,666,000	0.23%
49	Vermont	10,566,000	0.18%
50	Wyoming	6,966,000	0.12%
	District of Columbia	4,109,000	0.07%

Source: U.S. Bureau of the Census
"1992 Census of Service Industries, Geographic Area Series, United States" (SC92-A-52)
*Includes only establishments subject to the federal income tax. See Facilities Chapter for establishments.

Receipts per Office or Clinic of Chiropractors in 1992

National Rate = $216,543 per Establishment*

ALPHA ORDER

RANK	STATE	PER ESTABLISHMENT
37	Alabama	$180,833
3	Alaska	308,465
28	Arizona	198,021
44	Arkansas	166,097
19	California	222,766
39	Colorado	170,879
4	Connecticut	293,876
7	Delaware	273,320
10	Florida	240,524
26	Georgia	202,738
2	Hawaii	326,286
42	Idaho	167,687
25	Illinois	202,772
16	Indiana	225,140
47	Iowa	152,897
34	Kansas	183,776
30	Kentucky	190,019
24	Louisiana	206,007
21	Maine	212,532
1	Maryland	330,303
6	Massachusetts	284,991
45	Michigan	165,984
29	Minnesota	195,381
40	Mississippi	169,938
48	Missouri	149,386
50	Montana	139,402
33	Nebraska	184,503
5	Nevada	287,090
27	New Hampshire	200,815
9	New Jersey	262,418
32	New Mexico	185,395
18	New York	223,060
15	North Carolina	225,777
43	North Dakota	166,578
8	Ohio	273,225
22	Oklahoma	210,304
49	Oregon	140,713
17	Pennsylvania	223,703
14	Rhode Island	227,430
31	South Carolina	188,981
38	South Dakota	177,178
23	Tennessee	208,183
13	Texas	232,411
36	Utah	181,137
46	Vermont	162,554
11	Virginia	240,518
35	Washington	183,056
12	West Virginia	232,781
20	Wisconsin	214,678
41	Wyoming	169,902

RANK ORDER

RANK	STATE	PER ESTABLISHMENT
1	Maryland	$330,303
2	Hawaii	326,286
3	Alaska	308,465
4	Connecticut	293,876
5	Nevada	287,090
6	Massachusetts	284,991
7	Delaware	273,320
8	Ohio	273,225
9	New Jersey	262,418
10	Florida	240,524
11	Virginia	240,518
12	West Virginia	232,781
13	Texas	232,411
14	Rhode Island	227,430
15	North Carolina	225,777
16	Indiana	225,140
17	Pennsylvania	223,703
18	New York	223,060
19	California	222,766
20	Wisconsin	214,678
21	Maine	212,532
22	Oklahoma	210,304
23	Tennessee	208,183
24	Louisiana	206,007
25	Illinois	202,772
26	Georgia	202,738
27	New Hampshire	200,815
28	Arizona	198,021
29	Minnesota	195,381
30	Kentucky	190,019
31	South Carolina	188,981
32	New Mexico	185,395
33	Nebraska	184,503
34	Kansas	183,776
35	Washington	183,056
36	Utah	181,137
37	Alabama	180,833
38	South Dakota	177,178
39	Colorado	170,879
40	Mississippi	169,938
41	Wyoming	169,902
42	Idaho	167,687
43	North Dakota	166,578
44	Arkansas	166,097
45	Michigan	165,984
46	Vermont	162,554
47	Iowa	152,897
48	Missouri	149,386
49	Oregon	140,713
50	Montana	139,402
	District of Columbia	316,077

Source: Morgan Quitno Press using data from U.S. Bureau of the Census
  "1992 Census of Service Industries, Geographic Area Series, United States" (SC92-A-52)
*Includes only establishments subject to the federal income tax. See Facilities Chapter for establishments.

Receipts of Offices and Clinics of Optometrists in 1992

National Total = $4,939,521,000*

ALPHA ORDER

RANK	STATE	RECEIPTS	% of USA
27	Alabama	$65,608,000	1.33%
47	Alaska	17,112,000	0.35%
31	Arizona	49,165,000	1.00%
29	Arkansas	56,672,000	1.15%
1	California	754,317,000	15.27%
24	Colorado	73,235,000	1.48%
23	Connecticut	73,960,000	1.50%
49	Delaware	12,873,000	0.26%
5	Florida	221,280,000	4.48%
13	Georgia	102,345,000	2.07%
39	Hawaii	27,647,000	0.56%
40	Idaho	24,607,000	0.50%
7	Illinois	213,734,000	4.33%
11	Indiana	133,059,000	2.69%
19	Iowa	79,034,000	1.60%
20	Kansas	78,371,000	1.59%
25	Kentucky	72,650,000	1.47%
32	Louisiana	48,393,000	0.98%
37	Maine	35,347,000	0.72%
21	Maryland	78,104,000	1.58%
15	Massachusetts	97,781,000	1.98%
8	Michigan	203,832,000	4.13%
26	Minnesota	71,690,000	1.45%
35	Mississippi	37,655,000	0.76%
18	Missouri	88,489,000	1.79%
41	Montana	24,435,000	0.49%
34	Nebraska	38,725,000	0.78%
36	Nevada	36,924,000	0.75%
45	New Hampshire	20,073,000	0.41%
9	New Jersey	147,976,000	3.00%
38	New Mexico	30,091,000	0.61%
4	New York	226,940,000	4.59%
10	North Carolina	146,551,000	2.97%
43	North Dakota	21,635,000	0.44%
6	Ohio	218,608,000	4.43%
22	Oklahoma	76,308,000	1.54%
30	Oregon	51,605,000	1.04%
3	Pennsylvania	246,226,000	4.98%
44	Rhode Island	21,103,000	0.43%
28	South Carolina	58,093,000	1.18%
46	South Dakota	19,165,000	0.39%
14	Tennessee	101,398,000	2.05%
2	Texas	329,294,000	6.67%
42	Utah	21,944,000	0.44%
50	Vermont	11,768,000	0.24%
12	Virginia	115,755,000	2.34%
16	Washington	95,398,000	1.93%
33	West Virginia	43,184,000	0.87%
17	Wisconsin	94,432,000	1.91%
48	Wyoming	15,714,000	0.32%

RANK ORDER

RANK	STATE	RECEIPTS	% of USA
1	California	$754,317,000	15.27%
2	Texas	329,294,000	6.67%
3	Pennsylvania	246,226,000	4.98%
4	New York	226,940,000	4.59%
5	Florida	221,280,000	4.48%
6	Ohio	218,608,000	4.43%
7	Illinois	213,734,000	4.33%
8	Michigan	203,832,000	4.13%
9	New Jersey	147,976,000	3.00%
10	North Carolina	146,551,000	2.97%
11	Indiana	133,059,000	2.69%
12	Virginia	115,755,000	2.34%
13	Georgia	102,345,000	2.07%
14	Tennessee	101,398,000	2.05%
15	Massachusetts	97,781,000	1.98%
16	Washington	95,398,000	1.93%
17	Wisconsin	94,432,000	1.91%
18	Missouri	88,489,000	1.79%
19	Iowa	79,034,000	1.60%
20	Kansas	78,371,000	1.59%
21	Maryland	78,104,000	1.58%
22	Oklahoma	76,308,000	1.54%
23	Connecticut	73,960,000	1.50%
24	Colorado	73,235,000	1.48%
25	Kentucky	72,650,000	1.47%
26	Minnesota	71,690,000	1.45%
27	Alabama	65,608,000	1.33%
28	South Carolina	58,093,000	1.18%
29	Arkansas	56,672,000	1.15%
30	Oregon	51,605,000	1.04%
31	Arizona	49,165,000	1.00%
32	Louisiana	48,393,000	0.98%
33	West Virginia	43,184,000	0.87%
34	Nebraska	38,725,000	0.78%
35	Mississippi	37,655,000	0.76%
36	Nevada	36,924,000	0.75%
37	Maine	35,347,000	0.72%
38	New Mexico	30,091,000	0.61%
39	Hawaii	27,647,000	0.56%
40	Idaho	24,607,000	0.50%
41	Montana	24,435,000	0.49%
42	Utah	21,944,000	0.44%
43	North Dakota	21,635,000	0.44%
44	Rhode Island	21,103,000	0.43%
45	New Hampshire	20,073,000	0.41%
46	South Dakota	19,165,000	0.39%
47	Alaska	17,112,000	0.35%
48	Wyoming	15,714,000	0.32%
49	Delaware	12,873,000	0.26%
50	Vermont	11,768,000	0.24%
	District of Columbia	9,216,000	0.19%

Source: U.S. Bureau of the Census
  "1992 Census of Service Industries, Geographic Area Series, United States" (SC92-A-52)
*Includes only establishments subject to the federal income tax. See Facilities Chapter for establishments.

Receipts per Office or Clinic of Optometrists in 1992

National Rate = $288,271 per Establishment*

ALPHA ORDER

RANK	STATE	PER ESTABLISHMENT
24	Alabama	$286,498
1	Alaska	388,909
41	Arizona	260,132
28	Arkansas	280,554
10	California	316,674
26	Colorado	284,961
6	Connecticut	324,386
7	Delaware	321,825
42	Florida	259,110
32	Georgia	274,383
30	Hawaii	279,263
39	Idaho	261,777
11	Illinois	306,209
21	Indiana	287,384
18	Iowa	292,719
9	Kansas	317,291
17	Kentucky	292,944
45	Louisiana	246,903
22	Maine	287,374
5	Maryland	332,357
38	Massachusetts	264,273
3	Michigan	335,802
43	Minnesota	255,125
44	Mississippi	254,426
14	Missouri	293,983
48	Montana	237,233
8	Nebraska	320,041
4	Nevada	335,673
34	New Hampshire	271,257
36	New Jersey	269,047
20	New Mexico	289,337
23	New York	286,903
13	North Carolina	294,279
2	North Dakota	338,047
40	Ohio	261,493
46	Oklahoma	240,719
50	Oregon	232,455
27	Pennsylvania	283,344
16	Rhode Island	293,097
15	South Carolina	293,399
47	South Dakota	239,563
31	Tennessee	278,566
12	Texas	299,358
35	Utah	270,914
49	Vermont	235,360
37	Virginia	265,493
29	Washington	279,760
25	West Virginia	285,987
33	Wisconsin	272,138
19	Wyoming	291,000

RANK ORDER

RANK	STATE	PER ESTABLISHMENT
1	Alaska	$388,909
2	North Dakota	338,047
3	Michigan	335,802
4	Nevada	335,673
5	Maryland	332,357
6	Connecticut	324,386
7	Delaware	321,825
8	Nebraska	320,041
9	Kansas	317,291
10	California	316,674
11	Illinois	306,209
12	Texas	299,358
13	North Carolina	294,279
14	Missouri	293,983
15	South Carolina	293,399
16	Rhode Island	293,097
17	Kentucky	292,944
18	Iowa	292,719
19	Wyoming	291,000
20	New Mexico	289,337
21	Indiana	287,384
22	Maine	287,374
23	New York	286,903
24	Alabama	286,498
25	West Virginia	285,987
26	Colorado	284,961
27	Pennsylvania	283,344
28	Arkansas	280,554
29	Washington	279,760
30	Hawaii	279,263
31	Tennessee	278,566
32	Georgia	274,383
33	Wisconsin	272,138
34	New Hampshire	271,257
35	Utah	270,914
36	New Jersey	269,047
37	Virginia	265,493
38	Massachusetts	264,273
39	Idaho	261,777
40	Ohio	261,493
41	Arizona	260,132
42	Florida	259,110
43	Minnesota	255,125
44	Mississippi	254,426
45	Louisiana	246,903
46	Oklahoma	240,719
47	South Dakota	239,563
48	Montana	237,233
49	Vermont	235,360
50	Oregon	232,455
	District of Columbia	384,000

Source: Morgan Quitno Press using data from U.S. Bureau of the Census
"1992 Census of Service Industries, Geographic Area Series, United States" (SC92-A-52)
*Includes only establishments subject to the federal income tax. See Facilities Chapter for establishments.

Receipts of Offices and Clinics of Podiatrists in 1992

National Total = $1,920,076,000*

ALPHA ORDER					RANK ORDER			
RANK	STATE	RECEIPTS	% of USA		RANK	STATE	RECEIPTS	% of USA
23	Alabama	$15,910,000	0.83%		1	California	$217,602,000	11.33%
46	Alaska	2,222,000	0.12%		2	New York	209,057,000	10.89%
18	Arizona	27,962,000	1.46%		3	Florida	147,168,000	7.66%
42	Arkansas	5,017,000	0.26%		4	Pennsylvania	118,882,000	6.19%
1	California	217,602,000	11.33%		5	Michigan	112,871,000	5.88%
22	Colorado	18,980,000	0.99%		6	Ohio	109,704,000	5.71%
11	Connecticut	48,830,000	2.54%		7	Illinois	105,745,000	5.51%
37	Delaware	6,801,000	0.35%		8	Texas	104,569,000	5.45%
3	Florida	147,168,000	7.66%		9	New Jersey	103,924,000	5.41%
12	Georgia	47,600,000	2.48%		10	Maryland	56,379,000	2.94%
43	Hawaii	3,871,000	0.20%		11	Connecticut	48,830,000	2.54%
40	Idaho	5,283,000	0.28%		12	Georgia	47,600,000	2.48%
7	Illinois	105,745,000	5.51%		13	Massachusetts	43,366,000	2.26%
14	Indiana	41,792,000	2.18%		14	Indiana	41,792,000	2.18%
24	Iowa	14,998,000	0.78%		15	Virginia	40,402,000	2.10%
29	Kansas	12,107,000	0.63%		16	North Carolina	35,032,000	1.82%
31	Kentucky	10,299,000	0.54%		17	Washington	31,204,000	1.63%
26	Louisiana	13,876,000	0.72%		18	Arizona	27,962,000	1.46%
38	Maine	6,464,000	0.34%		19	Wisconsin	27,720,000	1.44%
10	Maryland	56,379,000	2.94%		20	Missouri	24,462,000	1.27%
13	Massachusetts	43,366,000	2.26%		21	Tennessee	23,034,000	1.20%
5	Michigan	112,871,000	5.88%		22	Colorado	18,980,000	0.99%
28	Minnesota	12,440,000	0.65%		23	Alabama	15,910,000	0.83%
44	Mississippi	3,801,000	0.20%		24	Iowa	14,998,000	0.78%
20	Missouri	24,462,000	1.27%		25	Oklahoma	14,850,000	0.77%
45	Montana	3,441,000	0.18%		26	Louisiana	13,876,000	0.72%
36	Nebraska	7,020,000	0.37%		27	Oregon	13,796,000	0.72%
35	Nevada	7,995,000	0.42%		28	Minnesota	12,440,000	0.65%
41	New Hampshire	5,180,000	0.27%		29	Kansas	12,107,000	0.63%
9	New Jersey	103,924,000	5.41%		30	Rhode Island	11,842,000	0.62%
34	New Mexico	8,215,000	0.43%		31	Kentucky	10,299,000	0.54%
2	New York	209,057,000	10.89%		32	South Carolina	9,906,000	0.52%
16	North Carolina	35,032,000	1.82%		33	Utah	9,326,000	0.49%
48	North Dakota	1,382,000	0.07%		34	New Mexico	8,215,000	0.43%
6	Ohio	109,704,000	5.71%		35	Nevada	7,995,000	0.42%
25	Oklahoma	14,850,000	0.77%		36	Nebraska	7,020,000	0.37%
27	Oregon	13,796,000	0.72%		37	Delaware	6,801,000	0.35%
4	Pennsylvania	118,882,000	6.19%		38	Maine	6,464,000	0.34%
30	Rhode Island	11,842,000	0.62%		39	West Virginia	5,602,000	0.29%
32	South Carolina	9,906,000	0.52%		40	Idaho	5,283,000	0.28%
47	South Dakota	1,774,000	0.09%		41	New Hampshire	5,180,000	0.27%
21	Tennessee	23,034,000	1.20%		42	Arkansas	5,017,000	0.26%
8	Texas	104,569,000	5.45%		43	Hawaii	3,871,000	0.20%
33	Utah	9,326,000	0.49%		44	Mississippi	3,801,000	0.20%
49	Vermont	1,157,000	0.06%		45	Montana	3,441,000	0.18%
15	Virginia	40,402,000	2.10%		46	Alaska	2,222,000	0.12%
17	Washington	31,204,000	1.63%		47	South Dakota	1,774,000	0.09%
39	West Virginia	5,602,000	0.29%		48	North Dakota	1,382,000	0.07%
19	Wisconsin	27,720,000	1.44%		49	Vermont	1,157,000	0.06%
50	Wyoming	1,035,000	0.05%		50	Wyoming	1,035,000	0.05%
						District of Columbia	8,181,000	0.43%

Source: U.S. Bureau of the Census
"1992 Census of Service Industries, Geographic Area Series, United States" (SC92-A-52)
*Includes only establishments subject to the federal income tax. See Facilities Chapter for establishments.

Receipts per Office or Clinic of Podiatrists in 1992

National Rate = $241,580 per Establishment*

ALPHA ORDER

RANK ORDER

RANK	STATE	PER ESTABLISHMENT		RANK	STATE	PER ESTABLISHMENT
3	Alabama	$324,694		1	Alaska	$444,400
1	Alaska	444,400		2	Georgia	342,446
28	Arizona	231,091		3	Alabama	324,694
17	Arkansas	250,850		4	Connecticut	321,250
25	California	233,981		5	Idaho	310,765
35	Colorado	215,682		6	Louisiana	289,083
4	Connecticut	321,250		7	Oklahoma	285,577
11	Delaware	272,040		8	Nevada	285,536
13	Florida	260,936		9	Michigan	282,178
2	Georgia	342,446		10	Texas	273,741
23	Hawaii	241,938		11	Delaware	272,040
5	Idaho	310,765		12	Maryland	267,199
15	Illinois	252,375		13	Florida	260,936
16	Indiana	251,759		14	Tennessee	255,933
46	Iowa	199,973		15	Illinois	252,375
33	Kansas	220,127		16	Indiana	251,759
30	Kentucky	223,891		17	Arkansas	250,850
6	Louisiana	289,083		18	North Carolina	250,229
48	Maine	179,556		19	Missouri	249,612
12	Maryland	267,199		20	New Mexico	248,939
41	Massachusetts	208,490		21	South Carolina	247,650
9	Michigan	282,178		22	Virginia	246,354
42	Minnesota	207,333		23	Hawaii	241,938
40	Mississippi	211,167		24	Rhode Island	236,840
19	Missouri	249,612		25	California	233,981
37	Montana	215,063		26	Wisconsin	232,941
44	Nebraska	206,471		27	New Jersey	231,457
8	Nevada	285,536		28	Arizona	231,091
34	New Hampshire	215,833		29	Oregon	226,164
27	New Jersey	231,457		30	Kentucky	223,891
20	New Mexico	248,939		31	Ohio	223,886
32	New York	222,875		32	New York	222,875
18	North Carolina	250,229		33	Kansas	220,127
47	North Dakota	197,429		34	New Hampshire	215,833
31	Ohio	223,886		35	Colorado	215,682
7	Oklahoma	285,577		36	West Virginia	215,462
29	Oregon	226,164		37	Montana	215,063
45	Pennsylvania	201,837		38	Washington	213,726
24	Rhode Island	236,840		39	Utah	211,955
21	South Carolina	247,650		40	Mississippi	211,167
50	South Dakota	126,714		41	Massachusetts	208,490
14	Tennessee	255,933		42	Minnesota	207,333
10	Texas	273,741		43	Wyoming	207,000
39	Utah	211,955		44	Nebraska	206,471
49	Vermont	128,556		45	Pennsylvania	201,837
22	Virginia	246,354		46	Iowa	199,973
38	Washington	213,726		47	North Dakota	197,429
36	West Virginia	215,462		48	Maine	179,556
26	Wisconsin	232,941		49	Vermont	128,556
43	Wyoming	207,000		50	South Dakota	126,714
					District of Columbia	255,656

Source: Morgan Quitno Press using data from U.S. Bureau of the Census
   "1992 Census of Service Industries, Geographic Area Series, United States" (SC92-A-52)
*Includes only establishments subject to the federal income tax. See Facilities Chapter for establishments.

Receipts of Offices and Clinics of Other Health Practitioners in 1992

National Total = $6,148,059,000*

ALPHA ORDER

RANK ORDER

RANK	STATE	RECEIPTS	% of USA		RANK	STATE	RECEIPTS	% of USA
29	Alabama	$52,156,000	0.85%		1	California	$1,034,853,000	16.83%
46	Alaska	12,434,000	0.20%		2	Texas	430,380,000	7.00%
21	Arizona	96,707,000	1.57%		3	Florida	426,622,000	6.94%
31	Arkansas	40,313,000	0.66%		4	Pennsylvania	374,184,000	6.09%
1	California	1,034,853,000	16.83%		5	New York	365,739,000	5.95%
17	Colorado	108,367,000	1.76%		6	Ohio	241,548,000	3.93%
16	Connecticut	109,057,000	1.77%		7	Illinois	224,938,000	3.66%
40	Delaware	24,546,000	0.40%		8	Michigan	212,093,000	3.45%
3	Florida	426,622,000	6.94%		9	New Jersey	211,576,000	3.44%
12	Georgia	161,961,000	2.63%		10	Maryland	179,434,000	2.92%
36	Hawaii	30,940,000	0.50%		11	Washington	162,891,000	2.65%
45	Idaho	14,480,000	0.24%		12	Georgia	161,961,000	2.63%
7	Illinois	224,938,000	3.66%		13	Massachusetts	158,543,000	2.58%
23	Indiana	84,829,000	1.38%		14	North Carolina	138,366,000	2.25%
32	Iowa	38,347,000	0.62%		15	Virginia	135,154,000	2.20%
33	Kansas	38,115,000	0.62%		16	Connecticut	109,057,000	1.77%
26	Kentucky	59,948,000	0.98%		17	Colorado	108,367,000	1.76%
24	Louisiana	80,487,000	1.31%		18	Minnesota	100,371,000	1.63%
41	Maine	23,413,000	0.38%		19	Missouri	99,140,000	1.61%
10	Maryland	179,434,000	2.92%		20	Tennessee	97,742,000	1.59%
13	Massachusetts	158,543,000	2.58%		21	Arizona	96,707,000	1.57%
8	Michigan	212,093,000	3.45%		22	Wisconsin	93,109,000	1.51%
18	Minnesota	100,371,000	1.63%		23	Indiana	84,829,000	1.38%
39	Mississippi	26,287,000	0.43%		24	Louisiana	80,487,000	1.31%
19	Missouri	99,140,000	1.61%		25	Oregon	71,873,000	1.17%
44	Montana	14,602,000	0.24%		26	Kentucky	59,948,000	0.98%
38	Nebraska	27,517,000	0.45%		27	Nevada	55,463,000	0.90%
27	Nevada	55,463,000	0.90%		28	Oklahoma	53,332,000	0.87%
34	New Hampshire	36,653,000	0.60%		29	Alabama	52,156,000	0.85%
9	New Jersey	211,576,000	3.44%		30	South Carolina	43,318,000	0.70%
37	New Mexico	30,081,000	0.49%		31	Arkansas	40,313,000	0.66%
5	New York	365,739,000	5.95%		32	Iowa	38,347,000	0.62%
14	North Carolina	138,366,000	2.25%		33	Kansas	38,115,000	0.62%
50	North Dakota	6,543,000	0.11%		34	New Hampshire	36,653,000	0.60%
6	Ohio	241,548,000	3.93%		35	Utah	36,264,000	0.59%
28	Oklahoma	53,332,000	0.87%		36	Hawaii	30,940,000	0.50%
25	Oregon	71,873,000	1.17%		37	New Mexico	30,081,000	0.49%
4	Pennsylvania	374,184,000	6.09%		38	Nebraska	27,517,000	0.45%
43	Rhode Island	16,002,000	0.26%		39	Mississippi	26,287,000	0.43%
30	South Carolina	43,318,000	0.70%		40	Delaware	24,546,000	0.40%
48	South Dakota	9,805,000	0.16%		41	Maine	23,413,000	0.38%
20	Tennessee	97,742,000	1.59%		42	West Virginia	18,885,000	0.31%
2	Texas	430,380,000	7.00%		43	Rhode Island	16,002,000	0.26%
35	Utah	36,264,000	0.59%		44	Montana	14,602,000	0.24%
47	Vermont	10,822,000	0.18%		45	Idaho	14,480,000	0.24%
15	Virginia	135,154,000	2.20%		46	Alaska	12,434,000	0.20%
11	Washington	162,891,000	2.65%		47	Vermont	10,822,000	0.18%
42	West Virginia	18,885,000	0.31%		48	South Dakota	9,805,000	0.16%
22	Wisconsin	93,109,000	1.51%		49	Wyoming	7,307,000	0.12%
49	Wyoming	7,307,000	0.12%		50	North Dakota	6,543,000	0.11%
						District of Columbia	20,522,000	0.33%

Source: U.S. Bureau of the Census
    "1992 Census of Service Industries, Geographic Area Series, United States" (SC92-A-52)
*Includes only establishments subject to the federal income tax. Includes health practitioners not otherwise
classified such as acupuncturists, midwives, nutritionists, physical and occupational therapists and psychologists.
See Facilities Chapter for establishments.

Receipts per Office or Clinic of Other Health Practitioners in 1992

National Rate = $276,193 per Establishment*

ALPHA ORDER				RANK ORDER		
RANK	STATE	PER ESTABLISHMENT		RANK	STATE	PER ESTABLISHMENT
11	Alabama	$299,747		1	Nevada	$426,638
44	Alaska	207,233		2	Pennsylvania	416,222
40	Arizona	216,347		3	Connecticut	349,542
29	Arkansas	258,417		4	Delaware	322,974
27	California	261,723		5	New Jersey	317,682
42	Colorado	210,421		6	Michigan	317,030
3	Connecticut	349,542		7	Illinois	311,548
4	Delaware	322,974		8	Indiana	308,469
28	Florida	259,502		9	Maryland	303,098
12	Georgia	297,722		10	Massachusetts	301,413
30	Hawaii	257,833		11	Alabama	299,747
47	Idaho	183,291		12	Georgia	297,722
7	Illinois	311,548		13	Tennessee	296,188
8	Indiana	308,469		14	New Hampshire	286,352
35	Iowa	245,814		15	Kentucky	282,774
37	Kansas	241,234		16	Ohio	280,870
15	Kentucky	282,774		17	Virginia	278,668
34	Louisiana	248,417		18	North Carolina	278,402
43	Maine	209,045		19	Minnesota	278,036
9	Maryland	303,098		20	Wisconsin	273,850
10	Massachusetts	301,413		21	West Virginia	273,696
6	Michigan	317,030		22	New York	272,127
19	Minnesota	278,036		23	Missouri	265,080
31	Mississippi	257,716		24	South Dakota	265,000
23	Missouri	265,080		25	Texas	263,068
49	Montana	169,791		26	Washington	262,727
32	Nebraska	257,168		27	California	261,723
1	Nevada	426,638		28	Florida	259,502
14	New Hampshire	286,352		29	Arkansas	258,417
5	New Jersey	317,682		30	Hawaii	257,833
48	New Mexico	180,126		31	Mississippi	257,716
22	New York	272,127		32	Nebraska	257,168
18	North Carolina	278,402		33	South Carolina	256,320
41	North Dakota	211,065		34	Louisiana	248,417
16	Ohio	280,870		35	Iowa	245,814
38	Oklahoma	233,912		36	Rhode Island	242,455
45	Oregon	199,094		37	Kansas	241,234
2	Pennsylvania	416,222		38	Oklahoma	233,912
36	Rhode Island	242,455		39	Utah	218,458
33	South Carolina	256,320		40	Arizona	216,347
24	South Dakota	265,000		41	North Dakota	211,065
13	Tennessee	296,188		42	Colorado	210,421
25	Texas	263,068		43	Maine	209,045
39	Utah	218,458		44	Alaska	207,233
50	Vermont	156,841		45	Oregon	199,094
17	Virginia	278,668		46	Wyoming	197,486
26	Washington	262,727		47	Idaho	183,291
21	West Virginia	273,696		48	New Mexico	180,126
20	Wisconsin	273,850		49	Montana	169,791
46	Wyoming	197,486		50	Vermont	156,841
					District of Columbia	301,794

Source: Morgan Quitno Press using data from U.S. Bureau of the Census
  "1992 Census of Service Industries, Geographic Area Series, United States" (SC92-A-52)
*Includes only establishments subject to the federal income tax. Includes health practitioners not otherwise classified such as acupuncturists, midwives, nutritionists, physical and occupational therapists and psychologists. See Facilities Chapter for establishments.

Receipts of Hospitals in 1992

National Total = $310,818,211,000*

ALPHA ORDER

RANK	STATE	RECEIPTS	% of USA
21	Alabama	$5,114,698,000	1.65%
NA	Alaska**	NA	NA
23	Arizona	4,064,528,000	1.31%
30	Arkansas	2,601,895,000	0.84%
1	California	34,552,067,000	11.12%
24	Colorado	3,876,008,000	1.25%
NA	Connecticut**	NA	NA
37	Delaware	903,055,000	0.29%
5	Florida	16,528,209,000	5.32%
11	Georgia	8,079,353,000	2.60%
NA	Hawaii**	NA	NA
38	Idaho	880,530,000	0.28%
6	Illinois	14,715,279,000	4.73%
16	Indiana	6,590,871,000	2.12%
NA	Iowa**	NA	NA
27	Kansas	2,856,257,000	0.92%
22	Kentucky	4,185,657,000	1.35%
17	Louisiana	5,658,657,000	1.82%
NA	Maine**	NA	NA
18	Maryland	5,440,457,000	1.75%
10	Massachusetts	9,714,787,000	3.13%
8	Michigan	11,444,321,000	3.68%
NA	Minnesota**	NA	NA
29	Mississippi	2,627,692,000	0.85%
13	Missouri	7,217,462,000	2.32%
39	Montana	864,812,000	0.28%
NA	Nebraska**	NA	NA
34	Nevada	1,296,942,000	0.42%
36	New Hampshire	1,250,889,000	0.40%
9	New Jersey	9,842,808,000	3.17%
33	New Mexico	1,558,035,000	0.50%
2	New York	27,722,480,000	8.92%
12	North Carolina	7,408,964,000	2.38%
NA	North Dakota**	NA	NA
7	Ohio	13,998,840,000	4.50%
26	Oklahoma	3,232,112,000	1.04%
28	Oregon	2,835,585,000	0.91%
4	Pennsylvania	18,019,449,000	5.80%
35	Rhode Island	1,257,773,000	0.40%
25	South Carolina	3,833,754,000	1.23%
NA	South Dakota**	NA	NA
15	Tennessee	6,770,631,000	2.18%
3	Texas	20,081,248,000	6.46%
32	Utah	1,626,872,000	0.52%
40	Vermont	545,676,000	0.18%
14	Virginia	6,793,601,000	2.19%
20	Washington	5,193,838,000	1.67%
31	West Virginia	2,243,147,000	0.72%
19	Wisconsin	5,262,803,000	1.69%
NA	Wyoming**	NA	NA

RANK ORDER

RANK	STATE	RECEIPTS	% of USA
1	California	$34,552,067,000	11.12%
2	New York	27,722,480,000	8.92%
3	Texas	20,081,248,000	6.46%
4	Pennsylvania	18,019,449,000	5.80%
5	Florida	16,528,209,000	5.32%
6	Illinois	14,715,279,000	4.73%
7	Ohio	13,998,840,000	4.50%
8	Michigan	11,444,321,000	3.68%
9	New Jersey	9,842,808,000	3.17%
10	Massachusetts	9,714,787,000	3.13%
11	Georgia	8,079,353,000	2.60%
12	North Carolina	7,408,964,000	2.38%
13	Missouri	7,217,462,000	2.32%
14	Virginia	6,793,601,000	2.19%
15	Tennessee	6,770,631,000	2.18%
16	Indiana	6,590,871,000	2.12%
17	Louisiana	5,658,657,000	1.82%
18	Maryland	5,440,457,000	1.75%
19	Wisconsin	5,262,803,000	1.69%
20	Washington	5,193,838,000	1.67%
21	Alabama	5,114,698,000	1.65%
22	Kentucky	4,185,657,000	1.35%
23	Arizona	4,064,528,000	1.31%
24	Colorado	3,876,008,000	1.25%
25	South Carolina	3,833,754,000	1.23%
26	Oklahoma	3,232,112,000	1.04%
27	Kansas	2,856,257,000	0.92%
28	Oregon	2,835,585,000	0.91%
29	Mississippi	2,627,692,000	0.85%
30	Arkansas	2,601,895,000	0.84%
31	West Virginia	2,243,147,000	0.72%
32	Utah	1,626,872,000	0.52%
33	New Mexico	1,558,035,000	0.50%
34	Nevada	1,296,942,000	0.42%
35	Rhode Island	1,257,773,000	0.40%
36	New Hampshire	1,250,889,000	0.40%
37	Delaware	903,055,000	0.29%
38	Idaho	880,530,000	0.28%
39	Montana	864,812,000	0.28%
40	Vermont	545,676,000	0.18%
NA	Alaska**	NA	NA
NA	Connecticut**	NA	NA
NA	Hawaii**	NA	NA
NA	Iowa**	NA	NA
NA	Maine**	NA	NA
NA	Minnesota**	NA	NA
NA	Nebraska**	NA	NA
NA	North Dakota**	NA	NA
NA	South Dakota**	NA	NA
NA	Wyoming**	NA	NA
	District of Columbia**	NA	NA

Source: Morgan Quitno Press using data from U.S. Bureau of the Census
   "1992 Census of Service Industries, Geographic Area Series, United States" (SC92-A-52)
*Includes establishments exempt from as well as subject to the federal income tax. Includes general medical and surgical hospitals, psychiatric hospitals and other specialty hospitals. Includes government owned hospitals.
**Not available.

Receipts per Hospital in 1992

National Rate = $43,654,243 per Hospital*

RANK	STATE	PER HOSPITAL
24	Alabama	$36,533,557
NA	Alaska**	NA
18	Arizona	40,645,280
34	Arkansas	25,508,775
9	California	57,205,409
21	Colorado	38,760,080
NA	Connecticut**	NA
10	Delaware	56,440,938
12	Florida	50,237,717
23	Georgia	38,473,110
NA	Hawaii**	NA
39	Idaho	16,306,111
8	Illinois	57,257,895
20	Indiana	40,434,791
NA	Iowa**	NA
38	Kansas	17,631,216
28	Kentucky	32,700,445
31	Louisiana	30,422,887
NA	Maine**	NA
3	Maryland	64,005,376
4	Massachusetts	60,717,419
11	Michigan	52,257,174
NA	Minnesota**	NA
36	Mississippi	22,268,576
16	Missouri	41,242,640
40	Montana	13,304,800
NA	Nebraska**	NA
19	Nevada	40,529,438
30	New Hampshire	30,509,488
2	New Jersey	72,909,689
35	New Mexico	23,254,254
1	New York	85,038,282
15	North Carolina	42,580,253
NA	North Dakota**	NA
6	Ohio	57,608,395
37	Oklahoma	21,547,413
25	Oregon	35,893,481
7	Pennsylvania	57,386,780
5	Rhode Island	59,893,952
17	South Carolina	41,223,161
NA	South Dakota**	NA
22	Tennessee	38,689,320
26	Texas	34,326,920
33	Utah	29,051,286
32	Vermont	30,315,333
13	Virginia	48,525,721
14	Washington	43,645,697
29	West Virginia	31,154,819
27	Wisconsin	33,521,038
NA	Wyoming**	NA

RANK ORDER

RANK	STATE	PER HOSPITAL
1	New York	$85,038,282
2	New Jersey	72,909,689
3	Maryland	64,005,376
4	Massachusetts	60,717,419
5	Rhode Island	59,893,952
6	Ohio	57,608,395
7	Pennsylvania	57,386,780
8	Illinois	57,257,895
9	California	57,205,409
10	Delaware	56,440,938
11	Michigan	52,257,174
12	Florida	50,237,717
13	Virginia	48,525,721
14	Washington	43,645,697
15	North Carolina	42,580,253
16	Missouri	41,242,640
17	South Carolina	41,223,161
18	Arizona	40,645,280
19	Nevada	40,529,438
20	Indiana	40,434,791
21	Colorado	38,760,080
22	Tennessee	38,689,320
23	Georgia	38,473,110
24	Alabama	36,533,557
25	Oregon	35,893,481
26	Texas	34,326,920
27	Wisconsin	33,521,038
28	Kentucky	32,700,445
29	West Virginia	31,154,819
30	New Hampshire	30,509,488
31	Louisiana	30,422,887
32	Vermont	30,315,333
33	Utah	29,051,286
34	Arkansas	25,508,775
35	New Mexico	23,254,254
36	Mississippi	22,268,576
37	Oklahoma	21,547,413
38	Kansas	17,631,216
39	Idaho	16,306,111
40	Montana	13,304,800
NA	Alaska**	NA
NA	Connecticut**	NA
NA	Hawaii**	NA
NA	Iowa**	NA
NA	Maine**	NA
NA	Minnesota**	NA
NA	Nebraska**	NA
NA	North Dakota**	NA
NA	South Dakota**	NA
NA	Wyoming**	NA
	District of Columbia**	NA

Source: Morgan Quitno Press using data from U.S. Bureau of the Census
   "1992 Census of Service Industries, Geographic Area Series, United States" (SC92-A-52)
*Calculated using Census Bureau count of 7,120 hospitals. Includes establishments exempt from as well as subject to the federal income tax. Includes general medical and surgical hospitals, psychiatric hospitals and other specialty hospitals. Includes government owned hospitals.
**Not available.

Uncompensated Care Expenses in Community Hospitals in 1992

National Total = $14,691,902,692

ALPHA ORDER

RANK	STATE	EXPENDITURES	% of USA		RANK	STATE	EXPENDITURES	% of USA
13	Alabama	$351,095,842	2.39%		1	California	$1,749,206,487	11.91%
45	Alaska	24,375,358	0.17%		2	Texas	1,566,829,829	10.66%
28	Arizona	145,956,397	0.99%		3	New York	1,111,077,206	7.56%
27	Arkansas	151,972,830	1.03%		4	Florida	889,185,169	6.05%
1	California	1,749,206,487	11.91%		5	New Jersey	809,838,266	5.51%
21	Colorado	190,349,245	1.30%		6	Illinois	690,349,440	4.70%
24	Connecticut	162,233,546	1.10%		7	Ohio	548,945,499	3.74%
36	Delaware	67,321,716	0.46%		8	Georgia	529,333,725	3.60%
4	Florida	889,185,169	6.05%		9	Massachusetts	515,229,143	3.51%
8	Georgia	529,333,725	3.60%		10	Pennsylvania	412,588,861	2.81%
43	Hawaii	32,924,191	0.22%		11	North Carolina	371,039,914	2.53%
47	Idaho	23,330,207	0.16%		12	Tennessee	370,874,408	2.52%
6	Illinois	690,349,440	4.70%		13	Alabama	351,095,842	2.39%
18	Indiana	277,941,471	1.89%		14	Missouri	333,946,598	2.27%
31	Iowa	114,462,867	0.78%		15	Virginia	325,204,129	2.21%
35	Kansas	79,861,499	0.54%		16	Maryland	321,800,126	2.19%
23	Kentucky	171,836,095	1.17%		17	Michigan	320,909,086	2.18%
20	Louisiana	221,501,951	1.51%		18	Indiana	277,941,471	1.89%
38	Maine	52,460,151	0.36%		19	South Carolina	231,851,479	1.58%
16	Maryland	321,800,126	2.19%		20	Louisiana	221,501,951	1.51%
9	Massachusetts	515,229,143	3.51%		21	Colorado	190,349,245	1.30%
17	Michigan	320,909,086	2.18%		22	Oklahoma	174,384,524	1.19%
33	Minnesota	95,883,389	0.65%		23	Kentucky	171,836,095	1.17%
25	Mississippi	162,207,782	1.10%		24	Connecticut	162,233,546	1.10%
14	Missouri	333,946,598	2.27%		25	Mississippi	162,207,782	1.10%
46	Montana	23,828,891	0.16%		26	Washington	158,806,874	1.08%
41	Nebraska	36,484,993	0.25%		27	Arkansas	151,972,830	1.03%
37	Nevada	64,441,467	0.44%		28	Arizona	145,956,397	0.99%
40	New Hampshire	49,940,964	0.34%		29	Oregon	129,882,254	0.88%
5	New Jersey	809,838,266	5.51%		30	West Virginia	118,024,511	0.80%
34	New Mexico	91,097,559	0.62%		31	Iowa	114,462,867	0.78%
3	New York	1,111,077,206	7.56%		32	Wisconsin	113,825,059	0.77%
11	North Carolina	371,039,914	2.53%		33	Minnesota	95,883,389	0.65%
50	North Dakota	15,359,749	0.10%		34	New Mexico	91,097,559	0.62%
7	Ohio	548,945,499	3.74%		35	Kansas	79,861,499	0.54%
22	Oklahoma	174,384,524	1.19%		36	Delaware	67,321,716	0.46%
29	Oregon	129,882,254	0.88%		37	Nevada	64,441,467	0.44%
10	Pennsylvania	412,588,861	2.81%		38	Maine	52,460,151	0.36%
42	Rhode Island	34,564,000	0.24%		39	Utah	51,850,984	0.35%
19	South Carolina	231,851,479	1.58%		40	New Hampshire	49,940,964	0.34%
49	South Dakota	16,035,925	0.11%		41	Nebraska	36,484,993	0.25%
12	Tennessee	370,874,408	2.52%		42	Rhode Island	34,564,000	0.24%
2	Texas	1,566,829,829	10.66%		43	Hawaii	32,924,191	0.22%
39	Utah	51,850,984	0.35%		44	Wyoming	26,505,671	0.18%
48	Vermont	17,802,967	0.12%		45	Alaska	24,375,358	0.17%
15	Virginia	325,204,129	2.21%		46	Montana	23,828,891	0.16%
26	Washington	158,806,874	1.08%		47	Idaho	23,330,207	0.16%
30	West Virginia	118,024,511	0.80%		48	Vermont	17,802,967	0.12%
32	Wisconsin	113,825,059	0.77%		49	South Dakota	16,035,925	0.11%
44	Wyoming	26,505,671	0.18%		50	North Dakota	15,359,749	0.10%
						District of Columbia	148,142,380	1.01%

Source: Health Insurance Association of America
"Source Book of Health Insurance Data 1994" (based on data from the American Hospital Association)

Medical Costs Due to Smoking in 1990

National Total = $36,446,000,000

ALPHA ORDER					RANK ORDER			

RANK	STATE	COSTS	% of USA		RANK	STATE	COSTS	% of USA
23	Alabama	$573,000,000	1.57%		1	California	$3,966,000,000	10.88%
49	Alaska	76,000,000	0.21%		2	New York	3,132,000,000	8.59%
24	Arizona	559,000,000	1.53%		3	Florida	2,302,000,000	6.32%
32	Arkansas	296,000,000	0.81%		4	Texas	2,007,000,000	5.51%
1	California	3,966,000,000	10.88%		5	Pennsylvania	1,982,000,000	5.44%
26	Colorado	504,000,000	1.38%		6	Ohio	1,643,000,000	4.51%
21	Connecticut	621,000,000	1.70%		7	Illinois	1,614,000,000	4.43%
43	Delaware	112,000,000	0.31%		8	Michigan	1,352,000,000	3.71%
3	Florida	2,302,000,000	6.32%		9	Massachusetts	1,330,000,000	3.65%
11	Georgia	880,000,000	2.41%		10	New Jersey	1,136,000,000	3.12%
41	Hawaii	129,000,000	0.35%		11	Georgia	880,000,000	2.41%
46	Idaho	84,000,000	0.23%		12	North Carolina	833,000,000	2.29%
7	Illinois	1,614,000,000	4.43%		13	Virginia	829,000,000	2.27%
19	Indiana	700,000,000	1.92%		14	Missouri	816,000,000	2.24%
30	Iowa	319,000,000	0.88%		15	Maryland	794,000,000	2.18%
31	Kansas	297,000,000	0.81%		16	Tennessee	782,000,000	2.15%
25	Kentucky	517,000,000	1.42%		17	Minnesota	722,000,000	1.98%
22	Louisiana	611,000,000	1.68%		18	Washington	706,000,000	1.94%
36	Maine	197,000,000	0.54%		19	Indiana	700,000,000	1.92%
15	Maryland	794,000,000	2.18%		20	Wisconsin	683,000,000	1.87%
9	Massachusetts	1,330,000,000	3.65%		21	Connecticut	621,000,000	1.70%
8	Michigan	1,352,000,000	3.71%		22	Louisiana	611,000,000	1.68%
17	Minnesota	722,000,000	1.98%		23	Alabama	573,000,000	1.57%
33	Mississippi	264,000,000	0.72%		24	Arizona	559,000,000	1.53%
14	Missouri	816,000,000	2.24%		25	Kentucky	517,000,000	1.42%
44	Montana	102,000,000	0.28%		26	Colorado	504,000,000	1.38%
38	Nebraska	174,000,000	0.48%		27	Oregon	407,000,000	1.12%
35	Nevada	198,000,000	0.54%		28	Oklahoma	390,000,000	1.07%
39	New Hampshire	172,000,000	0.47%		28	South Carolina	390,000,000	1.07%
10	New Jersey	1,136,000,000	3.12%		30	Iowa	319,000,000	0.88%
40	New Mexico	170,000,000	0.47%		31	Kansas	297,000,000	0.81%
2	New York	3,132,000,000	8.59%		32	Arkansas	296,000,000	0.81%
12	North Carolina	833,000,000	2.29%		33	Mississippi	264,000,000	0.72%
45	North Dakota	87,000,000	0.24%		34	West Virginia	260,000,000	0.71%
6	Ohio	1,643,000,000	4.51%		35	Nevada	198,000,000	0.54%
28	Oklahoma	390,000,000	1.07%		36	Maine	197,000,000	0.54%
27	Oregon	407,000,000	1.12%		37	Rhode Island	186,000,000	0.51%
5	Pennsylvania	1,982,000,000	5.44%		38	Nebraska	174,000,000	0.48%
37	Rhode Island	186,000,000	0.51%		39	New Hampshire	172,000,000	0.47%
28	South Carolina	390,000,000	1.07%		40	New Mexico	170,000,000	0.47%
47	South Dakota	82,000,000	0.22%		41	Hawaii	129,000,000	0.35%
16	Tennessee	782,000,000	2.15%		42	Utah	114,000,000	0.31%
4	Texas	2,007,000,000	5.51%		43	Delaware	112,000,000	0.31%
42	Utah	114,000,000	0.31%		44	Montana	102,000,000	0.28%
48	Vermont	80,000,000	0.22%		45	North Dakota	87,000,000	0.24%
13	Virginia	829,000,000	2.27%		46	Idaho	84,000,000	0.23%
18	Washington	706,000,000	1.94%		47	South Dakota	82,000,000	0.22%
34	West Virginia	260,000,000	0.71%		48	Vermont	80,000,000	0.22%
20	Wisconsin	683,000,000	1.87%		49	Alaska	76,000,000	0.21%
50	Wyoming	51,000,000	0.14%		50	Wyoming	51,000,000	0.14%
						District of Columbia	215,000,000	0.59%

Source: U.S. Department of Health and Human Services, Center for Disease Control and Prevention
"State Tobacco Control Highlights 1996" (Publication No. 099-4895)

V. INCIDENCE OF DISEASE

V. INCIDENCE OF DISEASE (Continued)

Estimated New Cancer Cases in 1998

National Estimated Total = 1,228,600 New Cases*

ALPHA ORDER

RANK	STATE	CASES	% of USA
20	Alabama	20,700	1.68%
50	Alaska	1,300	0.11%
24	Arizona	19,500	1.59%
30	Arkansas	14,000	1.14%
1	California	113,300	9.22%
31	Colorado	13,200	1.07%
28	Connecticut	15,400	1.25%
45	Delaware	3,800	0.31%
2	Florida	88,100	7.17%
13	Georgia	28,300	2.30%
43	Hawaii	4,300	0.35%
42	Idaho	4,400	0.36%
6	Illinois	58,100	4.73%
14	Indiana	28,100	2.29%
29	Iowa	14,800	1.20%
33	Kansas	11,900	0.97%
21	Kentucky	20,600	1.68%
22	Louisiana	20,500	1.67%
37	Maine	7,300	0.59%
19	Maryland	22,900	1.86%
11	Massachusetts	31,500	2.56%
8	Michigan	44,900	3.65%
23	Minnesota	19,600	1.60%
31	Mississippi	13,200	1.07%
14	Missouri	28,100	2.29%
44	Montana	4,100	0.33%
36	Nebraska	7,500	0.61%
35	Nevada	7,600	0.62%
39	New Hampshire	5,600	0.46%
9	New Jersey	40,500	3.30%
38	New Mexico	6,200	0.50%
3	New York	83,600	6.80%
10	North Carolina	35,100	2.86%
47	North Dakota	3,200	0.26%
7	Ohio	56,500	4.60%
27	Oklahoma	15,600	1.27%
26	Oregon	15,900	1.29%
5	Pennsylvania	68,800	5.60%
40	Rhode Island	5,200	0.42%
25	South Carolina	17,600	1.43%
46	South Dakota	3,500	0.28%
16	Tennessee	25,800	2.10%
4	Texas	77,500	6.31%
40	Utah	5,200	0.42%
48	Vermont	2,600	0.21%
12	Virginia	28,900	2.35%
18	Washington	24,100	1.96%
34	West Virginia	10,700	0.87%
17	Wisconsin	24,500	1.99%
49	Wyoming	1,800	0.15%

RANK ORDER

RANK	STATE	CASES	% of USA
1	California	113,300	9.22%
2	Florida	88,100	7.17%
3	New York	83,600	6.80%
4	Texas	77,500	6.31%
5	Pennsylvania	68,800	5.60%
6	Illinois	58,100	4.73%
7	Ohio	56,500	4.60%
8	Michigan	44,900	3.65%
9	New Jersey	40,500	3.30%
10	North Carolina	35,100	2.86%
11	Massachusetts	31,500	2.56%
12	Virginia	28,900	2.35%
13	Georgia	28,300	2.30%
14	Indiana	28,100	2.29%
14	Missouri	28,100	2.29%
16	Tennessee	25,800	2.10%
17	Wisconsin	24,500	1.99%
18	Washington	24,100	1.96%
19	Maryland	22,900	1.86%
20	Alabama	20,700	1.68%
21	Kentucky	20,600	1.68%
22	Louisiana	20,500	1.67%
23	Minnesota	19,600	1.60%
24	Arizona	19,500	1.59%
25	South Carolina	17,600	1.43%
26	Oregon	15,900	1.29%
27	Oklahoma	15,600	1.27%
28	Connecticut	15,400	1.25%
29	Iowa	14,800	1.20%
30	Arkansas	14,000	1.14%
31	Colorado	13,200	1.07%
31	Mississippi	13,200	1.07%
33	Kansas	11,900	0.97%
34	West Virginia	10,700	0.87%
35	Nevada	7,600	0.62%
36	Nebraska	7,500	0.61%
37	Maine	7,300	0.59%
38	New Mexico	6,200	0.50%
39	New Hampshire	5,600	0.46%
40	Rhode Island	5,200	0.42%
40	Utah	5,200	0.42%
42	Idaho	4,400	0.36%
43	Hawaii	4,300	0.35%
44	Montana	4,100	0.33%
45	Delaware	3,800	0.31%
46	South Dakota	3,500	0.28%
47	North Dakota	3,200	0.26%
48	Vermont	2,600	0.21%
49	Wyoming	1,800	0.15%
50	Alaska	1,300	0.11%
	District of Columbia	3,100	0.25%

Source: American Cancer Society

"Cancer Facts & Figures-1998" (Copyright 1998, Reprinted with permission from the American Cancer Society) *These estimates are offered as a rough guide and should not be regarded as definitive. They are calculated according to the distribution of estimated 1998 cancer deaths by state. Totals do not include carcinoma in situ or basal and squamous cell skin cancers.

Estimated Rate of New Cancer Cases in 1998

National Estimated Rate = 459.0 News Cases per 100,000 Population*

ALPHA ORDER

RANK	STATE	RATE
19	Alabama	479.3
50	Alaska	213.4
39	Arizona	428.1
5	Arkansas	554.9
47	California	351.1
48	Colorado	339.1
26	Connecticut	471.0
9	Delaware	519.4
1	Florida	601.2
42	Georgia	378.0
45	Hawaii	362.4
44	Idaho	363.6
16	Illinois	488.4
20	Indiana	479.2
10	Iowa	518.9
32	Kansas	458.6
6	Kentucky	527.1
25	Louisiana	471.1
3	Maine	587.7
35	Maryland	449.5
11	Massachusetts	514.9
31	Michigan	459.4
40	Minnesota	418.3
17	Mississippi	483.4
8	Missouri	520.2
29	Montana	466.5
34	Nebraska	452.7
33	Nevada	453.2
21	New Hampshire	477.5
13	New Jersey	502.9
46	New Mexico	358.4
30	New York	460.9
24	North Carolina	472.7
14	North Dakota	499.3
12	Ohio	505.1
27	Oklahoma	470.3
15	Oregon	490.2
4	Pennsylvania	572.4
7	Rhode Island	526.6
28	South Carolina	468.1
22	South Dakota	474.3
18	Tennessee	480.6
41	Texas	398.7
49	Utah	252.5
36	Vermont	441.4
38	Virginia	429.2
37	Washington	429.6
2	West Virginia	589.3
23	Wisconsin	473.9
43	Wyoming	375.2

RANK ORDER

RANK	STATE	RATE
1	Florida	601.2
2	West Virginia	589.3
3	Maine	587.7
4	Pennsylvania	572.4
5	Arkansas	554.9
6	Kentucky	527.1
7	Rhode Island	526.6
8	Missouri	520.2
9	Delaware	519.4
10	Iowa	518.9
11	Massachusetts	514.9
12	Ohio	505.1
13	New Jersey	502.9
14	North Dakota	499.3
15	Oregon	490.2
16	Illinois	488.4
17	Mississippi	483.4
18	Tennessee	480.6
19	Alabama	479.3
20	Indiana	479.2
21	New Hampshire	477.5
22	South Dakota	474.3
23	Wisconsin	473.9
24	North Carolina	472.7
25	Louisiana	471.1
26	Connecticut	471.0
27	Oklahoma	470.3
28	South Carolina	468.1
29	Montana	466.5
30	New York	460.9
31	Michigan	459.4
32	Kansas	458.6
33	Nevada	453.2
34	Nebraska	452.7
35	Maryland	449.5
36	Vermont	441.4
37	Washington	429.6
38	Virginia	429.2
39	Arizona	428.1
40	Minnesota	418.3
41	Texas	398.7
42	Georgia	378.0
43	Wyoming	375.2
44	Idaho	363.6
45	Hawaii	362.4
46	New Mexico	358.4
47	California	351.1
48	Colorado	339.1
49	Utah	252.5
50	Alaska	213.4

| | District of Columbia | 586.1 |

Source: Morgan Quitno Press using data from American Cancer Society
"Cancer Facts & Figures-1998" (Copyright 1998, Reprinted with permission from the American Cancer Society)
*These estimates are offered as a rough guide and should not be regarded as definitive. They are calculated according to the distribution of estimated 1998 cancer deaths by state. Totals do not include carcinoma in situ or basal and squamous cell skin cancers. Rates calculated using 1997 Census resident population estimates.

Estimated New Cases of Bladder Cancer in 1998

National Estimated Total = 54,400 New Cases*

ALPHA ORDER

RANK	STATE	CASES	% of USA
23	Alabama	700	1.29%
NA	Alaska**	NA	NA
19	Arizona	900	1.65%
32	Arkansas	500	0.92%
1	California	5,200	9.56%
27	Colorado	600	1.10%
23	Connecticut	700	1.29%
39	Delaware	200	0.37%
2	Florida	4,300	7.90%
19	Georgia	900	1.65%
39	Hawaii	200	0.37%
39	Idaho	200	0.37%
6	Illinois	2,500	4.60%
11	Indiana	1,300	2.39%
23	Iowa	700	1.29%
32	Kansas	500	0.92%
23	Kentucky	700	1.29%
27	Louisiana	600	1.10%
34	Maine	400	0.74%
16	Maryland	1,100	2.02%
10	Massachusetts	1,700	3.13%
8	Michigan	2,300	4.23%
22	Minnesota	800	1.47%
35	Mississippi	300	0.55%
11	Missouri	1,300	2.39%
39	Montana	200	0.37%
39	Nebraska	200	0.37%
35	Nevada	300	0.55%
35	New Hampshire	300	0.55%
9	New Jersey	2,200	4.04%
39	New Mexico	200	0.37%
3	New York	4,200	7.72%
11	North Carolina	1,300	2.39%
39	North Dakota	200	0.37%
7	Ohio	2,400	4.41%
27	Oklahoma	600	1.10%
27	Oregon	600	1.10%
4	Pennsylvania	3,000	5.51%
35	Rhode Island	300	0.55%
19	South Carolina	900	1.65%
39	South Dakota	200	0.37%
18	Tennessee	1,000	1.84%
5	Texas	2,900	5.33%
39	Utah	200	0.37%
48	Vermont	100	0.18%
11	Virginia	1,300	2.39%
16	Washington	1,100	2.02%
27	West Virginia	600	1.10%
15	Wisconsin	1,200	2.21%
NA	Wyoming**	NA	NA

RANK ORDER

RANK	STATE	CASES	% of USA
1	California	5,200	9.56%
2	Florida	4,300	7.90%
3	New York	4,200	7.72%
4	Pennsylvania	3,000	5.51%
5	Texas	2,900	5.33%
6	Illinois	2,500	4.60%
7	Ohio	2,400	4.41%
8	Michigan	2,300	4.23%
9	New Jersey	2,200	4.04%
10	Massachusetts	1,700	3.13%
11	Indiana	1,300	2.39%
11	Missouri	1,300	2.39%
11	North Carolina	1,300	2.39%
11	Virginia	1,300	2.39%
15	Wisconsin	1,200	2.21%
16	Maryland	1,100	2.02%
16	Washington	1,100	2.02%
18	Tennessee	1,000	1.84%
19	Arizona	900	1.65%
19	Georgia	900	1.65%
19	South Carolina	900	1.65%
22	Minnesota	800	1.47%
23	Alabama	700	1.29%
23	Connecticut	700	1.29%
23	Iowa	700	1.29%
23	Kentucky	700	1.29%
27	Colorado	600	1.10%
27	Louisiana	600	1.10%
27	Oklahoma	600	1.10%
27	Oregon	600	1.10%
27	West Virginia	600	1.10%
32	Arkansas	500	0.92%
32	Kansas	500	0.92%
34	Maine	400	0.74%
35	Mississippi	300	0.55%
35	Nevada	300	0.55%
35	New Hampshire	300	0.55%
35	Rhode Island	300	0.55%
39	Delaware	200	0.37%
39	Hawaii	200	0.37%
39	Idaho	200	0.37%
39	Montana	200	0.37%
39	Nebraska	200	0.37%
39	New Mexico	200	0.37%
39	North Dakota	200	0.37%
39	South Dakota	200	0.37%
39	Utah	200	0.37%
48	Vermont	100	0.18%
NA	Alaska**	NA	NA
NA	Wyoming**	NA	NA
	District of Columbia	100	0.18%

Source: American Cancer Society
   "Cancer Facts & Figures-1998" (Copyright 1998, Reprinted with permission from the American Cancer Society)
*These estimates are offered as a rough guide and should be interpreted with caution. They are calculated according to the distribution of estimated 1998 cancer deaths by state.
**Fewer than 50 cases.

Estimated Rate of New Cases of Bladder Cancer in 1998

National Estimated Rate = 20.3 New Cases per 100,000 Population*

ALPHA ORDER

RANK	STATE	RATE
39	Alabama	16.2
NA	Alaska**	NA
24	Arizona	19.8
24	Arkansas	19.8
40	California	16.1
41	Colorado	15.4
22	Connecticut	21.4
7	Delaware	27.3
5	Florida	29.3
45	Georgia	12.0
37	Hawaii	16.9
38	Idaho	16.5
23	Illinois	21.0
19	Indiana	22.2
12	Iowa	24.5
27	Kansas	19.3
32	Kentucky	17.9
43	Louisiana	13.8
2	Maine	32.2
20	Maryland	21.6
6	Massachusetts	27.8
15	Michigan	23.5
35	Minnesota	17.1
47	Mississippi	11.0
13	Missouri	24.1
18	Montana	22.8
44	Nebraska	12.1
32	Nevada	17.9
10	New Hampshire	25.6
7	New Jersey	27.3
46	New Mexico	11.6
16	New York	23.2
34	North Carolina	17.5
3	North Dakota	31.2
21	Ohio	21.5
31	Oklahoma	18.1
30	Oregon	18.5
11	Pennsylvania	25.0
4	Rhode Island	30.4
14	South Carolina	23.9
9	South Dakota	27.1
29	Tennessee	18.6
42	Texas	14.9
48	Utah	9.7
36	Vermont	17.0
27	Virginia	19.3
26	Washington	19.6
1	West Virginia	33.0
16	Wisconsin	23.2
NA	Wyoming**	NA

RANK ORDER

RANK	STATE	RATE
1	West Virginia	33.0
2	Maine	32.2
3	North Dakota	31.2
4	Rhode Island	30.4
5	Florida	29.3
6	Massachusetts	27.8
7	Delaware	27.3
7	New Jersey	27.3
9	South Dakota	27.1
10	New Hampshire	25.6
11	Pennsylvania	25.0
12	Iowa	24.5
13	Missouri	24.1
14	South Carolina	23.9
15	Michigan	23.5
16	New York	23.2
16	Wisconsin	23.2
18	Montana	22.8
19	Indiana	22.2
20	Maryland	21.6
21	Ohio	21.5
22	Connecticut	21.4
23	Illinois	21.0
24	Arizona	19.8
24	Arkansas	19.8
26	Washington	19.6
27	Kansas	19.3
27	Virginia	19.3
29	Tennessee	18.6
30	Oregon	18.5
31	Oklahoma	18.1
32	Kentucky	17.9
32	Nevada	17.9
34	North Carolina	17.5
35	Minnesota	17.1
36	Vermont	17.0
37	Hawaii	16.9
38	Idaho	16.5
39	Alabama	16.2
40	California	16.1
41	Colorado	15.4
42	Texas	14.9
43	Louisiana	13.8
44	Nebraska	12.1
45	Georgia	12.0
46	New Mexico	11.6
47	Mississippi	11.0
48	Utah	9.7
NA	Alaska**	NA
NA	Wyoming**	NA

District of Columbia   18.9

Source: Morgan Quitno Press using data from American Cancer Society
    "Cancer Facts & Figures-1998" (Copyright 1998, Reprinted with permission from the American Cancer Society)
*These estimates are offered as a rough guide and should not be regarded as definitive. They are calculated according to the distribution of estimated 1998 cancer deaths by state. Rates calculated using 1997 Census resident population estimates.
**Fewer than 50 cases.

Estimated New Female Breast Cancer Cases in 1998

National Estimated Total = 178,700 New Cases*

ALPHA ORDER

RANK	STATE	CASES	% of USA
24	Alabama	2,600	1.45%
50	Alaska	200	0.11%
21	Arizona	2,900	1.62%
31	Arkansas	1,800	1.01%
1	California	17,600	9.85%
29	Colorado	2,000	1.12%
29	Connecticut	2,000	1.12%
44	Delaware	500	0.28%
3	Florida	11,800	6.60%
13	Georgia	4,000	2.24%
44	Hawaii	500	0.28%
42	Idaho	700	0.39%
6	Illinois	8,900	4.98%
13	Indiana	4,000	2.24%
26	Iowa	2,400	1.34%
32	Kansas	1,700	0.95%
21	Kentucky	2,900	1.62%
20	Louisiana	3,100	1.73%
36	Maine	1,000	0.56%
17	Maryland	3,500	1.96%
11	Massachusetts	4,500	2.52%
8	Michigan	6,300	3.53%
23	Minnesota	2,800	1.57%
32	Mississippi	1,700	0.95%
18	Missouri	3,400	1.90%
43	Montana	600	0.34%
35	Nebraska	1,100	0.62%
36	Nevada	1,000	0.56%
38	New Hampshire	900	0.50%
9	New Jersey	6,200	3.47%
39	New Mexico	800	0.45%
2	New York	13,400	7.50%
10	North Carolina	4,700	2.63%
44	North Dakota	500	0.28%
7	Ohio	8,600	4.81%
27	Oklahoma	2,300	1.29%
28	Oregon	2,100	1.18%
5	Pennsylvania	10,800	6.04%
39	Rhode Island	800	0.45%
25	South Carolina	2,500	1.40%
44	South Dakota	500	0.28%
15	Tennessee	3,900	2.18%
4	Texas	11,300	6.32%
39	Utah	800	0.45%
48	Vermont	300	0.17%
12	Virginia	4,300	2.41%
19	Washington	3,200	1.79%
34	West Virginia	1,200	0.67%
16	Wisconsin	3,600	2.01%
48	Wyoming	300	0.17%

RANK ORDER

RANK	STATE	CASES	% of USA
1	California	17,600	9.85%
2	New York	13,400	7.50%
3	Florida	11,800	6.60%
4	Texas	11,300	6.32%
5	Pennsylvania	10,800	6.04%
6	Illinois	8,900	4.98%
7	Ohio	8,600	4.81%
8	Michigan	6,300	3.53%
9	New Jersey	6,200	3.47%
10	North Carolina	4,700	2.63%
11	Massachusetts	4,500	2.52%
12	Virginia	4,300	2.41%
13	Georgia	4,000	2.24%
13	Indiana	4,000	2.24%
15	Tennessee	3,900	2.18%
16	Wisconsin	3,600	2.01%
17	Maryland	3,500	1.96%
18	Missouri	3,400	1.90%
19	Washington	3,200	1.79%
20	Louisiana	3,100	1.73%
21	Arizona	2,900	1.62%
21	Kentucky	2,900	1.62%
23	Minnesota	2,800	1.57%
24	Alabama	2,600	1.45%
25	South Carolina	2,500	1.40%
26	Iowa	2,400	1.34%
27	Oklahoma	2,300	1.29%
28	Oregon	2,100	1.18%
29	Colorado	2,000	1.12%
29	Connecticut	2,000	1.12%
31	Arkansas	1,800	1.01%
32	Kansas	1,700	0.95%
32	Mississippi	1,700	0.95%
34	West Virginia	1,200	0.67%
35	Nebraska	1,100	0.62%
36	Maine	1,000	0.56%
36	Nevada	1,000	0.56%
38	New Hampshire	900	0.50%
39	New Mexico	800	0.45%
39	Rhode Island	800	0.45%
39	Utah	800	0.45%
42	Idaho	700	0.39%
43	Montana	600	0.34%
44	Delaware	500	0.28%
44	Hawaii	500	0.28%
44	North Dakota	500	0.28%
44	South Dakota	500	0.28%
48	Vermont	300	0.17%
48	Wyoming	300	0.17%
50	Alaska	200	0.11%
	District of Columbia	500	0.28%

Source: American Cancer Society
"Cancer Facts & Figures-1998" (Copyright 1998, Reprinted with permission from the American Cancer Society)
*These estimates are offered as a rough guide and should be interpreted with caution. They are calculated according to the distribution of estimated 1998 cancer deaths by state. National total does not include an estimated 1,600 new male breast cancer cases.

Estimated Rate of New Female Breast Cancer Cases in 1998

National Estimated Rate = 131.9 New Cases per 100,000 Female Population*

ALPHA ORDER

RANK ORDER

RANK	STATE	RATE		RANK	STATE	RATE
40	Alabama	117.2		1	Pennsylvania	172.8
50	Alaska	69.5		2	Iowa	164.1
27	Arizona	129.7		3	Florida	159.3
15	Arkansas	138.9		4	Maine	157.2
43	California	110.6		5	Rhode Island	155.7
45	Colorado	103.8		6	North Dakota	155.2
37	Connecticut	118.9		7	New Hampshire	152.5
21	Delaware	134.6		8	New Jersey	150.8
3	Florida	159.3		9	Ohio	149.2
44	Georgia	106.1		10	Illinois	146.8
48	Hawaii	85.3		11	Kentucky	145.2
39	Idaho	117.7		12	Massachusetts	142.8
10	Illinois	146.8		13	New York	142.2
23	Indiana	133.6		14	Tennessee	142.0
2	Iowa	164.1		15	Arkansas	138.9
26	Kansas	130.2		16	Louisiana	137.6
11	Kentucky	145.2		17	Wisconsin	137.3
16	Louisiana	137.6		18	Oklahoma	136.4
4	Maine	157.2		19	Montana	136.0
22	Maryland	134.5		20	South Dakota	134.7
12	Massachusetts	142.8		21	Delaware	134.6
29	Michigan	128.1		22	Maryland	134.5
38	Minnesota	118.7		23	Indiana	133.6
36	Mississippi	120.4		24	South Carolina	130.8
35	Missouri	123.1		25	Nebraska	130.5
19	Montana	136.0		26	Kansas	130.2
25	Nebraska	130.5		27	Arizona	129.7
30	Nevada	127.3		28	Oregon	129.6
7	New Hampshire	152.5		29	Michigan	128.1
8	New Jersey	150.8		30	Nevada	127.3
47	New Mexico	92.2		31	West Virginia	127.1
13	New York	142.2		32	Virginia	126.3
34	North Carolina	124.9		33	Wyoming	125.5
6	North Dakota	155.2		34	North Carolina	124.9
9	Ohio	149.2		35	Missouri	123.1
18	Oklahoma	136.4		36	Mississippi	120.4
28	Oregon	129.6		37	Connecticut	118.9
1	Pennsylvania	172.8		38	Minnesota	118.7
5	Rhode Island	155.7		39	Idaho	117.7
24	South Carolina	130.8		40	Alabama	117.2
20	South Dakota	134.7		41	Texas	116.8
14	Tennessee	142.0		42	Washington	115.2
41	Texas	116.8		43	California	110.6
49	Utah	79.7		44	Georgia	106.1
46	Vermont	100.5		45	Colorado	103.8
32	Virginia	126.3		46	Vermont	100.5
42	Washington	115.2		47	New Mexico	92.2
31	West Virginia	127.1		48	Hawaii	85.3
17	Wisconsin	137.3		49	Utah	79.7
33	Wyoming	125.5		50	Alaska	69.5
					District of Columbia	173.1

Source: Morgan Quitno Press using data from American Cancer Society
    "Cancer Facts & Figures-1998" (Copyright 1998, Reprinted with permission from the American Cancer Society)
*These estimates are offered as a rough guide and should be interpreted with caution. They are calculated
according to the distribution of estimated 1998 cancer deaths by state. Rates calculated using 1996 Census female
resident population estimates.

Percent of Women Age 50 and Older
Who Had a Breast Exam Within the Past Two Years: 1996
National Median = 75.12% of Women 50 Years and Older

ALPHA ORDER

RANK	STATE	PERCENT
43	Alabama	68.39
5	Alaska	82.55
4	Arizona	82.68
47	Arkansas	65.34
17	California	77.76
21	Colorado	77.15
27	Connecticut	74.67
9	Delaware	80.22
11	Florida	79.77
1	Georgia	87.06
NA	Hawaii*	NA
40	Idaho	69.33
34	Illinois	70.99
48	Indiana	65.15
49	Iowa	64.27
23	Kansas	75.72
37	Kentucky	70.18
45	Louisiana	66.95
13	Maine	78.70
2	Maryland	83.71
3	Massachusetts	82.74
31	Michigan	74.01
24	Minnesota	75.44
46	Mississippi	66.17
44	Missouri	67.30
14	Montana	78.59
29	Nebraska	74.42
32	Nevada	71.90
16	New Hampshire	78.03
41	New Jersey	69.28
35	New Mexico	70.57
7	New York	81.35
8	North Carolina	80.24
26	North Dakota	74.72
10	Ohio	79.89
19	Oklahoma	77.56
12	Oregon	79.49
42	Pennsylvania	68.76
15	Rhode Island	78.45
6	South Carolina	82.05
36	South Dakota	70.34
33	Tennessee	71.75
39	Texas	69.53
25	Utah	74.79
28	Vermont	74.63
18	Virginia	77.65
20	Washington	77.35
30	West Virginia	74.23
22	Wisconsin	77.13
38	Wyoming	69.55

RANK ORDER

RANK	STATE	PERCENT
1	Georgia	87.06
2	Maryland	83.71
3	Massachusetts	82.74
4	Arizona	82.68
5	Alaska	82.55
6	South Carolina	82.05
7	New York	81.35
8	North Carolina	80.24
9	Delaware	80.22
10	Ohio	79.89
11	Florida	79.77
12	Oregon	79.49
13	Maine	78.70
14	Montana	78.59
15	Rhode Island	78.45
16	New Hampshire	78.03
17	California	77.76
18	Virginia	77.65
19	Oklahoma	77.56
20	Washington	77.35
21	Colorado	77.15
22	Wisconsin	77.13
23	Kansas	75.72
24	Minnesota	75.44
25	Utah	74.79
26	North Dakota	74.72
27	Connecticut	74.67
28	Vermont	74.63
29	Nebraska	74.42
30	West Virginia	74.23
31	Michigan	74.01
32	Nevada	71.90
33	Tennessee	71.75
34	Illinois	70.99
35	New Mexico	70.57
36	South Dakota	70.34
37	Kentucky	70.18
38	Wyoming	69.55
39	Texas	69.53
40	Idaho	69.33
41	New Jersey	69.28
42	Pennsylvania	68.76
43	Alabama	68.39
44	Missouri	67.30
45	Louisiana	66.95
46	Mississippi	66.17
47	Arkansas	65.34
48	Indiana	65.15
49	Iowa	64.27
NA	Hawaii*	NA

District of Columbia 83.41

Source: U.S. Department of Health and Human Services, Centers for Disease Control and Prevention
"1996 Behavioral Risk Factor Surveillance Summary Prevalence Report" (January 8, 1998)
*Not available.

Estimated New Colon and Rectum Cancer Cases in 1998

National Estimated Total = 131,600 New Cases*

ALPHA ORDER

RANK ORDER

RANK	STATE	CASES	% of USA		RANK	STATE	CASES	% of USA
28	Alabama	1,600	1.22%		1	California	11,600	8.81%
49	Alaska	200	0.15%		2	New York	9,700	7.37%
22	Arizona	2,000	1.52%		3	Florida	9,400	7.14%
29	Arkansas	1,500	1.14%		4	Texas	8,500	6.46%
1	California	11,600	8.81%		5	Pennsylvania	7,900	6.00%
30	Colorado	1,400	1.06%		6	Illinois	6,400	4.86%
26	Connecticut	1,700	1.29%		7	Ohio	6,100	4.64%
44	Delaware	400	0.30%		8	Michigan	5,000	3.80%
3	Florida	9,400	7.14%		9	New Jersey	4,800	3.65%
17	Georgia	2,600	1.98%		10	Massachusetts	3,700	2.81%
42	Hawaii	500	0.38%		10	North Carolina	3,700	2.81%
44	Idaho	400	0.30%		12	Virginia	3,100	2.36%
6	Illinois	6,400	4.86%		13	Indiana	3,000	2.28%
13	Indiana	3,000	2.28%		13	Missouri	3,000	2.28%
24	Iowa	1,900	1.44%		15	Tennessee	2,800	2.13%
32	Kansas	1,300	0.99%		16	Maryland	2,700	2.05%
20	Kentucky	2,200	1.67%		17	Georgia	2,600	1.98%
21	Louisiana	2,100	1.60%		18	Wisconsin	2,500	1.90%
36	Maine	800	0.61%		19	Washington	2,300	1.75%
16	Maryland	2,700	2.05%		20	Kentucky	2,200	1.67%
10	Massachusetts	3,700	2.81%		21	Louisiana	2,100	1.60%
8	Michigan	5,000	3.80%		22	Arizona	2,000	1.52%
24	Minnesota	1,900	1.44%		22	South Carolina	2,000	1.52%
33	Mississippi	1,200	0.91%		24	Iowa	1,900	1.44%
13	Missouri	3,000	2.28%		24	Minnesota	1,900	1.44%
42	Montana	500	0.38%		26	Connecticut	1,700	1.29%
35	Nebraska	900	0.68%		26	Oklahoma	1,700	1.29%
36	Nevada	800	0.61%		28	Alabama	1,600	1.22%
38	New Hampshire	600	0.46%		29	Arkansas	1,500	1.14%
9	New Jersey	4,800	3.65%		30	Colorado	1,400	1.06%
38	New Mexico	600	0.46%		30	Oregon	1,400	1.06%
2	New York	9,700	7.37%		32	Kansas	1,300	0.99%
10	North Carolina	3,700	2.81%		33	Mississippi	1,200	0.91%
44	North Dakota	400	0.30%		34	West Virginia	1,100	0.84%
7	Ohio	6,100	4.64%		35	Nebraska	900	0.68%
26	Oklahoma	1,700	1.29%		36	Maine	800	0.61%
30	Oregon	1,400	1.06%		36	Nevada	800	0.61%
5	Pennsylvania	7,900	6.00%		38	New Hampshire	600	0.46%
38	Rhode Island	600	0.46%		38	New Mexico	600	0.46%
22	South Carolina	2,000	1.52%		38	Rhode Island	600	0.46%
47	South Dakota	300	0.23%		38	Utah	600	0.46%
15	Tennessee	2,800	2.13%		42	Hawaii	500	0.38%
4	Texas	8,500	6.46%		42	Montana	500	0.38%
38	Utah	600	0.46%		44	Delaware	400	0.30%
47	Vermont	300	0.23%		44	Idaho	400	0.30%
12	Virginia	3,100	2.36%		44	North Dakota	400	0.30%
19	Washington	2,300	1.75%		47	South Dakota	300	0.23%
34	West Virginia	1,100	0.84%		47	Vermont	300	0.23%
18	Wisconsin	2,500	1.90%		49	Alaska	200	0.15%
49	Wyoming	200	0.15%		49	Wyoming	200	0.15%
						District of Columbia	300	0.23%

Source: American Cancer Society
"Cancer Facts & Figures-1998" (Copyright 1998, Reprinted with permission from the American Cancer Society)
*These estimates are offered as a rough guide and should be interpreted with caution. They are calculated according to the distribution of estimated 1998 cancer deaths by state.

Estimated Rate of New Colon and Rectum Cancer Cases in 1998

National Estimated Rate = 49.2 New Cases per 100,000 Population*

ALPHA ORDER

RANK	STATE	RATE
43	Alabama	37.0
49	Alaska	32.8
34	Arizona	43.9
10	Arkansas	59.5
45	California	35.9
44	Colorado	36.0
22	Connecticut	52.0
14	Delaware	54.7
4	Florida	64.1
46	Georgia	34.7
38	Hawaii	42.1
48	Idaho	33.1
17	Illinois	53.8
23	Indiana	51.2
1	Iowa	66.6
28	Kansas	50.1
12	Kentucky	56.3
31	Louisiana	48.3
3	Maine	64.4
20	Maryland	53.0
8	Massachusetts	60.5
23	Michigan	51.2
42	Minnesota	40.6
34	Mississippi	43.9
13	Missouri	55.5
11	Montana	56.9
16	Nebraska	54.3
32	Nevada	47.7
23	New Hampshire	51.2
9	New Jersey	59.6
46	New Mexico	34.7
18	New York	53.5
29	North Carolina	49.8
5	North Dakota	62.4
15	Ohio	54.5
23	Oklahoma	51.2
37	Oregon	43.2
2	Pennsylvania	65.7
6	Rhode Island	60.8
19	South Carolina	53.2
41	South Dakota	40.7
21	Tennessee	52.2
36	Texas	43.7
50	Utah	29.1
27	Vermont	50.9
33	Virginia	46.0
40	Washington	41.0
7	West Virginia	60.6
30	Wisconsin	48.4
39	Wyoming	41.7

RANK ORDER

RANK	STATE	RATE
1	Iowa	66.6
2	Pennsylvania	65.7
3	Maine	64.4
4	Florida	64.1
5	North Dakota	62.4
6	Rhode Island	60.8
7	West Virginia	60.6
8	Massachusetts	60.5
9	New Jersey	59.6
10	Arkansas	59.5
11	Montana	56.9
12	Kentucky	56.3
13	Missouri	55.5
14	Delaware	54.7
15	Ohio	54.5
16	Nebraska	54.3
17	Illinois	53.8
18	New York	53.5
19	South Carolina	53.2
20	Maryland	53.0
21	Tennessee	52.2
22	Connecticut	52.0
23	Indiana	51.2
23	Michigan	51.2
23	New Hampshire	51.2
23	Oklahoma	51.2
27	Vermont	50.9
28	Kansas	50.1
29	North Carolina	49.8
30	Wisconsin	48.4
31	Louisiana	48.3
32	Nevada	47.7
33	Virginia	46.0
34	Arizona	43.9
34	Mississippi	43.9
36	Texas	43.7
37	Oregon	43.2
38	Hawaii	42.1
39	Wyoming	41.7
40	Washington	41.0
41	South Dakota	40.7
42	Minnesota	40.6
43	Alabama	37.0
44	Colorado	36.0
45	California	35.9
46	Georgia	34.7
46	New Mexico	34.7
48	Idaho	33.1
49	Alaska	32.8
50	Utah	29.1

District of Columbia 56.7

Source: Morgan Quitno Press using data from American Cancer Society
"Cancer Facts & Figures-1998" (Copyright 1998, Reprinted with permission from the American Cancer Society)
*These estimates are offered as a rough guide and should not be regarded as definitive. They are calculated according to the distribution of estimated 1998 cancer deaths by state. Rates calculated using 1997 Census resident population estimates.

Estimated New Lung Cancer Cases in 1998

National Estimated Total = 171,500 New Cases*

ALPHA ORDER					RANK ORDER			
RANK	STATE	CASES	% of USA		RANK	STATE	CASES	% of USA
21	Alabama	3,000	1.75%		1	California	14,700	8.57%
50	Alaska	200	0.12%		2	Florida	12,900	7.52%
22	Arizona	2,800	1.63%		3	Texas	11,600	6.76%
27	Arkansas	2,300	1.34%		4	New York	10,900	6.36%
1	California	14,700	8.57%		5	Pennsylvania	9,100	5.31%
33	Colorado	1,600	0.93%		6	Ohio	8,200	4.78%
29	Connecticut	2,000	1.17%		7	Illinois	7,800	4.55%
41	Delaware	600	0.35%		8	Michigan	6,400	3.73%
2	Florida	12,900	7.52%		9	North Carolina	5,400	3.15%
12	Georgia	4,200	2.45%		10	New Jersey	4,900	2.86%
43	Hawaii	500	0.29%		11	Missouri	4,300	2.51%
41	Idaho	600	0.35%		12	Georgia	4,200	2.45%
7	Illinois	7,800	4.55%		12	Indiana	4,200	2.45%
12	Indiana	4,200	2.45%		12	Tennessee	4,200	2.45%
29	Iowa	2,000	1.17%		15	Massachusetts	4,100	2.39%
33	Kansas	1,600	0.93%		16	Virginia	4,000	2.33%
17	Kentucky	3,600	2.10%		17	Kentucky	3,600	2.10%
20	Louisiana	3,100	1.81%		18	Washington	3,400	1.98%
36	Maine	1,000	0.58%		19	Maryland	3,200	1.87%
19	Maryland	3,200	1.87%		20	Louisiana	3,100	1.81%
15	Massachusetts	4,100	2.39%		21	Alabama	3,000	1.75%
8	Michigan	6,400	3.73%		22	Arizona	2,800	1.63%
26	Minnesota	2,400	1.40%		22	Wisconsin	2,800	1.63%
31	Mississippi	1,800	1.05%		24	South Carolina	2,600	1.52%
11	Missouri	4,300	2.51%		25	Oklahoma	2,500	1.46%
43	Montana	500	0.29%		26	Minnesota	2,400	1.40%
36	Nebraska	1,000	0.58%		27	Arkansas	2,300	1.34%
35	Nevada	1,200	0.70%		27	Oregon	2,300	1.34%
39	New Hampshire	700	0.41%		29	Connecticut	2,000	1.17%
10	New Jersey	4,900	2.86%		29	Iowa	2,000	1.17%
39	New Mexico	700	0.41%		31	Mississippi	1,800	1.05%
4	New York	10,900	6.36%		32	West Virginia	1,700	0.99%
9	North Carolina	5,400	3.15%		33	Colorado	1,600	0.93%
48	North Dakota	300	0.17%		33	Kansas	1,600	0.93%
6	Ohio	8,200	4.78%		35	Nevada	1,200	0.70%
25	Oklahoma	2,500	1.46%		36	Maine	1,000	0.58%
27	Oregon	2,300	1.34%		36	Nebraska	1,000	0.58%
5	Pennsylvania	9,100	5.31%		38	Rhode Island	800	0.47%
38	Rhode Island	800	0.47%		39	New Hampshire	700	0.41%
24	South Carolina	2,600	1.52%		39	New Mexico	700	0.41%
45	South Dakota	400	0.23%		41	Delaware	600	0.35%
12	Tennessee	4,200	2.45%		41	Idaho	600	0.35%
3	Texas	11,600	6.76%		43	Hawaii	500	0.29%
45	Utah	400	0.23%		43	Montana	500	0.29%
45	Vermont	400	0.23%		45	South Dakota	400	0.23%
16	Virginia	4,000	2.33%		45	Utah	400	0.23%
18	Washington	3,400	1.98%		45	Vermont	400	0.23%
32	West Virginia	1,700	0.99%		48	North Dakota	300	0.17%
22	Wisconsin	2,800	1.63%		48	Wyoming	300	0.17%
48	Wyoming	300	0.17%		50	Alaska	200	0.12%
						District of Columbia	400	0.23%

Source: American Cancer Society
"Cancer Facts & Figures-1998" (Copyright 1998, Reprinted with permission from the American Cancer Society)
*These estimates are offered as a rough guide and should be interpreted with caution. They are calculated according to the distribution of estimated 1998 cancer deaths by state.

Estimated Rate of New Lung Cancer Cases in 1998

National Estimated Rate = 64.1 New Cases per 100,000 Population*

ALPHA ORDER

RANK ORDER

RANK	STATE	RATE	RANK	STATE	RATE
19	Alabama	69.5	1	West Virginia	93.6
49	Alaska	32.8	2	Kentucky	92.1
29	Arizona	61.5	3	Arkansas	91.2
3	Arkansas	91.2	4	Florida	88.0
45	California	45.6	5	Delaware	82.0
47	Colorado	41.1	6	Rhode Island	81.0
30	Connecticut	61.2	7	Maine	80.5
5	Delaware	82.0	8	Missouri	79.6
4	Florida	88.0	9	Tennessee	78.2
39	Georgia	56.1	10	Pennsylvania	75.7
46	Hawaii	42.1	11	Oklahoma	75.4
43	Idaho	49.6	12	Ohio	73.3
24	Illinois	65.6	13	North Carolina	72.7
14	Indiana	71.6	14	Indiana	71.6
18	Iowa	70.1	14	Nevada	71.6
28	Kansas	61.7	16	Louisiana	71.2
2	Kentucky	92.1	17	Oregon	70.9
16	Louisiana	71.2	18	Iowa	70.1
7	Maine	80.5	19	Alabama	69.5
26	Maryland	62.8	20	South Carolina	69.1
22	Massachusetts	67.0	21	Vermont	67.9
25	Michigan	65.5	22	Massachusetts	67.0
42	Minnesota	51.2	23	Mississippi	65.9
23	Mississippi	65.9	24	Illinois	65.6
8	Missouri	79.6	25	Michigan	65.5
38	Montana	56.9	26	Maryland	62.8
33	Nebraska	60.4	27	Wyoming	62.5
14	Nevada	71.6	28	Kansas	61.7
35	New Hampshire	59.7	29	Arizona	61.5
31	New Jersey	60.8	30	Connecticut	61.2
48	New Mexico	40.5	31	New Jersey	60.8
34	New York	60.1	32	Washington	60.6
13	North Carolina	72.7	33	Nebraska	60.4
44	North Dakota	46.8	34	New York	60.1
12	Ohio	73.3	35	New Hampshire	59.7
11	Oklahoma	75.4	35	Texas	59.7
17	Oregon	70.9	37	Virginia	59.4
10	Pennsylvania	75.7	38	Montana	56.9
6	Rhode Island	81.0	39	Georgia	56.1
20	South Carolina	69.1	40	South Dakota	54.2
40	South Dakota	54.2	40	Wisconsin	54.2
9	Tennessee	78.2	42	Minnesota	51.2
35	Texas	59.7	43	Idaho	49.6
50	Utah	19.4	44	North Dakota	46.8
21	Vermont	67.9	45	California	45.6
37	Virginia	59.4	46	Hawaii	42.1
32	Washington	60.6	47	Colorado	41.1
1	West Virginia	93.6	48	New Mexico	40.5
40	Wisconsin	54.2	49	Alaska	32.8
27	Wyoming	62.5	50	Utah	19.4
				District of Columbia	75.6

Source: Morgan Quitno Press using data from American Cancer Society
"Cancer Facts & Figures-1998" (Copyright 1998, Reprinted with permission from the American Cancer Society)
*These estimates are offered as a rough guide and should not be regarded as definitive. They are calculated according to the distribution of estimated 1998 cancer deaths by state. Rates calculated using 1997 Census resident population estimates.

Estimated New Non-Hodgkin's Lymphoma Cases in 1998

National Estimated Total = 55,400 New Cases*

ALPHA ORDER					RANK ORDER			
RANK	STATE	CASES	% of USA		RANK	STATE	CASES	% of USA
20	Alabama	900	1.62%		1	California	4,900	8.84%
NA	Alaska**	NA	NA		2	New York	4,100	7.40%
20	Arizona	900	1.62%		3	Florida	3,900	7.04%
32	Arkansas	500	0.90%		4	Texas	3,800	6.86%
1	California	4,900	8.84%		5	Pennsylvania	3,200	5.78%
28	Colorado	700	1.26%		6	Ohio	2,700	4.87%
28	Connecticut	700	1.26%		7	Illinois	2,600	4.69%
43	Delaware	200	0.36%		8	Michigan	2,100	3.79%
3	Florida	3,900	7.04%		9	New Jersey	1,800	3.25%
19	Georgia	1,000	1.81%		10	Massachusetts	1,500	2.71%
36	Hawaii	300	0.54%		11	North Carolina	1,400	2.53%
43	Idaho	200	0.36%		12	Wisconsin	1,300	2.35%
7	Illinois	2,600	4.69%		13	Indiana	1,200	2.17%
13	Indiana	1,200	2.17%		13	Minnesota	1,200	2.17%
23	Iowa	800	1.44%		13	Missouri	1,200	2.17%
30	Kansas	600	1.08%		13	Virginia	1,200	2.17%
23	Kentucky	800	1.44%		17	Tennessee	1,100	1.99%
23	Louisiana	800	1.44%		17	Washington	1,100	1.99%
36	Maine	300	0.54%		19	Georgia	1,000	1.81%
20	Maryland	900	1.62%		20	Alabama	900	1.62%
10	Massachusetts	1,500	2.71%		20	Arizona	900	1.62%
8	Michigan	2,100	3.79%		20	Maryland	900	1.62%
13	Minnesota	1,200	2.17%		23	Iowa	800	1.44%
32	Mississippi	500	0.90%		23	Kentucky	800	1.44%
13	Missouri	1,200	2.17%		23	Louisiana	800	1.44%
43	Montana	200	0.36%		23	Oklahoma	800	1.44%
36	Nebraska	300	0.54%		23	Oregon	800	1.44%
36	Nevada	300	0.54%		28	Colorado	700	1.26%
36	New Hampshire	300	0.54%		28	Connecticut	700	1.26%
9	New Jersey	1,800	3.25%		30	Kansas	600	1.08%
36	New Mexico	300	0.54%		30	South Carolina	600	1.08%
2	New York	4,100	7.40%		32	Arkansas	500	0.90%
11	North Carolina	1,400	2.53%		32	Mississippi	500	0.90%
43	North Dakota	200	0.36%		34	Utah	400	0.72%
6	Ohio	2,700	4.87%		34	West Virginia	400	0.72%
23	Oklahoma	800	1.44%		36	Hawaii	300	0.54%
23	Oregon	800	1.44%		36	Maine	300	0.54%
5	Pennsylvania	3,200	5.78%		36	Nebraska	300	0.54%
36	Rhode Island	300	0.54%		36	Nevada	300	0.54%
30	South Carolina	600	1.08%		36	New Hampshire	300	0.54%
47	South Dakota	100	0.18%		36	New Mexico	300	0.54%
17	Tennessee	1,100	1.99%		36	Rhode Island	300	0.54%
4	Texas	3,800	6.86%		43	Delaware	200	0.36%
34	Utah	400	0.72%		43	Idaho	200	0.36%
47	Vermont	100	0.18%		43	Montana	200	0.36%
13	Virginia	1,200	2.17%		43	North Dakota	200	0.36%
17	Washington	1,100	1.99%		47	South Dakota	100	0.18%
34	West Virginia	400	0.72%		47	Vermont	100	0.18%
12	Wisconsin	1,300	2.35%		47	Wyoming	100	0.18%
47	Wyoming	100	0.18%		NA	Alaska**	NA	NA
						District of Columbia	100	0.18%

Source: American Cancer Society

"Cancer Facts & Figures-1998" (Copyright 1998, Reprinted with permission from the American Cancer Society)
*These estimates are offered as a rough guide and should be interpreted with caution. They are calculated according to the distribution of estimated 1998 cancer deaths by state.
**Fewer than 50 cases.

Estimated Rate of New Non-Hodgkin's Lymphoma Cases in 1998

National Estimated Rate = 20.7 New Cases per 100,000 Population*

ALPHA ORDER

RANK	STATE	RATE
25	Alabama	20.8
NA	Alaska**	NA
30	Arizona	19.8
30	Arkansas	19.8
47	California	15.2
39	Colorado	18.0
24	Connecticut	21.4
4	Delaware	27.3
5	Florida	26.6
49	Georgia	13.4
9	Hawaii	25.3
45	Idaho	16.5
22	Illinois	21.9
27	Indiana	20.5
3	Iowa	28.0
16	Kansas	23.1
27	Kentucky	20.5
36	Louisiana	18.4
13	Maine	24.2
42	Maryland	17.7
12	Massachusetts	24.5
23	Michigan	21.5
7	Minnesota	25.6
37	Mississippi	18.3
20	Missouri	22.2
17	Montana	22.8
38	Nebraska	18.1
40	Nevada	17.9
7	New Hampshire	25.6
19	New Jersey	22.4
43	New Mexico	17.3
18	New York	22.6
35	North Carolina	18.9
1	North Dakota	31.2
14	Ohio	24.1
14	Oklahoma	24.1
11	Oregon	24.7
5	Pennsylvania	26.6
2	Rhode Island	30.4
46	South Carolina	16.0
48	South Dakota	13.6
27	Tennessee	20.5
33	Texas	19.5
34	Utah	19.4
44	Vermont	17.0
41	Virginia	17.8
32	Washington	19.6
21	West Virginia	22.0
10	Wisconsin	25.1
25	Wyoming	20.8

RANK ORDER

RANK	STATE	RATE
1	North Dakota	31.2
2	Rhode Island	30.4
3	Iowa	28.0
4	Delaware	27.3
5	Florida	26.6
5	Pennsylvania	26.6
7	Minnesota	25.6
7	New Hampshire	25.6
9	Hawaii	25.3
10	Wisconsin	25.1
11	Oregon	24.7
12	Massachusetts	24.5
13	Maine	24.2
14	Ohio	24.1
14	Oklahoma	24.1
16	Kansas	23.1
17	Montana	22.8
18	New York	22.6
19	New Jersey	22.4
20	Missouri	22.2
21	West Virginia	22.0
22	Illinois	21.9
23	Michigan	21.5
24	Connecticut	21.4
25	Alabama	20.8
25	Wyoming	20.8
27	Indiana	20.5
27	Kentucky	20.5
27	Tennessee	20.5
30	Arizona	19.8
30	Arkansas	19.8
32	Washington	19.6
33	Texas	19.5
34	Utah	19.4
35	North Carolina	18.9
36	Louisiana	18.4
37	Mississippi	18.3
38	Nebraska	18.1
39	Colorado	18.0
40	Nevada	17.9
41	Virginia	17.8
42	Maryland	17.7
43	New Mexico	17.3
44	Vermont	17.0
45	Idaho	16.5
46	South Carolina	16.0
47	California	15.2
48	South Dakota	13.6
49	Georgia	13.4
NA	Alaska**	NA
	District of Columbia	18.9

Source: Morgan Quitno Press using data from American Cancer Society
 "Cancer Facts & Figures-1998" (Copyright 1998, Reprinted with permission from the American Cancer Society)
*These estimates are offered as a rough guide and should not be regarded as definitive. They are calculated according to the distribution of estimated 1998 cancer deaths by state. Rates calculated using 1997 Census resident population estimates.
**Fewer than 50 cases.

Estimated New Ovarian Cancer Cases in 1998

National Estimated Total = 25,400 New Cases*

ALPHA ORDER

RANK ORDER

RANK	STATE	CASES	% of USA	RANK	STATE	CASES	% of USA
20	Alabama	400	1.57%	1	California	2,600	10.24%
NA	Alaska**	NA	NA	2	Florida	1,900	7.48%
16	Arizona	500	1.97%	3	New York	1,800	7.09%
25	Arkansas	300	1.18%	4	Pennsylvania	1,500	5.91%
1	California	2,600	10.24%	4	Texas	1,500	5.91%
32	Colorado	200	0.79%	6	Illinois	1,200	4.72%
25	Connecticut	300	1.18%	7	New Jersey	1,000	3.94%
38	Delaware	100	0.39%	7	Ohio	1,000	3.94%
2	Florida	1,900	7.48%	9	Michigan	800	3.15%
10	Georgia	600	2.36%	10	Georgia	600	2.36%
38	Hawaii	100	0.39%	10	Indiana	600	2.36%
38	Idaho	100	0.39%	10	Massachusetts	600	2.36%
6	Illinois	1,200	4.72%	10	North Carolina	600	2.36%
10	Indiana	600	2.36%	10	Washington	600	2.36%
25	Iowa	300	1.18%	10	Wisconsin	600	2.36%
25	Kansas	300	1.18%	16	Arizona	500	1.97%
20	Kentucky	400	1.57%	16	Missouri	500	1.97%
25	Louisiana	300	1.18%	16	Tennessee	500	1.97%
32	Maine	200	0.79%	16	Virginia	500	1.97%
25	Maryland	300	1.18%	20	Alabama	400	1.57%
10	Massachusetts	600	2.36%	20	Kentucky	400	1.57%
9	Michigan	800	3.15%	20	Minnesota	400	1.57%
20	Minnesota	400	1.57%	20	Oregon	400	1.57%
32	Mississippi	200	0.79%	20	South Carolina	400	1.57%
16	Missouri	500	1.97%	25	Arkansas	300	1.18%
38	Montana	100	0.39%	25	Connecticut	300	1.18%
32	Nebraska	200	0.79%	25	Iowa	300	1.18%
38	Nevada	100	0.39%	25	Kansas	300	1.18%
38	New Hampshire	100	0.39%	25	Louisiana	300	1.18%
7	New Jersey	1,000	3.94%	25	Maryland	300	1.18%
38	New Mexico	100	0.39%	25	Oklahoma	300	1.18%
3	New York	1,800	7.09%	32	Colorado	200	0.79%
10	North Carolina	600	2.36%	32	Maine	200	0.79%
38	North Dakota	100	0.39%	32	Mississippi	200	0.79%
7	Ohio	1,000	3.94%	32	Nebraska	200	0.79%
25	Oklahoma	300	1.18%	32	Utah	200	0.79%
20	Oregon	400	1.57%	32	West Virginia	200	0.79%
4	Pennsylvania	1,500	5.91%	38	Delaware	100	0.39%
38	Rhode Island	100	0.39%	38	Hawaii	100	0.39%
20	South Carolina	400	1.57%	38	Idaho	100	0.39%
38	South Dakota	100	0.39%	38	Montana	100	0.39%
16	Tennessee	500	1.97%	38	Nevada	100	0.39%
4	Texas	1,500	5.91%	38	New Hampshire	100	0.39%
32	Utah	200	0.79%	38	New Mexico	100	0.39%
38	Vermont	100	0.39%	38	North Dakota	100	0.39%
16	Virginia	500	1.97%	38	Rhode Island	100	0.39%
10	Washington	600	2.36%	38	South Dakota	100	0.39%
32	West Virginia	200	0.79%	38	Vermont	100	0.39%
10	Wisconsin	600	2.36%	NA	Alaska**	NA	NA
NA	Wyoming**	NA	NA	NA	Wyoming**	NA	NA
					District of Columbia	100	0.39%

Source: American Cancer Society
"Cancer Facts & Figures-1998" (Copyright 1998, Reprinted with permission from the American Cancer Society)
*These estimates are offered as a rough guide and should be interpreted with caution. They are calculated according to the distribution of estimated 1998 cancer deaths by state.
**Fewer than 50 cases.

Estimated Rate of New Ovarian Cancer Cases in 1998

National Estimated Rate = 18.7 New Cases per 100,000 Female Population*

ALPHA ORDER

RANK	STATE	RATE
29	Alabama	18.0
NA	Alaska**	NA
15	Arizona	22.4
11	Arkansas	23.2
37	California	16.3
48	Colorado	10.4
30	Connecticut	17.8
4	Delaware	26.9
6	Florida	25.7
39	Georgia	15.9
33	Hawaii	17.1
36	Idaho	16.8
23	Illinois	19.8
20	Indiana	20.0
19	Iowa	20.5
12	Kansas	23.0
20	Kentucky	20.0
44	Louisiana	13.3
2	Maine	31.4
46	Maryland	11.5
26	Massachusetts	19.0
37	Michigan	16.3
34	Minnesota	17.0
43	Mississippi	14.2
28	Missouri	18.1
14	Montana	22.7
10	Nebraska	23.7
45	Nevada	12.7
35	New Hampshire	16.9
8	New Jersey	24.3
46	New Mexico	11.5
25	New York	19.1
39	North Carolina	15.9
3	North Dakota	31.0
32	Ohio	17.4
30	Oklahoma	17.8
7	Oregon	24.7
9	Pennsylvania	24.0
24	Rhode Island	19.5
18	South Carolina	20.9
4	South Dakota	26.9
27	Tennessee	18.2
41	Texas	15.5
22	Utah	19.9
1	Vermont	33.5
42	Virginia	14.7
16	Washington	21.6
17	West Virginia	21.2
13	Wisconsin	22.9
NA	Wyoming**	NA

RANK ORDER

RANK	STATE	RATE
1	Vermont	33.5
2	Maine	31.4
3	North Dakota	31.0
4	Delaware	26.9
4	South Dakota	26.9
6	Florida	25.7
7	Oregon	24.7
8	New Jersey	24.3
9	Pennsylvania	24.0
10	Nebraska	23.7
11	Arkansas	23.2
12	Kansas	23.0
13	Wisconsin	22.9
14	Montana	22.7
15	Arizona	22.4
16	Washington	21.6
17	West Virginia	21.2
18	South Carolina	20.9
19	Iowa	20.5
20	Indiana	20.0
20	Kentucky	20.0
22	Utah	19.9
23	Illinois	19.8
24	Rhode Island	19.5
25	New York	19.1
26	Massachusetts	19.0
27	Tennessee	18.2
28	Missouri	18.1
29	Alabama	18.0
30	Connecticut	17.8
30	Oklahoma	17.8
32	Ohio	17.4
33	Hawaii	17.1
34	Minnesota	17.0
35	New Hampshire	16.9
36	Idaho	16.8
37	California	16.3
37	Michigan	16.3
39	Georgia	15.9
39	North Carolina	15.9
41	Texas	15.5
42	Virginia	14.7
43	Mississippi	14.2
44	Louisiana	13.3
45	Nevada	12.7
46	Maryland	11.5
46	New Mexico	11.5
48	Colorado	10.4
NA	Alaska**	NA
NA	Wyoming**	NA
	District of Columbia	34.6

Source: Morgan Quitno Press using data from American Cancer Society
   "Cancer Facts & Figures-1998" (Copyright 1998, Reprinted with permission from the American Cancer Society)
*These estimates are offered as a rough guide and should be interpreted with caution. They are calculated
according to the distribution of estimated 1998 cancer deaths by state. Rates calculated using 1996 Census female
resident population estimates.
**Fewer than 50 cases.

Estimated New Prostate Cancer Cases in 1998

National Estimated Total = 184,500 New Cases*

ALPHA ORDER

RANK	STATE	CASES	% of USA
23	Alabama	3,000	1.63%
50	Alaska	200	0.11%
20	Arizona	3,200	1.73%
26	Arkansas	2,400	1.30%
1	California	17,200	9.32%
30	Colorado	2,200	1.19%
30	Connecticut	2,200	1.19%
47	Delaware	500	0.27%
2	Florida	14,100	7.64%
11	Georgia	4,500	2.44%
42	Hawaii	600	0.33%
39	Idaho	900	0.49%
6	Illinois	8,300	4.50%
16	Indiana	3,600	1.95%
27	Iowa	2,300	1.25%
33	Kansas	1,900	1.03%
25	Kentucky	2,500	1.36%
21	Louisiana	3,100	1.68%
39	Maine	900	0.49%
17	Maryland	3,500	1.90%
14	Massachusetts	4,300	2.33%
8	Michigan	6,600	3.58%
21	Minnesota	3,100	1.68%
27	Mississippi	2,300	1.25%
15	Missouri	3,900	2.11%
41	Montana	700	0.38%
35	Nebraska	1,100	0.60%
35	Nevada	1,100	0.60%
42	New Hampshire	600	0.33%
9	New Jersey	5,700	3.09%
35	New Mexico	1,100	0.60%
4	New York	11,800	6.40%
10	North Carolina	5,600	3.04%
42	North Dakota	600	0.33%
7	Ohio	8,200	4.44%
30	Oklahoma	2,200	1.19%
27	Oregon	2,300	1.25%
5	Pennsylvania	10,400	5.64%
42	Rhode Island	600	0.33%
23	South Carolina	3,000	1.63%
42	South Dakota	600	0.33%
19	Tennessee	3,300	1.79%
3	Texas	11,900	6.45%
38	Utah	1,000	0.54%
48	Vermont	300	0.16%
12	Virginia	4,400	2.38%
17	Washington	3,500	1.90%
34	West Virginia	1,500	0.81%
12	Wisconsin	4,400	2.38%
48	Wyoming	300	0.16%

RANK ORDER

RANK	STATE	CASES	% of USA
1	California	17,200	9.32%
2	Florida	14,100	7.64%
3	Texas	11,900	6.45%
4	New York	11,800	6.40%
5	Pennsylvania	10,400	5.64%
6	Illinois	8,300	4.50%
7	Ohio	8,200	4.44%
8	Michigan	6,600	3.58%
9	New Jersey	5,700	3.09%
10	North Carolina	5,600	3.04%
11	Georgia	4,500	2.44%
12	Virginia	4,400	2.38%
12	Wisconsin	4,400	2.38%
14	Massachusetts	4,300	2.33%
15	Missouri	3,900	2.11%
16	Indiana	3,600	1.95%
17	Maryland	3,500	1.90%
17	Washington	3,500	1.90%
19	Tennessee	3,300	1.79%
20	Arizona	3,200	1.73%
21	Louisiana	3,100	1.68%
21	Minnesota	3,100	1.68%
23	Alabama	3,000	1.63%
23	South Carolina	3,000	1.63%
25	Kentucky	2,500	1.36%
26	Arkansas	2,400	1.30%
27	Iowa	2,300	1.25%
27	Mississippi	2,300	1.25%
27	Oregon	2,300	1.25%
30	Colorado	2,200	1.19%
30	Connecticut	2,200	1.19%
30	Oklahoma	2,200	1.19%
33	Kansas	1,900	1.03%
34	West Virginia	1,500	0.81%
35	Nebraska	1,100	0.60%
35	Nevada	1,100	0.60%
35	New Mexico	1,100	0.60%
38	Utah	1,000	0.54%
39	Idaho	900	0.49%
39	Maine	900	0.49%
41	Montana	700	0.38%
42	Hawaii	600	0.33%
42	New Hampshire	600	0.33%
42	North Dakota	600	0.33%
42	Rhode Island	600	0.33%
42	South Dakota	600	0.33%
47	Delaware	500	0.27%
48	Vermont	300	0.16%
48	Wyoming	300	0.16%
50	Alaska	200	0.11%
	District of Columbia	600	0.33%

Source: American Cancer Society
"Cancer Facts & Figures-1998" (Copyright 1998, Reprinted with permission from the American Cancer Society)
*These estimates are offered as a rough guide and should be interpreted with caution. They are calculated according to the distribution of estimated 1998 cancer deaths by state.

Estimated Rate of New Prostate Cancer Cases in 1998

National Estimated Rate = 142.1 New Cases per 100,000 Male Population*

<table>
<tr><td colspan="3">ALPHA ORDER</td><td colspan="3">RANK ORDER</td></tr>
<tr><td>RANK</td><td>STATE</td><td>RATE</td><td>RANK</td><td>STATE</td><td>RATE</td></tr>
<tr><td>21</td><td>Alabama</td><td>146.0</td><td>1</td><td>Florida</td><td>201.6</td></tr>
<tr><td>50</td><td>Alaska</td><td>62.6</td><td>2</td><td>Arkansas</td><td>197.7</td></tr>
<tr><td>22</td><td>Arizona</td><td>145.9</td><td>3</td><td>North Dakota</td><td>186.7</td></tr>
<tr><td>2</td><td>Arkansas</td><td>197.7</td><td>4</td><td>Pennsylvania</td><td>179.2</td></tr>
<tr><td>45</td><td>California</td><td>107.7</td><td>5</td><td>Mississippi</td><td>176.3</td></tr>
<tr><td>44</td><td>Colorado</td><td>116.0</td><td>6</td><td>Wisconsin</td><td>173.3</td></tr>
<tr><td>28</td><td>Connecticut</td><td>138.2</td><td>7</td><td>West Virginia</td><td>170.2</td></tr>
<tr><td>26</td><td>Delaware</td><td>141.5</td><td>8</td><td>South Carolina</td><td>167.9</td></tr>
<tr><td>1</td><td>Florida</td><td>201.6</td><td>9</td><td>South Dakota</td><td>166.2</td></tr>
<tr><td>42</td><td>Georgia</td><td>125.6</td><td>10</td><td>Iowa</td><td>165.5</td></tr>
<tr><td>48</td><td>Hawaii</td><td>100.4</td><td>11</td><td>Montana</td><td>159.8</td></tr>
<tr><td>14</td><td>Idaho</td><td>151.4</td><td>12</td><td>North Carolina</td><td>157.4</td></tr>
<tr><td>24</td><td>Illinois</td><td>143.5</td><td>13</td><td>Ohio</td><td>151.6</td></tr>
<tr><td>39</td><td>Indiana</td><td>126.5</td><td>14</td><td>Idaho</td><td>151.4</td></tr>
<tr><td>10</td><td>Iowa</td><td>165.5</td><td>15</td><td>Kansas</td><td>150.1</td></tr>
<tr><td>15</td><td>Kansas</td><td>150.1</td><td>15</td><td>Missouri</td><td>150.1</td></tr>
<tr><td>35</td><td>Kentucky</td><td>132.5</td><td>17</td><td>Maine</td><td>148.2</td></tr>
<tr><td>18</td><td>Louisiana</td><td>147.8</td><td>18</td><td>Louisiana</td><td>147.8</td></tr>
<tr><td>17</td><td>Maine</td><td>148.2</td><td>19</td><td>New Jersey</td><td>147.1</td></tr>
<tr><td>25</td><td>Maryland</td><td>141.7</td><td>20</td><td>Massachusetts</td><td>146.2</td></tr>
<tr><td>20</td><td>Massachusetts</td><td>146.2</td><td>21</td><td>Alabama</td><td>146.0</td></tr>
<tr><td>27</td><td>Michigan</td><td>141.1</td><td>22</td><td>Arizona</td><td>145.9</td></tr>
<tr><td>31</td><td>Minnesota</td><td>134.9</td><td>23</td><td>Oregon</td><td>145.2</td></tr>
<tr><td>5</td><td>Mississippi</td><td>176.3</td><td>24</td><td>Illinois</td><td>143.5</td></tr>
<tr><td>15</td><td>Missouri</td><td>150.1</td><td>25</td><td>Maryland</td><td>141.7</td></tr>
<tr><td>11</td><td>Montana</td><td>159.8</td><td>26</td><td>Delaware</td><td>141.5</td></tr>
<tr><td>30</td><td>Nebraska</td><td>135.9</td><td>27</td><td>Michigan</td><td>141.1</td></tr>
<tr><td>33</td><td>Nevada</td><td>134.6</td><td>28</td><td>Connecticut</td><td>138.2</td></tr>
<tr><td>46</td><td>New Hampshire</td><td>104.8</td><td>29</td><td>Oklahoma</td><td>136.2</td></tr>
<tr><td>19</td><td>New Jersey</td><td>147.1</td><td>30</td><td>Nebraska</td><td>135.9</td></tr>
<tr><td>36</td><td>New Mexico</td><td>130.1</td><td>31</td><td>Minnesota</td><td>134.9</td></tr>
<tr><td>32</td><td>New York</td><td>134.7</td><td>32</td><td>New York</td><td>134.7</td></tr>
<tr><td>12</td><td>North Carolina</td><td>157.4</td><td>33</td><td>Nevada</td><td>134.6</td></tr>
<tr><td>3</td><td>North Dakota</td><td>186.7</td><td>34</td><td>Virginia</td><td>134.5</td></tr>
<tr><td>13</td><td>Ohio</td><td>151.6</td><td>35</td><td>Kentucky</td><td>132.5</td></tr>
<tr><td>29</td><td>Oklahoma</td><td>136.2</td><td>36</td><td>New Mexico</td><td>130.1</td></tr>
<tr><td>23</td><td>Oregon</td><td>145.2</td><td>37</td><td>Tennessee</td><td>128.3</td></tr>
<tr><td>4</td><td>Pennsylvania</td><td>179.2</td><td>38</td><td>Washington</td><td>127.0</td></tr>
<tr><td>40</td><td>Rhode Island</td><td>125.9</td><td>39</td><td>Indiana</td><td>126.5</td></tr>
<tr><td>8</td><td>South Carolina</td><td>167.9</td><td>40</td><td>Rhode Island</td><td>125.9</td></tr>
<tr><td>9</td><td>South Dakota</td><td>166.2</td><td>40</td><td>Texas</td><td>125.9</td></tr>
<tr><td>37</td><td>Tennessee</td><td>128.3</td><td>42</td><td>Georgia</td><td>125.6</td></tr>
<tr><td>40</td><td>Texas</td><td>125.9</td><td>43</td><td>Wyoming</td><td>123.8</td></tr>
<tr><td>49</td><td>Utah</td><td>100.3</td><td>44</td><td>Colorado</td><td>116.0</td></tr>
<tr><td>47</td><td>Vermont</td><td>103.4</td><td>45</td><td>California</td><td>107.7</td></tr>
<tr><td>34</td><td>Virginia</td><td>134.5</td><td>46</td><td>New Hampshire</td><td>104.8</td></tr>
<tr><td>38</td><td>Washington</td><td>127.0</td><td>47</td><td>Vermont</td><td>103.4</td></tr>
<tr><td>7</td><td>West Virginia</td><td>170.2</td><td>48</td><td>Hawaii</td><td>100.4</td></tr>
<tr><td>6</td><td>Wisconsin</td><td>173.3</td><td>49</td><td>Utah</td><td>100.3</td></tr>
<tr><td>43</td><td>Wyoming</td><td>123.8</td><td>50</td><td>Alaska</td><td>62.6</td></tr>
<tr><td></td><td></td><td></td><td></td><td>District of Columbia</td><td>235.9</td></tr>
</table>

Source: Morgan Quitno Press using data from American Cancer Society
"Cancer Facts & Figures-1998" (Copyright 1998, Reprinted with permission from the American Cancer Society)
*These estimates are offered as a rough guide and should be interpreted with caution. They are calculated according to the distribution of estimated 1998 cancer deaths by state. Rates calculated using 1996 Census male resident population estimates.

Estimated New Skin Melanoma Cases in 1998

National Estimated Total = 41,600 New Cases*

ALPHA ORDER

RANK ORDER

RANK	STATE	CASES	% of USA
17	Alabama	800	1.92%
NA	Alaska**	NA	NA
17	Arizona	800	1.92%
34	Arkansas	300	0.72%
1	California	4,500	10.82%
20	Colorado	700	1.68%
25	Connecticut	600	1.44%
43	Delaware	100	0.24%
2	Florida	2,900	6.97%
14	Georgia	1,000	2.40%
43	Hawaii	100	0.24%
37	Idaho	200	0.48%
6	Illinois	1,900	4.57%
15	Indiana	900	2.16%
31	Iowa	400	0.96%
25	Kansas	600	1.44%
17	Kentucky	800	1.92%
25	Louisiana	600	1.44%
37	Maine	200	0.48%
20	Maryland	700	1.68%
9	Massachusetts	1,300	3.13%
10	Michigan	1,200	2.88%
28	Minnesota	500	1.20%
37	Mississippi	200	0.48%
15	Missouri	900	2.16%
43	Montana	100	0.24%
37	Nebraska	200	0.48%
34	Nevada	300	0.72%
37	New Hampshire	200	0.48%
8	New Jersey	1,400	3.37%
31	New Mexico	400	0.96%
4	New York	2,300	5.53%
13	North Carolina	1,100	2.64%
43	North Dakota	100	0.24%
7	Ohio	1,600	3.85%
28	Oklahoma	500	1.20%
20	Oregon	700	1.68%
5	Pennsylvania	2,200	5.29%
43	Rhode Island	100	0.24%
28	South Carolina	500	1.20%
43	South Dakota	100	0.24%
10	Tennessee	1,200	2.88%
3	Texas	2,800	6.73%
34	Utah	300	0.72%
37	Vermont	200	0.48%
10	Virginia	1,200	2.88%
20	Washington	700	1.68%
31	West Virginia	400	0.96%
20	Wisconsin	700	1.68%
43	Wyoming	100	0.24%

RANK	STATE	CASES	% of USA
1	California	4,500	10.82%
2	Florida	2,900	6.97%
3	Texas	2,800	6.73%
4	New York	2,300	5.53%
5	Pennsylvania	2,200	5.29%
6	Illinois	1,900	4.57%
7	Ohio	1,600	3.85%
8	New Jersey	1,400	3.37%
9	Massachusetts	1,300	3.13%
10	Michigan	1,200	2.88%
10	Tennessee	1,200	2.88%
10	Virginia	1,200	2.88%
13	North Carolina	1,100	2.64%
14	Georgia	1,000	2.40%
15	Indiana	900	2.16%
15	Missouri	900	2.16%
17	Alabama	800	1.92%
17	Arizona	800	1.92%
17	Kentucky	800	1.92%
20	Colorado	700	1.68%
20	Maryland	700	1.68%
20	Oregon	700	1.68%
20	Washington	700	1.68%
20	Wisconsin	700	1.68%
25	Connecticut	600	1.44%
25	Kansas	600	1.44%
25	Louisiana	600	1.44%
28	Minnesota	500	1.20%
28	Oklahoma	500	1.20%
28	South Carolina	500	1.20%
31	Iowa	400	0.96%
31	New Mexico	400	0.96%
31	West Virginia	400	0.96%
34	Arkansas	300	0.72%
34	Nevada	300	0.72%
34	Utah	300	0.72%
37	Idaho	200	0.48%
37	Maine	200	0.48%
37	Mississippi	200	0.48%
37	Nebraska	200	0.48%
37	New Hampshire	200	0.48%
37	Vermont	200	0.48%
43	Delaware	100	0.24%
43	Hawaii	100	0.24%
43	Montana	100	0.24%
43	North Dakota	100	0.24%
43	Rhode Island	100	0.24%
43	South Dakota	100	0.24%
43	Wyoming	100	0.24%
NA	Alaska**	NA	NA
	District of Columbia**	NA	NA

Source: American Cancer Society

"Cancer Facts & Figures-1998" (Copyright 1998, Reprinted with permission from the American Cancer Society)
*These estimates are offered as a rough guide and should be interpreted with caution. They are calculated according to the distribution of estimated 1998 cancer deaths by state.
**Fewer than 50 cases.

Estimated Rate of New Skin Melanoma Cases in 1998

National Estimated Rate = 15.5 New Cases per 100,000 Population*

<table>
<tr><td colspan="3">ALPHA ORDER</td><td colspan="3">RANK ORDER</td></tr>
<tr><td>RANK</td><td>STATE</td><td>RATE</td><td>RANK</td><td>STATE</td><td>RATE</td></tr>
<tr><td>11</td><td>Alabama</td><td>18.5</td><td>1</td><td>Vermont</td><td>34.0</td></tr>
<tr><td>NA</td><td>Alaska**</td><td>NA</td><td>2</td><td>Kansas</td><td>23.1</td></tr>
<tr><td>17</td><td>Arizona</td><td>17.6</td><td>2</td><td>New Mexico</td><td>23.1</td></tr>
<tr><td>44</td><td>Arkansas</td><td>11.9</td><td>4</td><td>Tennessee</td><td>22.4</td></tr>
<tr><td>32</td><td>California</td><td>13.9</td><td>5</td><td>West Virginia</td><td>22.0</td></tr>
<tr><td>14</td><td>Colorado</td><td>18.0</td><td>6</td><td>Oregon</td><td>21.6</td></tr>
<tr><td>12</td><td>Connecticut</td><td>18.3</td><td>7</td><td>Massachusetts</td><td>21.3</td></tr>
<tr><td>34</td><td>Delaware</td><td>13.7</td><td>8</td><td>Wyoming</td><td>20.8</td></tr>
<tr><td>10</td><td>Florida</td><td>19.8</td><td>9</td><td>Kentucky</td><td>20.5</td></tr>
<tr><td>38</td><td>Georgia</td><td>13.4</td><td>10</td><td>Florida</td><td>19.8</td></tr>
<tr><td>48</td><td>Hawaii</td><td>8.4</td><td>11</td><td>Alabama</td><td>18.5</td></tr>
<tr><td>21</td><td>Idaho</td><td>16.5</td><td>12</td><td>Connecticut</td><td>18.3</td></tr>
<tr><td>23</td><td>Illinois</td><td>16.0</td><td>12</td><td>Pennsylvania</td><td>18.3</td></tr>
<tr><td>25</td><td>Indiana</td><td>15.3</td><td>14</td><td>Colorado</td><td>18.0</td></tr>
<tr><td>31</td><td>Iowa</td><td>14.0</td><td>15</td><td>Nevada</td><td>17.9</td></tr>
<tr><td>2</td><td>Kansas</td><td>23.1</td><td>16</td><td>Virginia</td><td>17.8</td></tr>
<tr><td>9</td><td>Kentucky</td><td>20.5</td><td>17</td><td>Arizona</td><td>17.6</td></tr>
<tr><td>33</td><td>Louisiana</td><td>13.8</td><td>18</td><td>New Jersey</td><td>17.4</td></tr>
<tr><td>22</td><td>Maine</td><td>16.1</td><td>19</td><td>New Hampshire</td><td>17.1</td></tr>
<tr><td>34</td><td>Maryland</td><td>13.7</td><td>20</td><td>Missouri</td><td>16.7</td></tr>
<tr><td>7</td><td>Massachusetts</td><td>21.3</td><td>21</td><td>Idaho</td><td>16.5</td></tr>
<tr><td>42</td><td>Michigan</td><td>12.3</td><td>22</td><td>Maine</td><td>16.1</td></tr>
<tr><td>46</td><td>Minnesota</td><td>10.7</td><td>23</td><td>Illinois</td><td>16.0</td></tr>
<tr><td>49</td><td>Mississippi</td><td>7.3</td><td>24</td><td>North Dakota</td><td>15.6</td></tr>
<tr><td>20</td><td>Missouri</td><td>16.7</td><td>25</td><td>Indiana</td><td>15.3</td></tr>
<tr><td>45</td><td>Montana</td><td>11.4</td><td>26</td><td>Oklahoma</td><td>15.1</td></tr>
<tr><td>43</td><td>Nebraska</td><td>12.1</td><td>27</td><td>North Carolina</td><td>14.8</td></tr>
<tr><td>15</td><td>Nevada</td><td>17.9</td><td>28</td><td>Utah</td><td>14.6</td></tr>
<tr><td>19</td><td>New Hampshire</td><td>17.1</td><td>29</td><td>Texas</td><td>14.4</td></tr>
<tr><td>18</td><td>New Jersey</td><td>17.4</td><td>30</td><td>Ohio</td><td>14.3</td></tr>
<tr><td>2</td><td>New Mexico</td><td>23.1</td><td>31</td><td>Iowa</td><td>14.0</td></tr>
<tr><td>40</td><td>New York</td><td>12.7</td><td>32</td><td>California</td><td>13.9</td></tr>
<tr><td>27</td><td>North Carolina</td><td>14.8</td><td>33</td><td>Louisiana</td><td>13.8</td></tr>
<tr><td>24</td><td>North Dakota</td><td>15.6</td><td>34</td><td>Delaware</td><td>13.7</td></tr>
<tr><td>30</td><td>Ohio</td><td>14.3</td><td>34</td><td>Maryland</td><td>13.7</td></tr>
<tr><td>26</td><td>Oklahoma</td><td>15.1</td><td>36</td><td>South Dakota</td><td>13.6</td></tr>
<tr><td>6</td><td>Oregon</td><td>21.6</td><td>37</td><td>Wisconsin</td><td>13.5</td></tr>
<tr><td>12</td><td>Pennsylvania</td><td>18.3</td><td>38</td><td>Georgia</td><td>13.4</td></tr>
<tr><td>47</td><td>Rhode Island</td><td>10.1</td><td>39</td><td>South Carolina</td><td>13.3</td></tr>
<tr><td>39</td><td>South Carolina</td><td>13.3</td><td>40</td><td>New York</td><td>12.7</td></tr>
<tr><td>36</td><td>South Dakota</td><td>13.6</td><td>41</td><td>Washington</td><td>12.5</td></tr>
<tr><td>4</td><td>Tennessee</td><td>22.4</td><td>42</td><td>Michigan</td><td>12.3</td></tr>
<tr><td>29</td><td>Texas</td><td>14.4</td><td>43</td><td>Nebraska</td><td>12.1</td></tr>
<tr><td>28</td><td>Utah</td><td>14.6</td><td>44</td><td>Arkansas</td><td>11.9</td></tr>
<tr><td>1</td><td>Vermont</td><td>34.0</td><td>45</td><td>Montana</td><td>11.4</td></tr>
<tr><td>16</td><td>Virginia</td><td>17.8</td><td>46</td><td>Minnesota</td><td>10.7</td></tr>
<tr><td>41</td><td>Washington</td><td>12.5</td><td>47</td><td>Rhode Island</td><td>10.1</td></tr>
<tr><td>5</td><td>West Virginia</td><td>22.0</td><td>48</td><td>Hawaii</td><td>8.4</td></tr>
<tr><td>37</td><td>Wisconsin</td><td>13.5</td><td>49</td><td>Mississippi</td><td>7.3</td></tr>
<tr><td>8</td><td>Wyoming</td><td>20.8</td><td>NA</td><td>Alaska**</td><td>NA</td></tr>
<tr><td></td><td></td><td></td><td></td><td>District of Columbia**</td><td>NA</td></tr>
</table>

Source: Morgan Quitno Press using data from American Cancer Society
"Cancer Facts & Figures-1998" (Copyright 1998, Reprinted with permission from the American Cancer Society)
These estimates are offered as a rough guide and should not be regarded as definitive. They are calculated according to the distribution of estimated 1998 cancer deaths by state. Rates calculated using 1997 Census resident population estimates.
**Fewer than 50 cases.*

Estimated New Cancer of the Uterus (Cervix) Cases in 1998

National Estimated Total = 13,700 New Cases*

ALPHA ORDER

RANK	STATE	CASES	% of USA
19	Alabama	200	1.46%
NA	Alaska**	NA	NA
19	Arizona	200	1.46%
19	Arkansas	200	1.46%
1	California	1,500	10.95%
19	Colorado	200	1.46%
29	Connecticut	100	0.73%
29	Delaware	100	0.73%
4	Florida	1,000	7.30%
12	Georgia	300	2.19%
NA	Hawaii**	NA	NA
NA	Idaho**	NA	NA
6	Illinois	600	4.38%
12	Indiana	300	2.19%
29	Iowa	100	0.73%
29	Kansas	100	0.73%
12	Kentucky	300	2.19%
19	Louisiana	200	1.46%
29	Maine	100	0.73%
12	Maryland	300	2.19%
19	Massachusetts	200	1.46%
8	Michigan	500	3.65%
29	Minnesota	100	0.73%
19	Mississippi	200	1.46%
9	Missouri	400	2.92%
NA	Montana**	NA	NA
NA	Nebraska**	NA	NA
29	Nevada	100	0.73%
29	New Hampshire	100	0.73%
9	New Jersey	400	2.92%
29	New Mexico	100	0.73%
3	New York	1,100	8.03%
12	North Carolina	300	2.19%
NA	North Dakota**	NA	NA
6	Ohio	600	4.38%
19	Oklahoma	200	1.46%
29	Oregon	100	0.73%
5	Pennsylvania	700	5.11%
NA	Rhode Island**	NA	NA
19	South Carolina	200	1.46%
NA	South Dakota**	NA	NA
9	Tennessee	400	2.92%
2	Texas	1,200	8.76%
29	Utah	100	0.73%
29	Vermont	100	0.73%
12	Virginia	300	2.19%
19	Washington	200	1.46%
29	West Virginia	100	0.73%
12	Wisconsin	300	2.19%
NA	Wyoming**	NA	NA

RANK ORDER

RANK	STATE	CASES	% of USA
1	California	1,500	10.95%
2	Texas	1,200	8.76%
3	New York	1,100	8.03%
4	Florida	1,000	7.30%
5	Pennsylvania	700	5.11%
6	Illinois	600	4.38%
6	Ohio	600	4.38%
8	Michigan	500	3.65%
9	Missouri	400	2.92%
9	New Jersey	400	2.92%
9	Tennessee	400	2.92%
12	Georgia	300	2.19%
12	Indiana	300	2.19%
12	Kentucky	300	2.19%
12	Maryland	300	2.19%
12	North Carolina	300	2.19%
12	Virginia	300	2.19%
12	Wisconsin	300	2.19%
19	Alabama	200	1.46%
19	Arizona	200	1.46%
19	Arkansas	200	1.46%
19	Colorado	200	1.46%
19	Louisiana	200	1.46%
19	Massachusetts	200	1.46%
19	Mississippi	200	1.46%
19	Oklahoma	200	1.46%
19	South Carolina	200	1.46%
19	Washington	200	1.46%
29	Connecticut	100	0.73%
29	Delaware	100	0.73%
29	Iowa	100	0.73%
29	Kansas	100	0.73%
29	Maine	100	0.73%
29	Minnesota	100	0.73%
29	Nevada	100	0.73%
29	New Hampshire	100	0.73%
29	New Mexico	100	0.73%
29	Oregon	100	0.73%
29	Utah	100	0.73%
29	Vermont	100	0.73%
29	West Virginia	100	0.73%
NA	Alaska**	NA	NA
NA	Hawaii**	NA	NA
NA	Idaho**	NA	NA
NA	Montana**	NA	NA
NA	Nebraska**	NA	NA
NA	North Dakota**	NA	NA
NA	Rhode Island**	NA	NA
NA	South Dakota**	NA	NA
NA	Wyoming**	NA	NA
	District of Columbia**	NA	NA

Source: American Cancer Society
"Cancer Facts & Figures-1998" (Copyright 1998, Reprinted with permission from the American Cancer Society)
*These estimates are offered as a rough guide and should be interpreted with caution. They are calculated according to the distribution of estimated 1998 cancer deaths by state.
**Fewer than 50 cases.

Estimated Rate of New Cancer of the Uterus (Cervix) Cases in 1998

National Estimated Rate = 10.1 New Cases per 100,000 Female Population*

ALPHA ORDER

RANK	STATE	RATE
29	Alabama	9.0
NA	Alaska**	NA
30	Arizona	8.9
5	Arkansas	15.4
28	California	9.4
21	Colorado	10.4
40	Connecticut	5.9
2	Delaware	26.9
10	Florida	13.5
33	Georgia	8.0
NA	Hawaii**	NA
NA	Idaho**	NA
26	Illinois	9.9
24	Indiana	10.0
37	Iowa	6.8
35	Kansas	7.7
6	Kentucky	15.0
30	Louisiana	8.9
4	Maine	15.7
15	Maryland	11.5
38	Massachusetts	6.3
23	Michigan	10.2
41	Minnesota	4.2
9	Mississippi	14.2
8	Missouri	14.5
NA	Montana**	NA
NA	Nebraska**	NA
11	Nevada	12.7
3	New Hampshire	16.9
27	New Jersey	9.7
15	New Mexico	11.5
14	New York	11.7
33	North Carolina	8.0
NA	North Dakota**	NA
21	Ohio	10.4
13	Oklahoma	11.9
39	Oregon	6.2
18	Pennsylvania	11.2
NA	Rhode Island**	NA
20	South Carolina	10.5
NA	South Dakota**	NA
7	Tennessee	14.6
12	Texas	12.4
24	Utah	10.0
1	Vermont	33.5
32	Virginia	8.8
36	Washington	7.2
19	West Virginia	10.6
17	Wisconsin	11.4
NA	Wyoming**	NA

RANK ORDER

RANK	STATE	RATE
1	Vermont	33.5
2	Delaware	26.9
3	New Hampshire	16.9
4	Maine	15.7
5	Arkansas	15.4
6	Kentucky	15.0
7	Tennessee	14.6
8	Missouri	14.5
9	Mississippi	14.2
10	Florida	13.5
11	Nevada	12.7
12	Texas	12.4
13	Oklahoma	11.9
14	New York	11.7
15	Maryland	11.5
15	New Mexico	11.5
17	Wisconsin	11.4
18	Pennsylvania	11.2
19	West Virginia	10.6
20	South Carolina	10.5
21	Colorado	10.4
21	Ohio	10.4
23	Michigan	10.2
24	Indiana	10.0
24	Utah	10.0
26	Illinois	9.9
27	New Jersey	9.7
28	California	9.4
29	Alabama	9.0
30	Arizona	8.9
30	Louisiana	8.9
32	Virginia	8.8
33	Georgia	8.0
33	North Carolina	8.0
35	Kansas	7.7
36	Washington	7.2
37	Iowa	6.8
38	Massachusetts	6.3
39	Oregon	6.2
40	Connecticut	5.9
41	Minnesota	4.2
NA	Alaska**	NA
NA	Hawaii**	NA
NA	Idaho**	NA
NA	Montana**	NA
NA	Nebraska**	NA
NA	North Dakota**	NA
NA	Rhode Island**	NA
NA	South Dakota**	NA
NA	Wyoming**	NA
	District of Columbia**	NA

Source: Morgan Quitno Press using data from American Cancer Society
"Cancer Facts & Figures-1998" (Copyright 1998, Reprinted with permission from the American Cancer Society)
*These estimates are offered as a rough guide and should be interpreted with caution. They are calculated according to the distribution of estimated 1998 cancer deaths by state. Rates calculated using 1996 Census female resident population estimates.
**Fewer than 50 cases.

Percent of Women 18 Years and Older
Who Had a Pap Smear Within the Past Three Years: 1996
National Median = 90.13% of Women 18 Years and Older*

ALPHA ORDER

RANK ORDER

RANK	STATE	PERCENT
34	Alabama	88.84
2	Alaska	95.74
10	Arizona	91.80
33	Arkansas	89.05
NA	California**	NA
3	Colorado	92.75
29	Connecticut	89.81
13	Delaware	91.33
31	Florida	89.65
1	Georgia	96.54
NA	Hawaii**	NA
41	Idaho	87.34
25	Illinois	90.03
45	Indiana	86.34
48	Iowa	84.01
11	Kansas	91.64
43	Kentucky	86.63
24	Louisiana	90.13
39	Maine	87.81
8	Maryland	92.10
16	Massachusetts	90.63
23	Michigan	90.15
6	Minnesota	92.36
35	Mississippi	88.83
15	Missouri	90.64
27	Montana	89.98
40	Nebraska	87.77
38	Nevada	88.23
22	New Hampshire	90.16
36	New Jersey	88.66
9	New Mexico	91.86
20	New York	90.44
7	North Carolina	92.18
44	North Dakota	86.38
14	Ohio	91.01
17	Oklahoma	90.61
21	Oregon	90.17
42	Pennsylvania	86.88
19	Rhode Island	90.51
5	South Carolina	92.38
37	South Dakota	88.42
18	Tennessee	90.55
28	Texas	89.97
32	Utah	89.59
12	Vermont	91.45
4	Virginia	92.54
30	Washington	89.72
47	West Virginia	85.83
26	Wisconsin	90.00
46	Wyoming	85.96

RANK	STATE	PERCENT
1	Georgia	96.54
2	Alaska	95.74
3	Colorado	92.75
4	Virginia	92.54
5	South Carolina	92.38
6	Minnesota	92.36
7	North Carolina	92.18
8	Maryland	92.10
9	New Mexico	91.86
10	Arizona	91.80
11	Kansas	91.64
12	Vermont	91.45
13	Delaware	91.33
14	Ohio	91.01
15	Missouri	90.64
16	Massachusetts	90.63
17	Oklahoma	90.61
18	Tennessee	90.55
19	Rhode Island	90.51
20	New York	90.44
21	Oregon	90.17
22	New Hampshire	90.16
23	Michigan	90.15
24	Louisiana	90.13
25	Illinois	90.03
26	Wisconsin	90.00
27	Montana	89.98
28	Texas	89.97
29	Connecticut	89.81
30	Washington	89.72
31	Florida	89.65
32	Utah	89.59
33	Arkansas	89.05
34	Alabama	88.84
35	Mississippi	88.83
36	New Jersey	88.66
37	South Dakota	88.42
38	Nevada	88.23
39	Maine	87.81
40	Nebraska	87.77
41	Idaho	87.34
42	Pennsylvania	86.88
43	Kentucky	86.63
44	North Dakota	86.38
45	Indiana	86.34
46	Wyoming	85.96
47	West Virginia	85.83
48	Iowa	84.01
NA	California**	NA
NA	Hawaii**	NA

District of Columbia 95.12

Source: U.S. Department of Health and Human Services, Centers for Disease Control and Prevention
"1996 Behavioral Risk Factor Surveillance Summary Prevalence Report" (January 8, 1998)
*A test for cancer, especially of the female genital tract. Named after George Papanicolaou (1883-1962), American anatomist.
**Not available.

AIDS Cases Reported in 1997

National Total = 62,649 New AIDS Cases*

ALPHA ORDER

RANK	STATE	CASES	% of USA
23	Alabama	521	0.83%
44	Alaska	44	0.07%
22	Arizona	532	0.85%
33	Arkansas	243	0.39%
2	California	8,177	13.05%
26	Colorado	432	0.69%
12	Connecticut	1,198	1.91%
30	Delaware	264	0.42%
3	Florida	6,725	10.73%
8	Georgia	2,108	3.36%
38	Hawaii	144	0.23%
44	Idaho	44	0.07%
9	Illinois	1,753	2.80%
21	Indiana	564	0.90%
40	Iowa	105	0.17%
35	Kansas	189	0.30%
27	Kentucky	405	0.65%
11	Louisiana	1,232	1.97%
43	Maine	55	0.09%
6	Maryland	2,175	3.47%
13	Massachusetts	1,126	1.80%
14	Michigan	949	1.51%
32	Minnesota	248	0.40%
25	Mississippi	448	0.72%
20	Missouri	691	1.10%
46	Montana	42	0.07%
41	Nebraska	99	0.16%
24	Nevada	466	0.74%
42	New Hampshire	68	0.11%
5	New Jersey	3,777	6.03%
34	New Mexico	229	0.37%
1	New York	12,525	19.99%
16	North Carolina	859	1.37%
49	North Dakota	10	0.02%
15	Ohio	930	1.48%
29	Oklahoma	288	0.46%
28	Oregon	357	0.57%
7	Pennsylvania	2,127	3.40%
36	Rhode Island	162	0.26%
17	South Carolina	815	1.30%
49	South Dakota	10	0.02%
18	Tennessee	796	1.27%
4	Texas	4,928	7.87%
37	Utah	159	0.25%
47	Vermont	32	0.05%
10	Virginia	1,255	2.00%
19	Washington	764	1.22%
39	West Virginia	113	0.18%
31	Wisconsin	253	0.40%
48	Wyoming	17	0.03%

RANK ORDER

RANK	STATE	CASES	% of USA
1	New York	12,525	19.99%
2	California	8,177	13.05%
3	Florida	6,725	10.73%
4	Texas	4,928	7.87%
5	New Jersey	3,777	6.03%
6	Maryland	2,175	3.47%
7	Pennsylvania	2,127	3.40%
8	Georgia	2,108	3.36%
9	Illinois	1,753	2.80%
10	Virginia	1,255	2.00%
11	Louisiana	1,232	1.97%
12	Connecticut	1,198	1.91%
13	Massachusetts	1,126	1.80%
14	Michigan	949	1.51%
15	Ohio	930	1.48%
16	North Carolina	859	1.37%
17	South Carolina	815	1.30%
18	Tennessee	796	1.27%
19	Washington	764	1.22%
20	Missouri	691	1.10%
21	Indiana	564	0.90%
22	Arizona	532	0.85%
23	Alabama	521	0.83%
24	Nevada	466	0.74%
25	Mississippi	448	0.72%
26	Colorado	432	0.69%
27	Kentucky	405	0.65%
28	Oregon	357	0.57%
29	Oklahoma	288	0.46%
30	Delaware	264	0.42%
31	Wisconsin	253	0.40%
32	Minnesota	248	0.40%
33	Arkansas	243	0.39%
34	New Mexico	229	0.37%
35	Kansas	189	0.30%
36	Rhode Island	162	0.26%
37	Utah	159	0.25%
38	Hawaii	144	0.23%
39	West Virginia	113	0.18%
40	Iowa	105	0.17%
41	Nebraska	99	0.16%
42	New Hampshire	68	0.11%
43	Maine	55	0.09%
44	Alaska	44	0.07%
44	Idaho	44	0.07%
46	Montana	42	0.07%
47	Vermont	32	0.05%
48	Wyoming	17	0.03%
49	North Dakota	10	0.02%
49	South Dakota	10	0.02%
	District of Columbia	1,196	1.91%

Source: U.S. Department of Health and Human Services, Centers for Disease Control and Prevention
   "HIV/AIDS Surveillance Report, 1997" (Mid-year Edition, Vol. 9, No. 1)
July 1996-June 1997. AIDS is Acquired Immunodeficiency Syndrome. It is a specific group of diseases or conditions which are indicative of severe immunosuppression related to infection with the Human Immunodeficiency Virus (HIV). National total does not include 2,210 cases in Puerto Rico, 56 cases in the Virgin Islands or 4 in other U.S. territories.

AIDS Rate in 1997

National Rate = 23.6 New AIDS Cases Reported per 100,000 Population*

<table>
<tr><td colspan="3">ALPHA ORDER</td><td colspan="3">RANK ORDER</td></tr>
<tr><td>RANK</td><td>STATE</td><td>RATE</td><td>RANK</td><td>STATE</td><td>RATE</td></tr>
<tr><td>23</td><td>Alabama</td><td>12.2</td><td>1</td><td>New York</td><td>68.9</td></tr>
<tr><td>37</td><td>Alaska</td><td>7.2</td><td>2</td><td>New Jersey</td><td>47.3</td></tr>
<tr><td>25</td><td>Arizona</td><td>12.0</td><td>3</td><td>Florida</td><td>46.7</td></tr>
<tr><td>31</td><td>Arkansas</td><td>9.7</td><td>4</td><td>Maryland</td><td>42.9</td></tr>
<tr><td>11</td><td>California</td><td>25.7</td><td>5</td><td>Connecticut</td><td>36.6</td></tr>
<tr><td>27</td><td>Colorado</td><td>11.3</td><td>6</td><td>Delaware</td><td>36.4</td></tr>
<tr><td>5</td><td>Connecticut</td><td>36.6</td><td>7</td><td>Nevada</td><td>29.1</td></tr>
<tr><td>6</td><td>Delaware</td><td>36.4</td><td>8</td><td>Georgia</td><td>28.7</td></tr>
<tr><td>3</td><td>Florida</td><td>46.7</td><td>9</td><td>Louisiana</td><td>28.3</td></tr>
<tr><td>8</td><td>Georgia</td><td>28.7</td><td>10</td><td>Texas</td><td>25.8</td></tr>
<tr><td>23</td><td>Hawaii</td><td>12.2</td><td>11</td><td>California</td><td>25.7</td></tr>
<tr><td>46</td><td>Idaho</td><td>3.7</td><td>12</td><td>South Carolina</td><td>22.0</td></tr>
<tr><td>19</td><td>Illinois</td><td>14.8</td><td>13</td><td>Virginia</td><td>18.8</td></tr>
<tr><td>31</td><td>Indiana</td><td>9.7</td><td>14</td><td>Massachusetts</td><td>18.5</td></tr>
<tr><td>46</td><td>Iowa</td><td>3.7</td><td>15</td><td>Pennsylvania</td><td>17.6</td></tr>
<tr><td>36</td><td>Kansas</td><td>7.3</td><td>16</td><td>Mississippi</td><td>16.5</td></tr>
<tr><td>29</td><td>Kentucky</td><td>10.4</td><td>17</td><td>Rhode Island</td><td>16.4</td></tr>
<tr><td>9</td><td>Louisiana</td><td>28.3</td><td>18</td><td>Tennessee</td><td>15.0</td></tr>
<tr><td>45</td><td>Maine</td><td>4.4</td><td>19</td><td>Illinois</td><td>14.8</td></tr>
<tr><td>4</td><td>Maryland</td><td>42.9</td><td>20</td><td>Washington</td><td>13.8</td></tr>
<tr><td>14</td><td>Massachusetts</td><td>18.5</td><td>21</td><td>New Mexico</td><td>13.4</td></tr>
<tr><td>30</td><td>Michigan</td><td>9.9</td><td>22</td><td>Missouri</td><td>12.9</td></tr>
<tr><td>42</td><td>Minnesota</td><td>5.3</td><td>23</td><td>Alabama</td><td>12.2</td></tr>
<tr><td>16</td><td>Mississippi</td><td>16.5</td><td>23</td><td>Hawaii</td><td>12.2</td></tr>
<tr><td>22</td><td>Missouri</td><td>12.9</td><td>25</td><td>Arizona</td><td>12.0</td></tr>
<tr><td>44</td><td>Montana</td><td>4.8</td><td>26</td><td>North Carolina</td><td>11.7</td></tr>
<tr><td>39</td><td>Nebraska</td><td>6.0</td><td>27</td><td>Colorado</td><td>11.3</td></tr>
<tr><td>7</td><td>Nevada</td><td>29.1</td><td>28</td><td>Oregon</td><td>11.1</td></tr>
<tr><td>40</td><td>New Hampshire</td><td>5.8</td><td>29</td><td>Kentucky</td><td>10.4</td></tr>
<tr><td>2</td><td>New Jersey</td><td>47.3</td><td>30</td><td>Michigan</td><td>9.9</td></tr>
<tr><td>21</td><td>New Mexico</td><td>13.4</td><td>31</td><td>Arkansas</td><td>9.7</td></tr>
<tr><td>1</td><td>New York</td><td>68.9</td><td>31</td><td>Indiana</td><td>9.7</td></tr>
<tr><td>26</td><td>North Carolina</td><td>11.7</td><td>33</td><td>Oklahoma</td><td>8.7</td></tr>
<tr><td>49</td><td>North Dakota</td><td>1.6</td><td>34</td><td>Ohio</td><td>8.3</td></tr>
<tr><td>34</td><td>Ohio</td><td>8.3</td><td>35</td><td>Utah</td><td>7.9</td></tr>
<tr><td>33</td><td>Oklahoma</td><td>8.7</td><td>36</td><td>Kansas</td><td>7.3</td></tr>
<tr><td>28</td><td>Oregon</td><td>11.1</td><td>37</td><td>Alaska</td><td>7.2</td></tr>
<tr><td>15</td><td>Pennsylvania</td><td>17.6</td><td>38</td><td>West Virginia</td><td>6.2</td></tr>
<tr><td>17</td><td>Rhode Island</td><td>16.4</td><td>39</td><td>Nebraska</td><td>6.0</td></tr>
<tr><td>12</td><td>South Carolina</td><td>22.0</td><td>40</td><td>New Hampshire</td><td>5.8</td></tr>
<tr><td>50</td><td>South Dakota</td><td>1.4</td><td>41</td><td>Vermont</td><td>5.4</td></tr>
<tr><td>18</td><td>Tennessee</td><td>15.0</td><td>42</td><td>Minnesota</td><td>5.3</td></tr>
<tr><td>10</td><td>Texas</td><td>25.8</td><td>43</td><td>Wisconsin</td><td>4.9</td></tr>
<tr><td>35</td><td>Utah</td><td>7.9</td><td>44</td><td>Montana</td><td>4.8</td></tr>
<tr><td>41</td><td>Vermont</td><td>5.4</td><td>45</td><td>Maine</td><td>4.4</td></tr>
<tr><td>13</td><td>Virginia</td><td>18.8</td><td>46</td><td>Idaho</td><td>3.7</td></tr>
<tr><td>20</td><td>Washington</td><td>13.8</td><td>46</td><td>Iowa</td><td>3.7</td></tr>
<tr><td>38</td><td>West Virginia</td><td>6.2</td><td>48</td><td>Wyoming</td><td>3.5</td></tr>
<tr><td>43</td><td>Wisconsin</td><td>4.9</td><td>49</td><td>North Dakota</td><td>1.6</td></tr>
<tr><td>48</td><td>Wyoming</td><td>3.5</td><td>50</td><td>South Dakota</td><td>1.4</td></tr>
<tr><td></td><td></td><td></td><td></td><td>District of Columbia</td><td>220.2</td></tr>
</table>

Source: U.S. Department of Health and Human Services, Centers for Disease Control and Prevention
    "HIV/AIDS Surveillance Report, 1997" (Mid-year Edition, Vol. 9, No. 1)
*July 1996-June 1997. AIDS is Acquired Immunodeficiency Syndrome. It is a specific group of diseases or conditions which are indicative of severe immunosuppression related to infection with the Human Immunodeficiency Virus (HIV). National rate does not include cases in U.S. territories.

AIDS Cases Reported Through June 1997

National Total = 591,775 Reported AIDS Cases*

ALPHA ORDER

RANK	STATE	CASES	% of USA
24	Alabama	4,504	0.76%
45	Alaska	385	0.07%
22	Arizona	5,258	0.89%
32	Arkansas	2,270	0.38%
2	California	101,569	17.16%
20	Colorado	5,962	1.01%
13	Connecticut	9,174	1.55%
34	Delaware	1,922	0.32%
3	Florida	62,200	10.51%
8	Georgia	17,985	3.04%
33	Hawaii	2,028	0.34%
44	Idaho	394	0.07%
6	Illinois	19,319	3.26%
23	Indiana	4,779	0.81%
39	Iowa	1,028	0.17%
35	Kansas	1,919	0.32%
31	Kentucky	2,401	0.41%
12	Louisiana	9,660	1.63%
42	Maine	783	0.13%
9	Maryland	16,223	2.74%
10	Massachusetts	12,523	2.12%
15	Michigan	8,770	1.48%
27	Minnesota	3,095	0.52%
28	Mississippi	3,050	0.52%
18	Missouri	7,487	1.27%
47	Montana	249	0.04%
40	Nebraska	843	0.14%
26	Nevada	3,300	0.56%
43	New Hampshire	729	0.12%
5	New Jersey	34,871	5.89%
37	New Mexico	1,522	0.26%
1	New York	113,549	19.19%
17	North Carolina	7,742	1.31%
50	North Dakota	85	0.01%
14	Ohio	9,109	1.54%
30	Oklahoma	2,886	0.49%
25	Oregon	4,021	0.68%
7	Pennsylvania	18,388	3.11%
36	Rhode Island	1,668	0.28%
19	South Carolina	6,661	1.13%
49	South Dakota	122	0.02%
21	Tennessee	5,947	1.00%
4	Texas	42,185	7.13%
38	Utah	1,449	0.24%
46	Vermont	316	0.05%
11	Virginia	9,699	1.64%
16	Washington	7,930	1.34%
41	West Virginia	801	0.14%
29	Wisconsin	2,916	0.49%
48	Wyoming	153	0.03%

RANK ORDER

RANK	STATE	CASES	% of USA
1	New York	113,549	19.19%
2	California	101,569	17.16%
3	Florida	62,200	10.51%
4	Texas	42,185	7.13%
5	New Jersey	34,871	5.89%
6	Illinois	19,319	3.26%
7	Pennsylvania	18,388	3.11%
8	Georgia	17,985	3.04%
9	Maryland	16,223	2.74%
10	Massachusetts	12,523	2.12%
11	Virginia	9,699	1.64%
12	Louisiana	9,660	1.63%
13	Connecticut	9,174	1.55%
14	Ohio	9,109	1.54%
15	Michigan	8,770	1.48%
16	Washington	7,930	1.34%
17	North Carolina	7,742	1.31%
18	Missouri	7,487	1.27%
19	South Carolina	6,661	1.13%
20	Colorado	5,962	1.01%
21	Tennessee	5,947	1.00%
22	Arizona	5,258	0.89%
23	Indiana	4,779	0.81%
24	Alabama	4,504	0.76%
25	Oregon	4,021	0.68%
26	Nevada	3,300	0.56%
27	Minnesota	3,095	0.52%
28	Mississippi	3,050	0.52%
29	Wisconsin	2,916	0.49%
30	Oklahoma	2,886	0.49%
31	Kentucky	2,401	0.41%
32	Arkansas	2,270	0.38%
33	Hawaii	2,028	0.34%
34	Delaware	1,922	0.32%
35	Kansas	1,919	0.32%
36	Rhode Island	1,668	0.28%
37	New Mexico	1,522	0.26%
38	Utah	1,449	0.24%
39	Iowa	1,028	0.17%
40	Nebraska	843	0.14%
41	West Virginia	801	0.14%
42	Maine	783	0.13%
43	New Hampshire	729	0.12%
44	Idaho	394	0.07%
45	Alaska	385	0.07%
46	Vermont	316	0.05%
47	Montana	249	0.04%
48	Wyoming	153	0.03%
49	South Dakota	122	0.02%
50	North Dakota	85	0.01%
	District of Columbia	9,946	1.68%

Source: U.S. Department of Health and Human Services, Centers for Disease Control and Prevention
    "HIV/AIDS Surveillance Report, 1997" (Mid-year Edition, Vol. 9, No. 1)
*Cumulative through June 1997. AIDS is Acquired Immunodeficiency Syndrome. It is a specific group of diseases or conditions which are indicative of severe immunosuppression related to infection with the Human Immunodeficiency Virus (HIV). National total does not include 19,583 cases in Puerto Rico, 330 cases in the Virgin Islands and 23 cases in other U.S. territories.

AIDS Cases in Children 12 Years and Younger Through June 1997

National Total = 7,525 Juvenile AIDS Cases*

ALPHA ORDER

RANK	STATE	CASES	% of USA
18	Alabama	63	0.84%
43	Alaska	5	0.07%
29	Arizona	21	0.28%
23	Arkansas	32	0.43%
4	California	549	7.30%
25	Colorado	27	0.36%
11	Connecticut	172	2.29%
34	Delaware	14	0.19%
2	Florida	1,270	16.88%
10	Georgia	177	2.35%
34	Hawaii	14	0.19%
48	Idaho	2	0.03%
8	Illinois	224	2.98%
22	Indiana	33	0.44%
40	Iowa	8	0.11%
37	Kansas	10	0.13%
29	Kentucky	21	0.28%
13	Louisiana	112	1.49%
38	Maine	9	0.12%
6	Maryland	268	3.56%
9	Massachusetts	192	2.55%
16	Michigan	89	1.18%
31	Minnesota	20	0.27%
21	Mississippi	44	0.58%
19	Missouri	50	0.66%
46	Montana	3	0.04%
38	Nebraska	9	0.12%
26	Nevada	25	0.33%
40	New Hampshire	8	0.11%
3	New Jersey	693	9.21%
43	New Mexico	5	0.07%
1	New York	2,008	26.68%
15	North Carolina	105	1.40%
50	North Dakota	0	0.00%
14	Ohio	108	1.44%
26	Oklahoma	25	0.33%
34	Oregon	14	0.19%
7	Pennsylvania	252	3.35%
33	Rhode Island	16	0.21%
17	South Carolina	69	0.92%
45	South Dakota	4	0.05%
20	Tennessee	46	0.61%
5	Texas	322	4.28%
31	Utah	20	0.27%
46	Vermont	3	0.04%
12	Virginia	151	2.01%
23	Washington	32	0.43%
40	West Virginia	8	0.11%
28	Wisconsin	24	0.32%
48	Wyoming	2	0.03%

RANK ORDER

RANK	STATE	CASES	% of USA
1	New York	2,008	26.68%
2	Florida	1,270	16.88%
3	New Jersey	693	9.21%
4	California	549	7.30%
5	Texas	322	4.28%
6	Maryland	268	3.56%
7	Pennsylvania	252	3.35%
8	Illinois	224	2.98%
9	Massachusetts	192	2.55%
10	Georgia	177	2.35%
11	Connecticut	172	2.29%
12	Virginia	151	2.01%
13	Louisiana	112	1.49%
14	Ohio	108	1.44%
15	North Carolina	105	1.40%
16	Michigan	89	1.18%
17	South Carolina	69	0.92%
18	Alabama	63	0.84%
19	Missouri	50	0.66%
20	Tennessee	46	0.61%
21	Mississippi	44	0.58%
22	Indiana	33	0.44%
23	Arkansas	32	0.43%
23	Washington	32	0.43%
25	Colorado	27	0.36%
26	Nevada	25	0.33%
26	Oklahoma	25	0.33%
28	Wisconsin	24	0.32%
29	Arizona	21	0.28%
29	Kentucky	21	0.28%
31	Minnesota	20	0.27%
31	Utah	20	0.27%
33	Rhode Island	16	0.21%
34	Delaware	14	0.19%
34	Hawaii	14	0.19%
34	Oregon	14	0.19%
37	Kansas	10	0.13%
38	Maine	9	0.12%
38	Nebraska	9	0.12%
40	Iowa	8	0.11%
40	New Hampshire	8	0.11%
40	West Virginia	8	0.11%
43	Alaska	5	0.07%
43	New Mexico	5	0.07%
45	South Dakota	4	0.05%
46	Montana	3	0.04%
46	Vermont	3	0.04%
48	Idaho	2	0.03%
48	Wyoming	2	0.03%
50	North Dakota	0	0.00%
	District of Columbia	147	1.95%

Source: U.S. Department of Health and Human Services, Centers for Disease Control and Prevention
    "HIV/AIDS Surveillance Report, 1997" (Mid-year Edition, Vol. 9, No. 1)
*Cumulative through June 1997. AIDS is Acquired Immunodeficiency Syndrome. It is a specific group of diseases or conditions which are indicative of severe immunosuppression related to infection with the Human Immunodeficiency Virus (HIV). National total does not include 363 cases in Puerto Rico and 13 cases in the Virgin Islands.

E-Coli Cases Reported in 1997

National Total = 2,457 Cases*

ALPHA ORDER

RANK	STATE	CASES	% of USA
35	Alabama	15	0.61%
41	Alaska	12	0.49%
25	Arizona*	30	1.22%
43	Arkansas	10	0.41%
2	California	185	7.53%
10	Colorado	83	3.38%
20	Connecticut	44	1.79%
48	Delaware	5	0.20%
17	Florida	49	1.99%
22	Georgia	41	1.67%
45	Hawaii*	9	0.37%
24	Idaho	38	1.55%
13	Illinois	71	2.89%
11	Indiana	81	3.30%
5	Iowa	119	4.84%
29	Kansas	26	1.06%
25	Kentucky	30	1.22%
37	Louisiana	14	0.57%
33	Maine	17	0.69%
29	Maryland	26	1.06%
7	Massachusetts	111	4.52%
3	Michigan	146	5.94%
1	Minnesota	214	8.71%
49	Mississippi	4	0.16%
16	Missouri	55	2.24%
31	Montana	24	0.98%
14	Nebraska	61	2.48%
42	Nevada	11	0.45%
37	New Hampshire	14	0.57%
27	New Jersey	29	1.18%
47	New Mexico	7	0.28%
6	New York	115	4.68%
12	North Carolina	74	3.01%
35	North Dakota	15	0.61%
8	Ohio	108	4.40%
39	Oklahoma	13	0.53%
9	Oregon	84	3.42%
32	Pennsylvania*	19	0.77%
43	Rhode Island	10	0.41%
39	South Carolina	13	0.53%
27	South Dakota	29	1.18%
19	Tennessee	47	1.91%
21	Texas	42	1.71%
15	Utah	59	2.40%
46	Vermont	8	0.33%
22	Virginia*	41	1.67%
4	Washington	130	5.29%
50	West Virginia*	1	0.04%
17	Wisconsin*	49	1.99%
33	Wyoming	17	0.69%

RANK ORDER

RANK	STATE	CASES	% of USA
1	Minnesota	214	8.71%
2	California	185	7.53%
3	Michigan	146	5.94%
4	Washington	130	5.29%
5	Iowa	119	4.84%
6	New York	115	4.68%
7	Massachusetts	111	4.52%
8	Ohio	108	4.40%
9	Oregon	84	3.42%
10	Colorado	83	3.38%
11	Indiana	81	3.30%
12	North Carolina	74	3.01%
13	Illinois	71	2.89%
14	Nebraska	61	2.48%
15	Utah	59	2.40%
16	Missouri	55	2.24%
17	Florida	49	1.99%
17	Wisconsin*	49	1.99%
19	Tennessee	47	1.91%
20	Connecticut	44	1.79%
21	Texas	42	1.71%
22	Georgia	41	1.67%
22	Virginia*	41	1.67%
24	Idaho	38	1.55%
25	Arizona*	30	1.22%
25	Kentucky	30	1.22%
27	New Jersey	29	1.18%
27	South Dakota	29	1.18%
29	Kansas	26	1.06%
29	Maryland	26	1.06%
31	Montana	24	0.98%
32	Pennsylvania*	19	0.77%
33	Maine	17	0.69%
33	Wyoming	17	0.69%
35	Alabama	15	0.61%
35	North Dakota	15	0.61%
37	Louisiana	14	0.57%
37	New Hampshire	14	0.57%
39	Oklahoma	13	0.53%
39	South Carolina	13	0.53%
41	Alaska	12	0.49%
42	Nevada	11	0.45%
43	Arkansas	10	0.41%
43	Rhode Island	10	0.41%
45	Hawaii*	9	0.37%
46	Vermont	8	0.33%
47	New Mexico	7	0.28%
48	Delaware	5	0.20%
49	Mississippi	4	0.16%
50	West Virginia*	1	0.04%
	District of Columbia	2	0.08%

Source: U.S. Department of Health and Human Services, National Center for Health Statistics
"Morbidity and Mortality Weekly Report" (January 9, 1998, Vol. 46, Nos. 52 & 53)

*Totals for Arizona, Hawaii, Pennsylvania, Virginia, West Virginia and Wisconsin are from the Public Health Laboratory Information System. All other states' data are from National Electronic Telecommunications System for Surveillance. Escherichia Coli is a common bacterium that normally inhabits the intestinal tracts of humans and animals but can cause infection in other parts of the body, especially the urinary tract. One strain, sometimes transmitted in hamburger meat, can cause serious infection resulting in diarrhea, anemia, kidney failure, and death.

E-Coli Rate in 1997

National Rate = 0.9 Cases per 100,000 Population*

ALPHA ORDER

RANK	STATE	RATE
43	Alabama	0.3
13	Alaska	2.0
30	Arizona*	0.7
39	Arkansas	0.4
33	California	0.6
12	Colorado	2.1
19	Connecticut	1.3
30	Delaware	0.7
43	Florida	0.3
37	Georgia	0.5
28	Hawaii*	0.8
6	Idaho	3.1
33	Illinois	0.6
16	Indiana	1.4
2	Iowa	4.2
21	Kansas	1.0
28	Kentucky	0.8
43	Louisiana	0.3
16	Maine	1.4
37	Maryland	0.5
14	Massachusetts	1.8
15	Michigan	1.5
1	Minnesota	4.6
49	Mississippi	0.1
21	Missouri	1.0
8	Montana	2.7
4	Nebraska	3.7
30	Nevada	0.7
20	New Hampshire	1.2
39	New Jersey	0.4
39	New Mexico	0.4
33	New York	0.6
21	North Carolina	1.0
10	North Dakota	2.3
21	Ohio	1.0
39	Oklahoma	0.4
9	Oregon	2.6
47	Pennsylvania*	0.2
21	Rhode Island	1.0
43	South Carolina	0.3
3	South Dakota	3.9
26	Tennessee	0.9
47	Texas	0.2
7	Utah	2.9
16	Vermont	1.4
33	Virginia*	0.6
10	Washington	2.3
49	West Virginia*	0.1
26	Wisconsin*	0.9
5	Wyoming	3.5

RANK ORDER

RANK	STATE	RATE
1	Minnesota	4.6
2	Iowa	4.2
3	South Dakota	3.9
4	Nebraska	3.7
5	Wyoming	3.5
6	Idaho	3.1
7	Utah	2.9
8	Montana	2.7
9	Oregon	2.6
10	North Dakota	2.3
10	Washington	2.3
12	Colorado	2.1
13	Alaska	2.0
14	Massachusetts	1.8
15	Michigan	1.5
16	Indiana	1.4
16	Maine	1.4
16	Vermont	1.4
19	Connecticut	1.3
20	New Hampshire	1.2
21	Kansas	1.0
21	Missouri	1.0
21	North Carolina	1.0
21	Ohio	1.0
21	Rhode Island	1.0
26	Tennessee	0.9
26	Wisconsin*	0.9
28	Hawaii*	0.8
28	Kentucky	0.8
30	Arizona*	0.7
30	Delaware	0.7
30	Nevada	0.7
33	California	0.6
33	Illinois	0.6
33	New York	0.6
33	Virginia*	0.6
37	Georgia	0.5
37	Maryland	0.5
39	Arkansas	0.4
39	New Jersey	0.4
39	New Mexico	0.4
39	Oklahoma	0.4
43	Alabama	0.3
43	Florida	0.3
43	Louisiana	0.3
43	South Carolina	0.3
47	Pennsylvania*	0.2
47	Texas	0.2
49	Mississippi	0.1
49	West Virginia*	0.1

District of Columbia		0.4

Source: Morgan Quitno Press using data from U.S. Dept. of Health & Human Serv's, National Center for Health Statistics
"Morbidity and Mortality Weekly Report" (January 9, 1998, Vol. 46, Nos. 52 & 53)
*Totals for Arizona, Hawaii, Pennsylvania, Virginia, West Virginia and Wisconsin are from the Public Health Laboratory Information System. All other states' data are from National Electronic Telecommunications System for Surveillance. Escherichia Coli is a common bacterium that normally inhabits the intestinal tracts of humans and animals but can cause infection in other parts of the body, especially the urinary tract. One strain, sometimes transmitted in hamburger meat, can cause serious infection resulting in diarrhea, anemia, kidney failure, and death.

German Measles (Rubella) Cases Reported in 1997

National Total = 161 Cases*

ALPHA ORDER

RANK ORDER

RANK	STATE	CASES	% of USA
17	Alabama	0	0.00%
17	Alaska	0	0.00%
6	Arizona	5	3.11%
17	Arkansas	0	0.00%
4	California	14	8.70%
17	Colorado	0	0.00%
13	Connecticut	1	0.62%
17	Delaware	0	0.00%
9	Florida	3	1.86%
17	Georgia	0	0.00%
5	Hawaii	8	4.97%
13	Idaho	1	0.62%
11	Illinois	2	1.24%
17	Indiana	0	0.00%
17	Iowa	0	0.00%
17	Kansas	0	0.00%
17	Kentucky	0	0.00%
17	Louisiana	0	0.00%
17	Maine	0	0.00%
17	Maryland	0	0.00%
13	Massachusetts	1	0.62%
17	Michigan	0	0.00%
17	Minnesota	0	0.00%
17	Mississippi	0	0.00%
11	Missouri	2	1.24%
17	Montana	0	0.00%
17	Nebraska	0	0.00%
17	Nevada	0	0.00%
17	New Hampshire	0	0.00%
17	New Jersey	0	0.00%
17	New Mexico	0	0.00%
2	New York	32	19.88%
1	North Carolina	59	36.65%
17	North Dakota	0	0.00%
17	Ohio	0	0.00%
17	Oklahoma	0	0.00%
17	Oregon	0	0.00%
17	Pennsylvania	0	0.00%
17	Rhode Island	0	0.00%
3	South Carolina	19	11.80%
17	South Dakota	0	0.00%
17	Tennessee	0	0.00%
8	Texas	4	2.48%
17	Utah	0	0.00%
17	Vermont	0	0.00%
13	Virginia	1	0.62%
6	Washington	5	3.11%
17	West Virginia	0	0.00%
9	Wisconsin	3	1.86%
17	Wyoming	0	0.00%

RANK	STATE	CASES	% of USA
1	North Carolina	59	36.65%
2	New York	32	19.88%
3	South Carolina	19	11.80%
4	California	14	8.70%
5	Hawaii	8	4.97%
6	Arizona	5	3.11%
6	Washington	5	3.11%
8	Texas	4	2.48%
9	Florida	3	1.86%
9	Wisconsin	3	1.86%
11	Illinois	2	1.24%
11	Missouri	2	1.24%
13	Connecticut	1	0.62%
13	Idaho	1	0.62%
13	Massachusetts	1	0.62%
13	Virginia	1	0.62%
17	Alabama	0	0.00%
17	Alaska	0	0.00%
17	Arkansas	0	0.00%
17	Colorado	0	0.00%
17	Delaware	0	0.00%
17	Georgia	0	0.00%
17	Indiana	0	0.00%
17	Iowa	0	0.00%
17	Kansas	0	0.00%
17	Kentucky	0	0.00%
17	Louisiana	0	0.00%
17	Maine	0	0.00%
17	Maryland	0	0.00%
17	Michigan	0	0.00%
17	Minnesota	0	0.00%
17	Mississippi	0	0.00%
17	Montana	0	0.00%
17	Nebraska	0	0.00%
17	Nevada	0	0.00%
17	New Hampshire	0	0.00%
17	New Jersey	0	0.00%
17	New Mexico	0	0.00%
17	North Dakota	0	0.00%
17	Ohio	0	0.00%
17	Oklahoma	0	0.00%
17	Oregon	0	0.00%
17	Pennsylvania	0	0.00%
17	Rhode Island	0	0.00%
17	South Dakota	0	0.00%
17	Tennessee	0	0.00%
17	Utah	0	0.00%
17	Vermont	0	0.00%
17	West Virginia	0	0.00%
17	Wyoming	0	0.00%
	District of Columbia	1	0.62%

Source: U.S. Department of Health and Human Services, National Center for Health Statistics
"Morbidity and Mortality Weekly Report" (January 9, 1998, Vol. 46, Nos. 52 & 53)
Provisional data. A mild, contagious, eruptive disease caused by a virus and capable of producing congenital defects in infants born to mothers infected during the first three months of pregnancy.

German Measles (Rubella) Rate in 1997

National Rate = 0.06 Cases per 100,000 Population*

ALPHA ORDER

RANK	STATE	RATE
17	Alabama	0.00
17	Alaska	0.00
5	Arizona	0.11
17	Arkansas	0.00
9	California	0.04
17	Colorado	0.00
11	Connecticut	0.03
17	Delaware	0.00
12	Florida	0.02
17	Georgia	0.00
2	Hawaii	0.67
7	Idaho	0.08
12	Illinois	0.02
17	Indiana	0.00
17	Iowa	0.00
17	Kansas	0.00
17	Kentucky	0.00
17	Louisiana	0.00
17	Maine	0.00
17	Maryland	0.00
12	Massachusetts	0.02
17	Michigan	0.00
17	Minnesota	0.00
17	Mississippi	0.00
9	Missouri	0.04
17	Montana	0.00
17	Nebraska	0.00
17	Nevada	0.00
17	New Hampshire	0.00
17	New Jersey	0.00
17	New Mexico	0.00
4	New York	0.18
1	North Carolina	0.79
17	North Dakota	0.00
17	Ohio	0.00
17	Oklahoma	0.00
17	Oregon	0.00
17	Pennsylvania	0.00
17	Rhode Island	0.00
3	South Carolina	0.51
17	South Dakota	0.00
17	Tennessee	0.00
12	Texas	0.02
17	Utah	0.00
17	Vermont	0.00
16	Virginia	0.01
6	Washington	0.09
17	West Virginia	0.00
8	Wisconsin	0.06
17	Wyoming	0.00

RANK ORDER

RANK	STATE	RATE
1	North Carolina	0.79
2	Hawaii	0.67
3	South Carolina	0.51
4	New York	0.18
5	Arizona	0.11
6	Washington	0.09
7	Idaho	0.08
8	Wisconsin	0.06
9	California	0.04
9	Missouri	0.04
11	Connecticut	0.03
12	Florida	0.02
12	Illinois	0.02
12	Massachusetts	0.02
12	Texas	0.02
16	Virginia	0.01
17	Alabama	0.00
17	Alaska	0.00
17	Arkansas	0.00
17	Colorado	0.00
17	Delaware	0.00
17	Georgia	0.00
17	Indiana	0.00
17	Iowa	0.00
17	Kansas	0.00
17	Kentucky	0.00
17	Louisiana	0.00
17	Maine	0.00
17	Maryland	0.00
17	Michigan	0.00
17	Minnesota	0.00
17	Mississippi	0.00
17	Montana	0.00
17	Nebraska	0.00
17	Nevada	0.00
17	New Hampshire	0.00
17	New Jersey	0.00
17	New Mexico	0.00
17	North Dakota	0.00
17	Ohio	0.00
17	Oklahoma	0.00
17	Oregon	0.00
17	Pennsylvania	0.00
17	Rhode Island	0.00
17	South Dakota	0.00
17	Tennessee	0.00
17	Utah	0.00
17	Vermont	0.00
17	West Virginia	0.00
17	Wyoming	0.00

District of Columbia — 0.19

Source: Morgan Quitno Press using data from U.S. Dept. of Health & Human Serv's, National Center for Health Statistics
"Morbidity and Mortality Weekly Report" (January 9, 1998, Vol. 46, Nos. 52 & 53)
*Provisional data. A mild, contagious, eruptive disease caused by a virus and capable of producing congenital defects in infants born to mothers infected during the first three months of pregnancy.

Hepatitis (Viral) Cases Reported in 1997

National Total = 36,548 Cases*

ALPHA ORDER

RANK	STATE	CASES	% of USA
36	Alabama	170	0.47%
44	Alaska	55	0.15%
3	Arizona	2,582	7.06%
29	Arkansas	284	0.78%
1	California	7,888	21.58%
16	Colorado	561	1.53%
35	Connecticut	190	0.52%
46	Delaware	37	0.10%
8	Florida	1,065	2.91%
12	Georgia	805	2.20%
38	Hawaii	146	0.40%
32	Idaho	204	0.56%
9	Illinois	933	2.55%
23	Indiana	415	1.14%
17	Iowa	539	1.47%
28	Kansas	290	0.79%
40	Kentucky	116	0.32%
24	Louisiana	410	1.12%
43	Maine	72	0.20%
24	Maryland	410	1.12%
27	Massachusetts	297	0.81%
5	Michigan	1,798	4.92%
30	Minnesota	240	0.66%
34	Mississippi	192	0.53%
7	Missouri	1,435	3.93%
41	Montana	84	0.23%
39	Nebraska	125	0.34%
19	Nevada	494	1.35%
45	New Hampshire	53	0.15%
18	New Jersey	509	1.39%
15	New Mexico	622	1.70%
4	New York	1,843	5.04%
21	North Carolina	476	1.30%
50	North Dakota	16	0.04%
22	Ohio	426	1.17%
6	Oklahoma	1,476	4.04%
20	Oregon	487	1.33%
10	Pennsylvania	880	2.41%
37	Rhode Island	148	0.40%
31	South Carolina	208	0.57%
47	South Dakota	28	0.08%
11	Tennessee	851	2.33%
2	Texas	4,533	12.40%
14	Utah	639	1.75%
49	Vermont	25	0.07%
26	Virginia	361	0.99%
13	Washington	753	2.06%
47	West Virginia	28	0.08%
33	Wisconsin	202	0.55%
42	Wyoming	81	0.22%

RANK ORDER

RANK	STATE	CASES	% of USA
1	California	7,888	21.58%
2	Texas	4,533	12.40%
3	Arizona	2,582	7.06%
4	New York	1,843	5.04%
5	Michigan	1,798	4.92%
6	Oklahoma	1,476	4.04%
7	Missouri	1,435	3.93%
8	Florida	1,065	2.91%
9	Illinois	933	2.55%
10	Pennsylvania	880	2.41%
11	Tennessee	851	2.33%
12	Georgia	805	2.20%
13	Washington	753	2.06%
14	Utah	639	1.75%
15	New Mexico	622	1.70%
16	Colorado	561	1.53%
17	Iowa	539	1.47%
18	New Jersey	509	1.39%
19	Nevada	494	1.35%
20	Oregon	487	1.33%
21	North Carolina	476	1.30%
22	Ohio	426	1.17%
23	Indiana	415	1.14%
24	Louisiana	410	1.12%
24	Maryland	410	1.12%
26	Virginia	361	0.99%
27	Massachusetts	297	0.81%
28	Kansas	290	0.79%
29	Arkansas	284	0.78%
30	Minnesota	240	0.66%
31	South Carolina	208	0.57%
32	Idaho	204	0.56%
33	Wisconsin	202	0.55%
34	Mississippi	192	0.53%
35	Connecticut	190	0.52%
36	Alabama	170	0.47%
37	Rhode Island	148	0.40%
38	Hawaii	146	0.40%
39	Nebraska	125	0.34%
40	Kentucky	116	0.32%
41	Montana	84	0.23%
42	Wyoming	81	0.22%
43	Maine	72	0.20%
44	Alaska	55	0.15%
45	New Hampshire	53	0.15%
46	Delaware	37	0.10%
47	South Dakota	28	0.08%
47	West Virginia	28	0.08%
49	Vermont	25	0.07%
50	North Dakota	16	0.04%
	District of Columbia	66	0.18%

Source: U.S. Department of Health and Human Services, National Center for Health Statistics
"Morbidity and Mortality Weekly Report" (January 9, 1998, Vol. 46, Nos. 52 & 53)
*Provisional data. An inflammation of the liver. Includes types A and B.

Hepatitis (Viral) Rate in 1997

National Rate = 13.7 Cases per 100,000 Population*

ALPHA ORDER

RANK	STATE	RATE
44	Alabama	3.9
25	Alaska	9.0
1	Arizona	56.7
19	Arkansas	11.3
7	California	24.4
16	Colorado	14.4
35	Connecticut	5.8
39	Delaware	5.1
29	Florida	7.3
21	Georgia	10.8
18	Hawaii	12.3
11	Idaho	16.9
27	Illinois	7.8
31	Indiana	7.1
9	Iowa	18.9
20	Kansas	11.2
48	Kentucky	3.0
24	Louisiana	9.4
35	Maine	5.8
26	Maryland	8.0
41	Massachusetts	4.9
10	Michigan	18.4
39	Minnesota	5.1
32	Mississippi	7.0
6	Missouri	26.6
23	Montana	9.6
28	Nebraska	7.5
5	Nevada	29.5
42	New Hampshire	4.5
34	New Jersey	6.3
3	New Mexico	36.0
22	New York	10.2
33	North Carolina	6.4
49	North Dakota	2.5
46	Ohio	3.8
2	Oklahoma	44.5
14	Oregon	15.0
29	Pennsylvania	7.3
14	Rhode Island	15.0
37	South Carolina	5.5
46	South Dakota	3.8
13	Tennessee	15.9
8	Texas	23.3
4	Utah	31.0
43	Vermont	4.2
38	Virginia	5.4
17	Washington	13.4
50	West Virginia	1.5
44	Wisconsin	3.9
11	Wyoming	16.9

RANK ORDER

RANK	STATE	RATE
1	Arizona	56.7
2	Oklahoma	44.5
3	New Mexico	36.0
4	Utah	31.0
5	Nevada	29.5
6	Missouri	26.6
7	California	24.4
8	Texas	23.3
9	Iowa	18.9
10	Michigan	18.4
11	Idaho	16.9
11	Wyoming	16.9
13	Tennessee	15.9
14	Oregon	15.0
14	Rhode Island	15.0
16	Colorado	14.4
17	Washington	13.4
18	Hawaii	12.3
19	Arkansas	11.3
20	Kansas	11.2
21	Georgia	10.8
22	New York	10.2
23	Montana	9.6
24	Louisiana	9.4
25	Alaska	9.0
26	Maryland	8.0
27	Illinois	7.8
28	Nebraska	7.5
29	Florida	7.3
29	Pennsylvania	7.3
31	Indiana	7.1
32	Mississippi	7.0
33	North Carolina	6.4
34	New Jersey	6.3
35	Connecticut	5.8
35	Maine	5.8
37	South Carolina	5.5
38	Virginia	5.4
39	Delaware	5.1
39	Minnesota	5.1
41	Massachusetts	4.9
42	New Hampshire	4.5
43	Vermont	4.2
44	Alabama	3.9
44	Wisconsin	3.9
46	Ohio	3.8
46	South Dakota	3.8
48	Kentucky	3.0
49	North Dakota	2.5
50	West Virginia	1.5

District of Columbia	12.5

Source: Morgan Quitno Press using data from U.S. Dept. of Health & Human Serv's, National Center for Health Statistics
"Morbidity and Mortality Weekly Report" (January 9, 1998, Vol. 46, Nos. 52 & 53)
*Provisional data. An inflammation of the liver. Includes types A and B.

Legionellosis Cases Reported in 1997

National Total = 1,054 Cases*

ALPHA ORDER

RANK	STATE	CASES	% of USA
34	Alabama	4	0.38%
47	Alaska	0	0.00%
25	Arizona	12	1.14%
47	Arkansas	0	0.00%
5	California	64	6.07%
18	Colorado	18	1.71%
15	Connecticut	20	1.90%
23	Delaware	13	1.23%
7	Florida	35	3.32%
39	Georgia	2	0.19%
44	Hawaii	1	0.09%
39	Idaho	2	0.19%
10	Illinois	28	2.66%
6	Indiana	54	5.12%
25	Iowa	12	1.14%
33	Kansas	6	0.57%
25	Kentucky	12	1.14%
29	Louisiana	8	0.76%
39	Maine	2	0.19%
10	Maryland	28	2.66%
12	Massachusetts	27	2.56%
3	Michigan	92	8.73%
36	Minnesota	3	0.28%
34	Mississippi	4	0.38%
9	Missouri	32	3.04%
44	Montana	1	0.09%
21	Nebraska	15	1.42%
31	Nevada	7	0.66%
31	New Hampshire	7	0.66%
15	New Jersey	20	1.90%
36	New Mexico	3	0.28%
4	New York	87	8.25%
22	North Carolina	14	1.33%
39	North Dakota	2	0.19%
1	Ohio	121	11.48%
36	Oklahoma	3	0.28%
47	Oregon	0	0.00%
2	Pennsylvania	120	11.39%
20	Rhode Island	16	1.52%
29	South Carolina	8	0.76%
39	South Dakota	2	0.19%
8	Tennessee	33	3.13%
14	Texas	23	2.18%
17	Utah	19	1.80%
23	Vermont	13	1.23%
12	Virginia	27	2.56%
28	Washington	10	0.95%
NA	West Virginia**	NA	NA
19	Wisconsin	17	1.61%
44	Wyoming	1	0.09%

RANK ORDER

RANK	STATE	CASES	% of USA
1	Ohio	121	11.48%
2	Pennsylvania	120	11.39%
3	Michigan	92	8.73%
4	New York	87	8.25%
5	California	64	6.07%
6	Indiana	54	5.12%
7	Florida	35	3.32%
8	Tennessee	33	3.13%
9	Missouri	32	3.04%
10	Illinois	28	2.66%
10	Maryland	28	2.66%
12	Massachusetts	27	2.56%
12	Virginia	27	2.56%
14	Texas	23	2.18%
15	Connecticut	20	1.90%
15	New Jersey	20	1.90%
17	Utah	19	1.80%
18	Colorado	18	1.71%
19	Wisconsin	17	1.61%
20	Rhode Island	16	1.52%
21	Nebraska	15	1.42%
22	North Carolina	14	1.33%
23	Delaware	13	1.23%
23	Vermont	13	1.23%
25	Arizona	12	1.14%
25	Iowa	12	1.14%
25	Kentucky	12	1.14%
28	Washington	10	0.95%
29	Louisiana	8	0.76%
29	South Carolina	8	0.76%
31	Nevada	7	0.66%
31	New Hampshire	7	0.66%
33	Kansas	6	0.57%
34	Alabama	4	0.38%
34	Mississippi	4	0.38%
36	Minnesota	3	0.28%
36	New Mexico	3	0.28%
36	Oklahoma	3	0.28%
39	Georgia	2	0.19%
39	Idaho	2	0.19%
39	Maine	2	0.19%
39	North Dakota	2	0.19%
39	South Dakota	2	0.19%
44	Hawaii	1	0.09%
44	Montana	1	0.09%
44	Wyoming	1	0.09%
47	Alaska	0	0.00%
47	Arkansas	0	0.00%
47	Oregon	0	0.00%
NA	West Virginia**	NA	NA
	District of Columbia	5	0.47%

*Source: U.S. Department of Health and Human Services, National Center for Health Statistics
"Morbidity and Mortality Weekly Report" (January 9, 1998, Vol. 46, Nos. 52 & 53)*
Provisional data. A pneumonia-like disease (Legionnaire's Disease).
**Not notifiable.*

Legionellosis Rate in 1997

National Rate = 0.4 Cases per 100,000 Population*

<u>ALPHA ORDER</u>

RANK	STATE	RATE
39	Alabama	0.1
46	Alaska	0.0
21	Arizona	0.3
46	Arkansas	0.0
26	California	0.2
14	Colorado	0.5
10	Connecticut	0.6
2	Delaware	1.8
26	Florida	0.2
46	Georgia	0.0
39	Hawaii	0.1
26	Idaho	0.2
26	Illinois	0.2
6	Indiana	0.9
17	Iowa	0.4
26	Kansas	0.2
21	Kentucky	0.3
26	Louisiana	0.2
26	Maine	0.2
14	Maryland	0.5
17	Massachusetts	0.4
6	Michigan	0.9
39	Minnesota	0.1
39	Mississippi	0.1
10	Missouri	0.6
39	Montana	0.1
6	Nebraska	0.9
17	Nevada	0.4
10	New Hampshire	0.6
26	New Jersey	0.2
26	New Mexico	0.2
14	New York	0.5
26	North Carolina	0.2
21	North Dakota	0.3
4	Ohio	1.1
39	Oklahoma	0.1
46	Oregon	0.0
5	Pennsylvania	1.0
3	Rhode Island	1.6
26	South Carolina	0.2
21	South Dakota	0.3
10	Tennessee	0.6
39	Texas	0.1
6	Utah	0.9
1	Vermont	2.2
17	Virginia	0.4
26	Washington	0.2
NA	West Virginia**	NA
21	Wisconsin	0.3
26	Wyoming	0.2

<u>RANK ORDER</u>

RANK	STATE	RATE
1	Vermont	2.2
2	Delaware	1.8
3	Rhode Island	1.6
4	Ohio	1.1
5	Pennsylvania	1.0
6	Indiana	0.9
6	Michigan	0.9
6	Nebraska	0.9
6	Utah	0.9
10	Connecticut	0.6
10	Missouri	0.6
10	New Hampshire	0.6
10	Tennessee	0.6
14	Colorado	0.5
14	Maryland	0.5
14	New York	0.5
17	Iowa	0.4
17	Massachusetts	0.4
17	Nevada	0.4
17	Virginia	0.4
21	Arizona	0.3
21	Kentucky	0.3
21	North Dakota	0.3
21	South Dakota	0.3
21	Wisconsin	0.3
26	California	0.2
26	Florida	0.2
26	Idaho	0.2
26	Illinois	0.2
26	Kansas	0.2
26	Louisiana	0.2
26	Maine	0.2
26	New Jersey	0.2
26	New Mexico	0.2
26	North Carolina	0.2
26	South Carolina	0.2
26	Washington	0.2
26	Wyoming	0.2
39	Alabama	0.1
39	Hawaii	0.1
39	Minnesota	0.1
39	Mississippi	0.1
39	Montana	0.1
39	Oklahoma	0.1
39	Texas	0.1
46	Alaska	0.0
46	Arkansas	0.0
46	Georgia	0.0
46	Oregon	0.0
NA	West Virginia**	NA
	District of Columbia	0.9

Source: Morgan Quitno Press using data from U.S. Dept. of Health & Human Serv's, National Center for Health Statistics "Morbidity and Mortality Weekly Report" (January 9, 1998, Vol. 46, Nos. 52 & 53)
*Provisional data. A pneumonia-like disease (Legionnaire's Disease).
**Not notifiable.

Lyme Disease Cases Reported in 1997

National Total = 10,979 Cases*

ALPHA ORDER

RANK	STATE	CASES	% of USA
25	Alabama	11	0.10%
40	Alaska	2	0.02%
36	Arizona	4	0.04%
20	Arkansas	25	0.23%
9	California	172	1.57%
32	Colorado	6	0.05%
2	Connecticut	2,184	19.89%
10	Delaware	105	0.96%
13	Florida	48	0.44%
31	Georgia	7	0.06%
46	Hawaii	0	0.00%
36	Idaho	4	0.04%
32	Illinois	6	0.05%
19	Indiana	29	0.26%
27	Iowa	10	0.09%
36	Kansas	4	0.04%
23	Kentucky	15	0.14%
32	Louisiana	6	0.05%
25	Maine	11	0.10%
5	Maryland	499	4.55%
7	Massachusetts	387	3.52%
46	Michigan	0	0.00%
8	Minnesota	196	1.79%
24	Mississippi	14	0.13%
22	Missouri	20	0.18%
46	Montana	0	0.00%
40	Nebraska	2	0.02%
40	Nevada	2	0.02%
15	New Hampshire	39	0.36%
4	New Jersey	1,639	14.93%
43	New Mexico	1	0.01%
1	New York	2,679	24.40%
17	North Carolina	34	0.31%
46	North Dakota	0	0.00%
12	Ohio	61	0.56%
17	Oklahoma	34	0.31%
21	Oregon	21	0.19%
3	Pennsylvania	2,103	19.15%
6	Rhode Island	409	3.73%
39	South Carolina	3	0.03%
43	South Dakota	1	0.01%
14	Tennessee	45	0.41%
16	Texas	35	0.32%
43	Utah	1	0.01%
30	Vermont	8	0.07%
11	Virginia	62	0.56%
27	Washington	10	0.09%
27	West Virginia	10	0.09%
NA	Wisconsin**	NA	NA
35	Wyoming	5	0.05%

RANK ORDER

RANK	STATE	CASES	% of USA
1	New York	2,679	24.40%
2	Connecticut	2,184	19.89%
3	Pennsylvania	2,103	19.15%
4	New Jersey	1,639	14.93%
5	Maryland	499	4.55%
6	Rhode Island	409	3.73%
7	Massachusetts	387	3.52%
8	Minnesota	196	1.79%
9	California	172	1.57%
10	Delaware	105	0.96%
11	Virginia	62	0.56%
12	Ohio	61	0.56%
13	Florida	48	0.44%
14	Tennessee	45	0.41%
15	New Hampshire	39	0.36%
16	Texas	35	0.32%
17	North Carolina	34	0.31%
17	Oklahoma	34	0.31%
19	Indiana	29	0.26%
20	Arkansas	25	0.23%
21	Oregon	21	0.19%
22	Missouri	20	0.18%
23	Kentucky	15	0.14%
24	Mississippi	14	0.13%
25	Alabama	11	0.10%
25	Maine	11	0.10%
27	Iowa	10	0.09%
27	Washington	10	0.09%
27	West Virginia	10	0.09%
30	Vermont	8	0.07%
31	Georgia	7	0.06%
32	Colorado	6	0.05%
32	Illinois	6	0.05%
32	Louisiana	6	0.05%
35	Wyoming	5	0.05%
36	Arizona	4	0.04%
36	Idaho	4	0.04%
36	Kansas	4	0.04%
39	South Carolina	3	0.03%
40	Alaska	2	0.02%
40	Nebraska	2	0.02%
40	Nevada	2	0.02%
43	New Mexico	1	0.01%
43	South Dakota	1	0.01%
43	Utah	1	0.01%
46	Hawaii	0	0.00%
46	Michigan	0	0.00%
46	Montana	0	0.00%
46	North Dakota	0	0.00%
NA	Wisconsin**	NA	NA
	District of Columbia	10	0.09%

*Source: U.S. Department of Health and Human Services, National Center for Health Statistics
"Morbidity and Mortality Weekly Report" (January 9, 1998, Vol. 46, Nos. 52 & 53)*
Provisional data. Caused by ticks-lesions, followed by arthritis of large joints, myalgia, malaise and neurologic and cardiac manifestations. Named after Old Lyme, CT, where the disease was first reported.
***Not available.*

Lyme Disease Rate in 1997

National Rate = 4.1 Cases per 100,000 Population*

ALPHA ORDER

RANK	STATE	RATE
28	Alabama	0.3
28	Alaska	0.3
36	Arizona	0.1
12	Arkansas	1.0
20	California	0.5
32	Colorado	0.2
1	Connecticut	66.8
6	Delaware	14.4
28	Florida	0.3
36	Georgia	0.1
45	Hawaii	0.0
28	Idaho	0.3
36	Illinois	0.1
20	Indiana	0.5
25	Iowa	0.4
32	Kansas	0.2
25	Kentucky	0.4
36	Louisiana	0.1
15	Maine	0.9
7	Maryland	9.8
8	Massachusetts	6.3
45	Michigan	0.0
9	Minnesota	4.2
20	Mississippi	0.5
25	Missouri	0.4
45	Montana	0.0
36	Nebraska	0.1
36	Nevada	0.1
10	New Hampshire	3.3
3	New Jersey	20.4
36	New Mexico	0.1
5	New York	14.8
20	North Carolina	0.5
45	North Dakota	0.0
20	Ohio	0.5
12	Oklahoma	1.0
18	Oregon	0.6
4	Pennsylvania	17.5
2	Rhode Island	41.4
36	South Carolina	0.1
36	South Dakota	0.1
17	Tennessee	0.8
32	Texas	0.2
45	Utah	0.0
11	Vermont	1.4
15	Virginia	0.9
32	Washington	0.2
18	West Virginia	0.6
NA	Wisconsin**	NA
12	Wyoming	1.0

RANK ORDER

RANK	STATE	RATE
1	Connecticut	66.8
2	Rhode Island	41.4
3	New Jersey	20.4
4	Pennsylvania	17.5
5	New York	14.8
6	Delaware	14.4
7	Maryland	9.8
8	Massachusetts	6.3
9	Minnesota	4.2
10	New Hampshire	3.3
11	Vermont	1.4
12	Arkansas	1.0
12	Oklahoma	1.0
12	Wyoming	1.0
15	Maine	0.9
15	Virginia	0.9
17	Tennessee	0.8
18	Oregon	0.6
18	West Virginia	0.6
20	California	0.5
20	Indiana	0.5
20	Mississippi	0.5
20	North Carolina	0.5
20	Ohio	0.5
25	Iowa	0.4
25	Kentucky	0.4
25	Missouri	0.4
28	Alabama	0.3
28	Alaska	0.3
28	Florida	0.3
28	Idaho	0.3
32	Colorado	0.2
32	Kansas	0.2
32	Texas	0.2
32	Washington	0.2
36	Arizona	0.1
36	Georgia	0.1
36	Illinois	0.1
36	Louisiana	0.1
36	Nebraska	0.1
36	Nevada	0.1
36	New Mexico	0.1
36	South Carolina	0.1
36	South Dakota	0.1
45	Hawaii	0.0
45	Michigan	0.0
45	Montana	0.0
45	North Dakota	0.0
45	Utah	0.0
NA	Wisconsin**	NA

District of Columbia   1.9

Source: Morgan Quitno Press using data from U.S. Dept. of Health & Human Serv's, National Center for Health Statistics
    "Morbidity and Mortality Weekly Report" (January 9, 1998, Vol. 46, Nos. 52 & 53)
*Provisional data. Caused by ticks-lesions, followed by arthritis of large joints, myalgia, malaise and neurologic
and cardiac manifestations. Named after Old Lyme, CT, where the disease was first reported.
**Not available.

Malaria Cases Reported in 1997

National Total = 1,772 Cases*

ALPHA ORDER

RANK ORDER

RANK	STATE	CASES	% of USA
28	Alabama	10	0.56%
37	Alaska	5	0.28%
25	Arizona	11	0.62%
37	Arkansas	5	0.28%
1	California	406	22.91%
14	Colorado	30	1.69%
11	Connecticut	42	2.37%
37	Delaware	5	0.28%
3	Florida	91	5.14%
8	Georgia	52	2.93%
31	Hawaii	9	0.51%
47	Idaho	1	0.06%
7	Illinois	55	3.10%
22	Indiana	16	0.90%
28	Iowa	10	0.56%
40	Kansas	4	0.23%
33	Kentucky	8	0.45%
20	Louisiana	18	1.02%
47	Maine	1	0.06%
4	Maryland	87	4.91%
14	Massachusetts	30	1.69%
10	Michigan	43	2.43%
12	Minnesota	36	2.03%
36	Mississippi	6	0.34%
24	Missouri	13	0.73%
44	Montana	2	0.11%
47	Nebraska	1	0.06%
31	Nevada	9	0.51%
28	New Hampshire	10	0.56%
5	New Jersey	78	4.40%
33	New Mexico	8	0.45%
2	New York	331	18.68%
18	North Carolina	21	1.19%
41	North Dakota	3	0.17%
19	Ohio	19	1.07%
33	Oklahoma	8	0.45%
17	Oregon	24	1.35%
13	Pennsylvania	33	1.86%
25	Rhode Island	11	0.62%
20	South Carolina	18	1.02%
41	South Dakota	3	0.17%
25	Tennessee	11	0.62%
16	Texas	28	1.58%
41	Utah	3	0.17%
44	Vermont	2	0.11%
6	Virginia	68	3.84%
9	Washington	49	2.77%
47	West Virginia	1	0.06%
23	Wisconsin	15	0.85%
44	Wyoming	2	0.11%

RANK	STATE	CASES	% of USA
1	California	406	22.91%
2	New York	331	18.68%
3	Florida	91	5.14%
4	Maryland	87	4.91%
5	New Jersey	78	4.40%
6	Virginia	68	3.84%
7	Illinois	55	3.10%
8	Georgia	52	2.93%
9	Washington	49	2.77%
10	Michigan	43	2.43%
11	Connecticut	42	2.37%
12	Minnesota	36	2.03%
13	Pennsylvania	33	1.86%
14	Colorado	30	1.69%
14	Massachusetts	30	1.69%
16	Texas	28	1.58%
17	Oregon	24	1.35%
18	North Carolina	21	1.19%
19	Ohio	19	1.07%
20	Louisiana	18	1.02%
20	South Carolina	18	1.02%
22	Indiana	16	0.90%
23	Wisconsin	15	0.85%
24	Missouri	13	0.73%
25	Arizona	11	0.62%
25	Rhode Island	11	0.62%
25	Tennessee	11	0.62%
28	Alabama	10	0.56%
28	Iowa	10	0.56%
28	New Hampshire	10	0.56%
31	Hawaii	9	0.51%
31	Nevada	9	0.51%
33	Kentucky	8	0.45%
33	New Mexico	8	0.45%
33	Oklahoma	8	0.45%
36	Mississippi	6	0.34%
37	Alaska	5	0.28%
37	Arkansas	5	0.28%
37	Delaware	5	0.28%
40	Kansas	4	0.23%
41	North Dakota	3	0.17%
41	South Dakota	3	0.17%
41	Utah	3	0.17%
44	Montana	2	0.11%
44	Vermont	2	0.11%
44	Wyoming	2	0.11%
47	Idaho	1	0.06%
47	Maine	1	0.06%
47	Nebraska	1	0.06%
47	West Virginia	1	0.06%
	District of Columbia	20	1.13%

Source: U.S. Department of Health and Human Services, National Center for Health Statistics
    "Morbidity and Mortality Weekly Report" (January 9, 1998, Vol. 46, Nos. 52 & 53)
*Provisional data. Infectious disease usually transmitted by bites of infected mosquitoes. Symptoms include high fever, shaking chills, sweating and anemia.

Malaria Rate in 1997

National Rate = 0.7 Cases per 100,000 Population*

ALPHA ORDER

RANK ORDER

RANK	STATE	RATE		RANK	STATE	RATE
34	Alabama	0.2		1	New York	1.8
10	Alaska	0.8		2	Maryland	1.7
34	Arizona	0.2		3	California	1.3
34	Arkansas	0.2		3	Connecticut	1.3
3	California	1.3		5	Rhode Island	1.1
10	Colorado	0.8		6	New Jersey	1.0
3	Connecticut	1.3		6	Virginia	1.0
14	Delaware	0.7		8	New Hampshire	0.9
17	Florida	0.6		8	Washington	0.9
14	Georgia	0.7		10	Alaska	0.8
10	Hawaii	0.8		10	Colorado	0.8
45	Idaho	0.1		10	Hawaii	0.8
18	Illinois	0.5		10	Minnesota	0.8
29	Indiana	0.3		14	Delaware	0.7
24	Iowa	0.4		14	Georgia	0.7
34	Kansas	0.2		14	Oregon	0.7
34	Kentucky	0.2		17	Florida	0.6
24	Louisiana	0.4		18	Illinois	0.5
45	Maine	0.1		18	Massachusetts	0.5
2	Maryland	1.7		18	Nevada	0.5
18	Massachusetts	0.5		18	New Mexico	0.5
24	Michigan	0.4		18	North Dakota	0.5
10	Minnesota	0.8		18	South Carolina	0.5
34	Mississippi	0.2		24	Iowa	0.4
34	Missouri	0.2		24	Louisiana	0.4
34	Montana	0.2		24	Michigan	0.4
45	Nebraska	0.1		24	South Dakota	0.4
18	Nevada	0.5		24	Wyoming	0.4
8	New Hampshire	0.9		29	Indiana	0.3
6	New Jersey	1.0		29	North Carolina	0.3
18	New Mexico	0.5		29	Pennsylvania	0.3
1	New York	1.8		29	Vermont	0.3
29	North Carolina	0.3		29	Wisconsin	0.3
18	North Dakota	0.5		34	Alabama	0.2
34	Ohio	0.2		34	Arizona	0.2
34	Oklahoma	0.2		34	Arkansas	0.2
14	Oregon	0.7		34	Kansas	0.2
29	Pennsylvania	0.3		34	Kentucky	0.2
5	Rhode Island	1.1		34	Mississippi	0.2
18	South Carolina	0.5		34	Missouri	0.2
24	South Dakota	0.4		34	Montana	0.2
34	Tennessee	0.2		34	Ohio	0.2
45	Texas	0.1		34	Oklahoma	0.2
45	Utah	0.1		34	Tennessee	0.2
29	Vermont	0.3		45	Idaho	0.1
6	Virginia	1.0		45	Maine	0.1
8	Washington	0.9		45	Nebraska	0.1
45	West Virginia	0.1		45	Texas	0.1
29	Wisconsin	0.3		45	Utah	0.1
24	Wyoming	0.4		45	West Virginia	0.1

District of Columbia   3.8

Source: Morgan Quitno Press using data from U.S. Dept. of Health & Human Serv's, National Center for Health Statistics
    "Morbidity and Mortality Weekly Report" (January 9, 1998, Vol. 46, Nos. 52 & 53)
*Provisional data. Infectious disease usually transmitted by bites of infected mosquitoes. Symptoms include high
fever, shaking chills, sweating and anemia.

Measles (Rubeola) Cases Reported in 1997

National Total = 135 Cases*

RANK	STATE	CASES	% of USA
28	Alabama	0	0.00%
28	Alaska	0	0.00%
10	Arizona	5	3.70%
28	Arkansas	0	0.00%
1	California	23	17.04%
28	Colorado	0	0.00%
18	Connecticut	1	0.74%
28	Delaware	0	0.00%
7	Florida	7	5.19%
18	Georgia	1	0.74%
11	Hawaii	4	2.96%
28	Idaho	0	0.00%
7	Illinois	7	5.19%
28	Indiana	0	0.00%
18	Iowa	1	0.74%
28	Kansas	0	0.00%
28	Kentucky	0	0.00%
28	Louisiana	0	0.00%
18	Maine	1	0.74%
13	Maryland	2	1.48%
2	Massachusetts	16	11.85%
13	Michigan	2	1.48%
4	Minnesota	8	5.93%
28	Mississippi	0	0.00%
18	Missouri	1	0.74%
28	Montana	0	0.00%
28	Nebraska	0	0.00%
13	Nevada	2	1.48%
18	New Hampshire	1	0.74%
12	New Jersey	3	2.22%
28	New Mexico	0	0.00%
2	New York	16	11.85%
13	North Carolina	2	1.48%
28	North Dakota	0	0.00%
28	Ohio	0	0.00%
18	Oklahoma	1	0.74%
28	Oregon	0	0.00%
4	Pennsylvania	8	5.93%
28	Rhode Island	0	0.00%
18	South Carolina	1	0.74%
4	South Dakota	8	5.93%
28	Tennessee	0	0.00%
7	Texas	7	5.19%
18	Utah	1	0.74%
28	Vermont	0	0.00%
18	Virginia	1	0.74%
13	Washington	2	1.48%
28	West Virginia	0	0.00%
28	Wisconsin	0	0.00%
28	Wyoming	0	0.00%

RANK	STATE	CASES	% of USA
1	California	23	17.04%
2	Massachusetts	16	11.85%
2	New York	16	11.85%
4	Minnesota	8	5.93%
4	Pennsylvania	8	5.93%
4	South Dakota	8	5.93%
7	Florida	7	5.19%
7	Illinois	7	5.19%
7	Texas	7	5.19%
10	Arizona	5	3.70%
11	Hawaii	4	2.96%
12	New Jersey	3	2.22%
13	Maryland	2	1.48%
13	Michigan	2	1.48%
13	Nevada	2	1.48%
13	North Carolina	2	1.48%
13	Washington	2	1.48%
18	Connecticut	1	0.74%
18	Georgia	1	0.74%
18	Iowa	1	0.74%
18	Maine	1	0.74%
18	Missouri	1	0.74%
18	New Hampshire	1	0.74%
18	Oklahoma	1	0.74%
18	South Carolina	1	0.74%
18	Utah	1	0.74%
18	Virginia	1	0.74%
28	Alabama	0	0.00%
28	Alaska	0	0.00%
28	Arkansas	0	0.00%
28	Colorado	0	0.00%
28	Delaware	0	0.00%
28	Idaho	0	0.00%
28	Indiana	0	0.00%
28	Kansas	0	0.00%
28	Kentucky	0	0.00%
28	Louisiana	0	0.00%
28	Mississippi	0	0.00%
28	Montana	0	0.00%
28	Nebraska	0	0.00%
28	New Mexico	0	0.00%
28	North Dakota	0	0.00%
28	Ohio	0	0.00%
28	Oregon	0	0.00%
28	Rhode Island	0	0.00%
28	Tennessee	0	0.00%
28	Vermont	0	0.00%
28	West Virginia	0	0.00%
28	Wisconsin	0	0.00%
28	Wyoming	0	0.00%
	District of Columbia	3	2.22%

Source: U.S. Department of Health and Human Services, National Center for Health Statistics
"Morbidity and Mortality Weekly Report" (January 9, 1998, Vol. 46, Nos. 52 & 53)
*Provisional data. Includes indigenous and imported cases.

Measles (Rubeola) Rate in 1997

National Rate = 0.05 Cases per 100,000 Population*

ALPHA ORDER

RANK	STATE	RATE
28	Alabama	0.00
28	Alaska	0.00
6	Arizona	0.11
28	Arkansas	0.00
10	California	0.07
28	Colorado	0.00
20	Connecticut	0.03
28	Delaware	0.00
13	Florida	0.05
26	Georgia	0.01
2	Hawaii	0.34
28	Idaho	0.00
12	Illinois	0.06
28	Indiana	0.00
15	Iowa	0.04
28	Kansas	0.00
28	Kentucky	0.00
28	Louisiana	0.00
9	Maine	0.08
15	Maryland	0.04
3	Massachusetts	0.26
24	Michigan	0.02
4	Minnesota	0.17
28	Mississippi	0.00
24	Missouri	0.02
28	Montana	0.00
28	Nebraska	0.00
5	Nevada	0.12
7	New Hampshire	0.09
15	New Jersey	0.04
28	New Mexico	0.00
7	New York	0.09
20	North Carolina	0.03
28	North Dakota	0.00
28	Ohio	0.00
20	Oklahoma	0.03
28	Oregon	0.00
10	Pennsylvania	0.07
28	Rhode Island	0.00
20	South Carolina	0.03
1	South Dakota	1.08
28	Tennessee	0.00
15	Texas	0.04
13	Utah	0.05
28	Vermont	0.00
26	Virginia	0.01
15	Washington	0.04
28	West Virginia	0.00
28	Wisconsin	0.00
28	Wyoming	0.00

RANK ORDER

RANK	STATE	RATE
1	South Dakota	1.08
2	Hawaii	0.34
3	Massachusetts	0.26
4	Minnesota	0.17
5	Nevada	0.12
6	Arizona	0.11
7	New Hampshire	0.09
7	New York	0.09
9	Maine	0.08
10	California	0.07
10	Pennsylvania	0.07
12	Illinois	0.06
13	Florida	0.05
13	Utah	0.05
15	Iowa	0.04
15	Maryland	0.04
15	New Jersey	0.04
15	Texas	0.04
15	Washington	0.04
20	Connecticut	0.03
20	North Carolina	0.03
20	Oklahoma	0.03
20	South Carolina	0.03
24	Michigan	0.02
24	Missouri	0.02
26	Georgia	0.01
26	Virginia	0.01
28	Alabama	0.00
28	Alaska	0.00
28	Arkansas	0.00
28	Colorado	0.00
28	Delaware	0.00
28	Idaho	0.00
28	Indiana	0.00
28	Kansas	0.00
28	Kentucky	0.00
28	Louisiana	0.00
28	Mississippi	0.00
28	Montana	0.00
28	Nebraska	0.00
28	New Mexico	0.00
28	North Dakota	0.00
28	Ohio	0.00
28	Oregon	0.00
28	Rhode Island	0.00
28	Tennessee	0.00
28	Vermont	0.00
28	West Virginia	0.00
28	Wisconsin	0.00
28	Wyoming	0.00

District of Columbia   0.57

Source: Morgan Quitno Press using data from U.S. Dept. of Health & Human Serv's, National Center for Health Statistics
"Morbidity and Mortality Weekly Report" (January 9, 1998, Vol. 46, Nos. 52 & 53)
*Provisional data. Includes indigenous and imported cases.

Meningococcal Infections Reported in 1997

National Total = 3,117 Cases*

ALPHA ORDER

RANK	STATE	CASES	% of USA
14	Alabama	85	2.73%
49	Alaska	3	0.10%
25	Arizona	46	1.48%
30	Arkansas	34	1.09%
1	California	396	12.70%
21	Colorado	51	1.64%
27	Connecticut	42	1.35%
46	Delaware	5	0.16%
3	Florida	162	5.20%
10	Georgia	106	3.40%
44	Hawaii	7	0.22%
41	Idaho	15	0.48%
5	Illinois	148	4.75%
18	Indiana	58	1.86%
22	Iowa	48	1.54%
33	Kansas	22	0.71%
22	Kentucky	48	1.54%
22	Louisiana	48	1.54%
37	Maine	18	0.58%
27	Maryland	42	1.35%
11	Massachusetts	102	3.27%
20	Michigan	53	1.70%
30	Minnesota	34	1.09%
35	Mississippi	19	0.61%
9	Missouri	109	3.50%
43	Montana	9	0.29%
42	Nebraska	14	0.45%
35	Nevada	19	0.61%
37	New Hampshire	18	0.58%
16	New Jersey	73	2.34%
32	New Mexico	30	0.96%
8	New York	121	3.88%
12	North Carolina	97	3.11%
50	North Dakota	2	0.06%
2	Ohio	164	5.26%
26	Oklahoma	45	1.44%
7	Oregon	126	4.04%
6	Pennsylvania	131	4.20%
34	Rhode Island	21	0.67%
17	South Carolina	61	1.96%
45	South Dakota	6	0.19%
14	Tennessee	85	2.73%
4	Texas	155	4.97%
40	Utah	16	0.51%
47	Vermont	4	0.13%
18	Virginia	58	1.86%
13	Washington	92	2.95%
37	West Virginia	18	0.58%
29	Wisconsin	38	1.22%
47	Wyoming	4	0.13%

RANK ORDER

RANK	STATE	CASES	% of USA
1	California	396	12.70%
2	Ohio	164	5.26%
3	Florida	162	5.20%
4	Texas	155	4.97%
5	Illinois	148	4.75%
6	Pennsylvania	131	4.20%
7	Oregon	126	4.04%
8	New York	121	3.88%
9	Missouri	109	3.50%
10	Georgia	106	3.40%
11	Massachusetts	102	3.27%
12	North Carolina	97	3.11%
13	Washington	92	2.95%
14	Alabama	85	2.73%
14	Tennessee	85	2.73%
16	New Jersey	73	2.34%
17	South Carolina	61	1.96%
18	Indiana	58	1.86%
18	Virginia	58	1.86%
20	Michigan	53	1.70%
21	Colorado	51	1.64%
22	Iowa	48	1.54%
22	Kentucky	48	1.54%
22	Louisiana	48	1.54%
25	Arizona	46	1.48%
26	Oklahoma	45	1.44%
27	Connecticut	42	1.35%
27	Maryland	42	1.35%
29	Wisconsin	38	1.22%
30	Arkansas	34	1.09%
30	Minnesota	34	1.09%
32	New Mexico	30	0.96%
33	Kansas	22	0.71%
34	Rhode Island	21	0.67%
35	Mississippi	19	0.61%
35	Nevada	19	0.61%
37	Maine	18	0.58%
37	New Hampshire	18	0.58%
37	West Virginia	18	0.58%
40	Utah	16	0.51%
41	Idaho	15	0.48%
42	Nebraska	14	0.45%
43	Montana	9	0.29%
44	Hawaii	7	0.22%
45	South Dakota	6	0.19%
46	Delaware	5	0.16%
47	Vermont	4	0.13%
47	Wyoming	4	0.13%
49	Alaska	3	0.10%
50	North Dakota	2	0.06%
	District of Columbia	9	0.29%

Source: U.S. Department of Health and Human Services, National Center for Health Statistics
"Morbidity and Mortality Weekly Report" (January 9, 1998, Vol. 46, Nos. 52 & 53)
*Provisional data. A bacterium (Neisseria meningitidis) that causes cerebrospinal meningitis.

Meningococcal Infection Rate in 1997

National Rate = 1.2 Cases per 100,000 Population*

ALPHA ORDER

RANK	STATE	RATE
3	Alabama	2.0
48	Alaska	0.5
28	Arizona	1.0
16	Arkansas	1.3
20	California	1.2
16	Colorado	1.3
16	Connecticut	1.3
41	Delaware	0.7
24	Florida	1.1
13	Georgia	1.4
47	Hawaii	0.6
20	Idaho	1.2
20	Illinois	1.2
28	Indiana	1.0
5	Iowa	1.7
34	Kansas	0.8
20	Kentucky	1.2
24	Louisiana	1.1
13	Maine	1.4
34	Maryland	0.8
5	Massachusetts	1.7
48	Michigan	0.5
41	Minnesota	0.7
41	Mississippi	0.7
3	Missouri	2.0
28	Montana	1.0
34	Nebraska	0.8
24	Nevada	1.1
11	New Hampshire	1.5
32	New Jersey	0.9
5	New Mexico	1.7
41	New York	0.7
16	North Carolina	1.3
50	North Dakota	0.3
11	Ohio	1.5
13	Oklahoma	1.4
1	Oregon	3.9
24	Pennsylvania	1.1
2	Rhode Island	2.1
8	South Carolina	1.6
34	South Dakota	0.8
8	Tennessee	1.6
34	Texas	0.8
34	Utah	0.8
41	Vermont	0.7
32	Virginia	0.9
8	Washington	1.6
28	West Virginia	1.0
41	Wisconsin	0.7
34	Wyoming	0.8

RANK ORDER

RANK	STATE	RATE
1	Oregon	3.9
2	Rhode Island	2.1
3	Alabama	2.0
3	Missouri	2.0
5	Iowa	1.7
5	Massachusetts	1.7
5	New Mexico	1.7
8	South Carolina	1.6
8	Tennessee	1.6
8	Washington	1.6
11	New Hampshire	1.5
11	Ohio	1.5
13	Georgia	1.4
13	Maine	1.4
13	Oklahoma	1.4
16	Arkansas	1.3
16	Colorado	1.3
16	Connecticut	1.3
16	North Carolina	1.3
20	California	1.2
20	Idaho	1.2
20	Illinois	1.2
20	Kentucky	1.2
24	Florida	1.1
24	Louisiana	1.1
24	Nevada	1.1
24	Pennsylvania	1.1
28	Arizona	1.0
28	Indiana	1.0
28	Montana	1.0
28	West Virginia	1.0
32	New Jersey	0.9
32	Virginia	0.9
34	Kansas	0.8
34	Maryland	0.8
34	Nebraska	0.8
34	South Dakota	0.8
34	Texas	0.8
34	Utah	0.8
34	Wyoming	0.8
41	Delaware	0.7
41	Minnesota	0.7
41	Mississippi	0.7
41	New York	0.7
41	Vermont	0.7
41	Wisconsin	0.7
47	Hawaii	0.6
48	Alaska	0.5
48	Michigan	0.5
50	North Dakota	0.3

District of Columbia	1.7

Source: Morgan Quitno Press using data from U.S. Dept. of Health & Human Serv's, National Center for Health Statistics
"Morbidity and Mortality Weekly Report" (January 9, 1998, Vol. 46, Nos. 52 & 53)
*Provisional data. A bacterium (Neisseria meningitidis) that causes cerebrospinal meningitis.

Mumps Cases Reported in 1997

National Total = 612 Cases*

ALPHA ORDER

RANK	STATE	CASES	% of USA
20	Alabama	9	1.47%
29	Alaska	4	0.65%
5	Arizona	34	5.56%
35	Arkansas	1	0.16%
1	California	147	24.02%
31	Colorado	3	0.49%
35	Connecticut	1	0.16%
39	Delaware	0	0.00%
7	Florida	23	3.76%
17	Georgia	10	1.63%
6	Hawaii	24	3.92%
26	Idaho	6	0.98%
14	Illinois	13	2.12%
13	Indiana	14	2.29%
17	Iowa	10	1.63%
39	Kansas	0	0.00%
31	Kentucky	3	0.49%
10	Louisiana	16	2.61%
39	Maine	0	0.00%
17	Maryland	10	1.63%
29	Massachusetts	4	0.65%
12	Michigan	15	2.45%
26	Minnesota	6	0.98%
20	Mississippi	9	1.47%
39	Missouri	0	0.00%
39	Montana	0	0.00%
34	Nebraska	2	0.33%
23	Nevada	7	1.14%
35	New Hampshire	1	0.16%
23	New Jersey	7	1.14%
NA	New Mexico**	NA	NA
10	New York	16	2.61%
15	North Carolina	12	1.96%
39	North Dakota	0	0.00%
4	Ohio	35	5.72%
39	Oklahoma	0	0.00%
NA	Oregon**	NA	NA
3	Pennsylvania	36	5.88%
26	Rhode Island	6	0.98%
16	South Carolina	11	1.80%
39	South Dakota	0	0.00%
23	Tennessee	7	1.14%
2	Texas	58	9.48%
22	Utah	8	1.31%
39	Vermont	0	0.00%
9	Virginia	19	3.10%
8	Washington	21	3.43%
39	West Virginia	0	0.00%
31	Wisconsin	3	0.49%
35	Wyoming	1	0.16%

RANK ORDER

RANK	STATE	CASES	% of USA
1	California	147	24.02%
2	Texas	58	9.48%
3	Pennsylvania	36	5.88%
4	Ohio	35	5.72%
5	Arizona	34	5.56%
6	Hawaii	24	3.92%
7	Florida	23	3.76%
8	Washington	21	3.43%
9	Virginia	19	3.10%
10	Louisiana	16	2.61%
10	New York	16	2.61%
12	Michigan	15	2.45%
13	Indiana	14	2.29%
14	Illinois	13	2.12%
15	North Carolina	12	1.96%
16	South Carolina	11	1.80%
17	Georgia	10	1.63%
17	Iowa	10	1.63%
17	Maryland	10	1.63%
20	Alabama	9	1.47%
20	Mississippi	9	1.47%
22	Utah	8	1.31%
23	Nevada	7	1.14%
23	New Jersey	7	1.14%
23	Tennessee	7	1.14%
26	Idaho	6	0.98%
26	Minnesota	6	0.98%
26	Rhode Island	6	0.98%
29	Alaska	4	0.65%
29	Massachusetts	4	0.65%
31	Colorado	3	0.49%
31	Kentucky	3	0.49%
31	Wisconsin	3	0.49%
34	Nebraska	2	0.33%
35	Arkansas	1	0.16%
35	Connecticut	1	0.16%
35	New Hampshire	1	0.16%
35	Wyoming	1	0.16%
39	Delaware	0	0.00%
39	Kansas	0	0.00%
39	Maine	0	0.00%
39	Missouri	0	0.00%
39	Montana	0	0.00%
39	North Dakota	0	0.00%
39	Oklahoma	0	0.00%
39	South Dakota	0	0.00%
39	Vermont	0	0.00%
39	West Virginia	0	0.00%
NA	New Mexico**	NA	NA
NA	Oregon**	NA	NA
	District of Columbia	0	0.00%

Source: U.S. Department of Health and Human Services, National Center for Health Statistics
"Morbidity and Mortality Weekly Report" (January 9, 1998, Vol. 46, Nos. 52 & 53)
Provisional data. An acute, inflammatory, contagious disease caused by a paramyxovirus and characterized by swelling of the salivary glands, especially the parotids, and sometimes of the pancreas, ovaries, or testes. This disease, mainly affecting children, can be prevented by vaccination.
**Mumps is not a notifiable disease in New Mexico or Oregon.*

Mumps Rate in 1997

National Rate = 0.23 Cases per 100,000 Population*

ALPHA ORDER

RANK	STATE	RATE
19	Alabama	0.21
3	Alaska	0.66
2	Arizona	0.75
37	Arkansas	0.04
6	California	0.46
33	Colorado	0.08
38	Connecticut	0.03
39	Delaware	0.00
22	Florida	0.16
25	Georgia	0.13
1	Hawaii	2.02
5	Idaho	0.50
29	Illinois	0.11
18	Indiana	0.24
11	Iowa	0.35
39	Kansas	0.00
33	Kentucky	0.08
9	Louisiana	0.37
39	Maine	0.00
21	Maryland	0.20
35	Massachusetts	0.07
24	Michigan	0.15
25	Minnesota	0.13
12	Mississippi	0.33
39	Missouri	0.00
39	Montana	0.00
28	Nebraska	0.12
7	Nevada	0.42
30	New Hampshire	0.09
30	New Jersey	0.09
NA	New Mexico**	NA
30	New York	0.09
22	North Carolina	0.16
39	North Dakota	0.00
13	Ohio	0.31
39	Oklahoma	0.00
NA	Oregon**	NA
14	Pennsylvania	0.30
4	Rhode Island	0.61
16	South Carolina	0.29
39	South Dakota	0.00
25	Tennessee	0.13
14	Texas	0.30
8	Utah	0.39
39	Vermont	0.00
17	Virginia	0.28
9	Washington	0.37
39	West Virginia	0.00
36	Wisconsin	0.06
19	Wyoming	0.21

RANK ORDER

RANK	STATE	RATE
1	Hawaii	2.02
2	Arizona	0.75
3	Alaska	0.66
4	Rhode Island	0.61
5	Idaho	0.50
6	California	0.46
7	Nevada	0.42
8	Utah	0.39
9	Louisiana	0.37
9	Washington	0.37
11	Iowa	0.35
12	Mississippi	0.33
13	Ohio	0.31
14	Pennsylvania	0.30
14	Texas	0.30
16	South Carolina	0.29
17	Virginia	0.28
18	Indiana	0.24
19	Alabama	0.21
19	Wyoming	0.21
21	Maryland	0.20
22	Florida	0.16
22	North Carolina	0.16
24	Michigan	0.15
25	Georgia	0.13
25	Minnesota	0.13
25	Tennessee	0.13
28	Nebraska	0.12
29	Illinois	0.11
30	New Hampshire	0.09
30	New Jersey	0.09
30	New York	0.09
33	Colorado	0.08
33	Kentucky	0.08
35	Massachusetts	0.07
36	Wisconsin	0.06
37	Arkansas	0.04
38	Connecticut	0.03
39	Delaware	0.00
39	Kansas	0.00
39	Maine	0.00
39	Missouri	0.00
39	Montana	0.00
39	North Dakota	0.00
39	Oklahoma	0.00
39	South Dakota	0.00
39	Vermont	0.00
39	West Virginia	0.00
NA	New Mexico**	NA
NA	Oregon**	NA

District of Columbia   0.00

Source: Morgan Quitno Press using data from U.S. Dept. of Health & Human Serv's, National Center for Health Statistics "Morbidity and Mortality Weekly Report" (January 9, 1998, Vol. 46, Nos. 52 & 53)
Provisional data. An acute, inflammatory, contagious disease caused by a paramyxovirus and characterized by swelling of the salivary glands, especially the parotids, and sometimes of the pancreas, ovaries, or testes. This disease, mainly affecting children, can be prevented by vaccination.
**Mumps is not a notifiable disease in New Mexico or Oregon.*

Rabies (Animal) Cases Reported in 1997

National Total = 7,853 Cases*

RANK	STATE	CASES	% of USA
21	Alabama	88	1.12%
33	Alaska	29	0.37%
28	Arizona	53	0.67%
27	Arkansas	55	0.70%
10	California	264	3.36%
34	Colorado	28	0.36%
5	Connecticut	545	6.94%
25	Delaware	67	0.85%
9	Florida	276	3.51%
6	Georgia	325	4.14%
47	Hawaii	0	0.00%
47	Idaho	0	0.00%
38	Illinois	20	0.25%
40	Indiana	13	0.17%
15	Iowa	158	2.01%
21	Kansas	88	1.12%
34	Kentucky	28	0.36%
44	Louisiana	5	0.06%
11	Maine	226	2.88%
4	Maryland	603	7.68%
8	Massachusetts	282	3.59%
34	Michigan	28	0.36%
26	Minnesota	61	0.78%
44	Mississippi	5	0.06%
37	Missouri	25	0.32%
29	Montana	52	0.66%
46	Nebraska	2	0.03%
42	Nevada	8	0.10%
30	New Hampshire	48	0.61%
12	New Jersey	190	2.42%
41	New Mexico	12	0.15%
1	New York	1,227	15.62%
2	North Carolina	893	11.37%
23	North Dakota	84	1.07%
17	Ohio	116	1.48%
19	Oklahoma	112	1.43%
39	Oregon	14	0.18%
7	Pennsylvania	302	3.85%
31	Rhode Island	41	0.52%
13	South Carolina	175	2.23%
24	South Dakota	74	0.94%
16	Tennessee	149	1.90%
14	Texas	169	2.15%
43	Utah	6	0.08%
18	Vermont	113	1.44%
3	Virginia	669	8.52%
47	Washington	0	0.00%
20	West Virginia	89	1.13%
47	Wisconsin	0	0.00%
32	Wyoming	31	0.39%

RANK	STATE	CASES	% of USA
1	New York	1,227	15.62%
2	North Carolina	893	11.37%
3	Virginia	669	8.52%
4	Maryland	603	7.68%
5	Connecticut	545	6.94%
6	Georgia	325	4.14%
7	Pennsylvania	302	3.85%
8	Massachusetts	282	3.59%
9	Florida	276	3.51%
10	California	264	3.36%
11	Maine	226	2.88%
12	New Jersey	190	2.42%
13	South Carolina	175	2.23%
14	Texas	169	2.15%
15	Iowa	158	2.01%
16	Tennessee	149	1.90%
17	Ohio	116	1.48%
18	Vermont	113	1.44%
19	Oklahoma	112	1.43%
20	West Virginia	89	1.13%
21	Alabama	88	1.12%
21	Kansas	88	1.12%
23	North Dakota	84	1.07%
24	South Dakota	74	0.94%
25	Delaware	67	0.85%
26	Minnesota	61	0.78%
27	Arkansas	55	0.70%
28	Arizona	53	0.67%
29	Montana	52	0.66%
30	New Hampshire	48	0.61%
31	Rhode Island	41	0.52%
32	Wyoming	31	0.39%
33	Alaska	29	0.37%
34	Colorado	28	0.36%
34	Kentucky	28	0.36%
34	Michigan	28	0.36%
37	Missouri	25	0.32%
38	Illinois	20	0.25%
39	Oregon	14	0.18%
40	Indiana	13	0.17%
41	New Mexico	12	0.15%
42	Nevada	8	0.10%
43	Utah	6	0.08%
44	Louisiana	5	0.06%
44	Mississippi	5	0.06%
46	Nebraska	2	0.03%
47	Hawaii	0	0.00%
47	Idaho	0	0.00%
47	Washington	0	0.00%
47	Wisconsin	0	0.00%
	District of Columbia	5	0.06%

Source: U.S. Department of Health and Human Services, National Center for Health Statistics "Morbidity and Mortality Weekly Report" (January 9, 1998, Vol. 46, Nos. 52 & 53)
Provisional data. An acute, infectious, often fatal viral disease of most warm-blooded animals, especially wolves, cats, and dogs, that attacks the central nervous system and is transmitted by the bite of infected animals.

Rabies (Animal) Rate in 1997

National Rate = 2.9 Cases per 100,000 Human Population*

ALPHA ORDER

RANK	STATE	RATE
27	Alabama	2.0
15	Alaska	4.8
30	Arizona	1.2
26	Arkansas	2.2
33	California	0.8
34	Colorado	0.7
3	Connecticut	16.7
9	Delaware	9.2
28	Florida	1.9
18	Georgia	4.3
47	Hawaii	0.0
47	Idaho	0.0
42	Illinois	0.2
42	Indiana	0.2
13	Iowa	5.5
21	Kansas	3.4
34	Kentucky	0.7
45	Louisiana	0.1
2	Maine	18.2
6	Maryland	11.8
17	Massachusetts	4.6
40	Michigan	0.3
29	Minnesota	1.3
42	Mississippi	0.2
37	Missouri	0.5
12	Montana	5.9
45	Nebraska	0.1
37	Nevada	0.5
20	New Hampshire	4.1
25	New Jersey	2.4
34	New Mexico	0.7
10	New York	6.8
5	North Carolina	12.0
4	North Dakota	13.1
31	Ohio	1.0
21	Oklahoma	3.4
39	Oregon	0.4
24	Pennsylvania	2.5
19	Rhode Island	4.2
16	South Carolina	4.7
7	South Dakota	10.0
23	Tennessee	2.8
32	Texas	0.9
40	Utah	0.3
1	Vermont	19.2
8	Virginia	9.9
47	Washington	0.0
14	West Virginia	4.9
47	Wisconsin	0.0
11	Wyoming	6.5

RANK ORDER

RANK	STATE	RATE
1	Vermont	19.2
2	Maine	18.2
3	Connecticut	16.7
4	North Dakota	13.1
5	North Carolina	12.0
6	Maryland	11.8
7	South Dakota	10.0
8	Virginia	9.9
9	Delaware	9.2
10	New York	6.8
11	Wyoming	6.5
12	Montana	5.9
13	Iowa	5.5
14	West Virginia	4.9
15	Alaska	4.8
16	South Carolina	4.7
17	Massachusetts	4.6
18	Georgia	4.3
19	Rhode Island	4.2
20	New Hampshire	4.1
21	Kansas	3.4
21	Oklahoma	3.4
23	Tennessee	2.8
24	Pennsylvania	2.5
25	New Jersey	2.4
26	Arkansas	2.2
27	Alabama	2.0
28	Florida	1.9
29	Minnesota	1.3
30	Arizona	1.2
31	Ohio	1.0
32	Texas	0.9
33	California	0.8
34	Colorado	0.7
34	Kentucky	0.7
34	New Mexico	0.7
37	Missouri	0.5
37	Nevada	0.5
39	Oregon	0.4
40	Michigan	0.3
40	Utah	0.3
42	Illinois	0.2
42	Indiana	0.2
42	Mississippi	0.2
45	Louisiana	0.1
45	Nebraska	0.1
47	Hawaii	0.0
47	Idaho	0.0
47	Washington	0.0
47	Wisconsin	0.0

| | District of Columbia | 0.9 |

Source: Morgan Quitno Press using data from U.S. Dept. of Health & Human Serv's, National Center for Health Statistics
"Morbidity and Mortality Weekly Report" (January 9, 1998, Vol. 46, Nos. 52 & 53)
*Provisional data. An acute, infectious, often fatal viral disease of most warm-blooded animals, especially wolves, cats, and dogs, that attacks the central nervous system and is transmitted by the bite of infected animals.

Salmonellosis Cases Reported in 1996

National Total = 45,471 Cases*

ALPHA ORDER

RANK	STATE	CASES	% of USA
28	Alabama	508	1.12%
48	Alaska	79	0.17%
20	Arizona	619	1.36%
30	Arkansas	455	1.00%
1	California	6,544	14.39%
18	Colorado	670	1.47%
22	Connecticut	590	1.30%
41	Delaware	151	0.33%
3	Florida	2,858	6.29%
10	Georgia	1,467	3.23%
31	Hawaii	428	0.94%
42	Idaho	135	0.30%
6	Illinois	1,972	4.34%
22	Indiana	590	1.30%
35	Iowa	335	0.74%
33	Kansas	419	0.92%
32	Kentucky	421	0.93%
21	Louisiana	616	1.35%
40	Maine	159	0.35%
13	Maryland	1,160	2.55%
7	Massachusetts	1,640	3.61%
14	Michigan	1,012	2.23%
19	Minnesota	653	1.44%
26	Mississippi	531	1.17%
24	Missouri	565	1.24%
46	Montana	101	0.22%
39	Nebraska	189	0.42%
37	Nevada	296	0.65%
43	New Hampshire	133	0.29%
9	New Jersey	1,580	3.47%
36	New Mexico	324	0.71%
2	New York	3,860	8.49%
11	North Carolina	1,466	3.22%
49	North Dakota	63	0.14%
8	Ohio	1,632	3.59%
25	Oklahoma	543	1.19%
34	Oregon	386	0.85%
5	Pennsylvania	2,030	4.46%
38	Rhode Island	198	0.44%
16	South Carolina	873	1.92%
45	South Dakota	119	0.26%
28	Tennessee	508	1.12%
4	Texas	2,800	6.16%
27	Utah	525	1.15%
46	Vermont	101	0.22%
12	Virginia	1,229	2.70%
17	Washington	734	1.61%
44	West Virginia	128	0.28%
15	Wisconsin	894	1.97%
50	Wyoming	57	0.13%

RANK ORDER

RANK	STATE	CASES	% of USA
1	California	6,544	14.39%
2	New York	3,860	8.49%
3	Florida	2,858	6.29%
4	Texas	2,800	6.16%
5	Pennsylvania	2,030	4.46%
6	Illinois	1,972	4.34%
7	Massachusetts	1,640	3.61%
8	Ohio	1,632	3.59%
9	New Jersey	1,580	3.47%
10	Georgia	1,467	3.23%
11	North Carolina	1,466	3.22%
12	Virginia	1,229	2.70%
13	Maryland	1,160	2.55%
14	Michigan	1,012	2.23%
15	Wisconsin	894	1.97%
16	South Carolina	873	1.92%
17	Washington	734	1.61%
18	Colorado	670	1.47%
19	Minnesota	653	1.44%
20	Arizona	619	1.36%
21	Louisiana	616	1.35%
22	Connecticut	590	1.30%
22	Indiana	590	1.30%
24	Missouri	565	1.24%
25	Oklahoma	543	1.19%
26	Mississippi	531	1.17%
27	Utah	525	1.15%
28	Alabama	508	1.12%
28	Tennessee	508	1.12%
30	Arkansas	455	1.00%
31	Hawaii	428	0.94%
32	Kentucky	421	0.93%
33	Kansas	419	0.92%
34	Oregon	386	0.85%
35	Iowa	335	0.74%
36	New Mexico	324	0.71%
37	Nevada	296	0.65%
38	Rhode Island	198	0.44%
39	Nebraska	189	0.42%
40	Maine	159	0.35%
41	Delaware	151	0.33%
42	Idaho	135	0.30%
43	New Hampshire	133	0.29%
44	West Virginia	128	0.28%
45	South Dakota	119	0.26%
46	Montana	101	0.22%
46	Vermont	101	0.22%
48	Alaska	79	0.17%
49	North Dakota	63	0.14%
50	Wyoming	57	0.13%
	District of Columbia	125	0.27%

Source: U.S. Department of Health and Human Services, National Center for Health Statistics
   "Morbidity and Mortality Weekly Report" (October 31, 1997, Vol. 45, No. 53)
*Final data. Any disease caused by a salmonella infection, which may be manifested as food poisoning with
acute gastroenteritis, vomiting and diarrhea.

Salmonellosis Rate in 1996

National Rate = 17.1 Cases per 100,000 Population*

ALPHA ORDER

RANK	STATE	RATE
38	Alabama	11.8
34	Alaska	13.1
31	Arizona	14.0
18	Arkansas	18.2
8	California	20.5
20	Colorado	17.6
19	Connecticut	18.1
7	Delaware	20.9
12	Florida	19.8
10	Georgia	20.0
1	Hawaii	36.2
43	Idaho	11.4
24	Illinois	16.6
47	Indiana	10.1
38	Iowa	11.8
26	Kansas	16.2
44	Kentucky	10.8
30	Louisiana	14.2
35	Maine	12.8
5	Maryland	22.9
2	Massachusetts	26.9
46	Michigan	10.4
31	Minnesota	14.0
14	Mississippi	19.6
45	Missouri	10.5
40	Montana	11.5
40	Nebraska	11.5
16	Nevada	18.5
40	New Hampshire	11.5
13	New Jersey	19.7
15	New Mexico	18.9
6	New York	21.3
9	North Carolina	20.1
48	North Dakota	9.8
29	Ohio	14.6
25	Oklahoma	16.5
36	Oregon	12.1
23	Pennsylvania	16.9
10	Rhode Island	20.0
4	South Carolina	23.5
27	South Dakota	16.1
49	Tennessee	9.6
28	Texas	14.7
3	Utah	26.0
22	Vermont	17.2
17	Virginia	18.4
33	Washington	13.3
50	West Virginia	7.0
21	Wisconsin	17.4
37	Wyoming	11.9

RANK ORDER

RANK	STATE	RATE
1	Hawaii	36.2
2	Massachusetts	26.9
3	Utah	26.0
4	South Carolina	23.5
5	Maryland	22.9
6	New York	21.3
7	Delaware	20.9
8	California	20.5
9	North Carolina	20.1
10	Georgia	20.0
10	Rhode Island	20.0
12	Florida	19.8
13	New Jersey	19.7
14	Mississippi	19.6
15	New Mexico	18.9
16	Nevada	18.5
17	Virginia	18.4
18	Arkansas	18.2
19	Connecticut	18.1
20	Colorado	17.6
21	Wisconsin	17.4
22	Vermont	17.2
23	Pennsylvania	16.9
24	Illinois	16.6
25	Oklahoma	16.5
26	Kansas	16.2
27	South Dakota	16.1
28	Texas	14.7
29	Ohio	14.6
30	Louisiana	14.2
31	Arizona	14.0
31	Minnesota	14.0
33	Washington	13.3
34	Alaska	13.1
35	Maine	12.8
36	Oregon	12.1
37	Wyoming	11.9
38	Alabama	11.8
38	Iowa	11.8
40	Montana	11.5
40	Nebraska	11.5
40	New Hampshire	11.5
43	Idaho	11.4
44	Kentucky	10.8
45	Missouri	10.5
46	Michigan	10.4
47	Indiana	10.1
48	North Dakota	9.8
49	Tennessee	9.6
50	West Virginia	7.0

District of Columbia 23.2

Source: Morgan Quitno Press using data from U.S. Dept. of Health & Human Serv's, National Center for Health Statistics "Morbidity and Mortality Weekly Report" (October 31, 1997, Vol. 45, No. 53)
*Final data. Any disease caused by a salmonella infection, which may be manifested as food poisoning with acute gastroenteritis, vomiting and diarrhea.

Shigellosis Cases Reported in 1996

National Total = 25,978 Cases*

ALPHA ORDER

RANK	STATE	CASES	% of USA
34	Alabama	144	0.55%
35	Alaska	116	0.45%
8	Arizona	1,124	4.33%
28	Arkansas	176	0.68%
1	California	3,952	15.21%
12	Colorado	660	2.54%
26	Connecticut	187	0.72%
32	Delaware	155	0.60%
3	Florida	2,057	7.92%
7	Georgia	1,125	4.33%
42	Hawaii	87	0.33%
37	Idaho	97	0.37%
11	Illinois	683	2.63%
31	Indiana	161	0.62%
33	Iowa	151	0.58%
36	Kansas	112	0.43%
5	Kentucky	1,151	4.43%
14	Louisiana	562	2.16%
48	Maine	16	0.06%
9	Maryland	985	3.79%
23	Massachusetts	265	1.02%
17	Michigan	451	1.74%
29	Minnesota	166	0.64%
27	Mississippi	178	0.69%
19	Missouri	387	1.49%
45	Montana	63	0.24%
44	Nebraska	70	0.27%
37	Nevada	97	0.37%
47	New Hampshire	20	0.08%
18	New Jersey	434	1.67%
16	New Mexico	473	1.82%
6	New York	1,130	4.35%
13	North Carolina	565	2.17%
43	North Dakota	80	0.31%
15	Ohio	559	2.15%
21	Oklahoma	318	1.22%
30	Oregon	163	0.63%
4	Pennsylvania	1,744	6.71%
46	Rhode Island	50	0.19%
24	South Carolina	212	0.82%
40	South Dakota	94	0.36%
25	Tennessee	210	0.81%
2	Texas	2,757	10.61%
22	Utah	307	1.18%
49	Vermont	12	0.05%
10	Virginia	746	2.87%
20	Washington	333	1.28%
39	West Virginia	96	0.37%
41	Wisconsin	89	0.34%
50	Wyoming	9	0.03%

RANK ORDER

RANK	STATE	CASES	% of USA
1	California	3,952	15.21%
2	Texas	2,757	10.61%
3	Florida	2,057	7.92%
4	Pennsylvania	1,744	6.71%
5	Kentucky	1,151	4.43%
6	New York	1,130	4.35%
7	Georgia	1,125	4.33%
8	Arizona	1,124	4.33%
9	Maryland	985	3.79%
10	Virginia	746	2.87%
11	Illinois	683	2.63%
12	Colorado	660	2.54%
13	North Carolina	565	2.17%
14	Louisiana	562	2.16%
15	Ohio	559	2.15%
16	New Mexico	473	1.82%
17	Michigan	451	1.74%
18	New Jersey	434	1.67%
19	Missouri	387	1.49%
20	Washington	333	1.28%
21	Oklahoma	318	1.22%
22	Utah	307	1.18%
23	Massachusetts	265	1.02%
24	South Carolina	212	0.82%
25	Tennessee	210	0.81%
26	Connecticut	187	0.72%
27	Mississippi	178	0.69%
28	Arkansas	176	0.68%
29	Minnesota	166	0.64%
30	Oregon	163	0.63%
31	Indiana	161	0.62%
32	Delaware	155	0.60%
33	Iowa	151	0.58%
34	Alabama	144	0.55%
35	Alaska	116	0.45%
36	Kansas	112	0.43%
37	Idaho	97	0.37%
37	Nevada	97	0.37%
39	West Virginia	96	0.37%
40	South Dakota	94	0.36%
41	Wisconsin	89	0.34%
42	Hawaii	87	0.33%
43	North Dakota	80	0.31%
44	Nebraska	70	0.27%
45	Montana	63	0.24%
46	Rhode Island	50	0.19%
47	New Hampshire	20	0.08%
48	Maine	16	0.06%
49	Vermont	12	0.05%
50	Wyoming	9	0.03%
	District of Columbia	199	0.77%

Source: U.S. Department of Health and Human Services, National Center for Health Statistics
"Morbidity and Mortality Weekly Report" (October 31, 1997, Vol. 45, No. 53)
*Final data. Dysentery caused by any of various species of shigellae, occurring most frequently in areas where poor sanitation and malnutrition are prevalent and commonly affecting children and infants.

Shigellosis Rate in 1996

National Rate = 9.8 Cases per 100,000 Population*

ALPHA ORDER

RANK	STATE	RATE
44	Alabama	3.4
6	Alaska	19.2
3	Arizona	25.3
24	Arkansas	7.0
15	California	12.4
7	Colorado	17.3
30	Connecticut	5.7
4	Delaware	21.4
12	Florida	14.3
8	Georgia	15.3
21	Hawaii	7.4
19	Idaho	8.2
29	Illinois	5.8
45	Indiana	2.8
33	Iowa	5.3
40	Kansas	4.3
1	Kentucky	29.6
13	Louisiana	12.9
50	Maine	1.3
5	Maryland	19.5
39	Massachusetts	4.4
38	Michigan	4.6
43	Minnesota	3.6
25	Mississippi	6.6
22	Missouri	7.2
22	Montana	7.2
41	Nebraska	4.2
27	Nevada	6.1
48	New Hampshire	1.7
32	New Jersey	5.4
2	New Mexico	27.6
26	New York	6.2
20	North Carolina	7.7
15	North Dakota	12.4
37	Ohio	5.0
18	Oklahoma	9.7
35	Oregon	5.1
10	Pennsylvania	14.5
35	Rhode Island	5.1
30	South Carolina	5.7
14	South Dakota	12.7
42	Tennessee	4.0
11	Texas	14.4
9	Utah	15.2
46	Vermont	2.0
17	Virginia	11.2
28	Washington	6.0
33	West Virginia	5.3
48	Wisconsin	1.7
47	Wyoming	1.9

RANK ORDER

RANK	STATE	RATE
1	Kentucky	29.6
2	New Mexico	27.6
3	Arizona	25.3
4	Delaware	21.4
5	Maryland	19.5
6	Alaska	19.2
7	Colorado	17.3
8	Georgia	15.3
9	Utah	15.2
10	Pennsylvania	14.5
11	Texas	14.4
12	Florida	14.3
13	Louisiana	12.9
14	South Dakota	12.7
15	California	12.4
15	North Dakota	12.4
17	Virginia	11.2
18	Oklahoma	9.7
19	Idaho	8.2
20	North Carolina	7.7
21	Hawaii	7.4
22	Missouri	7.2
22	Montana	7.2
24	Arkansas	7.0
25	Mississippi	6.6
26	New York	6.2
27	Nevada	6.1
28	Washington	6.0
29	Illinois	5.8
30	Connecticut	5.7
30	South Carolina	5.7
32	New Jersey	5.4
33	Iowa	5.3
33	West Virginia	5.3
35	Oregon	5.1
35	Rhode Island	5.1
37	Ohio	5.0
38	Michigan	4.6
39	Massachusetts	4.4
40	Kansas	4.3
41	Nebraska	4.2
42	Tennessee	4.0
43	Minnesota	3.6
44	Alabama	3.4
45	Indiana	2.8
46	Vermont	2.0
47	Wyoming	1.9
48	New Hampshire	1.7
48	Wisconsin	1.7
50	Maine	1.3

District of Columbia 36.9

Source: Morgan Quitno Press using data from U.S. Dept. of Health & Human Serv's, National Center for Health Statistics
"Morbidity and Mortality Weekly Report" (October 31, 1997, Vol. 45, No. 53)
*Final data. Dysentery caused by any of various species of shigellae, occurring most frequently in areas where poor sanitation and malnutrition are prevalent and commonly affecting children and infants.

Tuberculosis Cases Reported in 1997

National Total = 17,158 Cases*

ALPHA ORDER

RANK	STATE	CASES	% of USA
9	Alabama	416	2.42%
33	Alaska	73	0.43%
16	Arizona	272	1.59%
24	Arkansas	179	1.04%
1	California	3,297	19.22%
32	Colorado	76	0.44%
31	Connecticut	119	0.69%
43	Delaware	18	0.10%
4	Florida	1,111	6.48%
7	Georgia	595	3.47%
28	Hawaii	150	0.87%
44	Idaho	17	0.10%
5	Illinois	755	4.40%
28	Indiana	150	0.87%
33	Iowa	73	0.43%
35	Kansas	72	0.42%
23	Kentucky	184	1.07%
15	Louisiana	277	1.61%
47	Maine	13	0.08%
13	Maryland	314	1.83%
20	Massachusetts	254	1.48%
12	Michigan	318	1.85%
26	Minnesota	158	0.92%
22	Mississippi	236	1.38%
21	Missouri	238	1.39%
44	Montana	17	0.10%
41	Nebraska	22	0.13%
38	Nevada	46	0.27%
44	New Hampshire	17	0.10%
6	New Jersey	701	4.09%
37	New Mexico	53	0.31%
2	New York	2,071	12.07%
8	North Carolina	464	2.70%
48	North Dakota	12	0.07%
17	Ohio	270	1.57%
25	Oklahoma	176	1.03%
27	Oregon	154	0.90%
10	Pennsylvania	408	2.38%
39	Rhode Island	36	0.21%
19	South Carolina	260	1.52%
42	South Dakota	19	0.11%
11	Tennessee	358	2.09%
3	Texas	1,817	10.59%
40	Utah	32	0.19%
49	Vermont	6	0.03%
14	Virginia	305	1.78%
18	Washington	264	1.54%
36	West Virginia	54	0.31%
30	Wisconsin	123	0.72%
50	Wyoming	2	0.01%

RANK ORDER

RANK	STATE	CASES	% of USA
1	California	3,297	19.22%
2	New York	2,071	12.07%
3	Texas	1,817	10.59%
4	Florida	1,111	6.48%
5	Illinois	755	4.40%
6	New Jersey	701	4.09%
7	Georgia	595	3.47%
8	North Carolina	464	2.70%
9	Alabama	416	2.42%
10	Pennsylvania	408	2.38%
11	Tennessee	358	2.09%
12	Michigan	318	1.85%
13	Maryland	314	1.83%
14	Virginia	305	1.78%
15	Louisiana	277	1.61%
16	Arizona	272	1.59%
17	Ohio	270	1.57%
18	Washington	264	1.54%
19	South Carolina	260	1.52%
20	Massachusetts	254	1.48%
21	Missouri	238	1.39%
22	Mississippi	236	1.38%
23	Kentucky	184	1.07%
24	Arkansas	179	1.04%
25	Oklahoma	176	1.03%
26	Minnesota	158	0.92%
27	Oregon	154	0.90%
28	Hawaii	150	0.87%
28	Indiana	150	0.87%
30	Wisconsin	123	0.72%
31	Connecticut	119	0.69%
32	Colorado	76	0.44%
33	Alaska	73	0.43%
33	Iowa	73	0.43%
35	Kansas	72	0.42%
36	West Virginia	54	0.31%
37	New Mexico	53	0.31%
38	Nevada	46	0.27%
39	Rhode Island	36	0.21%
40	Utah	32	0.19%
41	Nebraska	22	0.13%
42	South Dakota	19	0.11%
43	Delaware	18	0.10%
44	Idaho	17	0.10%
44	Montana	17	0.10%
44	New Hampshire	17	0.10%
47	Maine	13	0.08%
48	North Dakota	12	0.07%
49	Vermont	6	0.03%
50	Wyoming	2	0.01%
	District of Columbia	106	0.62%

Source: U.S. Department of Health and Human Services, National Center for Health Statistics
"Morbidity and Mortality Weekly Report" (January 9, 1998, Vol. 46, Nos. 52 & 53)
*Provisional data. An infectious disease caused by the tubercle bacillus and causing the formation of tubercles on the lungs and other tissues of the body, often developing long after the initial infection. Characterized by the coughing up of mucus and sputum, fever, weight loss, and chest pain.

Tuberculosis Rate in 1997

National Rate = 6.4 Cases per 100,000 Population*

ALPHA ORDER

RANK	STATE	RATE
5	Alabama	9.6
2	Alaska	12.0
18	Arizona	6.0
11	Arkansas	7.1
4	California	10.2
41	Colorado	2.0
26	Connecticut	3.6
38	Delaware	2.5
10	Florida	7.6
9	Georgia	7.9
1	Hawaii	12.6
45	Idaho	1.4
15	Illinois	6.3
35	Indiana	2.6
35	Iowa	2.6
33	Kansas	2.8
20	Kentucky	4.7
14	Louisiana	6.4
48	Maine	1.0
16	Maryland	6.2
25	Massachusetts	4.2
30	Michigan	3.3
28	Minnesota	3.4
8	Mississippi	8.6
24	Missouri	4.4
42	Montana	1.9
47	Nebraska	1.3
34	Nevada	2.7
45	New Hampshire	1.4
7	New Jersey	8.7
31	New Mexico	3.1
3	New York	11.4
16	North Carolina	6.2
42	North Dakota	1.9
39	Ohio	2.4
19	Oklahoma	5.3
20	Oregon	4.7
28	Pennsylvania	3.4
26	Rhode Island	3.6
12	South Carolina	6.9
35	South Dakota	2.6
13	Tennessee	6.7
6	Texas	9.3
44	Utah	1.6
48	Vermont	1.0
23	Virginia	4.5
20	Washington	4.7
32	West Virginia	3.0
39	Wisconsin	2.4
50	Wyoming	0.4

RANK ORDER

RANK	STATE	RATE
1	Hawaii	12.6
2	Alaska	12.0
3	New York	11.4
4	California	10.2
5	Alabama	9.6
6	Texas	9.3
7	New Jersey	8.7
8	Mississippi	8.6
9	Georgia	7.9
10	Florida	7.6
11	Arkansas	7.1
12	South Carolina	6.9
13	Tennessee	6.7
14	Louisiana	6.4
15	Illinois	6.3
16	Maryland	6.2
16	North Carolina	6.2
18	Arizona	6.0
19	Oklahoma	5.3
20	Kentucky	4.7
20	Oregon	4.7
20	Washington	4.7
23	Virginia	4.5
24	Missouri	4.4
25	Massachusetts	4.2
26	Connecticut	3.6
26	Rhode Island	3.6
28	Minnesota	3.4
28	Pennsylvania	3.4
30	Michigan	3.3
31	New Mexico	3.1
32	West Virginia	3.0
33	Kansas	2.8
34	Nevada	2.7
35	Indiana	2.6
35	Iowa	2.6
35	South Dakota	2.6
38	Delaware	2.5
39	Ohio	2.4
39	Wisconsin	2.4
41	Colorado	2.0
42	Montana	1.9
42	North Dakota	1.9
44	Utah	1.6
45	Idaho	1.4
45	New Hampshire	1.4
47	Nebraska	1.3
48	Maine	1.0
48	Vermont	1.0
50	Wyoming	0.4
	District of Columbia	20.0

Source: Morgan Quitno Press using data from U.S. Dept. of Health & Human Serv's, National Center for Health Statistics
"Morbidity and Mortality Weekly Report" (January 9, 1998, Vol. 46, Nos. 52 & 53)
*Provisional data. An infectious disease caused by the tubercle bacillus and causing the formation of tubercles on the lungs and other tissues of the body, often developing long after the initial infection. Characterized by the coughing up of mucus and sputum, fever, weight loss, and chest pain.

Whooping Cough (Pertussis) Cases Reported in 1997

National Total = 5,519 Cases*

ALPHA ORDER

RANK ORDER

RANK	STATE	CASES	% of USA
30	Alabama	35	0.63%
37	Alaska	14	0.25%
27	Arizona	45	0.82%
24	Arkansas	60	1.09%
4	California	403	7.30%
6	Colorado	348	6.31%
30	Connecticut	35	0.63%
50	Delaware	1	0.02%
19	Florida	85	1.54%
37	Georgia	14	0.25%
37	Hawaii	14	0.25%
1	Idaho	570	10.33%
14	Illinois	126	2.28%
19	Indiana	85	1.54%
17	Iowa	113	2.05%
41	Kansas	13	0.24%
23	Kentucky	61	1.11%
34	Louisiana	20	0.36%
42	Maine	11	0.20%
15	Maryland	125	2.26%
2	Massachusetts	522	9.46%
22	Michigan	62	1.12%
5	Minnesota	384	6.96%
45	Mississippi	8	0.14%
21	Missouri	68	1.23%
35	Montana	19	0.34%
37	Nebraska	14	0.25%
29	Nevada	39	0.71%
13	New Hampshire	143	2.59%
42	New Jersey	11	0.20%
9	New Mexico	198	3.59%
8	New York	223	4.04%
16	North Carolina	118	2.14%
49	North Dakota	2	0.04%
12	Ohio	165	2.99%
26	Oklahoma	49	0.89%
44	Oregon	10	0.18%
10	Pennsylvania	175	3.17%
36	Rhode Island	17	0.31%
32	South Carolina	30	0.54%
48	South Dakota	5	0.09%
28	Tennessee	40	0.72%
11	Texas	167	3.03%
33	Utah	26	0.47%
7	Vermont	262	4.75%
25	Virginia	56	1.01%
3	Washington	406	7.36%
47	West Virginia	6	0.11%
18	Wisconsin	106	1.92%
46	Wyoming	7	0.13%

RANK	STATE	CASES	% of USA
1	Idaho	570	10.33%
2	Massachusetts	522	9.46%
3	Washington	406	7.36%
4	California	403	7.30%
5	Minnesota	384	6.96%
6	Colorado	348	6.31%
7	Vermont	262	4.75%
8	New York	223	4.04%
9	New Mexico	198	3.59%
10	Pennsylvania	175	3.17%
11	Texas	167	3.03%
12	Ohio	165	2.99%
13	New Hampshire	143	2.59%
14	Illinois	126	2.28%
15	Maryland	125	2.26%
16	North Carolina	118	2.14%
17	Iowa	113	2.05%
18	Wisconsin	106	1.92%
19	Florida	85	1.54%
19	Indiana	85	1.54%
21	Missouri	68	1.23%
22	Michigan	62	1.12%
23	Kentucky	61	1.11%
24	Arkansas	60	1.09%
25	Virginia	56	1.01%
26	Oklahoma	49	0.89%
27	Arizona	45	0.82%
28	Tennessee	40	0.72%
29	Nevada	39	0.71%
30	Alabama	35	0.63%
30	Connecticut	35	0.63%
32	South Carolina	30	0.54%
33	Utah	26	0.47%
34	Louisiana	20	0.36%
35	Montana	19	0.34%
36	Rhode Island	17	0.31%
37	Alaska	14	0.25%
37	Georgia	14	0.25%
37	Hawaii	14	0.25%
37	Nebraska	14	0.25%
41	Kansas	13	0.24%
42	Maine	11	0.20%
42	New Jersey	11	0.20%
44	Oregon	10	0.18%
45	Mississippi	8	0.14%
46	Wyoming	7	0.13%
47	West Virginia	6	0.11%
48	South Dakota	5	0.09%
49	North Dakota	2	0.04%
50	Delaware	1	0.02%
	District of Columbia	3	0.05%

*Source: U.S. Department of Health and Human Services, National Center for Health Statistics
"Morbidity and Mortality Weekly Report" (January 9, 1998, Vol. 46, Nos. 52 & 53)
Provisional data. Acute, highly contagious infection of respiratory tract.

Whooping Cough (Pertussis) Rate in 1997

National Rate = 2.1 Cases per 100,000 Population*

ALPHA ORDER

RANK	STATE	RATE
34	Alabama	0.8
12	Alaska	2.3
31	Arizona	1.0
11	Arkansas	2.4
26	California	1.2
5	Colorado	8.9
29	Connecticut	1.1
49	Delaware	0.1
40	Florida	0.6
48	Georgia	0.2
26	Hawaii	1.2
1	Idaho	47.1
29	Illinois	1.1
23	Indiana	1.4
9	Iowa	4.0
42	Kansas	0.5
17	Kentucky	1.6
42	Louisiana	0.5
32	Maine	0.9
10	Maryland	2.5
6	Massachusetts	8.5
40	Michigan	0.6
7	Minnesota	8.2
44	Mississippi	0.3
24	Missouri	1.3
14	Montana	2.2
34	Nebraska	0.8
12	Nevada	2.3
3	New Hampshire	12.2
49	New Jersey	0.1
4	New Mexico	11.4
26	New York	1.2
17	North Carolina	1.6
44	North Dakota	0.3
19	Ohio	1.5
19	Oklahoma	1.5
44	Oregon	0.3
19	Pennsylvania	1.5
16	Rhode Island	1.7
34	South Carolina	0.8
38	South Dakota	0.7
38	Tennessee	0.7
32	Texas	0.9
24	Utah	1.3
2	Vermont	44.5
34	Virginia	0.8
8	Washington	7.2
44	West Virginia	0.3
15	Wisconsin	2.1
19	Wyoming	1.5

RANK ORDER

RANK	STATE	RATE
1	Idaho	47.1
2	Vermont	44.5
3	New Hampshire	12.2
4	New Mexico	11.4
5	Colorado	8.9
6	Massachusetts	8.5
7	Minnesota	8.2
8	Washington	7.2
9	Iowa	4.0
10	Maryland	2.5
11	Arkansas	2.4
12	Alaska	2.3
12	Nevada	2.3
14	Montana	2.2
15	Wisconsin	2.1
16	Rhode Island	1.7
17	Kentucky	1.6
17	North Carolina	1.6
19	Ohio	1.5
19	Oklahoma	1.5
19	Pennsylvania	1.5
19	Wyoming	1.5
23	Indiana	1.4
24	Missouri	1.3
24	Utah	1.3
26	California	1.2
26	Hawaii	1.2
26	New York	1.2
29	Connecticut	1.1
29	Illinois	1.1
31	Arizona	1.0
32	Maine	0.9
32	Texas	0.9
34	Alabama	0.8
34	Nebraska	0.8
34	South Carolina	0.8
34	Virginia	0.8
38	South Dakota	0.7
38	Tennessee	0.7
40	Florida	0.6
40	Michigan	0.6
42	Kansas	0.5
42	Louisiana	0.5
44	Mississippi	0.3
44	North Dakota	0.3
44	Oregon	0.3
44	West Virginia	0.3
48	Georgia	0.2
49	Delaware	0.1
49	New Jersey	0.1

District of Columbia	0.6

Source: Morgan Quitno Press using data from U.S. Dept. of Health & Human Serv's, National Center for Health Statistics
"Morbidity and Mortality Weekly Report" (January 9, 1998, Vol. 46, Nos. 52 & 53)
*Provisional data. Acute, highly contagious infection of respiratory tract.

Percent of Children Aged 19 to 35 Months Fully Immunized in 1997

National Percent = 76%*

ALPHA ORDER

RANK	STATE	PERCENT
21	Alabama	78
42	Alaska	72
47	Arizona	69
31	Arkansas	75
31	California	75
39	Colorado	73
1	Connecticut	88
19	Delaware	79
26	Florida	77
13	Georgia	80
13	Hawaii	80
50	Idaho	67
30	Illinois	76
45	Indiana	71
13	Iowa	80
26	Kansas	77
26	Kentucky	77
6	Louisiana	82
3	Maine	85
21	Maryland	78
2	Massachusetts	86
39	Michigan	73
5	Minnesota	83
10	Mississippi	81
36	Missouri	74
21	Montana	78
21	Nebraska	78
46	Nevada	70
6	New Hampshire	82
39	New Jersey	73
31	New Mexico	75
36	New York	74
13	North Carolina	80
13	North Dakota	80
31	Ohio	75
47	Oklahoma	69
42	Oregon	72
6	Pennsylvania	82
10	Rhode Island	81
6	South Carolina	82
26	South Dakota	77
21	Tennessee	78
42	Texas	72
49	Utah	68
4	Vermont	84
31	Virginia	75
10	Washington	81
13	West Virginia	80
19	Wisconsin	79
36	Wyoming	74

RANK ORDER

RANK	STATE	PERCENT
1	Connecticut	88
2	Massachusetts	86
3	Maine	85
4	Vermont	84
5	Minnesota	83
6	Louisiana	82
6	New Hampshire	82
6	Pennsylvania	82
6	South Carolina	82
10	Mississippi	81
10	Rhode Island	81
10	Washington	81
13	Georgia	80
13	Hawaii	80
13	Iowa	80
13	North Carolina	80
13	North Dakota	80
13	West Virginia	80
19	Delaware	79
19	Wisconsin	79
21	Alabama	78
21	Maryland	78
21	Montana	78
21	Nebraska	78
21	Tennessee	78
26	Florida	77
26	Kansas	77
26	Kentucky	77
26	South Dakota	77
30	Illinois	76
31	Arkansas	75
31	California	75
31	New Mexico	75
31	Ohio	75
31	Virginia	75
36	Missouri	74
36	New York	74
36	Wyoming	74
39	Colorado	73
39	Michigan	73
39	New Jersey	73
42	Alaska	72
42	Oregon	72
42	Texas	72
45	Indiana	71
46	Nevada	70
47	Arizona	69
47	Oklahoma	69
49	Utah	68
50	Idaho	67
	District of Columbia**	NA

Source: U.S. Department of Health and Human Services, Centers for Disease Control and Prevention
   "State Vaccination Coverage Levels" (Morbidity and Mortality Weekly Report, Vol. 47, No. 6, 02/20/98)
As of June 1997. Fully immunized children received four doses of DTP/DT (Diphtheria, Tetanus, Pertussis (Whooping Cough)), three doses of OPV (Poliovirus), one dose of MCV (Measles Containing Vaccine) and three doses of Hib (Haemophilus influenzae type b).
**Not available.

Sexually Transmitted Diseases in 1996

National Total = 827,736 Cases*

ALPHA ORDER

RANK	STATE	CASES	% of USA
13	Alabama	22,003	2.66%
42	Alaska	1,826	0.22%
21	Arizona	14,505	1.75%
30	Arkansas	7,430	0.90%
1	California	80,721	9.75%
28	Colorado	8,675	1.05%
26	Connecticut	9,760	1.18%
36	Delaware	3,762	0.45%
4	Florida	44,315	5.35%
9	Georgia	34,050	4.11%
40	Hawaii	2,316	0.28%
44	Idaho	1,626	0.20%
5	Illinois	42,915	5.18%
19	Indiana	17,180	2.08%
33	Iowa	5,333	0.64%
31	Kansas	6,523	0.79%
25	Kentucky	11,188	1.35%
17	Louisiana	20,926	2.53%
47	Maine	1,023	0.12%
12	Maryland	24,224	2.93%
27	Massachusetts	9,113	1.10%
7	Michigan	35,178	4.25%
29	Minnesota	8,320	1.01%
23	Mississippi	11,913	1.44%
18	Missouri	20,601	2.49%
45	Montana	1,162	0.14%
37	Nebraska	3,648	0.44%
35	Nevada	3,892	0.47%
48	New Hampshire	887	0.11%
16	New Jersey	21,175	2.56%
34	New Mexico	4,900	0.59%
3	New York	47,455	5.73%
8	North Carolina	34,373	4.15%
46	North Dakota	1,053	0.13%
6	Ohio	36,189	4.37%
22	Oklahoma	12,455	1.50%
32	Oregon	6,353	0.77%
10	Pennsylvania	30,242	3.65%
39	Rhode Island	2,323	0.28%
14	South Carolina	21,462	2.59%
43	South Dakota	1,714	0.21%
11	Tennessee	25,686	3.10%
2	Texas	67,082	8.10%
41	Utah	1,878	0.23%
50	Vermont	445	0.05%
15	Virginia	21,443	2.59%
24	Washington	11,266	1.36%
38	West Virginia	3,068	0.37%
20	Wisconsin	14,949	1.81%
49	Wyoming	664	0.08%

RANK ORDER

RANK	STATE	CASES	% of USA
1	California	80,721	9.75%
2	Texas	67,082	8.10%
3	New York	47,455	5.73%
4	Florida	44,315	5.35%
5	Illinois	42,915	5.18%
6	Ohio	36,189	4.37%
7	Michigan	35,178	4.25%
8	North Carolina	34,373	4.15%
9	Georgia	34,050	4.11%
10	Pennsylvania	30,242	3.65%
11	Tennessee	25,686	3.10%
12	Maryland	24,224	2.93%
13	Alabama	22,003	2.66%
14	South Carolina	21,462	2.59%
15	Virginia	21,443	2.59%
16	New Jersey	21,175	2.56%
17	Louisiana	20,926	2.53%
18	Missouri	20,601	2.49%
19	Indiana	17,180	2.08%
20	Wisconsin	14,949	1.81%
21	Arizona	14,505	1.75%
22	Oklahoma	12,455	1.50%
23	Mississippi	11,913	1.44%
24	Washington	11,266	1.36%
25	Kentucky	11,188	1.35%
26	Connecticut	9,760	1.18%
27	Massachusetts	9,113	1.10%
28	Colorado	8,675	1.05%
29	Minnesota	8,320	1.01%
30	Arkansas	7,430	0.90%
31	Kansas	6,523	0.79%
32	Oregon	6,353	0.77%
33	Iowa	5,333	0.64%
34	New Mexico	4,900	0.59%
35	Nevada	3,892	0.47%
36	Delaware	3,762	0.45%
37	Nebraska	3,648	0.44%
38	West Virginia	3,068	0.37%
39	Rhode Island	2,323	0.28%
40	Hawaii	2,316	0.28%
41	Utah	1,878	0.23%
42	Alaska	1,826	0.22%
43	South Dakota	1,714	0.21%
44	Idaho	1,626	0.20%
45	Montana	1,162	0.14%
46	North Dakota	1,053	0.13%
47	Maine	1,023	0.12%
48	New Hampshire	887	0.11%
49	Wyoming	664	0.08%
50	Vermont	445	0.05%
	District of Columbia	6,546	0.79%

Source: Morgan Quitno Press using data from U.S. Dept. of Health and Human Services, Nat'l Center for Health Statistics "Sexually Transmitted Disease Surveillance 1996" (http://wonder.cdc.gov/wonder/STD/STDD006.PCW.html)
Includes chancroid, chlamydia, gonorrhea and primary and secondary syphilis.

Sexually Transmitted Disease Rate in 1996

National Rate = 323.0 Cases per 100,000 Population*

ALPHA ORDER

RANK	STATE	RATE
3	Alabama	517.3
20	Alaska	302.5
16	Arizona	343.9
21	Arkansas	299.1
28	California	255.5
34	Colorado	231.6
22	Connecticut	298.0
2	Delaware	524.5
19	Florida	312.8
9	Georgia	472.9
38	Hawaii	195.2
44	Idaho	139.7
14	Illinois	362.8
23	Indiana	296.1
39	Iowa	187.7
30	Kansas	254.3
26	Kentucky	289.9
5	Louisiana	481.9
48	Maine	82.4
6	Maryland	480.4
43	Massachusetts	150.0
13	Michigan	368.3
40	Minnesota	180.4
10	Mississippi	441.7
11	Missouri	387.1
46	Montana	133.6
35	Nebraska	222.9
29	Nevada	254.4
49	New Hampshire	77.3
27	New Jersey	266.6
25	New Mexico	290.7
8	New York	477.6
7	North Carolina	477.8
42	North Dakota	164.2
17	Ohio	324.5
12	Oklahoma	380.0
37	Oregon	202.3
31	Pennsylvania	250.6
33	Rhode Island	234.7
1	South Carolina	584.3
32	South Dakota	235.1
4	Tennessee	488.7
15	Texas	358.3
47	Utah	96.3
50	Vermont	76.1
18	Virginia	323.9
36	Washington	207.5
41	West Virginia	167.9
24	Wisconsin	291.8
45	Wyoming	138.2

RANK ORDER

RANK	STATE	RATE
1	South Carolina	584.3
2	Delaware	524.5
3	Alabama	517.3
4	Tennessee	488.7
5	Louisiana	481.9
6	Maryland	480.4
7	North Carolina	477.8
8	New York	477.6
9	Georgia	472.9
10	Mississippi	441.7
11	Missouri	387.1
12	Oklahoma	380.0
13	Michigan	368.3
14	Illinois	362.8
15	Texas	358.3
16	Arizona	343.9
17	Ohio	324.5
18	Virginia	323.9
19	Florida	312.8
20	Alaska	302.5
21	Arkansas	299.1
22	Connecticut	298.0
23	Indiana	296.1
24	Wisconsin	291.8
25	New Mexico	290.7
26	Kentucky	289.9
27	New Jersey	266.6
28	California	255.5
29	Nevada	254.4
30	Kansas	254.3
31	Pennsylvania	250.6
32	South Dakota	235.1
33	Rhode Island	234.7
34	Colorado	231.6
35	Nebraska	222.9
36	Washington	207.5
37	Oregon	202.3
38	Hawaii	195.2
39	Iowa	187.7
40	Minnesota	180.4
41	West Virginia	167.9
42	North Dakota	164.2
43	Massachusetts	150.0
44	Idaho	139.7
45	Wyoming	138.2
46	Montana	133.6
47	Utah	96.3
48	Maine	82.4
49	New Hampshire	77.3
50	Vermont	76.1

District of Columbia   1,213.8

Source: Morgan Quitno Press using data from U.S. Dept. of Health and Human Services, Nat'l Center for Health Statistics "Sexually Transmitted Disease Surveillance 1996" (http://wonder.cdc.gov/wonder/STD/STDD006.PCW.html)
*Includes chancroid, chlamydia, gonorrhea and primary and secondary syphilis.

Chancroid Cases Reported in 1996

National Total = 386 Cases*

ALPHA ORDER

RANK	STATE	CASES	% of USA
23	Alabama	0	0.00%
23	Alaska	0	0.00%
11	Arizona	2	0.52%
17	Arkansas	1	0.26%
6	California	8	2.07%
23	Colorado	0	0.00%
23	Connecticut	0	0.00%
23	Delaware	0	0.00%
10	Florida	3	0.78%
23	Georgia	0	0.00%
23	Hawaii	0	0.00%
23	Idaho	0	0.00%
4	Illinois	20	5.18%
17	Indiana	1	0.26%
23	Iowa	0	0.00%
11	Kansas	2	0.52%
23	Kentucky	0	0.00%
3	Louisiana	58	15.03%
23	Maine	0	0.00%
11	Maryland	2	0.52%
11	Massachusetts	2	0.52%
23	Michigan	0	0.00%
23	Minnesota	0	0.00%
17	Mississippi	1	0.26%
23	Missouri	0	0.00%
23	Montana	0	0.00%
23	Nebraska	0	0.00%
23	Nevada	0	0.00%
17	New Hampshire	1	0.26%
9	New Jersey	4	1.04%
23	New Mexico	0	0.00%
1	New York	182	47.15%
5	North Carolina	14	3.63%
23	North Dakota	0	0.00%
8	Ohio	6	1.55%
23	Oklahoma	0	0.00%
23	Oregon	0	0.00%
23	Pennsylvania	0	0.00%
23	Rhode Island	0	0.00%
6	South Carolina	8	2.07%
23	South Dakota	0	0.00%
11	Tennessee	2	0.52%
2	Texas	65	16.84%
23	Utah	0	0.00%
23	Vermont	0	0.00%
17	Virginia	1	0.26%
17	Washington	1	0.26%
23	West Virginia	0	0.00%
11	Wisconsin	2	0.52%
23	Wyoming	0	0.00%

RANK ORDER

RANK	STATE	CASES	% of USA
1	New York	182	47.15%
2	Texas	65	16.84%
3	Louisiana	58	15.03%
4	Illinois	20	5.18%
5	North Carolina	14	3.63%
6	California	8	2.07%
6	South Carolina	8	2.07%
8	Ohio	6	1.55%
9	New Jersey	4	1.04%
10	Florida	3	0.78%
11	Arizona	2	0.52%
11	Kansas	2	0.52%
11	Maryland	2	0.52%
11	Massachusetts	2	0.52%
11	Tennessee	2	0.52%
11	Wisconsin	2	0.52%
17	Arkansas	1	0.26%
17	Indiana	1	0.26%
17	Mississippi	1	0.26%
17	New Hampshire	1	0.26%
17	Virginia	1	0.26%
17	Washington	1	0.26%
23	Alabama	0	0.00%
23	Alaska	0	0.00%
23	Colorado	0	0.00%
23	Connecticut	0	0.00%
23	Delaware	0	0.00%
23	Georgia	0	0.00%
23	Hawaii	0	0.00%
23	Idaho	0	0.00%
23	Iowa	0	0.00%
23	Kentucky	0	0.00%
23	Maine	0	0.00%
23	Michigan	0	0.00%
23	Minnesota	0	0.00%
23	Missouri	0	0.00%
23	Montana	0	0.00%
23	Nebraska	0	0.00%
23	Nevada	0	0.00%
23	New Mexico	0	0.00%
23	North Dakota	0	0.00%
23	Oklahoma	0	0.00%
23	Oregon	0	0.00%
23	Pennsylvania	0	0.00%
23	Rhode Island	0	0.00%
23	South Dakota	0	0.00%
23	Utah	0	0.00%
23	Vermont	0	0.00%
23	West Virginia	0	0.00%
23	Wyoming	0	0.00%
	District of Columbia	0	0.00%

Source: U.S. Department of Health and Human Services, National Center for Health Statistics
   "Sexually Transmitted Disease Surveillance 1996" (http://wonder.cdc.gov/wonder/std/stdd146/table_40.html)
*A soft, highly infectious, nonsyphilitic venereal ulcer of the genital region, caused by the bacillus Hemophilus ducreyi. Also called soft chancre.

Chancroid Rate in 1996

National Rate = 0.15 Cases per 100,000 Population*

ALPHA ORDER

RANK	STATE	RATE
23	Alabama	0.00
23	Alaska	0.00
9	Arizona	0.05
12	Arkansas	0.04
17	California	0.03
23	Colorado	0.00
23	Connecticut	0.00
23	Delaware	0.00
19	Florida	0.02
23	Georgia	0.00
23	Hawaii	0.00
23	Idaho	0.00
6	Illinois	0.17
19	Indiana	0.02
23	Iowa	0.00
8	Kansas	0.08
23	Kentucky	0.00
1	Louisiana	1.34
23	Maine	0.00
12	Maryland	0.04
17	Massachusetts	0.03
23	Michigan	0.00
23	Minnesota	0.00
12	Mississippi	0.04
23	Missouri	0.00
23	Montana	0.00
23	Nebraska	0.00
23	Nevada	0.00
7	New Hampshire	0.09
9	New Jersey	0.05
23	New Mexico	0.00
2	New York	1.00
5	North Carolina	0.19
23	North Dakota	0.00
9	Ohio	0.05
23	Oklahoma	0.00
23	Oregon	0.00
23	Pennsylvania	0.00
23	Rhode Island	0.00
4	South Carolina	0.22
23	South Dakota	0.00
12	Tennessee	0.04
3	Texas	0.34
23	Utah	0.00
23	Vermont	0.00
19	Virginia	0.02
19	Washington	0.02
23	West Virginia	0.00
12	Wisconsin	0.04
23	Wyoming	0.00

RANK ORDER

RANK	STATE	RATE
1	Louisiana	1.34
2	New York	1.00
3	Texas	0.34
4	South Carolina	0.22
5	North Carolina	0.19
6	Illinois	0.17
7	New Hampshire	0.09
8	Kansas	0.08
9	Arizona	0.05
9	New Jersey	0.05
9	Ohio	0.05
12	Arkansas	0.04
12	Maryland	0.04
12	Mississippi	0.04
12	Tennessee	0.04
12	Wisconsin	0.04
17	California	0.03
17	Massachusetts	0.03
19	Florida	0.02
19	Indiana	0.02
19	Virginia	0.02
19	Washington	0.02
23	Alabama	0.00
23	Alaska	0.00
23	Colorado	0.00
23	Connecticut	0.00
23	Delaware	0.00
23	Georgia	0.00
23	Hawaii	0.00
23	Idaho	0.00
23	Iowa	0.00
23	Kentucky	0.00
23	Maine	0.00
23	Michigan	0.00
23	Minnesota	0.00
23	Missouri	0.00
23	Montana	0.00
23	Nebraska	0.00
23	Nevada	0.00
23	New Mexico	0.00
23	North Dakota	0.00
23	Oklahoma	0.00
23	Oregon	0.00
23	Pennsylvania	0.00
23	Rhode Island	0.00
23	South Dakota	0.00
23	Utah	0.00
23	Vermont	0.00
23	West Virginia	0.00
23	Wyoming	0.00
	District of Columbia	0.00

Source: Morgan Quitno Press using data from U.S. Dept. of Health and Human Services, Nat'l Center for Health Statistics
"Sexually Transmitted Disease Surveillance 1996" (http://wonder.cdc.gov/wonder/std/stdd146/table_40.html)
*A soft, highly infectious, nonsyphilitic venereal ulcer of the genital region, caused by the bacillus Hemophilus ducreyi. Also called soft chancre.

Chlamydia Cases Reported in 1996

National Total = 490,080 Cases*

ALPHA ORDER					RANK ORDER			
RANK	STATE		CASES	% of USA	RANK	STATE	CASES	% of USA
22	Alabama		8,306	1.69%	1	California	61,555	12.56%
44	Alaska		1,360	0.28%	2	Texas	43,003	8.77%
17	Arizona		10,692	2.18%	3	New York	26,455	5.40%
38	Arkansas		2,111	0.43%	4	Florida	24,763	5.05%
1	California		61,555	12.56%	5	Illinois	24,430	4.98%
24	Colorado		7,282	1.49%	6	Ohio	20,653	4.21%
27	Connecticut		6,269	1.28%	7	Michigan	19,865	4.05%
37	Delaware		2,271	0.46%	8	Pennsylvania	19,275	3.93%
4	Florida		24,763	5.05%	9	North Carolina	15,078	3.08%
10	Georgia		13,555	2.77%	10	Georgia	13,555	2.77%
40	Hawaii		1,816	0.37%	11	Tennessee	13,125	2.68%
43	Idaho		1,524	0.31%	12	New Jersey	12,273	2.50%
5	Illinois		24,430	4.98%	13	Missouri	11,959	2.44%
18	Indiana		10,334	2.11%	14	Maryland	11,901	2.43%
32	Iowa		4,165	0.85%	15	Virginia	11,756	2.40%
30	Kansas		4,449	0.91%	16	Louisiana	11,020	2.25%
26	Kentucky		6,805	1.39%	17	Arizona	10,692	2.18%
16	Louisiana		11,020	2.25%	18	Indiana	10,334	2.11%
47	Maine		967	0.20%	19	Wisconsin	10,290	2.10%
14	Maryland		11,901	2.43%	20	South Carolina	9,391	1.92%
25	Massachusetts		6,837	1.40%	21	Washington	9,236	1.88%
7	Michigan		19,865	4.05%	22	Alabama	8,306	1.69%
28	Minnesota		5,607	1.14%	23	Oklahoma	7,379	1.51%
31	Mississippi		4,351	0.89%	24	Colorado	7,282	1.49%
13	Missouri		11,959	2.44%	25	Massachusetts	6,837	1.40%
45	Montana		1,124	0.23%	26	Kentucky	6,805	1.39%
35	Nebraska		2,478	0.51%	27	Connecticut	6,269	1.28%
34	Nevada		2,847	0.58%	28	Minnesota	5,607	1.14%
48	New Hampshire		732	0.15%	29	Oregon	5,457	1.11%
12	New Jersey		12,273	2.50%	30	Kansas	4,449	0.91%
33	New Mexico		4,007	0.82%	31	Mississippi	4,351	0.89%
3	New York		26,455	5.40%	32	Iowa	4,165	0.85%
9	North Carolina		15,078	3.08%	33	New Mexico	4,007	0.82%
46	North Dakota		1,016	0.21%	34	Nevada	2,847	0.58%
6	Ohio		20,653	4.21%	35	Nebraska	2,478	0.51%
23	Oklahoma		7,379	1.51%	36	West Virginia	2,325	0.47%
29	Oregon		5,457	1.11%	37	Delaware	2,271	0.46%
8	Pennsylvania		19,275	3.93%	38	Arkansas	2,111	0.43%
39	Rhode Island		1,833	0.37%	39	Rhode Island	1,833	0.37%
20	South Carolina		9,391	1.92%	40	Hawaii	1,816	0.37%
42	South Dakota		1,538	0.31%	41	Utah	1,598	0.33%
11	Tennessee		13,125	2.68%	42	South Dakota	1,538	0.31%
2	Texas		43,003	8.77%	43	Idaho	1,524	0.31%
41	Utah		1,598	0.33%	44	Alaska	1,360	0.28%
50	Vermont		398	0.08%	45	Montana	1,124	0.23%
15	Virginia		11,756	2.40%	46	North Dakota	1,016	0.21%
21	Washington		9,236	1.88%	47	Maine	967	0.20%
36	West Virginia		2,325	0.47%	48	New Hampshire	732	0.15%
19	Wisconsin		10,290	2.10%	49	Wyoming	621	0.13%
49	Wyoming		621	0.13%	50	Vermont	398	0.08%
						District of Columbia	1,998	0.41%

Source: U.S. Department of Health and Human Services, National Center for Health Statistics
"Sexually Transmitted Disease Surveillance 1996" (http://wonder.cdc.gov/wonder/STD/STDD009/Table_5.html)
*Any of several common, often asymptomatic, sexually transmitted diseases caused by the microorganism Chlamydia trachomatis,, including nonspecific urethritis in men.

Chlamydia Rate in 1996

National Rate = 194.5 Cases per 100,000 Population*

ALPHA ORDER

RANK ORDER

RANK	STATE	RATE		RANK	STATE	RATE
18	Alabama	195.3		1	New York	361.8
10	Alaska	225.3		2	Delaware	316.6
5	Arizona	253.5		3	South Carolina	255.7
46	Arkansas	85.0		4	Louisiana	253.8
19	California	194.9		5	Arizona	253.5
20	Colorado	194.4		6	Tennessee	249.7
21	Connecticut	191.4		7	New Mexico	237.7
2	Delaware	316.6		8	Maryland	236.0
29	Florida	174.8		9	Texas	229.7
22	Georgia	188.2		10	Alaska	225.3
37	Hawaii	153.0		11	Oklahoma	225.1
40	Idaho	131.0		12	Missouri	224.7
16	Illinois	206.5		13	South Dakota	211.0
26	Indiana	178.1		14	North Carolina	209.6
39	Iowa	146.6		15	Michigan	208.0
31	Kansas	173.4		16	Illinois	206.5
28	Kentucky	176.3		17	Wisconsin	200.9
4	Louisiana	253.8		18	Alabama	195.3
48	Maine	77.9		19	California	194.9
8	Maryland	236.0		20	Colorado	194.4
45	Massachusetts	112.6		21	Connecticut	191.4
15	Michigan	208.0		22	Georgia	188.2
44	Minnesota	121.6		23	Nevada	186.1
33	Mississippi	161.3		24	Ohio	185.2
12	Missouri	224.7		24	Rhode Island	185.2
42	Montana	129.2		26	Indiana	178.1
38	Nebraska	151.4		27	Virginia	177.6
23	Nevada	186.1		28	Kentucky	176.3
50	New Hampshire	63.8		29	Florida	174.8
36	New Jersey	154.5		30	Oregon	173.8
7	New Mexico	237.7		31	Kansas	173.4
1	New York	361.8		32	Washington	170.1
14	North Carolina	209.6		33	Mississippi	161.3
35	North Dakota	158.4		34	Pennsylvania	159.7
24	Ohio	185.2		35	North Dakota	158.4
11	Oklahoma	225.1		36	New Jersey	154.5
30	Oregon	173.8		37	Hawaii	153.0
34	Pennsylvania	159.7		38	Nebraska	151.4
24	Rhode Island	185.2		39	Iowa	146.6
3	South Carolina	255.7		40	Idaho	131.0
13	South Dakota	211.0		41	Wyoming	129.3
6	Tennessee	249.7		42	Montana	129.2
9	Texas	229.7		43	West Virginia	127.2
47	Utah	81.9		44	Minnesota	121.6
49	Vermont	68.1		45	Massachusetts	112.6
27	Virginia	177.6		46	Arkansas	85.0
32	Washington	170.1		47	Utah	81.9
43	West Virginia	127.2		48	Maine	77.9
17	Wisconsin	200.9		49	Vermont	68.1
41	Wyoming	129.3		50	New Hampshire	63.8
					District of Columbia	370.5

Source: U.S. Department of Health and Human Services, National Center for Health Statistics
"Sexually Transmitted Disease Surveillance 1996" (http://wonder.cdc.gov/wonder/STD/STDD009/Table_5.html)
*Any of several common, often asymptomatic, sexually transmitted diseases caused by the microorganism Chlamydia trachomatis,, including nonspecific urethritis in men.

Gonorrhea Cases Reported in 1996

National Total = 325,883 Cases*

ALPHA ORDER

RANK ORDER

RANK	STATE	CASES	% of USA		RANK	STATE	CASES	% of USA
10	Alabama	13,169	4.04%		1	Texas	23,124	7.10%
41	Alaska	466	0.14%		2	New York	20,604	6.32%
25	Arizona	3,709	1.14%		3	Georgia	19,806	6.08%
21	Arkansas	5,056	1.55%		4	Florida	19,181	5.89%
5	California	18,652	5.72%		5	California	18,652	5.72%
32	Colorado	1,367	0.42%		6	North Carolina	18,229	5.59%
26	Connecticut	3,388	1.04%		7	Illinois	17,964	5.51%
31	Delaware	1,456	0.45%		8	Michigan	15,130	4.64%
4	Florida	19,181	5.89%		9	Ohio	14,946	4.59%
3	Georgia	19,806	6.08%		10	Alabama	13,169	4.04%
39	Hawaii	497	0.15%		11	Tennessee	11,709	3.59%
45	Idaho	98	0.03%		12	South Carolina	11,661	3.58%
7	Illinois	17,964	5.51%		13	Maryland	11,592	3.56%
20	Indiana	6,638	2.04%		14	Pennsylvania	10,803	3.31%
34	Iowa	1,145	0.35%		15	Louisiana	9,315	2.86%
29	Kansas	2,044	0.63%		16	Virginia	9,293	2.85%
24	Kentucky	4,229	1.30%		17	New Jersey	8,721	2.68%
15	Louisiana	9,315	2.86%		18	Missouri	8,421	2.58%
46	Maine	55	0.02%		19	Mississippi	6,742	2.07%
13	Maryland	11,592	3.56%		20	Indiana	6,638	2.04%
28	Massachusetts	2,189	0.67%		21	Arkansas	5,056	1.55%
8	Michigan	15,130	4.64%		22	Oklahoma	4,897	1.50%
27	Minnesota	2,697	0.83%		23	Wisconsin	4,481	1.38%
19	Mississippi	6,742	2.07%		24	Kentucky	4,229	1.30%
18	Missouri	8,421	2.58%		25	Arizona	3,709	1.14%
49	Montana	38	0.01%		26	Connecticut	3,388	1.04%
33	Nebraska	1,164	0.36%		27	Minnesota	2,697	0.83%
35	Nevada	1,025	0.31%		28	Massachusetts	2,189	0.67%
44	New Hampshire	153	0.05%		29	Kansas	2,044	0.63%
17	New Jersey	8,721	2.68%		30	Washington	2,020	0.62%
36	New Mexico	890	0.27%		31	Delaware	1,456	0.45%
2	New York	20,604	6.32%		32	Colorado	1,367	0.42%
6	North Carolina	18,229	5.59%		33	Nebraska	1,164	0.36%
50	North Dakota	37	0.01%		34	Iowa	1,145	0.35%
9	Ohio	14,946	4.59%		35	Nevada	1,025	0.31%
22	Oklahoma	4,897	1.50%		36	New Mexico	890	0.27%
37	Oregon	887	0.27%		37	Oregon	887	0.27%
14	Pennsylvania	10,803	3.31%		38	West Virginia	736	0.23%
40	Rhode Island	486	0.15%		39	Hawaii	497	0.15%
12	South Carolina	11,661	3.58%		40	Rhode Island	486	0.15%
43	South Dakota	176	0.05%		41	Alaska	466	0.14%
11	Tennessee	11,709	3.59%		42	Utah	277	0.08%
1	Texas	23,124	7.10%		43	South Dakota	176	0.05%
42	Utah	277	0.08%		44	New Hampshire	153	0.05%
47	Vermont	47	0.01%		45	Idaho	98	0.03%
16	Virginia	9,293	2.85%		46	Maine	55	0.02%
30	Washington	2,020	0.62%		47	Vermont	47	0.01%
38	West Virginia	736	0.23%		48	Wyoming	41	0.01%
23	Wisconsin	4,481	1.38%		49	Montana	38	0.01%
48	Wyoming	41	0.01%		50	North Dakota	37	0.01%
						District of Columbia	4,432	1.36%

Source: U.S. Department of Health and Human Services, National Center for Health Statistics
   "Sexually Transmitted Disease Surveillance 1996" (http://wonder.cdc.gov/wonder/STD/STDD010/Table_14.html)
*Gonorrhea is a sexually transmitted disease caused by gonococcal bacteria that affects the mucous membrane chiefly of the genital and urinary tracts and is characterized by an acute purulent discharge and painful or difficult urination, though women often have no symptoms.

Gonorrhea Rate in 1996

National Rate = 124.0 Cases per 100,000 Population*

ALPHA ORDER

RANK STATE

RANK	STATE	RATE
2	Alabama	309.6
28	Alaska	77.2
25	Arizona	87.9
9	Arkansas	203.6
31	California	59.0
39	Colorado	36.5
23	Connecticut	103.5
10	Delaware	203.0
16	Florida	135.4
3	Georgia	275.1
35	Hawaii	41.9
46	Idaho	8.4
13	Illinois	151.9
19	Indiana	114.4
36	Iowa	40.3
27	Kansas	79.7
22	Kentucky	109.6
8	Louisiana	214.5
49	Maine	4.4
6	Maryland	229.9
40	Massachusetts	36.0
11	Michigan	158.4
32	Minnesota	58.5
5	Mississippi	250.0
12	Missouri	158.2
49	Montana	4.4
29	Nebraska	71.1
30	Nevada	67.0
44	New Hampshire	13.3
21	New Jersey	109.8
33	New Mexico	52.8
20	New York	113.6
4	North Carolina	253.4
48	North Dakota	5.8
17	Ohio	134.0
14	Oklahoma	149.4
41	Oregon	28.2
24	Pennsylvania	89.5
34	Rhode Island	49.1
1	South Carolina	317.5
42	South Dakota	24.1
7	Tennessee	222.8
18	Texas	123.5
43	Utah	14.2
47	Vermont	8.0
15	Virginia	140.4
38	Washington	37.2
36	West Virginia	40.3
26	Wisconsin	87.5
45	Wyoming	8.5

RANK ORDER

RANK STATE

RANK	STATE	RATE
1	South Carolina	317.5
2	Alabama	309.6
3	Georgia	275.1
4	North Carolina	253.4
5	Mississippi	250.0
6	Maryland	229.9
7	Tennessee	222.8
8	Louisiana	214.5
9	Arkansas	203.6
10	Delaware	203.0
11	Michigan	158.4
12	Missouri	158.2
13	Illinois	151.9
14	Oklahoma	149.4
15	Virginia	140.4
16	Florida	135.4
17	Ohio	134.0
18	Texas	123.5
19	Indiana	114.4
20	New York	113.6
21	New Jersey	109.8
22	Kentucky	109.6
23	Connecticut	103.5
24	Pennsylvania	89.5
25	Arizona	87.9
26	Wisconsin	87.5
27	Kansas	79.7
28	Alaska	77.2
29	Nebraska	71.1
30	Nevada	67.0
31	California	59.0
32	Minnesota	58.5
33	New Mexico	52.8
34	Rhode Island	49.1
35	Hawaii	41.9
36	Iowa	40.3
36	West Virginia	40.3
38	Washington	37.2
39	Colorado	36.5
40	Massachusetts	36.0
41	Oregon	28.2
42	South Dakota	24.1
43	Utah	14.2
44	New Hampshire	13.3
45	Wyoming	8.5
46	Idaho	8.4
47	Vermont	8.0
48	North Dakota	5.8
49	Maine	4.4
49	Montana	4.4

District of Columbia — 821.8

Source: U.S. Department of Health and Human Services, National Center for Health Statistics
"Sexually Transmitted Disease Surveillance 1996" (http://wonder.cdc.gov/wonder/STD/STDD010/Table_14.html)
*Gonorrhea is a sexually transmitted disease caused by gonococcal bacteria that affects the mucous membrane chiefly of the genital and urinary tracts and is characterized by an acute purulent discharge and painful or difficult urination, though women often have no symptoms.

Syphilis Cases Reported in 1996

National Total = 11,387 Cases*

ALPHA ORDER

RANK	STATE	CASES	% of USA
9	Alabama	528	4.64%
46	Alaska	0	0.00%
26	Arizona	102	0.90%
15	Arkansas	262	2.30%
10	California	506	4.44%
30	Colorado	26	0.23%
25	Connecticut	103	0.90%
28	Delaware	35	0.31%
14	Florida	368	3.23%
6	Georgia	689	6.05%
40	Hawaii	3	0.03%
38	Idaho	4	0.04%
11	Illinois	501	4.40%
18	Indiana	207	1.82%
31	Iowa	23	0.20%
29	Kansas	28	0.25%
24	Kentucky	154	1.35%
8	Louisiana	533	4.68%
44	Maine	1	0.01%
5	Maryland	729	6.40%
27	Massachusetts	85	0.75%
19	Michigan	183	1.61%
33	Minnesota	16	0.14%
4	Mississippi	819	7.19%
16	Missouri	221	1.94%
46	Montana	0	0.00%
37	Nebraska	6	0.05%
32	Nevada	20	0.18%
44	New Hampshire	1	0.01%
21	New Jersey	177	1.55%
40	New Mexico	3	0.03%
17	New York	214	1.88%
1	North Carolina	1,052	9.24%
46	North Dakota	0	0.00%
7	Ohio	584	5.13%
20	Oklahoma	179	1.57%
34	Oregon	9	0.08%
23	Pennsylvania	164	1.44%
38	Rhode Island	4	0.04%
12	South Carolina	402	3.53%
46	South Dakota	0	0.00%
3	Tennessee	850	7.46%
2	Texas	890	7.82%
40	Utah	3	0.03%
46	Vermont	0	0.00%
13	Virginia	393	3.45%
34	Washington	9	0.08%
36	West Virginia	7	0.06%
22	Wisconsin	176	1.55%
43	Wyoming	2	0.02%

RANK ORDER

RANK	STATE	CASES	% of USA
1	North Carolina	1,052	9.24%
2	Texas	890	7.82%
3	Tennessee	850	7.46%
4	Mississippi	819	7.19%
5	Maryland	729	6.40%
6	Georgia	689	6.05%
7	Ohio	584	5.13%
8	Louisiana	533	4.68%
9	Alabama	528	4.64%
10	California	506	4.44%
11	Illinois	501	4.40%
12	South Carolina	402	3.53%
13	Virginia	393	3.45%
14	Florida	368	3.23%
15	Arkansas	262	2.30%
16	Missouri	221	1.94%
17	New York	214	1.88%
18	Indiana	207	1.82%
19	Michigan	183	1.61%
20	Oklahoma	179	1.57%
21	New Jersey	177	1.55%
22	Wisconsin	176	1.55%
23	Pennsylvania	164	1.44%
24	Kentucky	154	1.35%
25	Connecticut	103	0.90%
26	Arizona	102	0.90%
27	Massachusetts	85	0.75%
28	Delaware	35	0.31%
29	Kansas	28	0.25%
30	Colorado	26	0.23%
31	Iowa	23	0.20%
32	Nevada	20	0.18%
33	Minnesota	16	0.14%
34	Oregon	9	0.08%
34	Washington	9	0.08%
36	West Virginia	7	0.06%
37	Nebraska	6	0.05%
38	Idaho	4	0.04%
38	Rhode Island	4	0.04%
40	Hawaii	3	0.03%
40	New Mexico	3	0.03%
40	Utah	3	0.03%
43	Wyoming	2	0.02%
44	Maine	1	0.01%
44	New Hampshire	1	0.01%
46	Alaska	0	0.00%
46	Montana	0	0.00%
46	North Dakota	0	0.00%
46	South Dakota	0	0.00%
46	Vermont	0	0.00%
	District of Columbia	116	1.02%

Source: U.S. Department of Health and Human Services, National Center for Health Statistics
"Sexually Transmitted Disease Surveillance 1996" (http://wonder.cdc.gov/wonder/STD/STDD023/Table_26.html)
*Includes only primary and secondary cases. Does not include 41,608 cases in other stages. A chronic infectious disease caused by a spirochete (Treponema pallidum), either transmitted by direct contact, usually in sexual intercourse, or passed from mother to child in utero, and progressing through three stages characterized respectively by local formation of chancres, ulcerous skin eruptions, and systemic infection leading to general paresis.

Syphilis Rate in 1996

National Rate = 4.3 Cases per 100,000 Population*

<table>
<tr><td colspan="3"><u>ALPHA ORDER</u></td><td colspan="3"><u>RANK ORDER</u></td></tr>
<tr><th>RANK</th><th>STATE</th><th>RATE</th><th>RANK</th><th>STATE</th><th>RATE</th></tr>
<tr><td>5</td><td>Alabama</td><td>12.4</td><td>1</td><td>Mississippi</td><td>30.4</td></tr>
<tr><td>46</td><td>Alaska</td><td>0.0</td><td>2</td><td>Tennessee</td><td>16.2</td></tr>
<tr><td>22</td><td>Arizona</td><td>2.4</td><td>3</td><td>North Carolina</td><td>14.6</td></tr>
<tr><td>8</td><td>Arkansas</td><td>10.5</td><td>4</td><td>Maryland</td><td>14.5</td></tr>
<tr><td>25</td><td>California</td><td>1.6</td><td>5</td><td>Alabama</td><td>12.4</td></tr>
<tr><td>32</td><td>Colorado</td><td>0.7</td><td>6</td><td>Louisiana</td><td>12.3</td></tr>
<tr><td>20</td><td>Connecticut</td><td>3.1</td><td>7</td><td>South Carolina</td><td>10.9</td></tr>
<tr><td>13</td><td>Delaware</td><td>4.9</td><td>8</td><td>Arkansas</td><td>10.5</td></tr>
<tr><td>21</td><td>Florida</td><td>2.6</td><td>9</td><td>Georgia</td><td>9.6</td></tr>
<tr><td>9</td><td>Georgia</td><td>9.6</td><td>10</td><td>Virginia</td><td>5.9</td></tr>
<tr><td>37</td><td>Hawaii</td><td>0.3</td><td>11</td><td>Oklahoma</td><td>5.5</td></tr>
<tr><td>37</td><td>Idaho</td><td>0.3</td><td>12</td><td>Ohio</td><td>5.2</td></tr>
<tr><td>15</td><td>Illinois</td><td>4.2</td><td>13</td><td>Delaware</td><td>4.9</td></tr>
<tr><td>18</td><td>Indiana</td><td>3.6</td><td>14</td><td>Texas</td><td>4.8</td></tr>
<tr><td>31</td><td>Iowa</td><td>0.8</td><td>15</td><td>Illinois</td><td>4.2</td></tr>
<tr><td>30</td><td>Kansas</td><td>1.1</td><td>15</td><td>Missouri</td><td>4.2</td></tr>
<tr><td>17</td><td>Kentucky</td><td>4.0</td><td>17</td><td>Kentucky</td><td>4.0</td></tr>
<tr><td>6</td><td>Louisiana</td><td>12.3</td><td>18</td><td>Indiana</td><td>3.6</td></tr>
<tr><td>44</td><td>Maine</td><td>0.1</td><td>19</td><td>Wisconsin</td><td>3.4</td></tr>
<tr><td>4</td><td>Maryland</td><td>14.5</td><td>20</td><td>Connecticut</td><td>3.1</td></tr>
<tr><td>26</td><td>Massachusetts</td><td>1.4</td><td>21</td><td>Florida</td><td>2.6</td></tr>
<tr><td>24</td><td>Michigan</td><td>1.9</td><td>22</td><td>Arizona</td><td>2.4</td></tr>
<tr><td>37</td><td>Minnesota</td><td>0.3</td><td>23</td><td>New Jersey</td><td>2.2</td></tr>
<tr><td>1</td><td>Mississippi</td><td>30.4</td><td>24</td><td>Michigan</td><td>1.9</td></tr>
<tr><td>15</td><td>Missouri</td><td>4.2</td><td>25</td><td>California</td><td>1.6</td></tr>
<tr><td>46</td><td>Montana</td><td>0.0</td><td>26</td><td>Massachusetts</td><td>1.4</td></tr>
<tr><td>33</td><td>Nebraska</td><td>0.4</td><td>26</td><td>Pennsylvania</td><td>1.4</td></tr>
<tr><td>28</td><td>Nevada</td><td>1.3</td><td>28</td><td>Nevada</td><td>1.3</td></tr>
<tr><td>44</td><td>New Hampshire</td><td>0.1</td><td>29</td><td>New York</td><td>1.2</td></tr>
<tr><td>23</td><td>New Jersey</td><td>2.2</td><td>30</td><td>Kansas</td><td>1.1</td></tr>
<tr><td>41</td><td>New Mexico</td><td>0.2</td><td>31</td><td>Iowa</td><td>0.8</td></tr>
<tr><td>29</td><td>New York</td><td>1.2</td><td>32</td><td>Colorado</td><td>0.7</td></tr>
<tr><td>3</td><td>North Carolina</td><td>14.6</td><td>33</td><td>Nebraska</td><td>0.4</td></tr>
<tr><td>46</td><td>North Dakota</td><td>0.0</td><td>33</td><td>Rhode Island</td><td>0.4</td></tr>
<tr><td>12</td><td>Ohio</td><td>5.2</td><td>33</td><td>West Virginia</td><td>0.4</td></tr>
<tr><td>11</td><td>Oklahoma</td><td>5.5</td><td>33</td><td>Wyoming</td><td>0.4</td></tr>
<tr><td>37</td><td>Oregon</td><td>0.3</td><td>37</td><td>Hawaii</td><td>0.3</td></tr>
<tr><td>26</td><td>Pennsylvania</td><td>1.4</td><td>37</td><td>Idaho</td><td>0.3</td></tr>
<tr><td>33</td><td>Rhode Island</td><td>0.4</td><td>37</td><td>Minnesota</td><td>0.3</td></tr>
<tr><td>7</td><td>South Carolina</td><td>10.9</td><td>37</td><td>Oregon</td><td>0.3</td></tr>
<tr><td>46</td><td>South Dakota</td><td>0.0</td><td>41</td><td>New Mexico</td><td>0.2</td></tr>
<tr><td>2</td><td>Tennessee</td><td>16.2</td><td>41</td><td>Utah</td><td>0.2</td></tr>
<tr><td>14</td><td>Texas</td><td>4.8</td><td>41</td><td>Washington</td><td>0.2</td></tr>
<tr><td>41</td><td>Utah</td><td>0.2</td><td>44</td><td>Maine</td><td>0.1</td></tr>
<tr><td>46</td><td>Vermont</td><td>0.0</td><td>44</td><td>New Hampshire</td><td>0.1</td></tr>
<tr><td>10</td><td>Virginia</td><td>5.9</td><td>46</td><td>Alaska</td><td>0.0</td></tr>
<tr><td>41</td><td>Washington</td><td>0.2</td><td>46</td><td>Montana</td><td>0.0</td></tr>
<tr><td>33</td><td>West Virginia</td><td>0.4</td><td>46</td><td>North Dakota</td><td>0.0</td></tr>
<tr><td>19</td><td>Wisconsin</td><td>3.4</td><td>46</td><td>South Dakota</td><td>0.0</td></tr>
<tr><td>33</td><td>Wyoming</td><td>0.4</td><td>46</td><td>Vermont</td><td>0.0</td></tr>
<tr><td></td><td></td><td></td><td></td><td>District of Columbia</td><td>21.5</td></tr>
</table>

Source: U.S. Department of Health and Human Services, National Center for Health Statistics
   "Sexually Transmitted Disease Surveillance 1996" (http://wonder.cdc.gov/wonder/STD/STDD023/Table_26.html)
*Includes only primary and secondary cases. Does not include 41,608 cases in other stages. A chronic infectious disease caused by a spirochete (Treponema pallidum), either transmitted by direct contact, usually in sexual intercourse, or passed from mother to child in utero, and progressing through three stages characterized respectively by local formation of chancres, ulcerous skin eruptions, and systemic infection leading to general paresis.

VI. PROVIDERS

VI. PROVIDERS (continued)

Physicians in 1996

National Total = 725,804 Physicians*

ALPHA ORDER

RANK	STATE	PHYSICIANS	% of USA
25	Alabama	9,038	1.25%
49	Alaska	1,146	0.16%
23	Arizona	10,790	1.49%
32	Arkansas	5,132	0.71%
1	California	89,766	12.37%
24	Colorado	10,202	1.41%
20	Connecticut	12,416	1.71%
46	Delaware	1,845	0.25%
4	Florida	40,450	5.57%
14	Georgia	16,782	2.31%
38	Hawaii	3,657	0.50%
43	Idaho	2,037	0.28%
6	Illinois	32,782	4.52%
21	Indiana	12,083	1.66%
31	Iowa	5,549	0.76%
30	Kansas	5,956	0.82%
26	Kentucky	8,526	1.17%
22	Louisiana	11,060	1.52%
40	Maine	3,085	0.43%
11	Maryland	21,514	2.96%
8	Massachusetts	26,249	3.62%
10	Michigan	22,971	3.16%
18	Minnesota	12,758	1.76%
33	Mississippi	4,721	0.65%
17	Missouri	13,103	1.81%
44	Montana	1,948	0.27%
37	Nebraska	3,814	0.53%
42	Nevada	3,033	0.42%
41	New Hampshire	3,042	0.42%
9	New Jersey	24,733	3.41%
35	New Mexico	4,156	0.57%
2	New York	72,532	9.99%
12	North Carolina	18,346	2.53%
47	North Dakota	1,507	0.21%
7	Ohio	27,972	3.85%
29	Oklahoma	6,067	0.84%
27	Oregon	8,283	1.14%
5	Pennsylvania	36,882	5.08%
39	Rhode Island	3,382	0.47%
27	South Carolina	8,283	1.14%
48	South Dakota	1,505	0.21%
16	Tennessee	13,826	1.90%
3	Texas	41,679	5.74%
34	Utah	4,414	0.61%
45	Vermont	1,918	0.26%
13	Virginia	17,840	2.46%
15	Washington	14,955	2.06%
36	West Virginia	4,141	0.57%
19	Wisconsin	12,714	1.75%
50	Wyoming	925	0.13%

RANK ORDER

RANK	STATE	PHYSICIANS	% of USA
1	California	89,766	12.37%
2	New York	72,532	9.99%
3	Texas	41,679	5.74%
4	Florida	40,450	5.57%
5	Pennsylvania	36,882	5.08%
6	Illinois	32,782	4.52%
7	Ohio	27,972	3.85%
8	Massachusetts	26,249	3.62%
9	New Jersey	24,733	3.41%
10	Michigan	22,971	3.16%
11	Maryland	21,514	2.96%
12	North Carolina	18,346	2.53%
13	Virginia	17,840	2.46%
14	Georgia	16,782	2.31%
15	Washington	14,955	2.06%
16	Tennessee	13,826	1.90%
17	Missouri	13,103	1.81%
18	Minnesota	12,758	1.76%
19	Wisconsin	12,714	1.75%
20	Connecticut	12,416	1.71%
21	Indiana	12,083	1.66%
22	Louisiana	11,060	1.52%
23	Arizona	10,790	1.49%
24	Colorado	10,202	1.41%
25	Alabama	9,038	1.25%
26	Kentucky	8,526	1.17%
27	Oregon	8,283	1.14%
27	South Carolina	8,283	1.14%
29	Oklahoma	6,067	0.84%
30	Kansas	5,956	0.82%
31	Iowa	5,549	0.76%
32	Arkansas	5,132	0.71%
33	Mississippi	4,721	0.65%
34	Utah	4,414	0.61%
35	New Mexico	4,156	0.57%
36	West Virginia	4,141	0.57%
37	Nebraska	3,814	0.53%
38	Hawaii	3,657	0.50%
39	Rhode Island	3,382	0.47%
40	Maine	3,085	0.43%
41	New Hampshire	3,042	0.42%
42	Nevada	3,033	0.42%
43	Idaho	2,037	0.28%
44	Montana	1,948	0.27%
45	Vermont	1,918	0.26%
46	Delaware	1,845	0.25%
47	North Dakota	1,507	0.21%
48	South Dakota	1,505	0.21%
49	Alaska	1,146	0.16%
50	Wyoming	925	0.13%
	District of Columbia	4,289	0.59%

Source: American Medical Association (Chicago, Illinois)
"Physician Characteristics and Distribution in the U.S." (1997-98 Edition)
*As of December 31, 1996. Comprised of federal and nonfederal physicians. Total does not include 11,960 physicians in the U.S. territories and possessions, at APO's and FPO's and whose addresses are unknown.

Male Physicians in 1996

National Total = 571,373 Physicians

Source: American Medical Association (Chicago, Illinois)
"Physician Characteristics and Distribution in the U.S." (1997-98 Edition)
*As of December 31, 1996. Comprised of federal and nonfederal physicians. Total does not include 9,004 male physicians in the U.S. territories and possessions, at APO's and FPO's and whose addresses are unknown.

Female Physicians in 1996

National Total = 154,431 Physicians*

ALPHA ORDER

RANK	STATE	PHYSICIANS	% of USA
27	Alabama	1,470	0.95%
46	Alaska	247	0.16%
23	Arizona	2,054	1.33%
33	Arkansas	815	0.53%
1	California	19,040	12.33%
21	Colorado	2,230	1.44%
17	Connecticut	2,781	1.80%
44	Delaware	425	0.28%
7	Florida	6,274	4.06%
14	Georgia	3,221	2.09%
35	Hawaii	750	0.49%
46	Idaho	247	0.16%
3	Illinois	8,314	5.38%
22	Indiana	2,190	1.42%
32	Iowa	930	0.60%
29	Kansas	1,162	0.75%
26	Kentucky	1,568	1.02%
24	Louisiana	2,028	1.31%
40	Maine	614	0.40%
10	Maryland	5,506	3.57%
6	Massachusetts	7,020	4.55%
11	Michigan	5,182	3.36%
16	Minnesota	2,793	1.81%
37	Mississippi	710	0.46%
18	Missouri	2,633	1.70%
45	Montana	276	0.18%
39	Nebraska	658	0.43%
42	Nevada	453	0.29%
41	New Hampshire	546	0.35%
8	New Jersey	6,114	3.96%
30	New Mexico	1,057	0.68%
2	New York	18,418	11.93%
13	North Carolina	3,634	2.35%
49	North Dakota	206	0.13%
9	Ohio	6,102	3.95%
31	Oklahoma	1,031	0.67%
25	Oregon	1,618	1.05%
5	Pennsylvania	8,228	5.33%
34	Rhode Island	791	0.51%
28	South Carolina	1,438	0.93%
48	South Dakota	221	0.14%
20	Tennessee	2,389	1.55%
4	Texas	8,278	5.36%
38	Utah	665	0.43%
43	Vermont	430	0.28%
12	Virginia	3,894	2.52%
15	Washington	3,128	2.03%
36	West Virginia	749	0.49%
19	Wisconsin	2,555	1.65%
50	Wyoming	117	0.08%

RANK ORDER

RANK	STATE	PHYSICIANS	% of USA
1	California	19,040	12.33%
2	New York	18,418	11.93%
3	Illinois	8,314	5.38%
4	Texas	8,278	5.36%
5	Pennsylvania	8,228	5.33%
6	Massachusetts	7,020	4.55%
7	Florida	6,274	4.06%
8	New Jersey	6,114	3.96%
9	Ohio	6,102	3.95%
10	Maryland	5,506	3.57%
11	Michigan	5,182	3.36%
12	Virginia	3,894	2.52%
13	North Carolina	3,634	2.35%
14	Georgia	3,221	2.09%
15	Washington	3,128	2.03%
16	Minnesota	2,793	1.81%
17	Connecticut	2,781	1.80%
18	Missouri	2,633	1.70%
19	Wisconsin	2,555	1.65%
20	Tennessee	2,389	1.55%
21	Colorado	2,230	1.44%
22	Indiana	2,190	1.42%
23	Arizona	2,054	1.33%
24	Louisiana	2,028	1.31%
25	Oregon	1,618	1.05%
26	Kentucky	1,568	1.02%
27	Alabama	1,470	0.95%
28	South Carolina	1,438	0.93%
29	Kansas	1,162	0.75%
30	New Mexico	1,057	0.68%
31	Oklahoma	1,031	0.67%
32	Iowa	930	0.60%
33	Arkansas	815	0.53%
34	Rhode Island	791	0.51%
35	Hawaii	750	0.49%
36	West Virginia	749	0.49%
37	Mississippi	710	0.46%
38	Utah	665	0.43%
39	Nebraska	658	0.43%
40	Maine	614	0.40%
41	New Hampshire	546	0.35%
42	Nevada	453	0.29%
43	Vermont	430	0.28%
44	Delaware	425	0.28%
45	Montana	276	0.18%
46	Alaska	247	0.16%
46	Idaho	247	0.16%
48	South Dakota	221	0.14%
49	North Dakota	206	0.13%
50	Wyoming	117	0.08%
	District of Columbia	1,231	0.80%

Source: American Medical Association (Chicago, Illinois)
"Physician Characteristics and Distribution in the U.S." (1997-98 Edition)
*As of December 31, 1996. Comprised of federal and nonfederal physicians. Total does not include 2,956 female physicians in the U.S. territories and possessions, at APO's and FPO's and whose addresses are unknown.

Percent of Physicians Who Are Female: 1996

National Percent = 21.3% of Physicians*

ALPHA ORDER

ALPHA ORDER

RANK ORDER

RANK	STATE	PERCENT		RANK	STATE	PERCENT
40	Alabama	16		1	Massachusetts	27
17	Alaska	22		2	Maryland	26
29	Arizona	19		3	Illinois	25
41	Arkansas	16		3	New Mexico	25
18	California	21		3	New York	25
13	Colorado	22		6	New Jersey	25
10	Connecticut	22		7	Rhode Island	23
8	Delaware	23		8	Delaware	23
42	Florida	16		9	Michigan	23
28	Georgia	19		10	Connecticut	22
20	Hawaii	21		10	Vermont	22
50	Idaho	12		12	Pennsylvania	22
3	Illinois	25		13	Colorado	22
32	Indiana	18		13	Minnesota	22
39	Iowa	17		15	Ohio	22
26	Kansas	20		15	Virginia	22
30	Kentucky	18		17	Alaska	22
31	Louisiana	18		18	California	21
23	Maine	20		19	Washington	21
2	Maryland	26		20	Hawaii	21
1	Massachusetts	27		21	Missouri	20
9	Michigan	23		21	Wisconsin	20
13	Minnesota	22		23	Maine	20
44	Mississippi	15		23	Texas	20
21	Missouri	20		25	North Carolina	20
47	Montana	14		26	Kansas	20
36	Nebraska	17		26	Oregon	20
45	Nevada	15		28	Georgia	19
34	New Hampshire	18		29	Arizona	19
6	New Jersey	25		30	Kentucky	18
3	New Mexico	25		31	Louisiana	18
3	New York	25		32	Indiana	18
25	North Carolina	20		32	West Virginia	18
48	North Dakota	14		34	New Hampshire	18
15	Ohio	22		35	South Carolina	17
38	Oklahoma	17		36	Nebraska	17
26	Oregon	20		36	Tennessee	17
12	Pennsylvania	22		38	Oklahoma	17
7	Rhode Island	23		39	Iowa	17
35	South Carolina	17		40	Alabama	16
46	South Dakota	15		41	Arkansas	16
36	Tennessee	17		42	Florida	16
23	Texas	20		43	Utah	15
43	Utah	15		44	Mississippi	15
10	Vermont	22		45	Nevada	15
15	Virginia	22		46	South Dakota	15
19	Washington	21		47	Montana	14
32	West Virginia	18		48	North Dakota	14
21	Wisconsin	20		49	Wyoming	13
49	Wyoming	13		50	Idaho	12
					District of Columbia	29

Source: Morgan Quitno Press using data from American Medical Association (Chicago, Illinois)
"Physician Characteristics and Distribution in the U.S." (1997-98 Edition)
*As of December 31, 1996. Comprised of federal and nonfederal physicians. National percent does not include physicians in the U.S. territories and possessions, at APO's and FPO's and whose addresses are unknown.

Physicians Under 35 Years Old in 1996

National Total = 131,205 Physicians*

ALPHA ORDER				
RANK	STATE	PHYSICIANS	% of USA	
23	Alabama	1,666	1.27%	
48	Alaska	130	0.10%	
26	Arizona	1,587	1.21%	
32	Arkansas	831	0.63%	
2	California	12,774	9.74%	
25	Colorado	1,598	1.22%	
20	Connecticut	2,246	1.71%	
43	Delaware	298	0.23%	
9	Florida	4,605	3.51%	
14	Georgia	3,031	2.31%	
39	Hawaii	539	0.41%	
46	Idaho	207	0.16%	
4	Illinois	7,558	5.76%	
21	Indiana	2,015	1.54%	
29	Iowa	1,045	0.80%	
28	Kansas	1,061	0.81%	
27	Kentucky	1,537	1.17%	
18	Louisiana	2,397	1.83%	
41	Maine	331	0.25%	
10	Maryland	4,095	3.12%	
7	Massachusetts	5,680	4.33%	
8	Michigan	5,134	3.91%	
17	Minnesota	2,521	1.92%	
33	Mississippi	785	0.60%	
15	Missouri	2,816	2.15%	
49	Montana	119	0.09%	
34	Nebraska	742	0.57%	
42	Nevada	318	0.24%	
40	New Hampshire	349	0.27%	
11	New Jersey	3,860	2.94%	
38	New Mexico	598	0.46%	
1	New York	15,800	12.04%	
12	North Carolina	3,716	2.83%	
45	North Dakota	239	0.18%	
6	Ohio	5,951	4.54%	
31	Oklahoma	943	0.72%	
30	Oregon	1,043	0.79%	
5	Pennsylvania	7,365	5.61%	
35	Rhode Island	732	0.56%	
24	South Carolina	1,632	1.24%	
47	South Dakota	178	0.14%	
16	Tennessee	2,573	1.96%	
3	Texas	8,318	6.34%	
36	Utah	726	0.55%	
44	Vermont	293	0.22%	
13	Virginia	3,279	2.50%	
22	Washington	1,988	1.52%	
37	West Virginia	712	0.54%	
19	Wisconsin	2,282	1.74%	
50	Wyoming	109	0.08%	

RANK ORDER				
RANK	STATE	PHYSICIANS	% of USA	
1	New York	15,800	12.04%	
2	California	12,774	9.74%	
3	Texas	8,318	6.34%	
4	Illinois	7,558	5.76%	
5	Pennsylvania	7,365	5.61%	
6	Ohio	5,951	4.54%	
7	Massachusetts	5,680	4.33%	
8	Michigan	5,134	3.91%	
9	Florida	4,605	3.51%	
10	Maryland	4,095	3.12%	
11	New Jersey	3,860	2.94%	
12	North Carolina	3,716	2.83%	
13	Virginia	3,279	2.50%	
14	Georgia	3,031	2.31%	
15	Missouri	2,816	2.15%	
16	Tennessee	2,573	1.96%	
17	Minnesota	2,521	1.92%	
18	Louisiana	2,397	1.83%	
19	Wisconsin	2,282	1.74%	
20	Connecticut	2,246	1.71%	
21	Indiana	2,015	1.54%	
22	Washington	1,988	1.52%	
23	Alabama	1,666	1.27%	
24	South Carolina	1,632	1.24%	
25	Colorado	1,598	1.22%	
26	Arizona	1,587	1.21%	
27	Kentucky	1,537	1.17%	
28	Kansas	1,061	0.81%	
29	Iowa	1,045	0.80%	
30	Oregon	1,043	0.79%	
31	Oklahoma	943	0.72%	
32	Arkansas	831	0.63%	
33	Mississippi	785	0.60%	
34	Nebraska	742	0.57%	
35	Rhode Island	732	0.56%	
36	Utah	726	0.55%	
37	West Virginia	712	0.54%	
38	New Mexico	598	0.46%	
39	Hawaii	539	0.41%	
40	New Hampshire	349	0.27%	
41	Maine	331	0.25%	
42	Nevada	318	0.24%	
43	Delaware	298	0.23%	
44	Vermont	293	0.22%	
45	North Dakota	239	0.18%	
46	Idaho	207	0.16%	
47	South Dakota	178	0.14%	
48	Alaska	130	0.10%	
49	Montana	119	0.09%	
50	Wyoming	109	0.08%	
	District of Columbia	853	0.65%	

Source: American Medical Association (Chicago, Illinois)
   "Physician Characteristics and Distribution in the U.S." (1997-98 Edition)
*As of December 31, 1996. Comprised of federal and nonfederal physicians. Total does not include 1,800 physicians in the U.S. territories and possessions, at APO's and FPO's and whose addresses are unknown.

Percent of Physicians Under 35 Years Old in 1996

National Percent = 18.1% of Physicians*

ALPHA ORDER

RANK	STATE	PERCENT
18	Alabama	18.4
46	Alaska	11.3
36	Arizona	14.7
29	Arkansas	16.2
39	California	14.2
32	Colorado	15.7
20	Connecticut	18.1
29	Delaware	16.2
45	Florida	11.4
20	Georgia	18.1
36	Hawaii	14.7
49	Idaho	10.2
1	Illinois	23.1
26	Indiana	16.7
16	Iowa	18.8
24	Kansas	17.8
22	Kentucky	18.0
4	Louisiana	21.7
47	Maine	10.7
15	Maryland	19.0
5	Massachusetts	21.6
2	Michigan	22.3
12	Minnesota	19.8
27	Mississippi	16.6
7	Missouri	21.5
50	Montana	6.1
14	Nebraska	19.5
48	Nevada	10.5
44	New Hampshire	11.5
33	New Jersey	15.6
38	New Mexico	14.4
3	New York	21.8
9	North Carolina	20.3
31	North Dakota	15.9
8	Ohio	21.3
34	Oklahoma	15.5
41	Oregon	12.6
10	Pennsylvania	20.0
5	Rhode Island	21.6
13	South Carolina	19.7
42	South Dakota	11.8
17	Tennessee	18.6
10	Texas	20.0
28	Utah	16.4
35	Vermont	15.3
18	Virginia	18.4
40	Washington	13.3
25	West Virginia	17.2
23	Wisconsin	17.9
42	Wyoming	11.8

RANK ORDER

RANK	STATE	PERCENT
1	Illinois	23.1
2	Michigan	22.3
3	New York	21.8
4	Louisiana	21.7
5	Massachusetts	21.6
5	Rhode Island	21.6
7	Missouri	21.5
8	Ohio	21.3
9	North Carolina	20.3
10	Pennsylvania	20.0
10	Texas	20.0
12	Minnesota	19.8
13	South Carolina	19.7
14	Nebraska	19.5
15	Maryland	19.0
16	Iowa	18.8
17	Tennessee	18.6
18	Alabama	18.4
18	Virginia	18.4
20	Connecticut	18.1
20	Georgia	18.1
22	Kentucky	18.0
23	Wisconsin	17.9
24	Kansas	17.8
25	West Virginia	17.2
26	Indiana	16.7
27	Mississippi	16.6
28	Utah	16.4
29	Arkansas	16.2
29	Delaware	16.2
31	North Dakota	15.9
32	Colorado	15.7
33	New Jersey	15.6
34	Oklahoma	15.5
35	Vermont	15.3
36	Arizona	14.7
36	Hawaii	14.7
38	New Mexico	14.4
39	California	14.2
40	Washington	13.3
41	Oregon	12.6
42	South Dakota	11.8
42	Wyoming	11.8
44	New Hampshire	11.5
45	Florida	11.4
46	Alaska	11.3
47	Maine	10.7
48	Nevada	10.5
49	Idaho	10.2
50	Montana	6.1

| | District of Columbia | 19.9 |

Source: Morgan Quitno Press using data from American Medical Association (Chicago, Illinois)
"Physician Characteristics and Distribution in the U.S." (1997-98 Edition)
*As of December 31, 1996. Comprised of federal and nonfederal physicians. National percent does not include physicians in the U.S. territories and possessions, at APO's and FPO's and whose addresses are unknown.

Physicians 35 to 44 Years Old in 1996

National Total = 209,150 Physicians*

RANK	STATE	PHYSICIANS	% of USA
25	Alabama	2,910	1.39%
49	Alaska	374	0.18%
24	Arizona	3,013	1.44%
32	Arkansas	1,632	0.78%
1	California	22,751	10.88%
23	Colorado	3,071	1.47%
21	Connecticut	3,604	1.72%
46	Delaware	517	0.25%
4	Florida	11,103	5.31%
13	Georgia	5,395	2.58%
37	Hawaii	1,099	0.53%
43	Idaho	594	0.28%
6	Illinois	9,221	4.41%
20	Indiana	3,727	1.78%
31	Iowa	1,635	0.78%
30	Kansas	1,687	0.81%
26	Kentucky	2,650	1.27%
22	Louisiana	3,126	1.49%
42	Maine	852	0.41%
10	Maryland	6,470	3.09%
8	Massachusetts	7,848	3.75%
11	Michigan	6,295	3.01%
19	Minnesota	3,980	1.90%
33	Mississippi	1,428	0.68%
17	Missouri	4,012	1.92%
44	Montana	585	0.28%
36	Nebraska	1,183	0.57%
39	Nevada	963	0.46%
41	New Hampshire	905	0.43%
9	New Jersey	7,282	3.48%
35	New Mexico	1,209	0.58%
2	New York	20,122	9.62%
12	North Carolina	5,915	2.83%
48	North Dakota	460	0.22%
7	Ohio	7,957	3.80%
29	Oklahoma	1,733	0.83%
28	Oregon	2,285	1.09%
5	Pennsylvania	11,028	5.27%
40	Rhode Island	962	0.46%
27	South Carolina	2,430	1.16%
47	South Dakota	494	0.24%
15	Tennessee	4,471	2.14%
3	Texas	12,237	5.85%
34	Utah	1,388	0.66%
45	Vermont	538	0.26%
14	Virginia	5,244	2.51%
16	Washington	4,385	2.10%
38	West Virginia	1,092	0.52%
18	Wisconsin	4,009	1.92%
50	Wyoming	263	0.13%

RANK	STATE	PHYSICIANS	% of USA
1	California	22,751	10.88%
2	New York	20,122	9.62%
3	Texas	12,237	5.85%
4	Florida	11,103	5.31%
5	Pennsylvania	11,028	5.27%
6	Illinois	9,221	4.41%
7	Ohio	7,957	3.80%
8	Massachusetts	7,848	3.75%
9	New Jersey	7,282	3.48%
10	Maryland	6,470	3.09%
11	Michigan	6,295	3.01%
12	North Carolina	5,915	2.83%
13	Georgia	5,395	2.58%
14	Virginia	5,244	2.51%
15	Tennessee	4,471	2.14%
16	Washington	4,385	2.10%
17	Missouri	4,012	1.92%
18	Wisconsin	4,009	1.92%
19	Minnesota	3,980	1.90%
20	Indiana	3,727	1.78%
21	Connecticut	3,604	1.72%
22	Louisiana	3,126	1.49%
23	Colorado	3,071	1.47%
24	Arizona	3,013	1.44%
25	Alabama	2,910	1.39%
26	Kentucky	2,650	1.27%
27	South Carolina	2,430	1.16%
28	Oregon	2,285	1.09%
29	Oklahoma	1,733	0.83%
30	Kansas	1,687	0.81%
31	Iowa	1,635	0.78%
32	Arkansas	1,632	0.78%
33	Mississippi	1,428	0.68%
34	Utah	1,388	0.66%
35	New Mexico	1,209	0.58%
36	Nebraska	1,183	0.57%
37	Hawaii	1,099	0.53%
38	West Virginia	1,092	0.52%
39	Nevada	963	0.46%
40	Rhode Island	962	0.46%
41	New Hampshire	905	0.43%
42	Maine	852	0.41%
43	Idaho	594	0.28%
44	Montana	585	0.28%
45	Vermont	538	0.26%
46	Delaware	517	0.25%
47	South Dakota	494	0.24%
48	North Dakota	460	0.22%
49	Alaska	374	0.18%
50	Wyoming	263	0.13%
	District of Columbia	1,016	0.49%

Source: American Medical Association (Chicago, Illinois)
   "Physician Characteristics and Distribution in the U.S." (1997-98 Edition)
As of December 31, 1996. Comprised of federal and nonfederal physicians. Total does not include 3,603 physicians in the U.S. territories and possessions, at APO's and FPO's and whose addresses are unknown.

Physicians 45 to 54 Years Old in 1996

National Total = 164,937 Physicians*

ALPHA ORDER

RANK ORDER

RANK	STATE	PHYSICIANS	% of USA
26	Alabama	2,012	1.22%
49	Alaska	343	0.21%
24	Arizona	2,359	1.43%
32	Arkansas	1,171	0.71%
1	California	22,612	13.71%
22	Colorado	2,538	1.54%
21	Connecticut	2,742	1.66%
46	Delaware	405	0.25%
4	Florida	8,733	5.29%
15	Georgia	3,795	2.30%
37	Hawaii	879	0.53%
44	Idaho	531	0.32%
6	Illinois	7,141	4.33%
20	Indiana	2,759	1.67%
31	Iowa	1,250	0.76%
30	Kansas	1,344	0.81%
27	Kentucky	1,931	1.17%
23	Louisiana	2,444	1.48%
39	Maine	785	0.48%
11	Maryland	4,976	3.02%
9	Massachusetts	5,786	3.51%
10	Michigan	5,018	3.04%
17	Minnesota	2,887	1.75%
36	Mississippi	1,018	0.62%
18	Missouri	2,792	1.69%
43	Montana	535	0.32%
38	Nebraska	835	0.51%
40	Nevada	762	0.46%
41	New Hampshire	759	0.46%
7	New Jersey	5,971	3.62%
34	New Mexico	1,102	0.67%
2	New York	15,013	9.10%
14	North Carolina	3,820	2.32%
48	North Dakota	377	0.23%
8	Ohio	5,910	3.58%
29	Oklahoma	1,469	0.89%
25	Oregon	2,202	1.34%
5	Pennsylvania	7,884	4.78%
42	Rhode Island	645	0.39%
28	South Carolina	1,841	1.12%
47	South Dakota	396	0.24%
16	Tennessee	3,124	1.89%
3	Texas	9,431	5.72%
33	Utah	1,109	0.67%
45	Vermont	461	0.28%
12	Virginia	4,077	2.47%
13	Washington	3,938	2.39%
35	West Virginia	1,046	0.63%
19	Wisconsin	2,769	1.68%
50	Wyoming	234	0.14%

RANK	STATE	PHYSICIANS	% of USA
1	California	22,612	13.71%
2	New York	15,013	9.10%
3	Texas	9,431	5.72%
4	Florida	8,733	5.29%
5	Pennsylvania	7,884	4.78%
6	Illinois	7,141	4.33%
7	New Jersey	5,971	3.62%
8	Ohio	5,910	3.58%
9	Massachusetts	5,786	3.51%
10	Michigan	5,018	3.04%
11	Maryland	4,976	3.02%
12	Virginia	4,077	2.47%
13	Washington	3,938	2.39%
14	North Carolina	3,820	2.32%
15	Georgia	3,795	2.30%
16	Tennessee	3,124	1.89%
17	Minnesota	2,887	1.75%
18	Missouri	2,792	1.69%
19	Wisconsin	2,769	1.68%
20	Indiana	2,759	1.67%
21	Connecticut	2,742	1.66%
22	Colorado	2,538	1.54%
23	Louisiana	2,444	1.48%
24	Arizona	2,359	1.43%
25	Oregon	2,202	1.34%
26	Alabama	2,012	1.22%
27	Kentucky	1,931	1.17%
28	South Carolina	1,841	1.12%
29	Oklahoma	1,469	0.89%
30	Kansas	1,344	0.81%
31	Iowa	1,250	0.76%
32	Arkansas	1,171	0.71%
33	Utah	1,109	0.67%
34	New Mexico	1,102	0.67%
35	West Virginia	1,046	0.63%
36	Mississippi	1,018	0.62%
37	Hawaii	879	0.53%
38	Nebraska	835	0.51%
39	Maine	785	0.48%
40	Nevada	762	0.46%
41	New Hampshire	759	0.46%
42	Rhode Island	645	0.39%
43	Montana	535	0.32%
44	Idaho	531	0.32%
45	Vermont	461	0.28%
46	Delaware	405	0.25%
47	South Dakota	396	0.24%
48	North Dakota	377	0.23%
49	Alaska	343	0.21%
50	Wyoming	234	0.14%
	District of Columbia	976	0.59%

Source: American Medical Association (Chicago, Illinois)
"Physician Characteristics and Distribution in the U.S." (1997-98 Edition)
*As of December 31, 1996. Comprised of federal and nonfederal physicians. Total does not include 2,409 physicians in the U.S. territories and possessions, at APO's and FPO's and whose addresses are unknown.

Physicians 55 to 64 Years Old in 1996

National Total = 97,949 Physicians*

ALPHA ORDER

RANK	STATE	PHYSICIANS	% of USA
27	Alabama	1,129	1.15%
49	Alaska	192	0.20%
22	Arizona	1,487	1.52%
31	Arkansas	696	0.71%
1	California	13,457	13.74%
24	Colorado	1,372	1.40%
18	Connecticut	1,646	1.68%
45	Delaware	286	0.29%
3	Florida	5,791	5.91%
13	Georgia	2,242	2.29%
37	Hawaii	479	0.49%
44	Idaho	304	0.31%
6	Illinois	4,310	4.40%
20	Indiana	1,568	1.60%
34	Iowa	655	0.67%
30	Kansas	784	0.80%
26	Kentucky	1,159	1.18%
23	Louisiana	1,447	1.48%
41	Maine	436	0.45%
11	Maryland	2,912	2.97%
9	Massachusetts	3,142	3.21%
10	Michigan	3,067	3.13%
21	Minnesota	1,489	1.52%
32	Mississippi	692	0.71%
16	Missouri	1,699	1.73%
43	Montana	314	0.32%
38	Nebraska	466	0.48%
39	Nevada	464	0.47%
42	New Hampshire	411	0.42%
7	New Jersey	3,673	3.75%
35	New Mexico	552	0.56%
2	New York	9,794	10.00%
14	North Carolina	2,126	2.17%
47	North Dakota	223	0.23%
8	Ohio	3,625	3.70%
29	Oklahoma	920	0.94%
25	Oregon	1,214	1.24%
5	Pennsylvania	4,560	4.66%
40	Rhode Island	453	0.46%
28	South Carolina	1,042	1.06%
48	South Dakota	193	0.20%
17	Tennessee	1,665	1.70%
4	Texas	5,473	5.59%
36	Utah	514	0.52%
46	Vermont	236	0.24%
12	Virginia	2,387	2.44%
15	Washington	1,993	2.03%
33	West Virginia	658	0.67%
19	Wisconsin	1,631	1.67%
50	Wyoming	143	0.15%

RANK ORDER

RANK	STATE	PHYSICIANS	% of USA
1	California	13,457	13.74%
2	New York	9,794	10.00%
3	Florida	5,791	5.91%
4	Texas	5,473	5.59%
5	Pennsylvania	4,560	4.66%
6	Illinois	4,310	4.40%
7	New Jersey	3,673	3.75%
8	Ohio	3,625	3.70%
9	Massachusetts	3,142	3.21%
10	Michigan	3,067	3.13%
11	Maryland	2,912	2.97%
12	Virginia	2,387	2.44%
13	Georgia	2,242	2.29%
14	North Carolina	2,126	2.17%
15	Washington	1,993	2.03%
16	Missouri	1,699	1.73%
17	Tennessee	1,665	1.70%
18	Connecticut	1,646	1.68%
19	Wisconsin	1,631	1.67%
20	Indiana	1,568	1.60%
21	Minnesota	1,489	1.52%
22	Arizona	1,487	1.52%
23	Louisiana	1,447	1.48%
24	Colorado	1,372	1.40%
25	Oregon	1,214	1.24%
26	Kentucky	1,159	1.18%
27	Alabama	1,129	1.15%
28	South Carolina	1,042	1.06%
29	Oklahoma	920	0.94%
30	Kansas	784	0.80%
31	Arkansas	696	0.71%
32	Mississippi	692	0.71%
33	West Virginia	658	0.67%
34	Iowa	655	0.67%
35	New Mexico	552	0.56%
36	Utah	514	0.52%
37	Hawaii	479	0.49%
38	Nebraska	466	0.48%
39	Nevada	464	0.47%
40	Rhode Island	453	0.46%
41	Maine	436	0.45%
42	New Hampshire	411	0.42%
43	Montana	314	0.32%
44	Idaho	304	0.31%
45	Delaware	286	0.29%
46	Vermont	236	0.24%
47	North Dakota	223	0.23%
48	South Dakota	193	0.20%
49	Alaska	192	0.20%
50	Wyoming	143	0.15%

| | District of Columbia | 778 | 0.79% |

Source: American Medical Association (Chicago, Illinois)
   "Physician Characteristics and Distribution in the U.S." (1997-98 Edition)
*As of December 31, 1996. Comprised of federal and nonfederal physicians. Total does not include 1,549 physicians in the U.S. territories and possessions, at APO's and FPO's and whose addresses are unknown.

Physicians 65 Years Old and Older in 1996

National Total = 122,563 Physicians*

ALPHA ORDER

RANK	STATE	PHYSICIANS	% of USA
27	Alabama	1,321	1.08%
50	Alaska	107	0.09%
15	Arizona	2,344	1.91%
32	Arkansas	802	0.65%
1	California	18,172	14.83%
24	Colorado	1,623	1.32%
17	Connecticut	2,178	1.78%
46	Delaware	339	0.28%
3	Florida	10,218	8.34%
16	Georgia	2,319	1.89%
37	Hawaii	661	0.54%
43	Idaho	401	0.33%
6	Illinois	4,552	3.71%
19	Indiana	2,014	1.64%
31	Iowa	964	0.79%
29	Kansas	1,080	0.88%
28	Kentucky	1,249	1.02%
23	Louisiana	1,646	1.34%
35	Maine	681	0.56%
11	Maryland	3,061	2.50%
9	Massachusetts	3,793	3.09%
10	Michigan	3,457	2.82%
21	Minnesota	1,881	1.53%
33	Mississippi	798	0.65%
22	Missouri	1,784	1.46%
44	Montana	395	0.32%
41	Nebraska	588	0.48%
42	Nevada	526	0.43%
39	New Hampshire	618	0.50%
8	New Jersey	3,947	3.22%
34	New Mexico	695	0.57%
2	New York	11,803	9.63%
13	North Carolina	2,769	2.26%
48	North Dakota	208	0.17%
7	Ohio	4,529	3.70%
30	Oklahoma	1,002	0.82%
25	Oregon	1,539	1.26%
5	Pennsylvania	6,045	4.93%
40	Rhode Island	590	0.48%
26	South Carolina	1,338	1.09%
47	South Dakota	244	0.20%
20	Tennessee	1,993	1.63%
4	Texas	6,220	5.07%
36	Utah	677	0.55%
45	Vermont	390	0.32%
12	Virginia	2,853	2.33%
14	Washington	2,651	2.16%
38	West Virginia	633	0.52%
18	Wisconsin	2,023	1.65%
49	Wyoming	176	0.14%

RANK ORDER

RANK	STATE	PHYSICIANS	% of USA
1	California	18,172	14.83%
2	New York	11,803	9.63%
3	Florida	10,218	8.34%
4	Texas	6,220	5.07%
5	Pennsylvania	6,045	4.93%
6	Illinois	4,552	3.71%
7	Ohio	4,529	3.70%
8	New Jersey	3,947	3.22%
9	Massachusetts	3,793	3.09%
10	Michigan	3,457	2.82%
11	Maryland	3,061	2.50%
12	Virginia	2,853	2.33%
13	North Carolina	2,769	2.26%
14	Washington	2,651	2.16%
15	Arizona	2,344	1.91%
16	Georgia	2,319	1.89%
17	Connecticut	2,178	1.78%
18	Wisconsin	2,023	1.65%
19	Indiana	2,014	1.64%
20	Tennessee	1,993	1.63%
21	Minnesota	1,881	1.53%
22	Missouri	1,784	1.46%
23	Louisiana	1,646	1.34%
24	Colorado	1,623	1.32%
25	Oregon	1,539	1.26%
26	South Carolina	1,338	1.09%
27	Alabama	1,321	1.08%
28	Kentucky	1,249	1.02%
29	Kansas	1,080	0.88%
30	Oklahoma	1,002	0.82%
31	Iowa	964	0.79%
32	Arkansas	802	0.65%
33	Mississippi	798	0.65%
34	New Mexico	695	0.57%
35	Maine	681	0.56%
36	Utah	677	0.55%
37	Hawaii	661	0.54%
38	West Virginia	633	0.52%
39	New Hampshire	618	0.50%
40	Rhode Island	590	0.48%
41	Nebraska	588	0.48%
42	Nevada	526	0.43%
43	Idaho	401	0.33%
44	Montana	395	0.32%
45	Vermont	390	0.32%
46	Delaware	339	0.28%
47	South Dakota	244	0.20%
48	North Dakota	208	0.17%
49	Wyoming	176	0.14%
50	Alaska	107	0.09%
	District of Columbia	666	0.54%

Source: American Medical Association (Chicago, Illinois)
"Physician Characteristics and Distribution in the U.S." (1997-98 Edition)
As of December 31, 1996. Comprised of federal and nonfederal physicians. Total does not include 2,599 physicians in the U.S. territories and possessions, at APO's and FPO's and whose addresses are unknown.

Percent of Physicians 65 Years Old and Older in 1996

National Percent = 16.9% of Physicians*

ALPHA ORDER				RANK ORDER		
RANK	STATE	PERCENT		RANK	STATE	PERCENT
41	Alabama	14.6		1	Florida	25.3
50	Alaska	9.3		2	Maine	22.1
3	Arizona	21.7		3	Arizona	21.7
32	Arkansas	15.6		4	Montana	20.3
7	California	20.2		4	New Hampshire	20.3
30	Colorado	15.9		4	Vermont	20.3
15	Connecticut	17.5		7	California	20.2
11	Delaware	18.4		8	Idaho	19.7
1	Florida	25.3		9	Wyoming	19.0
47	Georgia	13.8		10	Oregon	18.6
12	Hawaii	18.1		11	Delaware	18.4
8	Idaho	19.7		12	Hawaii	18.1
46	Illinois	13.9		12	Kansas	18.1
20	Indiana	16.7		14	Washington	17.7
16	Iowa	17.4		15	Connecticut	17.5
12	Kansas	18.1		16	Iowa	17.4
41	Kentucky	14.6		16	Rhode Island	17.4
38	Louisiana	14.9		18	Nevada	17.3
2	Maine	22.1		19	Mississippi	16.9
45	Maryland	14.2		20	Indiana	16.7
43	Massachusetts	14.5		20	New Mexico	16.7
37	Michigan	15.0		22	Oklahoma	16.5
40	Minnesota	14.7		23	Pennsylvania	16.4
19	Mississippi	16.9		24	New York	16.3
49	Missouri	13.6		25	Ohio	16.2
4	Montana	20.3		25	South Carolina	16.2
33	Nebraska	15.4		25	South Dakota	16.2
18	Nevada	17.3		28	New Jersey	16.0
4	New Hampshire	20.3		28	Virginia	16.0
28	New Jersey	16.0		30	Colorado	15.9
20	New Mexico	16.7		30	Wisconsin	15.9
24	New York	16.3		32	Arkansas	15.6
36	North Carolina	15.1		33	Nebraska	15.4
47	North Dakota	13.8		34	Utah	15.3
25	Ohio	16.2		34	West Virginia	15.3
22	Oklahoma	16.5		36	North Carolina	15.1
10	Oregon	18.6		37	Michigan	15.0
23	Pennsylvania	16.4		38	Louisiana	14.9
16	Rhode Island	17.4		38	Texas	14.9
25	South Carolina	16.2		40	Minnesota	14.7
25	South Dakota	16.2		41	Alabama	14.6
44	Tennessee	14.4		41	Kentucky	14.6
38	Texas	14.9		43	Massachusetts	14.5
34	Utah	15.3		44	Tennessee	14.4
4	Vermont	20.3		45	Maryland	14.2
28	Virginia	16.0		46	Illinois	13.9
14	Washington	17.7		47	Georgia	13.8
34	West Virginia	15.3		47	North Dakota	13.8
30	Wisconsin	15.9		49	Missouri	13.6
9	Wyoming	19.0		50	Alaska	9.3
					District of Columbia	15.5

Source: Morgan Quitno Press using data from American Medical Association (Chicago, Illinois)
"Physician Characteristics and Distribution in the U.S." (1997-98 Edition)
*As of December 31, 1996. Comprised of federal and nonfederal physicians. National percent does not include physicians in the U.S. territories and possessions, at APO's and FPO's and whose addresses are unknown.

Federal Physicians in 1996

National Total = 19,132 Physicians*

RANK	STATE	PHYSICIANS	% of USA
29	Alabama	170	0.89%
31	Alaska	153	0.80%
16	Arizona	326	1.70%
37	Arkansas	84	0.44%
1	California	2,173	11.36%
10	Colorado	554	2.90%
25	Connecticut	206	1.08%
47	Delaware	33	0.17%
8	Florida	735	3.84%
5	Georgia	838	4.38%
14	Hawaii	348	1.82%
45	Idaho	41	0.21%
7	Illinois	788	4.12%
35	Indiana	107	0.56%
40	Iowa	70	0.37%
30	Kansas	154	0.80%
21	Kentucky	256	1.34%
22	Louisiana	221	1.16%
47	Maine	33	0.17%
3	Maryland	2,058	10.76%
19	Massachusetts	299	1.56%
27	Michigan	193	1.01%
20	Minnesota	282	1.47%
18	Mississippi	300	1.57%
26	Missouri	196	1.02%
46	Montana	35	0.18%
31	Nebraska	153	0.80%
36	Nevada	91	0.48%
44	New Hampshire	53	0.28%
17	New Jersey	324	1.69%
28	New Mexico	176	0.92%
6	New York	814	4.25%
12	North Carolina	463	2.42%
39	North Dakota	79	0.41%
11	Ohio	515	2.69%
31	Oklahoma	153	0.80%
34	Oregon	129	0.67%
13	Pennsylvania	405	2.12%
43	Rhode Island	57	0.30%
23	South Carolina	219	1.14%
41	South Dakota	58	0.30%
15	Tennessee	337	1.76%
2	Texas	2,123	11.10%
38	Utah	83	0.43%
50	Vermont	23	0.12%
4	Virginia	970	5.07%
9	Washington	636	3.32%
41	West Virginia	58	0.30%
24	Wisconsin	210	1.10%
49	Wyoming	29	0.15%

RANK	STATE	PHYSICIANS	% of USA
1	California	2,173	11.36%
2	Texas	2,123	11.10%
3	Maryland	2,058	10.76%
4	Virginia	970	5.07%
5	Georgia	838	4.38%
6	New York	814	4.25%
7	Illinois	788	4.12%
8	Florida	735	3.84%
9	Washington	636	3.32%
10	Colorado	554	2.90%
11	Ohio	515	2.69%
12	North Carolina	463	2.42%
13	Pennsylvania	405	2.12%
14	Hawaii	348	1.82%
15	Tennessee	337	1.76%
16	Arizona	326	1.70%
17	New Jersey	324	1.69%
18	Mississippi	300	1.57%
19	Massachusetts	299	1.56%
20	Minnesota	282	1.47%
21	Kentucky	256	1.34%
22	Louisiana	221	1.16%
23	South Carolina	219	1.14%
24	Wisconsin	210	1.10%
25	Connecticut	206	1.08%
26	Missouri	196	1.02%
27	Michigan	193	1.01%
28	New Mexico	176	0.92%
29	Alabama	170	0.89%
30	Kansas	154	0.80%
31	Alaska	153	0.80%
31	Nebraska	153	0.80%
31	Oklahoma	153	0.80%
34	Oregon	129	0.67%
35	Indiana	107	0.56%
36	Nevada	91	0.48%
37	Arkansas	84	0.44%
38	Utah	83	0.43%
39	North Dakota	79	0.41%
40	Iowa	70	0.37%
41	South Dakota	58	0.30%
41	West Virginia	58	0.30%
43	Rhode Island	57	0.30%
44	New Hampshire	53	0.28%
45	Idaho	41	0.21%
46	Montana	35	0.18%
47	Delaware	33	0.17%
47	Maine	33	0.17%
49	Wyoming	29	0.15%
50	Vermont	23	0.12%
	District of Columbia	321	1.68%

Source: American Medical Association (Chicago, Illinois)
"Physician Characteristics and Distribution in the U.S." (1997-98 Edition)
*As of December 31, 1996. Total does not include 1,297 physicians in U.S. territories and possessions.

Rate of Federal Physicians in 1996

National Rate = 7.2 Physicians per 100,000 Population*

ALPHA ORDER

RANK	STATE	RATE
37	Alabama	4.0
3	Alaska	25.3
14	Arizona	7.4
44	Arkansas	3.4
15	California	6.8
5	Colorado	14.5
18	Connecticut	6.3
30	Delaware	4.6
27	Florida	5.1
8	Georgia	11.4
2	Hawaii	29.4
43	Idaho	3.5
16	Illinois	6.7
50	Indiana	1.8
48	Iowa	2.5
22	Kansas	6.0
17	Kentucky	6.6
27	Louisiana	5.1
47	Maine	2.7
1	Maryland	40.7
29	Massachusetts	4.9
49	Michigan	2.0
21	Minnesota	6.1
9	Mississippi	11.1
42	Missouri	3.7
37	Montana	4.0
12	Nebraska	9.3
26	Nevada	5.7
30	New Hampshire	4.6
37	New Jersey	4.0
11	New Mexico	10.3
34	New York	4.5
18	North Carolina	6.3
6	North Dakota	12.3
30	Ohio	4.6
30	Oklahoma	4.6
37	Oregon	4.0
44	Pennsylvania	3.4
25	Rhode Island	5.8
24	South Carolina	5.9
13	South Dakota	7.9
18	Tennessee	6.3
9	Texas	11.1
35	Utah	4.1
41	Vermont	3.9
4	Virginia	14.6
7	Washington	11.5
46	West Virginia	3.2
35	Wisconsin	4.1
22	Wyoming	6.0

RANK ORDER

RANK	STATE	RATE
1	Maryland	40.7
2	Hawaii	29.4
3	Alaska	25.3
4	Virginia	14.6
5	Colorado	14.5
6	North Dakota	12.3
7	Washington	11.5
8	Georgia	11.4
9	Mississippi	11.1
9	Texas	11.1
11	New Mexico	10.3
12	Nebraska	9.3
13	South Dakota	7.9
14	Arizona	7.4
15	California	6.8
16	Illinois	6.7
17	Kentucky	6.6
18	Connecticut	6.3
18	North Carolina	6.3
18	Tennessee	6.3
21	Minnesota	6.1
22	Kansas	6.0
22	Wyoming	6.0
24	South Carolina	5.9
25	Rhode Island	5.8
26	Nevada	5.7
27	Florida	5.1
27	Louisiana	5.1
29	Massachusetts	4.9
30	Delaware	4.6
30	New Hampshire	4.6
30	Ohio	4.6
30	Oklahoma	4.6
34	New York	4.5
35	Utah	4.1
35	Wisconsin	4.1
37	Alabama	4.0
37	Montana	4.0
37	New Jersey	4.0
37	Oregon	4.0
41	Vermont	3.9
42	Missouri	3.7
43	Idaho	3.5
44	Arkansas	3.4
44	Pennsylvania	3.4
46	West Virginia	3.2
47	Maine	2.7
48	Iowa	2.5
49	Michigan	2.0
50	Indiana	1.8

District of Columbia 59.5

Source: Morgan Quitno Press using data from American Medical Association (Chicago, Illinois) "Physician Characteristics and Distribution in the U.S." (1997-98 Edition)
As of December 31, 1996. National rate does not include physicians in U.S. territories and possessions.

Nonfederal Physicians in 1996

National Total = 706,672 Physicians*

ALPHA ORDER

RANK	STATE	PHYSICIANS	% of USA
25	Alabama	8,868	1.25%
49	Alaska	993	0.14%
23	Arizona	10,464	1.48%
32	Arkansas	5,048	0.71%
1	California	87,593	12.40%
24	Colorado	9,648	1.37%
20	Connecticut	12,210	1.73%
46	Delaware	1,812	0.26%
3	Florida	39,715	5.62%
14	Georgia	15,944	2.26%
39	Hawaii	3,309	0.47%
43	Idaho	1,996	0.28%
6	Illinois	31,994	4.53%
21	Indiana	11,976	1.69%
31	Iowa	5,479	0.78%
30	Kansas	5,802	0.82%
26	Kentucky	8,270	1.17%
22	Louisiana	10,839	1.53%
40	Maine	3,052	0.43%
11	Maryland	19,456	2.75%
8	Massachusetts	25,950	3.67%
10	Michigan	22,778	3.22%
19	Minnesota	12,476	1.77%
33	Mississippi	4,421	0.63%
17	Missouri	12,907	1.83%
44	Montana	1,913	0.27%
37	Nebraska	3,661	0.52%
42	Nevada	2,942	0.42%
41	New Hampshire	2,989	0.42%
9	New Jersey	24,409	3.45%
36	New Mexico	3,980	0.56%
2	New York	71,718	10.15%
12	North Carolina	17,883	2.53%
48	North Dakota	1,428	0.20%
7	Ohio	27,457	3.89%
29	Oklahoma	5,914	0.84%
27	Oregon	8,154	1.15%
5	Pennsylvania	36,477	5.16%
38	Rhode Island	3,325	0.47%
28	South Carolina	8,064	1.14%
47	South Dakota	1,447	0.20%
16	Tennessee	13,489	1.91%
4	Texas	39,556	5.60%
34	Utah	4,331	0.61%
45	Vermont	1,895	0.27%
13	Virginia	16,870	2.39%
15	Washington	14,319	2.03%
35	West Virginia	4,083	0.58%
18	Wisconsin	12,504	1.77%
50	Wyoming	896	0.13%

RANK ORDER

RANK	STATE	PHYSICIANS	% of USA
1	California	87,593	12.40%
2	New York	71,718	10.15%
3	Florida	39,715	5.62%
4	Texas	39,556	5.60%
5	Pennsylvania	36,477	5.16%
6	Illinois	31,994	4.53%
7	Ohio	27,457	3.89%
8	Massachusetts	25,950	3.67%
9	New Jersey	24,409	3.45%
10	Michigan	22,778	3.22%
11	Maryland	19,456	2.75%
12	North Carolina	17,883	2.53%
13	Virginia	16,870	2.39%
14	Georgia	15,944	2.26%
15	Washington	14,319	2.03%
16	Tennessee	13,489	1.91%
17	Missouri	12,907	1.83%
18	Wisconsin	12,504	1.77%
19	Minnesota	12,476	1.77%
20	Connecticut	12,210	1.73%
21	Indiana	11,976	1.69%
22	Louisiana	10,839	1.53%
23	Arizona	10,464	1.48%
24	Colorado	9,648	1.37%
25	Alabama	8,868	1.25%
26	Kentucky	8,270	1.17%
27	Oregon	8,154	1.15%
28	South Carolina	8,064	1.14%
29	Oklahoma	5,914	0.84%
30	Kansas	5,802	0.82%
31	Iowa	5,479	0.78%
32	Arkansas	5,048	0.71%
33	Mississippi	4,421	0.63%
34	Utah	4,331	0.61%
35	West Virginia	4,083	0.58%
36	New Mexico	3,980	0.56%
37	Nebraska	3,661	0.52%
38	Rhode Island	3,325	0.47%
39	Hawaii	3,309	0.47%
40	Maine	3,052	0.43%
41	New Hampshire	2,989	0.42%
42	Nevada	2,942	0.42%
43	Idaho	1,996	0.28%
44	Montana	1,913	0.27%
45	Vermont	1,895	0.27%
46	Delaware	1,812	0.26%
47	South Dakota	1,447	0.20%
48	North Dakota	1,428	0.20%
49	Alaska	993	0.14%
50	Wyoming	896	0.13%
	District of Columbia	3,968	0.56%

Source: American Medical Association (Chicago, Illinois)
"Physician Characteristics and Distribution in the U.S." (1997-98 Edition)
As of December 31, 1996. Total does not include 9,352 nonfederal physicians in U.S. territories and possessions.

Rate of Nonfederal Physicians in 1996

National Rate = 268 Physicians per 100,000 Population*

ALPHA ORDER			RANK ORDER		
RANK	**STATE**	**RATE**	**RANK**	**STATE**	**RATE**
39	Alabama	208	1	Massachusetts	426
48	Alaska	169	2	New York	395
27	Arizona	237	3	Maryland	387
42	Arkansas	202	4	Connecticut	374
11	California	276	5	Rhode Island	337
18	Colorado	254	6	Vermont	322
4	Connecticut	374	7	New Jersey	306
20	Delaware	251	8	Pennsylvania	303
10	Florida	277	9	Hawaii	291
35	Georgia	219	10	Florida	277
9	Hawaii	291	11	California	276
49	Idaho	168	12	Illinois	271
12	Illinois	271	13	Minnesota	268
41	Indiana	205	14	Washington	261
44	Iowa	192	15	Virginia	259
30	Kansas	227	16	New Hampshire	257
38	Kentucky	214	17	Oregon	255
21	Louisiana	250	18	Colorado	254
23	Maine	246	18	Tennessee	254
3	Maryland	387	20	Delaware	251
1	Massachusetts	426	21	Louisiana	250
27	Michigan	237	22	North Carolina	248
13	Minnesota	268	23	Maine	246
50	Mississippi	164	23	Ohio	246
26	Missouri	241	25	Wisconsin	242
35	Montana	219	26	Missouri	241
33	Nebraska	223	27	Arizona	237
46	Nevada	184	27	Michigan	237
16	New Hampshire	257	29	New Mexico	234
7	New Jersey	306	30	Kansas	227
29	New Mexico	234	31	North Dakota	225
2	New York	395	32	West Virginia	224
22	North Carolina	248	33	Nebraska	223
31	North Dakota	225	34	South Carolina	220
23	Ohio	246	35	Georgia	219
47	Oklahoma	181	35	Montana	219
17	Oregon	255	37	Utah	217
8	Pennsylvania	303	38	Kentucky	214
5	Rhode Island	337	39	Alabama	208
34	South Carolina	220	39	Texas	208
43	South Dakota	198	41	Indiana	205
18	Tennessee	254	42	Arkansas	202
39	Texas	208	43	South Dakota	198
37	Utah	217	44	Iowa	192
6	Vermont	322	45	Wyoming	187
15	Virginia	259	46	Nevada	184
14	Washington	261	47	Oklahoma	181
32	West Virginia	224	48	Alaska	169
25	Wisconsin	242	49	Idaho	168
45	Wyoming	187	50	Mississippi	164
				District of Columbia	738

Source: American Medical Association (Chicago, Illinois)
    "Physician Characteristics and Distribution in the U.S." (1997-98 Edition)
*As of December 31, 1996.

Nonfederal Physicians in Patient Care in 1996

National Total = 572,945 Physicians*

ALPHA ORDER

RANK	STATE	PHYSICIANS	% of USA
25	Alabama	7,517	1.31%
49	Alaska	861	0.15%
23	Arizona	8,005	1.40%
32	Arkansas	4,221	0.74%
1	California	68,730	12.00%
24	Colorado	7,725	1.35%
21	Connecticut	9,733	1.70%
45	Delaware	1,482	0.26%
4	Florida	30,159	5.26%
14	Georgia	13,403	2.34%
39	Hawaii	2,657	0.46%
43	Idaho	1,643	0.29%
6	Illinois	26,758	4.67%
20	Indiana	9,987	1.74%
31	Iowa	4,374	0.76%
30	Kansas	4,706	0.82%
26	Kentucky	7,022	1.23%
22	Louisiana	9,210	1.61%
42	Maine	2,371	0.41%
11	Maryland	15,063	2.63%
8	Massachusetts	20,550	3.59%
10	Michigan	18,762	3.27%
19	Minnesota	10,066	1.76%
33	Mississippi	3,735	0.65%
17	Missouri	10,808	1.89%
44	Montana	1,535	0.27%
37	Nebraska	3,036	0.53%
40	Nevada	2,433	0.42%
41	New Hampshire	2,391	0.42%
9	New Jersey	20,127	3.51%
36	New Mexico	3,147	0.55%
2	New York	58,292	10.17%
12	North Carolina	14,577	2.54%
48	North Dakota	1,212	0.21%
7	Ohio	22,740	3.97%
29	Oklahoma	4,951	0.86%
28	Oregon	6,396	1.12%
5	Pennsylvania	29,859	5.21%
38	Rhode Island	2,721	0.47%
27	South Carolina	6,735	1.18%
47	South Dakota	1,225	0.21%
15	Tennessee	11,395	1.99%
3	Texas	33,156	5.79%
34	Utah	3,502	0.61%
46	Vermont	1,458	0.25%
13	Virginia	13,845	2.42%
16	Washington	11,243	1.96%
35	West Virginia	3,399	0.59%
18	Wisconsin	10,299	1.80%
50	Wyoming	714	0.12%

RANK ORDER

RANK	STATE	PHYSICIANS	% of USA
1	California	68,730	12.00%
2	New York	58,292	10.17%
3	Texas	33,156	5.79%
4	Florida	30,159	5.26%
5	Pennsylvania	29,859	5.21%
6	Illinois	26,758	4.67%
7	Ohio	22,740	3.97%
8	Massachusetts	20,550	3.59%
9	New Jersey	20,127	3.51%
10	Michigan	18,762	3.27%
11	Maryland	15,063	2.63%
12	North Carolina	14,577	2.54%
13	Virginia	13,845	2.42%
14	Georgia	13,403	2.34%
15	Tennessee	11,395	1.99%
16	Washington	11,243	1.96%
17	Missouri	10,808	1.89%
18	Wisconsin	10,299	1.80%
19	Minnesota	10,066	1.76%
20	Indiana	9,987	1.74%
21	Connecticut	9,733	1.70%
22	Louisiana	9,210	1.61%
23	Arizona	8,005	1.40%
24	Colorado	7,725	1.35%
25	Alabama	7,517	1.31%
26	Kentucky	7,022	1.23%
27	South Carolina	6,735	1.18%
28	Oregon	6,396	1.12%
29	Oklahoma	4,951	0.86%
30	Kansas	4,706	0.82%
31	Iowa	4,374	0.76%
32	Arkansas	4,221	0.74%
33	Mississippi	3,735	0.65%
34	Utah	3,502	0.61%
35	West Virginia	3,399	0.59%
36	New Mexico	3,147	0.55%
37	Nebraska	3,036	0.53%
38	Rhode Island	2,721	0.47%
39	Hawaii	2,657	0.46%
40	Nevada	2,433	0.42%
41	New Hampshire	2,391	0.42%
42	Maine	2,371	0.41%
43	Idaho	1,643	0.29%
44	Montana	1,535	0.27%
45	Delaware	1,482	0.26%
46	Vermont	1,458	0.25%
47	South Dakota	1,225	0.21%
48	North Dakota	1,212	0.21%
49	Alaska	861	0.15%
50	Wyoming	714	0.12%
	District of Columbia	3,009	0.53%

Source: American Medical Association (Chicago, Illinois)
"Physician Characteristics and Distribution in the U.S." (1997-98 Edition)
As of December 31, 1996. Total does not include 7,761 physicians in U.S. territories and possessions.

Rate of Nonfederal Physicians in Patient Care in 1996

National Rate = 216 Physicians per 100,000 Population*

ALPHA ORDER

RANK	STATE	RATE
37	Alabama	175
48	Alaska	142
34	Arizona	181
42	Arkansas	168
12	California	216
21	Colorado	202
3	Connecticut	298
18	Delaware	205
15	Florida	209
32	Georgia	183
10	Hawaii	225
49	Idaho	138
9	Illinois	226
41	Indiana	171
44	Iowa	154
33	Kansas	182
34	Kentucky	181
14	Louisiana	212
27	Maine	191
3	Maryland	298
1	Massachusetts	338
26	Michigan	193
11	Minnesota	217
49	Mississippi	138
21	Missouri	202
37	Montana	175
30	Nebraska	184
45	Nevada	152
17	New Hampshire	206
6	New Jersey	252
30	New Mexico	184
2	New York	321
25	North Carolina	199
28	North Dakota	189
19	Ohio	204
46	Oklahoma	150
23	Oregon	200
8	Pennsylvania	248
5	Rhode Island	275
34	South Carolina	181
43	South Dakota	166
13	Tennessee	215
39	Texas	174
39	Utah	174
7	Vermont	249
16	Virginia	208
19	Washington	204
29	West Virginia	187
23	Wisconsin	200
47	Wyoming	149

RANK ORDER

RANK	STATE	RATE
1	Massachusetts	338
2	New York	321
3	Connecticut	298
3	Maryland	298
5	Rhode Island	275
6	New Jersey	252
7	Vermont	249
8	Pennsylvania	248
9	Illinois	226
10	Hawaii	225
11	Minnesota	217
12	California	216
13	Tennessee	215
14	Louisiana	212
15	Florida	209
16	Virginia	208
17	New Hampshire	206
18	Delaware	205
19	Ohio	204
19	Washington	204
21	Colorado	202
21	Missouri	202
23	Oregon	200
23	Wisconsin	200
25	North Carolina	199
26	Michigan	193
27	Maine	191
28	North Dakota	189
29	West Virginia	187
30	Nebraska	184
30	New Mexico	184
32	Georgia	183
33	Kansas	182
34	Arizona	181
34	Kentucky	181
34	South Carolina	181
37	Alabama	175
37	Montana	175
39	Texas	174
39	Utah	174
41	Indiana	171
42	Arkansas	168
43	South Dakota	166
44	Iowa	154
45	Nevada	152
46	Oklahoma	150
47	Wyoming	149
48	Alaska	142
49	Idaho	138
49	Mississippi	138

District of Columbia 558

Source: Morgan Quitno Press using data from American Medical Association (Chicago, Illinois)
"Physician Characteristics and Distribution in the U.S." (1997-98 Edition)
*As of December 31, 1996. National rate does not include physicians in U.S. territories and possessions.

Physicians in Primary Care in 1996

National Total = 245,821 Physicians*

ALPHA ORDER

RANK	STATE	PHYSICIANS	% of USA
25	Alabama	3,283	1.34%
49	Alaska	479	0.19%
24	Arizona	3,459	1.41%
32	Arkansas	1,888	0.77%
1	California	29,536	12.02%
23	Colorado	3,499	1.42%
21	Connecticut	4,057	1.65%
46	Delaware	610	0.25%
5	Florida	11,953	4.86%
14	Georgia	5,890	2.40%
38	Hawaii	1,337	0.54%
43	Idaho	747	0.30%
4	Illinois	12,399	5.04%
20	Indiana	4,349	1.77%
31	Iowa	1,898	0.77%
30	Kansas	2,108	0.86%
26	Kentucky	3,038	1.24%
22	Louisiana	3,683	1.50%
40	Maine	1,065	0.43%
11	Maryland	6,638	2.70%
10	Massachusetts	8,046	3.27%
9	Michigan	8,077	3.29%
17	Minnesota	4,708	1.92%
33	Mississippi	1,724	0.70%
19	Missouri	4,358	1.77%
45	Montana	655	0.27%
36	Nebraska	1,441	0.59%
41	Nevada	1,035	0.42%
42	New Hampshire	1,028	0.42%
8	New Jersey	8,738	3.55%
35	New Mexico	1,496	0.61%
2	New York	24,549	9.99%
13	North Carolina	6,210	2.53%
48	North Dakota	595	0.24%
7	Ohio	9,688	3.94%
29	Oklahoma	2,164	0.88%
28	Oregon	2,809	1.14%
6	Pennsylvania	11,808	4.80%
39	Rhode Island	1,155	0.47%
27	South Carolina	3,019	1.23%
47	South Dakota	600	0.24%
16	Tennessee	4,796	1.95%
3	Texas	14,035	5.71%
37	Utah	1,430	0.58%
44	Vermont	663	0.27%
12	Virginia	6,238	2.54%
15	Washington	5,071	2.06%
34	West Virginia	1,517	0.62%
18	Wisconsin	4,549	1.85%
50	Wyoming	383	0.16%

RANK ORDER

RANK	STATE	PHYSICIANS	% of USA
1	California	29,536	12.02%
2	New York	24,549	9.99%
3	Texas	14,035	5.71%
4	Illinois	12,399	5.04%
5	Florida	11,953	4.86%
6	Pennsylvania	11,808	4.80%
7	Ohio	9,688	3.94%
8	New Jersey	8,738	3.55%
9	Michigan	8,077	3.29%
10	Massachusetts	8,046	3.27%
11	Maryland	6,638	2.70%
12	Virginia	6,238	2.54%
13	North Carolina	6,210	2.53%
14	Georgia	5,890	2.40%
15	Washington	5,071	2.06%
16	Tennessee	4,796	1.95%
17	Minnesota	4,708	1.92%
18	Wisconsin	4,549	1.85%
19	Missouri	4,358	1.77%
20	Indiana	4,349	1.77%
21	Connecticut	4,057	1.65%
22	Louisiana	3,683	1.50%
23	Colorado	3,499	1.42%
24	Arizona	3,459	1.41%
25	Alabama	3,283	1.34%
26	Kentucky	3,038	1.24%
27	South Carolina	3,019	1.23%
28	Oregon	2,809	1.14%
29	Oklahoma	2,164	0.88%
30	Kansas	2,108	0.86%
31	Iowa	1,898	0.77%
32	Arkansas	1,888	0.77%
33	Mississippi	1,724	0.70%
34	West Virginia	1,517	0.62%
35	New Mexico	1,496	0.61%
36	Nebraska	1,441	0.59%
37	Utah	1,430	0.58%
38	Hawaii	1,337	0.54%
39	Rhode Island	1,155	0.47%
40	Maine	1,065	0.43%
41	Nevada	1,035	0.42%
42	New Hampshire	1,028	0.42%
43	Idaho	747	0.30%
44	Vermont	663	0.27%
45	Montana	655	0.27%
46	Delaware	610	0.25%
47	South Dakota	600	0.24%
48	North Dakota	595	0.24%
49	Alaska	479	0.19%
50	Wyoming	383	0.16%
	District of Columbia	1,320	0.54%

Source: American Medical Association (Chicago, Illinois)
   "Physician Characteristics and Distribution in the U.S." (1997-98 Edition)
Federal and nonfederal physicians as of December 31, 1996. National total does not include 4,768 physicians in U.S. territories and possessions. Primary Care Specialties include Family Practice, General Practice, Internal Medicine, Obstetrics/Gynecology and Pediatrics.

Rate of Physicians in Primary Care in 1996

National Rate = 93 Physicians per 100,000 Population*

RANK	STATE	RATE		RANK	STATE	RATE
40	Alabama	77		1	New York	135
37	Alaska	79		2	Massachusetts	132
38	Arizona	78		3	Maryland	131
41	Arkansas	75		4	Connecticut	124
13	California	93		5	Rhode Island	117
15	Colorado	92		6	Hawaii	113
4	Connecticut	124		6	Vermont	113
27	Delaware	84		8	New Jersey	109
28	Florida	83		9	Illinois	105
35	Georgia	80		10	Minnesota	101
6	Hawaii	113		11	Pennsylvania	98
50	Idaho	63		12	Virginia	94
9	Illinois	105		13	California	93
41	Indiana	75		13	North Dakota	93
46	Iowa	67		15	Colorado	92
31	Kansas	82		15	Washington	92
38	Kentucky	78		17	Tennessee	90
25	Louisiana	85		18	New Hampshire	89
24	Maine	86		19	Oregon	88
3	Maryland	131		19	Wisconsin	88
2	Massachusetts	132		21	Nebraska	87
28	Michigan	83		21	New Mexico	87
10	Minnesota	101		21	Ohio	87
49	Mississippi	64		24	Maine	86
32	Missouri	81		25	Louisiana	85
41	Montana	75		25	North Carolina	85
21	Nebraska	87		27	Delaware	84
48	Nevada	65		28	Florida	83
18	New Hampshire	89		28	Michigan	83
8	New Jersey	109		28	West Virginia	83
21	New Mexico	87		31	Kansas	82
1	New York	135		32	Missouri	81
25	North Carolina	85		32	South Carolina	81
13	North Dakota	93		32	South Dakota	81
21	Ohio	87		35	Georgia	80
47	Oklahoma	66		35	Wyoming	80
19	Oregon	88		37	Alaska	79
11	Pennsylvania	98		38	Arizona	78
5	Rhode Island	117		38	Kentucky	78
32	South Carolina	81		40	Alabama	77
32	South Dakota	81		41	Arkansas	75
17	Tennessee	90		41	Indiana	75
44	Texas	74		41	Montana	75
45	Utah	71		44	Texas	74
6	Vermont	113		45	Utah	71
12	Virginia	94		46	Iowa	67
15	Washington	92		47	Oklahoma	66
28	West Virginia	83		48	Nevada	65
19	Wisconsin	88		49	Mississippi	64
35	Wyoming	80		50	Idaho	63

	District of Columbia	245

Source: Morgan Quitno Press using data from American Medical Association (Chicago, Illinois)
"Physician Characteristics and Distribution in the U.S." (1997-98 Edition)
*Federal and nonfederal physicians as of January 1, 1996. National rate does not include physicians in U.S.
territories and possessions. Primary Care Specialties include Family Practice, General Practice, Internal Medicine,
Obstetrics/Gynecology and Pediatrics.

Percent of Physicians in Primary Care in 1996

National Percent = 33.9% of Physicians*

RANK	STATE	PERCENT	RANK	STATE	PERCENT
14	Alabama	36.3	1	Alaska	41.8
1	Alaska	41.8	2	Wyoming	41.4
46	Arizona	32.1	3	South Dakota	39.9
8	Arkansas	36.8	4	North Dakota	39.5
43	California	32.9	5	Illinois	37.8
29	Colorado	34.3	5	Nebraska	37.8
44	Connecticut	32.7	7	Minnesota	36.9
42	Delaware	33.1	8	Arkansas	36.8
50	Florida	29.6	9	Idaho	36.7
23	Georgia	35.1	10	Hawaii	36.6
10	Hawaii	36.6	10	West Virginia	36.6
9	Idaho	36.7	12	Mississippi	36.5
5	Illinois	37.8	13	South Carolina	36.4
15	Indiana	36.0	14	Alabama	36.3
30	Iowa	34.2	15	Indiana	36.0
20	Kansas	35.4	15	New Mexico	36.0
19	Kentucky	35.6	17	Wisconsin	35.8
40	Louisiana	33.3	18	Oklahoma	35.7
28	Maine	34.5	19	Kentucky	35.6
48	Maryland	30.9	20	Kansas	35.4
49	Massachusetts	30.7	21	New Jersey	35.3
22	Michigan	35.2	22	Michigan	35.2
7	Minnesota	36.9	23	Georgia	35.1
12	Mississippi	36.5	24	Virginia	35.0
40	Missouri	33.3	25	Tennessee	34.7
39	Montana	33.6	26	Ohio	34.6
5	Nebraska	37.8	26	Vermont	34.6
32	Nevada	34.1	28	Maine	34.5
35	New Hampshire	33.8	29	Colorado	34.3
21	New Jersey	35.3	30	Iowa	34.2
15	New Mexico	36.0	30	Rhode Island	34.2
35	New York	33.8	32	Nevada	34.1
35	North Carolina	33.8	33	Oregon	33.9
4	North Dakota	39.5	33	Washington	33.9
26	Ohio	34.6	35	New Hampshire	33.8
18	Oklahoma	35.7	35	New York	33.8
33	Oregon	33.9	35	North Carolina	33.8
47	Pennsylvania	32.0	38	Texas	33.7
30	Rhode Island	34.2	39	Montana	33.6
13	South Carolina	36.4	40	Louisiana	33.3
3	South Dakota	39.9	40	Missouri	33.3
25	Tennessee	34.7	42	Delaware	33.1
38	Texas	33.7	43	California	32.9
45	Utah	32.4	44	Connecticut	32.7
26	Vermont	34.6	45	Utah	32.4
24	Virginia	35.0	46	Arizona	32.1
33	Washington	33.9	47	Pennsylvania	32.0
10	West Virginia	36.6	48	Maryland	30.9
17	Wisconsin	35.8	49	Massachusetts	30.7
2	Wyoming	41.4	50	Florida	29.6
				District of Columbia	30.8

Source: Morgan Quitno Press using data from American Medical Association (Chicago, Illinois)
"Physician Characteristics and Distribution in the U.S." (1997-98 Edition)
Federal and nonfederal physicians as of January 1, 1996. National rate does not include physicians in U.S. territories and possessions. Primary Care Specialties include Family Practice, General Practice, Internal Medicine, Obstetrics/Gynecology and Pediatrics.

Percent of Population Lacking Access to Primary Care in 1996

National Percent = 10.1% of Population*

ALPHA ORDER

RANK	STATE	RATE
5	Alabama	16.6
12	Alaska	13.4
44	Arizona	5.8
15	Arkansas	12.5
34	California	7.7
33	Colorado	8.0
39	Connecticut	7.2
47	Delaware	4.8
40	Florida	6.7
11	Georgia	13.6
50	Hawaii	2.9
8	Idaho	14.1
36	Illinois	7.5
29	Indiana	9.2
35	Iowa	7.6
28	Kansas	9.3
14	Kentucky	12.7
1	Louisiana	24.5
31	Maine	8.6
49	Maryland	3.6
42	Massachusetts	6.1
13	Michigan	12.8
48	Minnesota	4.3
2	Mississippi	23.2
19	Missouri	11.1
24	Montana	10.1
32	Nebraska	8.5
18	Nevada	11.7
43	New Hampshire	5.9
46	New Jersey	5.0
4	New Mexico	18.5
23	New York	10.8
17	North Carolina	11.8
7	North Dakota	14.4
37	Ohio	7.4
21	Oklahoma	11.0
25	Oregon	9.7
45	Pennsylvania	5.4
27	Rhode Island	9.6
8	South Carolina	14.1
3	South Dakota	19.3
25	Tennessee	9.7
22	Texas	10.9
16	Utah	12.1
37	Vermont	7.4
41	Virginia	6.3
29	Washington	9.2
10	West Virginia	13.8
19	Wisconsin	11.1
6	Wyoming	14.9

RANK ORDER

RANK	STATE	RATE
1	Louisiana	24.5
2	Mississippi	23.2
3	South Dakota	19.3
4	New Mexico	18.5
5	Alabama	16.6
6	Wyoming	14.9
7	North Dakota	14.4
8	Idaho	14.1
8	South Carolina	14.1
10	West Virginia	13.8
11	Georgia	13.6
12	Alaska	13.4
13	Michigan	12.8
14	Kentucky	12.7
15	Arkansas	12.5
16	Utah	12.1
17	North Carolina	11.8
18	Nevada	11.7
19	Missouri	11.1
19	Wisconsin	11.1
21	Oklahoma	11.0
22	Texas	10.9
23	New York	10.8
24	Montana	10.1
25	Oregon	9.7
25	Tennessee	9.7
27	Rhode Island	9.6
28	Kansas	9.3
29	Indiana	9.2
29	Washington	9.2
31	Maine	8.6
32	Nebraska	8.5
33	Colorado	8.0
34	California	7.7
35	Iowa	7.6
36	Illinois	7.5
37	Ohio	7.4
37	Vermont	7.4
39	Connecticut	7.2
40	Florida	6.7
41	Virginia	6.3
42	Massachusetts	6.1
43	New Hampshire	5.9
44	Arizona	5.8
45	Pennsylvania	5.4
46	New Jersey	5.0
47	Delaware	4.8
48	Minnesota	4.3
49	Maryland	3.6
50	Hawaii	2.9
	District of Columbia**	NA

Source: U.S. Department of Health and Human Services, Division of Shortage Designation
    "Selected Statistics on Health Manpower Shortage Areas" (March 31, 1997)
Percent of population considered under-served by primary medical practitioners (Family & General Practice doctors, Internists, Ob/Gyns and Pediatricians). An under-served population does not have primary medical care within reasonable economic and geographic bounds.
***Not available.*

Nonfederal Physicians in General/Family Practice in 1996

National Total = 75,216 Physicians*

ALPHA ORDER

RANK	STATE	PHYSICIANS	% of USA
22	Alabama	1,157	1.54%
47	Alaska	211	0.28%
20	Arizona	1,210	1.61%
28	Arkansas	1,003	1.33%
1	California	9,228	12.27%
18	Colorado	1,395	1.85%
35	Connecticut	571	0.76%
49	Delaware	204	0.27%
3	Florida	4,066	5.41%
15	Georgia	1,732	2.30%
45	Hawaii	279	0.37%
39	Idaho	445	0.59%
6	Illinois	3,382	4.50%
11	Indiana	2,134	2.84%
27	Iowa	1,031	1.37%
30	Kansas	977	1.30%
21	Kentucky	1,199	1.59%
25	Louisiana	1,094	1.45%
38	Maine	460	0.61%
24	Maryland	1,111	1.48%
26	Massachusetts	1,081	1.44%
8	Michigan	2,303	3.06%
10	Minnesota	2,240	2.98%
33	Mississippi	690	0.92%
23	Missouri	1,124	1.49%
44	Montana	319	0.42%
32	Nebraska	744	0.99%
40	Nevada	343	0.46%
42	New Hampshire	341	0.45%
17	New Jersey	1,449	1.93%
36	New Mexico	557	0.74%
5	New York	3,536	4.70%
12	North Carolina	2,099	2.79%
43	North Dakota	332	0.44%
7	Ohio	3,040	4.04%
31	Oklahoma	921	1.22%
29	Oregon	988	1.31%
4	Pennsylvania	3,688	4.90%
50	Rhode Island	197	0.26%
19	South Carolina	1,292	1.72%
41	South Dakota	342	0.45%
16	Tennessee	1,575	2.09%
2	Texas	5,047	6.71%
37	Utah	525	0.70%
46	Vermont	221	0.29%
13	Virginia	2,056	2.73%
9	Washington	2,300	3.06%
34	West Virginia	633	0.84%
14	Wisconsin	1,988	2.64%
48	Wyoming	209	0.28%

RANK ORDER

RANK	STATE	PHYSICIANS	% of USA
1	California	9,228	12.27%
2	Texas	5,047	6.71%
3	Florida	4,066	5.41%
4	Pennsylvania	3,688	4.90%
5	New York	3,536	4.70%
6	Illinois	3,382	4.50%
7	Ohio	3,040	4.04%
8	Michigan	2,303	3.06%
9	Washington	2,300	3.06%
10	Minnesota	2,240	2.98%
11	Indiana	2,134	2.84%
12	North Carolina	2,099	2.79%
13	Virginia	2,056	2.73%
14	Wisconsin	1,988	2.64%
15	Georgia	1,732	2.30%
16	Tennessee	1,575	2.09%
17	New Jersey	1,449	1.93%
18	Colorado	1,395	1.85%
19	South Carolina	1,292	1.72%
20	Arizona	1,210	1.61%
21	Kentucky	1,199	1.59%
22	Alabama	1,157	1.54%
23	Missouri	1,124	1.49%
24	Maryland	1,111	1.48%
25	Louisiana	1,094	1.45%
26	Massachusetts	1,081	1.44%
27	Iowa	1,031	1.37%
28	Arkansas	1,003	1.33%
29	Oregon	988	1.31%
30	Kansas	977	1.30%
31	Oklahoma	921	1.22%
32	Nebraska	744	0.99%
33	Mississippi	690	0.92%
34	West Virginia	633	0.84%
35	Connecticut	571	0.76%
36	New Mexico	557	0.74%
37	Utah	525	0.70%
38	Maine	460	0.61%
39	Idaho	445	0.59%
40	Nevada	343	0.46%
41	South Dakota	342	0.45%
42	New Hampshire	341	0.45%
43	North Dakota	332	0.44%
44	Montana	319	0.42%
45	Hawaii	279	0.37%
46	Vermont	221	0.29%
47	Alaska	211	0.28%
48	Wyoming	209	0.28%
49	Delaware	204	0.27%
50	Rhode Island	197	0.26%
	District of Columbia	147	0.20%

Source: American Medical Association (Chicago, Illinois)
"Physician Characteristics and Distribution in the U.S." (1997-98 Edition)
As of December 31, 1996. Total does not include 1,978 physicians in U.S. territories and possessions.

Rate of Nonfederal Physicians in General/Family Practice in 1996

National Rate = 28 Physicians per 100,000 Population*

ALPHA ORDER

RANK ORDER

RANK	STATE	RATE
33	Alabama	27
17	Alaska	35
33	Arizona	27
7	Arkansas	40
26	California	29
11	Colorado	37
50	Connecticut	17
30	Delaware	28
30	Florida	28
40	Georgia	24
40	Hawaii	24
11	Idaho	37
26	Illinois	29
11	Indiana	37
15	Iowa	36
9	Kansas	38
21	Kentucky	31
38	Louisiana	25
11	Maine	37
43	Maryland	22
48	Massachusetts	18
40	Michigan	24
2	Minnesota	48
38	Mississippi	25
44	Missouri	21
15	Montana	36
4	Nebraska	45
44	Nevada	21
26	New Hampshire	29
48	New Jersey	18
20	New Mexico	33
47	New York	19
26	North Carolina	29
1	North Dakota	52
33	Ohio	27
30	Oklahoma	28
21	Oregon	31
21	Pennsylvania	31
46	Rhode Island	20
17	South Carolina	35
3	South Dakota	46
25	Tennessee	30
36	Texas	26
36	Utah	26
9	Vermont	38
21	Virginia	31
6	Washington	42
17	West Virginia	35
8	Wisconsin	39
5	Wyoming	44

RANK	STATE	RATE
1	North Dakota	52
2	Minnesota	48
3	South Dakota	46
4	Nebraska	45
5	Wyoming	44
6	Washington	42
7	Arkansas	40
8	Wisconsin	39
9	Kansas	38
9	Vermont	38
11	Colorado	37
11	Idaho	37
11	Indiana	37
11	Maine	37
15	Iowa	36
15	Montana	36
17	Alaska	35
17	South Carolina	35
17	West Virginia	35
20	New Mexico	33
21	Kentucky	31
21	Oregon	31
21	Pennsylvania	31
21	Virginia	31
25	Tennessee	30
26	California	29
26	Illinois	29
26	New Hampshire	29
26	North Carolina	29
30	Delaware	28
30	Florida	28
30	Oklahoma	28
33	Alabama	27
33	Arizona	27
33	Ohio	27
36	Texas	26
36	Utah	26
38	Louisiana	25
38	Mississippi	25
40	Georgia	24
40	Hawaii	24
40	Michigan	24
43	Maryland	22
44	Missouri	21
44	Nevada	21
46	Rhode Island	20
47	New York	19
48	Massachusetts	18
48	New Jersey	18
50	Connecticut	17

District of Columbia   27

Source: Morgan Quitno Press using data from American Medical Association (Chicago, Illinois)
    "Physician Characteristics and Distribution in the U.S." (1997-98 Edition)
*As of December 31, 1996. National rate does not include physicians in U.S. territories and possessions.

Percent of Family Physicians Who Practice Pediatrics in 1998

National Percent = 87.9% of Family Physicians*

ALPHA ORDER

RANK ORDER

RANK	STATE	PERCENT		RANK	STATE	PERCENT
37	Alabama	86.7		1	South Dakota	97.1
33	Alaska	87.5		2	Nebraska	95.2
38	Arizona	86.4		3	Wisconsin	93.8
33	Arkansas	87.5		4	New Hampshire	93.5
42	California	85.8		5	Colorado	93.1
5	Colorado	93.1		5	Utah	93.1
36	Connecticut	87.1		7	Washington	92.8
22	Delaware	89.7		8	Minnesota	92.2
50	Florida	76.5		9	Massachusetts	92.1
38	Georgia	86.4		9	Montana	92.1
21	Hawaii	89.8		11	Idaho	91.9
11	Idaho	91.9		12	Indiana	91.8
32	Illinois	87.6		13	Iowa	91.6
12	Indiana	91.8		14	Vermont	91.4
13	Iowa	91.6		15	Kansas	91.3
15	Kansas	91.3		16	Maine	90.7
26	Kentucky	89.0		16	Rhode Island	90.7
41	Louisiana	86.0		18	New Mexico	90.1
16	Maine	90.7		19	Oklahoma	90.0
49	Maryland	82.1		20	Oregon	89.9
9	Massachusetts	92.1		21	Hawaii	89.8
26	Michigan	89.0		22	Delaware	89.7
8	Minnesota	92.2		23	Pennsylvania	89.4
35	Mississippi	87.3		24	Virginia	89.3
30	Missouri	87.8		25	Ohio	89.1
9	Montana	92.1		26	Kentucky	89.0
2	Nebraska	95.2		26	Michigan	89.0
28	Nevada	88.8		28	Nevada	88.8
4	New Hampshire	93.5		29	North Carolina	87.9
43	New Jersey	85.6		30	Missouri	87.8
18	New Mexico	90.1		30	North Dakota	87.8
45	New York	83.5		32	Illinois	87.6
29	North Carolina	87.9		33	Alaska	87.5
30	North Dakota	87.8		33	Arkansas	87.5
25	Ohio	89.1		35	Mississippi	87.3
19	Oklahoma	90.0		36	Connecticut	87.1
20	Oregon	89.9		37	Alabama	86.7
23	Pennsylvania	89.4		38	Arizona	86.4
16	Rhode Island	90.7		38	Georgia	86.4
43	South Carolina	85.6		38	Tennessee	86.4
1	South Dakota	97.1		41	Louisiana	86.0
38	Tennessee	86.4		42	California	85.8
47	Texas	82.5		43	New Jersey	85.6
5	Utah	93.1		43	South Carolina	85.6
14	Vermont	91.4		45	New York	83.5
24	Virginia	89.3		46	West Virginia	82.6
7	Washington	92.8		47	Texas	82.5
46	West Virginia	82.6		47	Wyoming	82.5
3	Wisconsin	93.8		49	Maryland	82.1
47	Wyoming	82.5		50	Florida	76.5

District of Columbia   80.0

Source: The American Academy of Family Physicians
      "Facts About Family Practice 1998"
As of January 1, 1998. Includes members of the Academy who are in direct patient care and who practice pediatrics "in some fashion".

Percent of Family Physicians Who Practice Obstetrics in 1998

National Percent = 30.4% of Family Physicians*

ALPHA ORDER

RANK ORDER

RANK	STATE	PERCENT
44	Alabama	12.9
3	Alaska	59.7
26	Arizona	26.0
30	Arkansas	23.0
30	California	23.0
14	Colorado	45.5
42	Connecticut	14.7
40	Delaware	15.5
50	Florida	6.3
36	Georgia	17.3
29	Hawaii	25.4
7	Idaho	53.7
23	Illinois	31.1
15	Indiana	44.0
11	Iowa	49.6
9	Kansas	51.9
47	Kentucky	12.6
38	Louisiana	16.3
18	Maine	39.8
46	Maryland	12.7
25	Massachusetts	28.1
19	Michigan	38.7
5	Minnesota	58.8
49	Mississippi	11.3
28	Missouri	25.7
8	Montana	52.5
4	Nebraska	59.4
48	Nevada	12.5
21	New Hampshire	34.1
41	New Jersey	14.8
22	New Mexico	33.8
26	New York	26.0
34	North Carolina	20.2
2	North Dakota	63.3
35	Ohio	18.1
16	Oklahoma	42.5
17	Oregon	42.0
39	Pennsylvania	16.1
24	Rhode Island	30.2
37	South Carolina	16.7
1	South Dakota	71.4
32	Tennessee	21.7
33	Texas	20.3
13	Utah	45.8
20	Vermont	37.0
44	Virginia	12.9
10	Washington	51.6
43	West Virginia	13.9
6	Wisconsin	58.4
12	Wyoming	49.2

RANK	STATE	PERCENT
1	South Dakota	71.4
2	North Dakota	63.3
3	Alaska	59.7
4	Nebraska	59.4
5	Minnesota	58.8
6	Wisconsin	58.4
7	Idaho	53.7
8	Montana	52.5
9	Kansas	51.9
10	Washington	51.6
11	Iowa	49.6
12	Wyoming	49.2
13	Utah	45.8
14	Colorado	45.5
15	Indiana	44.0
16	Oklahoma	42.5
17	Oregon	42.0
18	Maine	39.8
19	Michigan	38.7
20	Vermont	37.0
21	New Hampshire	34.1
22	New Mexico	33.8
23	Illinois	31.1
24	Rhode Island	30.2
25	Massachusetts	28.1
26	Arizona	26.0
26	New York	26.0
28	Missouri	25.7
29	Hawaii	25.4
30	Arkansas	23.0
30	California	23.0
32	Tennessee	21.7
33	Texas	20.3
34	North Carolina	20.2
35	Ohio	18.1
36	Georgia	17.3
37	South Carolina	16.7
38	Louisiana	16.3
39	Pennsylvania	16.1
40	Delaware	15.5
41	New Jersey	14.8
42	Connecticut	14.7
43	West Virginia	13.9
44	Alabama	12.9
44	Virginia	12.9
46	Maryland	12.7
47	Kentucky	12.6
48	Nevada	12.5
49	Mississippi	11.3
50	Florida	6.3

District of Columbia   20.0

Source: The American Academy of Family Physicians
"Facts About Family Practice 1998"

*As of January 1, 1998. Includes members of the Academy who are in direct patient care and who practice obstetrics "in some fashion".

Nonfederal Physicians in Medical Specialties in 1996

National Total = 215,426 Physicians*

RANK	STATE	PHYSICIANS	% of USA
24	Alabama	2,680	1.24%
49	Alaska	210	0.10%
23	Arizona	2,733	1.27%
33	Arkansas	1,222	0.57%
2	California	25,266	11.73%
25	Colorado	2,517	1.17%
15	Connecticut	4,418	2.05%
43	Delaware	527	0.24%
4	Florida	11,042	5.13%
14	Georgia	4,648	2.16%
38	Hawaii	1,040	0.48%
46	Idaho	360	0.17%
6	Illinois	10,692	4.96%
22	Indiana	3,040	1.41%
31	Iowa	1,261	0.59%
30	Kansas	1,388	0.64%
26	Kentucky	2,259	1.05%
21	Louisiana	3,203	1.49%
42	Maine	744	0.35%
11	Maryland	6,751	3.13%
7	Massachusetts	9,725	4.51%
10	Michigan	7,142	3.32%
19	Minnesota	3,408	1.58%
35	Mississippi	1,083	0.50%
16	Missouri	4,356	2.02%
45	Montana	412	0.19%
39	Nebraska	887	0.41%
40	Nevada	815	0.38%
41	New Hampshire	798	0.37%
8	New Jersey	9,308	4.32%
37	New Mexico	1,047	0.49%
1	New York	26,970	12.52%
12	North Carolina	5,210	2.42%
48	North Dakota	312	0.14%
9	Ohio	8,401	3.90%
29	Oklahoma	1,549	0.72%
27	Oregon	2,149	1.00%
3	Pennsylvania	11,180	5.19%
32	Rhode Island	1,250	0.58%
28	South Carolina	2,010	0.93%
47	South Dakota	324	0.15%
17	Tennessee	4,077	1.89%
5	Texas	11,004	5.11%
34	Utah	1,150	0.53%
44	Vermont	525	0.24%
13	Virginia	4,859	2.26%
18	Washington	3,470	1.61%
36	West Virginia	1,075	0.50%
20	Wisconsin	3,344	1.55%
50	Wyoming	161	0.07%

RANK	STATE	PHYSICIANS	% of USA
1	New York	26,970	12.52%
2	California	25,266	11.73%
3	Pennsylvania	11,180	5.19%
4	Florida	11,042	5.13%
5	Texas	11,004	5.11%
6	Illinois	10,692	4.96%
7	Massachusetts	9,725	4.51%
8	New Jersey	9,308	4.32%
9	Ohio	8,401	3.90%
10	Michigan	7,142	3.32%
11	Maryland	6,751	3.13%
12	North Carolina	5,210	2.42%
13	Virginia	4,859	2.26%
14	Georgia	4,648	2.16%
15	Connecticut	4,418	2.05%
16	Missouri	4,356	2.02%
17	Tennessee	4,077	1.89%
18	Washington	3,470	1.61%
19	Minnesota	3,408	1.58%
20	Wisconsin	3,344	1.55%
21	Louisiana	3,203	1.49%
22	Indiana	3,040	1.41%
23	Arizona	2,733	1.27%
24	Alabama	2,680	1.24%
25	Colorado	2,517	1.17%
26	Kentucky	2,259	1.05%
27	Oregon	2,149	1.00%
28	South Carolina	2,010	0.93%
29	Oklahoma	1,549	0.72%
30	Kansas	1,388	0.64%
31	Iowa	1,261	0.59%
32	Rhode Island	1,250	0.58%
33	Arkansas	1,222	0.57%
34	Utah	1,150	0.53%
35	Mississippi	1,083	0.50%
36	West Virginia	1,075	0.50%
37	New Mexico	1,047	0.49%
38	Hawaii	1,040	0.48%
39	Nebraska	887	0.41%
40	Nevada	815	0.38%
41	New Hampshire	798	0.37%
42	Maine	744	0.35%
43	Delaware	527	0.24%
44	Vermont	525	0.24%
45	Montana	412	0.19%
46	Idaho	360	0.17%
47	South Dakota	324	0.15%
48	North Dakota	312	0.14%
49	Alaska	210	0.10%
50	Wyoming	161	0.07%
	District of Columbia	1,424	0.66%

Source: American Medical Association (Chicago, Illinois)
  "Physician Characteristics and Distribution in the U.S." (1997-98 Edition)
*As of December 31, 1996. Total does not include 2,527 physicians in U.S. territories and possessions. Medical Specialties are Allergy/Immunology, Cardiovascular Diseases, Dermatology, Gastroenterology, Internal Medicine, Pediatrics, Pediatric Cardiology and Pulmonary Diseases.

Rate of Nonfederal Physicians in Medical Specialties in 1996

National Rate = 81 Physicians per 100,000 Population*

ALPHA ORDER

RANK	STATE	RATE
26	Alabama	63
48	Alaska	35
29	Arizona	62
41	Arkansas	49
12	California	79
24	Colorado	66
3	Connecticut	135
17	Delaware	73
13	Florida	77
26	Georgia	63
10	Hawaii	88
50	Idaho	30
8	Illinois	90
39	Indiana	52
45	Iowa	44
36	Kansas	54
33	Kentucky	58
16	Louisiana	74
31	Maine	60
4	Maryland	133
1	Massachusetts	160
17	Michigan	73
17	Minnesota	73
47	Mississippi	40
11	Missouri	81
43	Montana	47
36	Nebraska	54
40	Nevada	51
22	New Hampshire	69
6	New Jersey	116
30	New Mexico	61
2	New York	149
21	North Carolina	71
41	North Dakota	49
15	Ohio	75
43	Oklahoma	47
23	Oregon	67
7	Pennsylvania	93
5	Rhode Island	126
36	South Carolina	54
45	South Dakota	44
13	Tennessee	77
33	Texas	58
35	Utah	57
8	Vermont	90
17	Virginia	73
26	Washington	63
32	West Virginia	59
25	Wisconsin	65
49	Wyoming	34

RANK ORDER

RANK	STATE	RATE
1	Massachusetts	160
2	New York	149
3	Connecticut	135
4	Maryland	133
5	Rhode Island	126
6	New Jersey	116
7	Pennsylvania	93
8	Illinois	90
8	Vermont	90
10	Hawaii	88
11	Missouri	81
12	California	79
13	Florida	77
13	Tennessee	77
15	Ohio	75
16	Louisiana	74
17	Delaware	73
17	Michigan	73
17	Minnesota	73
17	Virginia	73
21	North Carolina	71
22	New Hampshire	69
23	Oregon	67
24	Colorado	66
25	Wisconsin	65
26	Alabama	63
26	Georgia	63
26	Washington	63
29	Arizona	62
30	New Mexico	61
31	Maine	60
32	West Virginia	59
33	Kentucky	58
33	Texas	58
35	Utah	57
36	Kansas	54
36	Nebraska	54
36	South Carolina	54
39	Indiana	52
40	Nevada	51
41	Arkansas	49
41	North Dakota	49
43	Montana	47
43	Oklahoma	47
45	Iowa	44
45	South Dakota	44
47	Mississippi	40
48	Alaska	35
49	Wyoming	34
50	Idaho	30

District of Columbia 264

Source: Morgan Quitno Press using data from American Medical Association (Chicago, Illinois)
"Physician Characteristics and Distribution in the U.S." (1997-98 Edition)
*As of December 31, 1996. National rate does not include physicians in U.S. territories and possessions.

Nonfederal Physicians in Internal Medicine in 1996

National Total = 116,157 Physicians*

ALPHA ORDER			
RANK	STATE	PHYSICIANS	% of USA
23	Alabama	1,460	1.26%
49	Alaska	103	0.09%
24	Arizona	1,336	1.15%
37	Arkansas	537	0.46%
2	California	13,141	11.31%
26	Colorado	1,244	1.07%
13	Connecticut	2,606	2.24%
44	Delaware	253	0.22%
6	Florida	5,366	4.62%
15	Georgia	2,443	2.10%
33	Hawaii	596	0.51%
46	Idaho	177	0.15%
3	Illinois	6,190	5.33%
22	Indiana	1,523	1.31%
32	Iowa	619	0.53%
30	Kansas	754	0.65%
27	Kentucky	1,128	0.97%
21	Louisiana	1,620	1.39%
42	Maine	407	0.35%
11	Maryland	3,750	3.23%
5	Massachusetts	5,870	5.05%
10	Michigan	4,073	3.51%
18	Minnesota	1,895	1.63%
36	Mississippi	545	0.47%
16	Missouri	2,399	2.07%
45	Montana	216	0.19%
40	Nebraska	439	0.38%
39	Nevada	457	0.39%
41	New Hampshire	426	0.37%
8	New Jersey	5,005	4.31%
35	New Mexico	546	0.47%
1	New York	15,743	13.55%
12	North Carolina	2,658	2.29%
48	North Dakota	172	0.15%
9	Ohio	4,398	3.79%
29	Oklahoma	799	0.69%
25	Oregon	1,292	1.11%
4	Pennsylvania	6,169	5.31%
31	Rhode Island	710	0.61%
28	South Carolina	989	0.85%
46	South Dakota	177	0.15%
17	Tennessee	2,128	1.83%
7	Texas	5,320	4.58%
38	Utah	514	0.44%
43	Vermont	305	0.26%
14	Virginia	2,514	2.16%
19	Washington	1,865	1.61%
34	West Virginia	585	0.50%
20	Wisconsin	1,820	1.57%
50	Wyoming	83	0.07%

RANK ORDER			
RANK	STATE	PHYSICIANS	% of USA
1	New York	15,743	13.55%
2	California	13,141	11.31%
3	Illinois	6,190	5.33%
4	Pennsylvania	6,169	5.31%
5	Massachusetts	5,870	5.05%
6	Florida	5,366	4.62%
7	Texas	5,320	4.58%
8	New Jersey	5,005	4.31%
9	Ohio	4,398	3.79%
10	Michigan	4,073	3.51%
11	Maryland	3,750	3.23%
12	North Carolina	2,658	2.29%
13	Connecticut	2,606	2.24%
14	Virginia	2,514	2.16%
15	Georgia	2,443	2.10%
16	Missouri	2,399	2.07%
17	Tennessee	2,128	1.83%
18	Minnesota	1,895	1.63%
19	Washington	1,865	1.61%
20	Wisconsin	1,820	1.57%
21	Louisiana	1,620	1.39%
22	Indiana	1,523	1.31%
23	Alabama	1,460	1.26%
24	Arizona	1,336	1.15%
25	Oregon	1,292	1.11%
26	Colorado	1,244	1.07%
27	Kentucky	1,128	0.97%
28	South Carolina	989	0.85%
29	Oklahoma	799	0.69%
30	Kansas	754	0.65%
31	Rhode Island	710	0.61%
32	Iowa	619	0.53%
33	Hawaii	596	0.51%
34	West Virginia	585	0.50%
35	New Mexico	546	0.47%
36	Mississippi	545	0.47%
37	Arkansas	537	0.46%
38	Utah	514	0.44%
39	Nevada	457	0.39%
40	Nebraska	439	0.38%
41	New Hampshire	426	0.37%
42	Maine	407	0.35%
43	Vermont	305	0.26%
44	Delaware	253	0.22%
45	Montana	216	0.19%
46	Idaho	177	0.15%
46	South Dakota	177	0.15%
48	North Dakota	172	0.15%
49	Alaska	103	0.09%
50	Wyoming	83	0.07%
	District of Columbia	792	0.68%

Source: American Medical Association (Chicago, Illinois)
   "Physician Characteristics and Distribution in the U.S." (1997-98 Edition)
*As of December 31, 1996. Total does not include 1,120 physicians in U.S. territories and possessions. Internal Medicine includes Diabetes, Endocrinology, Geriatrics, Hematology, Infectious Diseases, Nephrology, Nutrition, Medical Oncology and Rheumatology.

Rate of Nonfederal Physicians in Internal Medicine in 1996

National Rate = 44 Physicians per 100,000 Population*

ALPHA ORDER

RANK	STATE	RATE
25	Alabama	34
48	Alaska	17
32	Arizona	30
46	Arkansas	21
13	California	41
27	Colorado	33
3	Connecticut	80
23	Delaware	35
19	Florida	37
27	Georgia	33
10	Hawaii	50
50	Idaho	15
7	Illinois	52
40	Indiana	26
45	Iowa	22
33	Kansas	29
33	Kentucky	29
19	Louisiana	37
27	Maine	33
4	Maryland	74
1	Massachusetts	96
12	Michigan	42
13	Minnesota	41
47	Mississippi	20
11	Missouri	45
41	Montana	25
37	Nebraska	27
33	Nevada	29
19	New Hampshire	37
6	New Jersey	63
30	New Mexico	32
2	New York	87
22	North Carolina	36
37	North Dakota	27
17	Ohio	39
43	Oklahoma	24
15	Oregon	40
9	Pennsylvania	51
5	Rhode Island	72
37	South Carolina	27
43	South Dakota	24
15	Tennessee	40
36	Texas	28
41	Utah	25
7	Vermont	52
18	Virginia	38
25	Washington	34
30	West Virginia	32
23	Wisconsin	35
48	Wyoming	17

RANK ORDER

RANK	STATE	RATE
1	Massachusetts	96
2	New York	87
3	Connecticut	80
4	Maryland	74
5	Rhode Island	72
6	New Jersey	63
7	Illinois	52
7	Vermont	52
9	Pennsylvania	51
10	Hawaii	50
11	Missouri	45
12	Michigan	42
13	California	41
13	Minnesota	41
15	Oregon	40
15	Tennessee	40
17	Ohio	39
18	Virginia	38
19	Florida	37
19	Louisiana	37
19	New Hampshire	37
22	North Carolina	36
23	Delaware	35
23	Wisconsin	35
25	Alabama	34
25	Washington	34
27	Colorado	33
27	Georgia	33
27	Maine	33
30	New Mexico	32
30	West Virginia	32
32	Arizona	30
33	Kansas	29
33	Kentucky	29
33	Nevada	29
36	Texas	28
37	Nebraska	27
37	North Dakota	27
37	South Carolina	27
40	Indiana	26
41	Montana	25
41	Utah	25
43	Oklahoma	24
43	South Dakota	24
45	Iowa	22
46	Arkansas	21
47	Mississippi	20
48	Alaska	17
48	Wyoming	17
50	Idaho	15

District of Columbia   147

Source: Morgan Quitno Press using data from American Medical Association (Chicago, Illinois)
"Physician Characteristics and Distribution in the U.S." (1997-98 Edition)
*As of December 31, 1996. National rate does not include physicians in U.S. territories and possessions. Internal Medicine includes Diabetes, Endocrinology, Geriatrics, Hematology, Infectious Diseases, Nephrology, Nutrition, Medical Oncology and Rheumatology.

Nonfederal Physicians in Pediatrics in 1996

National Total = 51,402 Physicians*

ALPHA ORDER					RANK ORDER			

RANK	STATE	PHYSICIANS	% of USA	RANK	STATE	PHYSICIANS	% of USA
25	Alabama	604	1.18%	1	California	6,411	12.47%
47	Alaska	70	0.14%	2	New York	6,174	12.01%
23	Arizona	690	1.34%	3	Texas	3,029	5.89%
30	Arkansas	355	0.69%	4	Florida	2,529	4.92%
1	California	6,411	12.47%	5	Illinois	2,437	4.74%
24	Colorado	670	1.30%	6	New Jersey	2,280	4.44%
17	Connecticut	923	1.80%	7	Pennsylvania	2,272	4.42%
42	Delaware	162	0.32%	8	Ohio	2,161	4.20%
4	Florida	2,529	4.92%	9	Massachusetts	1,953	3.80%
14	Georgia	1,158	2.25%	10	Michigan	1,652	3.21%
37	Hawaii	269	0.52%	11	Maryland	1,641	3.19%
46	Idaho	77	0.15%	12	North Carolina	1,317	2.56%
5	Illinois	2,437	4.74%	13	Virginia	1,270	2.47%
22	Indiana	724	1.41%	14	Georgia	1,158	2.25%
33	Iowa	289	0.56%	15	Tennessee	1,035	2.01%
32	Kansas	321	0.62%	16	Missouri	955	1.86%
26	Kentucky	587	1.14%	17	Connecticut	923	1.80%
19	Louisiana	805	1.57%	18	Washington	829	1.61%
41	Maine	177	0.34%	19	Louisiana	805	1.57%
11	Maryland	1,641	3.19%	20	Wisconsin	781	1.52%
9	Massachusetts	1,953	3.80%	21	Minnesota	727	1.41%
10	Michigan	1,652	3.21%	22	Indiana	724	1.41%
21	Minnesota	727	1.41%	23	Arizona	690	1.34%
35	Mississippi	280	0.54%	24	Colorado	670	1.30%
16	Missouri	955	1.86%	25	Alabama	604	1.18%
45	Montana	82	0.16%	26	Kentucky	587	1.14%
39	Nebraska	212	0.41%	27	South Carolina	531	1.03%
43	Nevada	143	0.28%	28	Oregon	428	0.83%
40	New Hampshire	195	0.38%	29	Oklahoma	361	0.70%
6	New Jersey	2,280	4.44%	30	Arkansas	355	0.69%
34	New Mexico	283	0.55%	31	Utah	341	0.66%
2	New York	6,174	12.01%	32	Kansas	321	0.62%
12	North Carolina	1,317	2.56%	33	Iowa	289	0.56%
48	North Dakota	67	0.13%	34	New Mexico	283	0.55%
8	Ohio	2,161	4.20%	35	Mississippi	280	0.54%
29	Oklahoma	361	0.70%	36	Rhode Island	277	0.54%
28	Oregon	428	0.83%	37	Hawaii	269	0.52%
7	Pennsylvania	2,272	4.42%	38	West Virginia	253	0.49%
36	Rhode Island	277	0.54%	39	Nebraska	212	0.41%
27	South Carolina	531	1.03%	40	New Hampshire	195	0.38%
49	South Dakota	62	0.12%	41	Maine	177	0.34%
15	Tennessee	1,035	2.01%	42	Delaware	162	0.32%
3	Texas	3,029	5.89%	43	Nevada	143	0.28%
31	Utah	341	0.66%	44	Vermont	134	0.26%
44	Vermont	134	0.26%	45	Montana	82	0.16%
13	Virginia	1,270	2.47%	46	Idaho	77	0.15%
18	Washington	829	1.61%	47	Alaska	70	0.14%
38	West Virginia	253	0.49%	48	North Dakota	67	0.13%
20	Wisconsin	781	1.52%	49	South Dakota	62	0.12%
50	Wyoming	41	0.08%	50	Wyoming	41	0.08%
					District of Columbia	378	0.74%

Source: American Medical Association (Chicago, Illinois)
    "Physician Characteristics and Distribution in the U.S." (1996-97 Edition)
*As of December 31, 1996. Total does not include 952 physicians in U.S. territories and possessions. Pediatrics includes Adolescent Medicine, Neonatal-Perinatal, Pediatric Allergy, Pediatric Endocrinology, Pediatric Pulmonology, Pediatric Hematology-Oncology and Pediatric Nephrology.

Rate of Nonfederal Physicians in Pediatrics in 1996

National Rate = 74 Physicians per 100,000 Population 17 Years and Younger*

ALPHA ORDER

RANK	STATE	RATE
32	Alabama	56
44	Alaska	38
24	Arizona	60
35	Arkansas	54
16	California	72
19	Colorado	67
5	Connecticut	116
7	Delaware	92
15	Florida	74
26	Georgia	59
9	Hawaii	88
50	Idaho	22
13	Illinois	77
38	Indiana	48
42	Iowa	40
40	Kansas	47
23	Kentucky	61
21	Louisiana	65
26	Maine	59
3	Maryland	128
1	Massachusetts	137
21	Michigan	65
28	Minnesota	58
45	Mississippi	37
18	Missouri	68
46	Montana	35
38	Nebraska	48
47	Nevada	34
20	New Hampshire	66
6	New Jersey	115
32	New Mexico	56
2	New York	136
16	North Carolina	72
42	North Dakota	40
14	Ohio	76
41	Oklahoma	41
36	Oregon	53
10	Pennsylvania	78
4	Rhode Island	118
31	South Carolina	57
49	South Dakota	30
10	Tennessee	78
32	Texas	56
37	Utah	50
8	Vermont	91
10	Virginia	78
28	Washington	58
24	West Virginia	60
28	Wisconsin	58
48	Wyoming	31

RANK ORDER

RANK	STATE	RATE
1	Massachusetts	137
2	New York	136
3	Maryland	128
4	Rhode Island	118
5	Connecticut	116
6	New Jersey	115
7	Delaware	92
8	Vermont	91
9	Hawaii	88
10	Pennsylvania	78
10	Tennessee	78
10	Virginia	78
13	Illinois	77
14	Ohio	76
15	Florida	74
16	California	72
16	North Carolina	72
18	Missouri	68
19	Colorado	67
20	New Hampshire	66
21	Louisiana	65
21	Michigan	65
23	Kentucky	61
24	Arizona	60
24	West Virginia	60
26	Georgia	59
26	Maine	59
28	Minnesota	58
28	Washington	58
28	Wisconsin	58
31	South Carolina	57
32	Alabama	56
32	New Mexico	56
32	Texas	56
35	Arkansas	54
36	Oregon	53
37	Utah	50
38	Indiana	48
38	Nebraska	48
40	Kansas	47
41	Oklahoma	41
42	Iowa	40
42	North Dakota	40
44	Alaska	38
45	Mississippi	37
46	Montana	35
47	Nevada	34
48	Wyoming	31
49	South Dakota	30
50	Idaho	22

District of Columbia   345

Source: Morgan Quitno Press using data from American Medical Association (Chicago, Illinois)
"Physician Characteristics and Distribution in the U.S." (1996-97 Edition)
*As of December 31, 1996. National rate does not include physicians in U.S. territories and possessions. Pediatrics includes Adolescent Medicine, Neonatal-Perinatal, Pediatric Allergy, Pediatric Endocrinology, Pediatric Pulmonology, Pediatric Hematology-Oncology and Pediatric Nephrology.

Nonfederal Physicians in Surgical Specialties in 1996

National Total = 144,306 Physicians*

ALPHA ORDER

RANK	STATE	PHYSICIANS	% of USA
23	Alabama	2,113	1.46%
49	Alaska	213	0.15%
24	Arizona	2,018	1.40%
33	Arkansas	1,038	0.72%
1	California	16,901	11.71%
25	Colorado	1,937	1.34%
19	Connecticut	2,458	1.70%
45	Delaware	366	0.25%
4	Florida	7,945	5.51%
12	Georgia	3,783	2.62%
39	Hawaii	670	0.46%
43	Idaho	446	0.31%
6	Illinois	6,317	4.38%
21	Indiana	2,400	1.66%
30	Iowa	1,145	0.79%
31	Kansas	1,131	0.78%
26	Kentucky	1,858	1.29%
17	Louisiana	2,756	1.91%
42	Maine	577	0.40%
13	Maryland	3,782	2.62%
10	Massachusetts	4,460	3.09%
9	Michigan	4,727	3.28%
22	Minnesota	2,231	1.55%
32	Mississippi	1,105	0.77%
16	Missouri	2,899	2.01%
44	Montana	415	0.29%
36	Nebraska	761	0.53%
40	Nevada	644	0.45%
41	New Hampshire	620	0.43%
8	New Jersey	4,967	3.44%
37	New Mexico	749	0.52%
2	New York	13,785	9.55%
11	North Carolina	3,919	2.72%
48	North Dakota	287	0.20%
7	Ohio	5,831	4.04%
29	Oklahoma	1,260	0.87%
28	Oregon	1,625	1.13%
5	Pennsylvania	7,467	5.17%
38	Rhode Island	676	0.47%
27	South Carolina	1,831	1.27%
47	South Dakota	296	0.21%
15	Tennessee	3,116	2.16%
3	Texas	8,879	6.15%
34	Utah	961	0.67%
46	Vermont	336	0.23%
14	Virginia	3,619	2.51%
18	Washington	2,655	1.84%
35	West Virginia	918	0.64%
20	Wisconsin	2,431	1.68%
50	Wyoming	181	0.13%

RANK ORDER

RANK	STATE	PHYSICIANS	% of USA
1	California	16,901	11.71%
2	New York	13,785	9.55%
3	Texas	8,879	6.15%
4	Florida	7,945	5.51%
5	Pennsylvania	7,467	5.17%
6	Illinois	6,317	4.38%
7	Ohio	5,831	4.04%
8	New Jersey	4,967	3.44%
9	Michigan	4,727	3.28%
10	Massachusetts	4,460	3.09%
11	North Carolina	3,919	2.72%
12	Georgia	3,783	2.62%
13	Maryland	3,782	2.62%
14	Virginia	3,619	2.51%
15	Tennessee	3,116	2.16%
16	Missouri	2,899	2.01%
17	Louisiana	2,756	1.91%
18	Washington	2,655	1.84%
19	Connecticut	2,458	1.70%
20	Wisconsin	2,431	1.68%
21	Indiana	2,400	1.66%
22	Minnesota	2,231	1.55%
23	Alabama	2,113	1.46%
24	Arizona	2,018	1.40%
25	Colorado	1,937	1.34%
26	Kentucky	1,858	1.29%
27	South Carolina	1,831	1.27%
28	Oregon	1,625	1.13%
29	Oklahoma	1,260	0.87%
30	Iowa	1,145	0.79%
31	Kansas	1,131	0.78%
32	Mississippi	1,105	0.77%
33	Arkansas	1,038	0.72%
34	Utah	961	0.67%
35	West Virginia	918	0.64%
36	Nebraska	761	0.53%
37	New Mexico	749	0.52%
38	Rhode Island	676	0.47%
39	Hawaii	670	0.46%
40	Nevada	644	0.45%
41	New Hampshire	620	0.43%
42	Maine	577	0.40%
43	Idaho	446	0.31%
44	Montana	415	0.29%
45	Delaware	366	0.25%
46	Vermont	336	0.23%
47	South Dakota	296	0.21%
48	North Dakota	287	0.20%
49	Alaska	213	0.15%
50	Wyoming	181	0.13%
	District of Columbia	801	0.56%

Source: American Medical Association (Chicago, Illinois)
    "Physician Characteristics and Distribution in the U.S." (1997-98 Edition)
As of December 31, 1996. Total does not include 1,504 physicians in U.S. territories and possessions. Surgical Specialties include Colon and Rectal, General, Neurological, Obstetrics & Gynecology, Ophthalmology, Orthopedic, Otolaryngology, Plastic, Thoracic and Urological Surgeries.

Rate of Nonfederal Physicians in Surgical Specialties in 1996

National Rate = 54 Physicians per 100,000 Population*

ALPHA ORDER

RANK	STATE	RATE
25	Alabama	49
50	Alaska	35
36	Arizona	46
41	Arkansas	41
16	California	53
21	Colorado	51
2	Connecticut	75
21	Delaware	51
12	Florida	55
19	Georgia	52
10	Hawaii	57
47	Idaho	38
16	Illinois	53
41	Indiana	41
44	Iowa	40
39	Kansas	44
28	Kentucky	48
6	Louisiana	63
32	Maine	47
2	Maryland	75
4	Massachusetts	73
25	Michigan	49
28	Minnesota	48
41	Mississippi	41
13	Missouri	54
32	Montana	47
36	Nebraska	46
44	Nevada	40
16	New Hampshire	53
7	New Jersey	62
39	New Mexico	44
1	New York	76
13	North Carolina	54
38	North Dakota	45
19	Ohio	52
47	Oklahoma	38
21	Oregon	51
7	Pennsylvania	62
5	Rhode Island	68
25	South Carolina	49
44	South Dakota	40
9	Tennessee	59
32	Texas	47
28	Utah	48
10	Vermont	57
13	Virginia	54
28	Washington	48
24	West Virginia	50
32	Wisconsin	47
47	Wyoming	38

RANK ORDER

RANK	STATE	RATE
1	New York	76
2	Connecticut	75
2	Maryland	75
4	Massachusetts	73
5	Rhode Island	68
6	Louisiana	63
7	New Jersey	62
7	Pennsylvania	62
9	Tennessee	59
10	Hawaii	57
10	Vermont	57
12	Florida	55
13	Missouri	54
13	North Carolina	54
13	Virginia	54
16	California	53
16	Illinois	53
16	New Hampshire	53
19	Georgia	52
19	Ohio	52
21	Colorado	51
21	Delaware	51
21	Oregon	51
24	West Virginia	50
25	Alabama	49
25	Michigan	49
25	South Carolina	49
28	Kentucky	48
28	Minnesota	48
28	Utah	48
28	Washington	48
32	Maine	47
32	Montana	47
32	Texas	47
32	Wisconsin	47
36	Arizona	46
36	Nebraska	46
38	North Dakota	45
39	Kansas	44
39	New Mexico	44
41	Arkansas	41
41	Indiana	41
41	Mississippi	41
44	Iowa	40
44	Nevada	40
44	South Dakota	40
47	Idaho	38
47	Oklahoma	38
47	Wyoming	38
50	Alaska	35

District of Columbia 149

Source: Morgan Quitno Press using data from American Medical Association (Chicago, Illinois)
    "Physician Characteristics and Distribution in the U.S." (1997-98 Edition)
*As of December 31, 1996. National rate does not include physicians in U.S. territories and possessions. Surgical Specialties include Colon and Rectal, General, Neurological, Obstetrics & Gynecology, Ophthalmology, Orthopedic, Otolaryngology, Plastic, Thoracic and Urological Surgeries.

Nonfederal Physicians in General Surgery in 1996

National Total = 36,054 Physicians*

ALPHA ORDER

RANK	STATE	PHYSICIANS	% of USA
22	Alabama	564	1.56%
49	Alaska	48	0.13%
25	Arizona	481	1.33%
34	Arkansas	262	0.73%
1	California	3,758	10.42%
27	Colorado	422	1.17%
19	Connecticut	592	1.64%
44	Delaware	97	0.27%
5	Florida	1,753	4.86%
12	Georgia	942	2.61%
42	Hawaii	153	0.42%
43	Idaho	102	0.28%
6	Illinois	1,604	4.45%
21	Indiana	582	1.61%
30	Iowa	309	0.86%
29	Kansas	322	0.89%
24	Kentucky	511	1.42%
17	Louisiana	701	1.94%
40	Maine	159	0.44%
13	Maryland	916	2.54%
10	Massachusetts	1,245	3.45%
9	Michigan	1,264	3.51%
23	Minnesota	521	1.45%
33	Mississippi	272	0.75%
16	Missouri	730	2.02%
44	Montana	97	0.27%
35	Nebraska	220	0.61%
40	Nevada	159	0.44%
39	New Hampshire	169	0.47%
8	New Jersey	1,270	3.52%
38	New Mexico	181	0.50%
2	New York	3,755	10.41%
11	North Carolina	946	2.62%
48	North Dakota	77	0.21%
7	Ohio	1,569	4.35%
31	Oklahoma	292	0.81%
28	Oregon	387	1.07%
3	Pennsylvania	2,090	5.80%
36	Rhode Island	188	0.52%
26	South Carolina	469	1.30%
47	South Dakota	88	0.24%
15	Tennessee	838	2.32%
4	Texas	2,069	5.74%
37	Utah	185	0.51%
46	Vermont	95	0.26%
14	Virginia	851	2.36%
18	Washington	607	1.68%
32	West Virginia	283	0.78%
20	Wisconsin	584	1.62%
50	Wyoming	45	0.12%

RANK ORDER

RANK	STATE	PHYSICIANS	% of USA
1	California	3,758	10.42%
2	New York	3,755	10.41%
3	Pennsylvania	2,090	5.80%
4	Texas	2,069	5.74%
5	Florida	1,753	4.86%
6	Illinois	1,604	4.45%
7	Ohio	1,569	4.35%
8	New Jersey	1,270	3.52%
9	Michigan	1,264	3.51%
10	Massachusetts	1,245	3.45%
11	North Carolina	946	2.62%
12	Georgia	942	2.61%
13	Maryland	916	2.54%
14	Virginia	851	2.36%
15	Tennessee	838	2.32%
16	Missouri	730	2.02%
17	Louisiana	701	1.94%
18	Washington	607	1.68%
19	Connecticut	592	1.64%
20	Wisconsin	584	1.62%
21	Indiana	582	1.61%
22	Alabama	564	1.56%
23	Minnesota	521	1.45%
24	Kentucky	511	1.42%
25	Arizona	481	1.33%
26	South Carolina	469	1.30%
27	Colorado	422	1.17%
28	Oregon	387	1.07%
29	Kansas	322	0.89%
30	Iowa	309	0.86%
31	Oklahoma	292	0.81%
32	West Virginia	283	0.78%
33	Mississippi	272	0.75%
34	Arkansas	262	0.73%
35	Nebraska	220	0.61%
36	Rhode Island	188	0.52%
37	Utah	185	0.51%
38	New Mexico	181	0.50%
39	New Hampshire	169	0.47%
40	Maine	159	0.44%
40	Nevada	159	0.44%
42	Hawaii	153	0.42%
43	Idaho	102	0.28%
44	Delaware	97	0.27%
44	Montana	97	0.27%
46	Vermont	95	0.26%
47	South Dakota	88	0.24%
48	North Dakota	77	0.21%
49	Alaska	48	0.13%
50	Wyoming	45	0.12%
	District of Columbia	230	0.64%

Source: American Medical Association (Chicago, Illinois)
"Physician Characteristics and Distribution in the U.S." (1997-98 Edition)
As of December 31, 1996. Total does not include 408 physicians in U.S. territories and possessions. General Surgery includes Abdominal, Cardiovascular, Hand, Head and Neck, Pediatric, Traumatic and Vascular Surgeries.

Rate of Nonfederal Physicians in General Surgery in 1996

National Rate = 13.6 Physicians per 100,000 Population*

ALPHA ORDER

RANK	STATE	RATE
18	Alabama	13.2
50	Alaska	7.9
38	Arizona	10.8
42	Arkansas	10.5
32	California	11.8
35	Colorado	11.1
4	Connecticut	18.1
16	Delaware	13.4
28	Florida	12.2
23	Georgia	12.8
21	Hawaii	12.9
49	Idaho	8.6
15	Illinois	13.5
43	Indiana	10.0
38	Iowa	10.8
27	Kansas	12.5
18	Kentucky	13.2
8	Louisiana	16.1
23	Maine	12.8
4	Maryland	18.1
2	Massachusetts	20.5
20	Michigan	13.0
34	Minnesota	11.2
43	Mississippi	10.0
14	Missouri	13.6
35	Montana	11.1
17	Nebraska	13.3
45	Nevada	9.9
12	New Hampshire	14.6
9	New Jersey	15.9
41	New Mexico	10.6
1	New York	20.7
21	North Carolina	12.9
30	North Dakota	12.0
13	Ohio	14.1
48	Oklahoma	8.9
29	Oregon	12.1
6	Pennsylvania	17.4
3	Rhode Island	19.0
26	South Carolina	12.6
31	South Dakota	11.9
10	Tennessee	15.8
38	Texas	10.8
47	Utah	9.2
7	Vermont	16.2
23	Virginia	12.8
37	Washington	11.0
11	West Virginia	15.5
33	Wisconsin	11.3
46	Wyoming	9.4

RANK ORDER

RANK	STATE	RATE
1	New York	20.7
2	Massachusetts	20.5
3	Rhode Island	19.0
4	Connecticut	18.1
4	Maryland	18.1
6	Pennsylvania	17.4
7	Vermont	16.2
8	Louisiana	16.1
9	New Jersey	15.9
10	Tennessee	15.8
11	West Virginia	15.5
12	New Hampshire	14.6
13	Ohio	14.1
14	Missouri	13.6
15	Illinois	13.5
16	Delaware	13.4
17	Nebraska	13.3
18	Alabama	13.2
18	Kentucky	13.2
20	Michigan	13.0
21	Hawaii	12.9
21	North Carolina	12.9
23	Georgia	12.8
23	Maine	12.8
23	Virginia	12.8
26	South Carolina	12.6
27	Kansas	12.5
28	Florida	12.2
29	Oregon	12.1
30	North Dakota	12.0
31	South Dakota	11.9
32	California	11.8
33	Wisconsin	11.3
34	Minnesota	11.2
35	Colorado	11.1
35	Montana	11.1
37	Washington	11.0
38	Arizona	10.8
38	Iowa	10.8
38	Texas	10.8
41	New Mexico	10.6
42	Arkansas	10.5
43	Indiana	10.0
43	Mississippi	10.0
45	Nevada	9.9
46	Wyoming	9.4
47	Utah	9.2
48	Oklahoma	8.9
49	Idaho	8.6
50	Alaska	7.9

District of Columbia	42.6

Source: Morgan Quitno Press using data from American Medical Association (Chicago, Illinois)
"Physician Characteristics and Distribution in the U.S." (1997-98 Edition)
*As of December 31, 1996. National rate does not include physicians in U.S. territories and possessions. General Surgery includes Abdominal, Cardiovascular, Hand, Head and Neck, Pediatric, Traumatic and Vascular Surgeries.

Nonfederal Physicians in Obstetrics and Gynecology in 1996

National Total = 37,242 Physicians*

ALPHA ORDER

RANK	STATE	PHYSICIANS	% of USA
24	Alabama	505	1.36%
49	Alaska	50	0.13%
21	Arizona	544	1.46%
33	Arkansas	219	0.59%
1	California	4,469	12.00%
23	Colorado	521	1.40%
17	Connecticut	692	1.86%
45	Delaware	83	0.22%
4	Florida	1,891	5.08%
10	Georgia	1,107	2.97%
34	Hawaii	217	0.58%
43	Idaho	95	0.26%
5	Illinois	1,799	4.83%
20	Indiana	572	1.54%
35	Iowa	209	0.56%
31	Kansas	253	0.68%
27	Kentucky	440	1.18%
18	Louisiana	687	1.84%
42	Maine	126	0.34%
11	Maryland	1,075	2.89%
11	Massachusetts	1,075	2.89%
9	Michigan	1,315	3.53%
26	Minnesota	476	1.28%
30	Mississippi	281	0.75%
16	Missouri	717	1.93%
44	Montana	84	0.23%
40	Nebraska	154	0.41%
38	Nevada	189	0.51%
40	New Hampshire	154	0.41%
8	New Jersey	1,419	3.81%
37	New Mexico	200	0.54%
2	New York	3,616	9.71%
13	North Carolina	1,051	2.82%
47	North Dakota	53	0.14%
7	Ohio	1,490	4.00%
29	Oklahoma	305	0.82%
28	Oregon	381	1.02%
6	Pennsylvania	1,769	4.75%
39	Rhode Island	170	0.46%
25	South Carolina	479	1.29%
48	South Dakota	52	0.14%
15	Tennessee	800	2.15%
3	Texas	2,448	6.57%
32	Utah	237	0.64%
46	Vermont	77	0.21%
14	Virginia	1,038	2.79%
19	Washington	632	1.70%
36	West Virginia	207	0.56%
22	Wisconsin	541	1.45%
50	Wyoming	46	0.12%

RANK ORDER

RANK	STATE	PHYSICIANS	% of USA
1	California	4,469	12.00%
2	New York	3,616	9.71%
3	Texas	2,448	6.57%
4	Florida	1,891	5.08%
5	Illinois	1,799	4.83%
6	Pennsylvania	1,769	4.75%
7	Ohio	1,490	4.00%
8	New Jersey	1,419	3.81%
9	Michigan	1,315	3.53%
10	Georgia	1,107	2.97%
11	Maryland	1,075	2.89%
11	Massachusetts	1,075	2.89%
13	North Carolina	1,051	2.82%
14	Virginia	1,038	2.79%
15	Tennessee	800	2.15%
16	Missouri	717	1.93%
17	Connecticut	692	1.86%
18	Louisiana	687	1.84%
19	Washington	632	1.70%
20	Indiana	572	1.54%
21	Arizona	544	1.46%
22	Wisconsin	541	1.45%
23	Colorado	521	1.40%
24	Alabama	505	1.36%
25	South Carolina	479	1.29%
26	Minnesota	476	1.28%
27	Kentucky	440	1.18%
28	Oregon	381	1.02%
29	Oklahoma	305	0.82%
30	Mississippi	281	0.75%
31	Kansas	253	0.68%
32	Utah	237	0.64%
33	Arkansas	219	0.59%
34	Hawaii	217	0.58%
35	Iowa	209	0.56%
36	West Virginia	207	0.56%
37	New Mexico	200	0.54%
38	Nevada	189	0.51%
39	Rhode Island	170	0.46%
40	Nebraska	154	0.41%
40	New Hampshire	154	0.41%
42	Maine	126	0.34%
43	Idaho	95	0.26%
44	Montana	84	0.23%
45	Delaware	83	0.22%
46	Vermont	77	0.21%
47	North Dakota	53	0.14%
48	South Dakota	52	0.14%
49	Alaska	50	0.13%
50	Wyoming	46	0.12%
	District of Columbia	232	0.62%

Source: American Medical Association (Chicago, Illinois)
   "Physician Characteristics and Distribution in the U.S." (1997-98 Edition)
*As of December 31, 1996. Total does not include 536 physicians in U.S. territories and possessions. Obstetrics and Gynecology includes Gynecology and Oncology, Maternal and Fetal Medicine and Reproductive Endocrinology.

Rate of Nonfederal Physicians in Obstetrics and Gynecology in 1996

National Rate = 27 Physicians per 100,000 Female Population*

RANK	STATE	RATE		RANK	STATE	RATE
29	Alabama	23		1	Connecticut	41
45	Alaska	17		1	Maryland	41
25	Arizona	24		3	New York	38
45	Arkansas	17		4	Hawaii	37
13	California	28		5	New Jersey	35
16	Colorado	27		6	Massachusetts	34
1	Connecticut	41		7	Rhode Island	33
32	Delaware	22		8	Illinois	30
18	Florida	26		8	Louisiana	30
11	Georgia	29		8	Virginia	30
4	Hawaii	37		11	Georgia	29
47	Idaho	16		11	Tennessee	29
8	Illinois	30		13	California	28
39	Indiana	19		13	North Carolina	28
49	Iowa	14		13	Pennsylvania	28
39	Kansas	19		16	Colorado	27
32	Kentucky	22		16	Michigan	27
8	Louisiana	30		18	Florida	26
36	Maine	20		18	Missouri	26
1	Maryland	41		18	New Hampshire	26
6	Massachusetts	34		18	Ohio	26
16	Michigan	27		18	Vermont	26
36	Minnesota	20		23	South Carolina	25
36	Mississippi	20		23	Texas	25
18	Missouri	26		25	Arizona	24
39	Montana	19		25	Nevada	24
43	Nebraska	18		25	Oregon	24
25	Nevada	24		25	Utah	24
18	New Hampshire	26		29	Alabama	23
5	New Jersey	35		29	New Mexico	23
29	New Mexico	23		29	Washington	23
3	New York	38		32	Delaware	22
13	North Carolina	28		32	Kentucky	22
47	North Dakota	16		32	West Virginia	22
18	Ohio	26		35	Wisconsin	21
43	Oklahoma	18		36	Maine	20
25	Oregon	24		36	Minnesota	20
13	Pennsylvania	28		36	Mississippi	20
7	Rhode Island	33		39	Indiana	19
23	South Carolina	25		39	Kansas	19
49	South Dakota	14		39	Montana	19
11	Tennessee	29		39	Wyoming	19
23	Texas	25		43	Nebraska	18
25	Utah	24		43	Oklahoma	18
18	Vermont	26		45	Alaska	17
8	Virginia	30		45	Arkansas	17
29	Washington	23		47	Idaho	16
32	West Virginia	22		47	North Dakota	16
35	Wisconsin	21		49	Iowa	14
39	Wyoming	19		49	South Dakota	14

District of Columbia   80

Source: Morgan Quitno Press using data from American Medical Association (Chicago, Illinois)
"Physician Characteristics and Distribution in the U.S." (1997-98 Edition)
As of December 31, 1996. National rate does not include physicians in U.S. territories and possessions. Obstetrics and Gynecology includes Gynecology and Oncology, Maternal and Fetal Medicine and Reproductive Endocrinology.

Nonfederal Physicians in Ophthalmology in 1996

National Total = 17,214 Physicians*

ALPHA ORDER

RANK	STATE	PHYSICIANS	% of USA
26	Alabama	206	1.20%
49	Alaska	26	0.15%
23	Arizona	254	1.48%
32	Arkansas	139	0.81%
1	California	2,083	12.10%
24	Colorado	235	1.37%
20	Connecticut	298	1.73%
45	Delaware	45	0.26%
3	Florida	1,080	6.27%
14	Georgia	387	2.25%
37	Hawaii	86	0.50%
43	Idaho	56	0.33%
6	Illinois	713	4.14%
22	Indiana	275	1.60%
29	Iowa	168	0.98%
30	Kansas	145	0.84%
27	Kentucky	199	1.16%
16	Louisiana	342	1.99%
40	Maine	68	0.40%
11	Maryland	471	2.74%
10	Massachusetts	538	3.13%
9	Michigan	550	3.20%
21	Minnesota	288	1.67%
33	Mississippi	135	0.78%
15	Missouri	343	1.99%
44	Montana	50	0.29%
36	Nebraska	91	0.53%
41	Nevada	66	0.38%
42	New Hampshire	64	0.37%
8	New Jersey	602	3.50%
38	New Mexico	78	0.45%
2	New York	1,789	10.39%
12	North Carolina	408	2.37%
47	North Dakota	37	0.21%
7	Ohio	626	3.64%
30	Oklahoma	145	0.84%
28	Oregon	196	1.14%
5	Pennsylvania	914	5.31%
39	Rhode Island	70	0.41%
25	South Carolina	216	1.25%
48	South Dakota	35	0.20%
17	Tennessee	333	1.93%
4	Texas	985	5.72%
34	Utah	114	0.66%
46	Vermont	39	0.23%
13	Virginia	393	2.28%
19	Washington	303	1.76%
35	West Virginia	102	0.59%
18	Wisconsin	321	1.86%
50	Wyoming	15	0.09%

RANK ORDER

RANK	STATE	PHYSICIANS	% of USA
1	California	2,083	12.10%
2	New York	1,789	10.39%
3	Florida	1,080	6.27%
4	Texas	985	5.72%
5	Pennsylvania	914	5.31%
6	Illinois	713	4.14%
7	Ohio	626	3.64%
8	New Jersey	602	3.50%
9	Michigan	550	3.20%
10	Massachusetts	538	3.13%
11	Maryland	471	2.74%
12	North Carolina	408	2.37%
13	Virginia	393	2.28%
14	Georgia	387	2.25%
15	Missouri	343	1.99%
16	Louisiana	342	1.99%
17	Tennessee	333	1.93%
18	Wisconsin	321	1.86%
19	Washington	303	1.76%
20	Connecticut	298	1.73%
21	Minnesota	288	1.67%
22	Indiana	275	1.60%
23	Arizona	254	1.48%
24	Colorado	235	1.37%
25	South Carolina	216	1.25%
26	Alabama	206	1.20%
27	Kentucky	199	1.16%
28	Oregon	196	1.14%
29	Iowa	168	0.98%
30	Kansas	145	0.84%
30	Oklahoma	145	0.84%
32	Arkansas	139	0.81%
33	Mississippi	135	0.78%
34	Utah	114	0.66%
35	West Virginia	102	0.59%
36	Nebraska	91	0.53%
37	Hawaii	86	0.50%
38	New Mexico	78	0.45%
39	Rhode Island	70	0.41%
40	Maine	68	0.40%
41	Nevada	66	0.38%
42	New Hampshire	64	0.37%
43	Idaho	56	0.33%
44	Montana	50	0.29%
45	Delaware	45	0.26%
46	Vermont	39	0.23%
47	North Dakota	37	0.21%
48	South Dakota	35	0.20%
49	Alaska	26	0.15%
50	Wyoming	15	0.09%
	District of Columbia	92	0.53%

Source: American Medical Association (Chicago, Illinois)
  "Physician Characteristics and Distribution in the U.S." (1997-98 Edition)
*As of December 31, 1996. Total does not include 178 physicians in U.S. territories and possessions.

Rate of Nonfederal Physicians in Ophthalmology in 1996

National Rate = 6.5 Physicians per 100,000 Population*

ALPHA ORDER

RANK	STATE	RATE
42	Alabama	4.8
48	Alaska	4.3
25	Arizona	5.7
33	Arkansas	5.5
12	California	6.5
15	Colorado	6.2
3	Connecticut	9.1
15	Delaware	6.2
7	Florida	7.5
38	Georgia	5.3
9	Hawaii	7.3
43	Idaho	4.7
20	Illinois	6.0
43	Indiana	4.7
21	Iowa	5.9
29	Kansas	5.6
40	Kentucky	5.1
5	Louisiana	7.9
33	Maine	5.5
2	Maryland	9.3
4	Massachusetts	8.8
25	Michigan	5.7
15	Minnesota	6.2
41	Mississippi	5.0
13	Missouri	6.4
25	Montana	5.7
33	Nebraska	5.5
49	Nevada	4.1
33	New Hampshire	5.5
7	New Jersey	7.5
46	New Mexico	4.6
1	New York	9.9
29	North Carolina	5.6
23	North Dakota	5.8
29	Ohio	5.6
47	Oklahoma	4.4
19	Oregon	6.1
6	Pennsylvania	7.6
10	Rhode Island	7.1
23	South Carolina	5.8
43	South Dakota	4.7
14	Tennessee	6.3
39	Texas	5.2
25	Utah	5.7
11	Vermont	6.7
21	Virginia	5.9
33	Washington	5.5
29	West Virginia	5.6
15	Wisconsin	6.2
50	Wyoming	3.1

RANK ORDER

RANK	STATE	RATE
1	New York	9.9
2	Maryland	9.3
3	Connecticut	9.1
4	Massachusetts	8.8
5	Louisiana	7.9
6	Pennsylvania	7.6
7	Florida	7.5
7	New Jersey	7.5
9	Hawaii	7.3
10	Rhode Island	7.1
11	Vermont	6.7
12	California	6.5
13	Missouri	6.4
14	Tennessee	6.3
15	Colorado	6.2
15	Delaware	6.2
15	Minnesota	6.2
15	Wisconsin	6.2
19	Oregon	6.1
20	Illinois	6.0
21	Iowa	5.9
21	Virginia	5.9
23	North Dakota	5.8
23	South Carolina	5.8
25	Arizona	5.7
25	Michigan	5.7
25	Montana	5.7
25	Utah	5.7
29	Kansas	5.6
29	North Carolina	5.6
29	Ohio	5.6
29	West Virginia	5.6
33	Arkansas	5.5
33	Maine	5.5
33	Nebraska	5.5
33	New Hampshire	5.5
33	Washington	5.5
38	Georgia	5.3
39	Texas	5.2
40	Kentucky	5.1
41	Mississippi	5.0
42	Alabama	4.8
43	Idaho	4.7
43	Indiana	4.7
43	South Dakota	4.7
46	New Mexico	4.6
47	Oklahoma	4.4
48	Alaska	4.3
49	Nevada	4.1
50	Wyoming	3.1

District of Columbia 17.1

Source: Morgan Quitno Press using data from American Medical Association (Chicago, Illinois)
"Physician Characteristics and Distribution in the U.S." (1997-98 Edition)
*As of December 31, 1996. National rate does not include physicians in U.S. territories and possessions.

Nonfederal Physicians in Orthopedic Surgery in 1996

National Total = 21,773 Physicians*

ALPHA ORDER

RANK	STATE	PHYSICIANS	% of USA
25	Alabama	318	1.46%
48	Alaska	47	0.22%
24	Arizona	325	1.49%
33	Arkansas	169	0.78%
1	California	2,767	12.71%
23	Colorado	361	1.66%
22	Connecticut	371	1.70%
46	Delaware	52	0.24%
4	Florida	1,215	5.58%
12	Georgia	541	2.48%
42	Hawaii	88	0.40%
42	Idaho	88	0.40%
7	Illinois	869	3.99%
20	Indiana	402	1.85%
32	Iowa	176	0.81%
30	Kansas	180	0.83%
28	Kentucky	273	1.25%
21	Louisiana	399	1.83%
39	Maine	111	0.51%
14	Maryland	520	2.39%
9	Massachusetts	658	3.02%
10	Michigan	615	2.82%
18	Minnesota	424	1.95%
34	Mississippi	151	0.69%
19	Missouri	422	1.94%
44	Montana	83	0.38%
36	Nebraska	131	0.60%
41	Nevada	89	0.41%
40	New Hampshire	109	0.50%
8	New Jersey	693	3.18%
35	New Mexico	145	0.67%
2	New York	1,762	8.09%
11	North Carolina	610	2.80%
50	North Dakota	41	0.19%
6	Ohio	878	4.03%
29	Oklahoma	208	0.96%
26	Oregon	283	1.30%
5	Pennsylvania	1,069	4.91%
37	Rhode Island	116	0.53%
27	South Carolina	281	1.29%
47	South Dakota	49	0.23%
17	Tennessee	439	2.02%
3	Texas	1,298	5.96%
31	Utah	178	0.82%
45	Vermont	63	0.29%
13	Virginia	539	2.48%
15	Washington	482	2.21%
38	West Virginia	114	0.52%
16	Wisconsin	449	2.06%
49	Wyoming	42	0.19%

RANK ORDER

RANK	STATE	PHYSICIANS	% of USA
1	California	2,767	12.71%
2	New York	1,762	8.09%
3	Texas	1,298	5.96%
4	Florida	1,215	5.58%
5	Pennsylvania	1,069	4.91%
6	Ohio	878	4.03%
7	Illinois	869	3.99%
8	New Jersey	693	3.18%
9	Massachusetts	658	3.02%
10	Michigan	615	2.82%
11	North Carolina	610	2.80%
12	Georgia	541	2.48%
13	Virginia	539	2.48%
14	Maryland	520	2.39%
15	Washington	482	2.21%
16	Wisconsin	449	2.06%
17	Tennessee	439	2.02%
18	Minnesota	424	1.95%
19	Missouri	422	1.94%
20	Indiana	402	1.85%
21	Louisiana	399	1.83%
22	Connecticut	371	1.70%
23	Colorado	361	1.66%
24	Arizona	325	1.49%
25	Alabama	318	1.46%
26	Oregon	283	1.30%
27	South Carolina	281	1.29%
28	Kentucky	273	1.25%
29	Oklahoma	208	0.96%
30	Kansas	180	0.83%
31	Utah	178	0.82%
32	Iowa	176	0.81%
33	Arkansas	169	0.78%
34	Mississippi	151	0.69%
35	New Mexico	145	0.67%
36	Nebraska	131	0.60%
37	Rhode Island	116	0.53%
38	West Virginia	114	0.52%
39	Maine	111	0.51%
40	New Hampshire	109	0.50%
41	Nevada	89	0.41%
42	Hawaii	88	0.40%
42	Idaho	88	0.40%
44	Montana	83	0.38%
45	Vermont	63	0.29%
46	Delaware	52	0.24%
47	South Dakota	49	0.23%
48	Alaska	47	0.22%
49	Wyoming	42	0.19%
50	North Dakota	41	0.19%
	District of Columbia	80	0.37%

Source: American Medical Association (Chicago, Illinois)
"Physician Characteristics and Distribution in the U.S." (1997-98 Edition)
As of December 31, 1996. Total does not include 115 physicians in U.S. territories and possessions.

Rate of Nonfederal Physicians in Orthopedic Surgery in 1996

National Rate = 8.2 Physicians per 100,000 Population*

RANK	STATE	RATE
31	Alabama	7.4
29	Alaska	7.8
35	Arizona	7.3
42	Arkansas	6.7
16	California	8.7
7	Colorado	9.5
2	Connecticut	11.4
37	Delaware	7.2
22	Florida	8.4
31	Georgia	7.4
31	Hawaii	7.4
31	Idaho	7.4
35	Illinois	7.3
40	Indiana	6.9
48	Iowa	6.2
38	Kansas	7.0
38	Kentucky	7.0
10	Louisiana	9.2
12	Maine	9.0
5	Maryland	10.3
3	Massachusetts	10.8
45	Michigan	6.3
11	Minnesota	9.1
49	Mississippi	5.6
26	Missouri	7.9
7	Montana	9.5
26	Nebraska	7.9
49	Nevada	5.6
9	New Hampshire	9.4
16	New Jersey	8.7
21	New Mexico	8.5
6	New York	9.7
23	North Carolina	8.3
44	North Dakota	6.4
26	Ohio	7.9
45	Oklahoma	6.3
13	Oregon	8.9
13	Pennsylvania	8.9
1	Rhode Island	11.7
30	South Carolina	7.6
43	South Dakota	6.6
23	Tennessee	8.3
41	Texas	6.8
15	Utah	8.8
4	Vermont	10.7
25	Virginia	8.1
16	Washington	8.7
45	West Virginia	6.3
16	Wisconsin	8.7
16	Wyoming	8.7

RANK	STATE	RATE
1	Rhode Island	11.7
2	Connecticut	11.4
3	Massachusetts	10.8
4	Vermont	10.7
5	Maryland	10.3
6	New York	9.7
7	Colorado	9.5
7	Montana	9.5
9	New Hampshire	9.4
10	Louisiana	9.2
11	Minnesota	9.1
12	Maine	9.0
13	Oregon	8.9
13	Pennsylvania	8.9
15	Utah	8.8
16	California	8.7
16	New Jersey	8.7
16	Washington	8.7
16	Wisconsin	8.7
16	Wyoming	8.7
21	New Mexico	8.5
22	Florida	8.4
23	North Carolina	8.3
23	Tennessee	8.3
25	Virginia	8.1
26	Missouri	7.9
26	Nebraska	7.9
26	Ohio	7.9
29	Alaska	7.8
30	South Carolina	7.6
31	Alabama	7.4
31	Georgia	7.4
31	Hawaii	7.4
31	Idaho	7.4
35	Arizona	7.3
35	Illinois	7.3
37	Delaware	7.2
38	Kansas	7.0
38	Kentucky	7.0
40	Indiana	6.9
41	Texas	6.8
42	Arkansas	6.7
43	South Dakota	6.6
44	North Dakota	6.4
45	Michigan	6.3
45	Oklahoma	6.3
45	West Virginia	6.3
48	Iowa	6.2
49	Mississippi	5.6
49	Nevada	5.6

District of Columbia	14.8

Source: Morgan Quitno Press using data from American Medical Association (Chicago, Illinois)
"Physician Characteristics and Distribution in the U.S." (1997-98 Edition)
*As of December 31, 1996. National rate does not include physicians in U.S. territories and possessions.

Nonfederal Physicians in Plastic Surgery in 1996

National Total = 5,789 Physicians*

ALPHA ORDER

RANK	STATE	PHYSICIANS	% of USA
23	Alabama	82	1.42%
46	Alaska	10	0.17%
18	Arizona	109	1.88%
34	Arkansas	30	0.52%
1	California	893	15.43%
20	Colorado	84	1.45%
22	Connecticut	83	1.43%
44	Delaware	17	0.29%
3	Florida	436	7.53%
14	Georgia	136	2.35%
33	Hawaii	31	0.54%
42	Idaho	18	0.31%
6	Illinois	215	3.71%
20	Indiana	84	1.45%
37	Iowa	25	0.43%
30	Kansas	47	0.81%
24	Kentucky	77	1.33%
19	Louisiana	89	1.54%
45	Maine	14	0.24%
11	Maryland	140	2.42%
10	Massachusetts	164	2.83%
9	Michigan	172	2.97%
25	Minnesota	73	1.26%
35	Mississippi	28	0.48%
15	Missouri	131	2.26%
42	Montana	18	0.31%
36	Nebraska	26	0.45%
32	Nevada	33	0.57%
38	New Hampshire	24	0.41%
8	New Jersey	176	3.04%
39	New Mexico	22	0.38%
2	New York	551	9.52%
11	North Carolina	140	2.42%
46	North Dakota	10	0.17%
7	Ohio	209	3.61%
31	Oklahoma	41	0.71%
28	Oregon	58	1.00%
5	Pennsylvania	245	4.23%
40	Rhode Island	20	0.35%
29	South Carolina	56	0.97%
49	South Dakota	6	0.10%
16	Tennessee	127	2.19%
4	Texas	401	6.93%
27	Utah	61	1.05%
48	Vermont	7	0.12%
13	Virginia	137	2.37%
17	Washington	111	1.92%
40	West Virginia	20	0.35%
25	Wisconsin	73	1.26%
50	Wyoming	3	0.05%

RANK ORDER

RANK	STATE	PHYSICIANS	% of USA
1	California	893	15.43%
2	New York	551	9.52%
3	Florida	436	7.53%
4	Texas	401	6.93%
5	Pennsylvania	245	4.23%
6	Illinois	215	3.71%
7	Ohio	209	3.61%
8	New Jersey	176	3.04%
9	Michigan	172	2.97%
10	Massachusetts	164	2.83%
11	Maryland	140	2.42%
11	North Carolina	140	2.42%
13	Virginia	137	2.37%
14	Georgia	136	2.35%
15	Missouri	131	2.26%
16	Tennessee	127	2.19%
17	Washington	111	1.92%
18	Arizona	109	1.88%
19	Louisiana	89	1.54%
20	Colorado	84	1.45%
20	Indiana	84	1.45%
22	Connecticut	83	1.43%
23	Alabama	82	1.42%
24	Kentucky	77	1.33%
25	Minnesota	73	1.26%
25	Wisconsin	73	1.26%
27	Utah	61	1.05%
28	Oregon	58	1.00%
29	South Carolina	56	0.97%
30	Kansas	47	0.81%
31	Oklahoma	41	0.71%
32	Nevada	33	0.57%
33	Hawaii	31	0.54%
34	Arkansas	30	0.52%
35	Mississippi	28	0.48%
36	Nebraska	26	0.45%
37	Iowa	25	0.43%
38	New Hampshire	24	0.41%
39	New Mexico	22	0.38%
40	Rhode Island	20	0.35%
40	West Virginia	20	0.35%
42	Idaho	18	0.31%
42	Montana	18	0.31%
44	Delaware	17	0.29%
45	Maine	14	0.24%
46	Alaska	10	0.17%
46	North Dakota	10	0.17%
48	Vermont	7	0.12%
49	South Dakota	6	0.10%
50	Wyoming	3	0.05%
	District of Columbia	26	0.45%

Source: American Medical Association (Chicago, Illinois)
   "Physician Characteristics and Distribution in the U.S." (1997-98 Edition)
*As of December 31, 1996. Total does not include 27 physicians in U.S. territories and possessions.

Rate of Nonfederal Physicians in Plastic Surgery in 1996

National Rate = 2.2 Physicians per 100,000 Population*

ALPHA ORDER

RANK	STATE	RATE
25	Alabama	1.9
33	Alaska	1.7
8	Arizona	2.5
42	Arkansas	1.2
4	California	2.8
13	Colorado	2.2
8	Connecticut	2.5
12	Delaware	2.3
1	Florida	3.0
25	Georgia	1.9
7	Hawaii	2.6
37	Idaho	1.5
29	Illinois	1.8
39	Indiana	1.4
48	Iowa	0.9
29	Kansas	1.8
21	Kentucky	2.0
15	Louisiana	2.1
45	Maine	1.1
4	Maryland	2.8
6	Massachusetts	2.7
29	Michigan	1.8
34	Minnesota	1.6
47	Mississippi	1.0
10	Missouri	2.4
15	Montana	2.1
34	Nebraska	1.6
15	Nevada	2.1
15	New Hampshire	2.1
13	New Jersey	2.2
41	New Mexico	1.3
1	New York	3.0
25	North Carolina	1.9
34	North Dakota	1.6
25	Ohio	1.9
42	Oklahoma	1.2
29	Oregon	1.8
21	Pennsylvania	2.0
21	Rhode Island	2.0
37	South Carolina	1.5
49	South Dakota	0.8
10	Tennessee	2.4
15	Texas	2.1
1	Utah	3.0
42	Vermont	1.2
15	Virginia	2.1
21	Washington	2.0
45	West Virginia	1.1
39	Wisconsin	1.4
50	Wyoming	0.6

RANK ORDER

RANK	STATE	RATE
1	Florida	3.0
1	New York	3.0
1	Utah	3.0
4	California	2.8
4	Maryland	2.8
6	Massachusetts	2.7
7	Hawaii	2.6
8	Arizona	2.5
8	Connecticut	2.5
10	Missouri	2.4
10	Tennessee	2.4
12	Delaware	2.3
13	Colorado	2.2
13	New Jersey	2.2
15	Louisiana	2.1
15	Montana	2.1
15	Nevada	2.1
15	New Hampshire	2.1
15	Texas	2.1
15	Virginia	2.1
21	Kentucky	2.0
21	Pennsylvania	2.0
21	Rhode Island	2.0
21	Washington	2.0
25	Alabama	1.9
25	Georgia	1.9
25	North Carolina	1.9
25	Ohio	1.9
29	Illinois	1.8
29	Kansas	1.8
29	Michigan	1.8
29	Oregon	1.8
33	Alaska	1.7
34	Minnesota	1.6
34	Nebraska	1.6
34	North Dakota	1.6
37	Idaho	1.5
37	South Carolina	1.5
39	Indiana	1.4
39	Wisconsin	1.4
41	New Mexico	1.3
42	Arkansas	1.2
42	Oklahoma	1.2
42	Vermont	1.2
45	Maine	1.1
45	West Virginia	1.1
47	Mississippi	1.0
48	Iowa	0.9
49	South Dakota	0.8
50	Wyoming	0.6

District of Columbia   4.8

Source: Morgan Quitno Press using data from American Medical Association (Chicago, Illinois)
    "Physician Characteristics and Distribution in the U.S." (1997-98 Edition)
*As of December 31, 1996. National rate does not include physicians in U.S. territories and possessions.

Nonfederal Physicians in Other Specialties in 1996

National Total = 180,397 Physicians*

ALPHA ORDER

RANK	STATE	PHYSICIANS	% of USA
27	Alabama	2,004	1.11%
49	Alaska	270	0.15%
23	Arizona	2,543	1.41%
32	Arkansas	1,170	0.65%
1	California	22,433	12.44%
24	Colorado	2,484	1.38%
18	Connecticut	3,236	1.79%
44	Delaware	491	0.27%
5	Florida	8,739	4.84%
14	Georgia	4,138	2.29%
37	Hawaii	840	0.47%
46	Idaho	430	0.24%
6	Illinois	8,239	4.57%
20	Indiana	3,002	1.66%
31	Iowa	1,270	0.70%
30	Kansas	1,484	0.82%
25	Kentucky	2,070	1.15%
22	Louisiana	2,696	1.49%
42	Maine	734	0.41%
11	Maryland	5,442	3.02%
7	Massachusetts	7,652	4.24%
9	Michigan	5,909	3.28%
21	Minnesota	2,936	1.63%
35	Mississippi	1,016	0.56%
17	Missouri	3,239	1.80%
45	Montana	442	0.25%
38	Nebraska	836	0.46%
41	Nevada	749	0.42%
40	New Hampshire	772	0.43%
10	New Jersey	5,864	3.25%
34	New Mexico	1,040	0.58%
2	New York	19,072	10.57%
12	North Carolina	4,470	2.48%
47	North Dakota	341	0.19%
8	Ohio	6,939	3.85%
29	Oklahoma	1,510	0.84%
26	Oregon	2,022	1.12%
4	Pennsylvania	9,968	5.53%
39	Rhode Island	831	0.46%
28	South Carolina	1,997	1.11%
48	South Dakota	309	0.17%
16	Tennessee	3,331	1.85%
3	Texas	10,355	5.74%
33	Utah	1,134	0.63%
43	Vermont	503	0.28%
13	Virginia	4,211	2.33%
15	Washington	3,661	2.03%
36	West Virginia	981	0.54%
19	Wisconsin	3,199	1.77%
50	Wyoming	206	0.11%

RANK ORDER

RANK	STATE	PHYSICIANS	% of USA
1	California	22,433	12.44%
2	New York	19,072	10.57%
3	Texas	10,355	5.74%
4	Pennsylvania	9,968	5.53%
5	Florida	8,739	4.84%
6	Illinois	8,239	4.57%
7	Massachusetts	7,652	4.24%
8	Ohio	6,939	3.85%
9	Michigan	5,909	3.28%
10	New Jersey	5,864	3.25%
11	Maryland	5,442	3.02%
12	North Carolina	4,470	2.48%
13	Virginia	4,211	2.33%
14	Georgia	4,138	2.29%
15	Washington	3,661	2.03%
16	Tennessee	3,331	1.85%
17	Missouri	3,239	1.80%
18	Connecticut	3,236	1.79%
19	Wisconsin	3,199	1.77%
20	Indiana	3,002	1.66%
21	Minnesota	2,936	1.63%
22	Louisiana	2,696	1.49%
23	Arizona	2,543	1.41%
24	Colorado	2,484	1.38%
25	Kentucky	2,070	1.15%
26	Oregon	2,022	1.12%
27	Alabama	2,004	1.11%
28	South Carolina	1,997	1.11%
29	Oklahoma	1,510	0.84%
30	Kansas	1,484	0.82%
31	Iowa	1,270	0.70%
32	Arkansas	1,170	0.65%
33	Utah	1,134	0.63%
34	New Mexico	1,040	0.58%
35	Mississippi	1,016	0.56%
36	West Virginia	981	0.54%
37	Hawaii	840	0.47%
38	Nebraska	836	0.46%
39	Rhode Island	831	0.46%
40	New Hampshire	772	0.43%
41	Nevada	749	0.42%
42	Maine	734	0.41%
43	Vermont	503	0.28%
44	Delaware	491	0.27%
45	Montana	442	0.25%
46	Idaho	430	0.24%
47	North Dakota	341	0.19%
48	South Dakota	309	0.17%
49	Alaska	270	0.15%
50	Wyoming	206	0.11%
	District of Columbia	1,187	0.66%

Source: American Medical Association (Chicago, Illinois)
"Physician Characteristics and Distribution in the U.S." (1997-98 Edition)

*As of December 31, 1996. Total does not include 2,172 physicians in U.S. territories and possessions. Other Specialties include Aerospace Medicine, Anesthesiology, Child Psychiatry, Diagnostic Radiology, Emergency Medicine, Forensic Pathology, Nuclear Medicine, Occupational Medicine, Neurology, Psychiatry, Public Health, Anatomic/Clinical Pathology, Radiology, Radiation Oncology and other specialties.

Rate of Nonfederal Physicians in Other Specialties in 1996

National Rate = 68 Physicians per 100,000 Population*

ALPHA ORDER

RANK	STATE	RATE
41	Alabama	47
45	Alaska	45
30	Arizona	57
41	Arkansas	47
10	California	70
15	Colorado	65
4	Connecticut	99
12	Delaware	68
23	Florida	61
31	Georgia	56
9	Hawaii	71
50	Idaho	36
10	Illinois	70
38	Indiana	52
45	Iowa	45
29	Kansas	58
36	Kentucky	53
20	Louisiana	62
28	Maine	59
2	Maryland	108
1	Massachusetts	126
23	Michigan	61
16	Minnesota	63
49	Mississippi	37
27	Missouri	60
40	Montana	50
39	Nebraska	51
41	Nevada	47
13	New Hampshire	67
8	New Jersey	73
23	New Mexico	61
3	New York	105
23	North Carolina	61
36	North Dakota	53
20	Ohio	62
44	Oklahoma	46
16	Oregon	63
7	Pennsylvania	83
6	Rhode Island	84
33	South Carolina	54
48	South Dakota	42
16	Tennessee	63
33	Texas	54
31	Utah	56
5	Vermont	86
16	Virginia	63
14	Washington	66
33	West Virginia	54
20	Wisconsin	62
47	Wyoming	43

RANK ORDER

RANK	STATE	RATE
1	Massachusetts	126
2	Maryland	108
3	New York	105
4	Connecticut	99
5	Vermont	86
6	Rhode Island	84
7	Pennsylvania	83
8	New Jersey	73
9	Hawaii	71
10	California	70
10	Illinois	70
12	Delaware	68
13	New Hampshire	67
14	Washington	66
15	Colorado	65
16	Minnesota	63
16	Oregon	63
16	Tennessee	63
16	Virginia	63
20	Louisiana	62
20	Ohio	62
20	Wisconsin	62
23	Florida	61
23	Michigan	61
23	New Mexico	61
23	North Carolina	61
27	Missouri	60
28	Maine	59
29	Kansas	58
30	Arizona	57
31	Georgia	56
31	Utah	56
33	South Carolina	54
33	Texas	54
33	West Virginia	54
36	Kentucky	53
36	North Dakota	53
38	Indiana	52
39	Nebraska	51
40	Montana	50
41	Alabama	47
41	Arkansas	47
41	Nevada	47
44	Oklahoma	46
45	Alaska	45
45	Iowa	45
47	Wyoming	43
48	South Dakota	42
49	Mississippi	37
50	Idaho	36

District of Columbia — 220

Source: Morgan Quitno Press using data from American Medical Association (Chicago, Illinois)
"Physician Characteristics and Distribution in the U.S." (1997-98 Edition)
*As of December 31, 1996. National rate does not include physicians in U.S. territories and possessions. Other Specialties include Aerospace Medicine, Anesthesiology, Child Psychiatry, Diagnostic Radiology, Emergency Medicine, Forensic Pathology, Nuclear Medicine, Occupational Medicine, Neurology, Psychiatry, Public Health, Anatomic/Clinical Pathology, Radiology, Radiation Oncology and other specialties.

Nonfederal Physicians in Anesthesiology in 1996

National Total = 32,290 Physicians*

ALPHA ORDER

ALPHA ORDER

RANK	STATE	PHYSICIANS	% of USA
26	Alabama	403	1.25%
48	Alaska	46	0.14%
19	Arizona	573	1.77%
33	Arkansas	212	0.66%
1	California	4,014	12.43%
24	Colorado	446	1.38%
21	Connecticut	477	1.48%
46	Delaware	59	0.18%
4	Florida	1,841	5.70%
13	Georgia	741	2.29%
40	Hawaii	128	0.40%
44	Idaho	76	0.24%
6	Illinois	1,550	4.80%
15	Indiana	692	2.14%
31	Iowa	258	0.80%
32	Kansas	236	0.73%
24	Kentucky	446	1.38%
23	Louisiana	448	1.39%
39	Maine	130	0.40%
10	Maryland	847	2.62%
8	Massachusetts	1,200	3.72%
11	Michigan	799	2.47%
22	Minnesota	453	1.40%
34	Mississippi	210	0.65%
20	Missouri	569	1.76%
42	Montana	100	0.31%
37	Nebraska	156	0.48%
35	Nevada	185	0.57%
41	New Hampshire	118	0.37%
9	New Jersey	1,168	3.62%
36	New Mexico	160	0.50%
2	New York	3,059	9.47%
14	North Carolina	702	2.17%
47	North Dakota	52	0.16%
7	Ohio	1,285	3.98%
29	Oklahoma	309	0.96%
27	Oregon	395	1.22%
5	Pennsylvania	1,585	4.91%
43	Rhode Island	88	0.27%
28	South Carolina	349	1.08%
49	South Dakota	41	0.13%
17	Tennessee	648	2.01%
3	Texas	2,341	7.25%
30	Utah	266	0.82%
45	Vermont	62	0.19%
16	Virginia	691	2.14%
12	Washington	791	2.45%
38	West Virginia	147	0.46%
18	Wisconsin	588	1.82%
50	Wyoming	40	0.12%

RANK ORDER

RANK	STATE	PHYSICIANS	% of USA
1	California	4,014	12.43%
2	New York	3,059	9.47%
3	Texas	2,341	7.25%
4	Florida	1,841	5.70%
5	Pennsylvania	1,585	4.91%
6	Illinois	1,550	4.80%
7	Ohio	1,285	3.98%
8	Massachusetts	1,200	3.72%
9	New Jersey	1,168	3.62%
10	Maryland	847	2.62%
11	Michigan	799	2.47%
12	Washington	791	2.45%
13	Georgia	741	2.29%
14	North Carolina	702	2.17%
15	Indiana	692	2.14%
16	Virginia	691	2.14%
17	Tennessee	648	2.01%
18	Wisconsin	588	1.82%
19	Arizona	573	1.77%
20	Missouri	569	1.76%
21	Connecticut	477	1.48%
22	Minnesota	453	1.40%
23	Louisiana	448	1.39%
24	Colorado	446	1.38%
24	Kentucky	446	1.38%
26	Alabama	403	1.25%
27	Oregon	395	1.22%
28	South Carolina	349	1.08%
29	Oklahoma	309	0.96%
30	Utah	266	0.82%
31	Iowa	258	0.80%
32	Kansas	236	0.73%
33	Arkansas	212	0.66%
34	Mississippi	210	0.65%
35	Nevada	185	0.57%
36	New Mexico	160	0.50%
37	Nebraska	156	0.48%
38	West Virginia	147	0.46%
39	Maine	130	0.40%
40	Hawaii	128	0.40%
41	New Hampshire	118	0.37%
42	Montana	100	0.31%
43	Rhode Island	88	0.27%
44	Idaho	76	0.24%
45	Vermont	62	0.19%
46	Delaware	59	0.18%
47	North Dakota	52	0.16%
48	Alaska	46	0.14%
49	South Dakota	41	0.13%
50	Wyoming	40	0.12%
	District of Columbia	110	0.34%

Source: American Medical Association (Chicago, Illinois)
"Physician Characteristics and Distribution in the U.S." (1997-98 Edition)
As of December 31, 1996. Total does not include 207 physicians in U.S. territories and possessions.

Rate of Nonfederal Physicians in Anesthesiology in 1996

National Rate = 12.2 Physicians per 100,000 Population*

ALPHA ORDER

RANK	STATE	RATE
34	Alabama	9.4
48	Alaska	7.6
10	Arizona	12.9
41	Arkansas	8.5
12	California	12.6
17	Colorado	11.7
4	Connecticut	14.6
43	Delaware	8.2
11	Florida	12.8
30	Georgia	10.1
23	Hawaii	10.8
49	Idaho	6.4
9	Illinois	13.1
16	Indiana	11.9
39	Iowa	9.1
38	Kansas	9.2
19	Kentucky	11.5
28	Louisiana	10.3
26	Maine	10.5
3	Maryland	16.7
1	Massachusetts	19.7
43	Michigan	8.2
31	Minnesota	9.7
47	Mississippi	7.7
24	Missouri	10.6
21	Montana	11.4
33	Nebraska	9.5
18	Nevada	11.6
29	New Hampshire	10.2
4	New Jersey	14.6
37	New Mexico	9.3
2	New York	16.9
32	North Carolina	9.6
45	North Dakota	8.1
19	Ohio	11.5
34	Oklahoma	9.4
13	Oregon	12.4
7	Pennsylvania	13.2
40	Rhode Island	8.9
34	South Carolina	9.4
50	South Dakota	5.6
15	Tennessee	12.2
14	Texas	12.3
7	Utah	13.2
24	Vermont	10.6
27	Virginia	10.4
6	Washington	14.3
45	West Virginia	8.1
21	Wisconsin	11.4
42	Wyoming	8.3

RANK ORDER

RANK	STATE	RATE
1	Massachusetts	19.7
2	New York	16.9
3	Maryland	16.7
4	Connecticut	14.6
4	New Jersey	14.6
6	Washington	14.3
7	Pennsylvania	13.2
7	Utah	13.2
9	Illinois	13.1
10	Arizona	12.9
11	Florida	12.8
12	California	12.6
13	Oregon	12.4
14	Texas	12.3
15	Tennessee	12.2
16	Indiana	11.9
17	Colorado	11.7
18	Nevada	11.6
19	Kentucky	11.5
19	Ohio	11.5
21	Montana	11.4
21	Wisconsin	11.4
23	Hawaii	10.8
24	Missouri	10.6
24	Vermont	10.6
26	Maine	10.5
27	Virginia	10.4
28	Louisiana	10.3
29	New Hampshire	10.2
30	Georgia	10.1
31	Minnesota	9.7
32	North Carolina	9.6
33	Nebraska	9.5
34	Alabama	9.4
34	Oklahoma	9.4
34	South Carolina	9.4
37	New Mexico	9.3
38	Kansas	9.2
39	Iowa	9.1
40	Rhode Island	8.9
41	Arkansas	8.5
42	Wyoming	8.3
43	Delaware	8.2
43	Michigan	8.2
45	North Dakota	8.1
45	West Virginia	8.1
47	Mississippi	7.7
48	Alaska	7.6
49	Idaho	6.4
50	South Dakota	5.6

District of Columbia 20.4

Source: Morgan Quitno Press using data from American Medical Association (Chicago, Illinois)
"Physician Characteristics and Distribution in the U.S." (1997-98 Edition)
*As of December 31, 1996. National rate does not include physicians in U.S. territories and possessions.

Nonfederal Physicians in Psychiatry in 1996

National Total = 36,548 Physicians*

ALPHA ORDER				RANK ORDER			
RANK	STATE	PHYSICIANS	% of USA	RANK	STATE	PHYSICIANS	% of USA
29	Alabama	289	0.79%	1	New York	5,479	14.99%
49	Alaska	57	0.16%	2	California	4,883	13.36%
23	Arizona	425	1.16%	3	Massachusetts	1,965	5.38%
34	Arkansas	191	0.52%	4	Pennsylvania	1,935	5.29%
2	California	4,883	13.36%	5	Texas	1,702	4.66%
20	Colorado	501	1.37%	6	Florida	1,510	4.13%
12	Connecticut	891	2.44%	7	Illinois	1,453	3.98%
44	Delaware	94	0.26%	8	Maryland	1,261	3.45%
6	Florida	1,510	4.13%	9	New Jersey	1,259	3.44%
15	Georgia	750	2.05%	10	Ohio	1,103	3.02%
36	Hawaii	189	0.52%	11	Michigan	1,062	2.91%
47	Idaho	61	0.17%	12	Connecticut	891	2.44%
7	Illinois	1,453	3.98%	13	North Carolina	861	2.36%
24	Indiana	417	1.14%	14	Virginia	806	2.21%
35	Iowa	190	0.52%	15	Georgia	750	2.05%
28	Kansas	342	0.94%	16	Washington	674	1.84%
27	Kentucky	351	0.96%	17	Wisconsin	547	1.50%
21	Louisiana	497	1.36%	18	Missouri	538	1.47%
37	Maine	172	0.47%	19	Tennessee	517	1.41%
8	Maryland	1,261	3.45%	20	Colorado	501	1.37%
3	Massachusetts	1,965	5.38%	21	Louisiana	497	1.36%
11	Michigan	1,062	2.91%	22	Minnesota	469	1.28%
22	Minnesota	469	1.28%	23	Arizona	425	1.16%
41	Mississippi	143	0.39%	24	Indiana	417	1.14%
18	Missouri	538	1.47%	25	South Carolina	410	1.12%
45	Montana	69	0.19%	26	Oregon	372	1.02%
40	Nebraska	150	0.41%	27	Kentucky	351	0.96%
43	Nevada	111	0.30%	28	Kansas	342	0.94%
33	New Hampshire	193	0.53%	29	Alabama	289	0.79%
9	New Jersey	1,259	3.44%	30	Oklahoma	244	0.67%
31	New Mexico	231	0.63%	31	New Mexico	231	0.63%
1	New York	5,479	14.99%	32	Rhode Island	205	0.56%
13	North Carolina	861	2.36%	33	New Hampshire	193	0.53%
46	North Dakota	65	0.18%	34	Arkansas	191	0.52%
10	Ohio	1,103	3.02%	35	Iowa	190	0.52%
30	Oklahoma	244	0.67%	36	Hawaii	189	0.52%
26	Oregon	372	1.02%	37	Maine	172	0.47%
4	Pennsylvania	1,935	5.29%	38	West Virginia	165	0.45%
32	Rhode Island	205	0.56%	39	Utah	156	0.43%
25	South Carolina	410	1.12%	40	Nebraska	150	0.41%
48	South Dakota	60	0.16%	41	Mississippi	143	0.39%
19	Tennessee	517	1.41%	42	Vermont	141	0.39%
5	Texas	1,702	4.66%	43	Nevada	111	0.30%
39	Utah	156	0.43%	44	Delaware	94	0.26%
42	Vermont	141	0.39%	45	Montana	69	0.19%
14	Virginia	806	2.21%	46	North Dakota	65	0.18%
16	Washington	674	1.84%	47	Idaho	61	0.17%
38	West Virginia	165	0.45%	48	South Dakota	60	0.16%
17	Wisconsin	547	1.50%	49	Alaska	57	0.16%
50	Wyoming	32	0.09%	50	Wyoming	32	0.09%
					District of Columbia	360	0.99%

Source: American Medical Association (Chicago, Illinois)
     "Physician Characteristics and Distribution in the U.S." (1997-98 Edition)
*As of December 31, 1996. Total does not include 361 physicians in U.S. territories and possessions. Psychiatry includes psychoanalysis.

466

Rate of Nonfederal Physicians in Psychiatry in 1996

National Rate = 13.8 Physicians per 100,000 Population*

ALPHA ORDER

RANK	STATE	RATE
46	Alabama	6.7
34	Alaska	9.4
33	Arizona	9.6
42	Arkansas	7.6
11	California	15.3
15	Colorado	13.1
3	Connecticut	27.3
16	Delaware	13.0
26	Florida	10.5
27	Georgia	10.2
9	Hawaii	16.0
50	Idaho	5.1
17	Illinois	12.3
44	Indiana	7.2
46	Iowa	6.7
14	Kansas	13.3
37	Kentucky	9.0
22	Louisiana	11.4
12	Maine	13.9
4	Maryland	24.9
1	Massachusetts	32.3
24	Michigan	10.9
28	Minnesota	10.1
49	Mississippi	5.3
30	Missouri	10.0
40	Montana	7.9
35	Nebraska	9.1
45	Nevada	6.9
7	New Hampshire	16.6
10	New Jersey	15.7
13	New Mexico	13.5
2	New York	30.2
20	North Carolina	11.8
28	North Dakota	10.1
31	Ohio	9.9
43	Oklahoma	7.4
21	Oregon	11.6
8	Pennsylvania	16.1
6	Rhode Island	20.7
23	South Carolina	11.0
39	South Dakota	8.1
32	Tennessee	9.7
38	Texas	8.9
41	Utah	7.7
5	Vermont	24.0
19	Virginia	12.1
18	Washington	12.2
35	West Virginia	9.1
25	Wisconsin	10.6
46	Wyoming	6.7

RANK ORDER

RANK	STATE	RATE
1	Massachusetts	32.3
2	New York	30.2
3	Connecticut	27.3
4	Maryland	24.9
5	Vermont	24.0
6	Rhode Island	20.7
7	New Hampshire	16.6
8	Pennsylvania	16.1
9	Hawaii	16.0
10	New Jersey	15.7
11	California	15.3
12	Maine	13.9
13	New Mexico	13.5
14	Kansas	13.3
15	Colorado	13.1
16	Delaware	13.0
17	Illinois	12.3
18	Washington	12.2
19	Virginia	12.1
20	North Carolina	11.8
21	Oregon	11.6
22	Louisiana	11.4
23	South Carolina	11.0
24	Michigan	10.9
25	Wisconsin	10.6
26	Florida	10.5
27	Georgia	10.2
28	Minnesota	10.1
28	North Dakota	10.1
30	Missouri	10.0
31	Ohio	9.9
32	Tennessee	9.7
33	Arizona	9.6
34	Alaska	9.4
35	Nebraska	9.1
35	West Virginia	9.1
37	Kentucky	9.0
38	Texas	8.9
39	South Dakota	8.1
40	Montana	7.9
41	Utah	7.7
42	Arkansas	7.6
43	Oklahoma	7.4
44	Indiana	7.2
45	Nevada	6.9
46	Alabama	6.7
46	Iowa	6.7
46	Wyoming	6.7
49	Mississippi	5.3
50	Idaho	5.1

District of Columbia 66.8

Source: Morgan Quitno Press using data from American Medical Association (Chicago, Illinois)
"Physician Characteristics and Distribution in the U.S." (1997-98 Edition)
*As of December 31, 1996. National rate does not include physicians in U.S. territories and possessions.
Psychiatry includes psychoanalysis.

Percent of Nonfederal Physicians Who Are Specialists in 1996

National Percent = 74.9% of Physicians*

<table>
<tr><td colspan="3">ALPHA ORDER</td><td colspan="3">RANK ORDER</td></tr>
<tr><th>RANK</th><th>STATE</th><th>PHYSICIANS</th><th>RANK</th><th>STATE</th><th>PHYSICIANS</th></tr>
<tr><td>16</td><td>Alabama</td><td>76.6</td><td>1</td><td>Massachusetts</td><td>84.2</td></tr>
<tr><td>36</td><td>Alaska</td><td>69.8</td><td>2</td><td>New York</td><td>83.4</td></tr>
<tr><td>38</td><td>Arizona</td><td>69.7</td><td>3</td><td>Rhode Island</td><td>82.9</td></tr>
<tr><td>42</td><td>Arkansas</td><td>67.9</td><td>4</td><td>Connecticut</td><td>82.8</td></tr>
<tr><td>24</td><td>California</td><td>73.8</td><td>5</td><td>New Jersey</td><td>82.5</td></tr>
<tr><td>31</td><td>Colorado</td><td>71.9</td><td>6</td><td>Maryland</td><td>82.1</td></tr>
<tr><td>4</td><td>Connecticut</td><td>82.8</td><td>7</td><td>Missouri</td><td>81.3</td></tr>
<tr><td>17</td><td>Delaware</td><td>76.4</td><td>8</td><td>Louisiana</td><td>79.9</td></tr>
<tr><td>36</td><td>Florida</td><td>69.8</td><td>9</td><td>Illinois</td><td>78.9</td></tr>
<tr><td>10</td><td>Georgia</td><td>78.8</td><td>10</td><td>Georgia</td><td>78.8</td></tr>
<tr><td>14</td><td>Hawaii</td><td>77.1</td><td>11</td><td>Pennsylvania</td><td>78.4</td></tr>
<tr><td>49</td><td>Idaho</td><td>61.9</td><td>12</td><td>Michigan</td><td>78.0</td></tr>
<tr><td>9</td><td>Illinois</td><td>78.9</td><td>12</td><td>Tennessee</td><td>78.0</td></tr>
<tr><td>35</td><td>Indiana</td><td>70.5</td><td>14</td><td>Hawaii</td><td>77.1</td></tr>
<tr><td>45</td><td>Iowa</td><td>67.1</td><td>14</td><td>Ohio</td><td>77.1</td></tr>
<tr><td>39</td><td>Kansas</td><td>69.0</td><td>16</td><td>Alabama</td><td>76.6</td></tr>
<tr><td>23</td><td>Kentucky</td><td>74.8</td><td>17</td><td>Delaware</td><td>76.4</td></tr>
<tr><td>8</td><td>Louisiana</td><td>79.9</td><td>17</td><td>Texas</td><td>76.4</td></tr>
<tr><td>44</td><td>Maine</td><td>67.3</td><td>19</td><td>North Carolina</td><td>76.0</td></tr>
<tr><td>6</td><td>Maryland</td><td>82.1</td><td>20</td><td>Virginia</td><td>75.2</td></tr>
<tr><td>1</td><td>Massachusetts</td><td>84.2</td><td>21</td><td>Nevada</td><td>75.1</td></tr>
<tr><td>12</td><td>Michigan</td><td>78.0</td><td>22</td><td>Utah</td><td>74.9</td></tr>
<tr><td>40</td><td>Minnesota</td><td>68.7</td><td>23</td><td>Kentucky</td><td>74.8</td></tr>
<tr><td>28</td><td>Mississippi</td><td>72.5</td><td>24</td><td>California</td><td>73.8</td></tr>
<tr><td>7</td><td>Missouri</td><td>81.3</td><td>25</td><td>New Hampshire</td><td>73.3</td></tr>
<tr><td>46</td><td>Montana</td><td>66.3</td><td>26</td><td>Oklahoma</td><td>73.0</td></tr>
<tr><td>42</td><td>Nebraska</td><td>67.9</td><td>27</td><td>West Virginia</td><td>72.8</td></tr>
<tr><td>21</td><td>Nevada</td><td>75.1</td><td>28</td><td>Mississippi</td><td>72.5</td></tr>
<tr><td>25</td><td>New Hampshire</td><td>73.3</td><td>29</td><td>South Carolina</td><td>72.4</td></tr>
<tr><td>5</td><td>New Jersey</td><td>82.5</td><td>30</td><td>Vermont</td><td>72.0</td></tr>
<tr><td>33</td><td>New Mexico</td><td>71.3</td><td>31</td><td>Colorado</td><td>71.9</td></tr>
<tr><td>2</td><td>New York</td><td>83.4</td><td>32</td><td>Wisconsin</td><td>71.8</td></tr>
<tr><td>19</td><td>North Carolina</td><td>76.0</td><td>33</td><td>New Mexico</td><td>71.3</td></tr>
<tr><td>47</td><td>North Dakota</td><td>65.8</td><td>34</td><td>Oregon</td><td>71.1</td></tr>
<tr><td>14</td><td>Ohio</td><td>77.1</td><td>35</td><td>Indiana</td><td>70.5</td></tr>
<tr><td>26</td><td>Oklahoma</td><td>73.0</td><td>36</td><td>Alaska</td><td>69.8</td></tr>
<tr><td>34</td><td>Oregon</td><td>71.1</td><td>36</td><td>Florida</td><td>69.8</td></tr>
<tr><td>11</td><td>Pennsylvania</td><td>78.4</td><td>38</td><td>Arizona</td><td>69.7</td></tr>
<tr><td>3</td><td>Rhode Island</td><td>82.9</td><td>39</td><td>Kansas</td><td>69.0</td></tr>
<tr><td>29</td><td>South Carolina</td><td>72.4</td><td>40</td><td>Minnesota</td><td>68.7</td></tr>
<tr><td>48</td><td>South Dakota</td><td>64.2</td><td>41</td><td>Washington</td><td>68.3</td></tr>
<tr><td>12</td><td>Tennessee</td><td>78.0</td><td>42</td><td>Arkansas</td><td>67.9</td></tr>
<tr><td>17</td><td>Texas</td><td>76.4</td><td>42</td><td>Nebraska</td><td>67.9</td></tr>
<tr><td>22</td><td>Utah</td><td>74.9</td><td>44</td><td>Maine</td><td>67.3</td></tr>
<tr><td>30</td><td>Vermont</td><td>72.0</td><td>45</td><td>Iowa</td><td>67.1</td></tr>
<tr><td>20</td><td>Virginia</td><td>75.2</td><td>46</td><td>Montana</td><td>66.3</td></tr>
<tr><td>41</td><td>Washington</td><td>68.3</td><td>47</td><td>North Dakota</td><td>65.8</td></tr>
<tr><td>27</td><td>West Virginia</td><td>72.8</td><td>48</td><td>South Dakota</td><td>64.2</td></tr>
<tr><td>32</td><td>Wisconsin</td><td>71.8</td><td>49</td><td>Idaho</td><td>61.9</td></tr>
<tr><td>50</td><td>Wyoming</td><td>61.2</td><td>50</td><td>Wyoming</td><td>61.2</td></tr>
<tr><td></td><td></td><td></td><td></td><td>District of Columbia</td><td>86.0</td></tr>
</table>

Source: Morgan Quitno Press using data from American Medical Association (Chicago, Illinois)
"Physician Characteristics and Distribution in the U.S." (1997-98 Edition)
*As of December 31, 1996. National rate does not include physicians in U.S. territories and possessions. Includes physicians in medical, surgical and other specialties.

International Medical School Graduates Practicing in the U.S. in 1996

National Total = 161,927 Nonfederal Physicians*

ALPHA ORDER

RANK	STATE	PHYSICIANS	% of USA
26	Alabama	1,048	0.65%
48	Alaska	61	0.04%
20	Arizona	1,602	0.99%
38	Arkansas	442	0.27%
2	California	17,902	11.06%
33	Colorado	540	0.33%
13	Connecticut	3,109	1.92%
36	Delaware	473	0.29%
3	Florida	13,059	8.06%
15	Georgia	2,429	1.50%
35	Hawaii	519	0.32%
49	Idaho	57	0.04%
4	Illinois	11,062	6.83%
16	Indiana	2,013	1.24%
30	Iowa	776	0.48%
27	Kansas	923	0.57%
23	Kentucky	1,386	0.86%
21	Louisiana	1,429	0.88%
41	Maine	336	0.21%
10	Maryland	5,363	3.31%
11	Massachusetts	4,861	3.00%
9	Michigan	6,885	4.25%
22	Minnesota	1,407	0.87%
39	Mississippi	392	0.24%
14	Missouri	2,518	1.56%
47	Montana	82	0.05%
42	Nebraska	325	0.20%
32	Nevada	544	0.34%
40	New Hampshire	377	0.23%
5	New Jersey	10,801	6.67%
37	New Mexico	454	0.28%
1	New York	29,784	18.39%
18	North Carolina	1,766	1.09%
43	North Dakota	257	0.16%
8	Ohio	7,028	4.34%
29	Oklahoma	855	0.53%
34	Oregon	524	0.32%
7	Pennsylvania	7,936	4.90%
28	Rhode Island	863	0.53%
31	South Carolina	721	0.45%
45	South Dakota	145	0.09%
19	Tennessee	1,709	1.06%
6	Texas	8,351	5.16%
44	Utah	240	0.15%
46	Vermont	126	0.08%
12	Virginia	3,175	1.96%
25	Washington	1,262	0.78%
24	West Virginia	1,377	0.85%
17	Wisconsin	1,823	1.13%
50	Wyoming	48	0.03%

RANK ORDER

RANK	STATE	PHYSICIANS	% of USA
1	New York	29,784	18.39%
2	California	17,902	11.06%
3	Florida	13,059	8.06%
4	Illinois	11,062	6.83%
5	New Jersey	10,801	6.67%
6	Texas	8,351	5.16%
7	Pennsylvania	7,936	4.90%
8	Ohio	7,028	4.34%
9	Michigan	6,885	4.25%
10	Maryland	5,363	3.31%
11	Massachusetts	4,861	3.00%
12	Virginia	3,175	1.96%
13	Connecticut	3,109	1.92%
14	Missouri	2,518	1.56%
15	Georgia	2,429	1.50%
16	Indiana	2,013	1.24%
17	Wisconsin	1,823	1.13%
18	North Carolina	1,766	1.09%
19	Tennessee	1,709	1.06%
20	Arizona	1,602	0.99%
21	Louisiana	1,429	0.88%
22	Minnesota	1,407	0.87%
23	Kentucky	1,386	0.86%
24	West Virginia	1,377	0.85%
25	Washington	1,262	0.78%
26	Alabama	1,048	0.65%
27	Kansas	923	0.57%
28	Rhode Island	863	0.53%
29	Oklahoma	855	0.53%
30	Iowa	776	0.48%
31	South Carolina	721	0.45%
32	Nevada	544	0.34%
33	Colorado	540	0.33%
34	Oregon	524	0.32%
35	Hawaii	519	0.32%
36	Delaware	473	0.29%
37	New Mexico	454	0.28%
38	Arkansas	442	0.27%
39	Mississippi	392	0.24%
40	New Hampshire	377	0.23%
41	Maine	336	0.21%
42	Nebraska	325	0.20%
43	North Dakota	257	0.16%
44	Utah	240	0.15%
45	South Dakota	145	0.09%
46	Vermont	126	0.08%
47	Montana	82	0.05%
48	Alaska	61	0.04%
49	Idaho	57	0.04%
50	Wyoming	48	0.03%
	District of Columbia	762	0.47%

Source: American Medical Association (Chicago, Illinois)
    "Physician Characteristics and Distribution in the U.S." (1997-98 Edition)
As of December 31, 1996. Total does not include 5,104 physicians in U.S. territories and possessions.

Rate of International Medical School Graduates Practicing in the U.S. in 1996

National Rate = 61 Nonfederal Physicians per 100,000 Population*

ALPHA ORDER			RANK ORDER		
RANK	STATE	RATE	RANK	STATE	RATE
35	Alabama	24	1	New York	164
47	Alaska	10	2	New Jersey	135
20	Arizona	36	3	Maryland	106
42	Arkansas	18	4	Connecticut	95
14	California	56	5	Illinois	93
44	Colorado	14	6	Florida	91
4	Connecticut	95	7	Rhode Island	87
12	Delaware	65	8	Massachusetts	80
6	Florida	91	9	West Virginia	76
26	Georgia	33	10	Michigan	71
17	Hawaii	44	11	Pennsylvania	66
50	Idaho	5	12	Delaware	65
5	Illinois	93	13	Ohio	63
23	Indiana	35	14	California	56
31	Iowa	27	15	Virginia	48
20	Kansas	36	16	Missouri	47
20	Kentucky	36	17	Hawaii	44
26	Louisiana	33	17	Texas	44
31	Maine	27	19	North Dakota	40
3	Maryland	106	20	Arizona	36
8	Massachusetts	80	20	Kansas	36
10	Michigan	71	20	Kentucky	36
30	Minnesota	30	23	Indiana	35
44	Mississippi	14	23	Wisconsin	35
16	Missouri	47	25	Nevada	34
49	Montana	9	26	Georgia	33
39	Nebraska	20	26	Louisiana	33
25	Nevada	34	28	New Hampshire	32
28	New Hampshire	32	28	Tennessee	32
2	New Jersey	135	30	Minnesota	30
31	New Mexico	27	31	Iowa	27
1	New York	164	31	Maine	27
35	North Carolina	24	31	New Mexico	27
19	North Dakota	40	34	Oklahoma	26
13	Ohio	63	35	Alabama	24
34	Oklahoma	26	35	North Carolina	24
43	Oregon	16	37	Washington	23
11	Pennsylvania	66	38	Vermont	21
7	Rhode Island	87	39	Nebraska	20
41	South Carolina	19	39	South Dakota	20
39	South Dakota	20	41	South Carolina	19
28	Tennessee	32	42	Arkansas	18
17	Texas	44	43	Oregon	16
46	Utah	12	44	Colorado	14
38	Vermont	21	44	Mississippi	14
15	Virginia	48	46	Utah	12
37	Washington	23	47	Alaska	10
9	West Virginia	76	47	Wyoming	10
23	Wisconsin	35	49	Montana	9
47	Wyoming	10	50	Idaho	5
				District of Columbia	141

Source: Morgan Quitno Press using data from American Medical Association (Chicago, Illinois)
"Physician Characteristics and Distribution in the U.S." (1997-98 Edition)
As of December 31, 1996. National rate does not include physicians in U.S. territories and possessions.

International Medical School Graduates
As a Percent of Nonfederal Physicians in 1996
National Percent = 22.9% of Nonfederal Physicians*

ALPHA ORDER

RANK	STATE	PERCENT
32	Alabama	11.8
45	Alaska	6.1
24	Arizona	15.3
41	Arkansas	8.8
14	California	20.4
46	Colorado	5.6
11	Connecticut	25.5
8	Delaware	26.1
5	Florida	32.9
25	Georgia	15.2
23	Hawaii	15.7
50	Idaho	2.9
3	Illinois	34.6
20	Indiana	16.8
28	Iowa	14.2
22	Kansas	15.9
20	Kentucky	16.8
29	Louisiana	13.2
35	Maine	11.0
7	Maryland	27.6
17	Massachusetts	18.7
6	Michigan	30.2
34	Minnesota	11.3
38	Mississippi	8.9
15	Missouri	19.5
49	Montana	4.3
38	Nebraska	8.9
18	Nevada	18.5
31	New Hampshire	12.6
1	New Jersey	44.3
33	New Mexico	11.4
2	New York	41.5
37	North Carolina	9.9
19	North Dakota	18.0
10	Ohio	25.6
27	Oklahoma	14.5
44	Oregon	6.4
12	Pennsylvania	21.8
9	Rhode Island	26.0
38	South Carolina	8.9
36	South Dakota	10.0
30	Tennessee	12.7
13	Texas	21.1
47	Utah	5.5
43	Vermont	6.6
16	Virginia	18.8
41	Washington	8.8
4	West Virginia	33.7
26	Wisconsin	14.6
48	Wyoming	5.4

RANK ORDER

RANK	STATE	PERCENT
1	New Jersey	44.3
2	New York	41.5
3	Illinois	34.6
4	West Virginia	33.7
5	Florida	32.9
6	Michigan	30.2
7	Maryland	27.6
8	Delaware	26.1
9	Rhode Island	26.0
10	Ohio	25.6
11	Connecticut	25.5
12	Pennsylvania	21.8
13	Texas	21.1
14	California	20.4
15	Missouri	19.5
16	Virginia	18.8
17	Massachusetts	18.7
18	Nevada	18.5
19	North Dakota	18.0
20	Indiana	16.8
20	Kentucky	16.8
22	Kansas	15.9
23	Hawaii	15.7
24	Arizona	15.3
25	Georgia	15.2
26	Wisconsin	14.6
27	Oklahoma	14.5
28	Iowa	14.2
29	Louisiana	13.2
30	Tennessee	12.7
31	New Hampshire	12.6
32	Alabama	11.8
33	New Mexico	11.4
34	Minnesota	11.3
35	Maine	11.0
36	South Dakota	10.0
37	North Carolina	9.9
38	Mississippi	8.9
38	Nebraska	8.9
38	South Carolina	8.9
41	Arkansas	8.8
41	Washington	8.8
43	Vermont	6.6
44	Oregon	6.4
45	Alaska	6.1
46	Colorado	5.6
47	Utah	5.5
48	Wyoming	5.4
49	Montana	4.3
50	Idaho	2.9

District of Columbia 19.2

Source: Morgan Quitno Press using data from American Medical Association (Chicago, Illinois)
"Physician Characteristics and Distribution in the U.S." (1997-98 Edition)
*As of December 31, 1996. National rate does not include physicians in U.S. territories and possessions.

Osteopathic Physicians in 1997

National Total = 40,324 Osteopathic Physicians*

<table>
<tr><td colspan="4">ALPHA ORDER</td><td colspan="4">RANK ORDER</td></tr>
<tr><td>RANK</td><td>STATE</td><td>OSTEOPATHS</td><td>% of USA</td><td>RANK</td><td>STATE</td><td>OSTEOPATHS</td><td>% of USA</td></tr>
<tr><td>28</td><td>Alabama</td><td>251</td><td>0.62%</td><td>1</td><td>Michigan</td><td>4,876</td><td>12.09%</td></tr>
<tr><td>45</td><td>Alaska</td><td>65</td><td>0.16%</td><td>2</td><td>Pennsylvania</td><td>4,815</td><td>11.94%</td></tr>
<tr><td>12</td><td>Arizona</td><td>1,120</td><td>2.78%</td><td>3</td><td>Ohio</td><td>3,269</td><td>8.11%</td></tr>
<tr><td>38</td><td>Arkansas</td><td>167</td><td>0.41%</td><td>4</td><td>Florida</td><td>2,842</td><td>7.05%</td></tr>
<tr><td>8</td><td>California</td><td>1,828</td><td>4.53%</td><td>5</td><td>Texas</td><td>2,438</td><td>6.05%</td></tr>
<tr><td>14</td><td>Colorado</td><td>669</td><td>1.66%</td><td>6</td><td>New Jersey</td><td>2,393</td><td>5.93%</td></tr>
<tr><td>31</td><td>Connecticut</td><td>188</td><td>0.47%</td><td>7</td><td>New York</td><td>2,236</td><td>5.55%</td></tr>
<tr><td>36</td><td>Delaware</td><td>171</td><td>0.42%</td><td>8</td><td>California</td><td>1,828</td><td>4.53%</td></tr>
<tr><td>4</td><td>Florida</td><td>2,842</td><td>7.05%</td><td>9</td><td>Missouri</td><td>1,750</td><td>4.34%</td></tr>
<tr><td>18</td><td>Georgia</td><td>484</td><td>1.20%</td><td>10</td><td>Illinois</td><td>1,610</td><td>3.99%</td></tr>
<tr><td>43</td><td>Hawaii</td><td>87</td><td>0.22%</td><td>11</td><td>Oklahoma</td><td>1,147</td><td>2.84%</td></tr>
<tr><td>39</td><td>Idaho</td><td>99</td><td>0.25%</td><td>12</td><td>Arizona</td><td>1,120</td><td>2.78%</td></tr>
<tr><td>10</td><td>Illinois</td><td>1,610</td><td>3.99%</td><td>13</td><td>Iowa</td><td>925</td><td>2.29%</td></tr>
<tr><td>15</td><td>Indiana</td><td>591</td><td>1.47%</td><td>14</td><td>Colorado</td><td>669</td><td>1.66%</td></tr>
<tr><td>13</td><td>Iowa</td><td>925</td><td>2.29%</td><td>15</td><td>Indiana</td><td>591</td><td>1.47%</td></tr>
<tr><td>16</td><td>Kansas</td><td>542</td><td>1.34%</td><td>16</td><td>Kansas</td><td>542</td><td>1.34%</td></tr>
<tr><td>32</td><td>Kentucky</td><td>184</td><td>0.46%</td><td>17</td><td>Washington</td><td>491</td><td>1.22%</td></tr>
<tr><td>42</td><td>Louisiana</td><td>91</td><td>0.23%</td><td>18</td><td>Georgia</td><td>484</td><td>1.20%</td></tr>
<tr><td>21</td><td>Maine</td><td>418</td><td>1.04%</td><td>19</td><td>West Virginia</td><td>455</td><td>1.13%</td></tr>
<tr><td>26</td><td>Maryland</td><td>274</td><td>0.68%</td><td>20</td><td>Wisconsin</td><td>432</td><td>1.07%</td></tr>
<tr><td>23</td><td>Massachusetts</td><td>389</td><td>0.96%</td><td>21</td><td>Maine</td><td>418</td><td>1.04%</td></tr>
<tr><td>1</td><td>Michigan</td><td>4,876</td><td>12.09%</td><td>22</td><td>Oregon</td><td>402</td><td>1.00%</td></tr>
<tr><td>30</td><td>Minnesota</td><td>208</td><td>0.52%</td><td>23</td><td>Massachusetts</td><td>389</td><td>0.96%</td></tr>
<tr><td>34</td><td>Mississippi</td><td>175</td><td>0.43%</td><td>24</td><td>Virginia</td><td>329</td><td>0.82%</td></tr>
<tr><td>9</td><td>Missouri</td><td>1,750</td><td>4.34%</td><td>25</td><td>Tennessee</td><td>312</td><td>0.77%</td></tr>
<tr><td>44</td><td>Montana</td><td>71</td><td>0.18%</td><td>26</td><td>Maryland</td><td>274</td><td>0.68%</td></tr>
<tr><td>46</td><td>Nebraska</td><td>63</td><td>0.16%</td><td>27</td><td>Nevada</td><td>257</td><td>0.64%</td></tr>
<tr><td>27</td><td>Nevada</td><td>257</td><td>0.64%</td><td>28</td><td>Alabama</td><td>251</td><td>0.62%</td></tr>
<tr><td>40</td><td>New Hampshire</td><td>97</td><td>0.24%</td><td>29</td><td>North Carolina</td><td>232</td><td>0.58%</td></tr>
<tr><td>6</td><td>New Jersey</td><td>2,393</td><td>5.93%</td><td>30</td><td>Minnesota</td><td>208</td><td>0.52%</td></tr>
<tr><td>32</td><td>New Mexico</td><td>184</td><td>0.46%</td><td>31</td><td>Connecticut</td><td>188</td><td>0.47%</td></tr>
<tr><td>7</td><td>New York</td><td>2,236</td><td>5.55%</td><td>32</td><td>Kentucky</td><td>184</td><td>0.46%</td></tr>
<tr><td>29</td><td>North Carolina</td><td>232</td><td>0.58%</td><td>32</td><td>New Mexico</td><td>184</td><td>0.46%</td></tr>
<tr><td>48</td><td>North Dakota</td><td>51</td><td>0.13%</td><td>34</td><td>Mississippi</td><td>175</td><td>0.43%</td></tr>
<tr><td>3</td><td>Ohio</td><td>3,269</td><td>8.11%</td><td>35</td><td>Rhode Island</td><td>174</td><td>0.43%</td></tr>
<tr><td>11</td><td>Oklahoma</td><td>1,147</td><td>2.84%</td><td>36</td><td>Delaware</td><td>171</td><td>0.42%</td></tr>
<tr><td>22</td><td>Oregon</td><td>402</td><td>1.00%</td><td>36</td><td>South Carolina</td><td>171</td><td>0.42%</td></tr>
<tr><td>2</td><td>Pennsylvania</td><td>4,815</td><td>11.94%</td><td>38</td><td>Arkansas</td><td>167</td><td>0.41%</td></tr>
<tr><td>35</td><td>Rhode Island</td><td>174</td><td>0.43%</td><td>39</td><td>Idaho</td><td>99</td><td>0.25%</td></tr>
<tr><td>36</td><td>South Carolina</td><td>171</td><td>0.42%</td><td>40</td><td>New Hampshire</td><td>97</td><td>0.24%</td></tr>
<tr><td>47</td><td>South Dakota</td><td>58</td><td>0.14%</td><td>41</td><td>Utah</td><td>93</td><td>0.23%</td></tr>
<tr><td>25</td><td>Tennessee</td><td>312</td><td>0.77%</td><td>42</td><td>Louisiana</td><td>91</td><td>0.23%</td></tr>
<tr><td>5</td><td>Texas</td><td>2,438</td><td>6.05%</td><td>43</td><td>Hawaii</td><td>87</td><td>0.22%</td></tr>
<tr><td>41</td><td>Utah</td><td>93</td><td>0.23%</td><td>44</td><td>Montana</td><td>71</td><td>0.18%</td></tr>
<tr><td>49</td><td>Vermont</td><td>50</td><td>0.12%</td><td>45</td><td>Alaska</td><td>65</td><td>0.16%</td></tr>
<tr><td>24</td><td>Virginia</td><td>329</td><td>0.82%</td><td>46</td><td>Nebraska</td><td>63</td><td>0.16%</td></tr>
<tr><td>17</td><td>Washington</td><td>491</td><td>1.22%</td><td>47</td><td>South Dakota</td><td>58</td><td>0.14%</td></tr>
<tr><td>19</td><td>West Virginia</td><td>455</td><td>1.13%</td><td>48</td><td>North Dakota</td><td>51</td><td>0.13%</td></tr>
<tr><td>20</td><td>Wisconsin</td><td>432</td><td>1.07%</td><td>49</td><td>Vermont</td><td>50</td><td>0.12%</td></tr>
<tr><td>50</td><td>Wyoming</td><td>34</td><td>0.08%</td><td>50</td><td>Wyoming</td><td>34</td><td>0.08%</td></tr>
<tr><td></td><td></td><td></td><td></td><td></td><td>District of Columbia</td><td>30</td><td>0.07%</td></tr>
</table>

Source: American Osteopathic Association
        "AOA Yearbook and Directory of Osteopathic Physicians 1998"
*Excludes retired, disabled, foreign and federal osteopaths. Osteopaths practice a system of medicine based on the theory that disturbances in the musculoskeletal system affect other body parts, causing many disorders that can be corrected by various manipulative techniques in conjunction with conventional medical, surgical, pharmacological, and other therapeutic procedures.

Rate of Osteopathic Physicians in 1997

National Rate = 15.1 Osteopaths per 1000,000 Population*

ALPHA ORDER

RANK	STATE	RATE
38	Alabama	5.8
21	Alaska	10.7
10	Arizona	24.6
34	Arkansas	6.6
40	California	5.7
15	Colorado	17.2
40	Connecticut	5.7
11	Delaware	23.4
13	Florida	19.4
35	Georgia	6.5
32	Hawaii	7.3
28	Idaho	8.2
17	Illinois	13.5
23	Indiana	10.1
5	Iowa	32.4
12	Kansas	20.9
44	Kentucky	4.7
50	Louisiana	2.1
4	Maine	33.7
42	Maryland	5.4
36	Massachusetts	6.4
1	Michigan	49.9
47	Minnesota	4.4
36	Mississippi	6.4
5	Missouri	32.4
29	Montana	8.1
48	Nebraska	3.8
16	Nevada	15.3
27	New Hampshire	8.3
7	New Jersey	29.7
22	New Mexico	10.6
20	New York	12.3
49	North Carolina	3.1
30	North Dakota	8.0
8	Ohio	29.2
3	Oklahoma	34.6
19	Oregon	12.4
2	Pennsylvania	40.1
14	Rhode Island	17.6
45	South Carolina	4.5
31	South Dakota	7.9
38	Tennessee	5.8
18	Texas	12.5
45	Utah	4.5
25	Vermont	8.5
43	Virginia	4.9
24	Washington	8.8
9	West Virginia	25.1
26	Wisconsin	8.4
33	Wyoming	7.1

RANK ORDER

RANK	STATE	RATE
1	Michigan	49.9
2	Pennsylvania	40.1
3	Oklahoma	34.6
4	Maine	33.7
5	Iowa	32.4
5	Missouri	32.4
7	New Jersey	29.7
8	Ohio	29.2
9	West Virginia	25.1
10	Arizona	24.6
11	Delaware	23.4
12	Kansas	20.9
13	Florida	19.4
14	Rhode Island	17.6
15	Colorado	17.2
16	Nevada	15.3
17	Illinois	13.5
18	Texas	12.5
19	Oregon	12.4
20	New York	12.3
21	Alaska	10.7
22	New Mexico	10.6
23	Indiana	10.1
24	Washington	8.8
25	Vermont	8.5
26	Wisconsin	8.4
27	New Hampshire	8.3
28	Idaho	8.2
29	Montana	8.1
30	North Dakota	8.0
31	South Dakota	7.9
32	Hawaii	7.3
33	Wyoming	7.1
34	Arkansas	6.6
35	Georgia	6.5
36	Massachusetts	6.4
36	Mississippi	6.4
38	Alabama	5.8
38	Tennessee	5.8
40	California	5.7
40	Connecticut	5.7
42	Maryland	5.4
43	Virginia	4.9
44	Kentucky	4.7
45	South Carolina	4.5
45	Utah	4.5
47	Minnesota	4.4
48	Nebraska	3.8
49	North Carolina	3.1
50	Louisiana	2.1
	District of Columbia	5.7

Source: Morgan Quitno Press using data from American Osteopathic Association
   "AOA Yearbook and Directory of Osteopathic Physicians 1998"
*Excludes retired, disabled, foreign and federal osteopaths. Osteopaths practice a system of medicine based on
the theory that disturbances in the musculoskeletal system affect other body parts, causing many disorders that can
be corrected by various manipulative techniques in conjunction with conventional medical, surgical,
pharmacological, and other therapeutic procedures.

Osteopathic Physicians in Primary Care in 1996

National Total = 21,638 Osteopathic Physicians*

ALPHA ORDER

RANK	STATE	OSTEOPATHS	% of USA
28	Alabama	132	0.61%
40	Alaska	52	0.24%
12	Arizona	546	2.52%
33	Arkansas	97	0.45%
8	California	1,041	4.81%
14	Colorado	428	1.98%
36	Connecticut	87	0.40%
29	Delaware	111	0.51%
4	Florida	1,425	6.59%
18	Georgia	286	1.32%
39	Hawaii	63	0.29%
42	Idaho	50	0.23%
10	Illinois	778	3.60%
17	Indiana	304	1.40%
13	Iowa	527	2.44%
16	Kansas	310	1.43%
37	Kentucky	84	0.39%
44	Louisiana	44	0.20%
21	Maine	253	1.17%
26	Maryland	139	0.64%
23	Massachusetts	203	0.94%
2	Michigan	2,363	10.92%
31	Minnesota	110	0.51%
34	Mississippi	93	0.43%
9	Missouri	943	4.36%
46	Montana	32	0.15%
45	Nebraska	36	0.17%
27	Nevada	135	0.62%
40	New Hampshire	52	0.24%
6	New Jersey	1,288	5.95%
29	New Mexico	111	0.51%
7	New York	1,213	5.61%
35	North Carolina	92	0.43%
50	North Dakota	12	0.06%
3	Ohio	1,625	7.51%
11	Oklahoma	677	3.13%
22	Oregon	228	1.05%
1	Pennsylvania	2,751	12.71%
32	Rhode Island	98	0.45%
38	South Carolina	81	0.37%
47	South Dakota	28	0.13%
25	Tennessee	160	0.74%
5	Texas	1,396	6.45%
43	Utah	47	0.22%
48	Vermont	25	0.12%
24	Virginia	196	0.91%
15	Washington	324	1.50%
19	West Virginia	273	1.26%
20	Wisconsin	256	1.18%
49	Wyoming	19	0.09%

RANK ORDER

RANK	STATE	OSTEOPATHS	% of USA
1	Pennsylvania	2,751	12.71%
2	Michigan	2,363	10.92%
3	Ohio	1,625	7.51%
4	Florida	1,425	6.59%
5	Texas	1,396	6.45%
6	New Jersey	1,288	5.95%
7	New York	1,213	5.61%
8	California	1,041	4.81%
9	Missouri	943	4.36%
10	Illinois	778	3.60%
11	Oklahoma	677	3.13%
12	Arizona	546	2.52%
13	Iowa	527	2.44%
14	Colorado	428	1.98%
15	Washington	324	1.50%
16	Kansas	310	1.43%
17	Indiana	304	1.40%
18	Georgia	286	1.32%
19	West Virginia	273	1.26%
20	Wisconsin	256	1.18%
21	Maine	253	1.17%
22	Oregon	228	1.05%
23	Massachusetts	203	0.94%
24	Virginia	196	0.91%
25	Tennessee	160	0.74%
26	Maryland	139	0.64%
27	Nevada	135	0.62%
28	Alabama	132	0.61%
29	Delaware	111	0.51%
29	New Mexico	111	0.51%
31	Minnesota	110	0.51%
32	Rhode Island	98	0.45%
33	Arkansas	97	0.45%
34	Mississippi	93	0.43%
35	North Carolina	92	0.43%
36	Connecticut	87	0.40%
37	Kentucky	84	0.39%
38	South Carolina	81	0.37%
39	Hawaii	63	0.29%
40	Alaska	52	0.24%
40	New Hampshire	52	0.24%
42	Idaho	50	0.23%
43	Utah	47	0.22%
44	Louisiana	44	0.20%
45	Nebraska	36	0.17%
46	Montana	32	0.15%
47	South Dakota	28	0.13%
48	Vermont	25	0.12%
49	Wyoming	19	0.09%
50	North Dakota	12	0.06%
	District of Columbia	14	0.06%

Source: Morgan Quitno Press using data from American Osteopathic Association
"AOA Biographical Records" (February 1997)

As of June 1, 1996. Excludes retired, disabled, foreign and federal osteopaths. Osteopaths practice a system of medicine based on the theory that disturbances in the musculoskeletal system affect other body parts, causing many disorders that can be corrected by various manipulative techniques in conjunction with conventional medical, surgical, pharmacological, and other therapeutic procedures.

Podiatric Physicians in 1995

National Total = 11,628 Podiatric Physicians*

<table>
<tr><td colspan="4"><u>ALPHA ORDER</u></td><td colspan="4"><u>RANK ORDER</u></td></tr>
<tr><th>RANK</th><th>STATE</th><th>PODIATRISTS</th><th>% of USA</th><th>RANK</th><th>STATE</th><th>PODIATRISTS</th><th>% of USA</th></tr>
<tr><td>31</td><td>Alabama</td><td>61</td><td>0.52%</td><td>1</td><td>California</td><td>1,415</td><td>12.17%</td></tr>
<tr><td>49</td><td>Alaska</td><td>15</td><td>0.13%</td><td>2</td><td>New York</td><td>1,154</td><td>9.92%</td></tr>
<tr><td>17</td><td>Arizona</td><td>199</td><td>1.71%</td><td>3</td><td>Pennsylvania</td><td>994</td><td>8.55%</td></tr>
<tr><td>39</td><td>Arkansas</td><td>39</td><td>0.34%</td><td>4</td><td>Florida</td><td>877</td><td>7.54%</td></tr>
<tr><td>1</td><td>California</td><td>1,415</td><td>12.17%</td><td>5</td><td>New Jersey</td><td>747</td><td>6.42%</td></tr>
<tr><td>24</td><td>Colorado</td><td>115</td><td>0.99%</td><td>6</td><td>Illinois</td><td>670</td><td>5.76%</td></tr>
<tr><td>12</td><td>Connecticut</td><td>282</td><td>2.43%</td><td>7</td><td>Ohio</td><td>490</td><td>4.21%</td></tr>
<tr><td>43</td><td>Delaware</td><td>37</td><td>0.32%</td><td>8</td><td>Michigan</td><td>457</td><td>3.93%</td></tr>
<tr><td>4</td><td>Florida</td><td>877</td><td>7.54%</td><td>9</td><td>Massachusetts</td><td>429</td><td>3.69%</td></tr>
<tr><td>13</td><td>Georgia</td><td>248</td><td>2.13%</td><td>10</td><td>Texas</td><td>422</td><td>3.63%</td></tr>
<tr><td>46</td><td>Hawaii</td><td>20</td><td>0.17%</td><td>11</td><td>Maryland</td><td>330</td><td>2.84%</td></tr>
<tr><td>37</td><td>Idaho</td><td>44</td><td>0.38%</td><td>12</td><td>Connecticut</td><td>282</td><td>2.43%</td></tr>
<tr><td>6</td><td>Illinois</td><td>670</td><td>5.76%</td><td>13</td><td>Georgia</td><td>248</td><td>2.13%</td></tr>
<tr><td>14</td><td>Indiana</td><td>227</td><td>1.95%</td><td>14</td><td>Indiana</td><td>227</td><td>1.95%</td></tr>
<tr><td>19</td><td>Iowa</td><td>148</td><td>1.27%</td><td>15</td><td>Virginia</td><td>209</td><td>1.80%</td></tr>
<tr><td>27</td><td>Kansas</td><td>86</td><td>0.74%</td><td>16</td><td>North Carolina</td><td>206</td><td>1.77%</td></tr>
<tr><td>28</td><td>Kentucky</td><td>82</td><td>0.71%</td><td>17</td><td>Arizona</td><td>199</td><td>1.71%</td></tr>
<tr><td>30</td><td>Louisiana</td><td>72</td><td>0.62%</td><td>18</td><td>Wisconsin</td><td>180</td><td>1.55%</td></tr>
<tr><td>34</td><td>Maine</td><td>54</td><td>0.46%</td><td>19</td><td>Iowa</td><td>148</td><td>1.27%</td></tr>
<tr><td>11</td><td>Maryland</td><td>330</td><td>2.84%</td><td>19</td><td>Washington</td><td>148</td><td>1.27%</td></tr>
<tr><td>9</td><td>Massachusetts</td><td>429</td><td>3.69%</td><td>21</td><td>Minnesota</td><td>130</td><td>1.12%</td></tr>
<tr><td>8</td><td>Michigan</td><td>457</td><td>3.93%</td><td>22</td><td>Tennessee</td><td>129</td><td>1.11%</td></tr>
<tr><td>21</td><td>Minnesota</td><td>130</td><td>1.12%</td><td>23</td><td>Missouri</td><td>128</td><td>1.10%</td></tr>
<tr><td>44</td><td>Mississippi</td><td>28</td><td>0.24%</td><td>24</td><td>Colorado</td><td>115</td><td>0.99%</td></tr>
<tr><td>23</td><td>Missouri</td><td>128</td><td>1.10%</td><td>25</td><td>Utah</td><td>99</td><td>0.85%</td></tr>
<tr><td>38</td><td>Montana</td><td>40</td><td>0.34%</td><td>26</td><td>Oregon</td><td>98</td><td>0.84%</td></tr>
<tr><td>32</td><td>Nebraska</td><td>56</td><td>0.48%</td><td>27</td><td>Kansas</td><td>86</td><td>0.74%</td></tr>
<tr><td>35</td><td>Nevada</td><td>53</td><td>0.46%</td><td>28</td><td>Kentucky</td><td>82</td><td>0.71%</td></tr>
<tr><td>33</td><td>New Hampshire</td><td>55</td><td>0.47%</td><td>29</td><td>Oklahoma</td><td>74</td><td>0.64%</td></tr>
<tr><td>5</td><td>New Jersey</td><td>747</td><td>6.42%</td><td>30</td><td>Louisiana</td><td>72</td><td>0.62%</td></tr>
<tr><td>41</td><td>New Mexico</td><td>38</td><td>0.33%</td><td>31</td><td>Alabama</td><td>61</td><td>0.52%</td></tr>
<tr><td>2</td><td>New York</td><td>1,154</td><td>9.92%</td><td>32</td><td>Nebraska</td><td>56</td><td>0.48%</td></tr>
<tr><td>16</td><td>North Carolina</td><td>206</td><td>1.77%</td><td>33</td><td>New Hampshire</td><td>55</td><td>0.47%</td></tr>
<tr><td>48</td><td>North Dakota</td><td>16</td><td>0.14%</td><td>34</td><td>Maine</td><td>54</td><td>0.46%</td></tr>
<tr><td>7</td><td>Ohio</td><td>490</td><td>4.21%</td><td>35</td><td>Nevada</td><td>53</td><td>0.46%</td></tr>
<tr><td>29</td><td>Oklahoma</td><td>74</td><td>0.64%</td><td>35</td><td>West Virginia</td><td>53</td><td>0.46%</td></tr>
<tr><td>26</td><td>Oregon</td><td>98</td><td>0.84%</td><td>37</td><td>Idaho</td><td>44</td><td>0.38%</td></tr>
<tr><td>3</td><td>Pennsylvania</td><td>994</td><td>8.55%</td><td>38</td><td>Montana</td><td>40</td><td>0.34%</td></tr>
<tr><td>39</td><td>Rhode Island</td><td>39</td><td>0.34%</td><td>39</td><td>Arkansas</td><td>39</td><td>0.34%</td></tr>
<tr><td>41</td><td>South Carolina</td><td>38</td><td>0.33%</td><td>39</td><td>Rhode Island</td><td>39</td><td>0.34%</td></tr>
<tr><td>45</td><td>South Dakota</td><td>24</td><td>0.21%</td><td>41</td><td>New Mexico</td><td>38</td><td>0.33%</td></tr>
<tr><td>22</td><td>Tennessee</td><td>129</td><td>1.11%</td><td>41</td><td>South Carolina</td><td>38</td><td>0.33%</td></tr>
<tr><td>10</td><td>Texas</td><td>422</td><td>3.63%</td><td>43</td><td>Delaware</td><td>37</td><td>0.32%</td></tr>
<tr><td>25</td><td>Utah</td><td>99</td><td>0.85%</td><td>44</td><td>Mississippi</td><td>28</td><td>0.24%</td></tr>
<tr><td>46</td><td>Vermont</td><td>20</td><td>0.17%</td><td>45</td><td>South Dakota</td><td>24</td><td>0.21%</td></tr>
<tr><td>15</td><td>Virginia</td><td>209</td><td>1.80%</td><td>46</td><td>Hawaii</td><td>20</td><td>0.17%</td></tr>
<tr><td>19</td><td>Washington</td><td>148</td><td>1.27%</td><td>46</td><td>Vermont</td><td>20</td><td>0.17%</td></tr>
<tr><td>35</td><td>West Virginia</td><td>53</td><td>0.46%</td><td>48</td><td>North Dakota</td><td>16</td><td>0.14%</td></tr>
<tr><td>18</td><td>Wisconsin</td><td>180</td><td>1.55%</td><td>49</td><td>Alaska</td><td>15</td><td>0.13%</td></tr>
<tr><td>50</td><td>Wyoming</td><td>10</td><td>0.09%</td><td>50</td><td>Wyoming</td><td>10</td><td>0.09%</td></tr>
<tr><td></td><td></td><td></td><td></td><td></td><td>District of Columbia</td><td>43</td><td>0.37%</td></tr>
</table>

Source: American Podiatric Medical Association, Inc.
  "Podiatric Physicians in Active Practice"
*As of December 1995. Includes only Podiatric physicians considered in "active practice." Podiatry deals with the diagnosis, treatment, and prevention of diseases of the human foot. National total does not include eight podiatrists in Puerto Rico.

Rate of Podiatric Physicians in 1995

National Rate = 4.4 Podiatrists per 100,000 Population*

ALPHA ORDER

RANK	STATE	RATE
48	Alabama	1.4
36	Alaska	2.5
14	Arizona	4.6
47	Arkansas	1.6
16	California	4.5
30	Colorado	3.1
2	Connecticut	8.6
9	Delaware	5.2
7	Florida	6.2
24	Georgia	3.4
45	Hawaii	1.7
21	Idaho	3.8
8	Illinois	5.7
19	Indiana	3.9
9	Iowa	5.2
24	Kansas	3.4
43	Kentucky	2.1
45	Louisiana	1.7
17	Maine	4.4
5	Maryland	6.5
4	Massachusetts	7.1
12	Michigan	4.8
34	Minnesota	2.8
49	Mississippi	1.0
39	Missouri	2.4
14	Montana	4.6
24	Nebraska	3.4
22	Nevada	3.5
12	New Hampshire	4.8
1	New Jersey	9.4
41	New Mexico	2.2
6	New York	6.3
32	North Carolina	2.9
36	North Dakota	2.5
17	Ohio	4.4
40	Oklahoma	2.3
30	Oregon	3.1
3	Pennsylvania	8.2
19	Rhode Island	3.9
49	South Carolina	1.0
28	South Dakota	3.3
36	Tennessee	2.5
41	Texas	2.2
11	Utah	5.1
24	Vermont	3.4
29	Virginia	3.2
35	Washington	2.7
32	West Virginia	2.9
22	Wisconsin	3.5
43	Wyoming	2.1

RANK ORDER

RANK	STATE	RATE
1	New Jersey	9.4
2	Connecticut	8.6
3	Pennsylvania	8.2
4	Massachusetts	7.1
5	Maryland	6.5
6	New York	6.3
7	Florida	6.2
8	Illinois	5.7
9	Delaware	5.2
9	Iowa	5.2
11	Utah	5.1
12	Michigan	4.8
12	New Hampshire	4.8
14	Arizona	4.6
14	Montana	4.6
16	California	4.5
17	Maine	4.4
17	Ohio	4.4
19	Indiana	3.9
19	Rhode Island	3.9
21	Idaho	3.8
22	Nevada	3.5
22	Wisconsin	3.5
24	Georgia	3.4
24	Kansas	3.4
24	Nebraska	3.4
24	Vermont	3.4
28	South Dakota	3.3
29	Virginia	3.2
30	Colorado	3.1
30	Oregon	3.1
32	North Carolina	2.9
32	West Virginia	2.9
34	Minnesota	2.8
35	Washington	2.7
36	Alaska	2.5
36	North Dakota	2.5
36	Tennessee	2.5
39	Missouri	2.4
40	Oklahoma	2.3
41	New Mexico	2.2
41	Texas	2.2
43	Kentucky	2.1
43	Wyoming	2.1
45	Hawaii	1.7
45	Louisiana	1.7
47	Arkansas	1.6
48	Alabama	1.4
49	Mississippi	1.0
49	South Carolina	1.0
	District of Columbia	7.7

Source: Morgan Quitno Press using data from American Podiatric Medical Association, Inc.
   "Podiatric Physicians in Active Practice"
*Includes only Podiatric physicians considered in "active practice." Podiatry deals with the diagnosis, treatment, and prevention of diseases of the human foot. National rate does not include podiatrists in Puerto Rico.

Doctors of Chiropractic in 1997

National Total = 75,282 Chiropractors*

ALPHA ORDER

RANK	STATE	CHIROPRACTORS	% of USA
28	Alabama	749	0.99%
49	Alaska	179	0.24%
9	Arizona	2,490	3.31%
33	Arkansas	532	0.71%
1	California	11,332	15.05%
11	Colorado	1,970	2.62%
26	Connecticut	869	1.15%
46	Delaware	212	0.28%
3	Florida	4,224	5.61%
10	Georgia	2,474	3.29%
35	Hawaii	502	0.67%
40	Idaho	328	0.44%
7	Illinois	2,835	3.77%
25	Indiana	905	1.20%
21	Iowa	1,363	1.81%
29	Kansas	623	0.83%
23	Kentucky	1,037	1.38%
32	Louisiana	559	0.74%
37	Maine	367	0.49%
34	Maryland	518	0.69%
16	Massachusetts	1,663	2.21%
8	Michigan	2,527	3.36%
17	Minnesota	1,622	2.15%
39	Mississippi	335	0.44%
13	Missouri	1,827	2.43%
44	Montana	256	0.34%
42	Nebraska	296	0.39%
38	Nevada	356	0.47%
36	New Hampshire	497	0.66%
6	New Jersey	3,160	4.20%
30	New Mexico	590	0.78%
2	New York	5,909	7.85%
19	North Carolina	1,399	1.86%
47	North Dakota	201	0.27%
12	Ohio	1,944	2.58%
24	Oklahoma	1,013	1.35%
20	Oregon	1,370	1.82%
5	Pennsylvania	3,490	4.64%
50	Rhode Island	171	0.23%
22	South Carolina	1,139	1.51%
41	South Dakota	324	0.43%
27	Tennessee	778	1.03%
4	Texas	3,960	5.26%
31	Utah	575	0.76%
45	Vermont	246	0.33%
18	Virginia	1,462	1.94%
15	Washington	1,803	2.39%
43	West Virginia	273	0.36%
14	Wisconsin	1,804	2.40%
48	Wyoming	182	0.24%

RANK ORDER

RANK	STATE	CHIROPRACTORS	% of USA
1	California	11,332	15.05%
2	New York	5,909	7.85%
3	Florida	4,224	5.61%
4	Texas	3,960	5.26%
5	Pennsylvania	3,490	4.64%
6	New Jersey	3,160	4.20%
7	Illinois	2,835	3.77%
8	Michigan	2,527	3.36%
9	Arizona	2,490	3.31%
10	Georgia	2,474	3.29%
11	Colorado	1,970	2.62%
12	Ohio	1,944	2.58%
13	Missouri	1,827	2.43%
14	Wisconsin	1,804	2.40%
15	Washington	1,803	2.39%
16	Massachusetts	1,663	2.21%
17	Minnesota	1,622	2.15%
18	Virginia	1,462	1.94%
19	North Carolina	1,399	1.86%
20	Oregon	1,370	1.82%
21	Iowa	1,363	1.81%
22	South Carolina	1,139	1.51%
23	Kentucky	1,037	1.38%
24	Oklahoma	1,013	1.35%
25	Indiana	905	1.20%
26	Connecticut	869	1.15%
27	Tennessee	778	1.03%
28	Alabama	749	0.99%
29	Kansas	623	0.83%
30	New Mexico	590	0.78%
31	Utah	575	0.76%
32	Louisiana	559	0.74%
33	Arkansas	532	0.71%
34	Maryland	518	0.69%
35	Hawaii	502	0.67%
36	New Hampshire	497	0.66%
37	Maine	367	0.49%
38	Nevada	356	0.47%
39	Mississippi	335	0.44%
40	Idaho	328	0.44%
41	South Dakota	324	0.43%
42	Nebraska	296	0.39%
43	West Virginia	273	0.36%
44	Montana	256	0.34%
45	Vermont	246	0.33%
46	Delaware	212	0.28%
47	North Dakota	201	0.27%
48	Wyoming	182	0.24%
49	Alaska	179	0.24%
50	Rhode Island	171	0.23%
	District of Columbia	42	0.06%

*Source: Federation of Chiropractic Licensing Boards
"1998-99 Official Directory"*
As of December 1997. Licensed active doctors. There is some duplication as some doctors are licensed in more than one state.

Rate of Doctors of Chiropractic in 1997

National Rate = 28 Chiropractors per 100,000 Population*

ALPHA ORDER

RANK	STATE	RATE
42	Alabama	17
23	Alaska	29
1	Arizona	55
37	Arkansas	21
11	California	35
2	Colorado	51
29	Connecticut	27
23	Delaware	29
23	Florida	29
16	Georgia	33
5	Hawaii	42
29	Idaho	27
34	Illinois	24
45	Indiana	15
3	Iowa	48
34	Kansas	24
29	Kentucky	27
48	Louisiana	13
21	Maine	30
50	Maryland	10
29	Massachusetts	27
33	Michigan	26
11	Minnesota	35
49	Mississippi	12
14	Missouri	34
23	Montana	29
41	Nebraska	18
37	Nevada	21
5	New Hampshire	42
9	New Jersey	39
14	New Mexico	34
16	New York	33
40	North Carolina	19
19	North Dakota	31
42	Ohio	17
19	Oklahoma	31
5	Oregon	42
23	Pennsylvania	29
42	Rhode Island	17
21	South Carolina	30
4	South Dakota	44
47	Tennessee	14
39	Texas	20
28	Utah	28
5	Vermont	42
36	Virginia	22
18	Washington	32
45	West Virginia	15
11	Wisconsin	35
10	Wyoming	38

RANK ORDER

RANK	STATE	RATE
1	Arizona	55
2	Colorado	51
3	Iowa	48
4	South Dakota	44
5	Hawaii	42
5	New Hampshire	42
5	Oregon	42
5	Vermont	42
9	New Jersey	39
10	Wyoming	38
11	California	35
11	Minnesota	35
11	Wisconsin	35
14	Missouri	34
14	New Mexico	34
16	Georgia	33
16	New York	33
18	Washington	32
19	North Dakota	31
19	Oklahoma	31
21	Maine	30
21	South Carolina	30
23	Alaska	29
23	Delaware	29
23	Florida	29
23	Montana	29
23	Pennsylvania	29
28	Utah	28
29	Connecticut	27
29	Idaho	27
29	Kentucky	27
29	Massachusetts	27
33	Michigan	26
34	Illinois	24
34	Kansas	24
36	Virginia	22
37	Arkansas	21
37	Nevada	21
39	Texas	20
40	North Carolina	19
41	Nebraska	18
42	Alabama	17
42	Ohio	17
42	Rhode Island	17
45	Indiana	15
45	West Virginia	15
47	Tennessee	14
48	Louisiana	13
49	Mississippi	12
50	Maryland	10

| | District of Columbia | 8 |

Source: Morgan Quitno Press using data from Federation of Chiropractic Licensing Boards
"1998-99 Official Directory"

*As of December 1997. Licensed active doctors. There is some duplication as some doctors are licensed in more than one state.

Physician Assistants in Clinical Practice in 1998

National Total = 31,301 Physician Assistants*

ALPHA ORDER

RANK	STATE	PA's	% of USA
36	Alabama	200	0.64%
32	Alaska	256	0.82%
17	Arizona	500	1.60%
49	Arkansas	45	0.14%
2	California	3,370	10.77%
12	Colorado	708	2.26%
14	Connecticut	632	2.02%
48	Delaware	65	0.21%
6	Florida	1,575	5.03%
8	Georgia	1,068	3.41%
47	Hawaii	78	0.25%
42	Idaho	133	0.42%
16	Illinois	576	1.84%
38	Indiana	190	0.61%
21	Iowa	385	1.23%
25	Kansas	352	1.12%
22	Kentucky	383	1.22%
37	Louisiana	195	0.62%
26	Maine	347	1.11%
9	Maryland	1,014	3.24%
13	Massachusetts	667	2.13%
7	Michigan	1,151	3.68%
22	Minnesota	383	1.22%
50	Mississippi	41	0.13%
34	Missouri	230	0.73%
43	Montana	119	0.38%
24	Nebraska	374	1.19%
40	Nevada	147	0.47%
41	New Hampshire	145	0.46%
29	New Jersey	290	0.93%
27	New Mexico	342	1.09%
1	New York	3,998	12.77%
4	North Carolina	1,675	5.35%
39	North Dakota	172	0.55%
11	Ohio	926	2.96%
19	Oklahoma	467	1.49%
30	Oregon	274	0.88%
5	Pennsylvania	1,652	5.28%
44	Rhode Island	115	0.37%
31	South Carolina	264	0.84%
35	South Dakota	202	0.65%
20	Tennessee	412	1.32%
3	Texas	1,915	6.12%
33	Utah	248	0.79%
45	Vermont	108	0.35%
18	Virginia	479	1.53%
10	Washington	1,008	3.22%
28	West Virginia	311	0.99%
15	Wisconsin	630	2.01%
46	Wyoming	90	0.29%

RANK ORDER

RANK	STATE	PA's	% of USA
1	New York	3,998	12.77%
2	California	3,370	10.77%
3	Texas	1,915	6.12%
4	North Carolina	1,675	5.35%
5	Pennsylvania	1,652	5.28%
6	Florida	1,575	5.03%
7	Michigan	1,151	3.68%
8	Georgia	1,068	3.41%
9	Maryland	1,014	3.24%
10	Washington	1,008	3.22%
11	Ohio	926	2.96%
12	Colorado	708	2.26%
13	Massachusetts	667	2.13%
14	Connecticut	632	2.02%
15	Wisconsin	630	2.01%
16	Illinois	576	1.84%
17	Arizona	500	1.60%
18	Virginia	479	1.53%
19	Oklahoma	467	1.49%
20	Tennessee	412	1.32%
21	Iowa	385	1.23%
22	Kentucky	383	1.22%
22	Minnesota	383	1.22%
24	Nebraska	374	1.19%
25	Kansas	352	1.12%
26	Maine	347	1.11%
27	New Mexico	342	1.09%
28	West Virginia	311	0.99%
29	New Jersey	290	0.93%
30	Oregon	274	0.88%
31	South Carolina	264	0.84%
32	Alaska	256	0.82%
33	Utah	248	0.79%
34	Missouri	230	0.73%
35	South Dakota	202	0.65%
36	Alabama	200	0.64%
37	Louisiana	195	0.62%
38	Indiana	190	0.61%
39	North Dakota	172	0.55%
40	Nevada	147	0.47%
41	New Hampshire	145	0.46%
42	Idaho	133	0.42%
43	Montana	119	0.38%
44	Rhode Island	115	0.37%
45	Vermont	108	0.35%
46	Wyoming	90	0.29%
47	Hawaii	78	0.25%
48	Delaware	65	0.21%
49	Arkansas	45	0.14%
50	Mississippi	41	0.13%
	District of Columbia	177	0.57%

Source: The American Academy of Physician Assistants
      "Number of PAs in Clinical Practice, January 1, 1998" (Information Update, October 27, 1997)
*Projected.

Rate of Physician Assistants in Clinical Practice in 1998

National Rate = 11.7 PA's per 100,000 Population*

ALPHA ORDER

RANK	STATE	RATE
44	Alabama	4.6
1	Alaska	42.0
27	Arizona	11.0
49	Arkansas	1.8
31	California	10.4
13	Colorado	18.2
10	Connecticut	19.3
34	Delaware	8.9
30	Florida	10.7
16	Georgia	14.3
42	Hawaii	6.6
27	Idaho	11.0
43	Illinois	4.8
48	Indiana	3.2
20	Iowa	13.5
19	Kansas	13.6
33	Kentucky	9.8
45	Louisiana	4.5
2	Maine	27.9
8	Maryland	19.9
29	Massachusetts	10.9
25	Michigan	11.8
38	Minnesota	8.2
50	Mississippi	1.5
46	Missouri	4.3
20	Montana	13.5
5	Nebraska	22.6
35	Nevada	8.8
22	New Hampshire	12.4
47	New Jersey	3.6
9	New Mexico	19.8
7	New York	22.0
5	North Carolina	22.6
4	North Dakota	26.8
37	Ohio	8.3
17	Oklahoma	14.1
36	Oregon	8.4
18	Pennsylvania	13.7
26	Rhode Island	11.6
41	South Carolina	7.0
3	South Dakota	27.4
39	Tennessee	7.7
32	Texas	9.9
24	Utah	12.0
12	Vermont	18.3
40	Virginia	7.1
14	Washington	18.0
15	West Virginia	17.1
23	Wisconsin	12.2
11	Wyoming	18.8

RANK ORDER

RANK	STATE	RATE
1	Alaska	42.0
2	Maine	27.9
3	South Dakota	27.4
4	North Dakota	26.8
5	Nebraska	22.6
5	North Carolina	22.6
7	New York	22.0
8	Maryland	19.9
9	New Mexico	19.8
10	Connecticut	19.3
11	Wyoming	18.8
12	Vermont	18.3
13	Colorado	18.2
14	Washington	18.0
15	West Virginia	17.1
16	Georgia	14.3
17	Oklahoma	14.1
18	Pennsylvania	13.7
19	Kansas	13.6
20	Iowa	13.5
20	Montana	13.5
22	New Hampshire	12.4
23	Wisconsin	12.2
24	Utah	12.0
25	Michigan	11.8
26	Rhode Island	11.6
27	Arizona	11.0
27	Idaho	11.0
29	Massachusetts	10.9
30	Florida	10.7
31	California	10.4
32	Texas	9.9
33	Kentucky	9.8
34	Delaware	8.9
35	Nevada	8.8
36	Oregon	8.4
37	Ohio	8.3
38	Minnesota	8.2
39	Tennessee	7.7
40	Virginia	7.1
41	South Carolina	7.0
42	Hawaii	6.6
43	Illinois	4.8
44	Alabama	4.6
45	Louisiana	4.5
46	Missouri	4.3
47	New Jersey	3.6
48	Indiana	3.2
49	Arkansas	1.8
50	Mississippi	1.5
	District of Columbia	33.5

Source: Morgan Quitno Press using data from The American Academy of Physician Assistants
   "Number of PAs in Clinical Practice, January 1, 1998" (Information Update, October 27, 1997)
*Projected.

Registered Nurses in 1995

National Total = 2,116,000 Registered Nurses*

ALPHA ORDER

RANK ORDER

RANK	STATE	NURSES	% of USA	RANK	STATE	NURSES	% of USA
22	Alabama	32,300	1.53%	1	California	180,300	8.52%
48	Alaska	5,900	0.28%	2	New York	165,700	7.83%
23	Arizona	31,900	1.51%	3	Pennsylvania	122,800	5.80%
33	Arkansas	17,100	0.81%	4	Texas	120,400	5.69%
1	California	180,300	8.52%	5	Florida	115,200	5.44%
25	Colorado	30,800	1.46%	6	Illinois	102,200	4.83%
21	Connecticut	33,700	1.59%	7	Ohio	99,800	4.72%
44	Delaware	7,600	0.36%	8	Michigan	78,300	3.70%
5	Florida	115,200	5.44%	9	Massachusetts	72,500	3.43%
13	Georgia	52,300	2.47%	10	New Jersey	67,400	3.19%
42	Hawaii	8,700	0.41%	11	North Carolina	58,200	2.75%
45	Idaho	6,900	0.33%	12	Virginia	52,700	2.49%
6	Illinois	102,200	4.83%	13	Georgia	52,300	2.47%
15	Indiana	45,500	2.15%	14	Missouri	49,900	2.36%
27	Iowa	28,200	1.33%	15	Indiana	45,500	2.15%
30	Kansas	20,700	0.98%	15	Tennessee	45,500	2.15%
26	Kentucky	29,000	1.37%	17	Wisconsin	45,200	2.14%
24	Louisiana	31,300	1.48%	18	Minnesota	44,000	2.08%
36	Maine	13,100	0.62%	19	Washington	42,900	2.03%
20	Maryland	42,700	2.02%	20	Maryland	42,700	2.02%
9	Massachusetts	72,500	3.43%	21	Connecticut	33,700	1.59%
8	Michigan	78,300	3.70%	22	Alabama	32,300	1.53%
18	Minnesota	44,000	2.08%	23	Arizona	31,900	1.51%
32	Mississippi	19,000	0.90%	24	Louisiana	31,300	1.48%
14	Missouri	49,900	2.36%	25	Colorado	30,800	1.46%
47	Montana	6,500	0.31%	26	Kentucky	29,000	1.37%
34	Nebraska	15,300	0.72%	27	Iowa	28,200	1.33%
41	Nevada	9,300	0.44%	28	South Carolina	25,700	1.21%
38	New Hampshire	11,400	0.54%	29	Oregon	25,300	1.20%
10	New Jersey	67,400	3.19%	30	Kansas	20,700	0.98%
38	New Mexico	11,400	0.54%	31	Oklahoma	19,200	0.91%
2	New York	165,700	7.83%	32	Mississippi	19,000	0.90%
11	North Carolina	58,200	2.75%	33	Arkansas	17,100	0.81%
45	North Dakota	6,900	0.33%	34	Nebraska	15,300	0.72%
7	Ohio	99,800	4.72%	35	West Virginia	14,500	0.69%
31	Oklahoma	19,200	0.91%	36	Maine	13,100	0.62%
29	Oregon	25,300	1.20%	37	Utah	12,600	0.60%
3	Pennsylvania	122,800	5.80%	38	New Hampshire	11,400	0.54%
40	Rhode Island	11,200	0.53%	38	New Mexico	11,400	0.54%
28	South Carolina	25,700	1.21%	40	Rhode Island	11,200	0.53%
43	South Dakota	7,800	0.37%	41	Nevada	9,300	0.44%
15	Tennessee	45,500	2.15%	42	Hawaii	8,700	0.41%
4	Texas	120,400	5.69%	43	South Dakota	7,800	0.37%
37	Utah	12,600	0.60%	44	Delaware	7,600	0.36%
49	Vermont	5,400	0.26%	45	Idaho	6,900	0.33%
12	Virginia	52,700	2.49%	45	North Dakota	6,900	0.33%
19	Washington	42,900	2.03%	47	Montana	6,500	0.31%
35	West Virginia	14,500	0.69%	48	Alaska	5,900	0.28%
17	Wisconsin	45,200	2.14%	49	Vermont	5,400	0.26%
50	Wyoming	3,800	0.18%	50	Wyoming	3,800	0.18%
					District of Columbia	9,300	0.44%

Source: U.S. Department of Health and Human Services, Health Resources and Services Administration unpublished data
As of December 1995.

Rate of Registered Nurses in 1995

National Rate = 805 Nurses per 100,000 Population*

ALPHA ORDER				RANK ORDER		
RANK	STATE	RATE		RANK	STATE	RATE
34	Alabama	758		1	Massachusetts	1,196
11	Alaska	981		2	Rhode Island	1,131
37	Arizona	740		3	North Dakota	1,076
43	Arkansas	689		4	Delaware	1,062
50	California	571		5	Maine	1,061
23	Colorado	823		5	South Dakota	1,061
7	Connecticut	1,032		7	Connecticut	1,032
4	Delaware	1,062		8	Pennsylvania	1,019
24	Florida	812		9	New Hampshire	994
39	Georgia	727		10	Iowa	993
38	Hawaii	738		11	Alaska	981
48	Idaho	592		12	Minnesota	955
20	Illinois	866		13	Missouri	937
33	Indiana	786		14	Nebraska	935
10	Iowa	993		15	Vermont	926
27	Kansas	806		16	New York	913
35	Kentucky	752		17	Ohio	896
40	Louisiana	723		18	Wisconsin	884
5	Maine	1,061		19	Tennessee	869
21	Maryland	849		20	Illinois	866
1	Massachusetts	1,196		21	Maryland	849
25	Michigan	811		22	New Jersey	847
12	Minnesota	955		23	Colorado	823
41	Mississippi	706		24	Florida	812
13	Missouri	937		25	Michigan	811
36	Montana	748		26	North Carolina	810
14	Nebraska	935		27	Kansas	806
47	Nevada	608		28	Oregon	805
9	New Hampshire	994		29	Virginia	798
22	New Jersey	847		30	West Virginia	796
44	New Mexico	676		31	Wyoming	794
16	New York	913		32	Washington	789
26	North Carolina	810		33	Indiana	786
3	North Dakota	1,076		34	Alabama	758
17	Ohio	896		35	Kentucky	752
49	Oklahoma	587		36	Montana	748
28	Oregon	805		37	Arizona	740
8	Pennsylvania	1,019		38	Hawaii	738
2	Rhode Island	1,131		39	Georgia	727
42	South Carolina	698		40	Louisiana	723
5	South Dakota	1,061		41	Mississippi	706
19	Tennessee	869		42	South Carolina	698
45	Texas	643		43	Arkansas	689
46	Utah	638		44	New Mexico	676
15	Vermont	926		45	Texas	643
29	Virginia	798		46	Utah	638
32	Washington	789		47	Nevada	608
30	West Virginia	796		48	Idaho	592
18	Wisconsin	884		49	Oklahoma	587
31	Wyoming	794		50	California	571
					District of Columbia	1,684

Source: Morgan Quitno Press using data from U.S. Dept. of Health & Human Services, Health Resources/Services Admn.
    unpublished data
*As of December 1995. Calculated with updated Census population estimates for July 1, 1995.

Dentists in 1997

National Total = 160,529 Dentists*

ALPHA ORDER

RANK	STATE	DENTISTS	% of USA
27	Alabama	1,697	1.06%
45	Alaska	338	0.21%
26	Arizona	1,878	1.17%
34	Arkansas	995	0.62%
1	California	20,676	12.88%
19	Colorado	2,501	1.56%
22	Connecticut	2,378	1.48%
48	Delaware	301	0.19%
6	Florida	6,740	4.20%
14	Georgia	3,024	1.88%
36	Hawaii	902	0.56%
40	Idaho	612	0.38%
4	Illinois	7,559	4.71%
18	Indiana	2,683	1.67%
30	Iowa	1,424	0.89%
32	Kansas	1,204	0.75%
25	Kentucky	1,912	1.19%
24	Louisiana	1,920	1.20%
41	Maine	586	0.37%
13	Maryland	3,136	1.95%
10	Massachusetts	4,462	2.78%
8	Michigan	5,736	3.57%
17	Minnesota	2,787	1.74%
35	Mississippi	986	0.61%
21	Missouri	2,461	1.53%
44	Montana	449	0.28%
33	Nebraska	997	0.62%
41	Nevada	586	0.37%
38	New Hampshire	664	0.41%
7	New Jersey	5,826	3.63%
39	New Mexico	645	0.40%
2	New York	12,864	8.01%
16	North Carolina	2,815	1.75%
49	North Dakota	285	0.18%
9	Ohio	5,662	3.53%
28	Oklahoma	1,483	0.92%
23	Oregon	2,049	1.28%
5	Pennsylvania	7,259	4.52%
43	Rhode Island	544	0.34%
29	South Carolina	1,459	0.91%
47	South Dakota	310	0.19%
20	Tennessee	2,492	1.55%
3	Texas	8,078	5.03%
31	Utah	1,237	0.77%
46	Vermont	328	0.20%
11	Virginia	3,330	2.07%
12	Washington	3,263	2.03%
37	West Virginia	765	0.48%
15	Wisconsin	2,889	1.80%
50	Wyoming	235	0.15%

RANK ORDER

RANK	STATE	DENTISTS	% of USA
1	California	20,676	12.88%
2	New York	12,864	8.01%
3	Texas	8,078	5.03%
4	Illinois	7,559	4.71%
5	Pennsylvania	7,259	4.52%
6	Florida	6,740	4.20%
7	New Jersey	5,826	3.63%
8	Michigan	5,736	3.57%
9	Ohio	5,662	3.53%
10	Massachusetts	4,462	2.78%
11	Virginia	3,330	2.07%
12	Washington	3,263	2.03%
13	Maryland	3,136	1.95%
14	Georgia	3,024	1.88%
15	Wisconsin	2,889	1.80%
16	North Carolina	2,815	1.75%
17	Minnesota	2,787	1.74%
18	Indiana	2,683	1.67%
19	Colorado	2,501	1.56%
20	Tennessee	2,492	1.55%
21	Missouri	2,461	1.53%
22	Connecticut	2,378	1.48%
23	Oregon	2,049	1.28%
24	Louisiana	1,920	1.20%
25	Kentucky	1,912	1.19%
26	Arizona	1,878	1.17%
27	Alabama	1,697	1.06%
28	Oklahoma	1,483	0.92%
29	South Carolina	1,459	0.91%
30	Iowa	1,424	0.89%
31	Utah	1,237	0.77%
32	Kansas	1,204	0.75%
33	Nebraska	997	0.62%
34	Arkansas	995	0.62%
35	Mississippi	986	0.61%
36	Hawaii	902	0.56%
37	West Virginia	765	0.48%
38	New Hampshire	664	0.41%
39	New Mexico	645	0.40%
40	Idaho	612	0.38%
41	Maine	586	0.37%
41	Nevada	586	0.37%
43	Rhode Island	544	0.34%
44	Montana	449	0.28%
45	Alaska	338	0.21%
46	Vermont	328	0.20%
47	South Dakota	310	0.19%
48	Delaware	301	0.19%
49	North Dakota	285	0.18%
50	Wyoming	235	0.15%
	District of Columbia	583	0.36%

Source: American Dental Association
    "1997 ADA Dentist Masterfile"
*National total includes 14,534 dentists working for the military, Public Health Service or whose address is unknown. These are not distributed among the states. Does not include 4,411 dental graduate students.

Rate of Dentists in 1997

National Rate = 60 Dentists per 100,000 Population*

ALPHA ORDER			RANK ORDER		
RANK	STATE	RATE	RANK	STATE	RATE
44	Alabama	39	1	Hawaii	76
20	Alaska	55	2	Connecticut	73
41	Arizona	41	2	Massachusetts	73
44	Arkansas	39	4	New Jersey	72
6	California	64	5	New York	71
6	Colorado	64	6	California	64
2	Connecticut	73	6	Colorado	64
41	Delaware	41	6	Illinois	64
30	Florida	46	9	Oregon	63
43	Georgia	40	10	Maryland	62
1	Hawaii	76	11	Nebraska	60
22	Idaho	51	11	Pennsylvania	60
6	Illinois	64	11	Utah	60
30	Indiana	46	14	Michigan	59
25	Iowa	50	14	Minnesota	59
30	Kansas	46	16	Washington	58
26	Kentucky	49	17	New Hampshire	57
36	Louisiana	44	18	Vermont	56
29	Maine	47	18	Wisconsin	56
10	Maryland	62	20	Alaska	55
2	Massachusetts	73	20	Rhode Island	55
14	Michigan	59	22	Idaho	51
14	Minnesota	59	22	Montana	51
49	Mississippi	36	22	Ohio	51
30	Missouri	46	25	Iowa	50
22	Montana	51	26	Kentucky	49
11	Nebraska	60	26	Virginia	49
50	Nevada	35	26	Wyoming	49
17	New Hampshire	57	29	Maine	47
4	New Jersey	72	30	Florida	46
48	New Mexico	37	30	Indiana	46
5	New York	71	30	Kansas	46
47	North Carolina	38	30	Missouri	46
36	North Dakota	44	30	Tennessee	46
22	Ohio	51	35	Oklahoma	45
35	Oklahoma	45	36	Louisiana	44
9	Oregon	63	36	North Dakota	44
11	Pennsylvania	60	38	South Dakota	42
20	Rhode Island	55	38	Texas	42
44	South Carolina	39	38	West Virginia	42
38	South Dakota	42	41	Arizona	41
30	Tennessee	46	41	Delaware	41
38	Texas	42	43	Georgia	40
11	Utah	60	44	Alabama	39
18	Vermont	56	44	Arkansas	39
26	Virginia	49	44	South Carolina	39
16	Washington	58	47	North Carolina	38
38	West Virginia	42	48	New Mexico	37
18	Wisconsin	56	49	Mississippi	36
26	Wyoming	49	50	Nevada	35
				District of Columbia	110

Source: Morgan Quitno Press using data from American Dental Association
    "1997 ADA Dentist Masterfile"
*National total includes dentists working for the military, Public Health Service or whose address is unknown.
These are not distributed among the states. Does not include dental graduate students.

Community Hospital Personnel in 1996

National Total = 3,217,002 Personnel*

ALPHA ORDER

RANK	STATE	PERSONNEL	% of USA
17	Alabama	65,794	2.05%
50	Alaska	3,914	0.12%
29	Arizona	37,419	1.16%
30	Arkansas	33,941	1.06%
2	California	267,108	8.30%
27	Colorado	38,251	1.19%
31	Connecticut	33,727	1.05%
47	Delaware	8,174	0.25%
4	Florida	182,801	5.68%
11	Georgia	90,010	2.80%
39	Hawaii	12,688	0.39%
44	Idaho	9,942	0.31%
7	Illinois	149,946	4.66%
15	Indiana	72,259	2.25%
28	Iowa	38,024	1.18%
32	Kansas	31,814	0.99%
20	Kentucky	51,587	1.60%
16	Louisiana	71,572	2.22%
38	Maine	14,690	0.46%
21	Maryland	51,149	1.59%
12	Massachusetts	87,302	2.71%
8	Michigan	121,385	3.77%
19	Minnesota	55,899	1.74%
26	Mississippi	41,793	1.30%
13	Missouri	81,235	2.53%
43	Montana	10,056	0.31%
35	Nebraska	23,191	0.72%
40	Nevada	11,999	0.37%
41	New Hampshire	11,302	0.35%
9	New Jersey	97,727	3.04%
37	New Mexico	18,057	0.56%
1	New York	299,305	9.30%
10	North Carolina	93,725	2.91%
45	North Dakota	9,400	0.29%
6	Ohio	153,570	4.77%
24	Oklahoma	42,561	1.32%
34	Oregon	27,628	0.86%
5	Pennsylvania	180,044	5.60%
42	Rhode Island	11,209	0.35%
25	South Carolina	42,251	1.31%
46	South Dakota	9,273	0.29%
14	Tennessee	77,984	2.42%
3	Texas	216,529	6.73%
36	Utah	18,256	0.57%
48	Vermont	5,564	0.17%
18	Virginia	64,192	2.00%
23	Washington	43,831	1.36%
33	West Virginia	28,453	0.88%
22	Wisconsin	45,683	1.42%
49	Wyoming	5,095	0.16%

RANK ORDER

RANK	STATE	PERSONNEL	% of USA
1	New York	299,305	9.30%
2	California	267,108	8.30%
3	Texas	216,529	6.73%
4	Florida	182,801	5.68%
5	Pennsylvania	180,044	5.60%
6	Ohio	153,570	4.77%
7	Illinois	149,946	4.66%
8	Michigan	121,385	3.77%
9	New Jersey	97,727	3.04%
10	North Carolina	93,725	2.91%
11	Georgia	90,010	2.80%
12	Massachusetts	87,302	2.71%
13	Missouri	81,235	2.53%
14	Tennessee	77,984	2.42%
15	Indiana	72,259	2.25%
16	Louisiana	71,572	2.22%
17	Alabama	65,794	2.05%
18	Virginia	64,192	2.00%
19	Minnesota	55,899	1.74%
20	Kentucky	51,587	1.60%
21	Maryland	51,149	1.59%
22	Wisconsin	45,683	1.42%
23	Washington	43,831	1.36%
24	Oklahoma	42,561	1.32%
25	South Carolina	42,251	1.31%
26	Mississippi	41,793	1.30%
27	Colorado	38,251	1.19%
28	Iowa	38,024	1.18%
29	Arizona	37,419	1.16%
30	Arkansas	33,941	1.06%
31	Connecticut	33,727	1.05%
32	Kansas	31,814	0.99%
33	West Virginia	28,453	0.88%
34	Oregon	27,628	0.86%
35	Nebraska	23,191	0.72%
36	Utah	18,256	0.57%
37	New Mexico	18,057	0.56%
38	Maine	14,690	0.46%
39	Hawaii	12,688	0.39%
40	Nevada	11,999	0.37%
41	New Hampshire	11,302	0.35%
42	Rhode Island	11,209	0.35%
43	Montana	10,056	0.31%
44	Idaho	9,942	0.31%
45	North Dakota	9,400	0.29%
46	South Dakota	9,273	0.29%
47	Delaware	8,174	0.25%
48	Vermont	5,564	0.17%
49	Wyoming	5,095	0.16%
50	Alaska	3,914	0.12%
	District of Columbia	17,693	0.55%

Source: American Hospital Association (Chicago, IL)
   "Hospital Statistics" (1998 edition)

*Includes physicians, dentists, nurses and other salaried personnel in federal and nonfederal hospitals. Community hospitals are all nonfederal, short-term, general and special hospitals whose facilities and services are available to the public.

Employment in Health Services Industries in 1995

National Total = 10,851,331 Employees*

ALPHA ORDER

RANK	STATE	EMPLOYEES	% of USA
22	Alabama	175,484	1.62%
49	Alaska	17,604	0.16%
25	Arizona	143,798	1.33%
33	Arkansas	96,770	0.89%
1	California	1,034,262	9.53%
26	Colorado	142,825	1.32%
23	Connecticut	167,777	1.55%
47	Delaware	31,025	0.29%
4	Florida	595,307	5.49%
12	Georgia	269,929	2.49%
42	Hawaii	38,531	0.36%
43	Idaho	36,485	0.34%
7	Illinois	491,296	4.53%
14	Indiana	244,241	2.25%
27	Iowa	132,792	1.22%
30	Kansas	118,234	1.09%
24	Kentucky	157,107	1.45%
19	Louisiana	203,445	1.87%
38	Maine	56,301	0.52%
20	Maryland	201,530	1.86%
9	Massachusetts	350,238	3.23%
8	Michigan	388,499	3.58%
15	Minnesota	232,287	2.14%
32	Mississippi	98,002	0.90%
13	Missouri	249,295	2.30%
46	Montana	32,811	0.30%
35	Nebraska	73,635	0.68%
41	Nevada	42,451	0.39%
40	New Hampshire	47,075	0.43%
10	New Jersey	332,626	3.07%
37	New Mexico	56,698	0.52%
2	New York	926,979	8.54%
11	North Carolina	272,058	2.51%
45	North Dakota	34,779	0.32%
6	Ohio	506,271	4.67%
28	Oklahoma	131,285	1.21%
31	Oregon	104,765	0.97%
5	Pennsylvania	571,865	5.27%
39	Rhode Island	50,303	0.46%
29	South Carolina	119,604	1.10%
44	South Dakota	36,187	0.33%
17	Tennessee	227,895	2.10%
3	Texas	706,643	6.51%
36	Utah	66,796	0.62%
48	Vermont	23,599	0.22%
16	Virginia	231,568	2.13%
21	Washington	200,638	1.85%
34	West Virginia	74,969	0.69%
18	Wisconsin	224,493	2.07%
50	Wyoming	16,176	0.15%

RANK ORDER

RANK	STATE	EMPLOYEES	% of USA
1	California	1,034,262	9.53%
2	New York	926,979	8.54%
3	Texas	706,643	6.51%
4	Florida	595,307	5.49%
5	Pennsylvania	571,865	5.27%
6	Ohio	506,271	4.67%
7	Illinois	491,296	4.53%
8	Michigan	388,499	3.58%
9	Massachusetts	350,238	3.23%
10	New Jersey	332,626	3.07%
11	North Carolina	272,058	2.51%
12	Georgia	269,929	2.49%
13	Missouri	249,295	2.30%
14	Indiana	244,241	2.25%
15	Minnesota	232,287	2.14%
16	Virginia	231,568	2.13%
17	Tennessee	227,895	2.10%
18	Wisconsin	224,493	2.07%
19	Louisiana	203,445	1.87%
20	Maryland	201,530	1.86%
21	Washington	200,638	1.85%
22	Alabama	175,484	1.62%
23	Connecticut	167,777	1.55%
24	Kentucky	157,107	1.45%
25	Arizona	143,798	1.33%
26	Colorado	142,825	1.32%
27	Iowa	132,792	1.22%
28	Oklahoma	131,285	1.21%
29	South Carolina	119,604	1.10%
30	Kansas	118,234	1.09%
31	Oregon	104,765	0.97%
32	Mississippi	98,002	0.90%
33	Arkansas	96,770	0.89%
34	West Virginia	74,969	0.69%
35	Nebraska	73,635	0.68%
36	Utah	66,796	0.62%
37	New Mexico	56,698	0.52%
38	Maine	56,301	0.52%
39	Rhode Island	50,303	0.46%
40	New Hampshire	47,075	0.43%
41	Nevada	42,451	0.39%
42	Hawaii	38,531	0.36%
43	Idaho	36,485	0.34%
44	South Dakota	36,187	0.33%
45	North Dakota	34,779	0.32%
46	Montana	32,811	0.30%
47	Delaware	31,025	0.29%
48	Vermont	23,599	0.22%
49	Alaska	17,604	0.16%
50	Wyoming	16,176	0.15%
	District of Columbia	66,098	0.61%

Source: U.S. Bureau of the Census
"1995 County Business Patterns"

Total of employment in 1995 at establishments classified in Standard Industrial Classification (S.I.C.) code 8000. An establishment is a single physical location at which business is conducted or where services or industrial operations are performed. It is not necessarily identical with a company or enterprise, which may consist of one establishment or more.

VII. PHYSICAL FITNESS

Users of Exercise Equipment in 1996

National Total = 46,075,000 Users

ALPHA ORDER

RANK	STATE	USERS	% of USA
26	Alabama	607,000	1.32%
NA	Alaska*	NA	NA
19	Arizona	878,000	1.91%
35	Arkansas	317,000	0.69%
1	California	5,617,000	12.19%
30	Colorado	490,000	1.06%
22	Connecticut	762,000	1.65%
46	Delaware	111,000	0.24%
4	Florida	2,408,000	5.23%
10	Georgia	1,380,000	3.00%
NA	Hawaii*	NA	NA
36	Idaho	313,000	0.68%
5	Illinois	2,327,000	5.05%
17	Indiana	944,000	2.05%
31	Iowa	427,000	0.93%
33	Kansas	375,000	0.81%
21	Kentucky	774,000	1.68%
23	Louisiana	754,000	1.64%
38	Maine	266,000	0.58%
16	Maryland	989,000	2.15%
13	Massachusetts	1,010,000	2.19%
8	Michigan	1,705,000	3.70%
20	Minnesota	836,000	1.81%
32	Mississippi	393,000	0.85%
15	Missouri	993,000	2.16%
41	Montana	215,000	0.47%
37	Nebraska	285,000	0.62%
39	Nevada	262,000	0.57%
42	New Hampshire	177,000	0.38%
9	New Jersey	1,472,000	3.19%
40	New Mexico	217,000	0.47%
2	New York	3,255,000	7.06%
11	North Carolina	1,316,000	2.86%
45	North Dakota	112,000	0.24%
7	Ohio	1,935,000	4.20%
28	Oklahoma	547,000	1.19%
25	Oregon	742,000	1.61%
6	Pennsylvania	2,089,000	4.53%
47	Rhode Island	85,000	0.18%
27	South Carolina	575,000	1.25%
44	South Dakota	116,000	0.25%
24	Tennessee	753,000	1.63%
3	Texas	3,111,000	6.75%
29	Utah	497,000	1.08%
48	Vermont	75,000	0.16%
14	Virginia	1,000,000	2.17%
12	Washington	1,095,000	2.38%
34	West Virginia	365,000	0.79%
18	Wisconsin	926,000	2.01%
43	Wyoming	129,000	0.28%

RANK ORDER

RANK	STATE	USERS	% of USA
1	California	5,617,000	12.19%
2	New York	3,255,000	7.06%
3	Texas	3,111,000	6.75%
4	Florida	2,408,000	5.23%
5	Illinois	2,327,000	5.05%
6	Pennsylvania	2,089,000	4.53%
7	Ohio	1,935,000	4.20%
8	Michigan	1,705,000	3.70%
9	New Jersey	1,472,000	3.19%
10	Georgia	1,380,000	3.00%
11	North Carolina	1,316,000	2.86%
12	Washington	1,095,000	2.38%
13	Massachusetts	1,010,000	2.19%
14	Virginia	1,000,000	2.17%
15	Missouri	993,000	2.16%
16	Maryland	989,000	2.15%
17	Indiana	944,000	2.05%
18	Wisconsin	926,000	2.01%
19	Arizona	878,000	1.91%
20	Minnesota	836,000	1.81%
21	Kentucky	774,000	1.68%
22	Connecticut	762,000	1.65%
23	Louisiana	754,000	1.64%
24	Tennessee	753,000	1.63%
25	Oregon	742,000	1.61%
26	Alabama	607,000	1.32%
27	South Carolina	575,000	1.25%
28	Oklahoma	547,000	1.19%
29	Utah	497,000	1.08%
30	Colorado	490,000	1.06%
31	Iowa	427,000	0.93%
32	Mississippi	393,000	0.85%
33	Kansas	375,000	0.81%
34	West Virginia	365,000	0.79%
35	Arkansas	317,000	0.69%
36	Idaho	313,000	0.68%
37	Nebraska	285,000	0.62%
38	Maine	266,000	0.58%
39	Nevada	262,000	0.57%
40	New Mexico	217,000	0.47%
41	Montana	215,000	0.47%
42	New Hampshire	177,000	0.38%
43	Wyoming	129,000	0.28%
44	South Dakota	116,000	0.25%
45	North Dakota	112,000	0.24%
46	Delaware	111,000	0.24%
47	Rhode Island	85,000	0.18%
48	Vermont	75,000	0.16%
NA	Alaska*	NA	NA
NA	Hawaii*	NA	NA
	District of Columbia*	NA	NA

Source: The National Sporting Goods Association
 "NSGA Sports Participation Survey, January-December 1996 (Copyright 1997, reprinted with permission)
*Not available.

Participants in Golf in 1996

National Total = 23,520,000 Golfers

RANK	STATE	GOLFERS	% of USA	RANK	STATE	GOLFERS	% of USA
31	Alabama	189,000	0.80%	1	California	2,590,000	11.01%
NA	Alaska*	NA	NA	2	New York	1,564,000	6.65%
19	Arizona	401,000	1.70%	3	Florida	1,444,000	6.14%
39	Arkansas	126,000	0.54%	4	Texas	1,402,000	5.96%
1	California	2,590,000	11.01%	5	Illinois	1,185,000	5.04%
23	Colorado	351,000	1.49%	6	Michigan	1,155,000	4.91%
22	Connecticut	352,000	1.50%	7	Ohio	1,073,000	4.56%
47	Delaware	49,000	0.21%	8	Pennsylvania	1,059,000	4.50%
3	Florida	1,444,000	6.14%	9	North Carolina	794,000	3.38%
15	Georgia	561,000	2.39%	10	Wisconsin	745,000	3.17%
NA	Hawaii*	NA	NA	11	New Jersey	706,000	3.00%
38	Idaho	134,000	0.57%	12	Minnesota	602,000	2.56%
5	Illinois	1,185,000	5.04%	13	Indiana	594,000	2.53%
13	Indiana	594,000	2.53%	14	Washington	579,000	2.46%
20	Iowa	393,000	1.67%	15	Georgia	561,000	2.39%
30	Kansas	232,000	0.99%	16	Virginia	498,000	2.12%
24	Kentucky	345,000	1.47%	17	Massachusetts	461,000	1.96%
33	Louisiana	158,000	0.67%	18	Missouri	449,000	1.91%
43	Maine	84,000	0.36%	19	Arizona	401,000	1.70%
27	Maryland	303,000	1.29%	20	Iowa	393,000	1.67%
17	Massachusetts	461,000	1.96%	21	South Carolina	379,000	1.61%
6	Michigan	1,155,000	4.91%	22	Connecticut	352,000	1.50%
12	Minnesota	602,000	2.56%	23	Colorado	351,000	1.49%
34	Mississippi	154,000	0.65%	24	Kentucky	345,000	1.47%
18	Missouri	449,000	1.91%	25	Utah	338,000	1.44%
32	Montana	161,000	0.68%	26	Tennessee	331,000	1.41%
28	Nebraska	276,000	1.17%	27	Maryland	303,000	1.29%
36	Nevada	150,000	0.64%	28	Nebraska	276,000	1.17%
43	New Hampshire	84,000	0.36%	29	Oregon	263,000	1.12%
11	New Jersey	706,000	3.00%	30	Kansas	232,000	0.99%
37	New Mexico	143,000	0.61%	31	Alabama	189,000	0.80%
2	New York	1,564,000	6.65%	32	Montana	161,000	0.68%
9	North Carolina	794,000	3.38%	33	Louisiana	158,000	0.67%
45	North Dakota	80,000	0.34%	34	Mississippi	154,000	0.65%
7	Ohio	1,073,000	4.56%	35	Oklahoma	153,000	0.65%
35	Oklahoma	153,000	0.65%	36	Nevada	150,000	0.64%
29	Oregon	263,000	1.12%	37	New Mexico	143,000	0.61%
8	Pennsylvania	1,059,000	4.50%	38	Idaho	134,000	0.57%
41	Rhode Island	104,000	0.44%	39	Arkansas	126,000	0.54%
21	South Carolina	379,000	1.61%	40	West Virginia	120,000	0.51%
48	South Dakota	48,000	0.20%	41	Rhode Island	104,000	0.44%
26	Tennessee	331,000	1.41%	42	Wyoming	85,000	0.36%
4	Texas	1,402,000	5.96%	43	Maine	84,000	0.36%
25	Utah	338,000	1.44%	43	New Hampshire	84,000	0.36%
46	Vermont	66,000	0.28%	45	North Dakota	80,000	0.34%
16	Virginia	498,000	2.12%	46	Vermont	66,000	0.28%
14	Washington	579,000	2.46%	47	Delaware	49,000	0.21%
40	West Virginia	120,000	0.51%	48	South Dakota	48,000	0.20%
10	Wisconsin	745,000	3.17%	NA	Alaska*	NA	NA
42	Wyoming	85,000	0.36%	NA	Hawaii*	NA	NA
					District of Columbia*	NA	NA

Source: The National Sporting Goods Association
"NSGA Sports Participation Survey, January-December 1996 (Copyright 1997, reprinted with permission)
Not available.

Participants in Running/Jogging in 1996

National Total = 21,437,000 Runners/Joggers

RANK	STATE	RUNNERS	% of USA
29	Alabama	269,000	1.25%
NA	Alaska*	NA	NA
17	Arizona	376,000	1.75%
36	Arkansas	151,000	0.70%
1	California	3,290,000	15.35%
25	Colorado	296,000	1.38%
33	Connecticut	201,000	0.94%
45	Delaware	73,000	0.34%
5	Florida	996,000	4.65%
8	Georgia	718,000	3.35%
NA	Hawaii*	NA	NA
37	Idaho	135,000	0.63%
4	Illinois	1,041,000	4.86%
18	Indiana	356,000	1.66%
28	Iowa	271,000	1.26%
32	Kansas	210,000	0.98%
25	Kentucky	296,000	1.38%
19	Louisiana	340,000	1.59%
44	Maine	75,000	0.35%
16	Maryland	433,000	2.02%
24	Massachusetts	298,000	1.39%
9	Michigan	656,000	3.06%
21	Minnesota	325,000	1.52%
31	Mississippi	214,000	1.00%
15	Missouri	436,000	2.03%
38	Montana	122,000	0.57%
34	Nebraska	173,000	0.81%
40	Nevada	111,000	0.52%
39	New Hampshire	114,000	0.53%
13	New Jersey	551,000	2.57%
41	New Mexico	107,000	0.50%
3	New York	1,399,000	6.53%
10	North Carolina	614,000	2.86%
46	North Dakota	60,000	0.28%
7	Ohio	780,000	3.64%
30	Oklahoma	231,000	1.08%
22	Oregon	304,000	1.42%
6	Pennsylvania	883,000	4.12%
43	Rhode Island	78,000	0.36%
27	South Carolina	290,000	1.35%
48	South Dakota	33,000	0.15%
14	Tennessee	447,000	2.09%
2	Texas	1,565,000	7.30%
23	Utah	299,000	1.39%
47	Vermont	46,000	0.21%
12	Virginia	582,000	2.71%
11	Washington	594,000	2.77%
35	West Virginia	155,000	0.72%
20	Wisconsin	337,000	1.57%
42	Wyoming	82,000	0.38%

RANK	STATE	RUNNERS	% of USA
1	California	3,290,000	15.35%
2	Texas	1,565,000	7.30%
3	New York	1,399,000	6.53%
4	Illinois	1,041,000	4.86%
5	Florida	996,000	4.65%
6	Pennsylvania	883,000	4.12%
7	Ohio	780,000	3.64%
8	Georgia	718,000	3.35%
9	Michigan	656,000	3.06%
10	North Carolina	614,000	2.86%
11	Washington	594,000	2.77%
12	Virginia	582,000	2.71%
13	New Jersey	551,000	2.57%
14	Tennessee	447,000	2.09%
15	Missouri	436,000	2.03%
16	Maryland	433,000	2.02%
17	Arizona	376,000	1.75%
18	Indiana	356,000	1.66%
19	Louisiana	340,000	1.59%
20	Wisconsin	337,000	1.57%
21	Minnesota	325,000	1.52%
22	Oregon	304,000	1.42%
23	Utah	299,000	1.39%
24	Massachusetts	298,000	1.39%
25	Colorado	296,000	1.38%
25	Kentucky	296,000	1.38%
27	South Carolina	290,000	1.35%
28	Iowa	271,000	1.26%
29	Alabama	269,000	1.25%
30	Oklahoma	231,000	1.08%
31	Mississippi	214,000	1.00%
32	Kansas	210,000	0.98%
33	Connecticut	201,000	0.94%
34	Nebraska	173,000	0.81%
35	West Virginia	155,000	0.72%
36	Arkansas	151,000	0.70%
37	Idaho	135,000	0.63%
38	Montana	122,000	0.57%
39	New Hampshire	114,000	0.53%
40	Nevada	111,000	0.52%
41	New Mexico	107,000	0.50%
42	Wyoming	82,000	0.38%
43	Rhode Island	78,000	0.36%
44	Maine	75,000	0.35%
45	Delaware	73,000	0.34%
46	North Dakota	60,000	0.28%
47	Vermont	46,000	0.21%
48	South Dakota	33,000	0.15%
NA	Alaska*	NA	NA
NA	Hawaii*	NA	NA
District of Columbia*		NA	NA

Source: The National Sporting Goods Association
"NSGA Sports Participation Survey, January-December 1996 (Copyright 1997, reprinted with permission)
Not available.

Participants in Soccer in 1996

National Total = 12,926,000 Soccer Players

Source: The National Sporting Goods Association
"NSGA Sports Participation Survey, January-December 1996 (Copyright 1997, reprinted with permission)
*Not available.

Participants in Swimming in 1996

National Total = 60,877,000 Swimmers

Source: The National Sporting Goods Association
"NSGA Sports Participation Survey, January-December 1996 (Copyright 1997, reprinted with permission)
*Not available.

ALPHA ORDER

RANK	STATE	SWIMMERS	% of USA
28	Alabama	763,000	1.25%
NA	Alaska*	NA	NA
16	Arizona	1,229,000	2.02%
35	Arkansas	484,000	0.80%
1	California	6,887,000	11.31%
30	Colorado	612,000	1.01%
23	Connecticut	853,000	1.40%
43	Delaware	187,000	0.31%
4	Florida	3,996,000	6.56%
12	Georgia	1,530,000	2.51%
NA	Hawaii*	NA	NA
39	Idaho	325,000	0.53%
7	Illinois	2,627,000	4.32%
19	Indiana	1,091,000	1.79%
29	Iowa	621,000	1.02%
31	Kansas	583,000	0.96%
20	Kentucky	1,057,000	1.74%
26	Louisiana	806,000	1.32%
38	Maine	346,000	0.57%
17	Maryland	1,184,000	1.94%
11	Massachusetts	1,573,000	2.58%
9	Michigan	2,104,000	3.46%
24	Minnesota	851,000	1.40%
34	Mississippi	552,000	0.91%
15	Missouri	1,268,000	2.08%
47	Montana	121,000	0.20%
37	Nebraska	383,000	0.63%
36	Nevada	389,000	0.64%
40	New Hampshire	283,000	0.46%
8	New Jersey	2,133,000	3.50%
45	New Mexico	151,000	0.25%
2	New York	4,870,000	8.00%
10	North Carolina	1,672,000	2.75%
48	North Dakota	92,000	0.15%
6	Ohio	2,729,000	4.48%
27	Oklahoma	770,000	1.26%
25	Oregon	815,000	1.34%
5	Pennsylvania	3,208,000	5.27%
41	Rhode Island	227,000	0.37%
22	South Carolina	878,000	1.44%
44	South Dakota	184,000	0.30%
14	Tennessee	1,274,000	2.09%
3	Texas	4,122,000	6.77%
33	Utah	561,000	0.92%
42	Vermont	226,000	0.37%
18	Virginia	1,181,000	1.94%
21	Washington	1,012,000	1.66%
32	West Virginia	563,000	0.92%
13	Wisconsin	1,326,000	2.18%
46	Wyoming	137,000	0.23%

RANK ORDER

RANK	STATE	SWIMMERS	% of USA
1	California	6,887,000	11.31%
2	New York	4,870,000	8.00%
3	Texas	4,122,000	6.77%
4	Florida	3,996,000	6.56%
5	Pennsylvania	3,208,000	5.27%
6	Ohio	2,729,000	4.48%
7	Illinois	2,627,000	4.32%
8	New Jersey	2,133,000	3.50%
9	Michigan	2,104,000	3.46%
10	North Carolina	1,672,000	2.75%
11	Massachusetts	1,573,000	2.58%
12	Georgia	1,530,000	2.51%
13	Wisconsin	1,326,000	2.18%
14	Tennessee	1,274,000	2.09%
15	Missouri	1,268,000	2.08%
16	Arizona	1,229,000	2.02%
17	Maryland	1,184,000	1.94%
18	Virginia	1,181,000	1.94%
19	Indiana	1,091,000	1.79%
20	Kentucky	1,057,000	1.74%
21	Washington	1,012,000	1.66%
22	South Carolina	878,000	1.44%
23	Connecticut	853,000	1.40%
24	Minnesota	851,000	1.40%
25	Oregon	815,000	1.34%
26	Louisiana	806,000	1.32%
27	Oklahoma	770,000	1.26%
28	Alabama	763,000	1.25%
29	Iowa	621,000	1.02%
30	Colorado	612,000	1.01%
31	Kansas	583,000	0.96%
32	West Virginia	563,000	0.92%
33	Utah	561,000	0.92%
34	Mississippi	552,000	0.91%
35	Arkansas	484,000	0.80%
36	Nevada	389,000	0.64%
37	Nebraska	383,000	0.63%
38	Maine	346,000	0.57%
39	Idaho	325,000	0.53%
40	New Hampshire	283,000	0.46%
41	Rhode Island	227,000	0.37%
42	Vermont	226,000	0.37%
43	Delaware	187,000	0.31%
44	South Dakota	184,000	0.30%
45	New Mexico	151,000	0.25%
46	Wyoming	137,000	0.23%
47	Montana	121,000	0.20%
48	North Dakota	92,000	0.15%
NA	Alaska*	NA	NA
NA	Hawaii*	NA	NA
	District of Columbia*	NA	NA

Participants in Tennis in 1996

National Total = 12,028,000 Tennis Players

ALPHA ORDER			
RANK	STATE	PLAYERS	% of USA
22	Alabama	169,000	1.41%
NA	Alaska*	NA	NA
24	Arizona	152,000	1.26%
43	Arkansas	41,000	0.34%
1	California	1,432,000	11.91%
27	Colorado	135,000	1.12%
21	Connecticut	170,000	1.41%
41	Delaware	44,000	0.37%
4	Florida	720,000	5.99%
9	Georgia	504,000	4.19%
NA	Hawaii*	NA	NA
45	Idaho	31,000	0.26%
6	Illinois	559,000	4.65%
23	Indiana	165,000	1.37%
30	Iowa	112,000	0.93%
29	Kansas	114,000	0.95%
17	Kentucky	211,000	1.75%
32	Louisiana	106,000	0.88%
46	Maine	22,000	0.18%
14	Maryland	264,000	2.19%
18	Massachusetts	208,000	1.73%
12	Michigan	379,000	3.15%
25	Minnesota	148,000	1.23%
34	Mississippi	75,000	0.62%
13	Missouri	267,000	2.22%
44	Montana	40,000	0.33%
33	Nebraska	78,000	0.65%
38	Nevada	55,000	0.46%
42	New Hampshire	43,000	0.36%
8	New Jersey	523,000	4.35%
36	New Mexico	71,000	0.59%
3	New York	870,000	7.23%
11	North Carolina	399,000	3.32%
48	North Dakota	6,000	0.05%
7	Ohio	545,000	4.53%
30	Oklahoma	112,000	0.93%
26	Oregon	138,000	1.15%
5	Pennsylvania	625,000	5.20%
34	Rhode Island	75,000	0.62%
19	South Carolina	173,000	1.44%
38	South Dakota	55,000	0.46%
20	Tennessee	171,000	1.42%
2	Texas	901,000	7.49%
28	Utah	134,000	1.11%
37	Vermont	58,000	0.48%
10	Virginia	407,000	3.38%
16	Washington	222,000	1.85%
40	West Virginia	53,000	0.44%
15	Wisconsin	233,000	1.94%
47	Wyoming	7,000	0.06%

RANK ORDER			
RANK	STATE	PLAYERS	% of USA
1	California	1,432,000	11.91%
2	Texas	901,000	7.49%
3	New York	870,000	7.23%
4	Florida	720,000	5.99%
5	Pennsylvania	625,000	5.20%
6	Illinois	559,000	4.65%
7	Ohio	545,000	4.53%
8	New Jersey	523,000	4.35%
9	Georgia	504,000	4.19%
10	Virginia	407,000	3.38%
11	North Carolina	399,000	3.32%
12	Michigan	379,000	3.15%
13	Missouri	267,000	2.22%
14	Maryland	264,000	2.19%
15	Wisconsin	233,000	1.94%
16	Washington	222,000	1.85%
17	Kentucky	211,000	1.75%
18	Massachusetts	208,000	1.73%
19	South Carolina	173,000	1.44%
20	Tennessee	171,000	1.42%
21	Connecticut	170,000	1.41%
22	Alabama	169,000	1.41%
23	Indiana	165,000	1.37%
24	Arizona	152,000	1.26%
25	Minnesota	148,000	1.23%
26	Oregon	138,000	1.15%
27	Colorado	135,000	1.12%
28	Utah	134,000	1.11%
29	Kansas	114,000	0.95%
30	Iowa	112,000	0.93%
30	Oklahoma	112,000	0.93%
32	Louisiana	106,000	0.88%
33	Nebraska	78,000	0.65%
34	Mississippi	75,000	0.62%
34	Rhode Island	75,000	0.62%
36	New Mexico	71,000	0.59%
37	Vermont	58,000	0.48%
38	Nevada	55,000	0.46%
38	South Dakota	55,000	0.46%
40	West Virginia	53,000	0.44%
41	Delaware	44,000	0.37%
42	New Hampshire	43,000	0.36%
43	Arkansas	41,000	0.34%
44	Montana	40,000	0.33%
45	Idaho	31,000	0.26%
46	Maine	22,000	0.18%
47	Wyoming	7,000	0.06%
48	North Dakota	6,000	0.05%
NA	Alaska*	NA	NA
NA	Hawaii*	NA	NA
	District of Columbia*	NA	NA

Source: The National Sporting Goods Association
   "NSGA Sports Participation Survey, January-December 1996 (Copyright 1997, reprinted with permission)
Not available.

Apparent Alcohol Consumption in 1996

National Total = 450,251,000 Gallons*

ALPHA ORDER

RANK	STATE	GALLONS	% of USA
25	Alabama	6,275,000	1.39%
48	Alaska	1,179,000	0.26%
16	Arizona	9,072,000	2.01%
34	Arkansas	3,531,000	0.78%
1	California	53,266,000	11.83%
23	Colorado	7,832,000	1.74%
27	Connecticut	5,534,000	1.23%
45	Delaware	1,556,000	0.35%
3	Florida	29,796,000	6.62%
10	Georgia	12,530,000	2.78%
39	Hawaii	2,196,000	0.49%
42	Idaho	1,802,000	0.40%
5	Illinois	21,349,000	4.74%
18	Indiana	8,768,000	1.95%
32	Iowa	4,257,000	0.95%
35	Kansas	3,439,000	0.76%
28	Kentucky	5,331,000	1.18%
20	Louisiana	8,258,000	1.83%
40	Maine	2,178,000	0.48%
21	Maryland	8,206,000	1.82%
11	Massachusetts	11,519,000	2.56%
8	Michigan	15,788,000	3.51%
19	Minnesota	8,547,000	1.90%
31	Mississippi	4,437,000	0.99%
17	Missouri	8,900,000	1.98%
44	Montana	1,660,000	0.37%
37	Nebraska	2,765,000	0.61%
29	Nevada	5,161,000	1.15%
33	New Hampshire	3,752,000	0.83%
9	New Jersey	13,865,000	3.08%
36	New Mexico	3,131,000	0.70%
4	New York	27,313,000	6.07%
12	North Carolina	11,260,000	2.50%
47	North Dakota	1,217,000	0.27%
7	Ohio	17,075,000	3.79%
30	Oklahoma	4,560,000	1.01%
26	Oregon	5,732,000	1.27%
6	Pennsylvania	18,065,000	4.01%
43	Rhode Island	1,796,000	0.40%
24	South Carolina	6,868,000	1.53%
46	South Dakota	1,256,000	0.28%
22	Tennessee	7,943,000	1.76%
2	Texas	33,277,000	7.39%
41	Utah	1,881,000	0.42%
49	Vermont	1,097,000	0.24%
14	Virginia	10,129,000	2.25%
15	Washington	9,241,000	2.05%
38	West Virginia	2,392,000	0.53%
13	Wisconsin	10,724,000	2.38%
50	Wyoming	890,000	0.20%

RANK ORDER

RANK	STATE	GALLONS	% of USA
1	California	53,266,000	11.83%
2	Texas	33,277,000	7.39%
3	Florida	29,796,000	6.62%
4	New York	27,313,000	6.07%
5	Illinois	21,349,000	4.74%
6	Pennsylvania	18,065,000	4.01%
7	Ohio	17,075,000	3.79%
8	Michigan	15,788,000	3.51%
9	New Jersey	13,865,000	3.08%
10	Georgia	12,530,000	2.78%
11	Massachusetts	11,519,000	2.56%
12	North Carolina	11,260,000	2.50%
13	Wisconsin	10,724,000	2.38%
14	Virginia	10,129,000	2.25%
15	Washington	9,241,000	2.05%
16	Arizona	9,072,000	2.01%
17	Missouri	8,900,000	1.98%
18	Indiana	8,768,000	1.95%
19	Minnesota	8,547,000	1.90%
20	Louisiana	8,258,000	1.83%
21	Maryland	8,206,000	1.82%
22	Tennessee	7,943,000	1.76%
23	Colorado	7,832,000	1.74%
24	South Carolina	6,868,000	1.53%
25	Alabama	6,275,000	1.39%
26	Oregon	5,732,000	1.27%
27	Connecticut	5,534,000	1.23%
28	Kentucky	5,331,000	1.18%
29	Nevada	5,161,000	1.15%
30	Oklahoma	4,560,000	1.01%
31	Mississippi	4,437,000	0.99%
32	Iowa	4,257,000	0.95%
33	New Hampshire	3,752,000	0.83%
34	Arkansas	3,531,000	0.78%
35	Kansas	3,439,000	0.76%
36	New Mexico	3,131,000	0.70%
37	Nebraska	2,765,000	0.61%
38	West Virginia	2,392,000	0.53%
39	Hawaii	2,196,000	0.49%
40	Maine	2,178,000	0.48%
41	Utah	1,881,000	0.42%
42	Idaho	1,802,000	0.40%
43	Rhode Island	1,796,000	0.40%
44	Montana	1,660,000	0.37%
45	Delaware	1,556,000	0.35%
46	South Dakota	1,256,000	0.28%
47	North Dakota	1,217,000	0.27%
48	Alaska	1,179,000	0.26%
49	Vermont	1,097,000	0.24%
50	Wyoming	890,000	0.20%
	District of Columbia	1,653,000	0.37%

Source: Distilled Spirits Council of the United States, Inc., Steve L. Barsby Assoc.'s & Beer Institute
  "1996 Statistical Information for the Distilled Spirits Industry" (August 1997)
*This is apparent consumption of actual alcohol, not entire volume of an alcoholic beverage (e.g. wine is roughly
11% absolute alcohol content). Apparent consumption is based on several sources which together approximate
sales but do not actually measure consumption. Reported state volumes reflect only in-state purchases.
Accordingly, figures for some states may be skewed by purchases by nonresidents.

Adult Per Capita Apparent Alcohol Consumption in 1996

National Per Capita = 2.43 Gallons Consumed per Adult Age 21 Years & Older*

ALPHA ORDER

RANK	STATE	PER CAPITA
43	Alabama	2.09
3	Alaska	3.00
6	Arizona	2.94
45	Arkansas	2.03
25	California	2.45
6	Colorado	2.94
33	Connecticut	2.34
4	Delaware	2.99
8	Florida	2.84
24	Georgia	2.46
14	Hawaii	2.66
34	Idaho	2.31
18	Illinois	2.60
38	Indiana	2.14
39	Iowa	2.12
48	Kansas	1.94
47	Kentucky	1.95
8	Louisiana	2.84
26	Maine	2.44
35	Maryland	2.28
20	Massachusetts	2.58
32	Michigan	2.37
15	Minnesota	2.65
27	Mississippi	2.43
31	Missouri	2.38
12	Montana	2.74
27	Nebraska	2.43
1	Nevada	4.57
2	New Hampshire	4.55
27	New Jersey	2.43
10	New Mexico	2.76
41	New York	2.11
36	North Carolina	2.17
12	North Dakota	2.74
36	Ohio	2.17
46	Oklahoma	2.01
22	Oregon	2.53
44	Pennsylvania	2.08
23	Rhode Island	2.50
16	South Carolina	2.64
21	South Dakota	2.54
42	Tennessee	2.10
18	Texas	2.60
50	Utah	1.57
17	Vermont	2.62
39	Virginia	2.12
30	Washington	2.39
49	West Virginia	1.81
5	Wisconsin	2.98
11	Wyoming	2.75

RANK ORDER

RANK	STATE	PER CAPITA
1	Nevada	4.57
2	New Hampshire	4.55
3	Alaska	3.00
4	Delaware	2.99
5	Wisconsin	2.98
6	Arizona	2.94
6	Colorado	2.94
8	Florida	2.84
8	Louisiana	2.84
10	New Mexico	2.76
11	Wyoming	2.75
12	Montana	2.74
12	North Dakota	2.74
14	Hawaii	2.66
15	Minnesota	2.65
16	South Carolina	2.64
17	Vermont	2.62
18	Illinois	2.60
18	Texas	2.60
20	Massachusetts	2.58
21	South Dakota	2.54
22	Oregon	2.53
23	Rhode Island	2.50
24	Georgia	2.46
25	California	2.45
26	Maine	2.44
27	Mississippi	2.43
27	Nebraska	2.43
27	New Jersey	2.43
30	Washington	2.39
31	Missouri	2.38
32	Michigan	2.37
33	Connecticut	2.34
34	Idaho	2.31
35	Maryland	2.28
36	North Carolina	2.17
36	Ohio	2.17
38	Indiana	2.14
39	Iowa	2.12
39	Virginia	2.12
41	New York	2.11
42	Tennessee	2.10
43	Alabama	2.09
44	Pennsylvania	2.08
45	Arkansas	2.03
46	Oklahoma	2.01
47	Kentucky	1.95
48	Kansas	1.94
49	West Virginia	1.81
50	Utah	1.57
	District of Columbia	3.97

Source: MQ Press using data from Steve L. Barsby & Assoc. & Beer Institute as published by the Distilled Spirits Council of the United States, Inc. "1996 Statistical Information for the Distilled Spirits Industry" (August 1997) and Census
*This is apparent consumption of actual alcohol, not the liquid volume of an alcoholic beverage (e.g. wine is roughly 11% absolute alcohol content). Apparent consumption is based on several sources which together approximate sales but do not actually measure consumption. Reported state volumes reflect only in-state purchases. Accordingly, figures for some states may be skewed by purchases by nonresidents.

Apparent Beer Consumption in 1996

National Total = 5,851,579,000 Gallons of Beer Consumed*

ALPHA ORDER

RANK	STATE	GALLONS	% of USA
25	Alabama	89,534,000	1.53%
49	Alaska	13,612,000	0.23%
16	Arizona	121,932,000	2.08%
33	Arkansas	50,321,000	0.86%
1	California	609,522,000	10.42%
23	Colorado	94,622,000	1.62%
32	Connecticut	56,369,000	0.96%
45	Delaware	17,838,000	0.30%
3	Florida	364,567,000	6.23%
9	Georgia	161,436,000	2.76%
39	Hawaii	30,042,000	0.51%
42	Idaho	24,477,000	0.42%
5	Illinois	271,621,000	4.64%
17	Indiana	118,596,000	2.03%
29	Iowa	65,868,000	1.13%
34	Kansas	48,698,000	0.83%
26	Kentucky	74,050,000	1.27%
18	Louisiana	115,389,000	1.97%
41	Maine	26,432,000	0.45%
22	Maryland	94,627,000	1.62%
14	Massachusetts	127,075,000	2.17%
8	Michigan	206,990,000	3.54%
21	Minnesota	104,404,000	1.78%
28	Mississippi	66,057,000	1.13%
15	Missouri	126,254,000	2.16%
43	Montana	23,491,000	0.40%
36	Nebraska	40,254,000	0.69%
31	Nevada	56,460,000	0.96%
38	New Hampshire	36,123,000	0.62%
11	New Jersey	145,996,000	2.49%
35	New Mexico	46,564,000	0.80%
4	New York	320,410,000	5.48%
10	North Carolina	154,430,000	2.64%
47	North Dakota	17,112,000	0.29%
7	Ohio	260,599,000	4.45%
30	Oklahoma	65,669,000	1.12%
27	Oregon	71,380,000	1.22%
6	Pennsylvania	269,542,000	4.61%
44	Rhode Island	21,448,000	0.37%
24	South Carolina	93,873,000	1.60%
46	South Dakota	17,789,000	0.30%
19	Tennessee	114,468,000	1.96%
2	Texas	519,248,000	8.87%
40	Utah	26,452,000	0.45%
48	Vermont	13,708,000	0.23%
13	Virginia	137,318,000	2.35%
20	Washington	111,326,000	1.90%
37	West Virginia	38,272,000	0.65%
12	Wisconsin	142,468,000	2.43%
50	Wyoming	11,832,000	0.20%

RANK ORDER

RANK	STATE	GALLONS	% of USA
1	California	609,522,000	10.42%
2	Texas	519,248,000	8.87%
3	Florida	364,567,000	6.23%
4	New York	320,410,000	5.48%
5	Illinois	271,621,000	4.64%
6	Pennsylvania	269,542,000	4.61%
7	Ohio	260,599,000	4.45%
8	Michigan	206,990,000	3.54%
9	Georgia	161,436,000	2.76%
10	North Carolina	154,430,000	2.64%
11	New Jersey	145,996,000	2.49%
12	Wisconsin	142,468,000	2.43%
13	Virginia	137,318,000	2.35%
14	Massachusetts	127,075,000	2.17%
15	Missouri	126,254,000	2.16%
16	Arizona	121,932,000	2.08%
17	Indiana	118,596,000	2.03%
18	Louisiana	115,389,000	1.97%
19	Tennessee	114,468,000	1.96%
20	Washington	111,326,000	1.90%
21	Minnesota	104,404,000	1.78%
22	Maryland	94,627,000	1.62%
23	Colorado	94,622,000	1.62%
24	South Carolina	93,873,000	1.60%
25	Alabama	89,534,000	1.53%
26	Kentucky	74,050,000	1.27%
27	Oregon	71,380,000	1.22%
28	Mississippi	66,057,000	1.13%
29	Iowa	65,868,000	1.13%
30	Oklahoma	65,669,000	1.12%
31	Nevada	56,460,000	0.96%
32	Connecticut	56,369,000	0.96%
33	Arkansas	50,321,000	0.86%
34	Kansas	48,698,000	0.83%
35	New Mexico	46,564,000	0.80%
36	Nebraska	40,254,000	0.69%
37	West Virginia	38,272,000	0.65%
38	New Hampshire	36,123,000	0.62%
39	Hawaii	30,042,000	0.51%
40	Utah	26,452,000	0.45%
41	Maine	26,432,000	0.45%
42	Idaho	24,477,000	0.42%
43	Montana	23,491,000	0.40%
44	Rhode Island	21,448,000	0.37%
45	Delaware	17,838,000	0.30%
46	South Dakota	17,789,000	0.30%
47	North Dakota	17,112,000	0.29%
48	Vermont	13,708,000	0.23%
49	Alaska	13,612,000	0.23%
50	Wyoming	11,832,000	0.20%
	District of Columbia	15,013,000	0.26%

Source: Beer Institute as published by the Distilled Spirits Council of the United States, Inc.
  "1996 Statistical Information for the Distilled Spirits Industry" (August 1997)
*Apparent consumption is based on several sources which together approximate sales but do not actually measure consumption. Reported state volumes reflect only in-state purchases. Accordingly, figures for some states may be skewed by purchases by nonresidents.

Adult Per Capita Apparent Beer Consumption in 1996

National Per Capita = 31.57 Gallons Consumed per Adult 21 Years and Older*

ALPHA ORDER

RANK	STATE	PER CAPITA
33	Alabama	29.78
18	Alaska	34.69
7	Arizona	39.46
38	Arkansas	28.93
43	California	28.04
15	Colorado	35.49
49	Connecticut	23.85
19	Delaware	34.25
17	Florida	34.79
26	Georgia	31.73
11	Hawaii	36.36
28	Idaho	31.44
22	Illinois	33.08
36	Indiana	29.01
23	Iowa	32.82
44	Kansas	27.48
45	Kentucky	27.05
5	Louisiana	39.70
35	Maine	29.56
46	Maryland	26.27
42	Massachusetts	28.51
29	Michigan	31.09
25	Minnesota	32.43
12	Mississippi	36.18
20	Missouri	33.73
8	Montana	38.77
16	Nebraska	35.44
1	Nevada	50.01
2	New Hampshire	43.76
47	New Jersey	25.56
3	New Mexico	41.07
48	New York	24.74
34	North Carolina	29.75
9	North Dakota	38.50
21	Ohio	33.15
39	Oklahoma	28.89
27	Oregon	31.54
30	Pennsylvania	30.97
32	Rhode Island	29.83
13	South Carolina	36.14
14	South Dakota	36.04
31	Tennessee	30.31
4	Texas	40.53
50	Utah	22.09
24	Vermont	32.72
40	Virginia	28.79
41	Washington	28.78
37	West Virginia	29.00
6	Wisconsin	39.61
10	Wyoming	36.53

RANK ORDER

RANK	STATE	PER CAPITA
1	Nevada	50.01
2	New Hampshire	43.76
3	New Mexico	41.07
4	Texas	40.53
5	Louisiana	39.70
6	Wisconsin	39.61
7	Arizona	39.46
8	Montana	38.77
9	North Dakota	38.50
10	Wyoming	36.53
11	Hawaii	36.36
12	Mississippi	36.18
13	South Carolina	36.14
14	South Dakota	36.04
15	Colorado	35.49
16	Nebraska	35.44
17	Florida	34.79
18	Alaska	34.69
19	Delaware	34.25
20	Missouri	33.73
21	Ohio	33.15
22	Illinois	33.08
23	Iowa	32.82
24	Vermont	32.72
25	Minnesota	32.43
26	Georgia	31.73
27	Oregon	31.54
28	Idaho	31.44
29	Michigan	31.09
30	Pennsylvania	30.97
31	Tennessee	30.31
32	Rhode Island	29.83
33	Alabama	29.78
34	North Carolina	29.75
35	Maine	29.56
36	Indiana	29.01
37	West Virginia	29.00
38	Arkansas	28.93
39	Oklahoma	28.89
40	Virginia	28.79
41	Washington	28.78
42	Massachusetts	28.51
43	California	28.04
44	Kansas	27.48
45	Kentucky	27.05
46	Maryland	26.27
47	New Jersey	25.56
48	New York	24.74
49	Connecticut	23.85
50	Utah	22.09
	District of Columbia	36.01

Source: Beer Institute as published by the Distilled Spirits Council of the United States, Inc.
   "1996 Statistical Information for the Distilled Spirits Industry" (August 1997)
Apparent consumption is based on several sources which together approximate sales but do not actually measure consumption. Reported state volumes reflect only in-state purchases. Accordingly, figures for some states may be skewed by purchases by nonresidents.

Apparent Wine Consumption in 1996

National Total = 497,931,000 Gallons of Wine Consumed*

ALPHA ORDER

RANK ORDER

RANK	STATE	GALLONS	% of USA
28	Alabama	4,074,000	0.82%
45	Alaska	1,224,000	0.25%
16	Arizona	9,379,000	1.88%
41	Arkansas	1,907,000	0.38%
1	California	94,301,000	18.94%
17	Colorado	9,259,000	1.86%
15	Connecticut	9,653,000	1.94%
39	Delaware	1,993,000	0.40%
3	Florida	34,558,000	6.94%
14	Georgia	10,915,000	2.19%
32	Hawaii	2,765,000	0.56%
38	Idaho	2,160,000	0.43%
5	Illinois	24,960,000	5.01%
23	Indiana	7,105,000	1.43%
37	Iowa	2,262,000	0.45%
36	Kansas	2,284,000	0.46%
30	Kentucky	3,108,000	0.62%
25	Louisiana	5,883,000	1.18%
34	Maine	2,575,000	0.52%
18	Maryland	9,174,000	1.84%
7	Massachusetts	18,559,000	3.73%
10	Michigan	13,047,000	2.62%
21	Minnesota	7,524,000	1.51%
43	Mississippi	1,477,000	0.30%
22	Missouri	7,273,000	1.46%
44	Montana	1,476,000	0.30%
40	Nebraska	1,930,000	0.39%
24	Nevada	6,013,000	1.21%
29	New Hampshire	3,973,000	0.80%
6	New Jersey	22,219,000	4.46%
35	New Mexico	2,369,000	0.48%
2	New York	41,862,000	8.41%
13	North Carolina	11,105,000	2.23%
49	North Dakota	523,000	0.11%
12	Ohio	12,398,000	2.49%
31	Oklahoma	2,847,000	0.57%
19	Oregon	8,865,000	1.78%
8	Pennsylvania	14,612,000	2.93%
33	Rhode Island	2,733,000	0.55%
27	South Carolina	5,047,000	1.01%
48	South Dakota	604,000	0.12%
26	Tennessee	5,461,000	1.10%
4	Texas	25,041,000	5.03%
46	Utah	1,168,000	0.23%
42	Vermont	1,683,000	0.34%
11	Virginia	12,510,000	2.51%
9	Washington	13,813,000	2.77%
47	West Virginia	1,121,000	0.23%
20	Wisconsin	7,871,000	1.58%
50	Wyoming	492,000	0.10%

RANK	STATE	GALLONS	% of USA
1	California	94,301,000	18.94%
2	New York	41,862,000	8.41%
3	Florida	34,558,000	6.94%
4	Texas	25,041,000	5.03%
5	Illinois	24,960,000	5.01%
6	New Jersey	22,219,000	4.46%
7	Massachusetts	18,559,000	3.73%
8	Pennsylvania	14,612,000	2.93%
9	Washington	13,813,000	2.77%
10	Michigan	13,047,000	2.62%
11	Virginia	12,510,000	2.51%
12	Ohio	12,398,000	2.49%
13	North Carolina	11,105,000	2.23%
14	Georgia	10,915,000	2.19%
15	Connecticut	9,653,000	1.94%
16	Arizona	9,379,000	1.88%
17	Colorado	9,259,000	1.86%
18	Maryland	9,174,000	1.84%
19	Oregon	8,865,000	1.78%
20	Wisconsin	7,871,000	1.58%
21	Minnesota	7,524,000	1.51%
22	Missouri	7,273,000	1.46%
23	Indiana	7,105,000	1.43%
24	Nevada	6,013,000	1.21%
25	Louisiana	5,883,000	1.18%
26	Tennessee	5,461,000	1.10%
27	South Carolina	5,047,000	1.01%
28	Alabama	4,074,000	0.82%
29	New Hampshire	3,973,000	0.80%
30	Kentucky	3,108,000	0.62%
31	Oklahoma	2,847,000	0.57%
32	Hawaii	2,765,000	0.56%
33	Rhode Island	2,733,000	0.55%
34	Maine	2,575,000	0.52%
35	New Mexico	2,369,000	0.48%
36	Kansas	2,284,000	0.46%
37	Iowa	2,262,000	0.45%
38	Idaho	2,160,000	0.43%
39	Delaware	1,993,000	0.40%
40	Nebraska	1,930,000	0.39%
41	Arkansas	1,907,000	0.38%
42	Vermont	1,683,000	0.34%
43	Mississippi	1,477,000	0.30%
44	Montana	1,476,000	0.30%
45	Alaska	1,224,000	0.25%
46	Utah	1,168,000	0.23%
47	West Virginia	1,121,000	0.23%
48	South Dakota	604,000	0.12%
49	North Dakota	523,000	0.11%
50	Wyoming	492,000	0.10%
	District of Columbia	2,716,000	0.55%

Source: Steve L. Barsby and Associates, Inc. as published by the Distilled Spirits Council of the United States, Inc.
"1996 Statistical Information for the Distilled Spirits Industry" (August 1997)
*Apparent consumption is based on several sources which together approximate sales but do not actually measure consumption. Reported state volumes reflect only in-state purchases. Accordingly, figures for some states may be skewed by purchases by nonresidents.

Adult Per Capita Apparent Wine Consumption in 1996

National Per Capita = 2.69 Gallons Consumed per Adult Age 21 Years and Older*

ALPHA ORDER

RANK	STATE	PER CAPITA
40	Alabama	1.36
16	Alaska	3.12
17	Arizona	3.04
47	Arkansas	1.10
3	California	4.34
12	Colorado	3.47
5	Connecticut	4.08
9	Delaware	3.83
14	Florida	3.30
26	Georgia	2.15
13	Hawaii	3.35
20	Idaho	2.77
17	Illinois	3.04
34	Indiana	1.75
46	Iowa	1.13
41	Kansas	1.29
45	Kentucky	1.14
29	Louisiana	2.02
19	Maine	2.88
22	Maryland	2.55
4	Massachusetts	4.16
30	Michigan	1.96
24	Minnesota	2.34
50	Mississippi	0.81
32	Missouri	1.94
23	Montana	2.44
35	Nebraska	1.70
1	Nevada	5.33
2	New Hampshire	4.81
8	New Jersey	3.89
28	New Mexico	2.09
15	New York	3.23
27	North Carolina	2.14
44	North Dakota	1.18
37	Ohio	1.58
42	Oklahoma	1.25
7	Oregon	3.92
36	Pennsylvania	1.68
10	Rhode Island	3.80
32	South Carolina	1.94
43	South Dakota	1.22
39	Tennessee	1.45
31	Texas	1.95
48	Utah	0.98
6	Vermont	4.02
21	Virginia	2.62
11	Washington	3.57
49	West Virginia	0.85
25	Wisconsin	2.19
38	Wyoming	1.52

RANK ORDER

RANK	STATE	PER CAPITA
1	Nevada	5.33
2	New Hampshire	4.81
3	California	4.34
4	Massachusetts	4.16
5	Connecticut	4.08
6	Vermont	4.02
7	Oregon	3.92
8	New Jersey	3.89
9	Delaware	3.83
10	Rhode Island	3.80
11	Washington	3.57
12	Colorado	3.47
13	Hawaii	3.35
14	Florida	3.30
15	New York	3.23
16	Alaska	3.12
17	Arizona	3.04
17	Illinois	3.04
19	Maine	2.88
20	Idaho	2.77
21	Virginia	2.62
22	Maryland	2.55
23	Montana	2.44
24	Minnesota	2.34
25	Wisconsin	2.19
26	Georgia	2.15
27	North Carolina	2.14
28	New Mexico	2.09
29	Louisiana	2.02
30	Michigan	1.96
31	Texas	1.95
32	Missouri	1.94
32	South Carolina	1.94
34	Indiana	1.75
35	Nebraska	1.70
36	Pennsylvania	1.68
37	Ohio	1.58
38	Wyoming	1.52
39	Tennessee	1.45
40	Alabama	1.36
41	Kansas	1.29
42	Oklahoma	1.25
43	South Dakota	1.22
44	North Dakota	1.18
45	Kentucky	1.14
46	Iowa	1.13
47	Arkansas	1.10
48	Utah	0.98
49	West Virginia	0.85
50	Mississippi	0.81
	District of Columbia	6.52

Source: Steve L. Barsby and Associates, Inc. as published by the Distilled Spirits Council of the United States, Inc. "1996 Statistical Information for the Distilled Spirits Industry" (August 1997)

Apparent consumption is based on several sources which together approximate sales but do not actually measure consumption. Reported state volumes reflect only in-state purchases. Accordingly, figures for some states may be skewed by purchases by nonresidents.

Apparent Distilled Spirits Consumption in 1996

National Total = 330,393,000 Gallons of Distilled Spirits Consumed*

ALPHA ORDER

RANK	STATE	GALLONS	% of USA
27	Alabama	4,493,000	1.36%
46	Alaska	1,080,000	0.33%
20	Arizona	6,383,000	1.93%
33	Arkansas	2,643,000	0.80%
1	California	38,662,000	11.70%
19	Colorado	6,390,000	1.93%
26	Connecticut	4,838,000	1.46%
42	Delaware	1,336,000	0.40%
2	Florida	23,973,000	7.26%
9	Georgia	10,161,000	3.08%
41	Hawaii	1,349,000	0.41%
44	Idaho	1,157,000	0.35%
5	Illinois	15,951,000	4.83%
17	Indiana	6,608,000	2.00%
34	Iowa	2,610,000	0.79%
35	Kansas	2,491,000	0.75%
29	Kentucky	4,143,000	1.25%
21	Louisiana	6,047,000	1.83%
38	Maine	1,762,000	0.53%
15	Maryland	7,346,000	2.22%
11	Massachusetts	9,397,000	2.84%
6	Michigan	12,595,000	3.81%
14	Minnesota	7,553,000	2.29%
31	Mississippi	3,254,000	0.98%
21	Missouri	6,047,000	1.83%
45	Montana	1,102,000	0.33%
37	Nebraska	1,852,000	0.56%
25	Nevada	4,897,000	1.48%
28	New Hampshire	4,224,000	1.28%
7	New Jersey	12,128,000	3.67%
36	New Mexico	1,938,000	0.59%
3	New York	20,725,000	6.27%
13	North Carolina	7,724,000	2.34%
47	North Dakota	973,000	0.29%
10	Ohio	9,960,000	3.01%
32	Oklahoma	3,230,000	0.98%
30	Oregon	3,862,000	1.17%
8	Pennsylvania	10,820,000	3.27%
43	Rhode Island	1,325,000	0.40%
24	South Carolina	5,221,000	1.58%
48	South Dakota	972,000	0.29%
23	Tennessee	5,479,000	1.66%
4	Texas	17,892,000	5.42%
39	Utah	1,405,000	0.43%
50	Vermont	738,000	0.22%
18	Virginia	6,435,000	1.95%
16	Washington	6,780,000	2.05%
40	West Virginia	1,367,000	0.41%
12	Wisconsin	8,618,000	2.61%
49	Wyoming	759,000	0.23%

RANK ORDER

RANK	STATE	GALLONS	% of USA
1	California	38,662,000	11.70%
2	Florida	23,973,000	7.26%
3	New York	20,725,000	6.27%
4	Texas	17,892,000	5.42%
5	Illinois	15,951,000	4.83%
6	Michigan	12,595,000	3.81%
7	New Jersey	12,128,000	3.67%
8	Pennsylvania	10,820,000	3.27%
9	Georgia	10,161,000	3.08%
10	Ohio	9,960,000	3.01%
11	Massachusetts	9,397,000	2.84%
12	Wisconsin	8,618,000	2.61%
13	North Carolina	7,724,000	2.34%
14	Minnesota	7,553,000	2.29%
15	Maryland	7,346,000	2.22%
16	Washington	6,780,000	2.05%
17	Indiana	6,608,000	2.00%
18	Virginia	6,435,000	1.95%
19	Colorado	6,390,000	1.93%
20	Arizona	6,383,000	1.93%
21	Louisiana	6,047,000	1.83%
21	Missouri	6,047,000	1.83%
23	Tennessee	5,479,000	1.66%
24	South Carolina	5,221,000	1.58%
25	Nevada	4,897,000	1.48%
26	Connecticut	4,838,000	1.46%
27	Alabama	4,493,000	1.36%
28	New Hampshire	4,224,000	1.28%
29	Kentucky	4,143,000	1.25%
30	Oregon	3,862,000	1.17%
31	Mississippi	3,254,000	0.98%
32	Oklahoma	3,230,000	0.98%
33	Arkansas	2,643,000	0.80%
34	Iowa	2,610,000	0.79%
35	Kansas	2,491,000	0.75%
36	New Mexico	1,938,000	0.59%
37	Nebraska	1,852,000	0.56%
38	Maine	1,762,000	0.53%
39	Utah	1,405,000	0.43%
40	West Virginia	1,367,000	0.41%
41	Hawaii	1,349,000	0.41%
42	Delaware	1,336,000	0.40%
43	Rhode Island	1,325,000	0.40%
44	Idaho	1,157,000	0.35%
45	Montana	1,102,000	0.33%
46	Alaska	1,080,000	0.33%
47	North Dakota	973,000	0.29%
48	South Dakota	972,000	0.29%
49	Wyoming	759,000	0.23%
50	Vermont	738,000	0.22%
	District of Columbia	1,695,000	0.51%

Source: Distilled Spirits Council of the United States, Inc.
  "1996 Statistical Information for the Distilled Spirits Industry" (August 1997)
*Apparent consumption is based on several sources which together approximate sales but do not actually measure consumption. Reported state volumes reflect only in-state purchases. Accordingly, figures for some states may be skewed by purchases by nonresidents.

Adult Per Capita Apparent Distilled Spirits Consumption in 1996

National Per Capita = 1.78 Gallons Consumed per Adult Age 21 and Older*

ALPHA ORDER

RANK	STATE	PER CAPITA
38	Alabama	1.49
3	Alaska	2.75
14	Arizona	2.07
36	Arkansas	1.52
25	California	1.78
5	Colorado	2.40
15	Connecticut	2.05
4	Delaware	2.57
9	Florida	2.29
18	Georgia	2.00
31	Hawaii	1.63
38	Idaho	1.49
21	Illinois	1.94
33	Indiana	1.62
46	Iowa	1.30
43	Kansas	1.41
37	Kentucky	1.51
13	Louisiana	2.08
19	Maine	1.97
16	Maryland	2.04
12	Massachusetts	2.11
22	Michigan	1.89
7	Minnesota	2.35
25	Mississippi	1.78
33	Missouri	1.62
24	Montana	1.82
31	Nebraska	1.63
2	Nevada	4.34
1	New Hampshire	5.12
11	New Jersey	2.12
29	New Mexico	1.71
35	New York	1.60
38	North Carolina	1.49
10	North Dakota	2.19
47	Ohio	1.27
42	Oklahoma	1.42
29	Oregon	1.71
48	Pennsylvania	1.24
23	Rhode Island	1.84
17	South Carolina	2.01
19	South Dakota	1.97
41	Tennessee	1.45
44	Texas	1.40
49	Utah	1.17
27	Vermont	1.76
45	Virginia	1.35
28	Washington	1.75
50	West Virginia	1.04
5	Wisconsin	2.40
8	Wyoming	2.34

RANK ORDER

RANK	STATE	PER CAPITA
1	New Hampshire	5.12
2	Nevada	4.34
3	Alaska	2.75
4	Delaware	2.57
5	Colorado	2.40
5	Wisconsin	2.40
7	Minnesota	2.35
8	Wyoming	2.34
9	Florida	2.29
10	North Dakota	2.19
11	New Jersey	2.12
12	Massachusetts	2.11
13	Louisiana	2.08
14	Arizona	2.07
15	Connecticut	2.05
16	Maryland	2.04
17	South Carolina	2.01
18	Georgia	2.00
19	Maine	1.97
19	South Dakota	1.97
21	Illinois	1.94
22	Michigan	1.89
23	Rhode Island	1.84
24	Montana	1.82
25	California	1.78
25	Mississippi	1.78
27	Vermont	1.76
28	Washington	1.75
29	New Mexico	1.71
29	Oregon	1.71
31	Hawaii	1.63
31	Nebraska	1.63
33	Indiana	1.62
33	Missouri	1.62
35	New York	1.60
36	Arkansas	1.52
37	Kentucky	1.51
38	Alabama	1.49
38	Idaho	1.49
38	North Carolina	1.49
41	Tennessee	1.45
42	Oklahoma	1.42
43	Kansas	1.41
44	Texas	1.40
45	Virginia	1.35
46	Iowa	1.30
47	Ohio	1.27
48	Pennsylvania	1.24
49	Utah	1.17
50	West Virginia	1.04
	District of Columbia	4.07

Source: Distilled Spirits Council of the United States, Inc.
"1996 Statistical Information for the Distilled Spirits Industry" (August 1997)
*Apparent consumption is based on several sources which together approximate sales but do not actually measure consumption. Reported state volumes reflect only in-state purchases. Accordingly, figures for some states may be skewed by purchases by nonresidents.

Percent of Adults Who Are Binge Drinkers in 1995

National Median = 13.93% of Adults Are Binge Drinkers*

ALPHA ORDER

RANK	STATE	PERCENT
28	Alabama	13.58
3	Alaska	19.20
30	Arizona	13.46
43	Arkansas	8.75
16	California	15.30
12	Colorado	16.30
19	Connecticut	14.41
45	Delaware	8.61
32	Florida	13.12
37	Georgia	11.99
36	Hawaii	12.37
33	Idaho	12.94
28	Illinois	13.58
34	Indiana	12.75
8	Iowa	17.95
27	Kansas	13.86
41	Kentucky	9.70
24	Louisiana	14.01
38	Maine	11.45
46	Maryland	8.21
9	Massachusetts	17.83
6	Michigan	18.26
7	Minnesota	18.01
44	Mississippi	8.67
22	Missouri	14.10
21	Montana	14.31
14	Nebraska	15.83
4	Nevada	18.97
11	New Hampshire	16.59
25	New Jersey	13.95
23	New Mexico	14.06
35	New York	12.39
49	North Carolina	5.76
10	North Dakota	16.97
40	Ohio	9.87
47	Oklahoma	6.69
26	Oregon	13.90
2	Pennsylvania	19.38
5	Rhode Island	18.70
42	South Carolina	9.17
20	South Dakota	14.36
50	Tennessee	5.22
17	Texas	15.27
39	Utah	9.93
13	Vermont	15.96
18	Virginia	14.46
31	Washington	13.44
48	West Virginia	5.92
1	Wisconsin	22.89
15	Wyoming	15.57

RANK ORDER

RANK	STATE	PERCENT
1	Wisconsin	22.89
2	Pennsylvania	19.38
3	Alaska	19.20
4	Nevada	18.97
5	Rhode Island	18.70
6	Michigan	18.26
7	Minnesota	18.01
8	Iowa	17.95
9	Massachusetts	17.83
10	North Dakota	16.97
11	New Hampshire	16.59
12	Colorado	16.30
13	Vermont	15.96
14	Nebraska	15.83
15	Wyoming	15.57
16	California	15.30
17	Texas	15.27
18	Virginia	14.46
19	Connecticut	14.41
20	South Dakota	14.36
21	Montana	14.31
22	Missouri	14.10
23	New Mexico	14.06
24	Louisiana	14.01
25	New Jersey	13.95
26	Oregon	13.90
27	Kansas	13.86
28	Alabama	13.58
28	Illinois	13.58
30	Arizona	13.46
31	Washington	13.44
32	Florida	13.12
33	Idaho	12.94
34	Indiana	12.75
35	New York	12.39
36	Hawaii	12.37
37	Georgia	11.99
38	Maine	11.45
39	Utah	9.93
40	Ohio	9.87
41	Kentucky	9.70
42	South Carolina	9.17
43	Arkansas	8.75
44	Mississippi	8.67
45	Delaware	8.61
46	Maryland	8.21
47	Oklahoma	6.69
48	West Virginia	5.92
49	North Carolina	5.76
50	Tennessee	5.22
	District of Columbia**	NA

Source: U.S. Department of Health and Human Services, Centers for Disease Control and Prevention
    "1995 Behavioral Risk Factor Surveillance Summary Prevalence Report" (December 10, 1996)
*Persons 18 and older reporting consumption of five or more alcoholic drinks on one or more occasions during the previous month.
**Not available.

Percent of Adults Who Smoke: 1996

National Median = 23.51% of Adults Smoke*

ALPHA ORDER

RANK	STATE	PERCENT
37	Alabama	22.42
7	Alaska	27.68
24	Arizona	23.71
13	Arkansas	25.29
48	California	18.60
34	Colorado	22.79
41	Connecticut	21.80
21	Delaware	24.22
40	Florida	21.81
47	Georgia	20.27
NA	Hawaii**	NA
43	Idaho	21.14
16	Illinois	24.80
2	Indiana	28.63
25	Iowa	23.59
39	Kansas	22.06
1	Kentucky	31.66
9	Louisiana	25.88
12	Maine	25.31
44	Maryland	20.90
29	Massachusetts	23.35
11	Michigan	25.63
46	Minnesota	20.58
31	Mississippi	23.24
6	Missouri	27.78
42	Montana	21.69
38	Nebraska	22.09
4	Nevada	28.16
15	New Hampshire	24.84
35	New Jersey	22.72
33	New Mexico	22.83
30	New York	23.25
10	North Carolina	25.69
28	North Dakota	23.38
3	Ohio	28.40
22	Oklahoma	24.08
27	Oregon	23.41
19	Pennsylvania	24.54
36	Rhode Island	22.51
20	South Carolina	24.46
45	South Dakota	20.66
5	Tennessee	27.98
32	Texas	22.91
49	Utah	15.91
23	Vermont	24.07
17	Virginia	24.79
26	Washington	23.44
8	West Virginia	26.63
14	Wisconsin	24.86
18	Wyoming	24.56

RANK ORDER

RANK	STATE	PERCENT
1	Kentucky	31.66
2	Indiana	28.63
3	Ohio	28.40
4	Nevada	28.16
5	Tennessee	27.98
6	Missouri	27.78
7	Alaska	27.68
8	West Virginia	26.63
9	Louisiana	25.88
10	North Carolina	25.69
11	Michigan	25.63
12	Maine	25.31
13	Arkansas	25.29
14	Wisconsin	24.86
15	New Hampshire	24.84
16	Illinois	24.80
17	Virginia	24.79
18	Wyoming	24.56
19	Pennsylvania	24.54
20	South Carolina	24.46
21	Delaware	24.22
22	Oklahoma	24.08
23	Vermont	24.07
24	Arizona	23.71
25	Iowa	23.59
26	Washington	23.44
27	Oregon	23.41
28	North Dakota	23.38
29	Massachusetts	23.35
30	New York	23.25
31	Mississippi	23.24
32	Texas	22.91
33	New Mexico	22.83
34	Colorado	22.79
35	New Jersey	22.72
36	Rhode Island	22.51
37	Alabama	22.42
38	Nebraska	22.09
39	Kansas	22.06
40	Florida	21.81
41	Connecticut	21.80
42	Montana	21.69
43	Idaho	21.14
44	Maryland	20.90
45	South Dakota	20.66
46	Minnesota	20.58
47	Georgia	20.27
48	California	18.60
49	Utah	15.91
NA	Hawaii**	NA
	District of Columbia	20.50

Source: U.S. Department of Health and Human Services, Centers for Disease Control and Prevention
"1996 Behavioral Risk Factor Surveillance Summary Prevalence Report" (January 8, 1998)
*Persons 18 and older who have ever smoked 100 cigarettes and currently smoke.
**Not available.

Percent of Men Who Smoke: 1996

National Median = 25.48% of Men*

ALPHA ORDER

RANK	STATE	PERCENT
37	Alabama	24.32
6	Alaska	30.79
17	Arizona	27.11
13	Arkansas	27.70
46	California	21.41
33	Colorado	24.47
42	Connecticut	22.75
28	Delaware	25.04
40	Florida	23.33
31	Georgia	24.67
NA	Hawaii**	NA
47	Idaho	21.24
27	Illinois	25.24
4	Indiana	31.53
21	Iowa	26.27
22	Kansas	26.05
1	Kentucky	33.96
3	Louisiana	31.58
9	Maine	28.88
43	Maryland	22.55
38	Massachusetts	23.91
19	Michigan	26.48
45	Minnesota	21.72
10	Mississippi	28.61
8	Missouri	28.96
48	Montana	20.54
25	Nebraska	25.47
11	Nevada	28.41
24	New Hampshire	25.48
30	New Jersey	24.88
29	New Mexico	24.91
41	New York	23.26
7	North Carolina	29.90
36	North Dakota	24.37
2	Ohio	33.91
20	Oklahoma	26.37
34	Oregon	24.41
39	Pennsylvania	23.83
23	Rhode Island	25.63
26	South Carolina	25.40
44	South Dakota	22.27
5	Tennessee	31.13
15	Texas	27.52
49	Utah	18.57
18	Vermont	26.55
14	Virginia	27.60
32	Washington	24.57
12	West Virginia	27.95
16	Wisconsin	27.51
35	Wyoming	24.40

RANK ORDER

RANK	STATE	PERCENT
1	Kentucky	33.96
2	Ohio	33.91
3	Louisiana	31.58
4	Indiana	31.53
5	Tennessee	31.13
6	Alaska	30.79
7	North Carolina	29.90
8	Missouri	28.96
9	Maine	28.88
10	Mississippi	28.61
11	Nevada	28.41
12	West Virginia	27.95
13	Arkansas	27.70
14	Virginia	27.60
15	Texas	27.52
16	Wisconsin	27.51
17	Arizona	27.11
18	Vermont	26.55
19	Michigan	26.48
20	Oklahoma	26.37
21	Iowa	26.27
22	Kansas	26.05
23	Rhode Island	25.63
24	New Hampshire	25.48
25	Nebraska	25.47
26	South Carolina	25.40
27	Illinois	25.24
28	Delaware	25.04
29	New Mexico	24.91
30	New Jersey	24.88
31	Georgia	24.67
32	Washington	24.57
33	Colorado	24.47
34	Oregon	24.41
35	Wyoming	24.40
36	North Dakota	24.37
37	Alabama	24.32
38	Massachusetts	23.91
39	Pennsylvania	23.83
40	Florida	23.33
41	New York	23.26
42	Connecticut	22.75
43	Maryland	22.55
44	South Dakota	22.27
45	Minnesota	21.72
46	California	21.41
47	Idaho	21.24
48	Montana	20.54
49	Utah	18.57
NA	Hawaii**	NA

	District of Columbia	23.95

Source: U.S. Department of Health and Human Services, Centers for Disease Control and Prevention
"1996 Behavioral Risk Factor Surveillance Summary Prevalence Report" (January 8, 1998)
*Men 18 and older who have ever smoked 100 cigarettes and currently smoke.
**Not available.

Percent of Women Who Smoke: 1996

National Median = 22.01% of Women*

ALPHA ORDER

RANK ORDER

RANK	STATE	PERCENT
36	Alabama	20.74
11	Alaska	24.22
37	Arizona	20.48
17	Arkansas	23.14
48	California	15.85
29	Colorado	21.19
32	Connecticut	20.93
13	Delaware	23.48
38	Florida	20.43
47	Georgia	16.25
NA	Hawaii**	NA
31	Idaho	21.05
13	Illinois	23.48
4	Indiana	26.00
30	Iowa	21.15
46	Kansas	18.34
1	Kentucky	29.57
34	Louisiana	20.86
25	Maine	22.04
41	Maryland	19.38
18	Massachusetts	22.85
8	Michigan	24.84
40	Minnesota	19.52
45	Mississippi	18.53
3	Missouri	26.73
19	Montana	22.78
43	Nebraska	18.96
2	Nevada	27.91
10	New Hampshire	24.24
35	New Jersey	20.76
33	New Mexico	20.88
16	New York	23.23
27	North Carolina	21.85
21	North Dakota	22.42
15	Ohio	23.47
26	Oklahoma	21.99
20	Oregon	22.47
6	Pennsylvania	25.16
39	Rhode Island	19.73
12	South Carolina	23.62
42	South Dakota	19.16
6	Tennessee	25.16
44	Texas	18.57
49	Utah	13.38
28	Vermont	21.76
24	Virginia	22.15
23	Washington	22.36
5	West Virginia	25.46
22	Wisconsin	22.39
9	Wyoming	24.72

RANK	STATE	PERCENT
1	Kentucky	29.57
2	Nevada	27.91
3	Missouri	26.73
4	Indiana	26.00
5	West Virginia	25.46
6	Pennsylvania	25.16
6	Tennessee	25.16
8	Michigan	24.84
9	Wyoming	24.72
10	New Hampshire	24.24
11	Alaska	24.22
12	South Carolina	23.62
13	Delaware	23.48
13	Illinois	23.48
15	Ohio	23.47
16	New York	23.23
17	Arkansas	23.14
18	Massachusetts	22.85
19	Montana	22.78
20	Oregon	22.47
21	North Dakota	22.42
22	Wisconsin	22.39
23	Washington	22.36
24	Virginia	22.15
25	Maine	22.04
26	Oklahoma	21.99
27	North Carolina	21.85
28	Vermont	21.76
29	Colorado	21.19
30	Iowa	21.15
31	Idaho	21.05
32	Connecticut	20.93
33	New Mexico	20.88
34	Louisiana	20.86
35	New Jersey	20.76
36	Alabama	20.74
37	Arizona	20.48
38	Florida	20.43
39	Rhode Island	19.73
40	Minnesota	19.52
41	Maryland	19.38
42	South Dakota	19.16
43	Nebraska	18.96
44	Texas	18.57
45	Mississippi	18.53
46	Kansas	18.34
47	Georgia	16.25
48	California	15.85
49	Utah	13.38
NA	Hawaii**	NA
	District of Columbia	17.58

Source: U.S. Department of Health and Human Services, Centers for Disease Control and Prevention
   "1996 Behavioral Risk Factor Surveillance Summary Prevalence Report" (January 8, 1998)
*Women 18 and older who have ever smoked 100 cigarettes and currently smoke.
**Not available.

Percent of Adults Overweight: 1996

National Median = 29.28% of Adults*

ALPHA ORDER

RANK	STATE	PERCENT
3	Alabama	33.89
23	Alaska	30.03
44	Arizona	26.28
13	Arkansas	31.83
36	California	27.73
49	Colorado	22.32
40	Connecticut	27.16
14	Delaware	31.78
20	Florida	30.54
48	Georgia	24.07
NA	Hawaii**	NA
25	Idaho	29.28
24	Illinois	29.84
12	Indiana	32.70
11	Iowa	32.73
45	Kansas	26.06
9	Kentucky	32.96
6	Louisiana	33.39
33	Maine	28.14
17	Maryland	30.78
43	Massachusetts	26.67
8	Michigan	33.03
34	Minnesota	27.91
2	Mississippi	34.52
7	Missouri	33.11
30	Montana	28.84
28	Nebraska	29.00
37	Nevada	27.67
46	New Hampshire	25.99
38	New Jersey	27.53
42	New Mexico	26.82
29	New York	28.96
19	North Carolina	30.65
10	North Dakota	32.87
5	Ohio	33.43
27	Oklahoma	29.05
25	Oregon	29.28
15	Pennsylvania	31.76
31	Rhode Island	28.48
1	South Carolina	34.68
22	South Dakota	30.10
18	Tennessee	30.77
16	Texas	31.34
47	Utah	25.93
41	Vermont	27.12
32	Virginia	28.33
39	Washington	27.34
4	West Virginia	33.46
20	Wisconsin	30.54
35	Wyoming	27.89

RANK ORDER

RANK	STATE	PERCENT
1	South Carolina	34.68
2	Mississippi	34.52
3	Alabama	33.89
4	West Virginia	33.46
5	Ohio	33.43
6	Louisiana	33.39
7	Missouri	33.11
8	Michigan	33.03
9	Kentucky	32.96
10	North Dakota	32.87
11	Iowa	32.73
12	Indiana	32.70
13	Arkansas	31.83
14	Delaware	31.78
15	Pennsylvania	31.76
16	Texas	31.34
17	Maryland	30.78
18	Tennessee	30.77
19	North Carolina	30.65
20	Florida	30.54
20	Wisconsin	30.54
22	South Dakota	30.10
23	Alaska	30.03
24	Illinois	29.84
25	Idaho	29.28
25	Oregon	29.28
27	Oklahoma	29.05
28	Nebraska	29.00
29	New York	28.96
30	Montana	28.84
31	Rhode Island	28.48
32	Virginia	28.33
33	Maine	28.14
34	Minnesota	27.91
35	Wyoming	27.89
36	California	27.73
37	Nevada	27.67
38	New Jersey	27.53
39	Washington	27.34
40	Connecticut	27.16
41	Vermont	27.12
42	New Mexico	26.82
43	Massachusetts	26.67
44	Arizona	26.28
45	Kansas	26.06
46	New Hampshire	25.99
47	Utah	25.93
48	Georgia	24.07
49	Colorado	22.32
NA	Hawaii**	NA
	District of Columbia	29.15

Source: U.S. Department of Health and Human Services, Centers for Disease Control and Prevention
"1996 Behavioral Risk Factor Surveillance Summary Prevalence Report" (January 8, 1998)
*Persons 18 and older. Overweight is defined as men with a Body Mass Index (BMI) of 27.8 or greater and women with an index of 27.3 or greater. BMI is a ratio of height to weight. As an example, a person 5' 8" and weighing 185 pounds has a BMI of 28. See http://www.warner-lambert.com/info/bmi.html.
**Not available.

Number of Days in the Past Month When Physical Health was "Not Good": 1996

National Median = 2.98 Days*

ALPHA ORDER

RANK	STATE	DAYS
10	Alabama	3.27
47	Alaska	2.10
45	Arizona	2.16
21	Arkansas	3.08
19	California	3.13
32	Colorado	2.90
42	Connecticut	2.53
37	Delaware	2.76
7	Florida	3.40
48	Georgia	2.04
NA	Hawaii**	NA
34	Idaho	2.84
18	Illinois	3.15
6	Indiana	3.42
35	Iowa	2.82
48	Kansas	2.04
2	Kentucky	3.60
29	Louisiana	2.92
33	Maine	2.89
43	Maryland	2.49
14	Massachusetts	3.19
35	Michigan	2.82
27	Minnesota	2.95
13	Mississippi	3.20
5	Missouri	3.48
40	Montana	2.62
30	Nebraska	2.91
25	Nevada	2.99
26	New Hampshire	2.96
24	New Jersey	3.00
1	New Mexico	3.72
19	New York	3.13
39	North Carolina	2.67
3	North Dakota	3.56
41	Ohio	2.56
46	Oklahoma	2.13
23	Oregon	3.02
15	Pennsylvania	3.16
4	Rhode Island	3.51
38	South Carolina	2.68
44	South Dakota	2.25
12	Tennessee	3.22
8	Texas	3.32
22	Utah	3.07
15	Vermont	3.16
30	Virginia	2.91
9	Washington	3.28
11	West Virginia	3.25
15	Wisconsin	3.16
27	Wyoming	2.95

RANK ORDER

RANK	STATE	DAYS
1	New Mexico	3.72
2	Kentucky	3.60
3	North Dakota	3.56
4	Rhode Island	3.51
5	Missouri	3.48
6	Indiana	3.42
7	Florida	3.40
8	Texas	3.32
9	Washington	3.28
10	Alabama	3.27
11	West Virginia	3.25
12	Tennessee	3.22
13	Mississippi	3.20
14	Massachusetts	3.19
15	Pennsylvania	3.16
15	Vermont	3.16
15	Wisconsin	3.16
18	Illinois	3.15
19	California	3.13
19	New York	3.13
21	Arkansas	3.08
22	Utah	3.07
23	Oregon	3.02
24	New Jersey	3.00
25	Nevada	2.99
26	New Hampshire	2.96
27	Minnesota	2.95
27	Wyoming	2.95
29	Louisiana	2.92
30	Nebraska	2.91
30	Virginia	2.91
32	Colorado	2.90
33	Maine	2.89
34	Idaho	2.84
35	Iowa	2.82
35	Michigan	2.82
37	Delaware	2.76
38	South Carolina	2.68
39	North Carolina	2.67
40	Montana	2.62
41	Ohio	2.56
42	Connecticut	2.53
43	Maryland	2.49
44	South Dakota	2.25
45	Arizona	2.16
46	Oklahoma	2.13
47	Alaska	2.10
48	Georgia	2.04
48	Kansas	2.04
NA	Hawaii**	NA
	District of Columbia	2.50

Source: U.S. Department of Health and Human Services, Centers for Disease Control and Prevention
"1996 Behavioral Risk Factor Surveillance Summary Prevalence Report" (January 8, 1998)
*Persons 18 and older.
**Not available.

Average Number of Days in the Past Month When Mental Health was "Not Good": 1996
National Median = 2.97 Days*

ALPHA ORDER

RANK	STATE	DAYS
4	Alabama	3.35
19	Alaska	3.03
44	Arizona	2.15
24	Arkansas	2.97
22	California	2.98
6	Colorado	3.31
27	Connecticut	2.93
41	Delaware	2.30
12	Florida	3.18
43	Georgia	2.16
NA	Hawaii**	NA
25	Idaho	2.96
17	Illinois	3.07
9	Indiana	3.28
31	Iowa	2.86
47	Kansas	1.99
1	Kentucky	4.59
16	Louisiana	3.10
27	Maine	2.93
40	Maryland	2.33
5	Massachusetts	3.34
10	Michigan	3.25
11	Minnesota	3.19
42	Mississippi	2.28
19	Missouri	3.03
39	Montana	2.45
22	Nebraska	2.98
6	Nevada	3.31
33	New Hampshire	2.81
18	New Jersey	3.05
3	New Mexico	3.42
26	New York	2.95
46	North Carolina	2.01
34	North Dakota	2.77
48	Ohio	1.85
45	Oklahoma	2.05
13	Oregon	3.16
30	Pennsylvania	2.90
15	Rhode Island	3.12
32	South Carolina	2.82
49	South Dakota	1.75
37	Tennessee	2.53
8	Texas	3.29
2	Utah	3.63
29	Vermont	2.91
36	Virginia	2.61
13	Washington	3.16
38	West Virginia	2.47
21	Wisconsin	3.00
35	Wyoming	2.62

RANK ORDER

RANK	STATE	DAYS
1	Kentucky	4.59
2	Utah	3.63
3	New Mexico	3.42
4	Alabama	3.35
5	Massachusetts	3.34
6	Colorado	3.31
6	Nevada	3.31
8	Texas	3.29
9	Indiana	3.28
10	Michigan	3.25
11	Minnesota	3.19
12	Florida	3.18
13	Oregon	3.16
13	Washington	3.16
15	Rhode Island	3.12
16	Louisiana	3.10
17	Illinois	3.07
18	New Jersey	3.05
19	Alaska	3.03
19	Missouri	3.03
21	Wisconsin	3.00
22	California	2.98
22	Nebraska	2.98
24	Arkansas	2.97
25	Idaho	2.96
26	New York	2.95
27	Connecticut	2.93
27	Maine	2.93
29	Vermont	2.91
30	Pennsylvania	2.90
31	Iowa	2.86
32	South Carolina	2.82
33	New Hampshire	2.81
34	North Dakota	2.77
35	Wyoming	2.62
36	Virginia	2.61
37	Tennessee	2.53
38	West Virginia	2.47
39	Montana	2.45
40	Maryland	2.33
41	Delaware	2.30
42	Mississippi	2.28
43	Georgia	2.16
44	Arizona	2.15
45	Oklahoma	2.05
46	North Carolina	2.01
47	Kansas	1.99
48	Ohio	1.85
49	South Dakota	1.75
NA	Hawaii**	NA
	District of Columbia	3.02

Source: U.S. Department of Health and Human Services, Centers for Disease Control and Prevention
"1996 Behavioral Risk Factor Surveillance Summary Prevalence Report" (January 8, 1998)
*Persons 18 and older.
**Not available.

Percent of Adults Who Have Ever Been Tested for AIDS: 1996

National Median = 41.26% of Adults*

ALPHA ORDER

RANK	STATE	PERCENT
11	Alabama	46.50
8	Alaska	48.56
16	Arizona	44.38
15	Arkansas	44.63
NA	California**	NA
13	Colorado	45.89
22	Connecticut	41.64
12	Delaware	46.05
2	Florida	53.64
41	Georgia	33.63
NA	Hawaii**	NA
20	Idaho	42.59
25	Illinois	41.17
30	Indiana	39.37
42	Iowa	32.94
45	Kansas	30.12
39	Kentucky	34.59
7	Louisiana	49.04
40	Maine	34.41
5	Maryland	50.44
35	Massachusetts	38.05
18	Michigan	43.04
43	Minnesota	31.43
10	Mississippi	47.57
29	Missouri	39.68
37	Montana	35.44
38	Nebraska	35.01
1	Nevada	54.68
36	New Hampshire	36.86
14	New Jersey	45.67
6	New Mexico	50.23
26	New York	41.05
33	North Carolina	38.69
46	North Dakota	28.97
47	Ohio	28.10
34	Oklahoma	38.58
21	Oregon	42.47
23	Pennsylvania	41.63
9	Rhode Island	47.61
19	South Carolina	43.03
48	South Dakota	27.31
27	Tennessee	40.03
4	Texas	51.12
32	Utah	38.98
28	Vermont	39.81
3	Virginia	53.23
17	Washington	44.14
44	West Virginia	30.72
24	Wisconsin	41.26
30	Wyoming	39.37

RANK ORDER

RANK	STATE	PERCENT
1	Nevada	54.68
2	Florida	53.64
3	Virginia	53.23
4	Texas	51.12
5	Maryland	50.44
6	New Mexico	50.23
7	Louisiana	49.04
8	Alaska	48.56
9	Rhode Island	47.61
10	Mississippi	47.57
11	Alabama	46.50
12	Delaware	46.05
13	Colorado	45.89
14	New Jersey	45.67
15	Arkansas	44.63
16	Arizona	44.38
17	Washington	44.14
18	Michigan	43.04
19	South Carolina	43.03
20	Idaho	42.59
21	Oregon	42.47
22	Connecticut	41.64
23	Pennsylvania	41.63
24	Wisconsin	41.26
25	Illinois	41.17
26	New York	41.05
27	Tennessee	40.03
28	Vermont	39.81
29	Missouri	39.68
30	Indiana	39.37
30	Wyoming	39.37
32	Utah	38.98
33	North Carolina	38.69
34	Oklahoma	38.58
35	Massachusetts	38.05
36	New Hampshire	36.86
37	Montana	35.44
38	Nebraska	35.01
39	Kentucky	34.59
40	Maine	34.41
41	Georgia	33.63
42	Iowa	32.94
43	Minnesota	31.43
44	West Virginia	30.72
45	Kansas	30.12
46	North Dakota	28.97
47	Ohio	28.10
48	South Dakota	27.31
NA	California**	NA
NA	Hawaii**	NA
	District of Columbia	61.29

Source: U.S. Department of Health and Human Services, Centers for Disease Control and Prevention
"1996 Behavioral Risk Factor Surveillance Summary Prevalence Report" (January 8, 1998)

*Persons 18 to 64 years old.

**Not available.

Percent of Adults Who Believe They Have a Chance of Getting AIDS: 1996

National Median = 6.46% of Adults*

ALPHA ORDER

RANK	STATE	PERCENT
27	Alabama	6.20
41	Alaska	5.16
17	Arizona	6.74
6	Arkansas	7.84
NA	California**	NA
29	Colorado	6.14
15	Connecticut	6.92
34	Delaware	5.54
10	Florida	7.49
47	Georgia	3.86
NA	Hawaii**	NA
42	Idaho	5.14
7	Illinois	7.62
32	Indiana	5.76
12	Iowa	7.28
8	Kansas	7.60
34	Kentucky	5.54
20	Louisiana	6.65
22	Maine	6.49
45	Maryland	4.55
39	Massachusetts	5.41
30	Michigan	6.13
10	Minnesota	7.49
14	Mississippi	6.93
18	Missouri	6.73
44	Montana	4.69
2	Nebraska	10.00
5	Nevada	8.42
37	New Hampshire	5.45
8	New Jersey	7.60
28	New Mexico	6.15
16	New York	6.83
48	North Carolina	1.19
19	North Dakota	6.72
43	Ohio	5.04
21	Oklahoma	6.63
40	Oregon	5.28
13	Pennsylvania	7.19
31	Rhode Island	5.80
33	South Carolina	5.68
46	South Dakota	4.44
3	Tennessee	9.84
4	Texas	9.22
36	Utah	5.51
26	Vermont	6.22
25	Virginia	6.30
38	Washington	5.44
1	West Virginia	14.01
23	Wisconsin	6.46
24	Wyoming	6.38

RANK ORDER

RANK	STATE	PERCENT
1	West Virginia	14.01
2	Nebraska	10.00
3	Tennessee	9.84
4	Texas	9.22
5	Nevada	8.42
6	Arkansas	7.84
7	Illinois	7.62
8	Kansas	7.60
8	New Jersey	7.60
10	Florida	7.49
10	Minnesota	7.49
12	Iowa	7.28
13	Pennsylvania	7.19
14	Mississippi	6.93
15	Connecticut	6.92
16	New York	6.83
17	Arizona	6.74
18	Missouri	6.73
19	North Dakota	6.72
20	Louisiana	6.65
21	Oklahoma	6.63
22	Maine	6.49
23	Wisconsin	6.46
24	Wyoming	6.38
25	Virginia	6.30
26	Vermont	6.22
27	Alabama	6.20
28	New Mexico	6.15
29	Colorado	6.14
30	Michigan	6.13
31	Rhode Island	5.80
32	Indiana	5.76
33	South Carolina	5.68
34	Delaware	5.54
34	Kentucky	5.54
36	Utah	5.51
37	New Hampshire	5.45
38	Washington	5.44
39	Massachusetts	5.41
40	Oregon	5.28
41	Alaska	5.16
42	Idaho	5.14
43	Ohio	5.04
44	Montana	4.69
45	Maryland	4.55
46	South Dakota	4.44
47	Georgia	3.86
48	North Carolina	1.19
NA	California**	NA
NA	Hawaii**	NA
	District of Columbia	11.11

Source: U.S. Department of Health and Human Services, Centers for Disease Control and Prevention
   "1996 Behavioral Risk Factor Surveillance Summary Prevalence Report" (January 8, 1998)
*For persons 18 to 64 years old who believe their chances of getting the AIDS virus are "medium" or "high."
**Not available.

Safety Belt Usage Rate in 1997

National Average = 64% Use Safety Belts*

ALPHA ORDER				RANK ORDER		
RANK	STATE	PERCENT		RANK	STATE	PERCENT
40	Alabama	54		1	California	87
17	Alaska	69		2	New Mexico	85
37	Arizona	56		3	Washington	84
45	Arkansas	48		4	North Carolina	82
1	California	87		4	Oregon	82
37	Colorado	56		6	Hawaii	80
26	Connecticut	62		7	Iowa	75
19	Delaware	68		8	New York	74
22	Florida	64		8	Texas	74
26	Georgia	62		10	Montana	73
6	Hawaii	80		11	Wyoming	72
40	Idaho	54		12	Michigan	71
22	Illinois	64		12	Nevada	71
26	Indiana	62		12	Pennsylvania	71
7	Iowa	75		15	Maryland	70
40	Kansas	54		15	Virginia	70
39	Kentucky	55		17	Alaska	69
19	Louisiana	68		17	Vermont	69
44	Maine	50		19	Delaware	68
15	Maryland	70		19	Louisiana	68
40	Massachusetts	54		21	Nebraska	65
12	Michigan	71		22	Florida	64
22	Minnesota	64		22	Illinois	64
48	Mississippi	46		22	Minnesota	64
26	Missouri	62		25	Tennessee	63
10	Montana	73		26	Connecticut	62
21	Nebraska	65		26	Georgia	62
12	Nevada	71		26	Indiana	62
NA	New Hampshire**	NA		26	Missouri	62
33	New Jersey	60		26	Ohio	62
2	New Mexico	85		31	South Carolina	61
8	New York	74		31	Wisconsin	61
4	North Carolina	82		33	New Jersey	60
49	North Dakota	43		33	Utah	60
26	Ohio	62		35	Rhode Island	58
45	Oklahoma	48		35	West Virginia	58
4	Oregon	82		37	Arizona	56
12	Pennsylvania	71		37	Colorado	56
35	Rhode Island	58		39	Kentucky	55
31	South Carolina	61		40	Alabama	54
47	South Dakota	47		40	Idaho	54
25	Tennessee	63		40	Kansas	54
8	Texas	74		40	Massachusetts	54
33	Utah	60		44	Maine	50
17	Vermont	69		45	Arkansas	48
15	Virginia	70		45	Oklahoma	48
3	Washington	84		47	South Dakota	47
35	West Virginia	58		48	Mississippi	46
31	Wisconsin	61		49	North Dakota	43
11	Wyoming	72		NA	New Hampshire**	NA
					District of Columbia	58

Source: U.S. Department of Transportation, National Highway Safety Traffic Safety Administration
     "Key Provisions of Safety Belt Use" (September 1997)
*As of January 1997. National average is a simple average of reporting states' rates.
**Not reported.

Percent of Adults Whose Children Use a Car Safety Seat: 1995

National Median = 96.51% of Adults*

ALPHA ORDER

RANK ORDER

RANK	STATE	PERCENT
27	Alabama	95.79
37	Alaska	94.24
41	Arizona	93.45
3	Arkansas	99.13
46	California	90.66
30	Colorado	95.62
49	Connecticut	89.08
2	Delaware	99.20
27	Florida	95.79
13	Georgia	98.12
7	Hawaii	98.83
43	Idaho	91.89
50	Illinois	88.04
1	Indiana	99.65
20	Iowa	96.91
17	Kansas	97.40
25	Kentucky	96.64
47	Louisiana	90.32
12	Maine	98.21
9	Maryland	98.52
4	Massachusetts	99.06
36	Michigan	94.47
19	Minnesota	96.98
26	Mississippi	96.38
44	Missouri	91.53
39	Montana	93.87
18	Nebraska	97.24
34	Nevada	94.69
21	New Hampshire	96.90
29	New Jersey	95.70
32	New Mexico	95.40
38	New York	93.93
6	North Carolina	98.84
24	North Dakota	96.80
10	Ohio	98.48
15	Oklahoma	97.97
42	Oregon	93.19
48	Pennsylvania	89.53
11	Rhode Island	98.24
8	South Carolina	98.57
23	South Dakota	96.89
16	Tennessee	97.85
33	Texas	95.33
35	Utah	94.52
5	Vermont	98.87
40	Virginia	93.76
21	Washington	96.90
14	West Virginia	98.03
45	Wisconsin	90.86
31	Wyoming	95.57

RANK	STATE	PERCENT
1	Indiana	99.65
2	Delaware	99.20
3	Arkansas	99.13
4	Massachusetts	99.06
5	Vermont	98.87
6	North Carolina	98.84
7	Hawaii	98.83
8	South Carolina	98.57
9	Maryland	98.52
10	Ohio	98.48
11	Rhode Island	98.24
12	Maine	98.21
13	Georgia	98.12
14	West Virginia	98.03
15	Oklahoma	97.97
16	Tennessee	97.85
17	Kansas	97.40
18	Nebraska	97.24
19	Minnesota	96.98
20	Iowa	96.91
21	New Hampshire	96.90
21	Washington	96.90
23	South Dakota	96.89
24	North Dakota	96.80
25	Kentucky	96.64
26	Mississippi	96.38
27	Alabama	95.79
27	Florida	95.79
29	New Jersey	95.70
30	Colorado	95.62
31	Wyoming	95.57
32	New Mexico	95.40
33	Texas	95.33
34	Nevada	94.69
35	Utah	94.52
36	Michigan	94.47
37	Alaska	94.24
38	New York	93.93
39	Montana	93.87
40	Virginia	93.76
41	Arizona	93.45
42	Oregon	93.19
43	Idaho	91.89
44	Missouri	91.53
45	Wisconsin	90.86
46	California	90.66
47	Louisiana	90.32
48	Pennsylvania	89.53
49	Connecticut	89.08
50	Illinois	88.04

District of Columbia**   NA

Source: U.S. Department of Health and Human Services, Centers for Disease Control and Prevention
"1995 Behavioral Risk Factor Surveillance Summary Prevalence Report" (December 10, 1996)
*Persons whose children under 5 years old "always or nearly always use a safety seat".
**Not available.

VIII. APPENDIX

Population Charts

Population in 1997

National Total = 267,636,061*

ALPHA ORDER

RANK	STATE	POPULATION	% of USA
23	Alabama	4,319,154	1.61%
48	Alaska	609,311	0.23%
21	Arizona	4,554,966	1.70%
33	Arkansas	2,522,819	0.94%
1	California	32,268,301	12.06%
25	Colorado	3,892,644	1.45%
28	Connecticut	3,269,858	1.22%
46	Delaware	731,581	0.27%
4	Florida	14,653,945	5.48%
10	Georgia	7,486,242	2.80%
41	Hawaii	1,186,602	0.44%
40	Idaho	1,210,232	0.45%
6	Illinois	11,895,849	4.44%
14	Indiana	5,864,108	2.19%
30	Iowa	2,852,423	1.07%
32	Kansas	2,594,840	0.97%
24	Kentucky	3,908,124	1.46%
22	Louisiana	4,351,769	1.63%
39	Maine	1,242,051	0.46%
19	Maryland	5,094,289	1.90%
13	Massachusetts	6,117,520	2.29%
8	Michigan	9,773,892	3.65%
20	Minnesota	4,685,549	1.75%
31	Mississippi	2,730,501	1.02%
16	Missouri	5,402,058	2.02%
44	Montana	878,810	0.33%
38	Nebraska	1,656,870	0.62%
37	Nevada	1,676,809	0.63%
42	New Hampshire	1,172,709	0.44%
9	New Jersey	8,052,849	3.01%
36	New Mexico	1,729,751	0.65%
3	New York	18,137,226	6.78%
11	North Carolina	7,425,183	2.77%
47	North Dakota	640,883	0.24%
7	Ohio	11,186,331	4.18%
27	Oklahoma	3,317,091	1.24%
29	Oregon	3,243,487	1.21%
5	Pennsylvania	12,019,661	4.49%
43	Rhode Island	987,429	0.37%
26	South Carolina	3,760,181	1.40%
45	South Dakota	737,973	0.28%
17	Tennessee	5,368,198	2.01%
2	Texas	19,439,337	7.26%
34	Utah	2,059,148	0.77%
49	Vermont	588,978	0.22%
12	Virginia	6,733,996	2.52%
15	Washington	5,610,362	2.10%
35	West Virginia	1,815,787	0.68%
18	Wisconsin	5,169,677	1.93%
50	Wyoming	479,743	0.18%

RANK ORDER

RANK	STATE	POPULATION	% of USA
1	California	32,268,301	12.06%
2	Texas	19,439,337	7.26%
3	New York	18,137,226	6.78%
4	Florida	14,653,945	5.48%
5	Pennsylvania	12,019,661	4.49%
6	Illinois	11,895,849	4.44%
7	Ohio	11,186,331	4.18%
8	Michigan	9,773,892	3.65%
9	New Jersey	8,052,849	3.01%
10	Georgia	7,486,242	2.80%
11	North Carolina	7,425,183	2.77%
12	Virginia	6,733,996	2.52%
13	Massachusetts	6,117,520	2.29%
14	Indiana	5,864,108	2.19%
15	Washington	5,610,362	2.10%
16	Missouri	5,402,058	2.02%
17	Tennessee	5,368,198	2.01%
18	Wisconsin	5,169,677	1.93%
19	Maryland	5,094,289	1.90%
20	Minnesota	4,685,549	1.75%
21	Arizona	4,554,966	1.70%
22	Louisiana	4,351,769	1.63%
23	Alabama	4,319,154	1.61%
24	Kentucky	3,908,124	1.46%
25	Colorado	3,892,644	1.45%
26	South Carolina	3,760,181	1.40%
27	Oklahoma	3,317,091	1.24%
28	Connecticut	3,269,858	1.22%
29	Oregon	3,243,487	1.21%
30	Iowa	2,852,423	1.07%
31	Mississippi	2,730,501	1.02%
32	Kansas	2,594,840	0.97%
33	Arkansas	2,522,819	0.94%
34	Utah	2,059,148	0.77%
35	West Virginia	1,815,787	0.68%
36	New Mexico	1,729,751	0.65%
37	Nevada	1,676,809	0.63%
38	Nebraska	1,656,870	0.62%
39	Maine	1,242,051	0.46%
40	Idaho	1,210,232	0.45%
41	Hawaii	1,186,602	0.44%
42	New Hampshire	1,172,709	0.44%
43	Rhode Island	987,429	0.37%
44	Montana	878,810	0.33%
45	South Dakota	737,973	0.28%
46	Delaware	731,581	0.27%
47	North Dakota	640,883	0.24%
48	Alaska	609,311	0.23%
49	Vermont	588,978	0.22%
50	Wyoming	479,743	0.18%
	District of Columbia	528,964	0.20%

Source: U.S. Bureau of the Census
    Press Release (CB97-213, December 30, 1997)
*As of July 1, 1997. Includes armed forces residing in each state.

Population in 1996

National Total = 265,179,411*

ALPHA ORDER

RANK	STATE	POPULATION	% of USA
23	Alabama	4,287,178	1.62%
48	Alaska	604,966	0.23%
21	Arizona	4,434,340	1.67%
33	Arkansas	2,506,293	0.95%
1	California	31,857,646	12.01%
25	Colorado	3,816,179	1.44%
28	Connecticut	3,267,293	1.23%
46	Delaware	723,475	0.27%
4	Florida	14,418,917	5.44%
10	Georgia	7,334,274	2.77%
41	Hawaii	1,182,948	0.45%
40	Idaho	1,187,597	0.45%
6	Illinois	11,845,316	4.47%
14	Indiana	5,828,090	2.20%
30	Iowa	2,848,033	1.07%
32	Kansas	2,579,149	0.97%
24	Kentucky	3,882,071	1.46%
22	Louisiana	4,340,818	1.64%
39	Maine	1,238,566	0.47%
19	Maryland	5,060,296	1.91%
13	Massachusetts	6,085,395	2.29%
8	Michigan	9,730,925	3.67%
20	Minnesota	4,648,596	1.75%
31	Mississippi	2,710,750	1.02%
16	Missouri	5,363,669	2.02%
44	Montana	876,684	0.33%
37	Nebraska	1,648,696	0.62%
38	Nevada	1,600,810	0.60%
42	New Hampshire	1,160,213	0.44%
9	New Jersey	8,001,850	3.02%
36	New Mexico	1,711,256	0.65%
3	New York	18,134,226	6.84%
11	North Carolina	7,309,055	2.76%
47	North Dakota	642,633	0.24%
7	Ohio	11,162,797	4.21%
27	Oklahoma	3,295,315	1.24%
29	Oregon	3,196,313	1.21%
5	Pennsylvania	12,040,084	4.54%
43	Rhode Island	988,283	0.37%
26	South Carolina	3,716,645	1.40%
45	South Dakota	737,561	0.28%
17	Tennessee	5,307,381	2.00%
2	Texas	19,091,207	7.20%
34	Utah	2,017,573	0.76%
49	Vermont	586,461	0.22%
12	Virginia	6,666,167	2.51%
15	Washington	5,519,525	2.08%
35	West Virginia	1,820,407	0.69%
18	Wisconsin	5,146,199	1.94%
50	Wyoming	480,011	0.18%

RANK ORDER

RANK	STATE	POPULATION	% of USA
1	California	31,857,646	12.01%
2	Texas	19,091,207	7.20%
3	New York	18,134,226	6.84%
4	Florida	14,418,917	5.44%
5	Pennsylvania	12,040,084	4.54%
6	Illinois	11,845,316	4.47%
7	Ohio	11,162,797	4.21%
8	Michigan	9,730,925	3.67%
9	New Jersey	8,001,850	3.02%
10	Georgia	7,334,274	2.77%
11	North Carolina	7,309,055	2.76%
12	Virginia	6,666,167	2.51%
13	Massachusetts	6,085,395	2.29%
14	Indiana	5,828,090	2.20%
15	Washington	5,519,525	2.08%
16	Missouri	5,363,669	2.02%
17	Tennessee	5,307,381	2.00%
18	Wisconsin	5,146,199	1.94%
19	Maryland	5,060,296	1.91%
20	Minnesota	4,648,596	1.75%
21	Arizona	4,434,340	1.67%
22	Louisiana	4,340,818	1.64%
23	Alabama	4,287,178	1.62%
24	Kentucky	3,882,071	1.46%
25	Colorado	3,816,179	1.44%
26	South Carolina	3,716,645	1.40%
27	Oklahoma	3,295,315	1.24%
28	Connecticut	3,267,293	1.23%
29	Oregon	3,196,313	1.21%
30	Iowa	2,848,033	1.07%
31	Mississippi	2,710,750	1.02%
32	Kansas	2,579,149	0.97%
33	Arkansas	2,506,293	0.95%
34	Utah	2,017,573	0.76%
35	West Virginia	1,820,407	0.69%
36	New Mexico	1,711,256	0.65%
37	Nebraska	1,648,696	0.62%
38	Nevada	1,600,810	0.60%
39	Maine	1,238,566	0.47%
40	Idaho	1,187,597	0.45%
41	Hawaii	1,182,948	0.45%
42	New Hampshire	1,160,213	0.44%
43	Rhode Island	988,283	0.37%
44	Montana	876,684	0.33%
45	South Dakota	737,561	0.28%
46	Delaware	723,475	0.27%
47	North Dakota	642,633	0.24%
48	Alaska	604,966	0.23%
49	Vermont	586,461	0.22%
50	Wyoming	480,011	0.18%
	District of Columbia	539,279	0.20%

Source: U.S. Bureau of the Census
   Press Release (CB97-213, December 30, 1997)
*Includes armed forces residing in each state. This updates earlier 1996 estimates.

Male Population in 1996

National Total = 129,810,215 Males

RANK	STATE	MALES	% of USA
23	Alabama	2,054,281	1.58%
48	Alaska	319,298	0.25%
21	Arizona	2,192,581	1.69%
33	Arkansas	1,214,148	0.94%
1	California	15,963,923	12.30%
24	Colorado	1,896,268	1.46%
28	Connecticut	1,591,547	1.23%
46	Delaware	353,257	0.27%
4	Florida	6,993,990	5.39%
10	Georgia	3,583,009	2.76%
40	Hawaii	597,342	0.46%
41	Idaho	594,604	0.46%
6	Illinois	5,784,530	4.46%
14	Indiana	2,846,191	2.19%
30	Iowa	1,389,670	1.07%
32	Kansas	1,266,212	0.98%
25	Kentucky	1,886,869	1.45%
22	Louisiana	2,097,558	1.62%
39	Maine	607,220	0.47%
19	Maryland	2,469,575	1.90%
13	Massachusetts	2,940,798	2.27%
8	Michigan	4,676,908	3.60%
20	Minnesota	2,298,010	1.77%
31	Mississippi	1,304,446	1.00%
16	Missouri	2,597,463	2.00%
44	Montana	438,111	0.34%
38	Nebraska	809,208	0.62%
37	Nevada	817,422	0.63%
42	New Hampshire	572,415	0.44%
9	New Jersey	3,875,876	2.99%
36	New Mexico	845,621	0.65%
3	New York	8,760,858	6.75%
11	North Carolina	3,558,460	2.74%
47	North Dakota	321,408	0.25%
7	Ohio	5,409,219	4.17%
27	Oklahoma	1,615,192	1.24%
29	Oregon	1,583,503	1.22%
5	Pennsylvania	5,804,443	4.47%
43	Rhode Island	476,535	0.37%
26	South Carolina	1,786,976	1.38%
45	South Dakota	361,074	0.28%
17	Tennessee	2,572,358	1.98%
2	Texas	9,450,785	7.28%
34	Utah	996,638	0.77%
49	Vermont	290,010	0.22%
12	Virginia	3,271,690	2.52%
15	Washington	2,756,056	2.12%
35	West Virginia	881,249	0.68%
18	Wisconsin	2,538,652	1.96%
50	Wyoming	242,375	0.19%

RANK	STATE	MALES	% of USA
1	California	15,963,923	12.30%
2	Texas	9,450,785	7.28%
3	New York	8,760,858	6.75%
4	Florida	6,993,990	5.39%
5	Pennsylvania	5,804,443	4.47%
6	Illinois	5,784,530	4.46%
7	Ohio	5,409,219	4.17%
8	Michigan	4,676,908	3.60%
9	New Jersey	3,875,876	2.99%
10	Georgia	3,583,009	2.76%
11	North Carolina	3,558,460	2.74%
12	Virginia	3,271,690	2.52%
13	Massachusetts	2,940,798	2.27%
14	Indiana	2,846,191	2.19%
15	Washington	2,756,056	2.12%
16	Missouri	2,597,463	2.00%
17	Tennessee	2,572,358	1.98%
18	Wisconsin	2,538,652	1.96%
19	Maryland	2,469,575	1.90%
20	Minnesota	2,298,010	1.77%
21	Arizona	2,192,581	1.69%
22	Louisiana	2,097,558	1.62%
23	Alabama	2,054,281	1.58%
24	Colorado	1,896,268	1.46%
25	Kentucky	1,886,869	1.45%
26	South Carolina	1,786,976	1.38%
27	Oklahoma	1,615,192	1.24%
28	Connecticut	1,591,547	1.23%
29	Oregon	1,583,503	1.22%
30	Iowa	1,389,670	1.07%
31	Mississippi	1,304,446	1.00%
32	Kansas	1,266,212	0.98%
33	Arkansas	1,214,148	0.94%
34	Utah	996,638	0.77%
35	West Virginia	881,249	0.68%
36	New Mexico	845,621	0.65%
37	Nevada	817,422	0.63%
38	Nebraska	809,208	0.62%
39	Maine	607,220	0.47%
40	Hawaii	597,342	0.46%
41	Idaho	594,604	0.46%
42	New Hampshire	572,415	0.44%
43	Rhode Island	476,535	0.37%
44	Montana	438,111	0.34%
45	South Dakota	361,074	0.28%
46	Delaware	353,257	0.27%
47	North Dakota	321,408	0.25%
48	Alaska	319,298	0.25%
49	Vermont	290,010	0.22%
50	Wyoming	242,375	0.19%
	District of Columbia	254,383	0.20%

Source: U.S. Bureau of the Census
"Estimates of the Population of the States by Selected Age Groups and Sex" (CB97-64, April 21, 1997)
(http://www.census.gov/population/estimates/state/96agesex.txt)

Female Population in 1996

National Total = 135,473,568 Females

ALPHA ORDER

RANK	STATE	FEMALES	% of USA
23	Alabama	2,218,803	1.64%
49	Alaska	287,709	0.21%
22	Arizona	2,235,487	1.65%
33	Arkansas	1,295,645	0.96%
1	California	15,914,311	11.75%
25	Colorado	1,926,408	1.42%
28	Connecticut	1,682,691	1.24%
45	Delaware	371,585	0.27%
4	Florida	7,405,995	5.47%
10	Georgia	3,770,216	2.78%
42	Hawaii	586,381	0.43%
40	Idaho	594,647	0.44%
6	Illinois	6,062,014	4.47%
14	Indiana	2,994,337	2.21%
30	Iowa	1,462,122	1.08%
32	Kansas	1,305,938	0.96%
24	Kentucky	1,996,854	1.47%
21	Louisiana	2,253,021	1.66%
39	Maine	636,096	0.47%
19	Maryland	2,602,029	1.92%
13	Massachusetts	3,151,554	2.33%
8	Michigan	4,917,442	3.63%
20	Minnesota	2,359,748	1.74%
31	Mississippi	1,411,669	1.04%
16	Missouri	2,761,229	2.04%
44	Montana	441,261	0.33%
37	Nebraska	842,885	0.62%
38	Nevada	785,741	0.58%
41	New Hampshire	590,066	0.44%
9	New Jersey	4,112,057	3.04%
36	New Mexico	867,786	0.64%
3	New York	9,423,916	6.96%
11	North Carolina	3,764,410	2.78%
47	North Dakota	322,131	0.24%
7	Ohio	5,763,563	4.25%
27	Oklahoma	1,685,710	1.24%
29	Oregon	1,620,232	1.20%
5	Pennsylvania	6,251,669	4.61%
43	Rhode Island	513,690	0.38%
26	South Carolina	1,911,770	1.41%
46	South Dakota	371,331	0.27%
17	Tennessee	2,747,296	2.03%
2	Texas	9,677,476	7.14%
34	Utah	1,003,856	0.74%
48	Vermont	298,644	0.22%
12	Virginia	3,403,761	2.51%
15	Washington	2,776,883	2.05%
35	West Virginia	944,505	0.70%
18	Wisconsin	2,621,143	1.93%
50	Wyoming	239,025	0.18%

RANK ORDER

RANK	STATE	FEMALES	% of USA
1	California	15,914,311	11.75%
2	Texas	9,677,476	7.14%
3	New York	9,423,916	6.96%
4	Florida	7,405,995	5.47%
5	Pennsylvania	6,251,669	4.61%
6	Illinois	6,062,014	4.47%
7	Ohio	5,763,563	4.25%
8	Michigan	4,917,442	3.63%
9	New Jersey	4,112,057	3.04%
10	Georgia	3,770,216	2.78%
11	North Carolina	3,764,410	2.78%
12	Virginia	3,403,761	2.51%
13	Massachusetts	3,151,554	2.33%
14	Indiana	2,994,337	2.21%
15	Washington	2,776,883	2.05%
16	Missouri	2,761,229	2.04%
17	Tennessee	2,747,296	2.03%
18	Wisconsin	2,621,143	1.93%
19	Maryland	2,602,029	1.92%
20	Minnesota	2,359,748	1.74%
21	Louisiana	2,253,021	1.66%
22	Arizona	2,235,487	1.65%
23	Alabama	2,218,803	1.64%
24	Kentucky	1,996,854	1.47%
25	Colorado	1,926,408	1.42%
26	South Carolina	1,911,770	1.41%
27	Oklahoma	1,685,710	1.24%
28	Connecticut	1,682,691	1.24%
29	Oregon	1,620,232	1.20%
30	Iowa	1,462,122	1.08%
31	Mississippi	1,411,669	1.04%
32	Kansas	1,305,938	0.96%
33	Arkansas	1,295,645	0.96%
34	Utah	1,003,856	0.74%
35	West Virginia	944,505	0.70%
36	New Mexico	867,786	0.64%
37	Nebraska	842,885	0.62%
38	Nevada	785,741	0.58%
39	Maine	636,096	0.47%
40	Idaho	594,647	0.44%
41	New Hampshire	590,066	0.44%
42	Hawaii	586,381	0.43%
43	Rhode Island	513,690	0.38%
44	Montana	441,261	0.33%
45	Delaware	371,585	0.27%
46	South Dakota	371,331	0.27%
47	North Dakota	322,131	0.24%
48	Vermont	298,644	0.22%
49	Alaska	287,709	0.21%
50	Wyoming	239,025	0.18%
	District of Columbia	288,830	0.21%

Source: U.S. Bureau of the Census
"Estimates of the Population of the States by Selected Age Groups and Sex" (CB97-64, April 21, 1997)
(http://www.census.gov/population/estimates/state/96agesex.txt)

Population in 1995

National Total = 262,760,639*

	ALPHA ORDER				RANK ORDER		
RANK	STATE	POPULATION	% of USA	RANK	STATE	POPULATION	% of USA
23	Alabama	4,261,963	1.62%	1	California	31,558,406	12.01%
48	Alaska	601,646	0.23%	2	Texas	18,737,574	7.13%
22	Arizona	4,308,188	1.64%	3	New York	18,145,847	6.91%
33	Arkansas	2,480,819	0.94%	4	Florida	14,181,147	5.40%
1	California	31,558,406	12.01%	5	Pennsylvania	12,045,956	4.58%
25	Colorado	3,741,575	1.42%	6	Illinois	11,794,631	4.49%
28	Connecticut	3,266,775	1.24%	7	Ohio	11,132,614	4.24%
46	Delaware	715,700	0.27%	8	Michigan	9,655,305	3.67%
4	Florida	14,181,147	5.40%	9	New Jersey	7,955,750	3.03%
10	Georgia	7,192,305	2.74%	10	Georgia	7,192,305	2.74%
40	Hawaii	1,178,824	0.45%	11	North Carolina	7,186,912	2.74%
41	Idaho	1,164,887	0.44%	12	Virginia	6,601,122	2.51%
6	Illinois	11,794,631	4.49%	13	Massachusetts	6,060,566	2.31%
14	Indiana	5,787,839	2.20%	14	Indiana	5,787,839	2.20%
30	Iowa	2,840,571	1.08%	15	Washington	5,435,893	2.07%
32	Kansas	2,569,619	0.98%	16	Missouri	5,324,825	2.03%
24	Kentucky	3,856,212	1.47%	17	Tennessee	5,235,358	1.99%
21	Louisiana	4,328,552	1.65%	18	Wisconsin	5,113,124	1.95%
39	Maine	1,234,115	0.47%	19	Maryland	5,027,451	1.91%
19	Maryland	5,027,451	1.91%	20	Minnesota	4,606,797	1.75%
13	Massachusetts	6,060,566	2.31%	21	Louisiana	4,328,552	1.65%
8	Michigan	9,655,305	3.67%	22	Arizona	4,308,188	1.64%
20	Minnesota	4,606,797	1.75%	23	Alabama	4,261,963	1.62%
31	Mississippi	2,690,563	1.02%	24	Kentucky	3,856,212	1.47%
16	Missouri	5,324,825	2.03%	25	Colorado	3,741,575	1.42%
44	Montana	868,748	0.33%	26	South Carolina	3,683,395	1.40%
37	Nebraska	1,636,275	0.62%	27	Oklahoma	3,271,413	1.25%
38	Nevada	1,529,549	0.58%	28	Connecticut	3,266,775	1.24%
42	New Hampshire	1,146,411	0.44%	29	Oregon	3,142,978	1.20%
9	New Jersey	7,955,750	3.03%	30	Iowa	2,840,571	1.08%
36	New Mexico	1,686,288	0.64%	31	Mississippi	2,690,563	1.02%
3	New York	18,145,847	6.91%	32	Kansas	2,569,619	0.98%
11	North Carolina	7,186,912	2.74%	33	Arkansas	2,480,819	0.94%
47	North Dakota	641,344	0.24%	34	Utah	1,974,363	0.75%
7	Ohio	11,132,614	4.24%	35	West Virginia	1,821,957	0.69%
27	Oklahoma	3,271,413	1.25%	36	New Mexico	1,686,288	0.64%
29	Oregon	3,142,978	1.20%	37	Nebraska	1,636,275	0.62%
5	Pennsylvania	12,045,956	4.58%	38	Nevada	1,529,549	0.58%
43	Rhode Island	989,871	0.38%	39	Maine	1,234,115	0.47%
26	South Carolina	3,683,395	1.40%	40	Hawaii	1,178,824	0.45%
45	South Dakota	734,932	0.28%	41	Idaho	1,164,887	0.44%
17	Tennessee	5,235,358	1.99%	42	New Hampshire	1,146,411	0.44%
2	Texas	18,737,574	7.13%	43	Rhode Island	989,871	0.38%
34	Utah	1,974,363	0.75%	44	Montana	868,748	0.33%
49	Vermont	582,848	0.22%	45	South Dakota	734,932	0.28%
12	Virginia	6,601,122	2.51%	46	Delaware	715,700	0.27%
15	Washington	5,435,893	2.07%	47	North Dakota	641,344	0.24%
35	West Virginia	1,821,957	0.69%	48	Alaska	601,646	0.23%
18	Wisconsin	5,113,124	1.95%	49	Vermont	582,848	0.22%
50	Wyoming	478,532	0.18%	50	Wyoming	478,532	0.18%
					District of Columbia	552,304	0.21%

Source: U.S. Bureau of the Census
  Press Release (CB97-213, December 30, 1997)
Includes armed forces residing in each state. This updates earlier 1995 estimates.

Population in 1993

National Total = 257,752,702*

ALPHA ORDER			
RANK	STATE	POPULATION	% of USA
22	Alabama	4,192,560	1.63%
48	Alaska	596,808	0.23%
23	Arizona	3,994,223	1.55%
33	Arkansas	2,424,010	0.94%
1	California	31,183,081	12.10%
26	Colorado	3,563,364	1.38%
27	Connecticut	3,273,395	1.27%
46	Delaware	698,253	0.27%
4	Florida	13,711,576	5.32%
11	Georgia	6,896,173	2.68%
40	Hawaii	1,160,403	0.45%
42	Idaho	1,101,086	0.43%
6	Illinois	11,675,123	4.53%
14	Indiana	5,700,243	2.21%
30	Iowa	2,820,102	1.09%
32	Kansas	2,534,668	0.98%
24	Kentucky	3,792,623	1.47%
21	Louisiana	4,285,043	1.66%
39	Maine	1,236,619	0.48%
19	Maryland	4,944,742	1.92%
13	Massachusetts	6,007,539	2.33%
8	Michigan	9,524,255	3.70%
20	Minnesota	4,523,992	1.76%
31	Mississippi	2,635,197	1.02%
16	Missouri	5,237,867	2.03%
44	Montana	840,023	0.33%
37	Nebraska	1,612,625	0.63%
38	Nevada	1,382,480	0.54%
41	New Hampshire	1,121,689	0.44%
9	New Jersey	7,868,516	3.05%
36	New Mexico	1,616,737	0.63%
2	New York	18,139,150	7.04%
10	North Carolina	6,947,919	2.70%
47	North Dakota	637,205	0.25%
7	Ohio	11,058,454	4.29%
28	Oklahoma	3,228,876	1.25%
29	Oregon	3,035,788	1.18%
5	Pennsylvania	12,022,378	4.66%
43	Rhode Island	998,284	0.39%
25	South Carolina	3,624,570	1.41%
45	South Dakota	722,653	0.28%
17	Tennessee	5,082,518	1.97%
3	Texas	18,035,131	7.00%
34	Utah	1,874,575	0.73%
49	Vermont	573,959	0.22%
12	Virginia	6,465,292	2.51%
15	Washington	5,250,176	2.04%
35	West Virginia	1,816,343	0.70%
18	Wisconsin	5,038,350	1.95%
50	Wyoming	469,076	0.18%

RANK ORDER			
RANK	STATE	POPULATION	% of USA
1	California	31,183,081	12.10%
2	New York	18,139,150	7.04%
3	Texas	18,035,131	7.00%
4	Florida	13,711,576	5.32%
5	Pennsylvania	12,022,378	4.66%
6	Illinois	11,675,123	4.53%
7	Ohio	11,058,454	4.29%
8	Michigan	9,524,255	3.70%
9	New Jersey	7,868,516	3.05%
10	North Carolina	6,947,919	2.70%
11	Georgia	6,896,173	2.68%
12	Virginia	6,465,292	2.51%
13	Massachusetts	6,007,539	2.33%
14	Indiana	5,700,243	2.21%
15	Washington	5,250,176	2.04%
16	Missouri	5,237,867	2.03%
17	Tennessee	5,082,518	1.97%
18	Wisconsin	5,038,350	1.95%
19	Maryland	4,944,742	1.92%
20	Minnesota	4,523,992	1.76%
21	Louisiana	4,285,043	1.66%
22	Alabama	4,192,560	1.63%
23	Arizona	3,994,223	1.55%
24	Kentucky	3,792,623	1.47%
25	South Carolina	3,624,570	1.41%
26	Colorado	3,563,364	1.38%
27	Connecticut	3,273,395	1.27%
28	Oklahoma	3,228,876	1.25%
29	Oregon	3,035,788	1.18%
30	Iowa	2,820,102	1.09%
31	Mississippi	2,635,197	1.02%
32	Kansas	2,534,668	0.98%
33	Arkansas	2,424,010	0.94%
34	Utah	1,874,575	0.73%
35	West Virginia	1,816,343	0.70%
36	New Mexico	1,616,737	0.63%
37	Nebraska	1,612,625	0.63%
38	Nevada	1,382,480	0.54%
39	Maine	1,236,619	0.48%
40	Hawaii	1,160,403	0.45%
41	New Hampshire	1,121,689	0.44%
42	Idaho	1,101,086	0.43%
43	Rhode Island	998,284	0.39%
44	Montana	840,023	0.33%
45	South Dakota	722,653	0.28%
46	Delaware	698,253	0.27%
47	North Dakota	637,205	0.25%
48	Alaska	596,808	0.23%
49	Vermont	573,959	0.22%
50	Wyoming	469,076	0.18%
	District of Columbia	576,990	0.22%

Source: U.S. Bureau of the Census
      Press Release (CB97-213, December 30, 1997)
*Includes armed forces residing in each state. This updates earlier 1993 estimates.

IX. SOURCES

American Academy of Family Physicians
8880 Ward Parkway
Kansas City, MO 64114-2797
816-333-9700
Internet: www.aafp.org

American Academy of Physicians Assistants
950 North Washington Street
Alexandria, VA 22314-1552
703-333-9700
Internet: www.aapa.org

American Association of Health Plans
1129 20th Street, NW., Suite 600
Washington, DC 20036-3421
202-778-3200
Internet: www.aahp.org

American Cancer Society, Inc.
1599 Clifton Road, NE.
Atlanta, GA 30329-4251
800-227-2345
Internet: http://www.cancer.org

American Dental Association
211 E. Chicago Ave.
Chicago, IL 60611
312-440-2500
Internet: www.ada.org

American Hospital Association
One North Franklin
Chicago, IL 60606-3401
312-422-3501
Internet: www.aha.org

American Medical Association
515 North State Street
Chicago, IL 60610
312-464-5000
Internet: http://www.ama-assn.org

American Osteopathic Association
142 East Ontario Street
Chicago, IL 60611
312-202-8000
Internet: www.am-osteo-assn.org

American Podiatric Medical Association
9312 Old Georgetown Road
Bethesda, MD 20814-1698
301-571-9200
Internet: www.apma.org

Census Bureau
3 Silver Hill and Suitland Roads
Suitland, MD 20746
301-457-2794
Internet: http://www.census.gov

Centers for Disease Control and Prevention
1600 Clifton Road, NE.
Atlanta, GA 30333
404-639-3286 (Public Affairs)
800-458-5231 (AIDS Clearinghouse)
Internet: http://www.cdc.gov

Distilled Spirits Council of the U.S., Inc.
1250 Eye Street, NW., Ste. 900
Washington, DC 20005
202-628-3544
Internet: http://www.discus.health.org

Federation of Chiropractic Licensing Boards
901 54th Ave., Ste. 101
Greeley, CO 80634
970-356-3500
Internet: www.sni.net/fclb/

Health Care Financing Administration
U.S. Department of Health and Human Services
7500 Security Boulevard
Baltimore, MD 21244
410-786-3000
Internet: http://www.hcfa.gov

Health Insurance Association of America
555 13th Street, NW., Suite 600 East
Washington, DC 20004
202-824-1600
Internet: www.hiaa.org

National Center for Health Statistics
U.S. Department of Health and Human Services
6525 Belcrest Road
Hyattsville, MD 20782
301-436-8951 (vital statistics division)
Internet: http://www.cdc.gov/nchswww/

National Sporting Goods Association
1699 Wall Street, Suite 700
Mt. Prospect, IL 60056-5780
847-439-4000
Internet: www.nsga.org

Smoking and Health Office
Centers for Disease Control and Prevention
4770 Buford Hwy, NE., Mail Stop K-50
Atlanta, GA 30341-3724
770-488-5705
www.cdc.gov/nccdphp/osh/oshresfa.htm

X. INDEX

X. INDEX (continued)

X. INDEX (continued)

CHAPTER INDEX

HOW TO USE THIS INDEX

Place left thumb on the outer edge of this page. To locate the desired entry, fold back the remaining page edges and align the index edge mark with the appropriate page edge mark.

Other books by Morgan Quitno Press:

- *State Rankings 1998 ($49.95)*
- *Crime State Rankings 1998 ($49.95)*
- *City Crime Rankings, 4th Edition ($37.95)*

Call toll free: 1-800-457-0742 or
visit us at http://www.morganquitno.com